Seventh Edition

Fundamentals of Periodontal Instrumentation

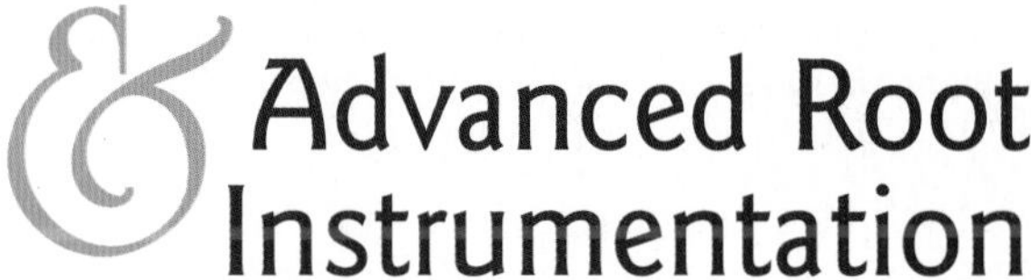

Jill S. Nield-Gehrig, RDH, MA

Dean Emeritus, Division of Allied Health & Public Service Education
Asheville-Buncombe Technical Community College
Asheville, North Carolina

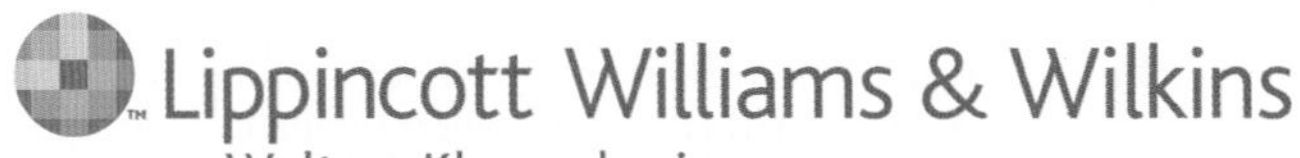

a Wolters Kluwer business

Philadelphia • Baltimore • New York • London
Buenos Aires • Hong Kong • Sydney • Tokyo

Senior Publisher: Julie Stegman
Product Manager: John Larkin
Marketing Manager: Shauna Kelley
Creative Director: Doug Smock
Compositor: Absolute Service, Inc.

Seventh Edition

351 West Camden Street
Baltimore, MD 21201

Two Commerce Square
2001 Market Street
Philadelphia, PA 19103

Printed in China

9 8 7 6 5 4 3 2 1

Library of Congress Cataloging-in-Publication Data

Nield-Gehrig, Jill S. (Jill Shiffer)
Fundamentals of periodontal instrumentation & advanced root instrumentation / Jill S. Nield-Gehrig. – 7th ed.
p. ; cm.
Fundamentals of periodontal instrumentation and advanced root instrumentation
Includes bibliographical references and index.
ISBN 978-1-60913-331-3 (alk. paper)
I. Title. II. Title: Fundamentals of periodontal instrumentation and advanced root instrumentation.
[DNLM: 1. Dental Prophylaxis–instrumentation. 2. Dental Prophylaxis–methods. 3. Root Planing–instrumentation. 4. Root Planing–methods. WU 113]
LC classification not assigned
617.6'01–dc23

2011032373

DISCLAIMER

Care has been taken to confirm the accuracy of the information present and to describe generally accepted practices. However, the authors, editors, and publisher are not responsible for errors or omissions or for any consequences from application of the information in this book and make no warranty, expressed or implied, with respect to the currency, completeness, or accuracy of the contents of the publication. Application of this information in a particular situation remains the professional responsibility of the practitioner; the clinical treatments described and recommended may not be considered absolute and universal recommendations.

The authors, editors, and publisher have exerted every effort to ensure that drug selection and dosage set forth in this text are in accordance with the current recommendations and practice at the time of publication. However, in view of ongoing research, changes in government regulations, and the constant flow of information relating to drug therapy and drug reactions, the reader is urged to check the package insert for each drug for any change in indications and dosage and for added warnings and precautions. This is particularly important when the recommended agent is a new or infrequently employed drug.

Some drugs and medical devices presented in this publication have Food and Drug Administration (FDA) clearance for limited use in restricted research settings. It is the responsibility of the healthcare provider to ascertain the FDA status of each drug or device planned for use in their clinical practice.

To purchase additional copies of this book, call our customer service department at **(800) 638-3030** or fax orders to **(301) 223-2320**. International customers should call **(301) 223-2300**.

Visit Lippincott Williams & Wilkins on the Internet: **http://www.lww.com.** Lippincott Williams & Wilkins customer service representatives are available from 8:30 a.m. to 6:00 p.m., EST.

Registered Trade Marks

American Eagle Instruments, Inc.
Gracey +3 Access Curettes
Gracey +3 Deep Pocket Curettes

DentalView, Inc.
Perioscopy Systems (dental endoscope)

DENTSPLY Preventive Care
Cavitron ultrasonic scalers
Prophy-Jet
JetShield

EMS (Electro Medical Systems)
Piezon Master 400

The Florida Probe

Hu-Friedy Mfg. Company, Inc.
After Five Curettes
After Five 11/12 Explorer
O'Hehir Debridement Curettes
Mini Five Curettes
Satin Steel instrument handle
Vision Curvette instrument series

KaVo America Corporation
KaVo Sonicflex scaler

Kilgore International, Inc.
Dental hygiene and periodontal typodonts
Acrylic tooth models
Dental manikin systems

Parkell USA
Burnett Power-Tip

SportsHealth Power Putty

SurgiTel/General Scientific Corporation
SurgiTel telescopic magnification system

Preface for Course Instructors

Fundamentals of Periodontal Instrumentation & Advanced Root Instrumentation, Seventh Edition is a detailed instructional guide to periodontal instrumentation that takes students from the basic skills—patient positioning, intraoral finger rests, and basic instrumentation—all the way to advanced techniques—assessment of periodontal patients and instrumentation of the root branches of multirooted teeth, root concavities, and furcation areas.

The foremost instructional goal of *Fundamentals* is to make it easy for students to learn and faculty to teach instrumentation. The seventh edition retains the features that have made it the market-leading textbook on periodontal instrumentation and adds many new features designed to facilitate learning and teaching.

Online Teaching/Learning Resources (thePoint)

Follow the steps below to access the online instructor resources.

Accessing Online Instructor Resources

1. Open an Internet browser and select: **http://thePoint.lww.com/GehrigFundamentals7e**
2. Existing users: Log on. Skip to step 4 in this list.
3. New users: Select "Register a New Account." Complete all required fields on the online access request form. Select the **Submit Adoption Form** button. Once the form is submitted in good order, you will receive an approval notice. US and Canadian educators, please allow 3 business days for a reply. Note: The access codes that come in the textbook provide students with access to the full online text only.
4. Locate **Fundamentals of Periodontal Instrumentation and Advanced Root Instrumentation**. Select "Instructor Resources."

Note: Students can access resources by selecting "Student Resources."

Online resources—available at thePoint **(http://thePoint.lww.com/GehrigFundamentals7e)**—include:

1. **PowerPoint Slides.** The PowerPoint slides were designed to be user friendly for a wide variety of software versions and equipment.
   - The PowerPoint presentations may be customized by saving the slides to your computer hard drive and using the formatting features of your slide presentation software, such as the slide design, slide color scheme, or slide background feature.
   - Special effects, such as progressive disclosure, may be added to the slide presentations using the custom animation features of your slide presentation software. In addition, individual slides may be deleted and new instructor-created slides added to the presentations.
2. **Videoclips.** Included in this edition are 20 videoclips available free of charge to both students and instructors online at thePoint. Students can view these clips in the classroom and at home while studying.
   - Clock Positions for Anterior Teeth: Right-Handed Clinicians
   - Clock Positions for Anterior Teeth: Left-Handed Clinicians
   - Clock Positions for Posterior Teeth: Right-Handed Clinicians
   - Clock Positions for Posterior Teeth: Left-Handed Clinicians
   - Instrument Grasp
   - Introduction to Mirror Use
   - Establishing a Finger Rest
   - Introduction to Adaptation
   - Activation, Handle Roll, and Adaptation
   - Periodontal Probe
   - The ODU 11/12 Explorer
   - The 17/23 Orban Explorer
   - Selecting the Correct Working-End
   - Calculus Removal Stroke
   - Sickle Scalers
   - Anterior Sickle Scaler
   - Universal Curets
   - The Columbia 13/14 Universal Curet
   - Area-Specific Curets
   - The Gracey 13/14 Area-Specific Curet
3. **Test Bank.** The test bank questions can be used for quizzes, combined to make up unit tests, or combined to create midterm and final examinations.
4. **Instructor Guide.** The instructor guide includes:
   - Suggestions for leading classroom discussions of the *Practical Focus* sections in the modules.
   - A list of phrases that facilitate the teaching of instrumentation.
   - Teaching tips for instruction, as well as sources for periodontal typodonts.
   - Guidelines for introduction of alternate and advanced techniques.
5. **Module Evaluation Forms.** Evaluation forms for instructor grading are now located online in two formats.
   - **Evaluations for Computerized Grading.** These forms are designed to allow the instructor to enter grades and comments directly on a computer. Computerized forms include evaluation forms for each module, a summative evaluation ("instrumentation final exam"), and a cumulative scores form. Instructions for use of these computerized forms can be found online at thePoint.
   - **Evaluations for Paper Grading.** These forms are designed to be printed out and used for "paper and pen" manual grading. Paper forms include evaluation forms for each module.

Textbook Features

1. **Module outlines.** Each chapter begins with a module outline that provides an overview of content and makes it easier to locate material within the module. The outline provides the reader with an organizational framework with which to approach new material.
2. **Learning objectives** assist students in recognizing and studying important concepts in each chapter.
3. **Step-by-step format.** The clear, step-by-step self-instructional format allows the learner to work independently, fostering student autonomy and decision-making skills. The learner is free to work at his or her own pace, spending more time on a skill that he or she finds difficult and moving on when a skill comes easily. The self-instructional format relieves the instructor from the task of endlessly repeating basic information, and frees him or her to demonstrate instrumentation techniques, observe student practice, and facilitate the process of skill acquisition.
4. **Key terms** are listed at the start of each module. One of the most challenging tasks for any student is learning a whole new dental vocabulary and gaining the confidence to use new terms with accuracy and ease. The key terms list assists students in this task by identifying important terminology and facilitating the study and review of terminology in each instructional module.
5. **Study aids**—boxes, tables, and flow charts—visually highlight and reinforce important content and permit quick reference during technique practice and at-home review.
6. **Critical thinking activities**—in the *Practical Focus* sections of the book—encourage students to apply concepts to clinical situations, facilitate classroom discussion, and promote the development of student problem-solving skills.
7. **Case-based patient experiences** allow students to apply instrumentation concepts to patient cases.
8. **The glossary of instrumentation terms** provides quick access to instrumentation terminology.
9. **Student self-evaluation checklists** guide student practice, promote student self-assessment skills, and provide benchmarks for faculty evaluation of skill attainment. Use of the student self-evaluation portion of the evaluation forms should be encouraged. The self-evaluation process helps students to develop the ability to assess their own level of competence rather than relying on instructor confirmation of skill attainment.

Module Format and Sequencing

The book is divided into four major content areas:

Part 1: Basic Skills
Part 2: Hand-Activated Instruments
Part 3: Powered Instrumentation
Part 4: Appendices

Mathematical Principles and Problem Identification

Appendices 1 and 2 contain two important modules in the book. Appendix 1 is Getting Ready for Instrumentation: Mathematical Principles and Anatomical Descriptors. Appendix 2 is Problem Identification: Difficulties in Instrumentation.

Online Modules 27 and 28

In addition to the Student and Instructor Resources, two modules are located online at thePoint website **(http://thePoint.lww.com/GehrigFundamentals7e)**. The two modules are Module 27: Debridement of Dental Implants and Module 28: Cosmetic Polishing Procedures. These modules may be studied online or printed out.

From an instructional viewpoint, it is important to note that *each major instrument classification is addressed in a stand-alone module*—sickle scalers, universal curets, and area-specific curets. Each stand-alone module provides complete step-by-step instruction in the use of an instrument classification. For example, the module on universal curets provides complete instruction on the use of universal curets. This chapter does not rely on the student having studied the previous module on sickle scalers before beginning the universal curet module. This stand-alone module structure means that it is not necessary to cover the instrument modules in any particular order or even to include all of the modules. If sickle scalers, for example, are not part of the school's instrument kit, this module does not need to be included in the course outline.

I appreciate the enthusiastic comments and suggestions from educators and students about previous editions of *Fundamentals*, and welcome continued input. Mastering the psychomotor skill of periodontal instrumentation is a very challenging process. It is my sincere hope that this textbook will help students to acquire the psychomotor skills that—combined with clinical experience—will lead to excellence in periodontal instrumentation.

Jill S. Nield-Gehrig, RDH, MA

Acknowledgments

It is gratifying to be a member of a profession that includes so many individuals who strive for excellence in teaching. I am most grateful to all of the outstanding educators who shared their comments and suggestions for improving this edition. I thank all who generously gave their time, ideas, and resources, and gratefully acknowledge the special contributions of the following individuals:

- **Charles D. Whitehead and Holly R. Fischer**, MFA, the highly skilled medical illustrators who created all the wonderful illustrations for the book.
- **Dee Robert Gehrig**, PE, Gehrig Photographic Studio—the talented individual who created the hundreds of photographs for this book.
- **Rebecca Sroda**, RDH, MS, **Darlene Saccuzzo**, RDH, BASHD, and **Christian Negron**, the highly talented individuals who created the online videoclips for this edition.
- **Sharon Logue**, RDH, MPH, for her suggestions for the improvement of this edition.
- The following individuals who were extremely generous with their time and knowledge—**Victoria Goodman, Karen Neiner, and Patricia Parker** of Hu-Friedy Manufacturing and **Tree Mainella** of Parkell USA. A very special "thank you" to **Craig Kilgore**, President, Kilgore International, Inc., for providing the periodontal typodonts used throughout the book.
- **Kevin Dietz**, a colleague and friend, for his vision and guidance for this book.
- And finally, and with great thanks, my wonderful team at Lippincott Williams & Wilkins, without whose guidance and support this book would not have been possible: **Pete Sabatini, John Larkin, and Jennifer Clements**.

Jill S. Nield-Gehrig

Contents

PART 2: HAND-ACTIVATED INSTRUMENTS

APPENDICES

ONLINE CHAPTERS

Contributors

Christine Dominick, CDA, RDH, MEd
Associate Professor, Forsyth School of Dental Hygiene
Massachusetts College of Pharmacy and Health Sciences
Boston, Massachusetts

Richard Foster, DMD
Dental Director
Guilford Technical Community College
Jamestown, North Carolina

Cynthia Biron Leisica, RDH, EMT, MS
President, DH Meth-Ed, Inc.
Dental Hygiene Methodology
Tallahassee, Florida

Sharon Logue, RDH, MPH
Virginia Department of Health
Division of Dental Health
Richmond, Virginia

Robin B. Matloff, RDH, BSDH, JD
Associate Professor, Dental Hygiene Program
Mount Ida College
Newton, Massachusetts

Lydia T. Pierce, LPT
Physical Medicine and Rehabilitation
Asheville, North Carolina

Darlene Saccuzzo, CDA, RDH, BASDH
Professor, Dental Education
South Florida Community College
Avon Park, Florida

Rebecca Sroda, RDH, MS
Associate Dean, Allied Health
South Florida Community College
Avon Park, Florida

Cherie M. Stevens, PhD
Professor, Computer Science
South Florida Community College
Avon Park, Florida

Donald E. Willmann, DDS, MS
Professor Emeritus, Department of Periodontics
University of Texas Health Science Center at San Antonio
San Antonio, Texas

Sueellen Nipper-Williams, RDH, BASDH, MHSc
Dental Education
South Florida Community College
Avon Park, Florida

Module 1

Principles of Positioning

Module Overview

This module introduces the principles of positioning for periodontal instrumentation. Correct positioning techniques help to (1) prevent clinician discomfort and injury, (2) permit a clear view of the tooth being worked on, (3) allow easy access to the teeth during instrumentation, and (4) facilitate efficient treatment of the patient.

Module Outline

Key Terms

Musculoskeletal disorder (MSD)
Repetitive task
Ergonomics
Neutral spine
Neutral seated position
Supine position
Semi-supine position
Chin-up position
Chin-down position
Co-axial illumination sources
Dental headlights
Magnification loupes
Working distance
Angle of declination
Depth of field
Field of view
Blind zone

Learning Objectives

1. Define the term musculoskeletal disorder (MSD).
2. Develop an appreciation of evidence-based knowledge of positioning in the dental environment.
3. Understand the relationship between neutral position and the prevention of musculoskeletal problems.
4. Identify MSDs commonly experienced by dental health professionals, their causes, and their prevention.
5. Demonstrate operation of the clinician stool and patient chair.
6. Discuss the elements of neutral seated position for the clinician.
7. Demonstrate correct patient position relative to the clinician.
8. State the reason why it is important that the top of the patient's head is even with top edge of the chair headrest. Demonstrate how to correctly position a short individual and a child in the dental chair so that (1) the patient is comfortable and (2) the clinician has good vision and access to the oral cavity.
9. Position equipment so that it enhances neutral positioning.
10. Recognize incorrect position and describe or demonstrate how to correct the problem.

Section 1
Foundational Skills for Periodontal Instrumentation

Periodontal instrumentation is a complex psychomotor skill that involves the precise execution of many individual component skills. Swinging a golf club is an everyday example of a complex psychomotor skill that involves many component skills, for example, proper stance, grip on the club handle, position of the golfer's head, and movement to swing the club.

1. **Foundational Building Blocks of Periodontal Instrumentation.** Many building blocks—individual skill components—are involved in periodontal instrumentation. These building blocks are discussed below and illustrated in Figure 1-1.
   A. **Building Block 1: Position.** The building block of "positioning" entails the proper use of equipment, as well as positioning the patient and clinician.
   B. **Building Block 2: Instrument Grasp.** This building block involves the way in which the clinician holds a periodontal instrument.
   C. **Building Block 3: Mirror Use.** A dental mirror allows a clinician to view tooth surfaces or other oral structures that are obscured from direct viewing.
   D. **Building Block 4: Finger Rests.** This building block entails the manner in which the clinician stabilizes his or her hand in the oral cavity during periodontal instrumentation.
   E. **Building Block 5: Stroke Production.** This building block refers to the manner in which the working-end of a periodontal instrument is moved against the tooth surface. Stroke production is a complex skill that involves several smaller component skills—activation, adaptation, and angulation—that are discussed later in this book.
2. **Significance of the Building Blocks for Periodontal Instrumentation**
   A. Precise Performance
      1. Precise, accurate performance of the building blocks is essential if periodontal instrumentation is to be effective, efficient, safe for the patient, and comfortable for the clinician.
      2. Research on psychomotor skill acquisition indicates that a high level of mastery in the performance of skill building blocks is essential to successful mastery of periodontal instrumentation.
         a. The building block skills are the foundation that "supports" successful periodontal instrumentation.
         b. These skills should be mastered one-by-one.
         c. Each skill should be over-learned until it can be performed easily and without hesitation. It is impossible to devote too much time to the practice of these building block skills.
         d. *If the building block skills are mastered, then the use of any periodontal instrument will be relatively easy to learn.* The building block skills are the same no matter which periodontal instrument is used.
   B. Faulty Performance. *Incorrect performance of even one of the building blocks means that, at the very least, periodontal instrumentation will be inefficient* (Fig. 1-2). Most likely, faulty performance results in ineffective calculus removal, unnecessary discomfort for the patient, and musculoskeletal stress to the clinician.

3. **Module Content Sequencing.** The modules in this book are sequenced to allow beginning clinicians to practice the building blocks to periodontal instrumentation one-by-one. Each building block should be practiced until it is easy to perform from memory before attempting the next building block in the skill sequence. This module presents the first building block: position.

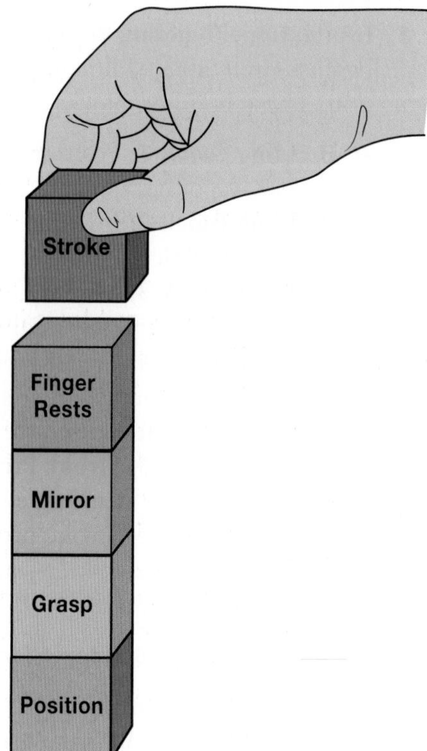

Figure 1-1. Building Blocks for Periodontal Instrumentation. Successful periodontal instrumentation requires the mastery of the skill building blocks of position, grasp, mirror use, finger rests, and stroke production.

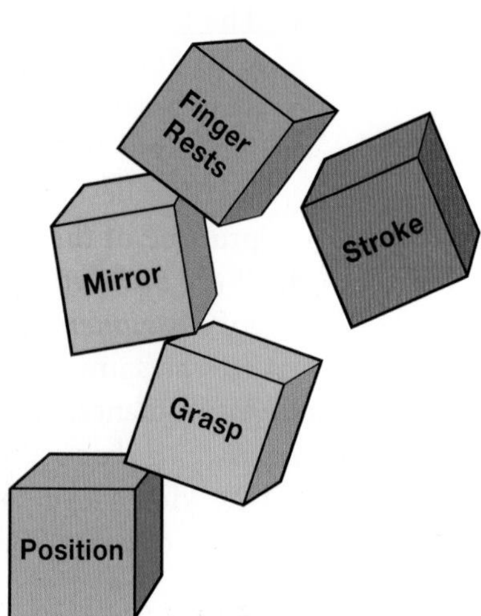

Figure 1-2. Faulty Execution of Building Blocks. Incorrect performance of even one of the building blocks means that periodontal instrumentation will be inefficient and, most likely, ineffective and uncomfortable for both the patient and clinician.

Section 2

Ergonomic Risk Factors Associated with Periodontal Instrumentation

INTRODUCTION TO MUSCULOSKELETAL DISORDERS

1. **Musculoskeletal Stresses and the Dental Professional**

   A. **Musculoskeletal Disorders.** The dental literature indicates that both dentists and hygienists are exposed to occupational risk factors that often lead to musculoskeletal disorders.[1–10]

      1. A musculoskeletal disorder (MSD) is a condition where parts of the musculoskeletal system—muscles, tendons, nerves—are injured over time.
         a. MSDs occur when too much stress is exerted on a body part, resulting in pain.
         b. When a body part is overused repeatedly, the constant stress causes damage.
         c. Examples of MSDs include carpal tunnel, rotator cuff injury, de Quervain's disease, trigger finger, tarsal tunnel, sciatica, tendinitis, and herniated spinal disc.
         d. Work activities that are frequent and repetitive or activities with awkward postures cause MSDs that may be painful during work or at rest (Fig. 1-3).
      2. Almost all work requires the use of the arms and hands. Therefore, most MSDs affect the hands, wrists, elbows, neck, and shoulders.
      3. The literature indicates that dentists and dental hygienists experience back, neck, and shoulder pain with an average incidence of over 60% having experienced musculoskeletal pain.[11]
      4. Musculoskeletal problems begin early, with dental and dental hygiene students in educational programs and recent graduates reporting pain and discomfort.[6,7,12]
      5. MSDs continue to be a major source of disability and lost work time in dental professionals.

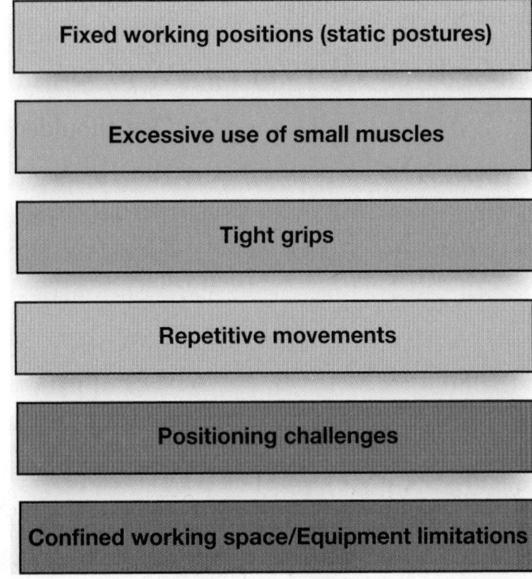

Figure 1-3. Risk Factors for Musculoskeletal Stress in Dental Professionals.

B. Causes of Musculoskeletal Pain in Dental Professionals. Given the high incidence of musculoskeletal pain, it is important for clinicians to understand the causes of MSDs and to take actions to prevent them. Boxes 1-1A and 1-1B summarize certain factors, including clinician posture and positioning factors, that are associated with increased risk of musculoskeletal symptoms for dentists and dental hygienists.[7]

1. Factors that appear to be instrumental in contributing to MSDs in dentists and dental hygienists include excessive use of small muscles, repetitive motions, tight grips, fixed working positions (staying in one position for extended periods), limited movements, and long-term static load on muscles (maintaining muscles in same position during application of force).[13]
2. The result is injury to the muscles, nerves, and tendon sheaths of the back, shoulders, neck, arms, elbows, wrists, and hands that can cause loss of strength, impairment of motor control, tingling, numbness, or pain.
3. The human body was not designed to maintain the same body position—prolonged static posture—or engage in fine hand movements hour after hour, day after day.
   a. Silverstein et al., in an article in the *American Journal of Industrial Medicine*, defined a repetitive task as a task that involves the same fundamental movement for more than 50% of the work cycle.[14]
   b. Periodontal instrumentation would certainly be categorized as a repetitive task under this definition.
   c. Periodontal instrumentation requires excessive upper-body immobility while the tendons and muscles of the forearms, hands, and fingers overwork.
4. ***The dental healthcare professional has a high risk of musculoskeletal injury when repetitive motions are combined with forceful movements, awkward postures, and insufficient recovery time.***[15–18]

Box 1-1A. Factors Associated with Decreased Risk of Injury[7,19]

- Stool adjusted for the clinician
- Torso aligned with long axis of the body
- Shoulders level
- Treatment room design permits clinician to move freely around the patient chair (in all "clock positions")
- Elbows resting at the clinician's sides during periodontal instrumentation
- Back of patient chair parallel to the floor for maxillary arch
- Unit light positioned close to the clinician's line of sight for maxillary treatment
- Limiting use of a 7:00 to 8:30 or 3:30 to 5:00 clock position as much as possible

Box 1-1B. Factors Associated with Increased Risk of Injury[7,19]

- Stool not adjusted for individual clinician
- Torso twisted
- One shoulder higher than the other
- Treatment room design does not permit clinician to move freely around the patient chair (unable to use all "clock positions")
- Elbows held above waist and away from the body
- Back of patient chair not parallel to the floor for maxillary arch
- Unit light positioned toward the patient's feet, away from the clinician's line of sight.
- Frequent use of a 7:00 to 8:30 or 3:30 to 5:00 clock position

2. **Prevention of Musculoskeletal Disorders.** Fortunately, injury to the muscles, tendons, and nerves can be prevented in most cases.

   A. Ergonomics is an applied science concerned with the "fit" between people and their technological tools and environments.
      1. In application, ergonomics is a discipline focused on making products and tasks comfortable and efficient for the user.
      2. A primary ergonomic principle is that equipment—such as computer keyboards and workstations—should be designed to fit the user instead of forcing the user to fit the equipment.
      3. Ergonomics is the science of making things efficient. Efficiency is quite simply making something easier to do.

   B. **Ergonomic Guidelines in Dentistry.** It is possible to define ergonomic guidelines for use of dental operatory equipment to minimize exposure of dental healthcare providers to musculoskeletal stress.[3,6,7,12,19–38] Postural and positional factors associated with decreased risk of musculoskeletal stress for dentists and dental hygienists are summarized in Box 1-1A.[7,19]

MUSCULOSKELETAL DISORDERS COMMON IN DENTAL HEALTHCARE PROVIDERS

MSDs commonly experienced by dentists and dental hygienists are illustrated in Figures 1-4 to 1-11.

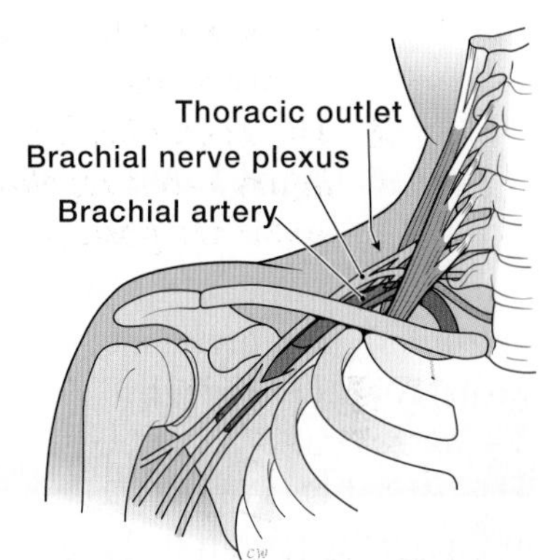

Figure 1-4. Thoracic Outlet Syndrome.

1. Definition
A painful disorder of the fingers, hand, and/or wrist due to the compression of the brachial nerve plexus and vessels between the neck and shoulder
2. Causes
Tilting the head forward, hunching the shoulders forward, and continuously reaching overhead
3. Symptoms
Numbness, tingling, and/or pain in the fingers, hand, or wrist

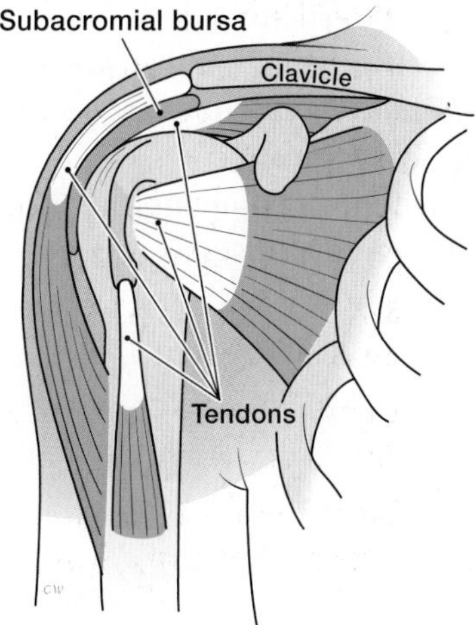

Figure 1-5. Rotator Cuff Tendinitis.

1. Definition
A painful inflammation of the muscle tendons in the shoulder region
2. Causes
Holding the elbow above waist level and holding the upper arm away from the body
3. Symptoms
Severe pain and impaired function of the shoulder joint

Figure 1-6. Pronator Syndrome.

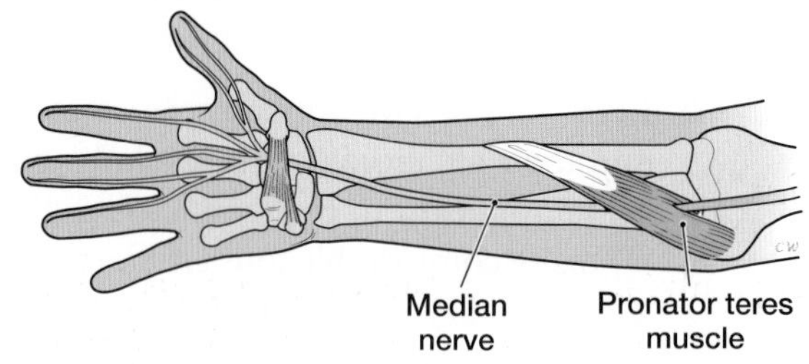

1. Definition
A painful disorder of the wrist and hand caused by compression of the median nerve between the two heads of the pronator teres muscle
2. Causes
Holding the lower arm away from the body
3. Symptoms
Similar to those of carpal tunnel syndrome

Figure 1-7. Extensor Wad Strain.

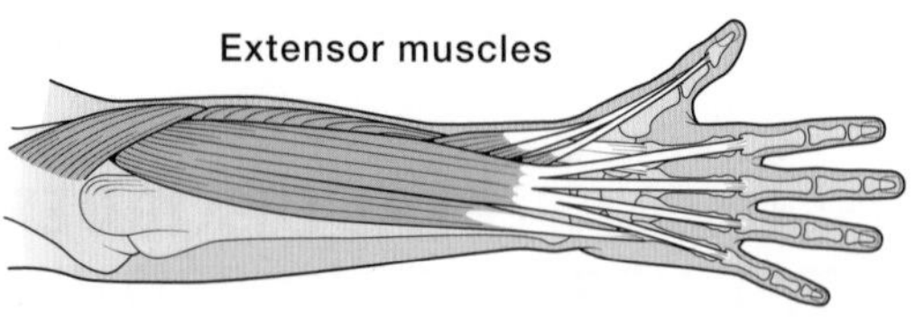

1. Definition
A painful disorder of the fingers due to injury of the extensor muscles of the thumb and fingers
2. Causes
Extending the fingers independently of each other
3. Symptoms
Numbness, pain, and loss of strength in the fingers

Figure 1-8. Carpal Tunnel Syndrome (CTS).

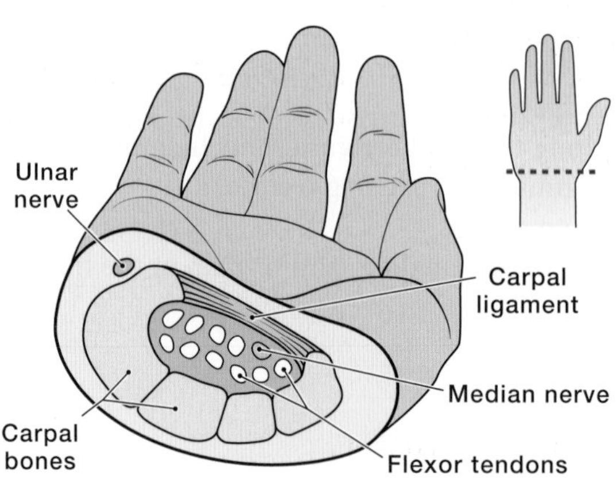

1. Definition
A painful disorder of the wrist and hand caused by compression of the median nerve within the carpal tunnel of the wrist
2. Causes
The nerve fibers of the median nerve originate in the spinal cord in the neck; therefore, poor posture can cause symptoms of CTS. Other causes include repeatedly bending the hand up, down, or from side-to-side at the wrist and continuously pinch-gripping an instrument without resting the muscles
3. Symptoms
Numbness, pain, and tingling in the thumb, index, and middle fingers

Figure 1-9. Ulnar Nerve Entrapment.

1. Definition
A painful disorder of the lower arm and wrist caused by compression of the ulnar nerve of the arm as it passes through the wrist
2. Causes
Bending the hand up, down, or from side-to-side at the wrist and holding the little finger a full span away from the hand
3. Symptoms
Numbness, tingling, and/or loss of strength in the lower arm or wrist

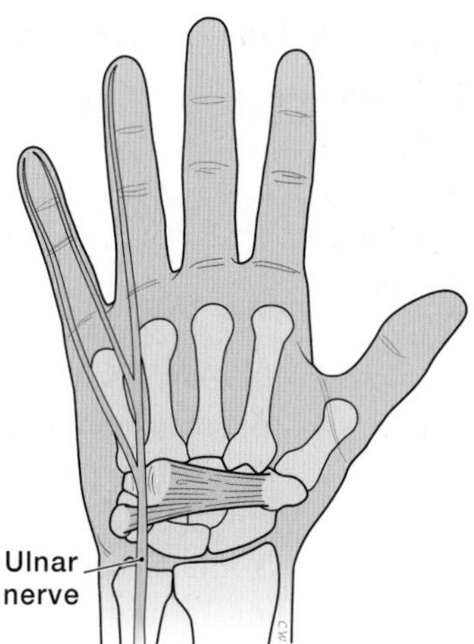

Figure 1-10. Tenosynovitis.

1. Definition
A painful inflammation of the tendons on the side of the wrist and at the base of the thumb
2. Causes
Hand twisting, forceful gripping, bending the hand back or to the side
3. Symptoms
Pain on the side of the wrist and the base of the thumb; sometimes movement of the wrist yields a crackling noise

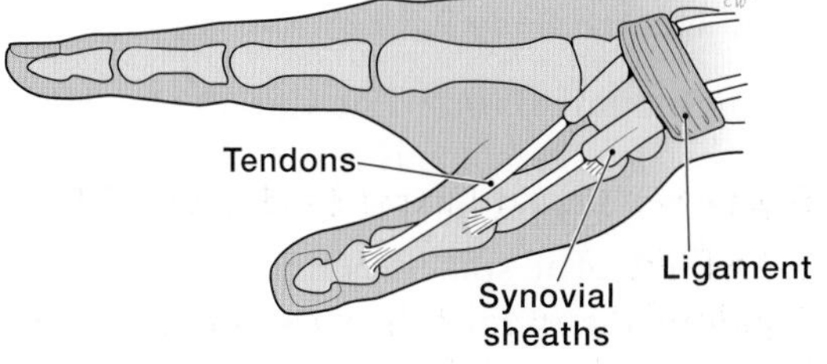

Figure 1-11. Tendinitis.

1. Definition
A painful inflammation of the tendons of the wrist resulting from strain
2. Causes
Repeatedly extending the hand up or down at the wrist
3. Symptoms
Pain in the wrist, especially on the outer edges of the hand, rather than through the center of the wrist

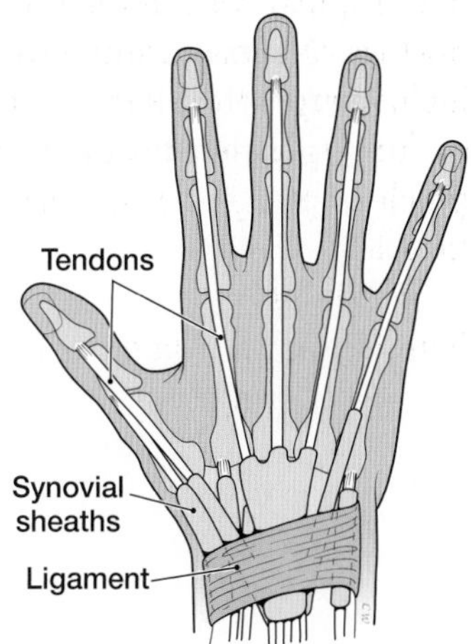

Section 3
Protecting Your Back: Neutral Seated Position

NEUTRAL POSITION FOR THE CLINICIAN

1. Ergonomic Dos and Don'ts

A. Ergonomic Don'ts
1. When a dental professional alters his or her body position or equipment in a manner that is uncomfortable or painful just to "get the job done," musculoskeletal stress is the result.
2. A mindset that it is acceptable to assume an uncomfortable position "just for 15 minutes while performing periodontal instrumentation on these two teeth" is destined to lead to MSDs.
3. Pain and injury result when the body's natural spinal curves are not maintained in a seated position.

B. Ergonomic Dos
1. ***For a healthy and productive career, the dental hygienist maintains a neutral, balanced body position and then alters the patient's chair and dental equipment to complete periodontal instrumentation.***
2. Good posture requires the seated dental hygienist to use a neutral spine position that maintains the natural curves of the spine (Fig. 1-12).

2. Neutral Body Position

A. Spine Basics: The Curves of a Healthy Back
1. The spine is made up of three segments: the cervical, thoracic, and lumbar sections.
2. The spine has three natural curves that form an S-shape.[39] When the three natural curves are properly aligned, the ears, shoulders, and hips are in a straight line.
   a. When viewed from the side, the cervical and lumbar segments have a slight inward curve (lordosis).
   b. When viewed from the side, the thoracic segment of the spine has a gentle outward curve (kyphosis).

B. **Neutral Body Position for the Clinician.** Figures 1-13 to 1-19 illustrate the characteristics of neutral body position for the clinician.

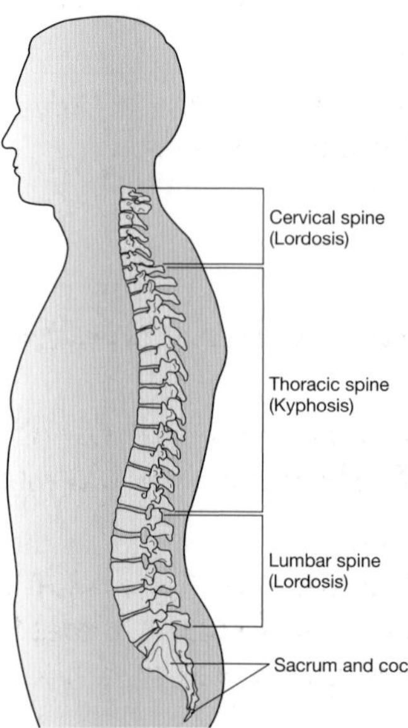

Figure 1-12. Three Curves of a Healthy Back. The spine has three natural curves: cervical, thoracic, and lumbar curves. The cervical and lumbar segments have a gentle inward curve. The thoracic segment has a slight outward curve.

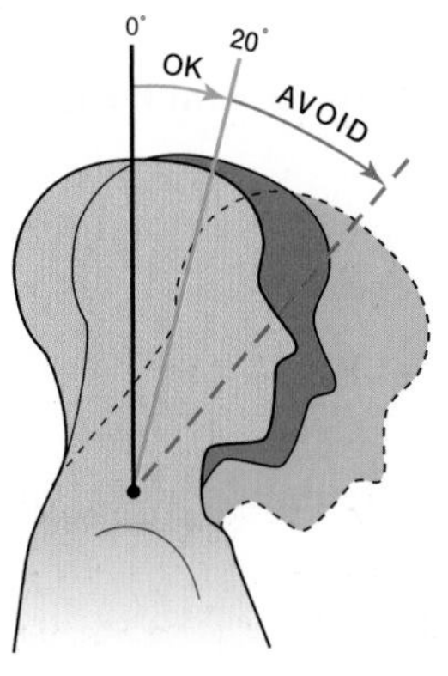

Figure 1-13. Neutral Neck Position.

Goal:
- Head tilt of 0° to 20°
- The line from eyes to the treatment area should be as near to vertical as possible

Avoid:
- Head tipped too far forward
- Head tilted to one side

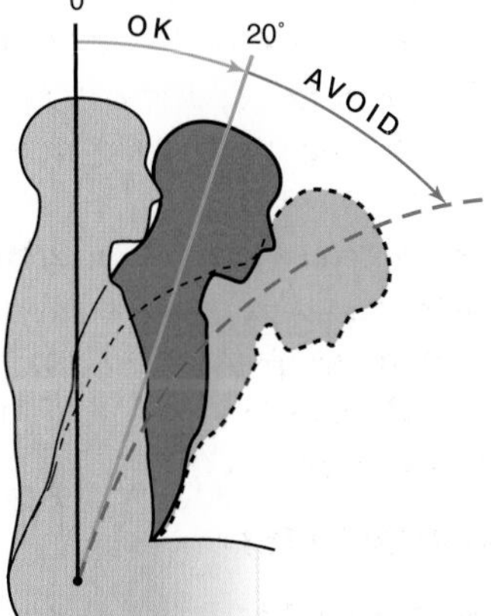

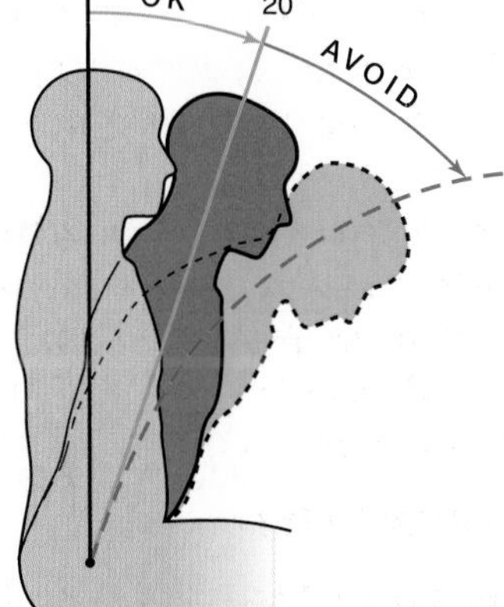

Figure 1-14. Neutral Back Position.

Goal:
- Lean forward slightly from the hips (hinge at hips)
- Trunk flexion of 0° to 20°

Avoid:
- Overflexion of the spine (curved back)

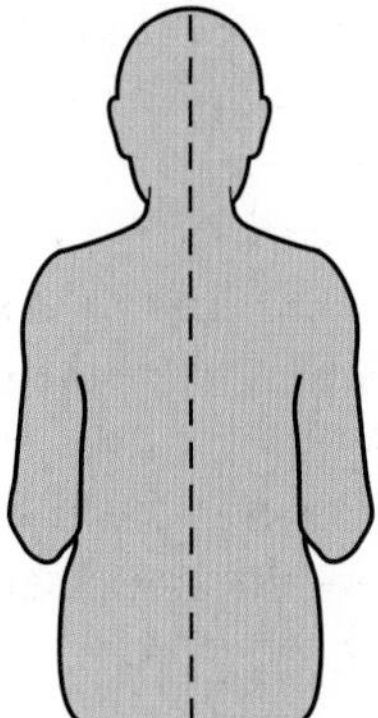

Figure 1-15. Neutral Torso Position.

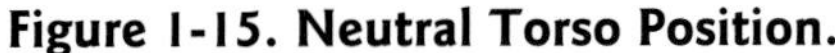

Goal:
- Torso in line with long axis of the body

Avoid:
- Leaning torso to one side
- Twisting the torso

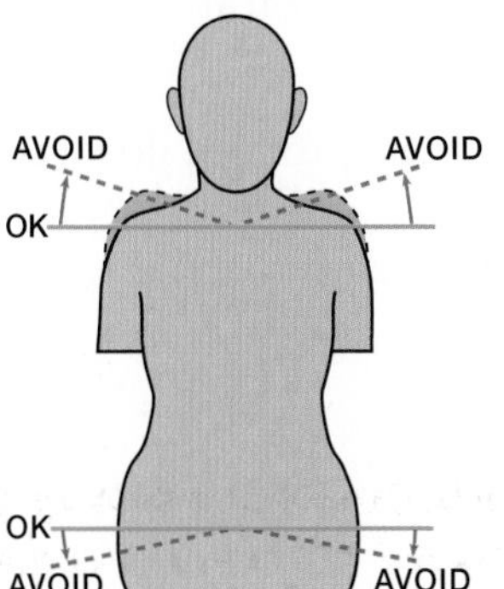

Figure 1-16. Neutral Shoulder Position.

Goal:
- Shoulders in horizontal line
- Weight evenly balanced when seated

Avoid:
- Shoulders lifted up toward ears
- Shoulders hunched forward
- Sitting with weight on one hip

Figure 1-17. Neutral Upper Arm Position.

Goal:

- Upper arms hang parallel to the long axis of torso
- Elbows at waist level held slightly away from body

Avoid:

- Greater than 20° of elbow abduction away from the body
- Elbows held above waist level

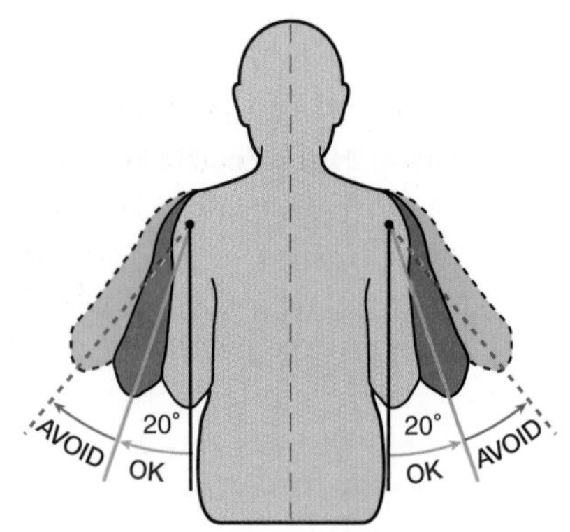

Figure 1-18. Neutral Forearm Position.

Goal:

- Forearm held parallel to the floor
- Forearm raised or lowered, if necessary, by pivoting at the elbow joint

Avoid:

- Angle between forearm and upper arm of less than 60°

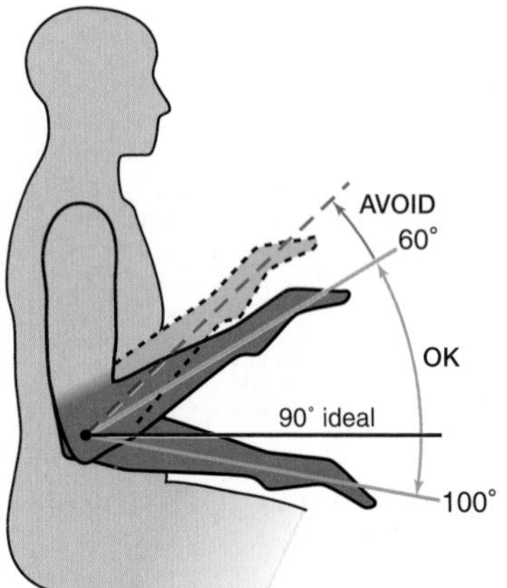

Figure 1-19. Neutral Hand Position.

Goal:

- Little finger-side of palm is slightly lower than thumb-side of palm
- Wrist aligned with forearm

Avoid:

- Thumb-side of palm rotated down so that palm is parallel to floor
- Hand and wrist bent up or down

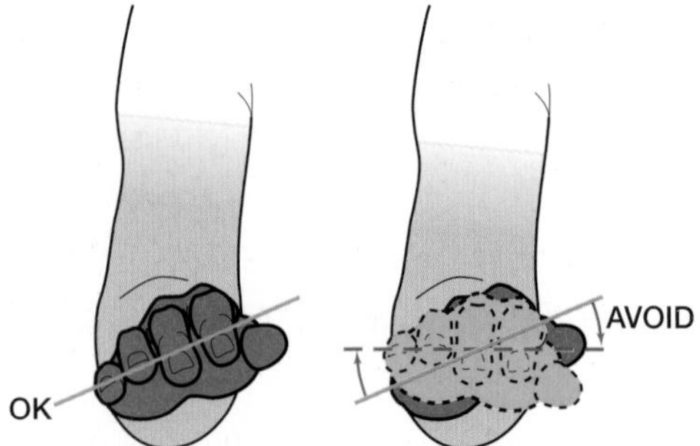

SELECTING A CLINICIAN STOOL

Dental professionals spend long hours sitting. Clinician stools cannot be a "one size fits all" design. Dentists and dental hygienists come in all sizes: tall or short with a delicate or round physique. A dental hygienist who is 6'4" in height certainly needs a different chair than a dental hygienist who is 5'1" in height. A stool that is adjusted correctly for clinician A may be uncomfortable for clinician B. Just as each driver of the family car must change the position of the driver's seat and mirrors, ***each clinician should adjust the stool height and seat back to conform to his or her own body proportions and height.*** Properly designed clinician seating is the foundation for a healthy neutral sitting position.[3,7,23,40] Table 1-1 provides evaluation criteria for assessment of clinician seating.

TABLE 1-1. Ergonomic Seating Evaluation Form

Evaluation Criteria	**Scale:** **U = Unacceptable** **A = Average** **E = Excellent**
A. Legs	
1. Five legs for stability	
2. Large casters for easy movement	
B. Stool Adjustments	
1. Stool seat height, backrest, and seat pan adjust independently to allow for comfortable seating.	
2. Stool seat height, backrest, and seat pan adjust easily while in a seated position.	
3. Seat height easily adjusts to accommodate both tall and short clinicians (range of 14–20 inches).	
4. Seat pan tilts slightly so that the seat back is an inch or so higher than the front.	
C. Seat Comfort	
1. Seat pan depth is comfortable and supportive. Seat pan is large enough to support the clinician's thighs and buttocks.	
2. Front edge of the seat pan has a waterfall shape (rounded front edge).	
3. When the clinician is seated with his or her back against the backrest, the seat pan does not impinge on the back of the clinician's knees, but allows a couple of inches between the edge and the back of the knee.	
D. Backrest Comfort	
1. The backrest adjusts in a vertical direction—up and down—to provide support to the lumbar region of the back for both short and tall clinicians.	
2. The backrest adjusts in a horizontal direction—closer or farther away from the seat—to provide lumbar support.	

IMPORTANT ELEMENTS OF THE SEATED POSITION

Figures 1-20 and 1-21 depict important elements of the seated clinician position.

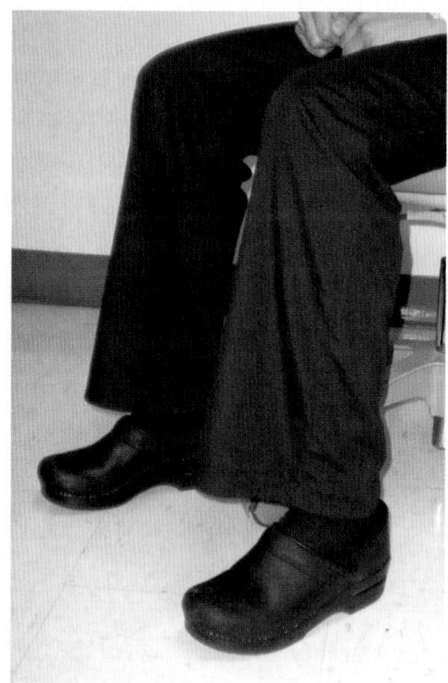

Figure 1-20. Correct Feet Position. The feet should be positioned to create a "wide base of support" for the seated clinician. That is, the feet should be flat on the floor about a shoulder's width apart for ideal balance while seated.

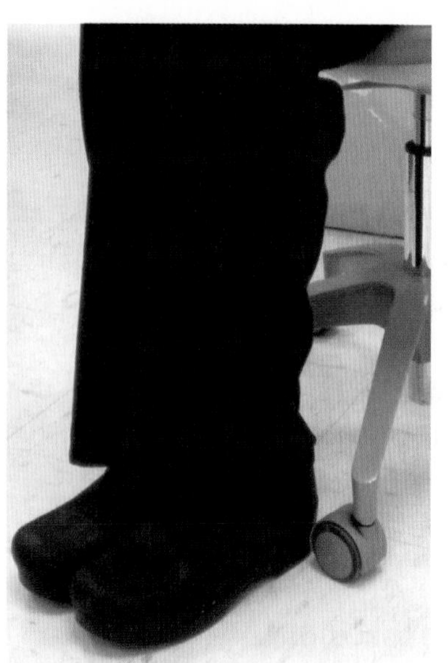

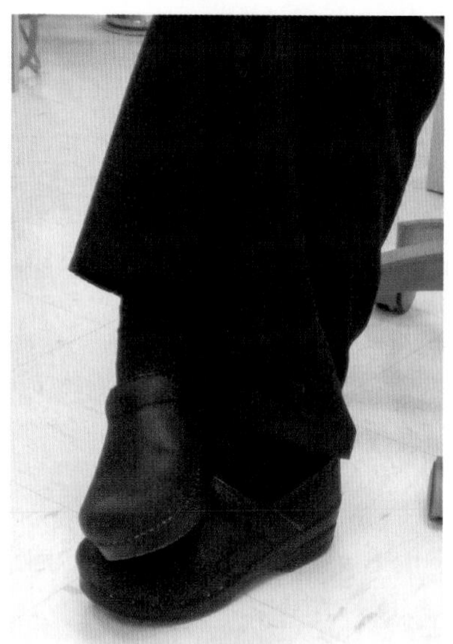

Figure 1-21. Incorrect Feet Position for Seated Clinician.

A. Narrow Base of Support. A narrow base of support with the feet together or tucked under the chair interferes with the clinician's balance and can limit his or her range of motion during instrumentation.

B. Crossed Legs. Crossing the legs at the knees or ankles restricts blood flow to the legs and feet. In addition, this position places more weight on one side of hips and interferes with the clinician's balance during periodontal instrumentation. (Photos courtesy of Dr. Richard Foster, Guilford Technical Community College, Jamestown, NC.)

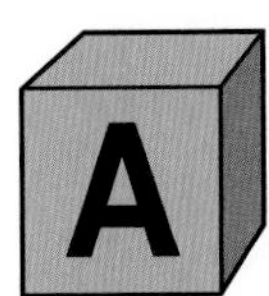

SKILL BUILDING. NEUTRAL SEATED POSITION FOR THE CLINICIAN

Directions: Practice the neutral clinician position by following the steps 1 to 9 as illustrated in Figures 1-22 to 1-30.

The ideal seated position for the clinician is called the neutral seated position. ***Adjust the clinician stool first. A common mistake clinicians make is positioning the patient first and then adjusting the clinician stool to accommodate the patient.***

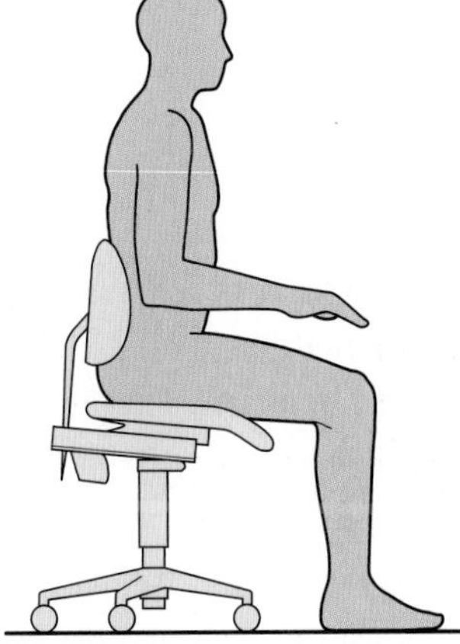

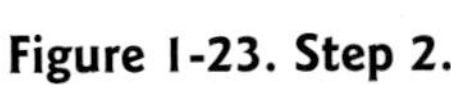

Figure 1-22. Step 1.

- Position the buttocks all the way back in the chair. Distribute the body's weight evenly on both hips.

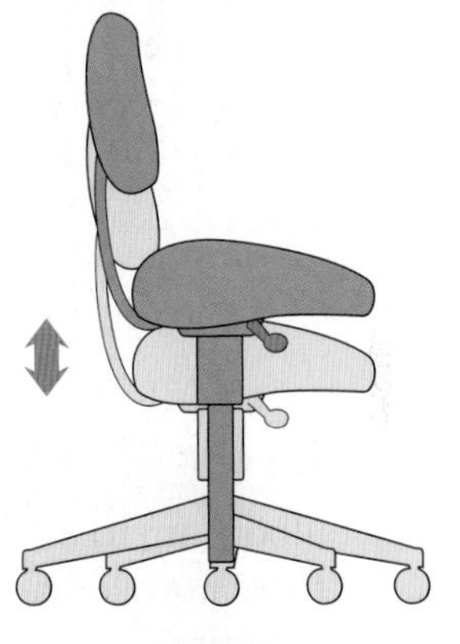

Figure 1-23. Step 2.

- Adjust seat height so the feet rest flat on the floor. Establish a "wide base of support" with feet on floor at least shoulder-width apart and in front of the hips.[3]
- Legs should not dangle or be crossed at the knees or ankles. Dangling legs or crossing them puts pressure on the back of the thighs and restricts blood flow.

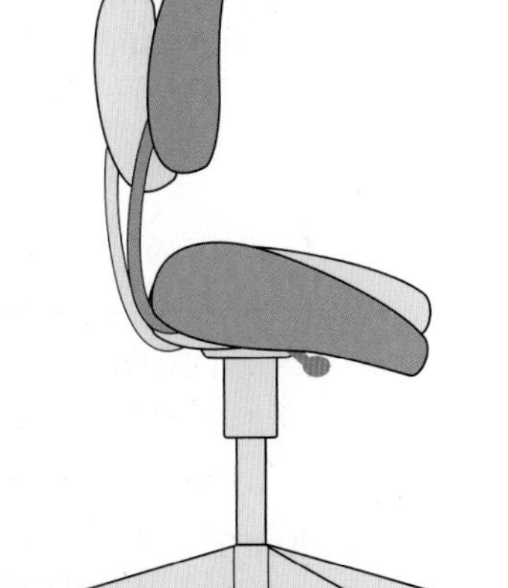

Figure 1-24. Step 3.

- Adjust the seat tilt so that the seat back is about an inch higher than the front (hips slightly higher than the knees).[3,7,19–25]
- The seat tilt helps to maintain the natural lower curve of the spine and relaxes the bend of the knees. The seat tilt should only be about 5°; overtilting it can cause too much low back curve.
- **Note:** Chairs without a tilt feature can be retrofitted with an ergonomic wedge-shaped cushion.

Steps continue on the next page. . .

Figure 1-25. Step 4.

- With buttocks seated all the way back in the chair, adjust the lumbar depth by moving the backrest closer or farther from the seat pan until the backrest nestles against the lower back.
- The unsupported lower back tends to straighten rather than maintain a healthy curve.[20,25]

Figure 1-26. Step 5. Adjust the lumbar height by moving the backrest up or down until it nestles in the natural lumbar curve of the lower back. This helps to support the natural curve of the spine.[20]

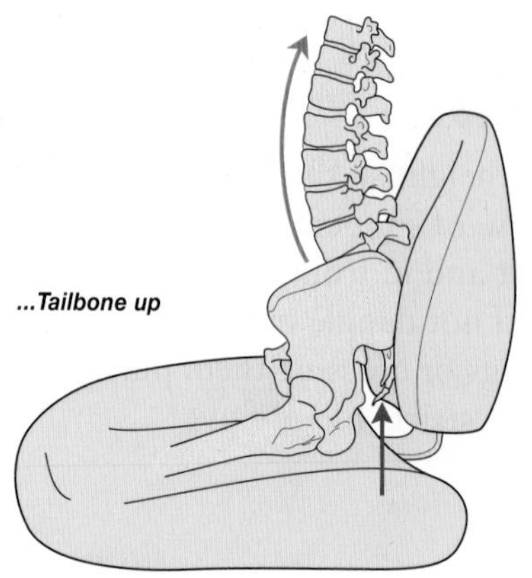

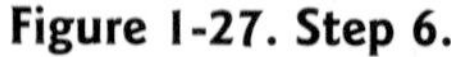

Figure 1-27. Step 6.

- Raise the tailbone up to establish correct spinal curves. All three normal back curves should be present while sitting.
- Studies of the seated body show that the position of the pelvis determines the shape of the spine.[24]

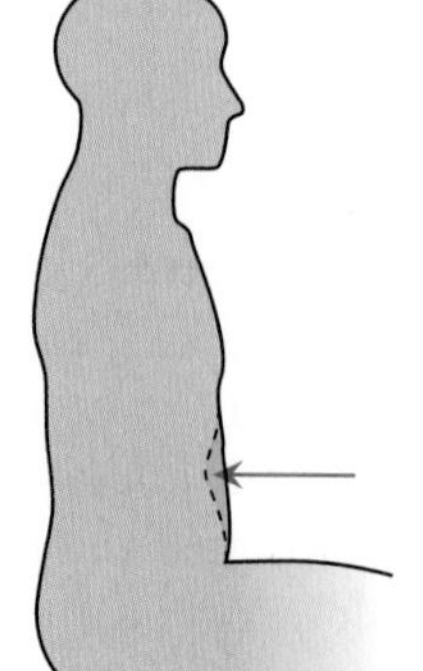

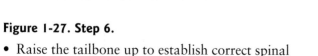

Figure 1-28. Step 7.

- Stabilize the low back curve by pulling the stomach muscles toward the spine.[25]

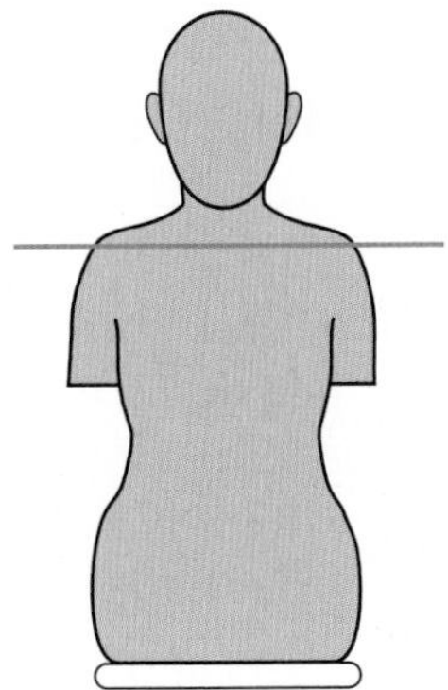

Figure 1-29. Step 8.

- Relax your shoulders so that they are down and back.[21]
- If your stool has armrests, adjust the height of each armrest so the arms are supported. This helps take weight off of the shoulders.

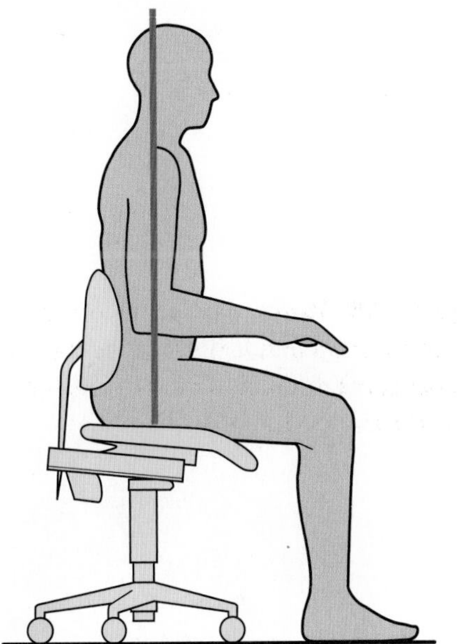

Figure 1-30. Step 9.

- Position the upper arms parallel to the long axis of the torso with elbows held near the body.
- Maintain a trunk position such that an imaginary straight line can be drawn connecting from the ear, shoulder, and hips.[3]

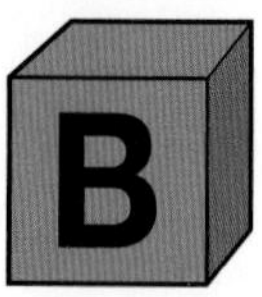

SKILL BUILDING. THE MASKING TAPE TRICK

An easy way to monitor back position while practicing instrumentation in preclinic is to use the masking tape trick. While sitting with your back in a neutral position, have a friend apply a strip of masking tape down the center of your back, along your spinal column. Figure 1-31 shows how the masking tape will appear when a clinician is seated in neutral position. If a clinician bends forward, out of neutral position, the masking tape breaks, as shown in Figure 1-32.

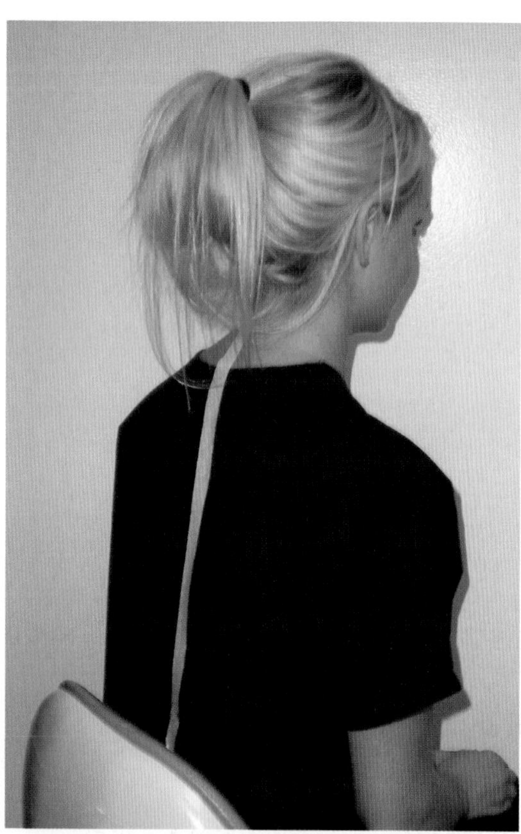

Figure 1-31. Correct Position—Neutral Back Position. Maintain a neutral back position while practicing positioning or periodontal instrumentation and the strip of masking tape remains intact and straight. (Photo courtesy of Dr. Richard Foster, Guilford Technical Community College, Jamestown, NC.)

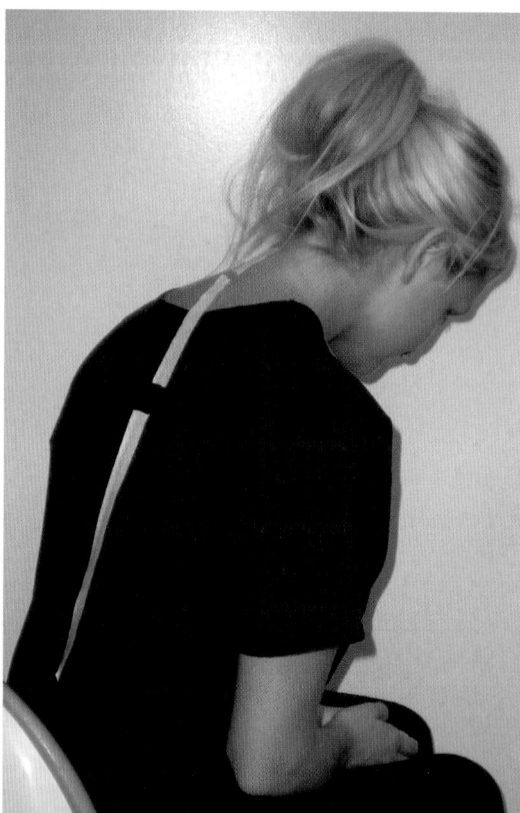

Figure 1-32. Incorrect Position—Rounded Back Position. The masking tape strip will tear if you bend over, rounding your back while practicing positioning or periodontal instrumentation. Torn masking tape will alert you to problems with your seated position. (Photo courtesy of Dr. Richard Foster, Guilford Technical Community College, Jamestown, NC.)

Section 4

Positioning the Patient

SUPINE AND SEMI-SUPINE PATIENT POSITION

The recommended patient position for dental treatment is with the patient lying on his or her back. For maxillary treatment areas, the back of the dental chair is nearly parallel to the floor in a supine position (Table 1-2). For mandibular treatment areas, the back of the dental chair is slightly upright in a semi-supine position (Table 1-3).

TABLE 1-2. Position for Maxillary Treatment Areas

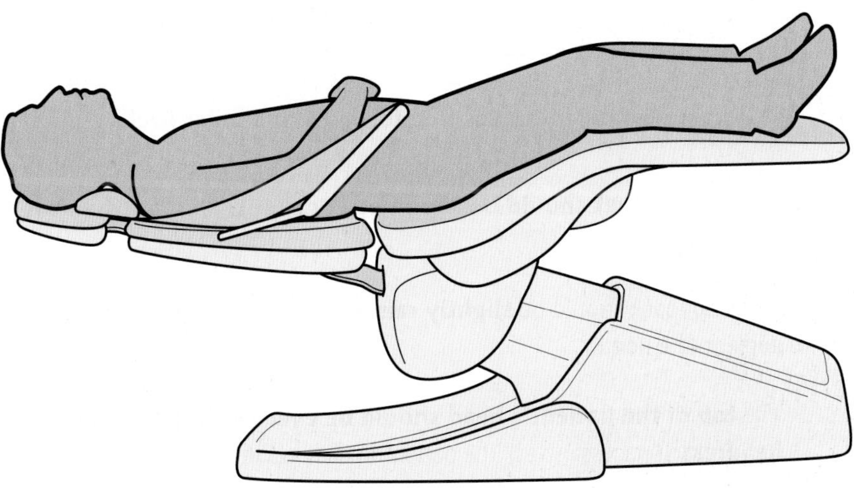

Figure 1-33. Patient Position for the Maxillary Arch.

Body	The patient's **feet should be even with or slightly higher than the tip of his or her nose**.
Chair Back	The chair back should be nearly **parallel to the floor** for maxillary treatment areas.
Head	The **top of the patient's head should be even with the upper edge of the headrest**. If necessary, ask the patient to slide up in the chair to assume this position.
Headrest	Adjust the headrest so that the patient's head is in a **chin-up position**, with the patient's nose and chin level. Patient head position is discussed in more detail later in this chapter.

TABLE 1-3. Position for Mandibular Treatment Areas

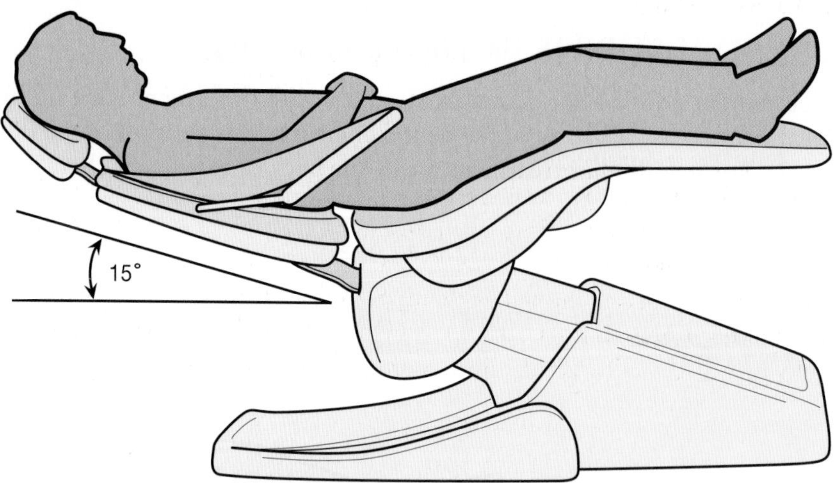

Figure 1-34. Patient Position for the Mandibular Arch.

Body	The patient's **feet should be even with or slightly higher than the tip of his or her nose**.
Chair Back	The chair back should be **slightly raised above the parallel position** at a 15°–20° angle to the floor.[25]
Head	The **top of the patient's head should be even with the upper edge of the headrest**. If necessary, ask the patient to slide up in the chair to assume this position.
Headrest	Raise the headrest slightly so that the patient's head is in a **chin-down position**, with the patient's chin lower than the nose. Patient head position is discussed in greater detail later in this chapter.

PATIENT HEAD POSITION

The patient's head position is an important factor in determining whether the clinician can see and access the teeth in a treatment area.

- Unfortunately, a clinician may ignore this important aspect of patient positioning, contorting his or her body into an uncomfortable position instead of asking the patient to change head positions. Working in this manner not only causes stress on the musculoskeletal system, but also makes it difficult to see the treatment area.
- Remember that the patient is only in the chair for a limited period of time, while the clinician spends hours at chairside day after day. The patient should be asked to adjust his or her head position to provide the clinician with the best view of the treatment area.
- The patient's head should be positioned at the upper edge of the headrest. This position permits maximal visibility and access to the oral cavity. Figures 1-35A and 1-35B depict correct patient head position for an adult and a young child. Incorrect head position is shown in Figure 1-36.

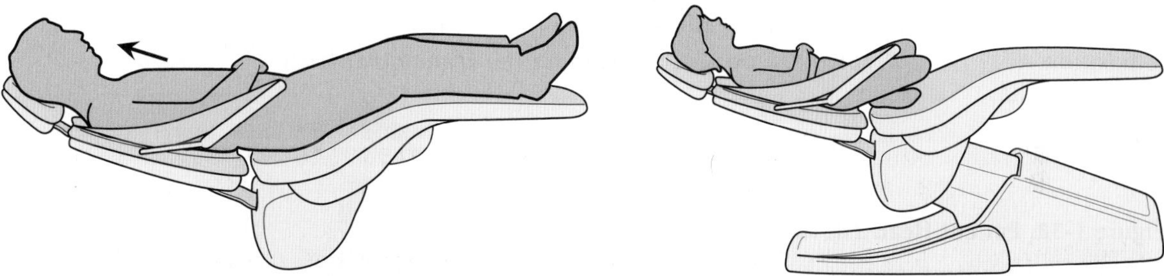

Figure 1-35. Correct Position.

A. Adult Patient. Once the patient chair is in a supine or semi-supine position, ask the patient to slide up until his or her head is even with the top edge of the headrest.

B. Young Child. Asking a young child to bend the knees and cross the legs may be helpful in keeping him or her from sliding down in the chair.

Figure 1-36. Incorrect Position. The patient may slide down in the chair when the patient chair is reclined. If the patient's head is not even with the upper edge of the headrest, access and visibility of the oral cavity are restricted.

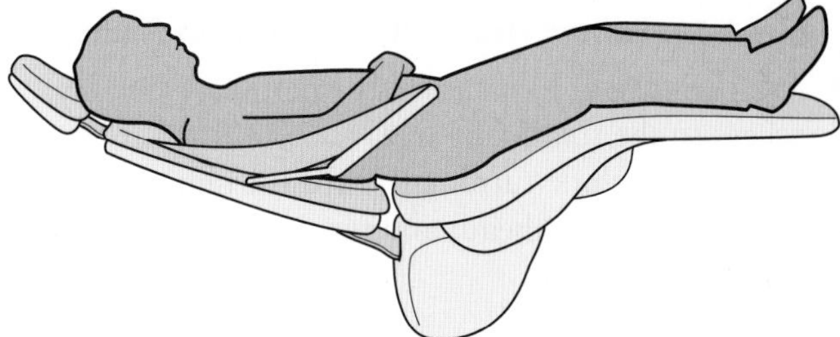

PATIENT HEAD ADJUSTMENT FOR OPTIMAL VISIBILITY

Once the patient is comfortably lying in a reclined position, the next objective is to ask the patient to adjust his or her head position to attain an optimal view of the treatment area. The patient can (1) tilt the head up or down, (2) rotate the head toward or away from the clinician, and (3) bend the head to the side (Figs. 1-37 to 1-40). Articulating headrests facilitate adjustment of the patient's head. Cervical rolls can be used with nonarticulating headrests to maintain patient head position.

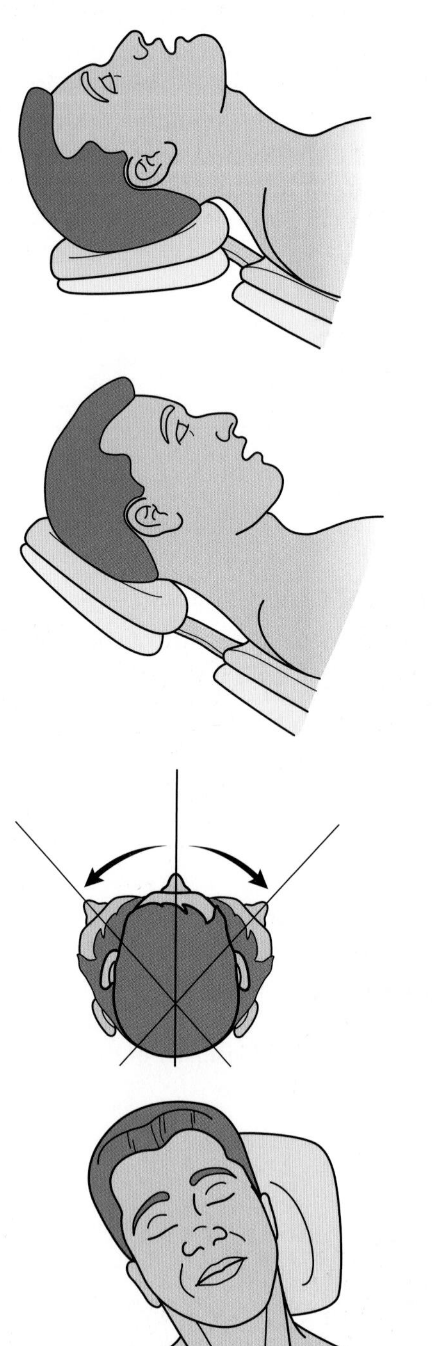

Figure 1-37. Patient Head Tilt for Maxillary Arch.

- Angle the headrest up into the back of the patient's head (occipital area) so that the nose and chin are approximately level.
- The upper arch needs to be angled backward past the vertical plane.
- This patient head position is known as the chin-up position.

Figure 1-38. Patient Head Tilt for Mandibular Arch.

- Angle the headrest forward and down, so that the chin is lower than nose level.
- The occlusal or incisal surfaces of the treatment area should be approximately parallel to the floor.
- This patient head position is known as the chin-down position.

Figure 1-39. Patient Head Rotation for Both Arches.

- Ask the patient to rotate his or her head for easy access to the treatment area.
- Positions include turning toward the clinician, looking straight ahead, and turning slightly away from the clinician.

Figure 1-40. Bending the Head to the Side.

- If the patient chair has a flat, nonarticulated headrest, it is helpful to ask the patient to side-bend the head toward the clinician and then turn his or her head for the treatment area.
- This technique can position the oral cavity 2 to 3 inches closer to the clinician and enhance viewing of the treatment area.

Section 5

Adjusting the Overhead Light and Instrument Tray

POSITIONING THE OVERHEAD DENTAL LIGHT

Ideally, the overhead dental light is positioned so that the light beam is parallel to the clinician's line of sight.[7,25]

- For mandibular treatment areas, the overhead dental light is positioned so that the light beam is approximately perpendicular to the floor (Fig. 1-41).
- For maxillary treatment areas, it is usually not possible to direct the light beam identically to the clinician's line of sight. For maxillary areas, it is often necessary to move the dental light above the patient's neck and angle the light beam into the mouth (Fig. 1-42).
- It is significant to note that dentists and dental hygienists whose overhead dental lights are positioned farther away from their sight lines (toward the patient's feet) for maxillary treatment are more likely to experience lower back pain.[7]

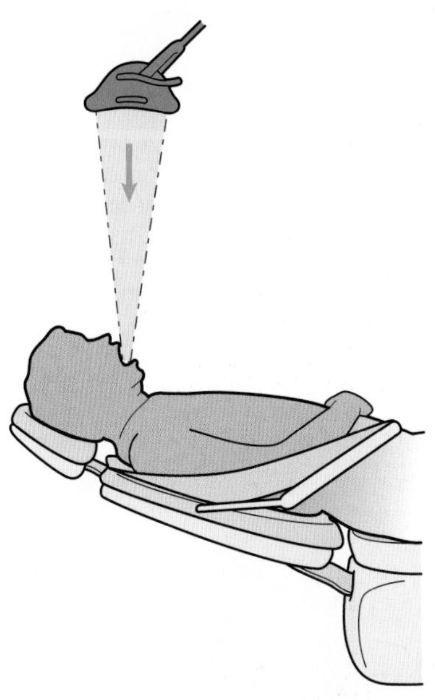

Figure 1-41. Light Position for Mandibular Arch.

- For the mandibular treatment areas, the overhead dental unit light is positioned directly over the oral cavity.
- Position the light **at arm's length** within comfortable reach. Avoid positioning the light close to the patient's head.
- The patient is in a chin-down head position.
- The light beam is directed approximately perpendicular to the floor.

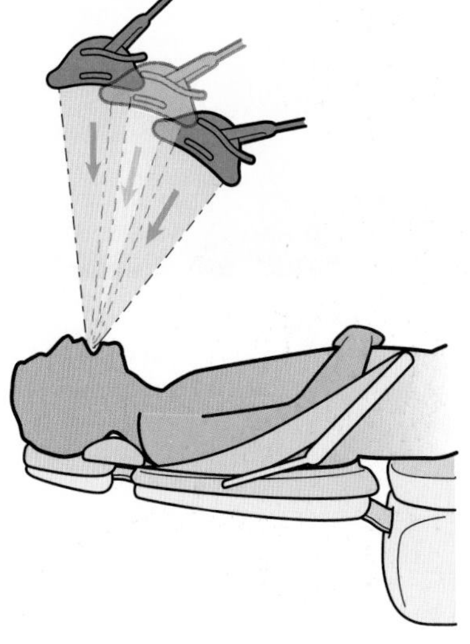

Figure 1-42. Light Position for Maxillary Arch.

- For the maxillary treatment areas, the position of the overhead dental unit light ranges from being directly over the oral cavity to a position over the patient's neck.
- Position the light **at arm's length** within comfortable reach.
- Ideally, the light beam always would be perpendicular to the floor, but this is not always possible using an overhead dental light. This is why a co-axial illumination source is ideal. Co-axial illumination is discussed later in this chapter.
- The patient is in a chin-up position.
- The direction of the light beam ranges from perpendicular to the floor to a 60° to 90° angle to the floor.

POSITIONING THE INSTRUMENT TRAY

The instrument tray should be positioned within easy reach of the clinician's dominant hand (Fig. 1-43). Incorrect positioning of the instrument tray as depicted in Figure 1-44 places unnecessary stress on the clinician.

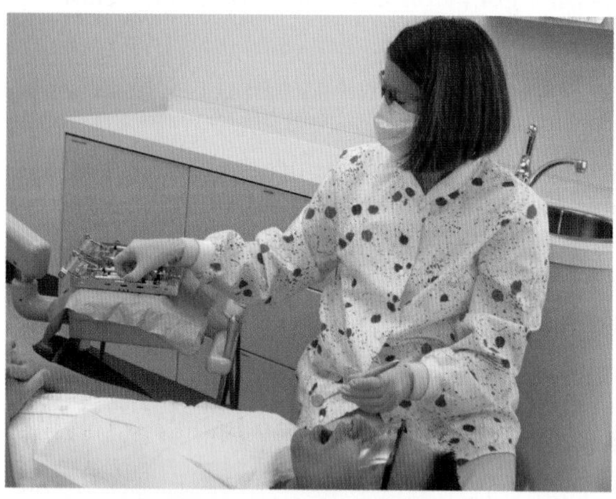

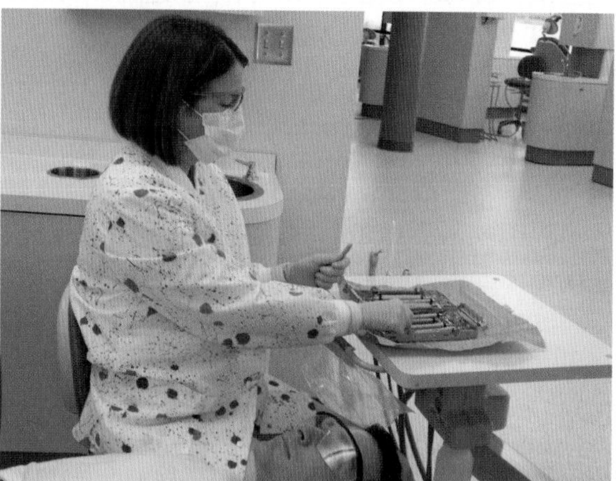

Figure 1-43. Correct Positioning of the Instrument Tray.

A. Front/Side Delivery. Instrument tray positioned correctly for front or side delivery within easy reach of the clinician's dominant hand.

B. Rear Delivery. Instrument tray positioned correctly for rear delivery within easy reach of the clinician's dominant hand.

Figure 1-44. Incorrect Positioning. A combination of positioning errors is demonstrated in this photo.

- The patient's oral cavity is positioned too high at mid-torso, instead of at the clinician's waist level.
- The bracket table is positioned too far from the clinician, causing her to have to stretch to reach the instrument.

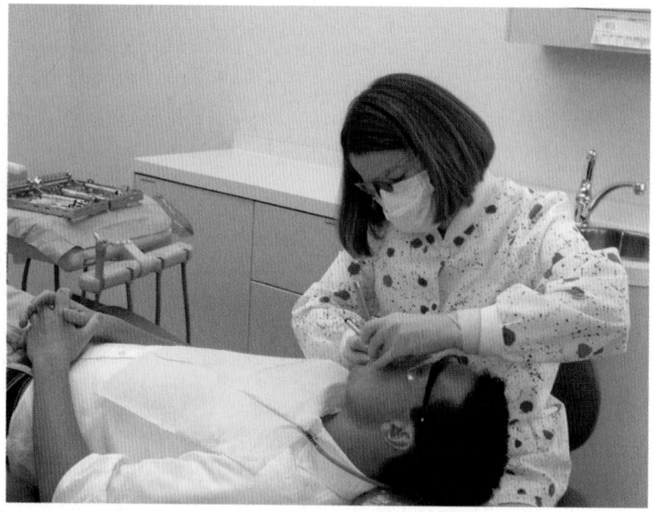

Section 6
Adjusting the Patient to Facilitate Neutral Seated Position

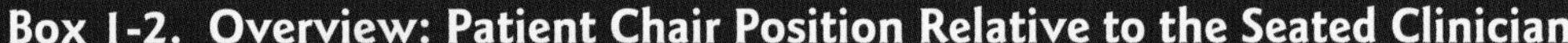

A major component in avoiding fatigue and injury is proper positioning of the patient and dental equipment in relation to the seated clinician.

- While working, the clinician must be able to gain access to the patient's mouth and the dental unit without bending, stretching, or holding his or her elbows above waist level.
- *The neutral seated position is established first, and then everything else—the patient chair, the patient's head, the dental unit light, and other dental equipment—is adjusted to facilitate maintenance of the neutral seated position.*
- Box 1-2 provides an overview of the relationship of the patient chair to the seated clinician.

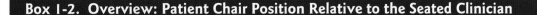

Box 1-2. Overview: Patient Chair Position Relative to the Seated Clinician

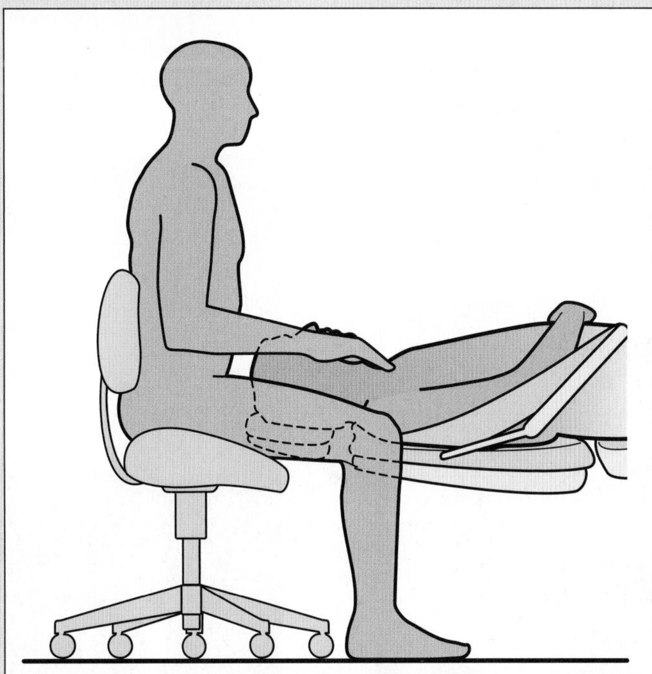

Figure 1-45

- Clinician assumes a neutral seated position.
- The clinician establishes a "wide base of support" with feet on floor at least shoulder-width apart and in front of the hips.
- The patient chair is lowered until the tip of the patient's nose is below the clinician's waist.
- The clinician should position his or her stool close to the patient to enhance vision of the treatment area and to minimize forward bending.
- Whenever possible, the clinician should straddle the headrest to facilitate neutral position.

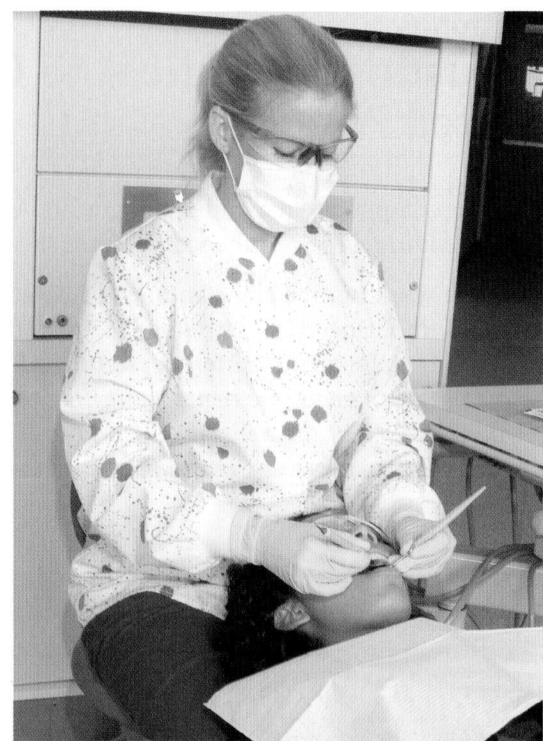

Figure 1-46. Correct Positioning. Here, the patient chair and patient's head are positioned at the correct height in relation to the clinician. Note that the clinician holds her upper arms parallel to her torso, her arms are not raised, and her shoulders are relaxed.

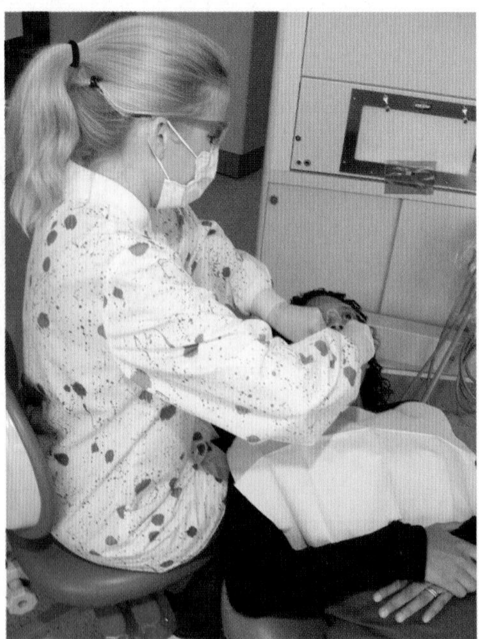

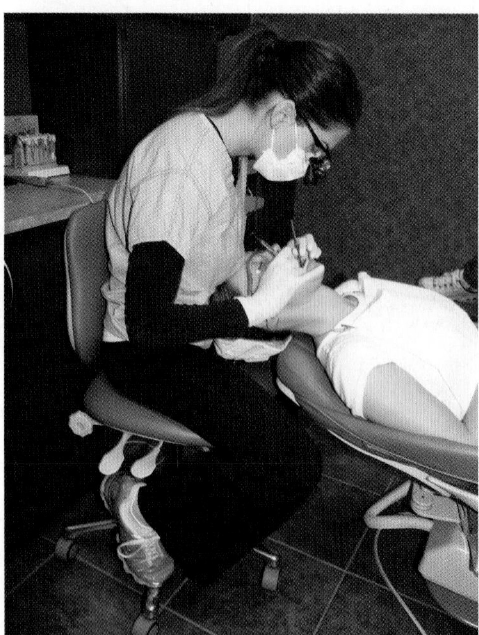

Figure 1-47. Incorrect Positioning—Patient Too High.

A. Note how this clinician must hold her elbows up in a stressful position in order to reach the patient's mouth. This error is often due to the misconception that the clinician sees better if the patient is closer. Actually, the reverse is true; the clinician has improved vision of the mouth when the patient is in a lower position.

B. In this example, the patient is positioned too high for the clinician, and as a result, the clinician's chair is too high, causing her to rest her feet on the rungs of the chair. (Courtesy of Sara Solomon, LPT, DMD, Toronto, Ontario, Canada.)

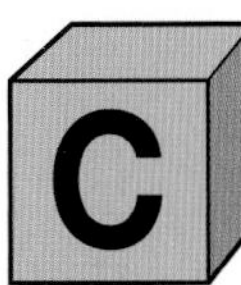

SKILL BUILDING. ESTABLISHING HEIGHT OF THE PATIENT CHAIR

Directions: Follow steps 1 to 5 shown in Figure 1-48 to practice establishing the correct height of the patient chair in relation to the seated clinician.

1. Assume a neutral seated position. Sit next to the patient with the forearms crossed at your waist.
2. Position the patient chair for the treatment area (maxillary: supine; mandibular: semi-supine).
3. Position the patient's head for the treatment area (chin-up or chin-down).
4. The patient's open mouth should be ***below*** the point of your elbow.
5. In this position, you will be able to reach the treatment area without raising your elbows above waist level.

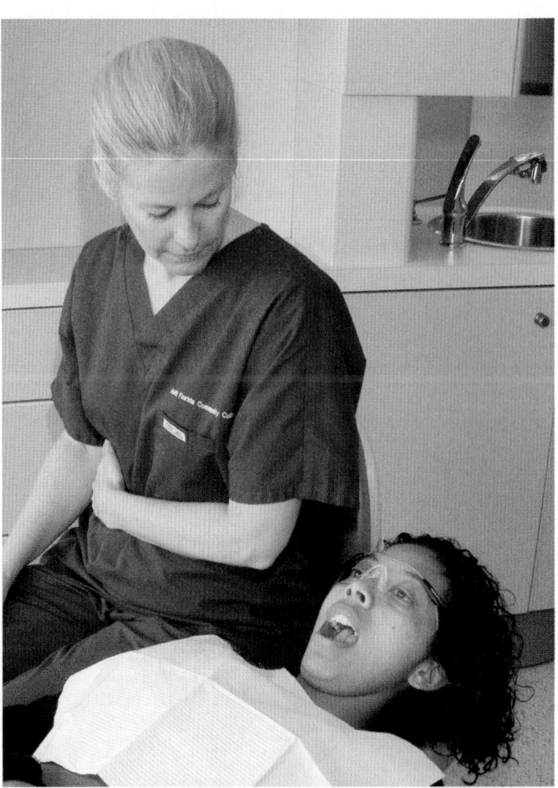

Figure 1-48

Section 7
Ancillary Equipment

Ancillary equipment that may be helpful to the clinician during periodontal instrumentation includes a co-axial illumination source and magnification loupes.

DENTAL HEADLIGHTS: CO-AXIAL ILLUMINATION

Adequate light must be present for human eyes to function effectively. In many instances, the clinician's hands or instruments block the light from the overhead dental light, causing the clinician to crane the neck and assume a poor working posture. Instead of using the overhead dental light for illumination, many clinicians use a light source attached to a headband or mounted to magnification loupes.

1. **Co-Axial Illumination**
   - Co-axial illumination sources are spectacle-mounted or headband-mounted miniature lights that provide a beam of light that is parallel to the clinician's sight line (Figs. 1-49 to 1-52). In everyday terms, co-axial illumination sources are called dental headlights.
2. **Advantages of Dental Headlights**
   - Co-axial illumination provides a light source that is parallel to the clinician's line of vision that eliminates shadows produced by hands and instruments.
   - Dental headlights provide the clinician with shadow-free light and facilitate improved posture.[41]
   - Dental professionals spend many hours per year adjusting traditional overhead dental lights. Dental headlights improve productivity because time is not wasted adjusting a traditional overhead dental light.[41]
   - Dental headlights are highly recommended for use when learning and performing periodontal instrumentation.

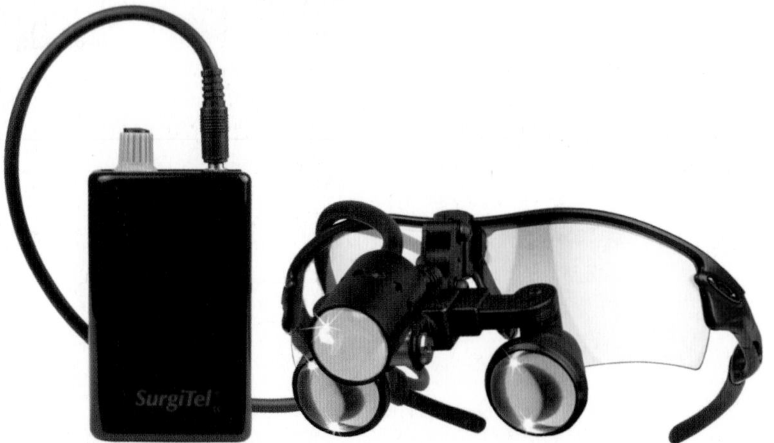

Figure 1-49. Co-Axial Illumination Source. A headlight mounted to eyeglass frames. Note also that magnification loupes are mounted to the lenses of the glasses. The battery power source for the headlight is shown on the left-hand side of the photo. (Courtesy of SurgiTel/General Scientific Corporation.)

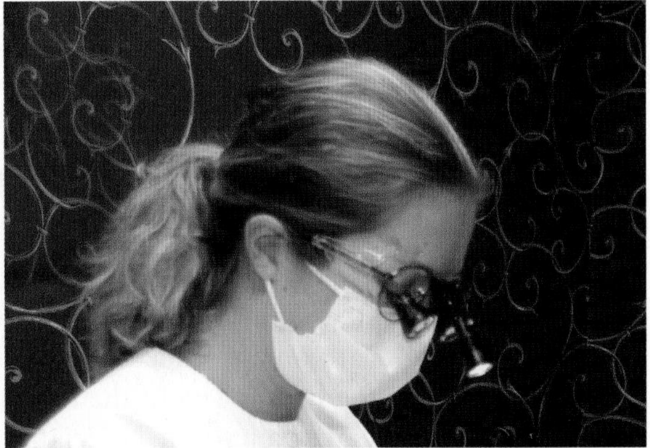

Figure 1-50. Dental Headlight. A dental hygienist wearing a spectacle-mounted dental headlight.

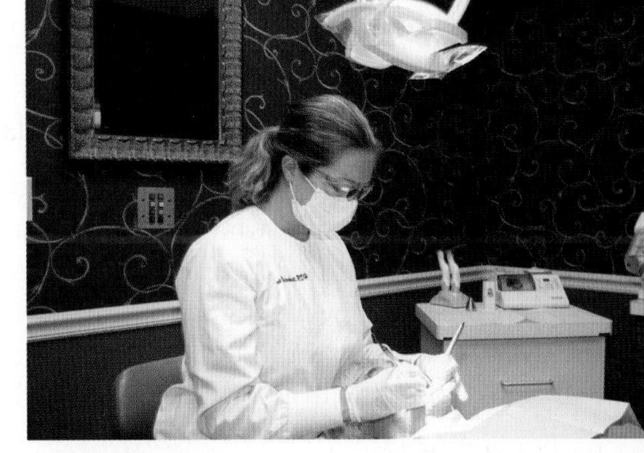

Figure 1-51. Illumination with an Overhead Light. Often, it is difficult to position an overhead light to achieve good illumination of the maxillary arch. Note that the hygienist's head is blocking the light beams.

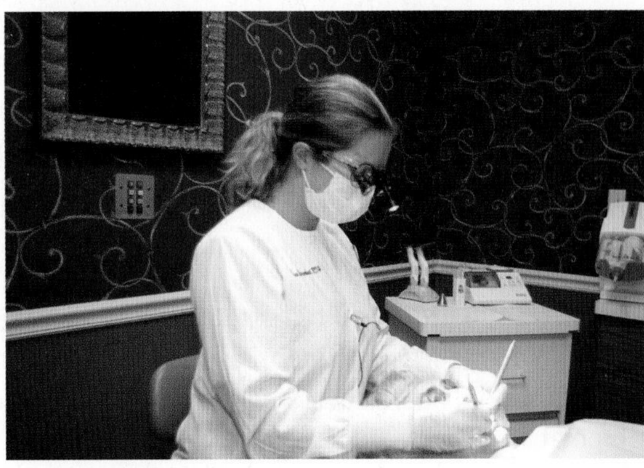

Figure 1-52. Co-Axial Illumination. The dental headlight provides a beam of light that is parallel to the clinician's line of sight. The headlight provides good illumination of maxillary and mandibular treatment areas. And, there is no need to reach up to adjust an overhead light!

MAGNIFICATION LOUPES

Magnification through surgical telescopes—known as magnification loupes—can be a technological aid during periodontal instrumentation (Figs. 1-53 and 1-54).

I. Magnification Loupes: Ergonomically Helpful or Harmful?

A. Benefits of Loupes

1. Clinicians using appropriate magnification loupes report decreased eyestrain and an improved visual sharpness.[7,41,42]
2. Magnification may reduce the tendency to lean forward in an attempt to obtain a better view of the treatment area and, therefore, reduce musculoskeletal strain to the clinician's neck, back, and shoulder muscles. For these reasons, some dental and dental hygiene programs have begun including magnification loops in their instrument kits.

B. Problems Associated with Loupes

1. As with most equipment, how the loupes are used determines whether this equipment is beneficial in reducing musculoskeletal strain. ***A poorly fitted or incorrectly used magnification system is more likely to exacerbate musculoskeletal problems than to solve them.***[10,43–45] It is important to make sure that the magnification system is properly fitted to the clinician.
2. According to B.J. Chang, PhD, President and Chief Scientist of SurgiTel/General Scientific Group, "Many clinicians think loupes solve ergonomic problems, but loupes can create ergonomic problems. The key is to find loupes that meet their ergonomic requirements."[43]
   a. Loupes with improper working distances and declination angles can actually cause chronic neck and upper back pain.[43,45–47]
   b. Misalignment of the two oculars can cause eyestrain, double vision, and headaches.
   c. Clinicians should try loupes before they buy and ensure the loupes are custom-fit.

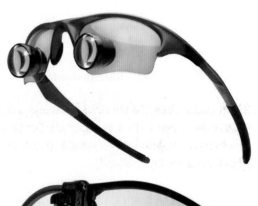

Figure 1-53. Through-the-Lens Style. Through-the-lens style compound lenses loupes provide low-to-medium magnification. (Courtesy of SurgiTel/General Scientific Corporation.)

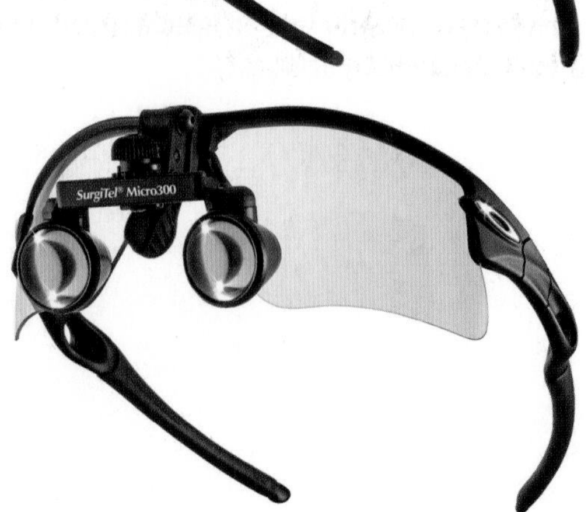

Figure 1-54. Flip-up Style. Flip-up styles have the magnification telescopes attached to the eyeglasses by a hinged bracket. The bracket allows the clinician to obtain nonmagnified vision by rotating the telescopes above the eyewear. (Courtesy of SurgiTel/General Scientific Corporation.)

2. Magnification Loupes for Periodontal Instrumentation

A. Ergonomic Criteria for Loupes Selection. Four essential considerations when selecting loupes for periodontal instrumentation are (1) working distance, (2) declination angle, (3) depth of field, and (4) frame size and weight.[43,47]

1. Working distance is the distance measured from the eyes to the teeth being treated. ***If the working distance measured for the loupes is too short, the clinician needs to assume a head-forward or hunching posture to see the treatment area.***
2. Angle of declination is the angle between the temple piece of the spectacle-mounted magnification system and the actual line of sight chosen by the clinician (Fig. 1-55).
   a. Declination angles among clinicians range from 15° to 44°.[47] Each clinician has a unique optimal declination angle determined by the individual's most balanced seated position.
   b. ***If the declination angle of the loupes is too small, the clinician will have to tip the head forward or use a hunching posture to view the treatment area through the loupes.***
   c. ***If the declination angle is too great, the clinician will have to tilt the head backward in order to view the treatment area through the loupes.***
3. **Depth of Field.** Depth of field is the distance range within which the object being viewed remains in sharp focus.
   a. Adequate depth of field allows the clinician to move his or her head without the treatment area going out of focus.
   b. ***Inadequate depth of field may cause the clinician to assume an awkward head position in order to clearly view the treatment area.***

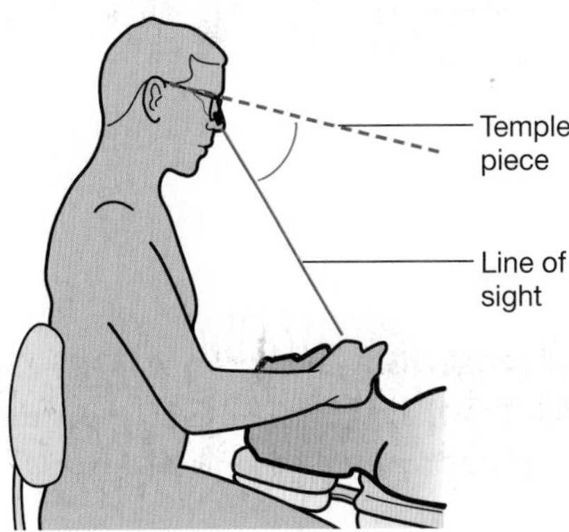

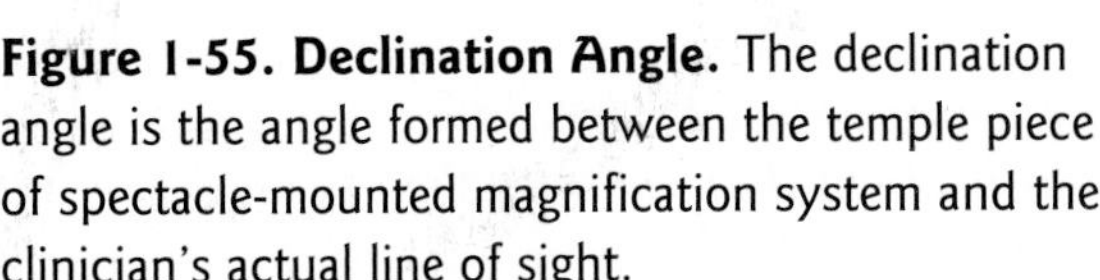

Figure 1-55. Declination Angle. The declination angle is the angle formed between the temple piece of spectacle-mounted magnification system and the clinician's actual line of sight.

4. **Sizes and Weight of Spectacle Frame**
   a. Large frames that sit low on the cheek allow better placement of the telescopes than narrow, oval frames. In general, the lower the telescopes are in relation to the clinician's pupils, the better the declination angle.
   b. The dental professional may wear magnification loupes for many hours each day. Therefore, it is important that the frames be as light and comfortable as possible.

3. Important Considerations for Preclinical Periodontal Instrumentation

A. Limitations on What Can Be Seen with Magnification

1. **Field of View with Magnification.** The field of view is the total size of the object that can be viewed through the loupes.
   a. The most popular magnification strengths for periodontal debridement are 2.0×, 2.5×, and 2.6×.[43] These magnifications allow the clinician to view the entire mouth at one time. Higher magnification levels result in a smaller field of view.
   b. The lowest level of magnification required should be selected. Lower magnification levels increase the depth of field and minimize the blind zone.[48]
   c. Too great a level of magnification makes it difficult to keep the treatment area steady in the field of vision.
2. **Blind Zone with Magnification.** The blind zone is an area of vision between the unmagnified peripheral field of vision and the magnified center of the field of vision.
   a. The blind zone presents the most difficulty when an instrument is being moved into or out of the magnified field of view. Injury to the patient or the clinician is a possibility as the instrument is moved through the blind spot. Most clinicians simply move the loupes aside until a stable fulcrum has been established with the instrument.
   b. The lowest magnification should be selected to minimize the size of the blind zone.

B. Criteria for Use of Magnification Loupes in Preclinical Setting

1. **Ability for Student Self-Assessment**
   a. When learning the skills of clinician position, patient position, clock positions, mirror use, and finger rests, it is vital that the student clinician is able to continuously self-assess the positioning of his or her body, arms, hands, and fingers.
   b. ***Self-assessment of these skills during the learning process means that the student clinician must have a visual field that includes the patient's head and the clinician's arms, hands, and fingers, as well as the patient's oral cavity.***
   c. Figure 1-56 shows the minimum field of vision needed by the student clinician while practicing and mastering the fundamental skills of patient position, clock positions, mirror use, and finger rests.
   d. Magnification loupes limit the clinician's field of vision to the oral cavity.[49] Figure 1-57 shows the clinician's field of vision using 2.5× magnification loupes. Once a clinician has mastered the fundamental skills of patient position, clock positions, mirror use, and finger rests, the loupes provide a field of vision that is adequate for instrumentation.
   e. ***This magnified field of vision, however, is too restrictive to permit self-evaluation of skills when acquiring the fundamental preclinical skills of positioning and finger rests.***

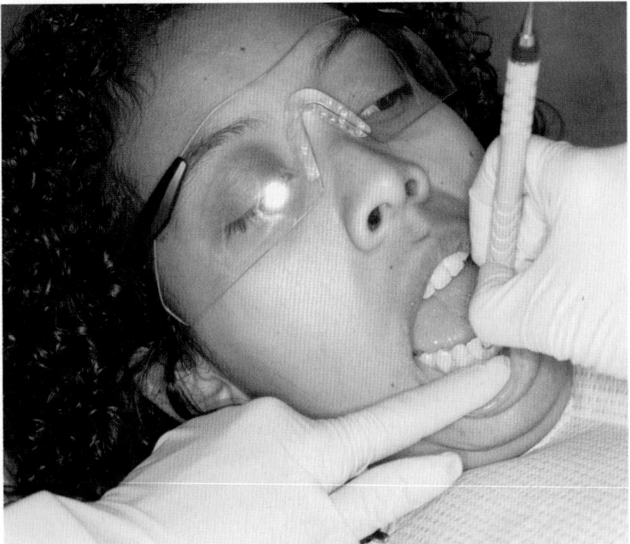

Figure 1-56. Field of View without Loupes. When learning and mastering the fundamental skills of positioning, mirror use, and finger rests, the student clinician needs a field of vision that allows him or her to continuously self-evaluate these skills.

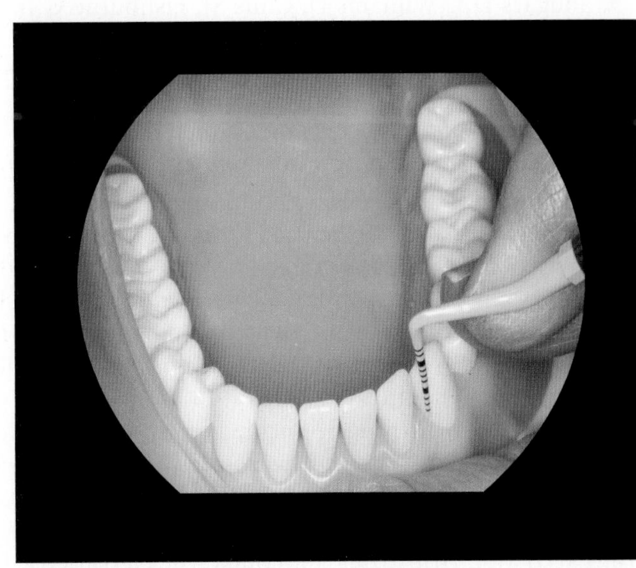

Figure 1-57. Field of View with Loupes. When wearing magnification loupes, the clinician's field of vision is limited to the oral cavity. This field of vision is too restrictive when practicing and perfecting the fundamental skills of positioning, mirror use, and finger rests.

Box 1-3. No Magnification, Please

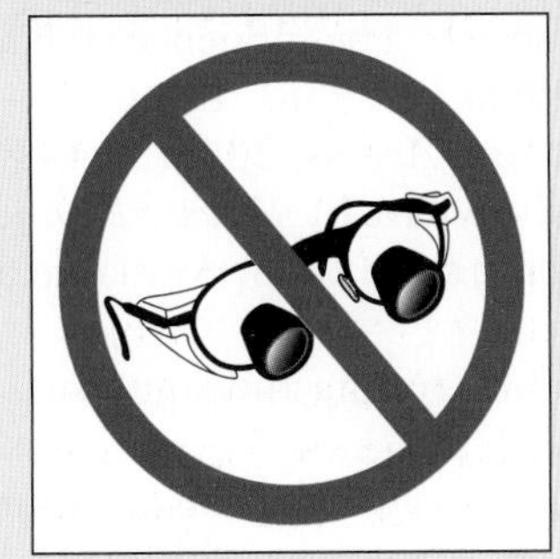

Magnification loupes should not be worn when first attempting, practicing, and perfecting certain fundamental skills of periodontal instrumentation. The limited field of vision created by magnification loupes makes it impossible for student clinicians to self-evaluate fundamental skills such as positioning, grasp, and finger rests.

REFERENCES

1. Beach JC, DeBiase CB. Assessment of ergonomic education in dental hygiene curricula. *J Dent Educ*. 1998;62:421–425.
2. Boyer EM, Elton J, Preston K. Precautionary procedures. Use in dental hygiene practice. *Dent Hyg (Chic)*. 1986;60:516–523.
3. Dylla J, Forrest JL. Fit to sit–strategies to maximize function and minimize occupational pain. *J Mich Dent Assoc*. 2008;90:38–45.
4. Gravois SL, Stringer RB. Survey of occupational health hazards in dental hygiene. *Dent Hyg (Chic)*. 1980;54:518–523.
5. Oberg T, Oberg U. Musculoskeletal complaints in dental hygiene: a survey study from a Swedish county. *J Dent Hyg*. 1993;67:257–261.
6. Rising DW, Bennett BC, Hursh K, Plesh O. Reports of body pain in a dental student population. *J Am Dent Assoc*. 2005;136:81–86.
7. Rucker LM, Sunell S. Ergonomic risk factors associated with clinical dentistry. *J Calif Dent Assoc*. 2002;30:139–148.
8. Rundcrantz BL, Johnsson B, Moritz U. Cervical pain and discomfort among dentists. Epidemiological, clinical and therapeutic aspects. Part 1. A survey of pain and discomfort. *Swed Dent J*. 1990;14:71–80.
9. Shugars DA, Williams D, Cline SJ, Fishburne C Jr. Musculoskeletal back pain among dentists. *Gen Dent*. 1984;32:481–485.
10. Sunell S, Rucker L. Surgical magnification in dental hygiene practice. *Int J Dent Hyg*. 2004;2:26–35.
11. Alexopoulos EC, Stathi IC, Charizani F. Prevalence of musculoskeletal disorders in dentists. *BMC Musculoskelet Disord*. 2004;5:16.
12. Barry RM, Woodall WR, Mahan JM. Postural changes in dental hygienists. Four-year longitudinal study. *J Dent Hyg*. 1992;66:147–150.
13. Meador HL. The biocentric technique: a guide to avoiding occupational pain. *J Dent Hyg*. 1993;67:38–51.
14. Silverstein BA, Stetson DS, Keyserling WM, Fine LJ. Work-related musculoskeletal disorders: comparison of data sources for surveillance. *Am J Ind Med*. 1997;31:600–608.
15. Silverstein BA, Fine LJ, Armstrong TJ. Hand wrist cumulative trauma disorders in industry. *Br J Ind Med*. 1986;43:779–784.
16. Kilbom S, Armstrong T, Buckle P, et al. Musculoskeletal disorders: work-related risk factors and prevention. *Int J Occup Environ Health*. 1996;2:239–246.
17. Silverstein BA, Fine LJ, Armstrong TJ. Occupational factors and carpal tunnel syndrome. *Am J Ind Med*. 1987;11:343–358.
18. Latko WA, Armstrong TJ, Foulke JA, Herrin GD, Rabourn RA, Ulin SS. Development and evaluation of an observational method for assessing repetition in hand tasks. *Am Ind Hyg Assoc J*. 1997;58:278–285.
19. Rucker L. Musculoskeletal health status in B.C. dentist and dental hygienists: evaluation the preventive impact of surgical ergonomics training and surgical magnification. 2000. Available at: http://www.worksafebc.com/about_us/library_services/reports_and_guides/wcb_research/Default.asp.
20. Andersson GB, Murphy RW, Ortengren R, Nachemson AL. The influence of backrest inclination and lumbar support on lumbar lordosis. *Spine (Phila Pa 1976)*. 1979;4:52–58.
21. Dylia J, Forrest JL. Training to sit, starting with structure. *Access*. 2006;20:42–44.
22. Dylia J, Forrest JL. Training to sit, starting with structure part II. *Access*. 2006;20:19–23.
23. Mandal AC. Balanced sitting posture on forward sloping seat. 2008. Available at: http://acmandal.com/.
24. Schoberth H. Correct workplace sitting, scientific studies, results and solutions. Der arbeitssitz in industriellen produktionsbereich. Berlin: Springer; 1970.
25. Valachi B, Valachi K. Preventing musculoskeletal disorders in clinical dentistry: strategies to address the mechanisms leading to musculoskeletal disorders. *J Am Dent Assoc*. 2003;134:1604–1612.
26. Akesson I, Johnsson B, Rylander L, Moritz U, Skerfving S. Musculoskeletal disorders among female dental personnel–clinical examination and a 5-year follow-up study of symptoms. *Int Arch Occup Environ Health*. 1999;72:395–403.

27. Anton D, Rosecrance J, Merlino L, Cook T. Prevalence of musculoskeletal symptoms and carpal tunnel syndrome among dental hygienists. *Am J Ind Med.* 2002;42:248–257.
28. de Carvalho MV, Soriano EP, de Franca Caldas A Jr, Campello RI, de Miranda HF, Cavalcanti FI. Work-related musculoskeletal disorders among Brazilian dental students. *J Dent Educ.* 2009;73:624–630.
29. Hayes M, Cockrell D, Smith DR. A systematic review of musculoskeletal disorders among dental professionals. *Int J Dent Hyg.* 2009;7:159–165.
30. Hayes MJ, Smith DR, Cockrell D. Prevalence and correlates of musculoskeletal disorders among Australian dental hygiene students. *Int J Dent Hyg.* 2009;7:176–181.
31. Melis M, Abou-Atme YS, Cottogno L, Pittau R. Upper body musculoskeletal symptoms in Sardinian dental students. *J Can Dent Assoc.* 2004;70:306–310.
32. Michalak-Turcotte C. Controlling dental hygiene work-related musculoskeletal disorders: the ergonomic process. *J Dent Hyg.* 2000;74:41–48.
33. Morse T, Bruneau H, Dussetschleger J. Musculoskeletal disorders of the neck and shoulder in the dental professions. *Work.* 2010;35:419–429.
34. Morse T, Bruneau H, Michalak-Turcotte C, et al. Musculoskeletal disorders of the neck and shoulder in dental hygienists and dental hygiene students. *J Dent Hyg.* 2007;81:10.
35. Samotoi A, Moffat SM, Thomson WM. Musculoskeletal symptoms in New Zealand dental therapists: prevalence and associated disability. *N Z Dent J.* 2008;104:49–53.
36. Thornton LJ, Barr AE, Stuart-Buttle C, et al. Perceived musculoskeletal symptoms among dental students in the clinic work environment. *Ergonomics.* 2008;51:573–586.
37. Warren N. Causes of musculoskeletal disorders in dental hygienists and dental hygiene students: a study of combined biomechanical and psychosocial risk factors. *Work.* 2010;35:441–454.
38. Yamalik N. Musculoskeletal disorders (MSDs) and dental practice. Part 2. Risk factors for dentistry, magnitude of the problem, prevention, and dental ergonomics. *Int Dent J.* 2007;57:45–54.
39. American Academy of Orthopedic Surgeons. Spine basics: spinal curves. American Academy of Orthopedic Surgeons. Available at: hppt://orthoinfo.aaso.org/topic.cfm?topic5A00575.
40. Valachi B, Valachi K. Mechanisms leading to musculoskeletal disorders in dentistry. *J Am Dent Assoc.* 2003;134:1344–1350.
41. Branson BG, Bray KK, Gadbury-Amyot C, et al. Effect of magnification lenses on student operator posture. *J Dent Educ.* 2004;68:384–389.
42. Maillet JP, Millar AM, Burke JM, Maillet MA, Maillet WA, Neish NR. Effect of magnification loupes on dental hygiene student posture. *J Dent Educ.* 2008;72:33–44.
43. Chang BJ. Ergonomic benefits of surgical telescope systems: selection guidelines. *J Calif Dent Assoc.* 2002;30:161–169.
44. Donaldson ME, Knight GW, Guenzel PJ. The effect of magnification on student performance in pediatric operative dentistry. *J Dent Educ.* 1998;62:905–910.
45. Rucker L. Surgical telescopes: posture maker or posture breaker? In: Murphy D, ed. *Ergonomics and the Dental Care Worker.* Washington, DC: American Public Health Association; 1998.
46. Chaffin DB. Localized muscle fatigue–definiton and measurement. *J Occup Med.* 1973;15:346–354.
47. Rucker LM, Beattie C, McGregor C, Sunell S, Ito Y. Declination angle and its role in selecting surgical telescopes. *J Am Dent Assoc.* 1999;130:1096–1100.
48. Rucker L, McGregor C. Effects of low-magnification surgical telescopes on preclinical operative dental performance. *J Dent Educ.* 1992;1:34.
49. Barbieri S. Magnification for the dental hygienist. *Dimen Dent Hyg.* 2006;4:28, 30–31.

RECOMMENDED READING

Branson BG, Williams KB, Bray KK, McLlnay SL, Dickey D. Validity and reliability of a dental operator posture assessment instrument (PAI). *J Dent Hyg.* 2002;76:255–261.

ONLINE MODULE SKILL EVALUATIONS

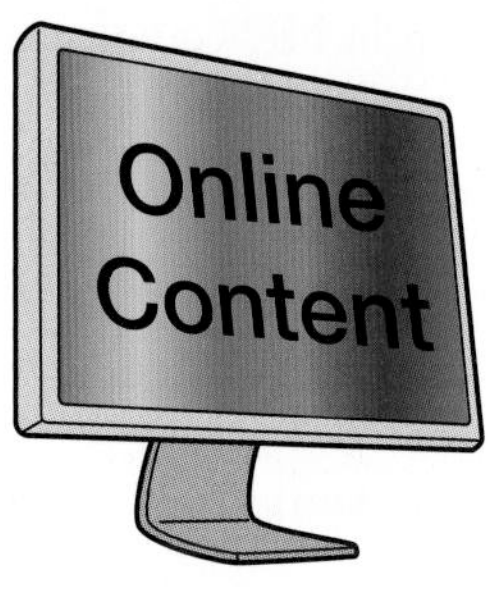

Module Skill Evaluations for instructor use can be downloaded at http://thepoint.lww.com/GehrigFundamentals7e

Module Skill Evaluations may be downloaded to a computer for use on a computer or printed out as paper copies.

- These computerized module evaluations automatically tabulate the percentage grade for each module evaluation.
- The computerized evaluation forms may be modified to meet each individual program's needs by adding or deleting criteria.
- In addition to the individual module evaluation forms, a summative evaluation form for use as a psychomotor final examination is available on thePoint website.
- For details, see the Instructor Resources section of the online materials at thePoint website (http://thepoint.lww.com/GehrigFundamentals7e).

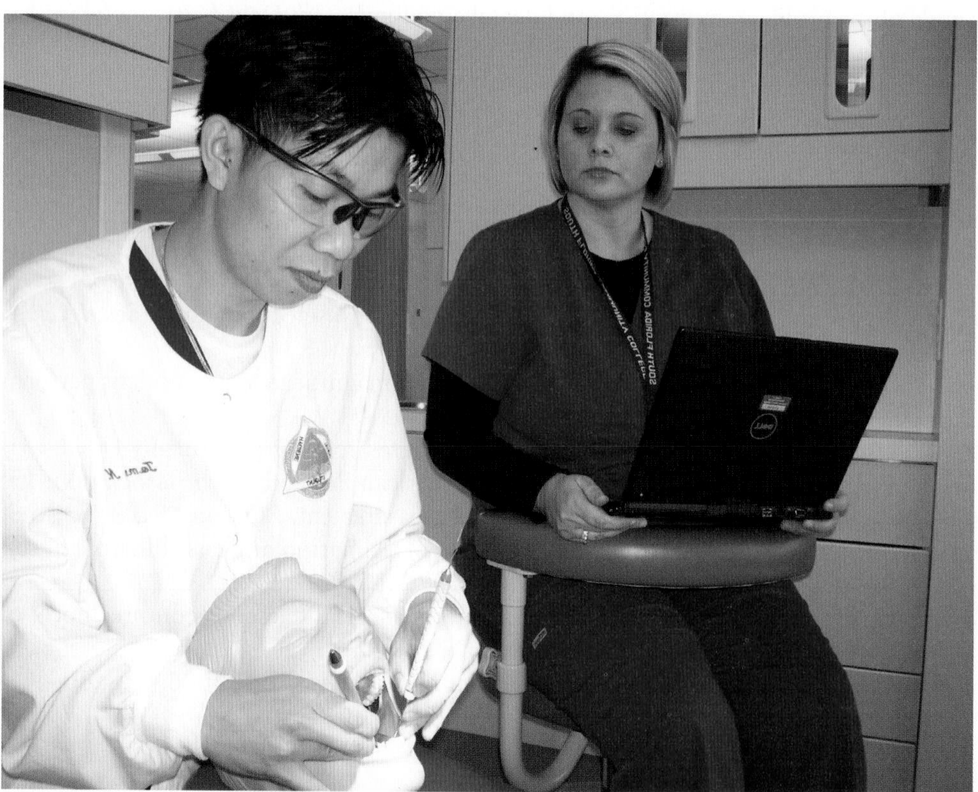

Figure 1-58. Computerized Module Skill Evaluation Forms. Skill Evaluation forms downloaded from thePoint website may be used on a computer during the preclinical evaluation process.

STUDENT SELF-EVALUATION MODULE 1 POSITION

Student: ______________________ Date: ______________________

DIRECTIONS: Self-evaluate your skill level in each treatment area as: **S** (satisfactory) or **U** (unsatisfactory).

Positioning/Ergonomics	Self-Evaluation
Adjusts clinician chair correctly	
Reclines patient chair and ensures that patient's head is even with top of headrest	
Positions instrument table within easy reach for front, side, or rear delivery as appropriate for operatory configuration	
Positions unit light at arm's length or dons dental headlight and adjusts it for use	
Positions backrest of patient chair for the specified arch	
Adjusts height of patient chair so that clinician's elbows remain at waist level when fingers touch teeth in treatment area	
Maintains neutral seated position	

Module 2

Clinician Clock Positions

Module Overview

The manner in which the seated clinician is positioned in relation to a treatment area is known as the clock position. This module introduces the traditional clock positions for periodontal instrumentation.

Module Outline

Online Content

Videos for this topic can be viewed at http://thepoint.lww.com/GehrigFundamentals7e

Key Terms

Clock positions

Anterior surfaces toward the clinician

Anterior surfaces away from the clinician

Posterior aspects facing toward the clinician

Posterior aspects facing away from the clinician

Learning Objectives

1. Demonstrate and maintain neutral seated position for each of the mandibular and maxillary treatment areas.
2. Demonstrate correct patient position relative to the clinician.
3. Demonstrate, from memory, the traditional clock position for each of the mandibular and maxillary treatment areas.
4. Demonstrate standing clinician position for the mandibular treatment areas.
5. Recognize incorrect position and describe or demonstrate how to correct the problem.

Section I
Clock Positions for Instrumentation

1. Range of Clinician Positions. During periodontal instrumentation, the seated clinician moves around the patient to maintain neutral body position.

A. Goal of Positioning. *Correct positioning of the seated clinician in relation to the treatment area (1) facilitates neutral positioning of the clinician's arms, wrists, and hands and (2) provides optimal vision of the tooth surfaces.*

B. Clock Positions

1. Instrumentation of the various treatment areas may be accomplished from a range of clinician positions (Fig. 2-1).
2. Using an analog clock face as a guide—with the patient's head being at 12 o'clock and the feet being at 6 o'clock—is a common method of identifying the clinician's position in relation to the patient's head (Fig. 2-2).
3. The positions that the clinician assumes in relation to the patient's head are known as "clock positions."

2. Range of Patient Head Positions. *In addition to assuming an optimal clock position, it is important to ask the patient to assume a head position that facilitates neutral arm, wrist, and hand position for the clinician* (Fig. 2-3).

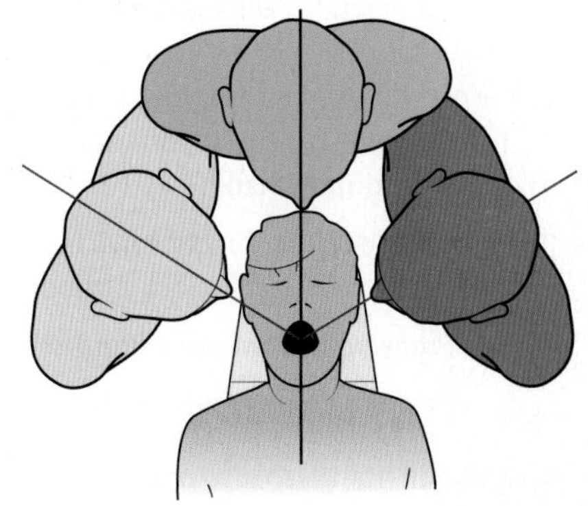

Figure 2-1. Movement around the Patient.

- The seated clinician can assume a range of positions around the patient during periodontal instrumentation.
- This illustration shows just three examples of possible seated positions in relation to the patient. The range of possible clock positions is from 8 to 4 o'clock.

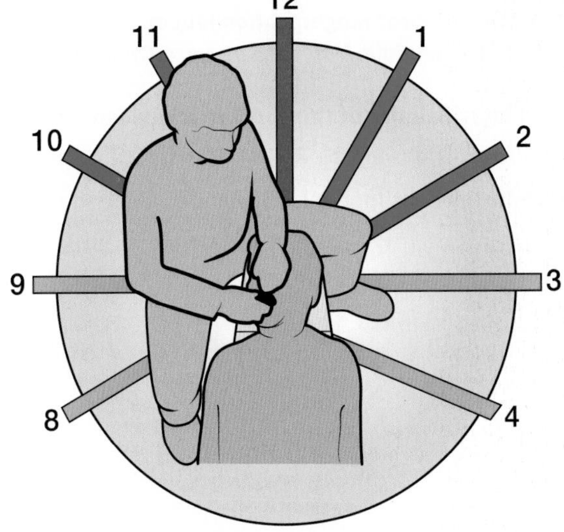

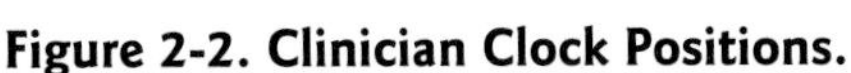

Figure 2-2. Clinician Clock Positions.

- Clinician clock positions are identified using the face of an analog clock as the guide.
- The patient's head is at the 12 o'clock position, and the feet are at the 6 o'clock position.

Figure 2-3. Patient Head Positions.

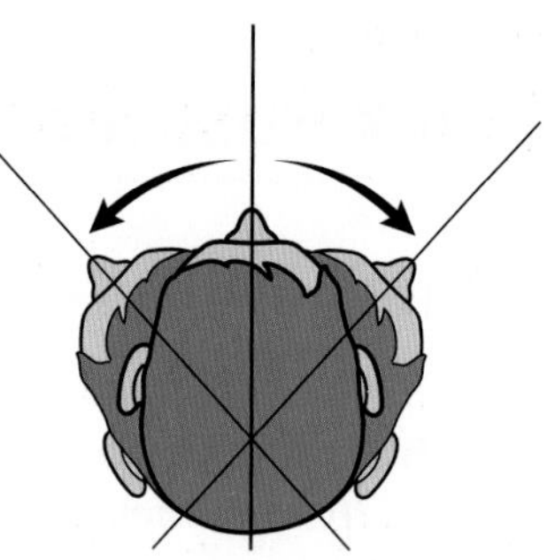

- The patient's head should be positioned to facilitate neutral arm, wrist, and hand position for the clinician. The patient's head may be neutral—straight—or turned toward or away from the clinician.
- The clinician should request that the patient position the head to facilitate visibility and access to the treatment area. The patient is only in the dental chair for 45 to 60 minutes, while the clinician works at chairside throughout an 8-hour day.

Box 2-1. Directions for Sections 2 and 3 of This Module

1. The next two sections of this module contain instructions for practicing the traditional clock positions for each treatment area of the mouth.
2. ***For this module, you should concentrate on mastering your positioning for each treatment area.***
   - ***Work without dental instruments and just concentrate on learning positioning.***
   - ***Before picking up a periodontal instrument, you should master the large motor skills of positioning yourself, your patient, and the dental equipment to facilitate neutral position.***
3. As you practice each clock position, position your arms and hands as described in this module.
   - You will use both of your hands for periodontal instrumentation; the periodontal instrument is held in your dominant hand, and the mirror is held in your **nondominant** hand.
   - For this module, practice placing the fingertips of your hands as shown in the illustration for each clock position.
     - ***Place your dominant hand on the teeth in the treatment area.***
     - ***Rest your nondominant hand on the patient's cheek or chin.***
4. You will not be able to obtain a clear view of all tooth surfaces as you practice positioning in this module. In Modules 3, 4, and 5, you will learn to use a dental mouth mirror to view these "hidden" tooth surfaces.
5. ***Do not wear magnification loupes when practicing and perfecting your positioning skills in this module. You need an unrestricted visual field for self-evaluation.***

The remainder of this module is divided into right- and left-handed sections.

- Instructions for the **RIGHT-Handed** clinician begin on the following page.
- Instructions for the **LEFT-Handed** clinician begin in Section 3 on page 54.

Section 2
Traditional Positioning for the RIGHT-Handed Clinician

This section depicts the traditional clock positions for the right-handed clinician. Traditional clock positions for the right-handed clinician range from 8 to 1 o'clock. *Modules 3, 4, and 5 present content on modified clock positions used for certain treatment areas of the mouth.*

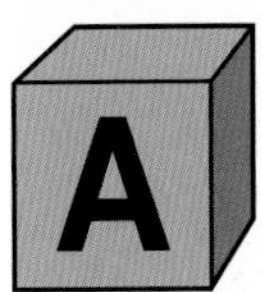

SKILL BUILDING. TRADITIONAL CLOCK POSITIONS FOR THE RIGHT-HANDED CLINICIAN

Directions: Practice each clock position by following the criteria outlined below.

8 O'clock Positions (To the Front of the Patient)

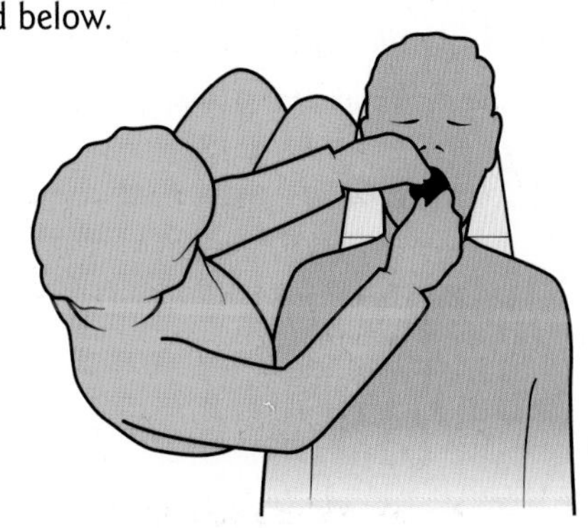

- **Torso Position.** Sit facing the patient with your hip in line with the patient's upper arm.
- **Leg Position.** Your thighs should rest against the side of the patient chair.
- **Arm Positions.** To reach the patient's mouth, hold your arms slightly away from your sides. Hold your lower right arm over the patient's chest. NOTE: Do not rest your arm on the patient's head or chest.
- **Line of Vision.** Your line of vision is straight ahead, into the patient's mouth.

Ergonomic Considerations: It is difficult to maintain neutral arm and torso position when seated in the 8 o'clock position. For this reason, use of the 8 o'clock position should be limited. The goal is to minimize postural abnormalities whenever possible.

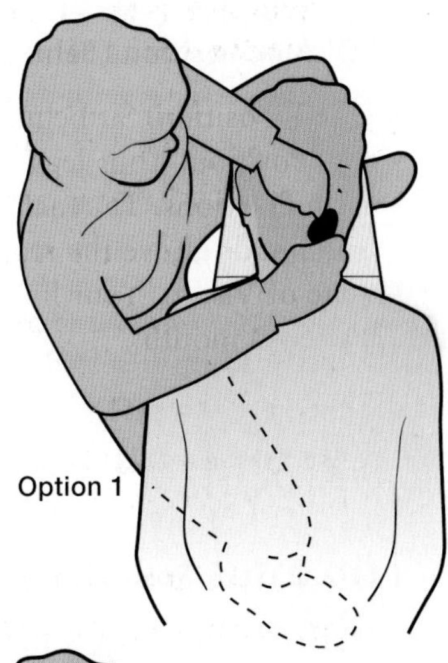
Option 1

9 O'clock Position (To the Side of the Patient)

- **Torso Position.** Sit facing the side of the patient's head. The midline of your torso is even with the patient's mouth.
- **Leg Position.** Your legs may be in either of two acceptable positions: (1) straddling the patient chair or (2) underneath the *headrest* of the patient chair. Neutral position is best achieved by straddling the chair; however, you should use the alternative position if you find straddling uncomfortable.
- **Arm Positions.** To reach the patient's mouth, hold the lower half of your right arm in approximate alignment with the patient's shoulder. Hold your left hand and wrist over the region of the patient's right eye.
- **Line of Vision.** Your line of vision is straight down into the mouth.

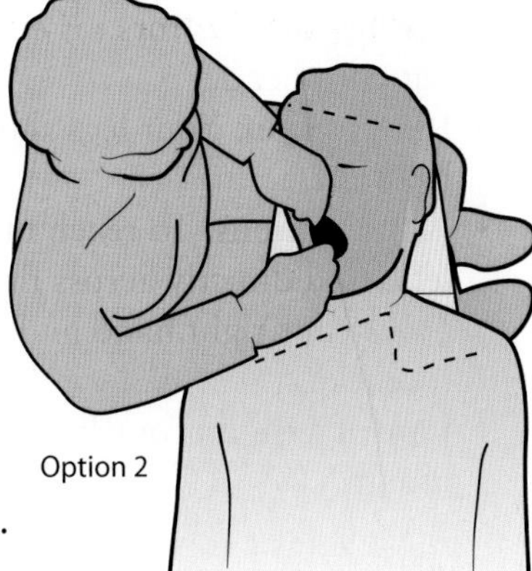
Option 2

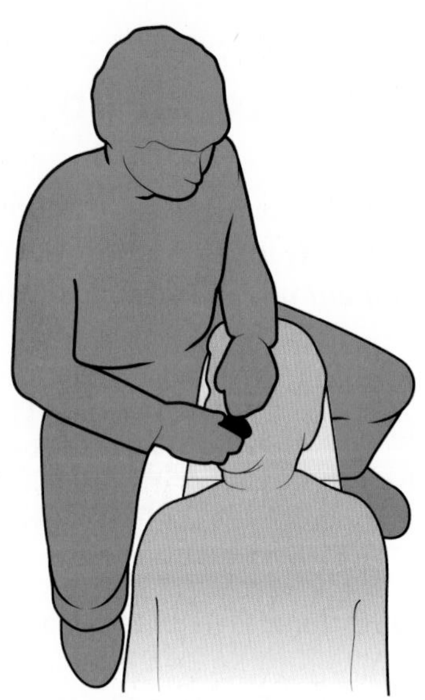

10 to 11 O'clock Position (Near Corner of Headrest)

- **Torso Position.** Sit at the top right corner of the headrest; the midline of your torso is even with the temple region of the patient's head.
- **Leg Position.** Your legs should straddle the corner of the headrest.
- **Arm Positions.** To reach the patient's mouth, hold your right hand directly across the corner of the patient's mouth. Hold your left hand and wrist above the patient's nose and forehead.
- **Line of Vision.** Your line of vision is straight down into the mouth.

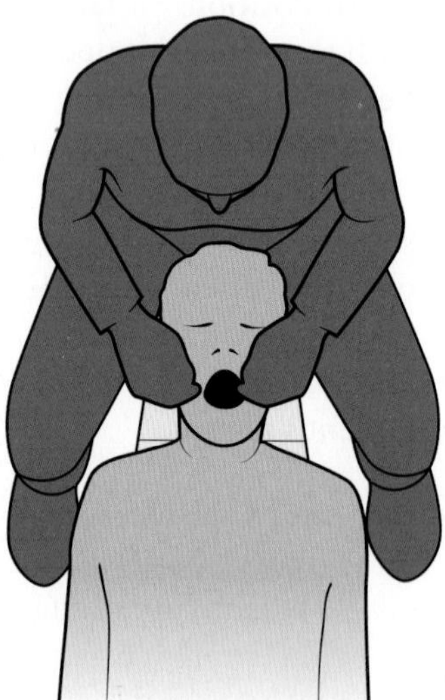

12 O'clock Position (Behind the Patient)

- **Torso Position.** Sit behind the patient's head.
- **Leg Position.** Your legs should straddle the headrest.
- **Arm Positions.** To reach the patient's mouth, hold your wrists and hands above the region of the patient's ears and cheeks.
- **Line of Vision.** Your line of vision is straight down into the patient's mouth.

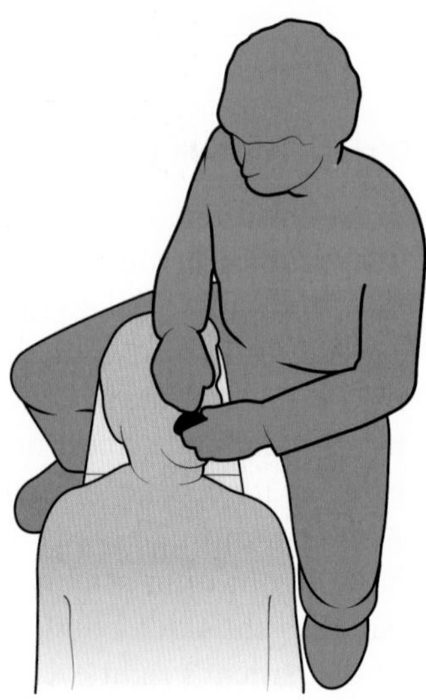

1 to 2 O'clock Position (Near Corner of Headrest)

- **Torso Position.** Sit at the top left corner of the headrest; the midline of your torso is even with the temple region of the patient's head.
- **Leg Position.** Your legs should straddle the corner of the headrest.
- **Arm Positions.** To reach the patient's mouth, hold your left hand directly across the corner of the patient's mouth. Hold your right hand and wrist above the patient's nose and forehead.
- **Line of Vision.** Your line of vision is straight down into the mouth.

FLOW CHART: SEQUENCE FOR PRACTICING POSITIONING

For successful periodontal instrumentation, it is important to proceed in a step-by-step manner. A useful saying to help you remember the step-by-step approach is "*Me, My Patient, My Light, My Nondominant Hand, My Dominant Hand*" (Fig. 2-4).

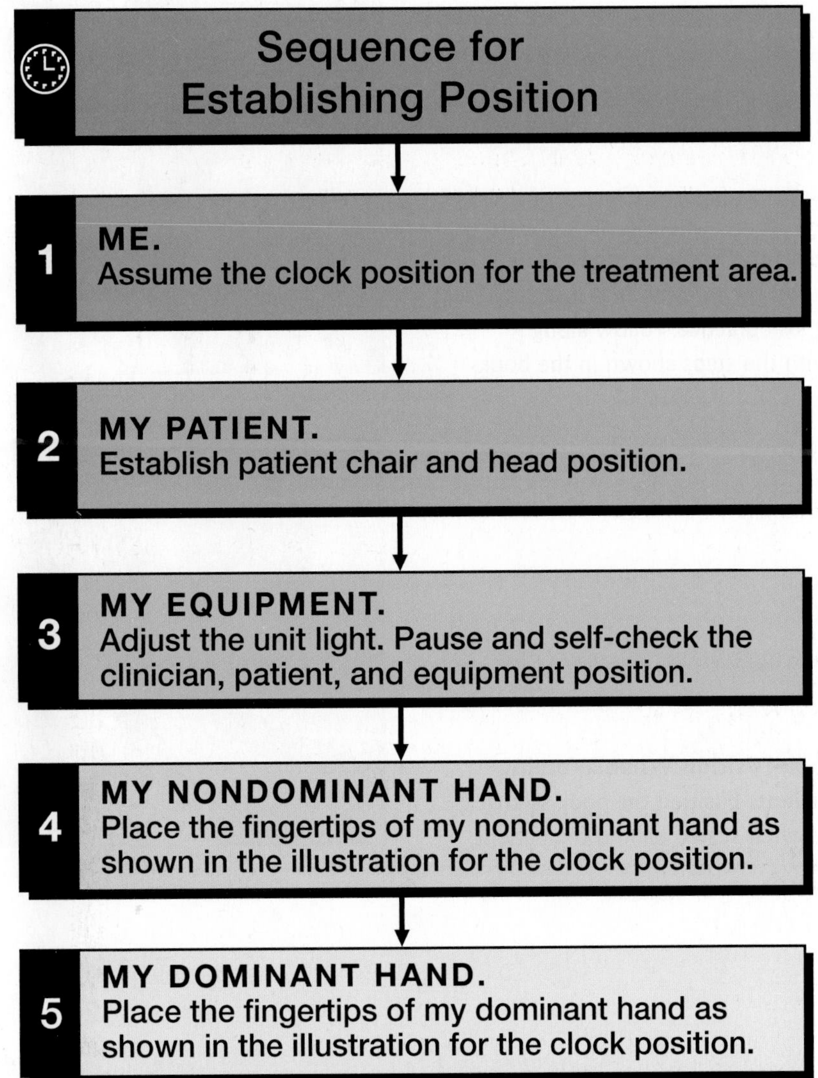
Sequence for Establishing Position
1 ME. Assume the clock position for the treatment area.
2 MY PATIENT. Establish patient chair and head position.
3 MY EQUIPMENT. Adjust the unit light. Pause and self-check the clinician, patient, and equipment position.
4 MY NONDOMINANT HAND. Place the fingertips of my nondominant hand as shown in the illustration for the clock position.
5 MY DOMINANT HAND. Place the fingertips of my dominant hand as shown in the illustration for the clock position.

Figure 2-4. Sequence for Establishing Position.

USE OF TEXTBOOK DURING SKILL PRACTICE

The Skill Building sections of each module are designed to lead the reader step-by-step through each skill practice. It is important to position the textbook for ease of viewing throughout each skill practice (Figs. 2-5 and 2-6).

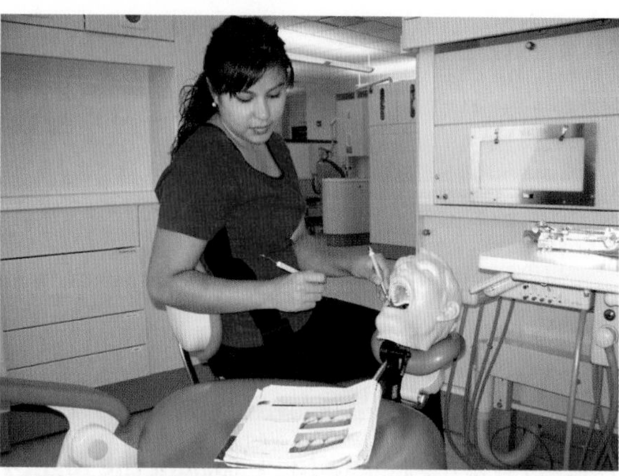

Figure 2-5. Position the Book for Ease of Viewing. Position the book so that it is easy to view during skill practice. Follow along step-by-step with the steps shown in the book.

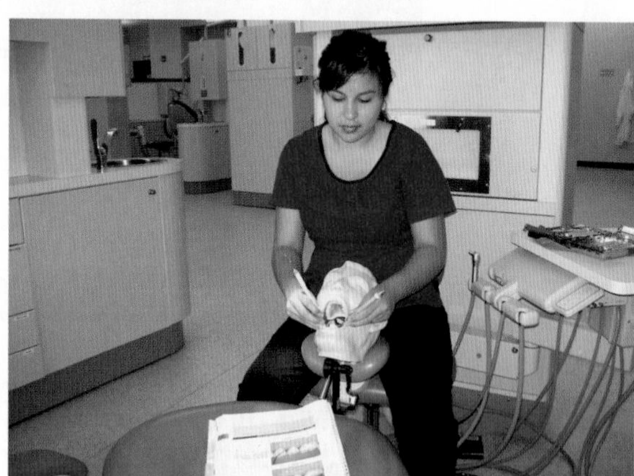

Figure 2-6. Book Position When Working behind the Patient. Position the book so that it is easy to view when seated behind the patient.

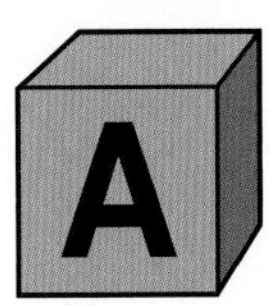

SKILL BUILDING. ANTERIOR SEXTANTS: QUICK START GUIDE TO TRADITIONAL CLOCK POSITIONS

There is no need to waste time memorizing the clock position for each treatment area. The clock positions are easy to remember if you learn to recognize the positioning pattern for the anterior teeth. For periodontal instrumentation of the anterior teeth, each tooth is divided in half at the midline.

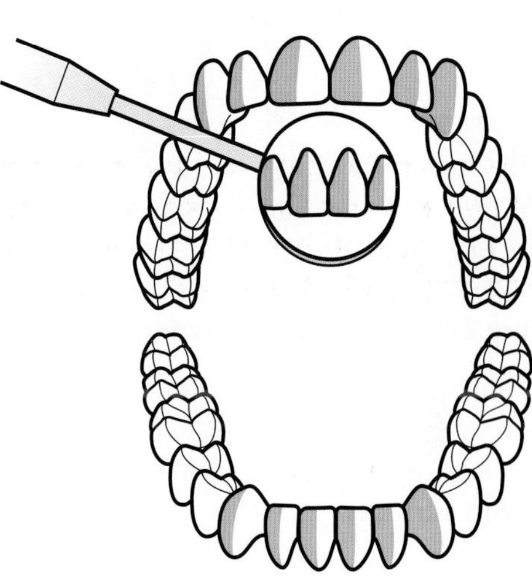

Figure 2-7. Anterior *Surfaces Toward* the Right-Handed Clinician.

- The anterior tooth surfaces shaded in yellow on this drawing are called the anterior surfaces toward the clinician.
- The **clock position** for the anterior surfaces toward the clinician ranges from **8 to 10 o'clock.**

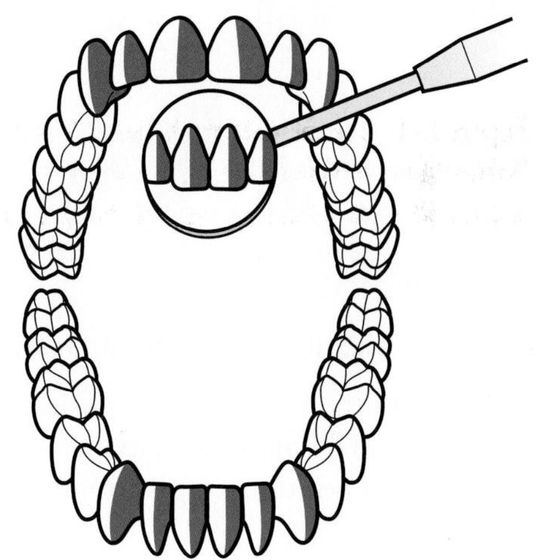

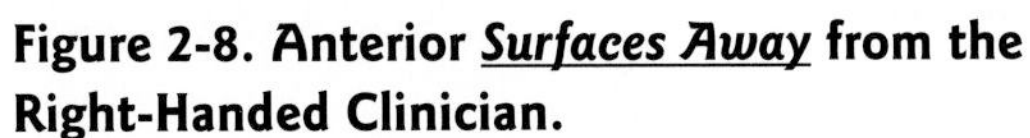

Figure 2-8. Anterior *Surfaces Away* from the Right-Handed Clinician.

- The anterior surfaces shaded in purple on this drawing are called the anterior surfaces away from the clinician.
- The **clock position** for anterior surfaces away from the clinician ranges from **11 to 1 o'clock.**

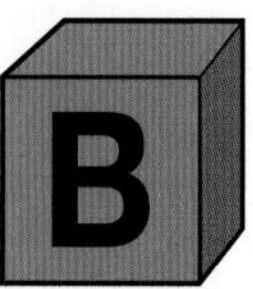

SKILL PRACTICE. TRADITIONAL POSITIONING FOR THE ANTERIOR SURFACES TOWARD

Practice the recommended clinician clock and patient head positions for the anterior surfaces toward by following the illustrations below.

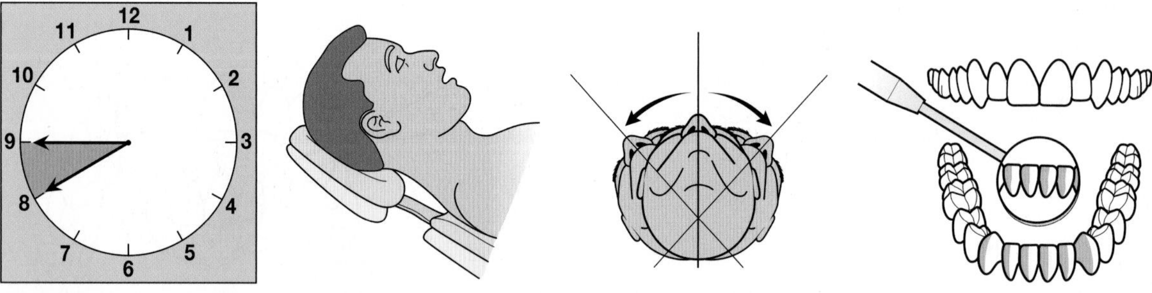

Figure 2-9. Mandibular Anterior Surfaces, TOWARD.

- Clinician in the 8 to 9 o'clock position.
- Patient chin DOWN; place the mandibular occlusal plane as parallel to the floor as possible.
- Patient head position ranges from neutral to turned to the right or left to facilitate vision of the tooth surfaces.

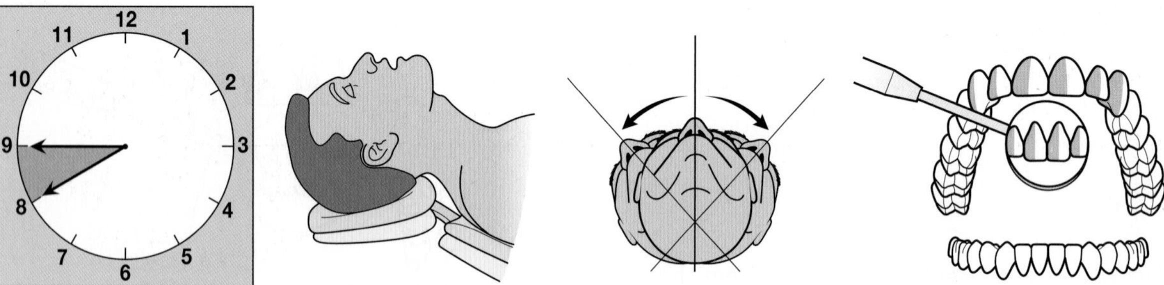

Figure 2-10. Maxillary Anterior Surfaces, TOWARD.

- Clinician in the 8 to 9 o'clock position.
- Patient chin UP; place the maxillary occlusal plane perpendicular to the floor.
- Patient head position ranges from neutral to turned to the right or left to facilitate vision of the tooth surfaces.

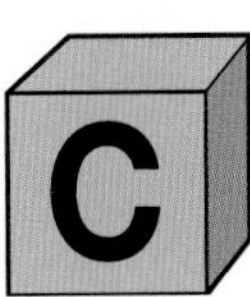

SKILL PRACTICE. TRADITIONAL POSITIONING FOR THE ANTERIOR

Practice the recommended clinician clock and patient head positions for the anterior surfaces away by following the illustrations below.

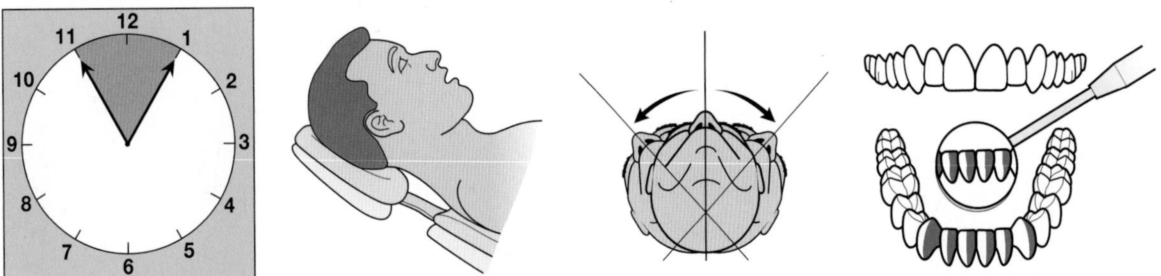

Figure 2-11. Mandibular Anterior Surfaces, AWAY.

- Clinician in the 11 to 1 o'clock position.
- Patient chin DOWN; place the mandibular occlusal plane as parallel to the floor as possible.
- Patient head position ranges from a neutral position to turning the head to the right or left to facilitate vision of the tooth surfaces.

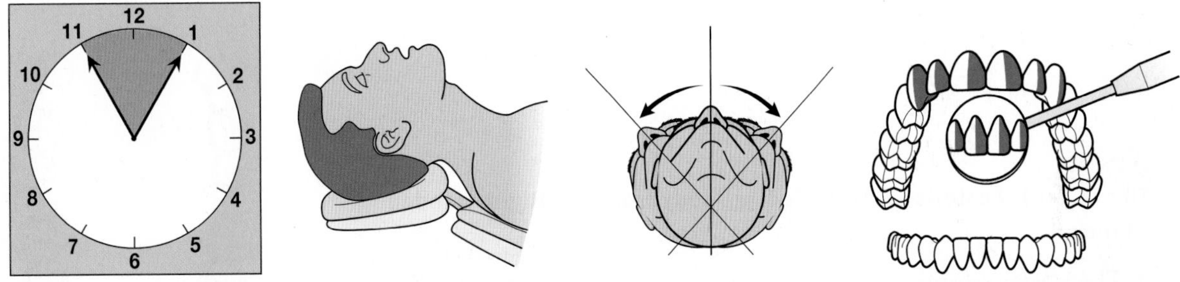

Figure 2-12. Maxillary Anterior Surfaces, AWAY.

- Clinician in the 11 to 1 o'clock position.
- Patient chin UP; place the maxillary occlusal plane perpendicular to the floor.
- Patient head position ranges from a neutral position to turning the head to the right or left to facilitate vision of the tooth surfaces.

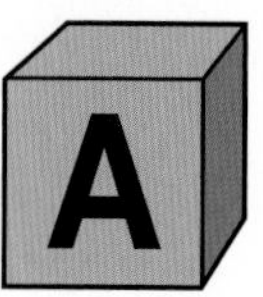

SKILL BUILDING. POSTERIOR SEXTANTS: QUICK START GUIDE TO TRADITIONAL CLOCK POSITIONS

There is no need to waste time memorizing the clock position for each posterior treatment area. The clock positions are easy to remember if you learn to recognize the positioning pattern for the posterior sextants. ***For periodontal instrumentation, each posterior sextant is divided into two aspects: (1) the facial aspect and (2) the lingual aspect of the sextant.***

Figure 2-13. Posterior *Aspects Facing Toward* the Right-Handed Clinician.

- The posterior surfaces shaded in yellow on this drawing are called the posterior aspects facing toward the clinician.
- The **clock position** for posterior aspects toward the clinician is 9 o'clock.

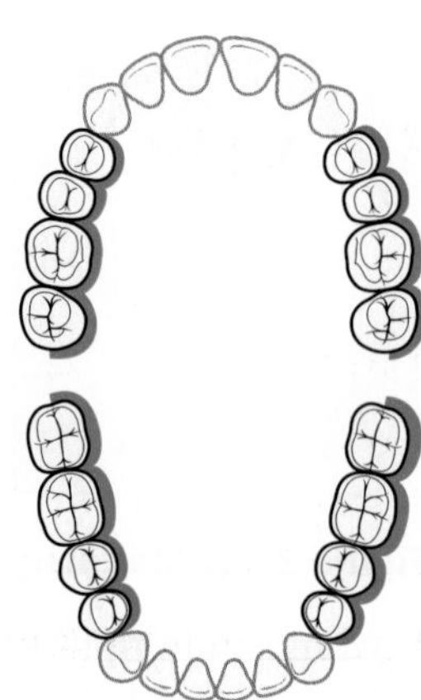

Figure 2-14. Posterior *Aspects Facing Away* from the Right-Handed Clinician.

- The posterior surfaces shaded in blue on this drawing are called the posterior aspects facing away from the clinician.
- The **clock position** for posterior aspects away from the clinician ranges from **10 to 11 o'clock.**

RIGHT-Handed Clinician

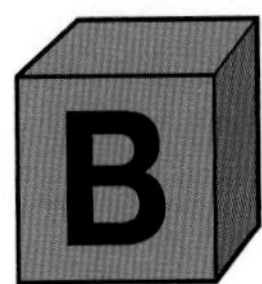

SKILL PRACTICE. TRADITIONAL POSITIONING FOR THE POSTERIOR SEXTANTS, ASPECTS FACING TOWARD THE CLINICIAN

Practice the recommended clinician clock and patient head positions for the posterior sextants facing toward the clinician by following the illustrations below.

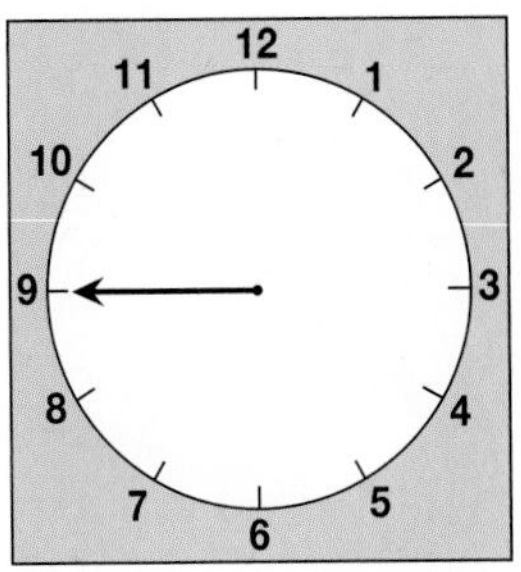

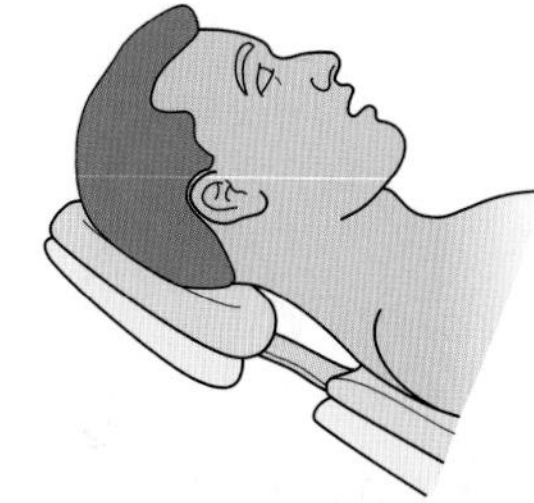
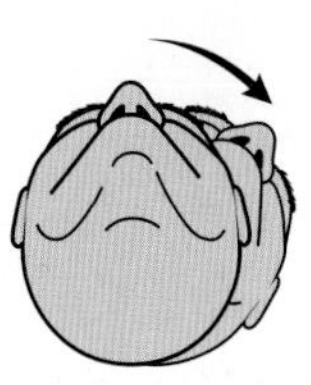
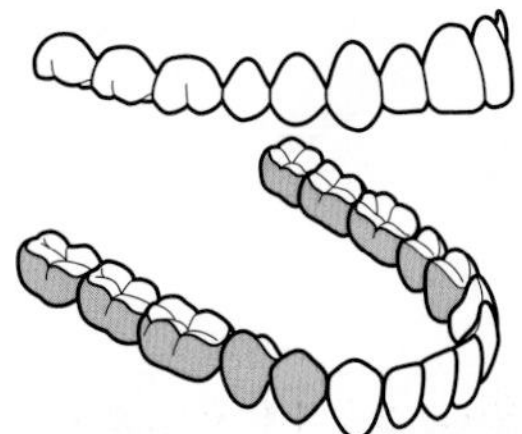

Figure 2-15. Mandibular Posterior Aspects Facing TOWARD.

- Clinician in the 9 o'clock position.
- Chin DOWN; place the mandibular occlusal plan as parallel to the floor as possible.
- Patient head position ranges from a neutral position to turning the head slightly away from the clinician.

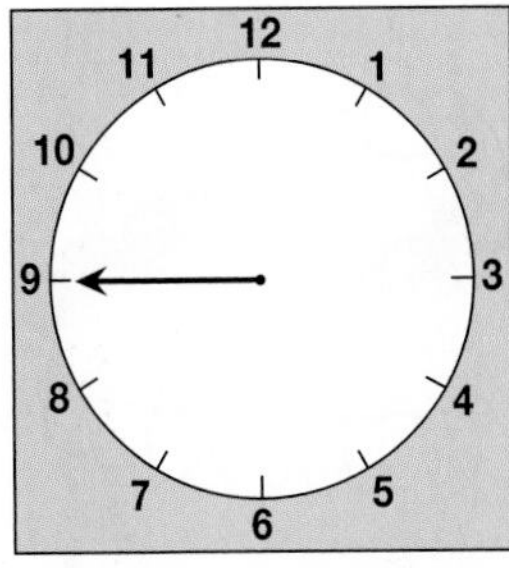

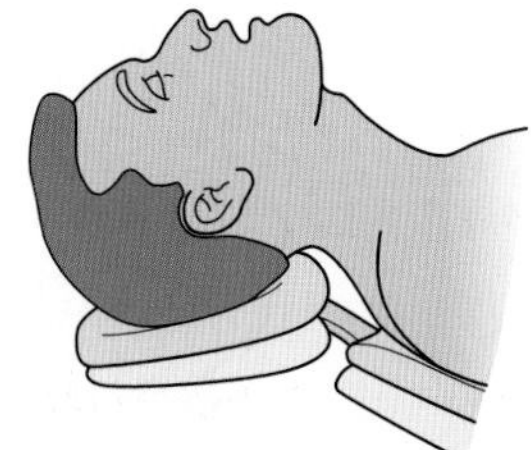
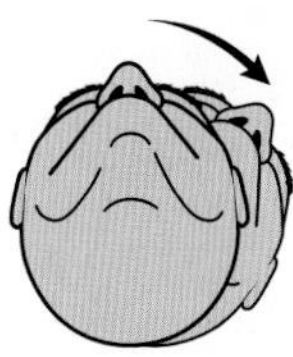
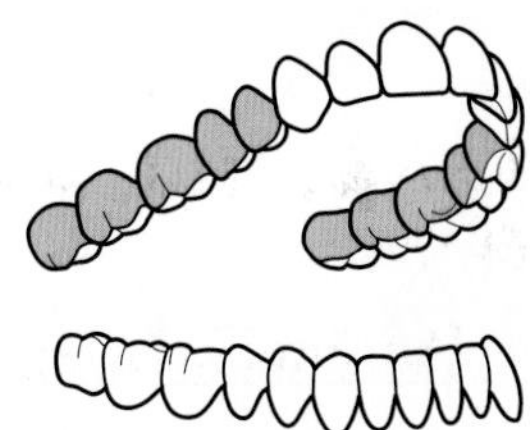

Figure 2-16. Maxillary Posterior Aspects Facing TOWARD.

- Clinician in the 9 o'clock position.
- Chin UP; place the maxillary occlusal plane perpendicular to the floor.
- Patient head position ranges from a neutral position to turning the head slightly away from the clinician.

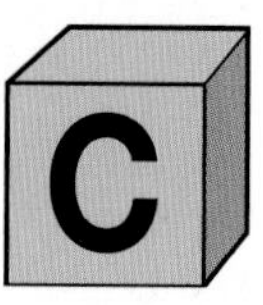

SKILL PRACTICE. TRADITIONAL POSITIONING FOR THE POSTERIOR SEXTANTS, ASPECTS FACING AWAY FROM THE CLINICIAN

Practice the recommended clinician clock and patient head positions for the posterior sextants facing away from the clinician by following the illustrations below.

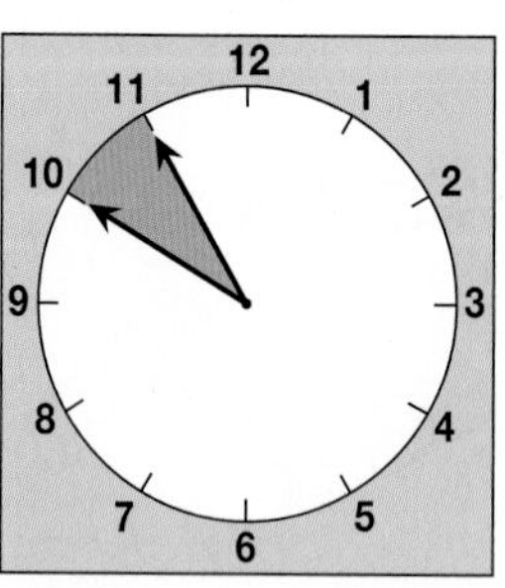

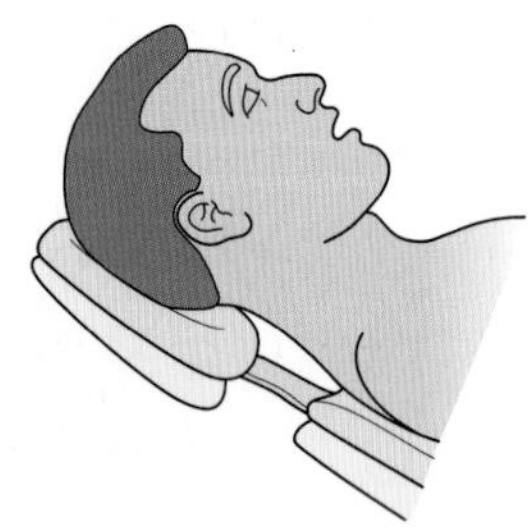
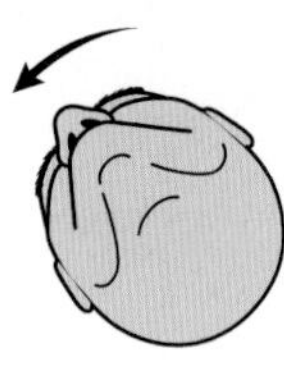
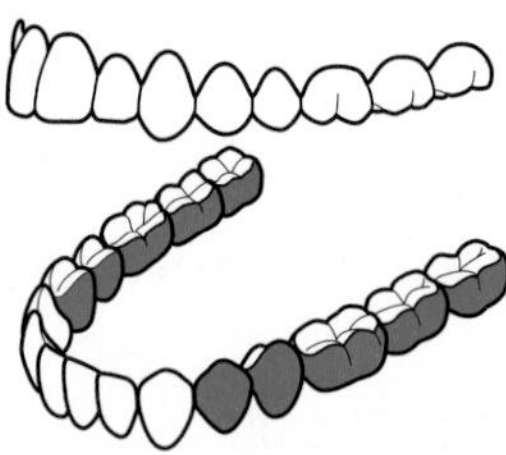

Figure 2-17. Mandibular Posterior Aspects Facing AWAY.

- Clinician seated in the 10 to 11 o'clock position.
- Chin DOWN; place the mandibular occlusal plan as parallel to the floor as possible.
- Patient head position is turned toward the clinician.

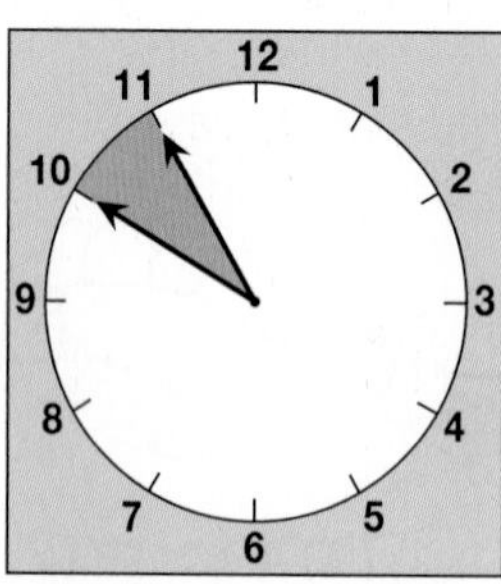

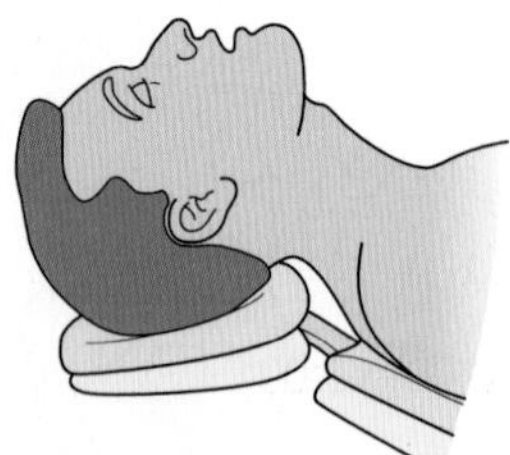
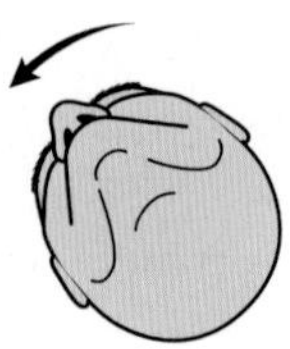
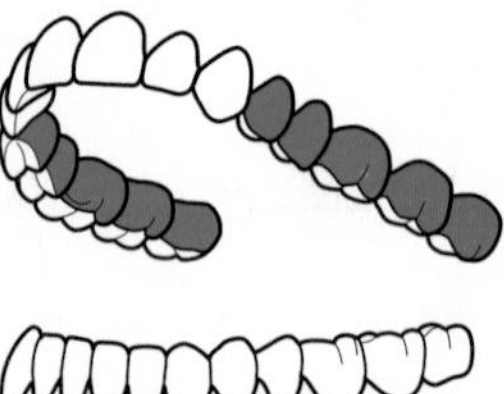

Figure 2-18. Maxillary Posterior Aspects Facing AWAY.

- Clinician seated in the 10 to 11 o'clock position.
- Chin UP; place the maxillary occlusal plane perpendicular to the floor.
- Patient head position is turned toward the clinician.

RIGHT-Handed Clinician

REFERENCE SHEET: POSITION FOR THE RIGHT-HANDED CLINICIAN

Table 2-1 summarizes the traditional clock positions for the right-handed clinician. Photocopy this page and use it for quick reference as you practice your positioning skills. Place the photocopied reference sheet in a plastic page protector for longer use.

TABLE 2-1. Traditional Clock Positions—Positioning Summary

Treatment Area	Clock Position	Patient Head Position
Mandibular Arch—Anterior surfaces toward	8:00–9:00	Chin down; neutral to turned right or left
Maxillary Arch—Anterior surfaces toward	8:00–9:00	Chin up; neutral to turned right or left
Mandibular Arch—Anterior surfaces away	11:00–1:00	Chin down; neutral to turned right or left
Maxillary Arch—Anterior surfaces away	11:00–1:00	Chin up; neutral to turned right or left
Mandibular Arch—Posterior aspects toward	9:00	Chin down; neutral
Maxillary Arch—Posterior aspects toward	9:00	Chin up; neutral to turned slightly away
Mandibular Arch—Posterior aspects away	10:00–11:00	Chin down; toward
Maxillary Arch—Posterior aspects away	10:00–11:00	Chin up; toward

RIGHT-Handed Clinicians: This ends Section 2 for the right-handed clinician. Please turn to page 65 for Section 4: Modified Positioning: Working from a Standing Position.

RIGHT-Handed Clinician

Section 3
Traditional Positioning for the LEFT-Handed Clinician

This section depicts the traditional clock positions for the left-handed clinician. Traditional clock positions for the left-handed clinician range from 11 to 4 o'clock. ***Modules 3, 4, and 5 present content on modified clock positions used for certain treatment areas of the mouth.***

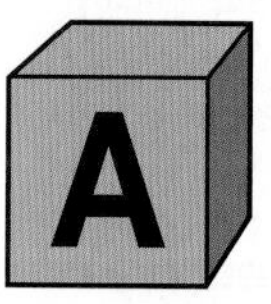

SKILL BUILDING. TRADITIONAL CLOCK POSITIONS FOR THE LEFT-HANDED CLINICIAN

Directions: Practice each clock position by following the criteria outlined below.

3 to 4 O'clock Position (To the Front of the Patient)

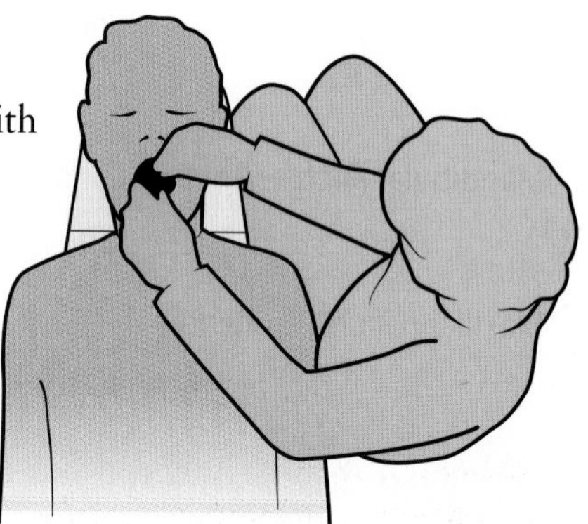

- **Torso Position.** Sit facing the patient with your hip in line with the patient's upper arm.
- **Leg Position.** Your thighs should rest against the side of the patient chair.
- **Arm Positions.** To reach the patient's mouth, hold your arms slightly away from your sides. Hold your lower left arm over the patient's chest. The side of your right hand rests in the area of the patient's right cheekbone and upper lip. NOTE: Do not rest your arm on the patient's head or chest.
- **Line of Vision.** Your line of vision is straight ahead, into the patient's mouth.

Ergonomic Considerations: It is difficult to maintain neutral arm and torso position when seated in the 4 o'clock position. For this reason, use of the 4 o'clock position should be limited. The goal is to minimize postural abnormalities whenever possible.

3 O'clock Position (To the Side)

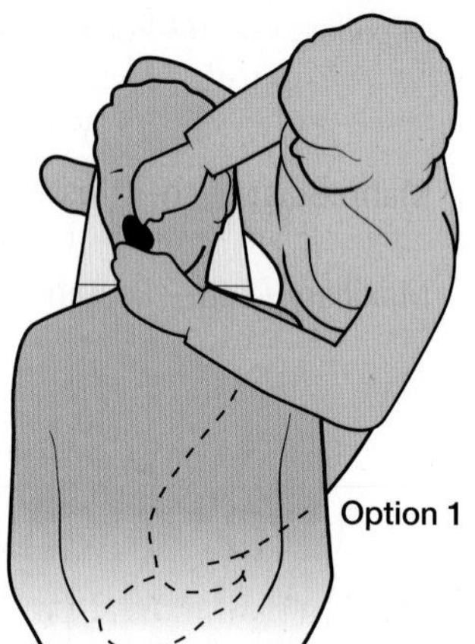

Option 1

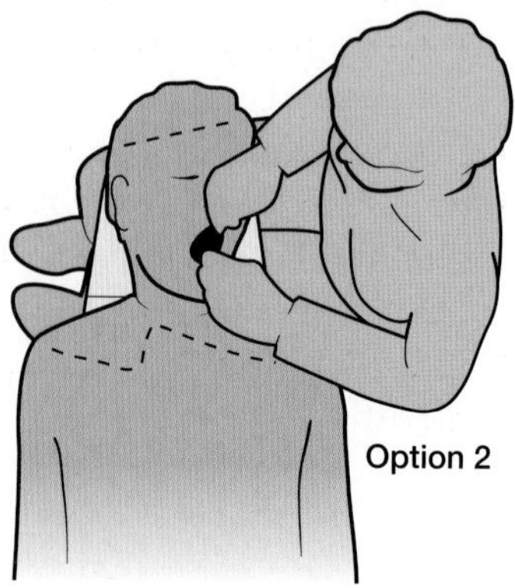

Option 2

- **Torso Position.** Sit facing the side of the patient's head. The midline of your torso is even with the patient's mouth.
- **Leg Position.** Your legs may be in either of two acceptable positions: (1) straddling the patient chair or (2) underneath the *headrest* of the patient chair. Neutral position is best achieved by straddling the chair; however, you should use the alternative position if you find straddling uncomfortable.
- **Arm Positions.** To reach the patient's mouth, hold the lower half of your left arm in approximate alignment with the patient's shoulder. Hold your right hand and wrist over the region of patient's left eye.
- **Hand Positions.** Rest your right hand in the area of the patient's left cheekbone. Rest the fingertips of your left hand on the premolar teeth of the mandibular left posterior sextant.
- **Line of Vision.** Your line of vision is straight down into the mouth.

LEFT-Handed Clinician

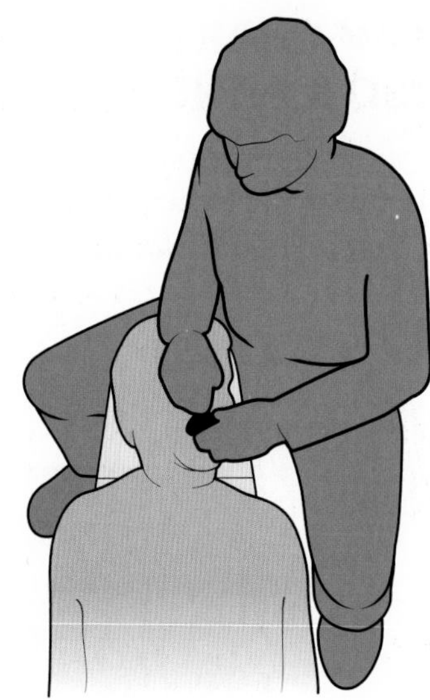

1 to 2 O'clock Position (Near Corner of Headrest)

- **Torso Position.** Sit at the top left corner of the headrest; the midline of your torso is even with the temple region of the patient's head.
- **Leg Position.** Your legs should straddle the corner of the headrest.
- **Arm Positions.** To reach the patient's mouth, hold your left hand directly across the corner of the patient's mouth. Hold your right hand and wrist above the patient's nose and forehead.
- **Line of Vision.** Your line of vision is straight down into the mouth.

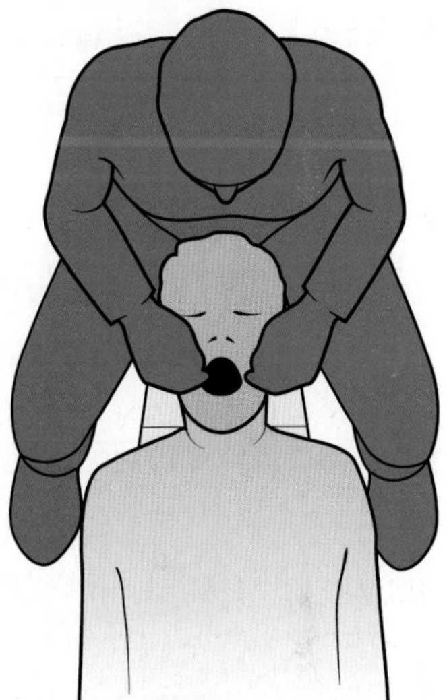

12 O'clock Position (Directly behind Patient)

- **Torso Position.** Sit directly behind the patient's head; you may sit anywhere from the left corner of the headrest to directly behind the headrest.
- **Leg Position.** Your legs should straddle the headrest.
- **Arm Positions.** To reach the patient's mouth, hold your wrists and hands above the region of the patient's ears and cheeks.
- **Line of Vision.** Your line of vision is straight down into the patient's mouth.

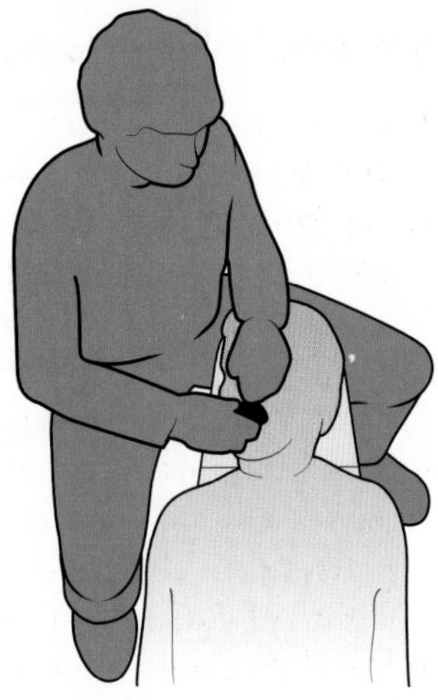

10 to 11 O'clock Position (Near Corner of Headrest)

- **Torso Position.** Sit at the top right corner of the headrest; the midline of your torso is even with the temple region of the patient's head.
- **Leg Position.** Your legs should straddle the corner of the headrest.
- **Arm Positions.** To reach the patient's mouth, hold your right hand directly across the corner of the patient's mouth. Hold your left hand and wrist above the patient's nose and forehead.
- **Line of Vision.** Your line of vision is straight down into the mouth.

FLOW CHART: SEQUENCE FOR PRACTICING POSITIONING

For successful periodontal instrumentation, it is important to proceed in a step-by-step manner. A useful saying to help you remember the step-by-step approach is "***Me, My Patient, My Light, My Nondominant Hand, My Dominant Hand.***"

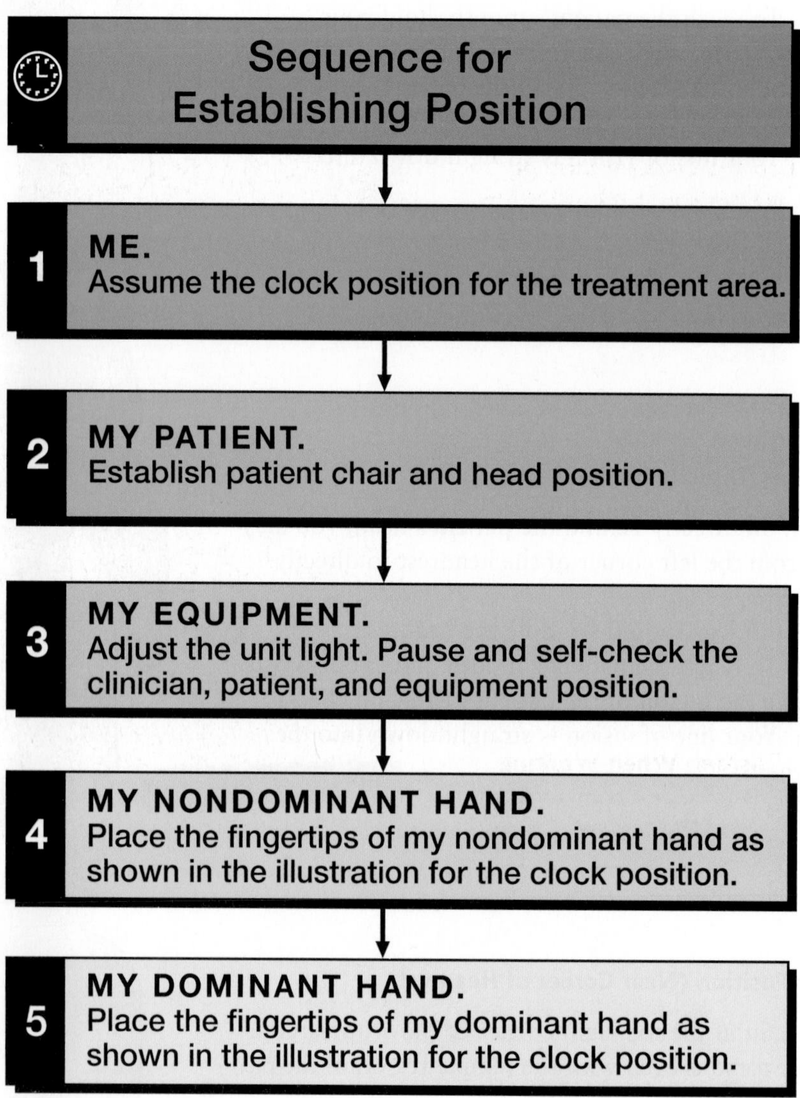

Sequence for Establishing Position
1
ME.
Assume the clock position for the treatment area.
2
MY PATIENT.
Establish patient chair and head position.
3
MY EQUIPMENT.
Adjust the unit light. Pause and self-check the clinician, patient, and equipment position.
4
MY NONDOMINANT HAND.
Place the fingertips of my nondominant hand as shown in the illustration for the clock position.
5
MY DOMINANT HAND.
Place the fingertips of my dominant hand as shown in the illustration for the clock position.

Figure 2-19. Sequence for Establishing Position.

USE OF TEXTBOOK DURING SKILL PRACTICE

The Skill Building sections of each module are designed to lead the reader step-by-step through each skill practice. It is important to position the textbook for ease of viewing throughout each skill practice.

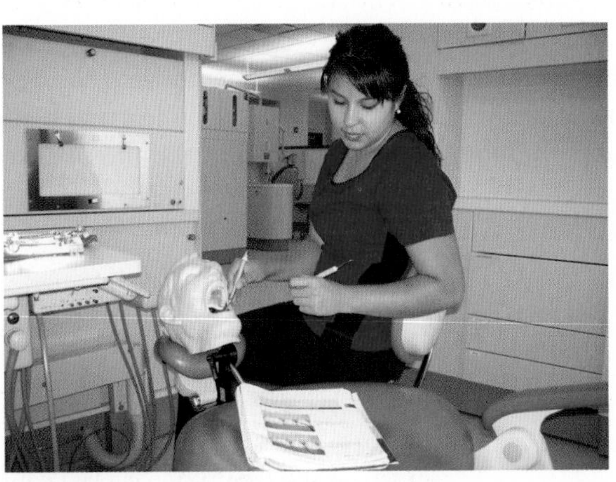

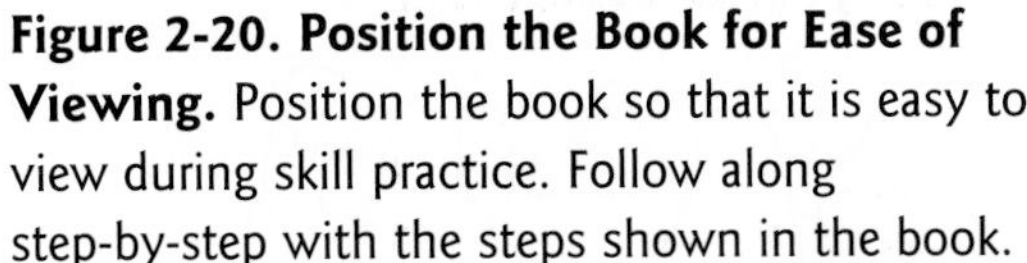

Figure 2-20. Position the Book for Ease of Viewing. Position the book so that it is easy to view during skill practice. Follow along step-by-step with the steps shown in the book.

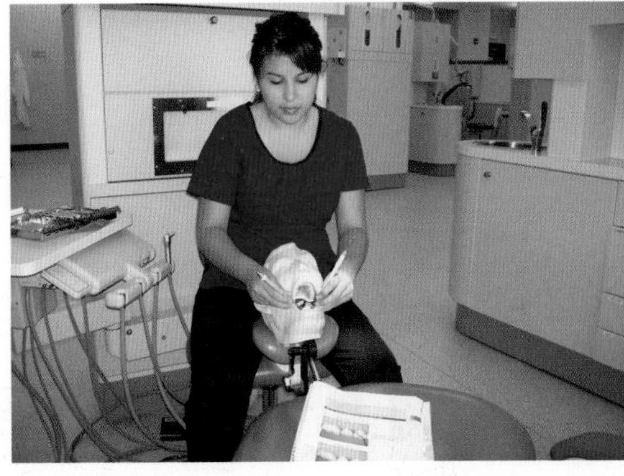

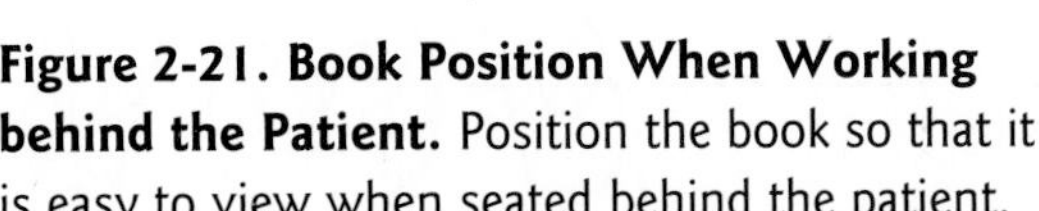

Figure 2-21. Book Position When Working behind the Patient. Position the book so that it is easy to view when seated behind the patient.

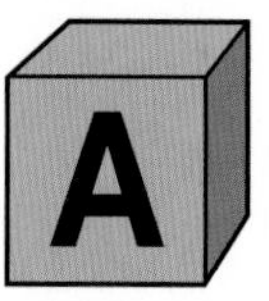

SKILL BUILDING: ANTERIOR SEXTANTS: QUICK START GUIDE TO TRADITIONAL CLOCK POSITIONS

There is no need to waste time memorizing the clock position for each treatment area. The clock positions are easy to remember if you learn to recognize the positioning pattern for the anterior teeth. For periodontal instrumentation of the anterior teeth, each tooth is divided in half at the midline.

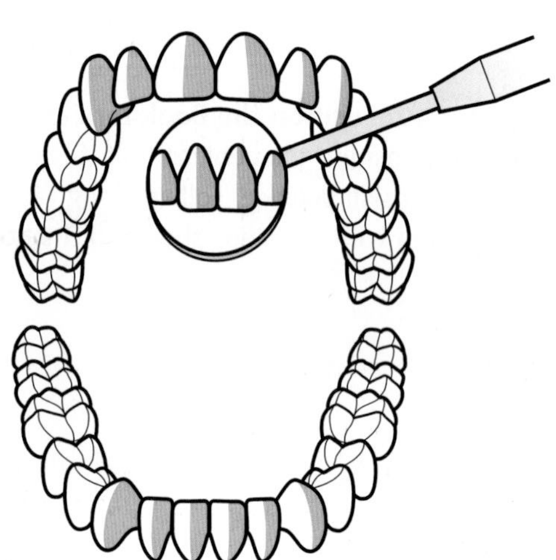

Figure 2-22. Anterior *Surfaces Toward* the Left-Handed Clinician.

- The anterior tooth surfaces shaded in yellow on this drawing are called the anterior surfaces toward the clinician.
- The **clock position** for the anterior surfaces toward the clinician ranges from **3 to 4 o'clock.**

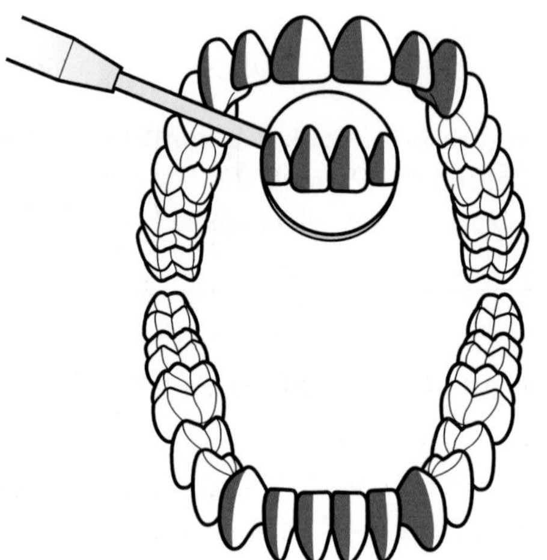

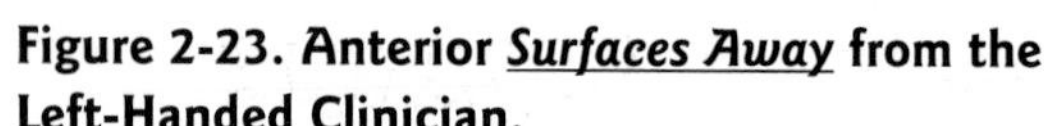

Figure 2-23. Anterior *Surfaces Away* from the Left-Handed Clinician.

- The anterior surfaces shaded in purple on this drawing are called the anterior surfaces away from the clinician.
- The **clock position** for the anterior surfaces away from the clinician ranges from **11 to 1 o'clock.**

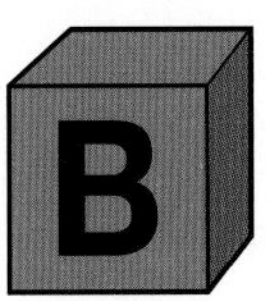

SKILL PRACTICE. TRADITIONAL POSITIONING FOR THE ANTERIOR SURFACES TOWARD

Practice the recommended clinician clock and patient head positions for the anterior surfaces toward by following the illustrations below.

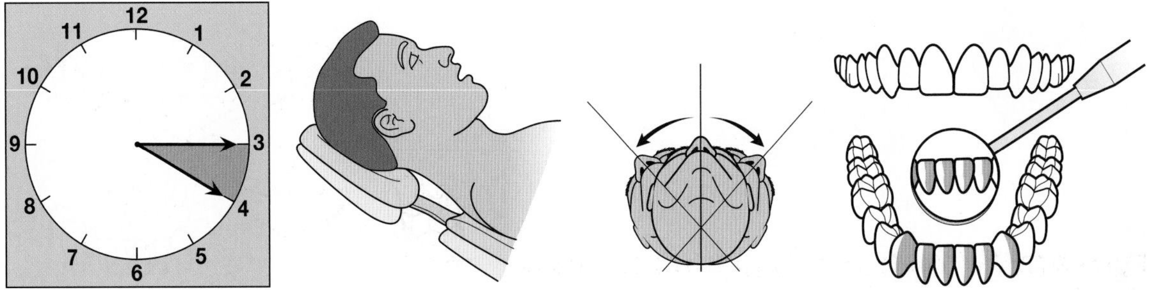

Figure 2-24. Mandibular Anterior Surfaces, TOWARD.

- Clinician seated in the 3 to 4 o'clock position.
- Patient chin DOWN; place the mandibular occlusal plane as parallel to the floor as possible.
- Patient head position ranges from neutral to turned to the right or left to facilitate vision of the tooth surfaces.

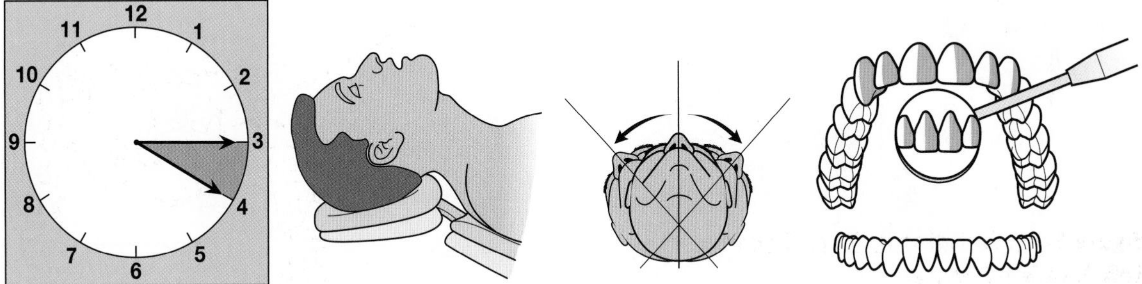

Figure 2-25. Maxillary Anterior Surfaces, TOWARD.

- Clinician in the 3 to 4 o'clock position.
- Patient chin UP; place the maxillary occlusal plane perpendicular to the floor.
- Patient head position ranges from neutral to turned to the right or left to facilitate vision of the tooth surfaces.

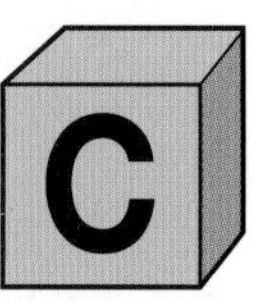

SKILL PRACTICE. TRADITIONAL POSITIONING FOR THE ANTERIOR SURFACES AWAY

Practice the recommended clinician clock and patient head positions for the anterior surfaces away by following the illustrations below.

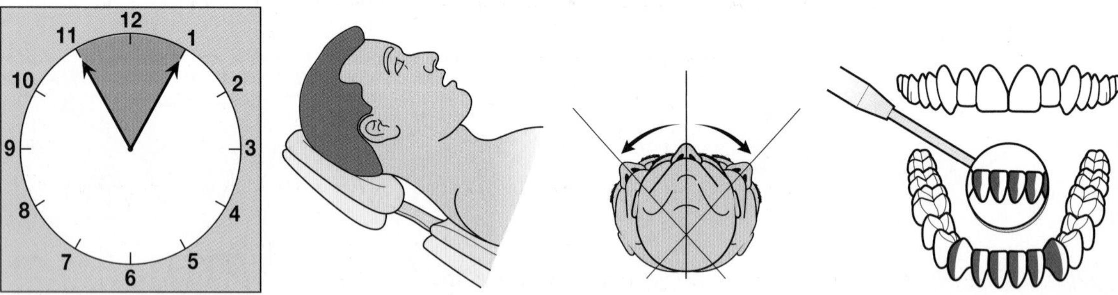

Figure 2-26. Mandibular Anterior Surfaces, AWAY.

- Clinician seated in the 11 to 1 o'clock position.
- Patient chin DOWN; place the mandibular occlusal plane as parallel to the floor as possible.
- Patient head position ranges from a neutral position to turning the head to the right or left to facilitate vision of the tooth surfaces.

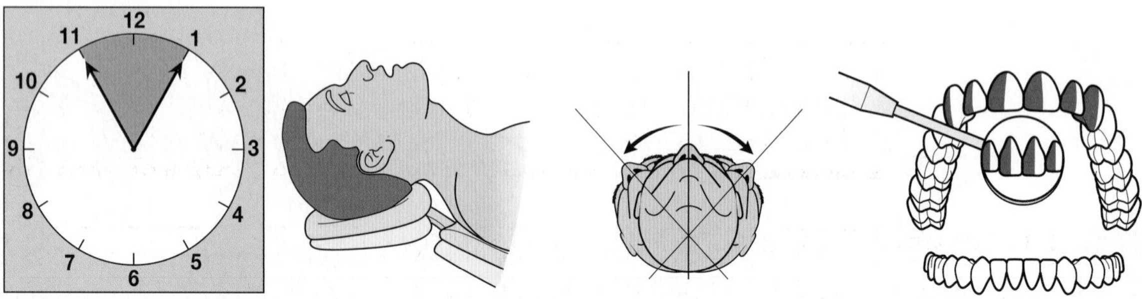

Figure 2-27. Maxillary Anterior Surfaces, AWAY.

- Clinician seated in the 11 to 1 o'clock position.
- Patient chin UP; place the maxillary occlusal plane perpendicular to the floor.
- Patient head position ranges from a neutral position to turning the head to the right or left to facilitate vision of the tooth surfaces.

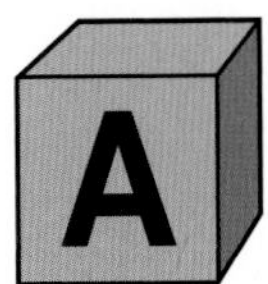

SKILL BUILDING. POSTERIOR SEXTANTS: QUICK START GUIDE TO TRADITIONAL CLOCK POSITIONS

There is no need to waste time memorizing the clock position for each posterior treatment area. The clock positions are easy to remember if you learn to recognize the positioning pattern for the posterior sextants. ***For periodontal instrumentation, each posterior sextant is divided into two aspects: (1) the facial aspect and (2) the lingual aspect of the sextant.***

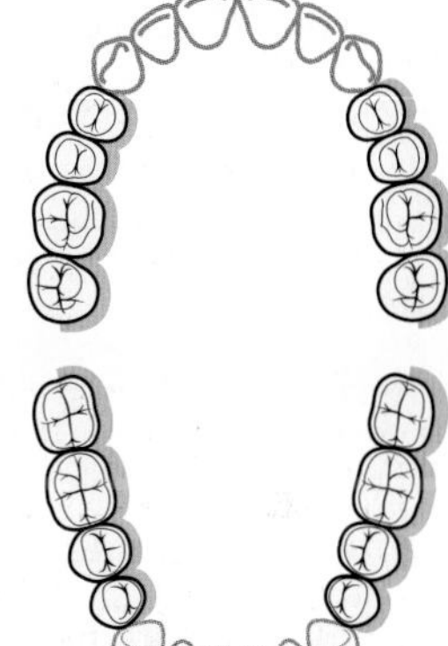

Figure 2-28. Posterior *Aspects Facing Toward* the Left-Handed Clinician.

- The posterior surfaces shaded in yellow on this drawing are called the posterior aspects facing toward the clinician.
- The **clock position** for the posterior aspects toward the clinician is **3 o'clock.**

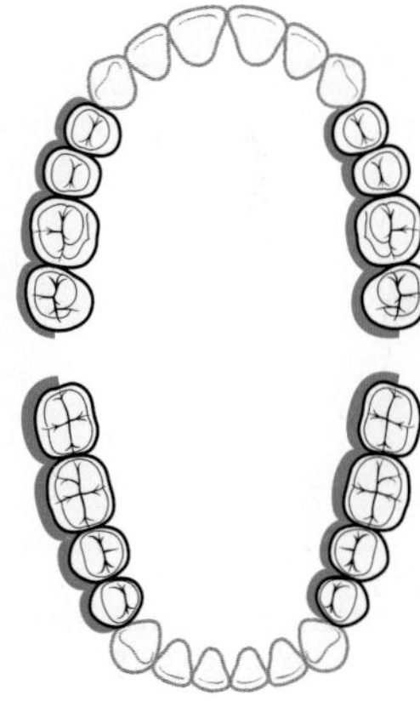

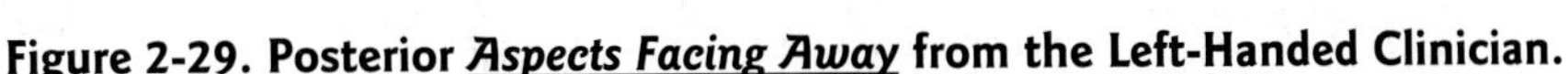

Figure 2-29. Posterior *Aspects Facing Away* from the Left-Handed Clinician.

- The posterior surfaces shaded in blue on this drawing are called the posterior aspects facing away from the clinician.
- The **clock position** for posterior aspects away from the clinician ranges from **1 to 2 o'clock.**

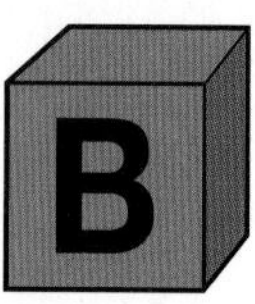

SKILL PRACTICE. TRADITIONAL POSITIONING FOR THE POSTERIOR SEXTANTS, ASPECTS FACING TOWARD THE CLINICIAN

Practice the recommended clinician clock and patient head positions for the posterior sextants facing toward the clinician by following the illustrations below.

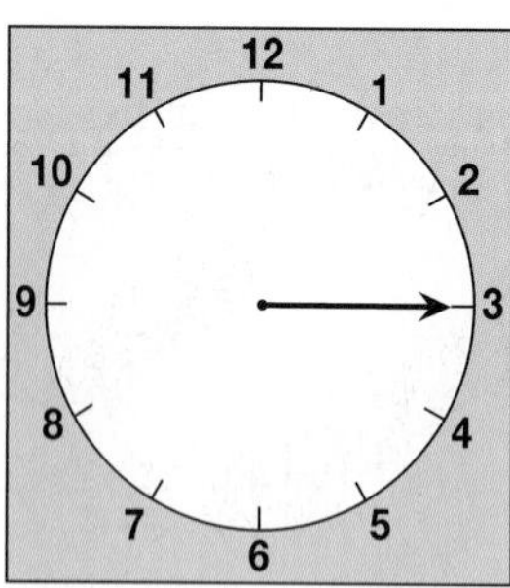

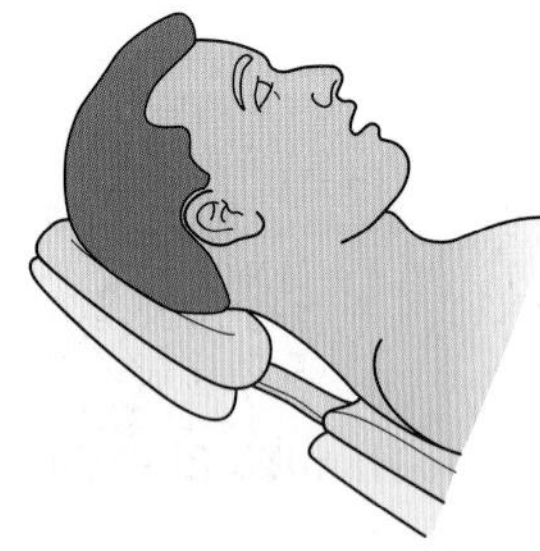

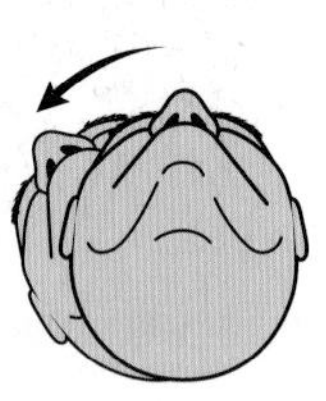

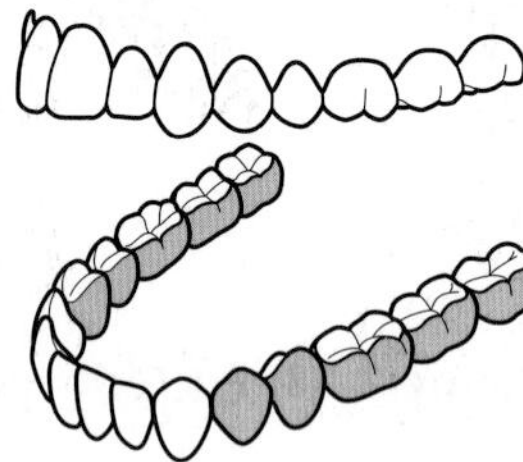

Figure 2-30. Mandibular Posterior Aspects Facing TOWARD.

- Clinician seated in the 3 o'clock position.
- Chin DOWN; place the mandibular occlusal plane as parallel to the floor as possible.
- Patient head position ranges from a neutral position to turning the head slightly away from the clinician.

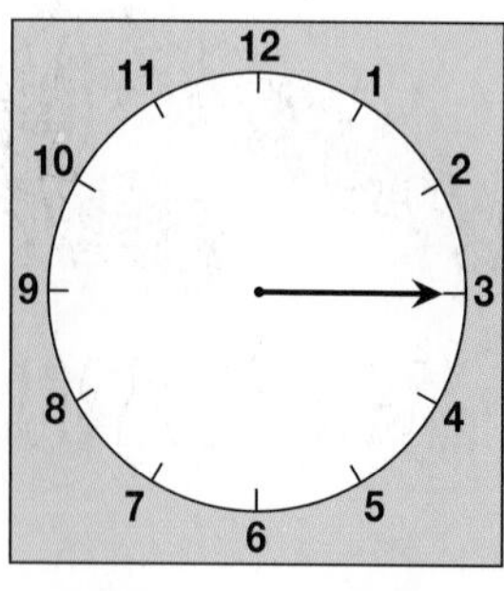

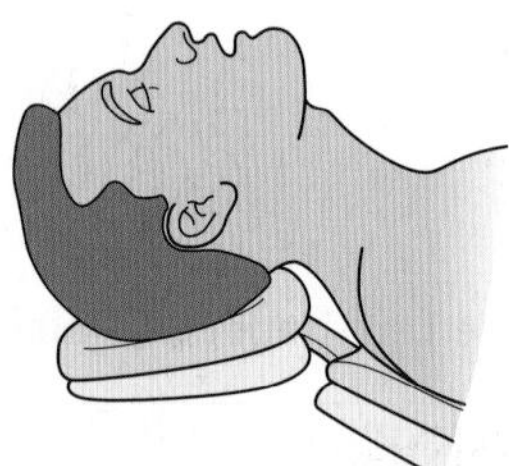

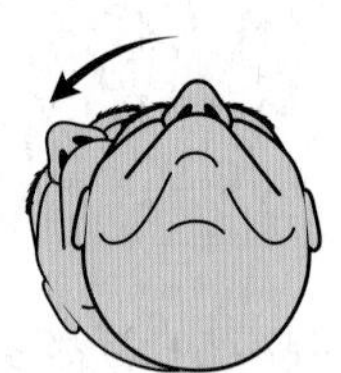

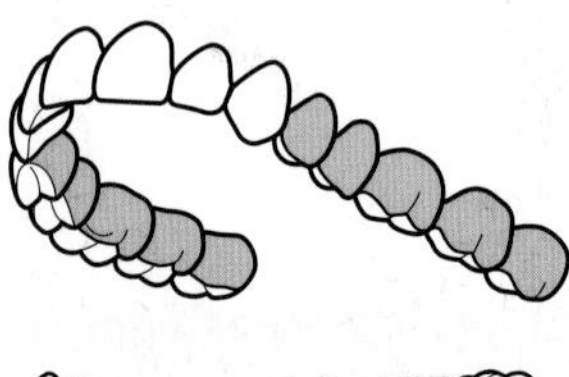

Figure 2-31. Maxillary Posterior Aspects Facing TOWARD.

- Clinician seated in the 3 o'clock position.
- Chin UP; place the maxillary occlusal plane perpendicular to the floor.
- Patient head position ranges from a neutral position to turning the head slightly away from the clinician.

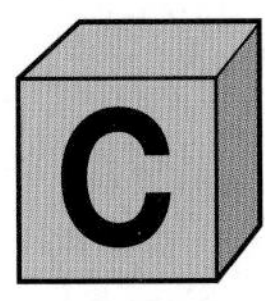

SKILL PRACTICE. TRADITIONAL POSITIONING FOR THE POSTERIOR SEXTANTS, ASPECTS FACING AWAY FROM THE CLINICIAN

Practice the recommended clinician clock and patient head positions for the posterior sextants facing away from the clinician by following the illustrations below.

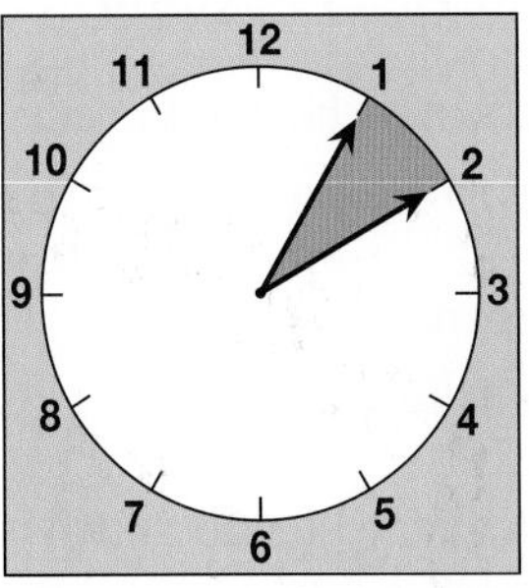

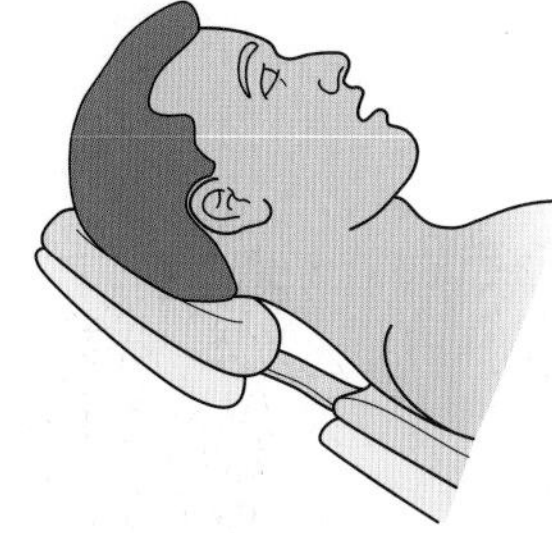
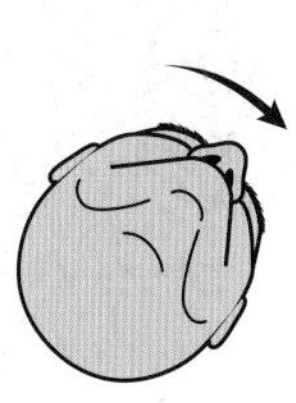
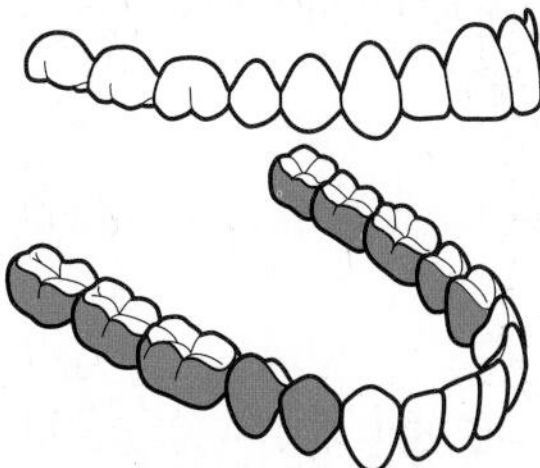

Figure 2-32. Mandibular Posterior Aspects Facing AWAY.

- Clinician seated in the 1 to 2 o'clock position.
- Chin DOWN; place the mandibular occlusal plane as parallel to the floor as possible.
- Patient head position is turned toward the clinician.

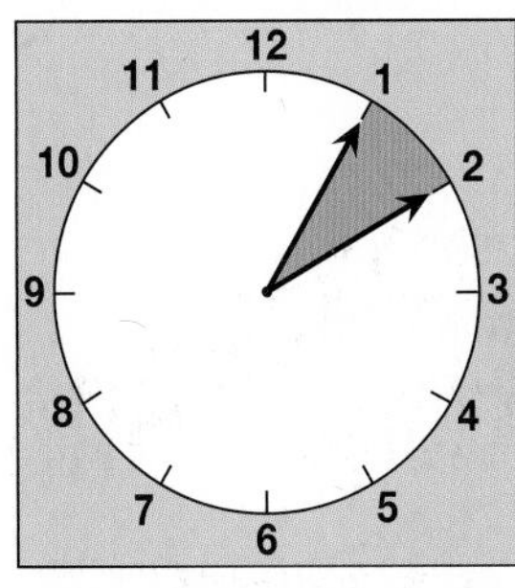

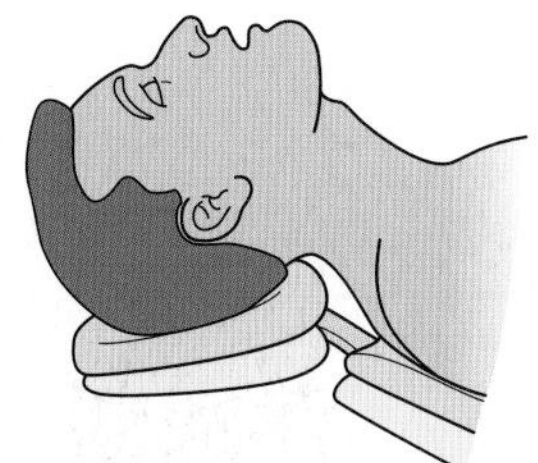
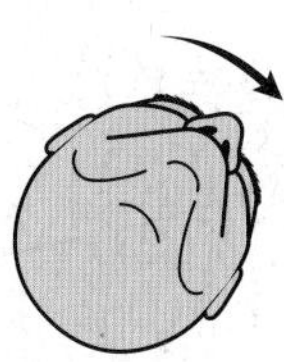
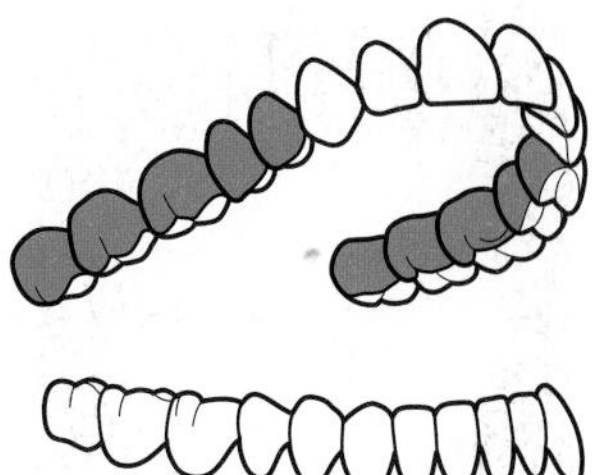

Figure 2-33. Maxillary Posterior Aspects Facing AWAY.

- Clinician seated in the 1 to 2 o'clock position.
- Chin UP; place the maxillary occlusal plane perpendicular to the floor.
- Patient head position is turned toward the clinician.

REFERENCE SHEET: POSITION FOR THE LEFT-HANDED CLINICIAN

Table 2-2 summarizes the traditional clock positions for the left-handed clinician. Photocopy this page and use it for quick reference as you practice your positioning skills. Place the photocopied reference sheet in a plastic page protector for longer use.

TABLE 2-2. Traditional Clock Positions—Positioning Summary

Treatment Area	Clock Position	Patient Head Position
Mandibular Arch—Anterior surfaces toward	3:00–4:00	Chin down; neutral to turned right or left
Maxillary Arch—Anterior surfaces toward	3:00–4:00	Chin up; neutral to turned right or left
Mandibular Arch—Anterior surfaces away	11:00–1:00	Chin down; neutral to turned right or left
Maxillary Arch—Anterior surfaces away	11:00–1:00	Chin up; neutral to turned right or left
Mandibular Arch—Posterior aspects toward	3:00	Chin down; neutral
Maxillary Arch—Posterior aspects toward	3:00	Chin up; neutral to turned slightly away
Mandibular Arch—Posterior aspects away	1:00–2:00	Chin down; toward
Maxillary Arch—Posterior aspects away	1:00–2:00	Chin up; toward

Note: This ends Section 3 for the left-handed clinician. Please turn to page 65 for Section 4: Modified Positioning: Working from a Standing Position.

LEFT-Handed Clinician

Section 4
Modified Positioning: Working from a Standing Position

At times, it may be helpful for the clinician to use a standing position, rather than a seated position, for periodontal instrumentation. A standing position can be used when there is difficulty accessing the treatment area, when the patient cannot be placed in a supine position due to medical or physical contraindications, or when working on mandibular treatment areas (Figs. 2-34 and 2-35).

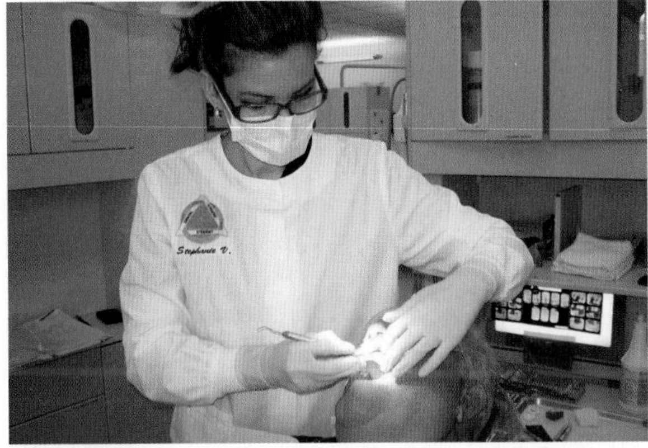

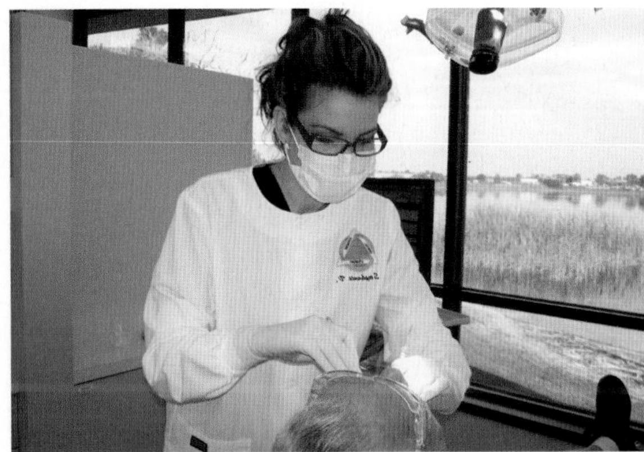

Figure 2-34. Correct Standing Clinician Position.

- A standing clinician position can be used to facilitate access to a treatment area or when a supine position is contraindicated for a patient due to medical or physical limitations.
- Notice that the clinician's shoulders are relaxed, the elbow of her dominant hand is at waist level, her torso is in neutral position, and she is not leaning over the patient.

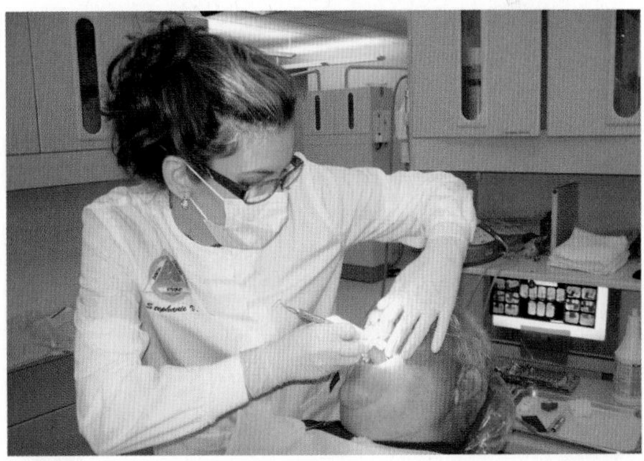

Figure 2-35. Incorrect Standing Clinician Position.

- This is an example of incorrect standing position.
- Note that the clinician's shoulders are hunched, her torso is tilted and twisted, and her elbows are raised.

Section 5
Skill Application

PRACTICAL FOCUS

Your course assignment is to visit a local dental office and photograph a clinician at work in order to assess position. Your photographs are shown below:

1. Evaluate each photograph for clinician, patient, and equipment position.
2. For each incorrect positioning element, describe: (a) what the problem is, (b) how the problem could be corrected, and (c) the musculoskeletal problems that could result from each positioning problem.

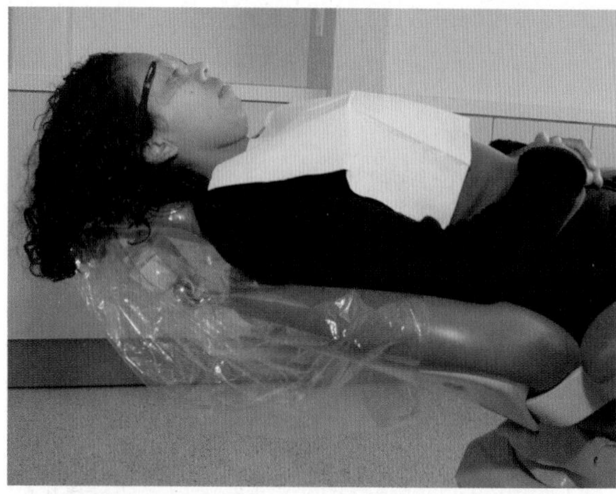

Figure 2-36. Photo 1.

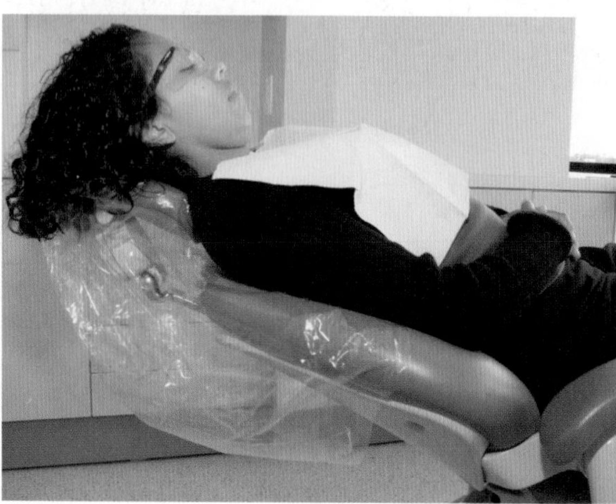

Figure 2-37. Photo 2.

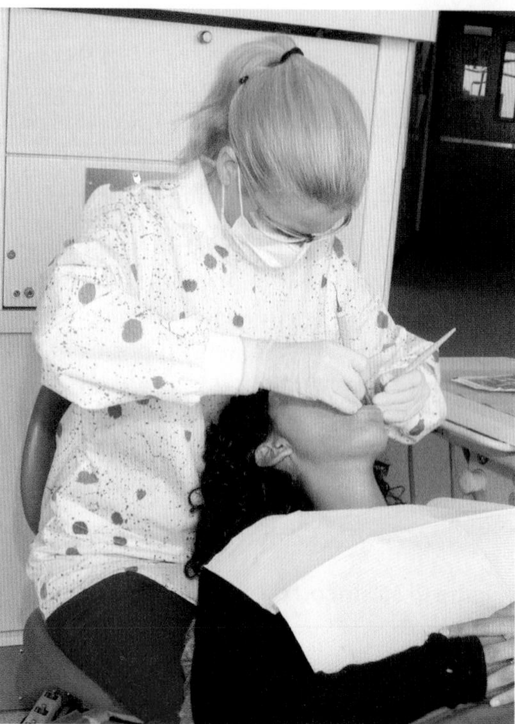

Figure 2-38. Photo 3.

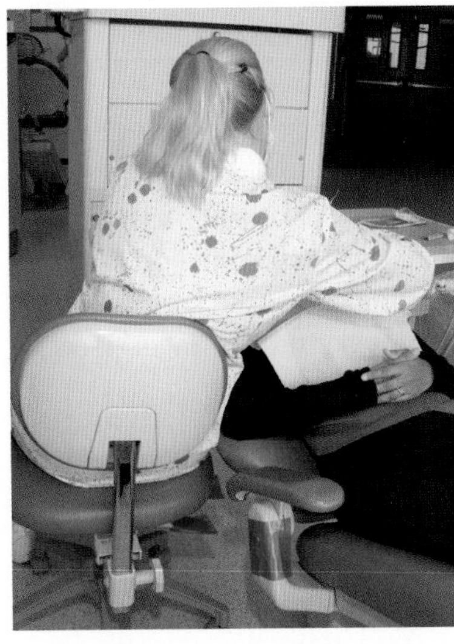

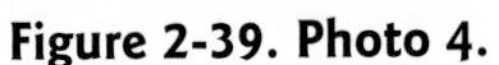

Figure 2-39. Photo 4.

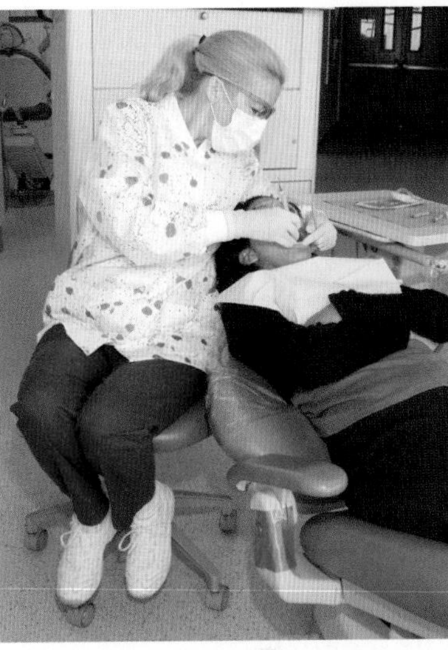

Figure 2-40. Photo 5.

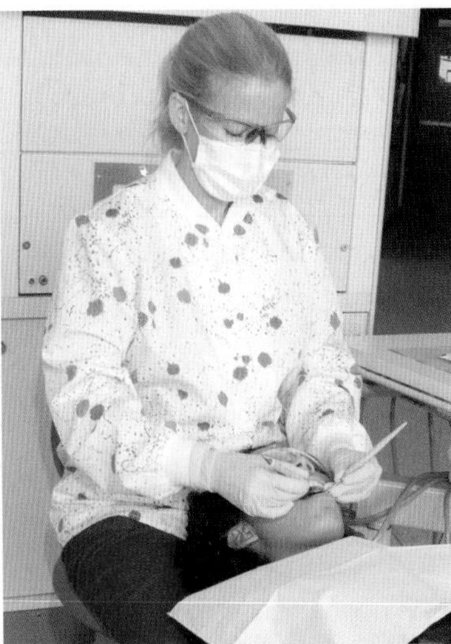

Figure 2-41. Photo 6.

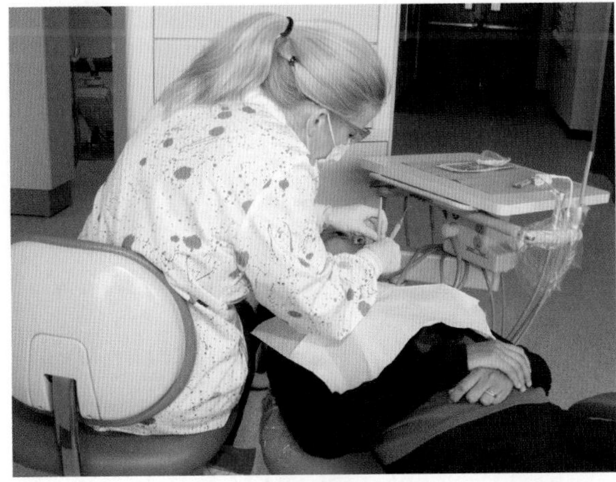

Figure 2-42. Photo 7.

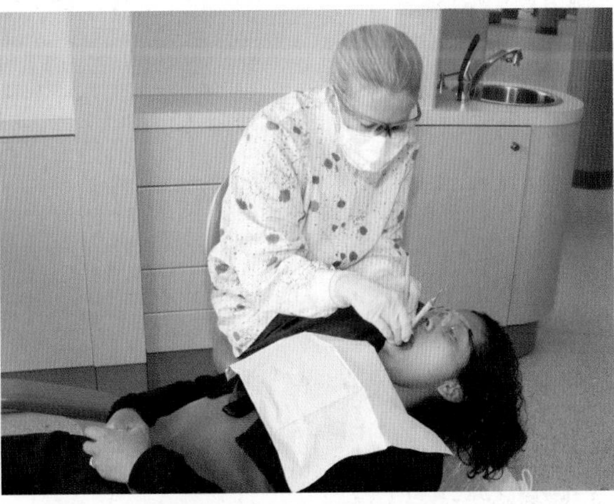

Figure 2-43. Photo 8.

Note to Course Instructors:
To download Module Evaluations for this textbook, go to http://thepoint.lww.com/GehrigFundamentals7e and log on to access the Instructor Resources for *Fundamentals of Periodontal Instrumentation and Advanced Root Instrumentation.*

STUDENT SELF-EVALUATION MODULE 2 POSITIONING AND CLOCK POSITIONS

Student: ______________________________

Date: ______________________________

Area 1 = anterior sextant, facial aspect
Area 2 = anterior sextant, lingual aspect
Area 3 = right posterior sextant, facial aspect
Area 4 = right posterior sextant, lingual aspect
Area 5 = left posterior sextant, facial aspect
Area 6 = left posterior sextant, lingual aspect

DIRECTIONS: Self-evaluate your skill level in each treatment area as: **S** (satisfactory) or **U** (unsatisfactory).

Criteria						
Positioning/Ergonomics	**Area 1**	**Area 2**	**Area 3**	**Area 4**	**Area 5**	**Area 6**
Adjusts clinician chair correctly						
Reclines patient chair and ensures that patient's head is even with top of headrest						
Positions instrument tray within easy reach for front, side, or rear delivery as appropriate for operatory configuration						
Positions unit light at arm's length or dons dental headlight and adjusts it for use						
Assumes the recommended clock position						
Positions backrest of patient chair for the specified arch and adjusts height of patient chair so that clinician's elbows remain at waist level when accessing the specified treatment area						
Asks patient to assume the head position that facilitates the clinician's view of the specified treatment area						
Maintains neutral position						
Directs light to illuminate the specified treatment area						

Criteria: Maxillary Arch						
Positioning/Ergonomics	**Area 1**	**Area 2**	**Area 3**	**Area 4**	**Area 5**	**Area 6**
Adjusts clinician chair correctly						
Reclines patient chair and ensures that patient's head is even with top of headrest						
Positions instrument tray within easy reach for front, side, or rear delivery as appropriate for operatory configuration						
Positions unit light at arm's length or dons dental headlight and adjusts it for use						
Assumes the recommended clock position						
Positions backrest of patient chair for the specified arch and adjusts height of patient chair so that clinician's elbows remain at waist level when accessing the specified treatment area						
Asks patient to assume the head position that facilitates the clinician's view of the specified treatment area						
Maintains neutral position						
Directs light to illuminate the specified treatment area						

Module 3

Instrument Grasp

Module Overview

Module 3 introduces the modified pen grasp for holding a periodontal instrument. The correct instrument grasp—called the modified pen grasp—allows precise control of the working-end of a periodontal instrument, permits a wide range of movement, and facilitates good tactile conduction (allows the clinician to feel rough areas on the tooth).

Module Outline

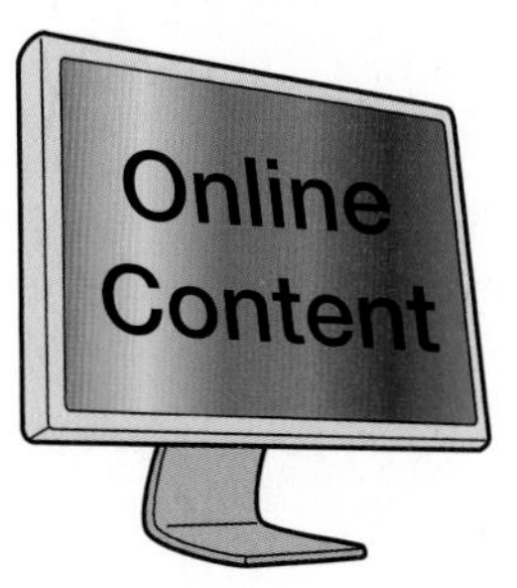

A video for this topic can be viewed online at http://thepoint.lww.com/GehrigFundamentals7e

Key Terms

Modified pen grasp
Handle
Shank
Working-end
Joint hypermobility
"Knuckles-up" position
"Knuckles-down" position

Learning Objectives

1. Given a variety of periodontal instruments, identify the parts of each instrument.
2. Identify the fingers of the hand as thumb, index, middle, ring, and little fingers.
3. Understand the relationship among correct finger position in the modified pen grasp, the prevention of musculoskeletal problems, and the control of a periodontal instrument during instrumentation.
4. Demonstrate the modified pen grasp using precise finger placement on the handle of a periodontal instrument:
   - Finger pads of thumb and index finger are opposite one another on handle.
   - Thumb and index finger do not overlap each other on the handle.
   - Pad of middle finger rests lightly on the shank.
   - Pad of middle finger touches the ring finger.
   - Thumb, index, and middle fingers are in a "knuckles-up" position.
   - Ring finger is straight and supports weight of the hand.
5. Describe the function each finger serves in the modified pen grasp.
6. Define joint hypermobility and describe how hyperextended joints in the modified pen grasp can affect periodontal instrumentation.
7. Recognize incorrect finger position in the modified pen grasp and describe how to correct the problem(s).
8. Select the correct glove size for your own hands and explain how the glove size selected meets the criteria for proper glove fit.
9. Understand the relationship between proper glove fit and the prevention of musculoskeletal problems in the hands.
10. Perform exercises for improved hand strength.

Section I

Grasp for Periodontal Instrumentation

THE MODIFIED PEN GRASP

The modified pen grasp is the recommended method for holding a periodontal instrument (Fig. 3-1).[1] The modified pen grasp facilitates precise control of the instrument as it moves over the tooth, allows the clinician to detect rough areas on the tooth surface, and lessens musculoskeletal stress to the clinician's fingers during periodontal instrumentation.

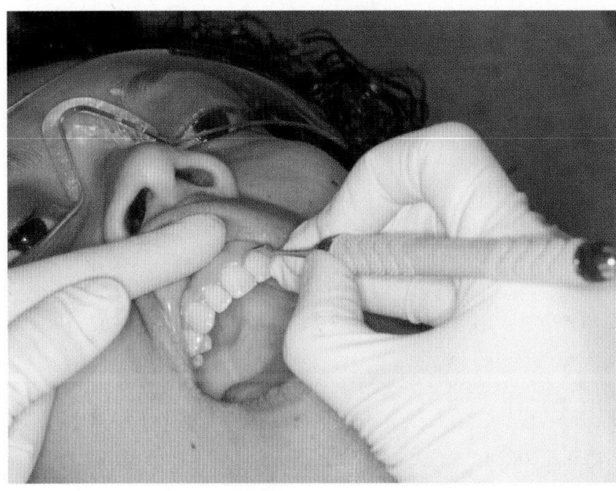

Figure 3-1. The Modified Pen Grasp. The **modified pen grasp** is the recommended grasp for holding a periodontal instrument.

PARTS OF THE PERIODONTAL INSTRUMENT

In order to master the modified pen grasp, the preclinical student must be able to identify the parts of a periodontal instrument (Fig. 3-2).

- Handle—the part of a periodontal instrument used for holding the instrument.
- Shank—a rod-shaped length of metal located between the handle and the working-end of a dental instrument. The shank generally is circular, smooth, and much smaller in diameter than the handle. The shank may be straight, or it may be bent in one or more places.
- Working-End—the part of a dental instrument that does the work of the instrument. The working-end begins where the instrument shank ends. On a periodontal instrument, the working-end may be shaped or flattened on some of its surfaces. The working-end could appear wire-like, look like a tiny ruler, or even be a small mirror. A single instrument may have one or two working-ends.

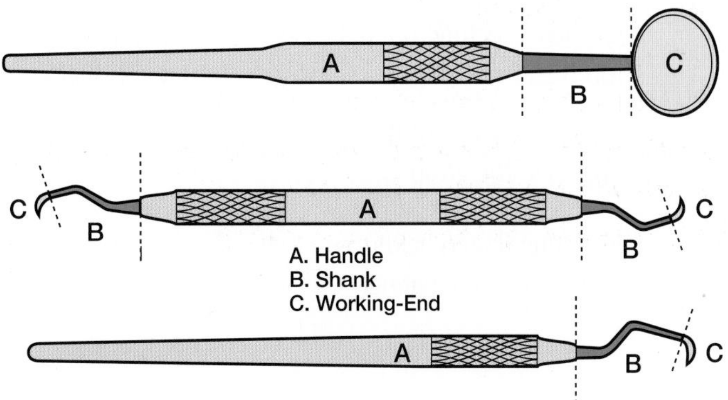

Figure 3-2. Parts of a Periodontal Instrument. The parts of a periodontal instrument are **(A)** the handle, **(B)** the shank, and **(C)** the working-end.

FINGER IDENTIFICATION FOR THE INSTRUMENT GRASP

The correct instrument grasp requires precise finger placement on the instrument.[2,3] Figure 3-3 shows how the fingers of the hand are identified for purposes of the modified pen grasp. Table 3-1 outlines the placement and function of each finger in the instrument grasp.

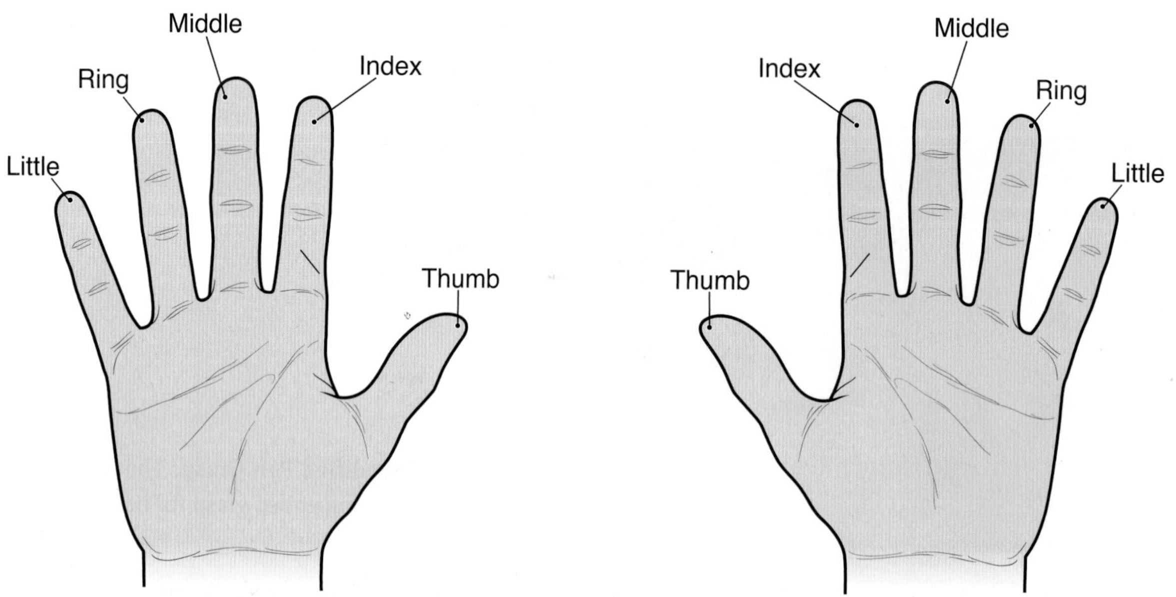

Figure 3-3. Finger Identification and Placement in Modified Pen Grasp.

TABLE 3-1. Finger Placement and Function

Digit(s)	Placement	Function
Index and Thumb	• On the instrument handle	• Hold the instrument
Middle Finger	• Rests lightly on the shank	• Helps to guide the working-end • Feels vibrations transmitted from the working-end to the shank[4]
Ring Finger	• On oral structure; often a tooth surface • Advances ahead of the other fingers in the grasp	• Stabilizes and supports the hand for control and strength
Little Finger	• Near ring finger; held in a natural, relaxed manner	• Has no function in the grasp

RIGHT-Handed Clinicians: Continue reading on the next page.
LEFT-Handed Clinicians: Turn to page 74 for the modified pen grasp for left-handed clinicians.

A SKILL BUILDING. MODIFIED PEN GRASP: RIGHT-HANDED CLINICIAN

Directions: Practice the modified pen grasp by referring to the criteria labeled in Figures 3-4 and 3-5.

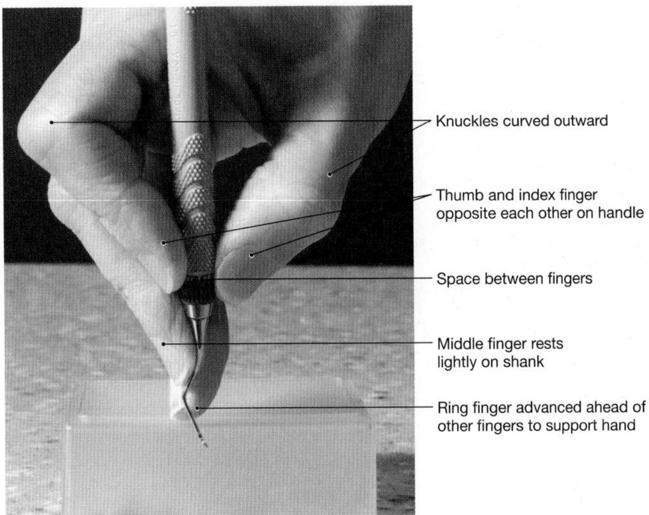

Figure 3-4. Modified Pen Grasp for Right-Handed Clinician (Side View). A side view of a right-handed clinician holding a periodontal instrument in a modified pen grasp.

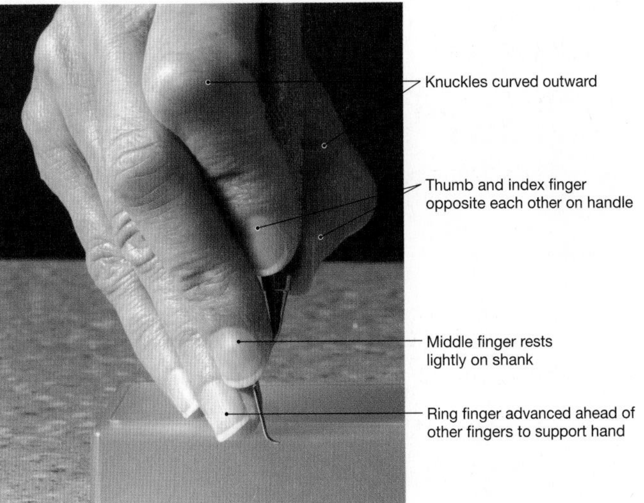

Figure 3-5. Modified Pen Grasp for Right-Handed Clinician (Front View). The front view of a right-handed clinician holding a periodontal instrument in a modified pen grasp.

A SKILL BUILDING. MODIFIED PEN GRASP: LEFT-HANDED CLINICIAN

Directions: Practice the modified pen grasp by referring to the criteria labeled in Figures 3-6 and 3-7.

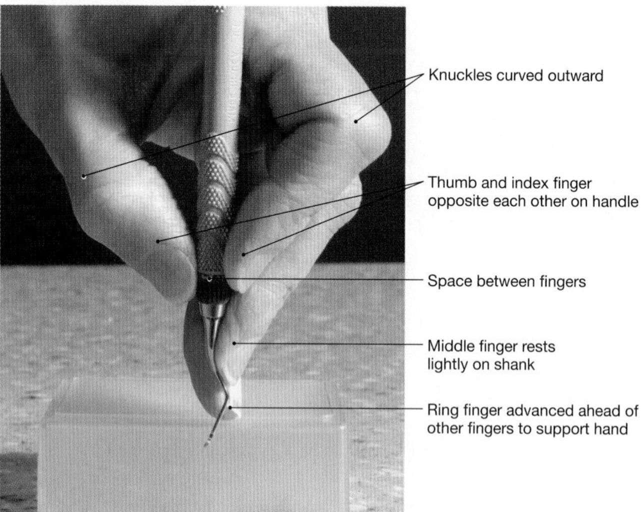

Figure 3-6. Modified Pen Grasp for Left-Handed Clinician (Side View). A side view of a left-handed clinician holding a periodontal instrument in a modified pen grasp.

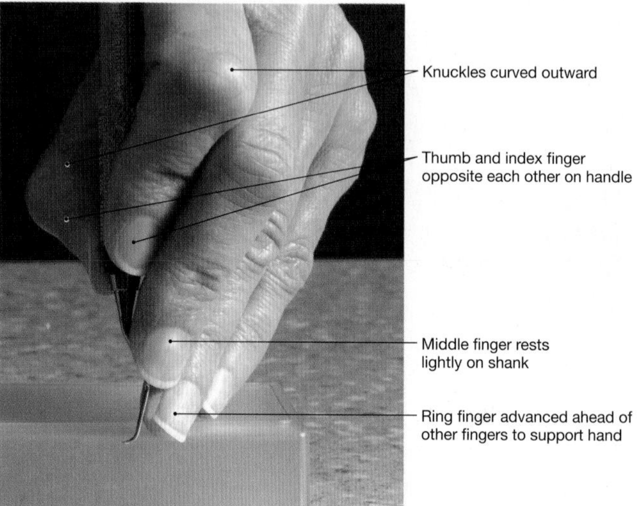

Figure 3-7. Modified Pen Grasp for Left-Handed Clinician (Front View). The front view of a left-handed clinician holding a periodontal instrument in a modified pen grasp.

FINE-TUNING YOUR GRASP

Precise finger placement in the modified pen grasp is critical to successful instrumentation.[1] Note that the finger placement for a modified pen grasp differs from that used when writing.

TABLE 3-2. Summary Sheet: Correct Finger Placement

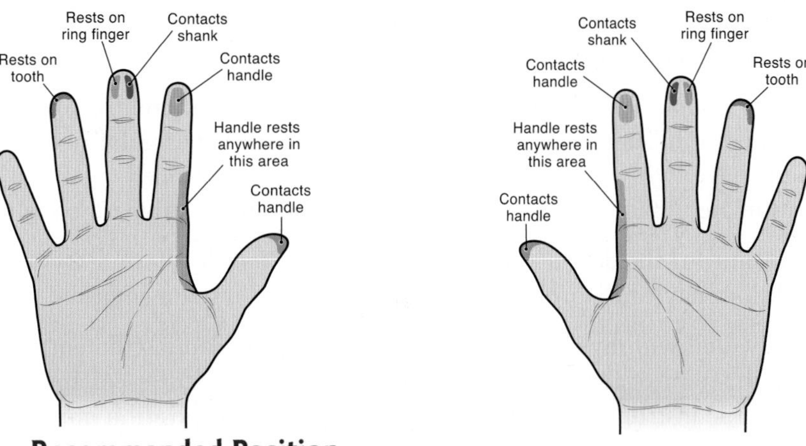

Digit	Recommended Position
Thumb and Index Finger	• The finger pads rest opposite each other at or near the junction of the handle and the shank.[3] • The fingers do not overlap; there is a tiny space between them.[3] • The fingers hold the handle in a relaxed manner. If your fingers are blanched, you are holding too tightly. • The index finger and thumb curve outward from the handle in a convex shape. This position places the finger pads on the handle in the best position for instrumentation. • The index finger and thumb should not collapse inward toward the handle in a concave shape. This collapsed shape causes the finger pads to lift off of the handle, making it difficult to roll the instrument during instrumentation.
Middle Finger	• One side of the finger pad rests lightly on the instrument shank. The other side of the finger pad rests against (or slightly overlaps) the ring finger. • Not used to hold the instrument. You should be able to lift your middle finger off of the shank without dropping the instrument. If you drop the instrument, then you are incorrectly using the middle finger to help hold the instrument.
Ring Finger	• Fingertip of the ring finger—not the pad—balances firmly on a tooth to support the weight of the hand and a periodontal instrument. • When grasping a dental mirror, the ring finger may rest on a tooth or against the patient's lip or cheek area. • The ring finger of the dominant hand advances ahead of the other fingers in the grasp. It is held straight and upright to act as a strong support beam for the hand. The finger should not feel tense, but it should not be held limply against a tooth.
Little Finger	• The little finger is held in a relaxed manner close to the ring finger.

Section 2
Joint Hypermobility of the Hand

WHAT IS JOINT HYPERMOBILITY?

1. Joint hypermobility is a condition that features joints that easily move beyond the normal range expected for a particular joint. Figure 3-8 shows an individual with joint hypermobility of the thumb.
   a. The term *double-jointed* often is used to describe hypermobility; however, the name is a misnomer because the individual with hypermobility does not actually have two separate joints where others have just one.[5]
   b. It is estimated that 10% to 15% of normal children have hypermobile joints.
2. It is important for the dental hygienist to recognize joint hypermobility because this condition may cause problems during periodontal instrumentation:
   a. An individual with hypermobility must learn to grasp an instrument without having the joint of the thumb or index finger hyperextend or collapse.
   b. Holding the instrument with joints in a hyperextended position impairs the ability to roll the instrument handle between the thumb and index finger in a precise, controlled manner. The tips of the finger pads should contact the instrument handle for precise control during rolling.
   c. In addition, performing periodontal instrumentation with the joints in a hyperextended position may cause injury to a hypermobile joint by overstretching it.[5]
3. ***A clinician with hypermobility needs to counteract joint hyperextension by bending the thumb and/or index finger in the modified pen grasp.***

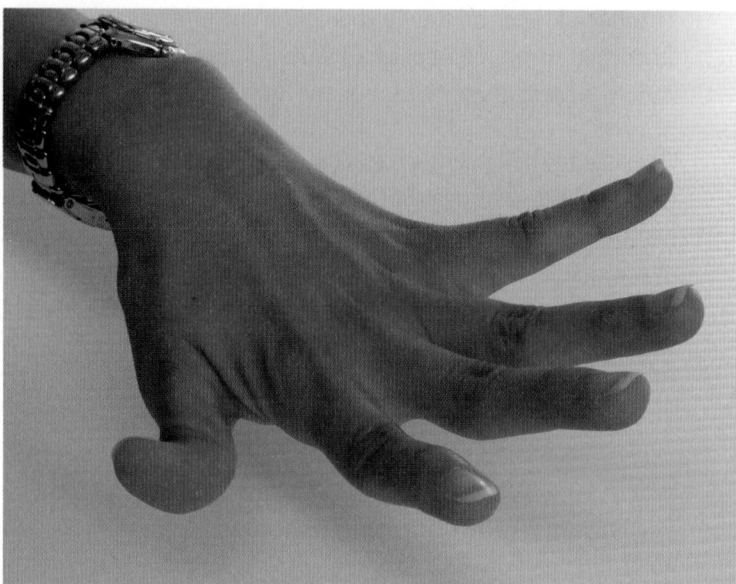

Figure 3-8. Joint Hypermobility of the Fingers. The individual pictured here has joint hypermobility, allowing her to bend her fingers back beyond the normal range of movement.

GRASP FOR PRECISE CONTROL

The correct grasp allows the clinician to achieve precise control of the working-end during instrumentation and reduce musculoskeletal stress to the hands and fingers.[1,2,6] The examples shown below illustrate how finger placement can facilitate or hinder instrumentation (Figs. 3-9 and 3-10).

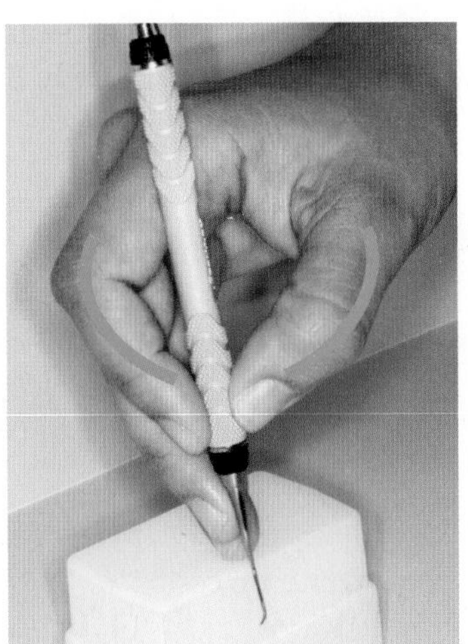

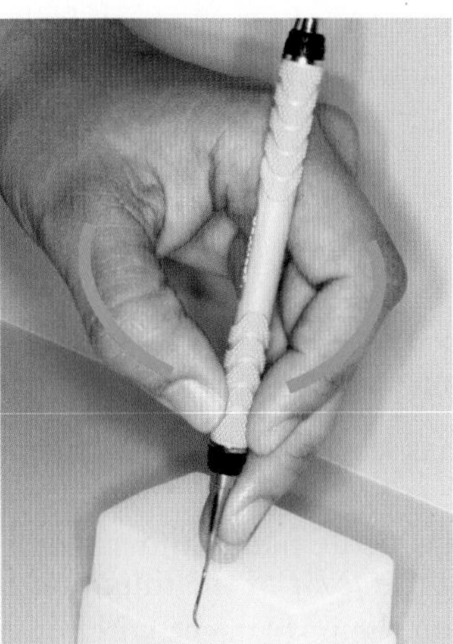

Figure 3-9. Ideal Grasp. The finger placement shown here facilitates precise control during periodontal instrumentation. This grasp—with tips of finger pads contacting the handle—enables the clinician to roll the instrument handle between the fingers in a controlled manner. The handle roll is used to position the working-end against the tooth surface in a precise manner.

- **Convex Finger Shape.** The index finger and thumb should be in a "knuckles-up" position.
- **Finger Pads.** The finger pads contact the handle to allow precise control of the instrument.

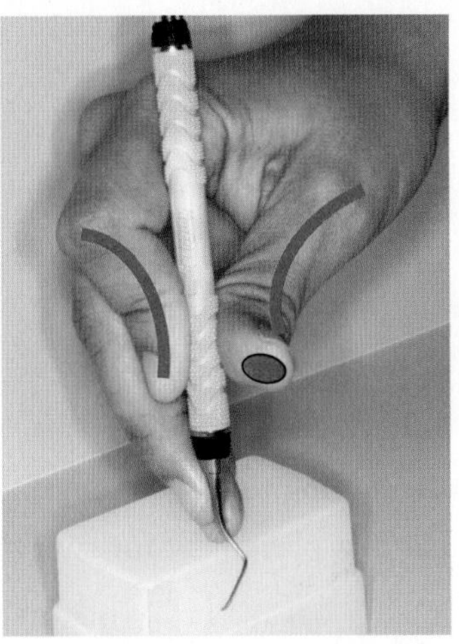

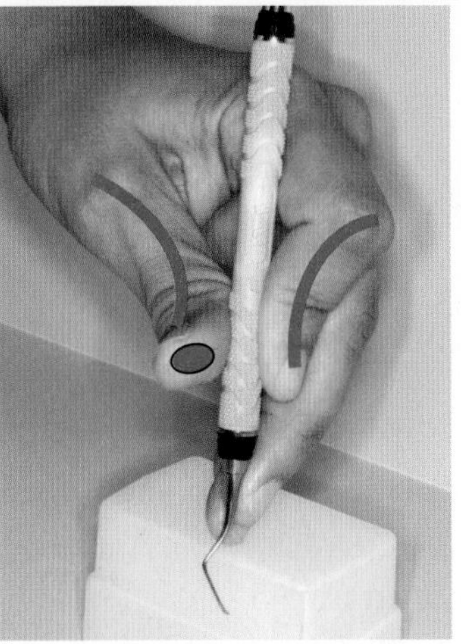

Figure 3-10. Incorrect Grasp. The finger placement shown here hinders control of a periodontal instrument. This grasp—with hyperextended joints—makes it extremely difficult to roll the instrument handle between the fingers. It will be difficult to control the position of the working-end with the fingers in this position.

- **Concave Finger Shape.** The index finger and thumb should NOT collapse inward toward the handle in a "knuckles-down" position as shown here.
- **Pads Not in Contact.** This collapsed finger position—with hyperextended joints—causes the finger pads to lift off of the handle, making it very difficult to roll the instrument handle between the fingers.

Section 3
Grasp Variations

FINGER LENGTH

A clinician's finger length determines the location where he or she grasps the instrument handle and establishes a finger rest. Figures 3-11 and 3-12 show two individuals with very different finger lengths.

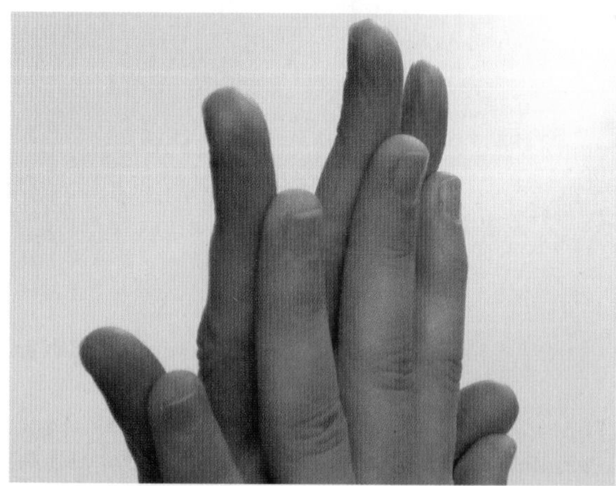

Figure 3-11. Finger Length.

- Clinician A has long fingers and a larger hand size.
- Clinician B has petite hands and a shorter finger length.

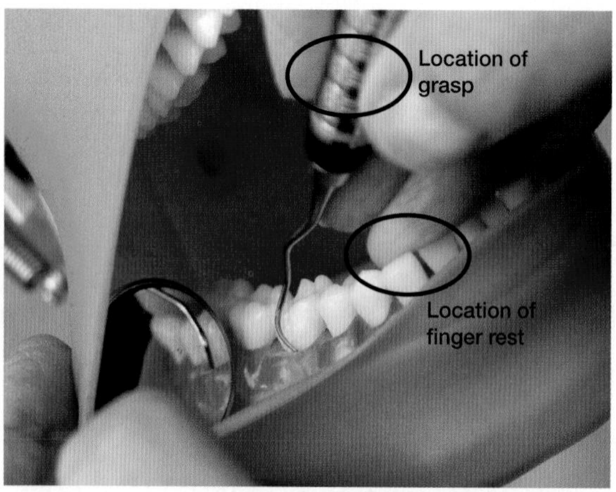

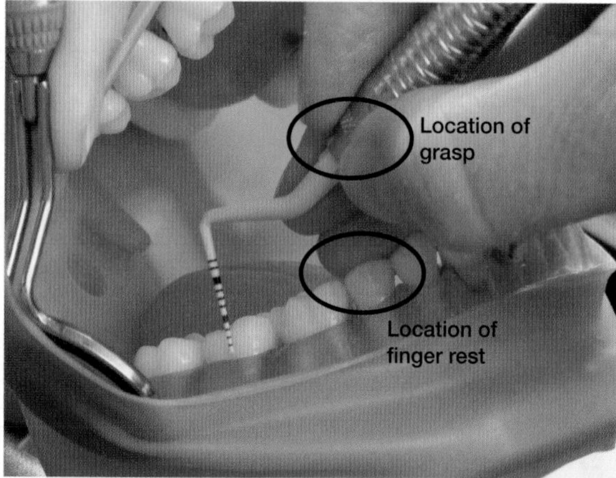

Figure 13-12. Variation in Grasp and Finger Rest Position According to Finger Length.

These two photographs show variations in grasp and finger rest placement for two clinicians with differing finger lengths.

- **Figure 13-12A. Clinician A: Long Finger Length (Photo on Left).**
  - Note that Clinician A establishes her grasp higher on the instrument handle than Clinician B.
  - Clinician A rests her ring finger on the canine.
- **Figure 13-12B. Clinician B: Short Finger Length (Photo on Right).**
  - Clinician B establishes her grasp low on the tapered portion of the instrument handle.
  - Clinician B rests her ring finger on the second premolar.

JOINT HYPERMOBILITY

Depending on the extent of joint hypermobility and the number of fingers involved, a clinician may need to modify the finger placement in the grasp (Fig. 3-13).

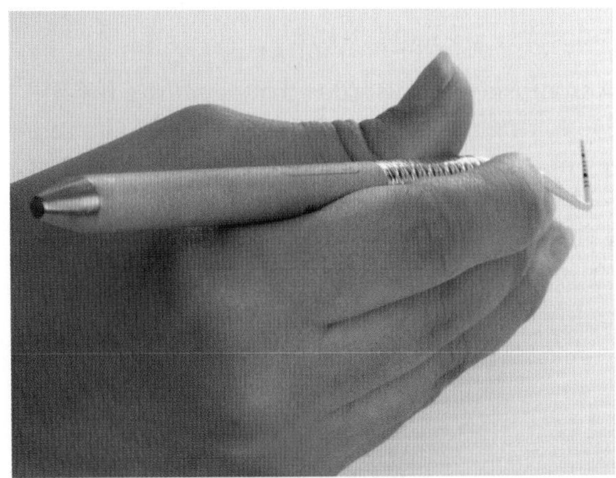

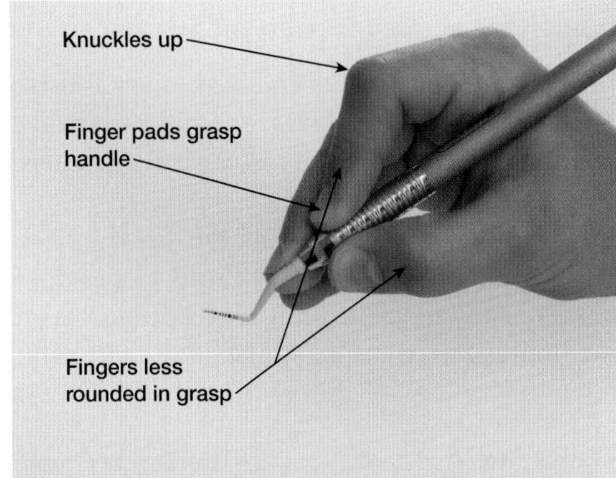

Figure 3-13. Modified Grasp for Clinician with Joint Hypermobility. This photo shows an example of a modified pen grasp for a clinician with joint hypermobility. Note that the fingers may be less rounded in the grasp than in a person without joint hypermobility; however, with the fingers in the "knuckles-up" position, the pads of the fingers grasp the instrument handle.

ARTHRITIS

A condition less commonly seen in dental hygiene students is arthritis of the hands. The clinician pictured in Figure 3-14 has arthritis of the joints of her hand.

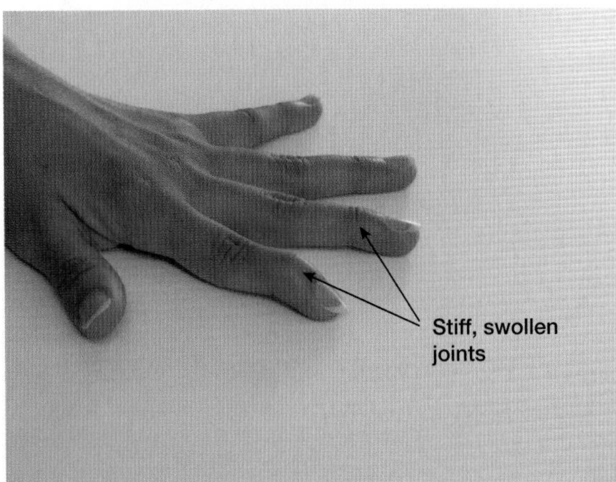

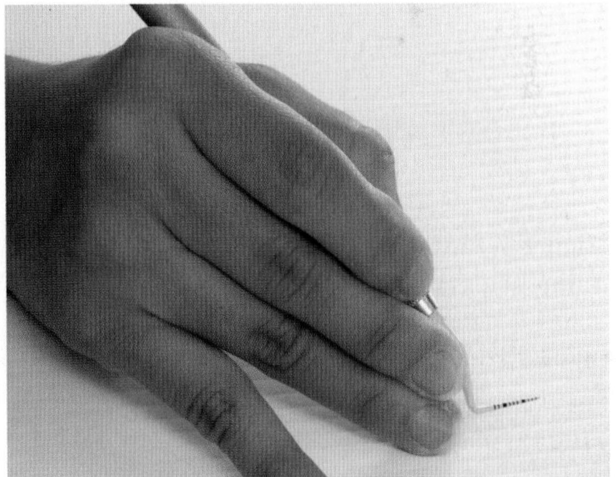

Figure 3-14. Modified Grasp for Clinician with Arthritis. This photo shows an example of a modified pen grasp for a clinician with arthritis.

Section 4
Proper Glove Fit for Instrumentation

Proper glove fit is important in avoiding muscle strain during instrumentation. Gloves should be loose fitting across the palm and wrist areas of the hand (Figs. 3-15 and 3-16).

- In fact, surgical glove–induced injury is a type of musculoskeletal disorder that is caused by improperly fitting gloves. Symptoms include numbness, tingling, or pain in the wrist, hand, and/or fingers. This disorder is caused by wearing gloves that are too tight or by wearing ambidextrous gloves (Fig. 3-17).
- It is best to wear right- and left-fitted gloves rather than ambidextrous gloves that are designed to fit either hand. Ambidextrous gloves do not fit as well as fitted gloves, causing them to exert greater force on the hands. Over time, this force could contribute to vascular constriction, nerve compression, muscle fatigue, and hand pain.[7]

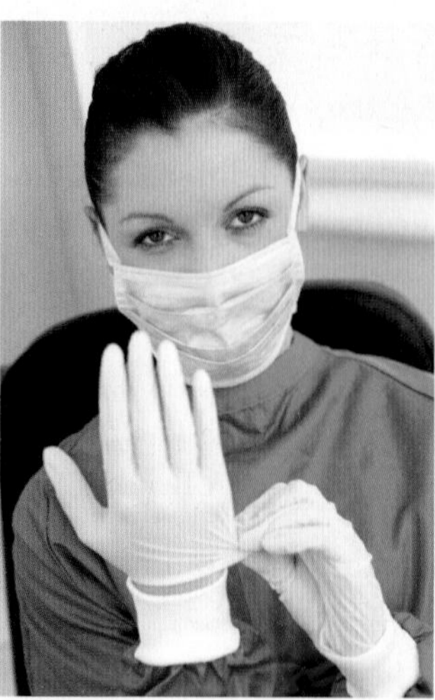

Figure 3-15. Glove Fit. Select a glove size that is loose fitting across the palm of the hand and wrist. Try gloves from several manufacturers to find the brand that fits best. Clinicians with long fingers need to find a brand that accommodates their finger length. Conversely, clinicians with shorter fingers should find a brand of gloves with fingers that do not hang over the fingertips. (Courtesy of Can Stock Photo Inc.)

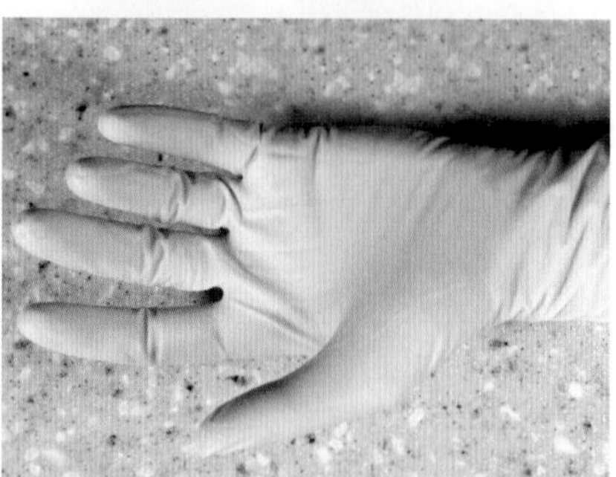

Figure 3-16. Correct Glove Fit. Gloves should be loose fitting across the palm and wrist areas of the hand. The index finger of your opposite hand should slip easily under the wrist area of the gloved hand.

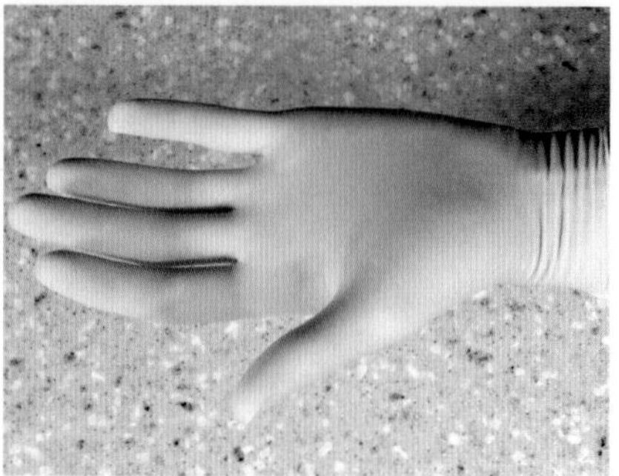

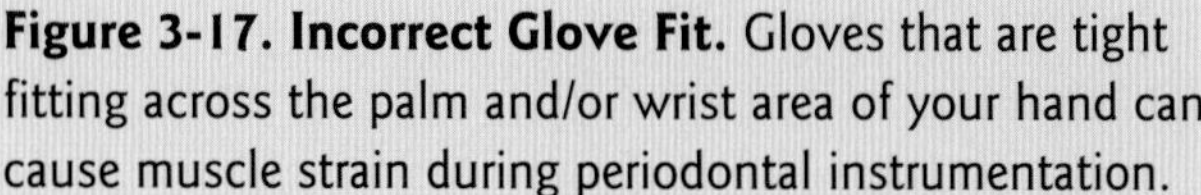

Figure 3-17. Incorrect Glove Fit. Gloves that are tight fitting across the palm and/or wrist area of your hand can cause muscle strain during periodontal instrumentation.

Section 5
Exercises for Improved Hand Strength

Well-conditioned hand muscles have improved control and endurance, allow for freer wrist movement, and reduce the likelihood of injury. The hand exercises shown here will help to develop and maintain muscle strength for periodontal instrumentation.

Directions: These exercises use Power Putty, a silicone rubber material that resists both squeezing and stretching forces. For each exercise illustrated, squeeze or stretch the Power Putty for the suggested number of repetitions. The exercise set, for both hands doing all nine exercises, should take no more than 10 to 20 minutes. When exercising, maintain your hands at waist level.

CAUTION: Not all exercise programs are suitable for everyone; discontinue any exercise that causes you discomfort and consult a medical expert. If you have or suspect that you may have a musculoskeletal injury, do not attempt these exercises without the permission of a physician. Any user assumes the risk of injury resulting from performing the exercises. The creators and authors disclaim any liabilities in connection with the exercises and advice herein.

1. Full Grip (flexor muscles). Squeeze putty with your fingers against the palm of your hand. Roll it over and around in your hand and repeat as rapidly and with as much strength as possible. Suggested Repetitions: 10

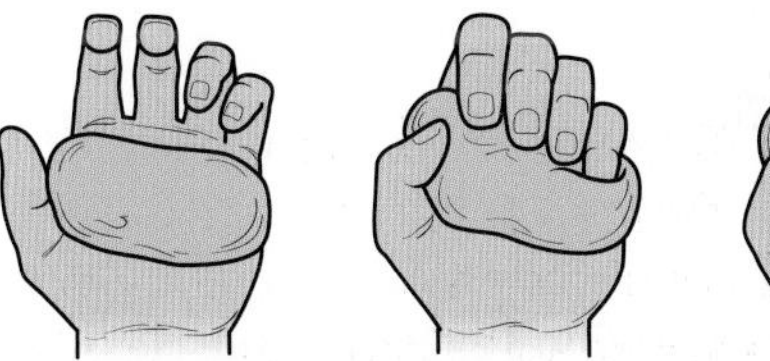
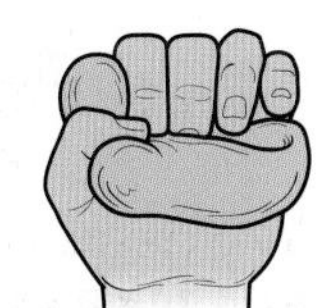

2. All Finger Spread (extensor and abductor muscles). Form putty into a thick pancake shape and place on a tabletop. Bunch fingertips together and place in putty. Spread fingers out as fast as possible. Suggested Repetitions: 3

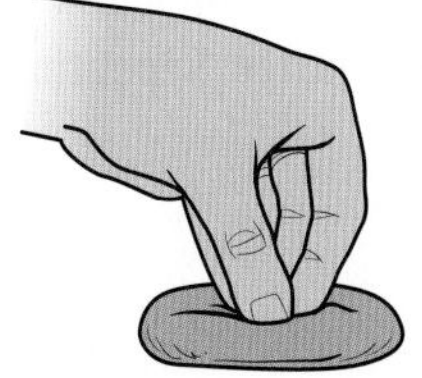
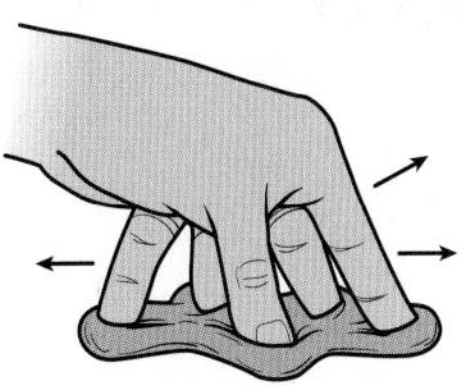

3. Fingers Dig (flexor muscles). Place putty in the palm of your hand and dig fingertips deep into the putty. Release the fingers, roll putty over, and repeat. Suggested Repetitions: 10

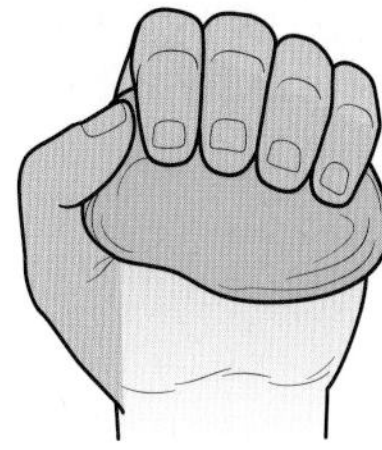
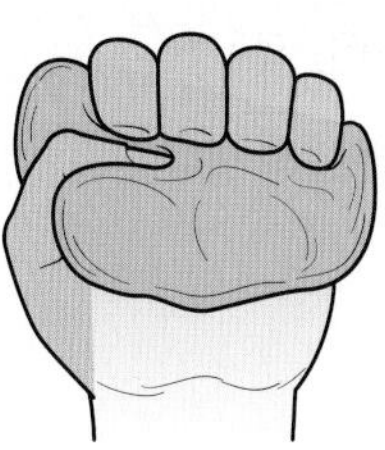

4. Finger Extension (extensor muscles). Close one finger into palm of hand. Wrap putty over tip of finger and hold loose ends with the other hand. As quickly as possible, extend finger to a fully opened position. Regulate difficulty by increasing or decreasing thickness of putty wrapped over the fingertip. Repeat with each finger. Suggested Repetitions: 3

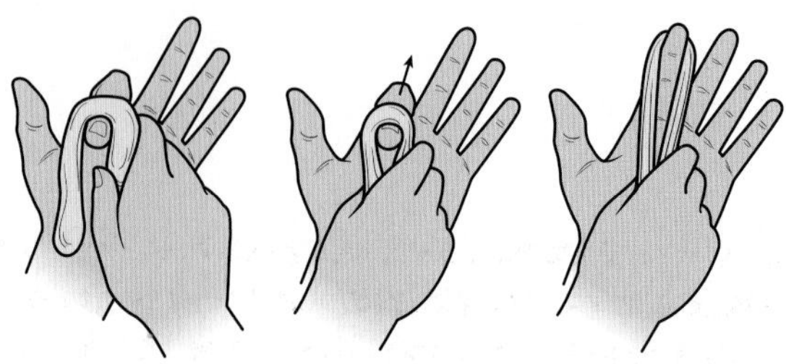

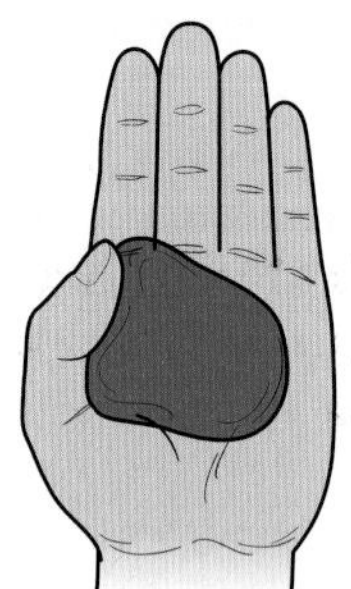

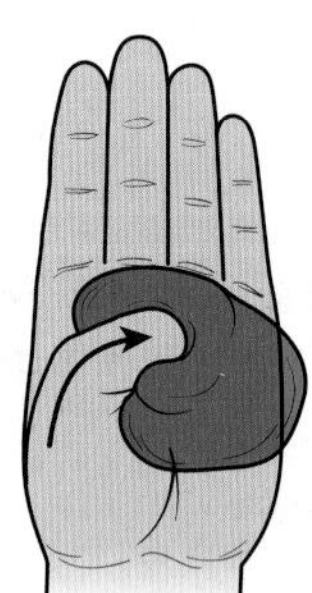

5. Thumb Press (flexor muscles). Form putty into a barrel shape and place in the palm of your hand. Press your thumb into the putty with as much force as you can. Reform putty and repeat. Suggested Repetitions: 5

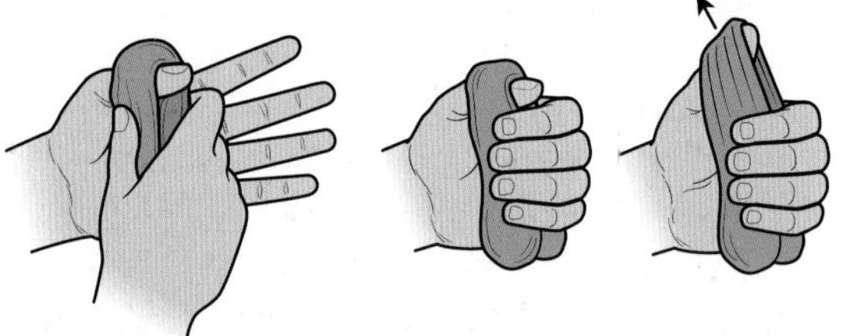

6. Thumb Extension (extensor muscles). Bend your thumb toward the palm of the hand; wrap putty over the thumb tip. Hold the loose ends down and extend the thumb open as quickly as possible. Regulate difficulty by increasing or decreasing the thickness of putty wrapped over tip of thumb. Suggested Repetitions: 3

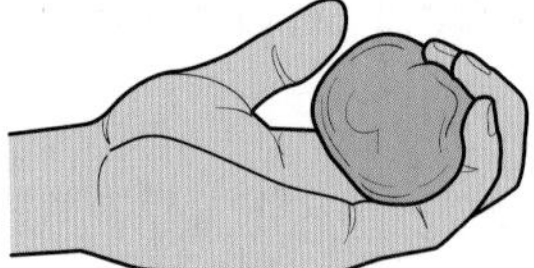

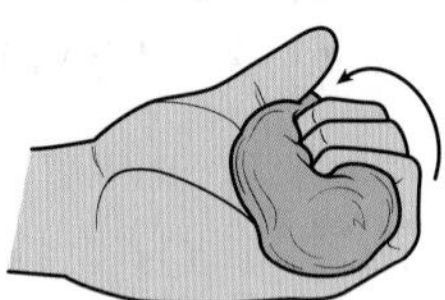

7. Fingers Only (flexor muscles). Lay putty across fingers and squeeze with fingertips only. Keep the palm of your hand flat and open. Rotate putty with thumb and repeat. Suggested Repetitions: 10

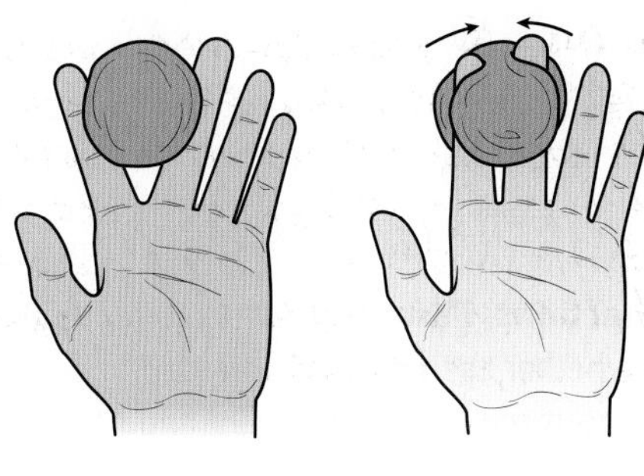

8. Finger Scissors (adductor muscles). Form putty into the shape of a ball and place between any two fingers. Squeeze fingers together in scissors-like motion. Repeat with each pair of fingers. Suggested Repetitions: 3

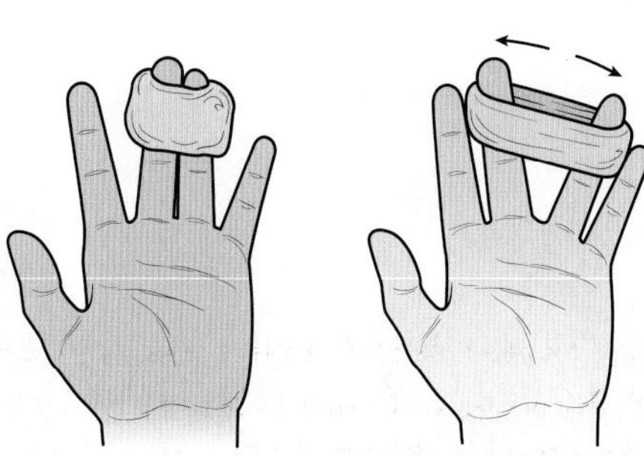

9. Finger Splits (abductor muscles). Mold putty around any two fingers while they are closed together. Spread fingers apart as quickly as possible. Repeat exercise with each pair of fingers. Suggested Repetitions: 3

Power Putty can be purchased in sport stores or directly from ***SportsHealth***, 527 West Windsor Road, Glendale, California 91204 USA, 818-240-7170; http://www.powerputty.com

REFERENCES

1. Canakci V, Orbak R, Tezel A, Canakci CF. Influence of different periodontal curette grips on the outcome of mechanical non-surgical therapy. *Int Dent J*. 2003;53:153–158.
2. Baur B, Furholzer W, Jasper I, Marquardt C, Hermsdorfer J. Effects of modified pen grip and handwriting training on writer's cramp. *Arch Phys Med Rehabil*. 2009;90:867–875.
3. Scaramucci M. Getting a grasp. *Dimen Dent Hyg*. 2008;5:24–26.
4. Rucker LM, Gibson G, McGregor C. Getting the "feel" of it: the non-visual component of dimensional accuracy during operative tooth preparation. *J Can Dent Assoc*. 1990;56:937–941.
5. Arthritis Research Campaign. Joint hypermobility: an information booklet. Available at http://www.arthritisresearchuk.org/Files/2019-Joint-hypermobility.pdf. Accessed September 27, 2010.
6. Chin DH, Jones NF. Repetitive motion hand disorders. *J Calif Dent Assoc*. 2002;30:149–160.
7. Powell BJ, Winkley GP, Brown JO, Etersque S. Evaluating the fit of ambidextrous and fitted gloves: implications for hand discomfort. *J Am Dent Assoc*. 1994;125:1235–1242.

RECOMMENDED READING

Gentilucci M, Caselli L, Secchi C. Finger control in the tripod grasp. *Exp Brain Res*. 2003;149:351–360.

Macdonald G, Wilson SG, Waldman KB. Physical characteristics of the hand and early clinical skills. Their relationship in a group of dental hygiene students. *J Dent Hyg*. 1991;65:380–384.

Section 6
Skill Application

PRACTICAL FOCUS

Directions, Part 1: Evaluate the modified pen grasp in the photographs in Figures 3-18 to 3-26. Indicate whether each grasp is correct or incorrect. For each incorrect grasp element, describe (1) what is incorrect about the finger placement and (2) what problems might result from the incorrect finger placement.

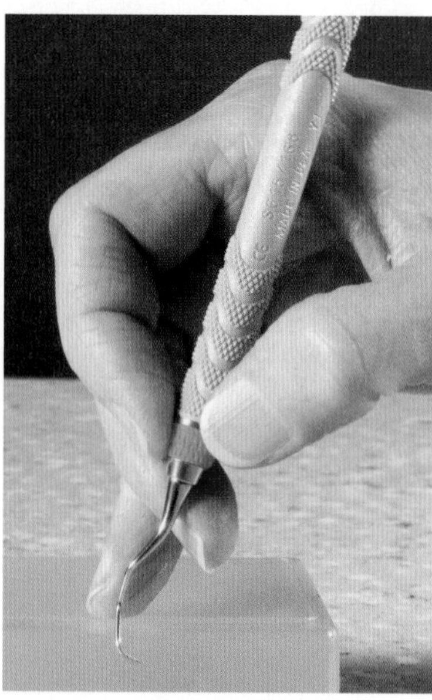

Figure 3-18

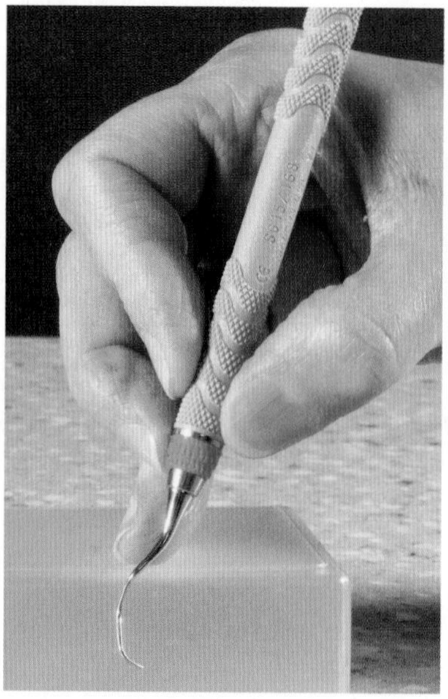

Figure 3-19

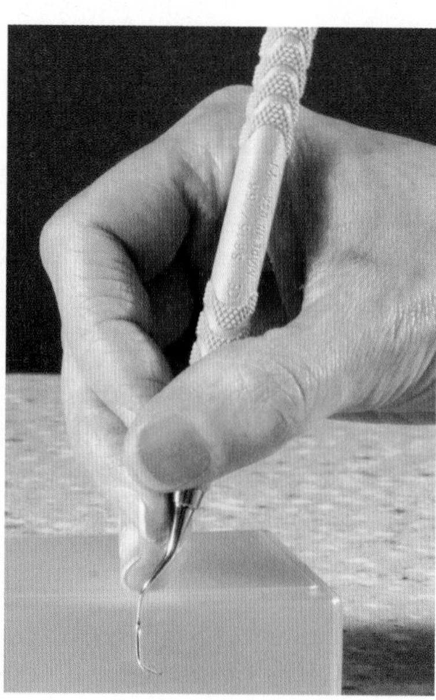

Figure 3-20

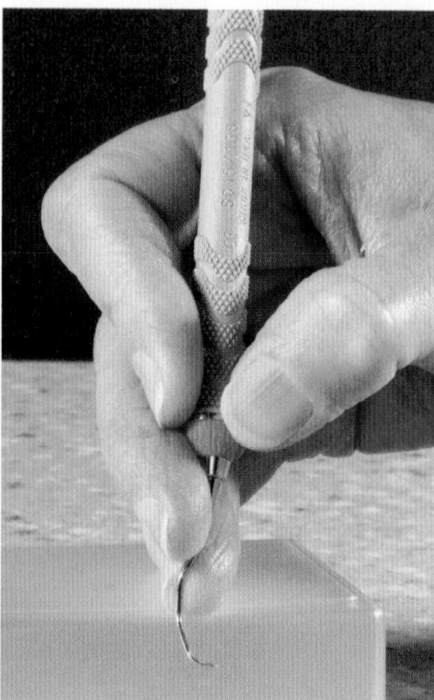

Figure 3-21

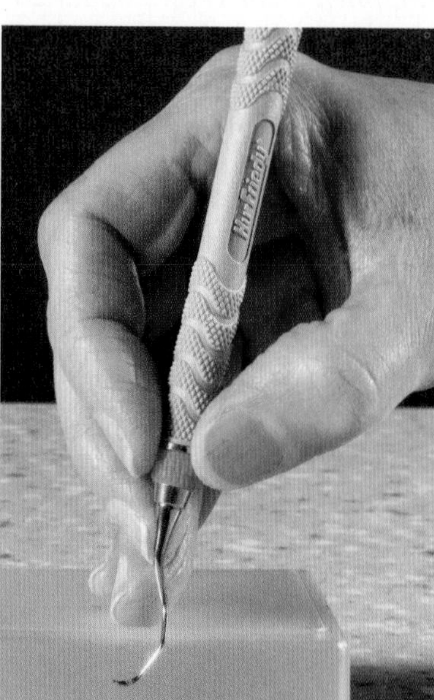

Figure 3-22

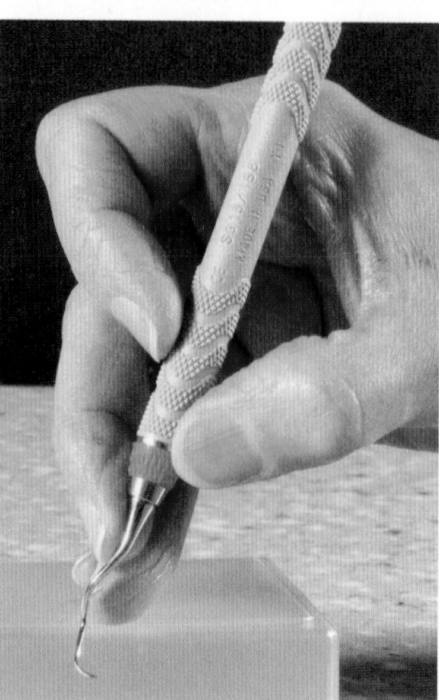

Figure 3-23

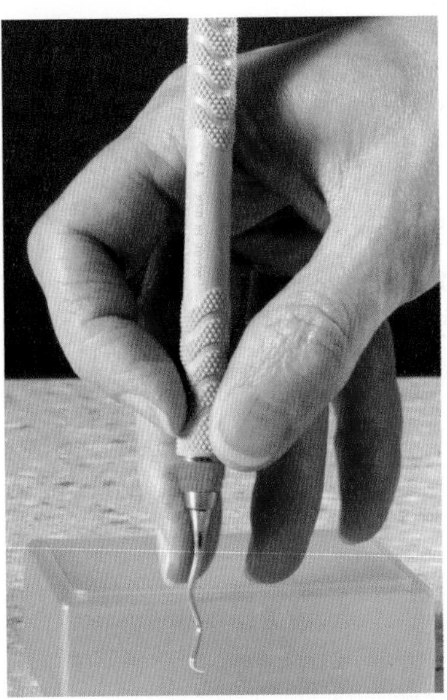

Figure 3-24

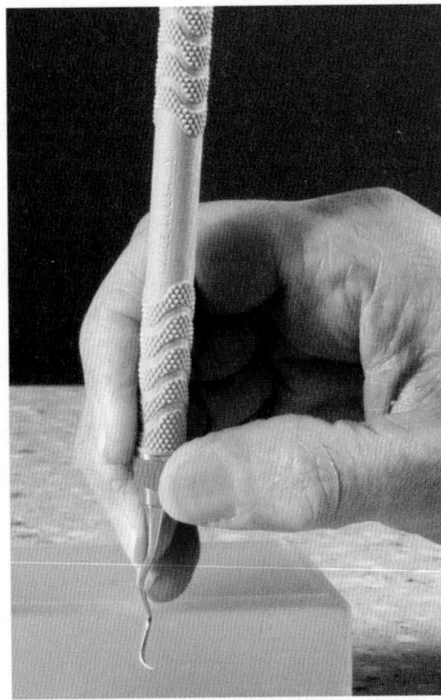

Figure 3-25

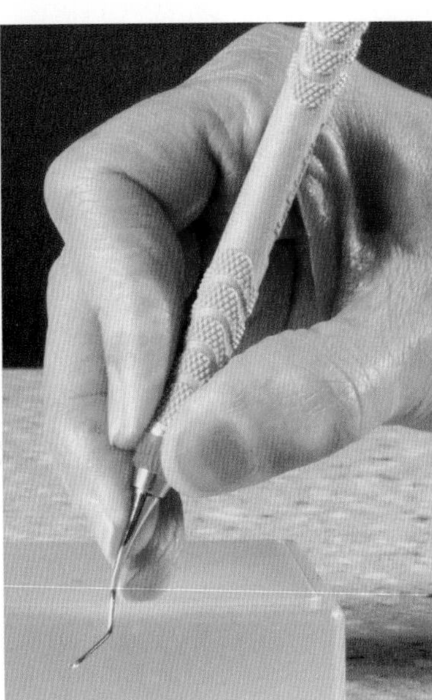

Figure 3-26

Directions, Part 2: Examine the gloved hands pictured in Figure 3-27 below. Evaluate the glove fit for the right and left hands pictured below.

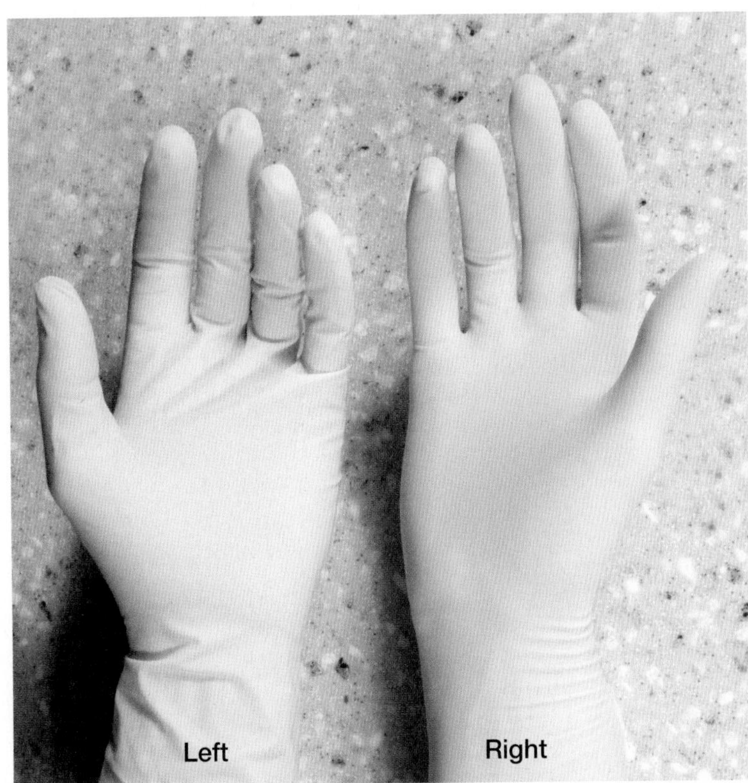

Figure 3-27

STUDENT SELF-EVALUATION MODULE 3 INSTRUMENT GRASP

Student: ______________________ 1 = Grasp with mirror hand

Date: ______________________ 2 = Grasp with instrument hand

DIRECTIONS: Self-evaluate your skill level as: **S** (satisfactory) or **U** (unsatisfactory)

Instrument Grasp	1	2
Identifies handle, shank, and working-end(s) of a mirror and periodontal instruments		
Describes the function each finger serves in the grasp		
Describes criteria for proper glove fit		
Grasps handle with tips of finger pads of index finger and thumb so that these fingers are opposite each other on the handle, but do NOT touch or overlap		
Rests pad of middle finger lightly on instrument shank; middle finger makes contact with the ring finger		
Positions the thumb, index, and middle fingers in the "knuckles-up" convex position; hyperextended joint position is avoided		
Holds ring finger straight so that it supports the weight of hand and instrument; ring finger position is "advanced ahead of" the other fingers in the grasp		
Keeps index, middle, ring, and little fingers in contact; "like fingers inside a mitten"		
Maintains a relaxed grasp; fingers are NOT blanched in grasp		

Module 4

Mirror and Finger Rests in Anterior Sextants

Module Overview

This module describes techniques for using a dental mirror and finger rests in the anterior treatment areas. Content in this module includes the topics of (1) fulcrums and finger rests, (2) the dental mirror and its uses, and (3) recommended wrist position and hand placement during periodontal instrumentation. A step-by-step technique practice for using a mirror and finger rests in the anterior treatment sextants is found in Sections 4 and 5.

Module Outline

Skill Application

Practical Focus

Student Self-Evaluation Module 4: Mirror and Finger Rests in Anterior Sextants

Key Terms

Fulcrum	Advanced fulcrum	Dental mirror	Indirect illumination
"Support beam"	"Out of the line of fire"	Indirect vision	Transillumination
Intraoral fulcrum	Neutral wrist position	Retraction	Finger-on-finger fulcrum
Extraoral fulcrum			

Learning Objectives

1. Name and describe three common types of dental mirrors.
2. Demonstrate use of a mirror for indirect vision, retraction, indirect illumination, and transillumination.
3. Demonstrate an extraoral and intraoral finger rest.
4. Position equipment so that it enhances neutral positioning.
5. Maintain neutral seated position while using the recommended clock position for each of the mandibular and maxillary anterior treatment areas.
6. While seated in the correct clock position for the treatment area, access the anterior teeth with optimum vision while maintaining neutral positioning.
7. Demonstrate correct mirror use, grasp, and finger rest in each of the anterior sextants while maintaining neutral positioning of your wrist.
8. Demonstrate finger rests using precise finger placement on the handle of a periodontal instrument:
   - Finger pads of thumb and index finger are opposite one another on handle.
   - Thumb and index finger do not overlap each other on the handle.
   - Pad of middle finger rests lightly on the shank.
   - Thumb, index, and middle fingers are in a "knuckles-up" position.
   - Ring finger is straight and supports weight of the hand.
9. Identify the correct wrist position when using an intraoral finger rest in the maxillary and mandibular anterior treatment areas.
10. Recognize incorrect mirror use, grasp, or finger rest and describe how to correct the problem(s).
11. Understand the relationship between proper stabilization of the dominant hand during instrumentation and the prevention of (1) musculoskeletal problems in the clinician's hands and (2) injury to the patient.
12. Understand the relationship between the large motor skills, such as positioning, and small motor skills, such as finger rests. Recognize the importance of initiating these skills in a step-by-step manner.

Section I
The Fulcrum

Fulcrum—a finger rest used to stabilize the clinician's hand during periodontal instrumentation. The fulcrum improves the precision of instrumentation strokes, prevents sudden movements that could injure the patient, and reduces muscle load to the clinician's hand (Box 4-1).[1–5]

1. Functions of the Fulcrum
   - a. Serves as a *"support beam"* for the hand during instrumentation.
   - b. Enables the hand and instrument to move as a unit as strokes are made against the tooth.
   - c. Allows precise control of stroke pressure and length during periodontal instrumentation.
2. Types of Fulcrums
   - a. Intraoral fulcrum—stabilization of the clinician's dominant hand by placing the pad of the ring finger on a tooth near the tooth being instrumented (Fig. 4-1, Table 4-1).
   - b. Extraoral fulcrum—stabilization of the clinician's nondominant hand outside the patient's mouth, usually on the chin or cheek. An extraoral fulcrum may be used with a mirror (Fig. 4-2).
   - c. Advanced fulcrum—variations of an intraoral or extraoral finger rest used to gain access to root surfaces within periodontal pockets.

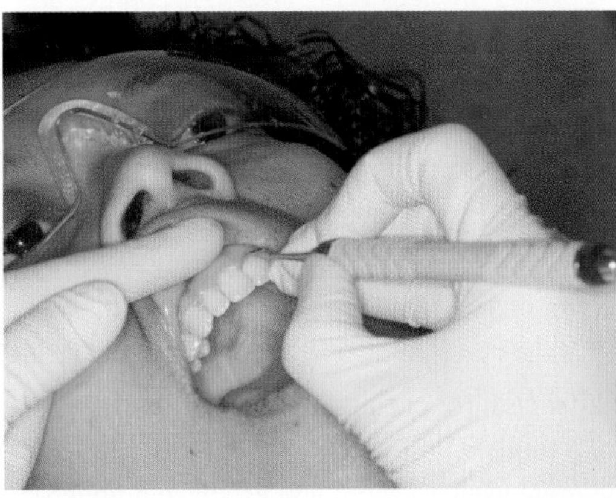

Figure 4-1. Intraoral Finger Rest. The pad of the ring finger is placed on a tooth near the tooth being instrumented. The intraoral finger rest is used with the dominant hand to stabilize a periodontal instrument in the oral cavity.

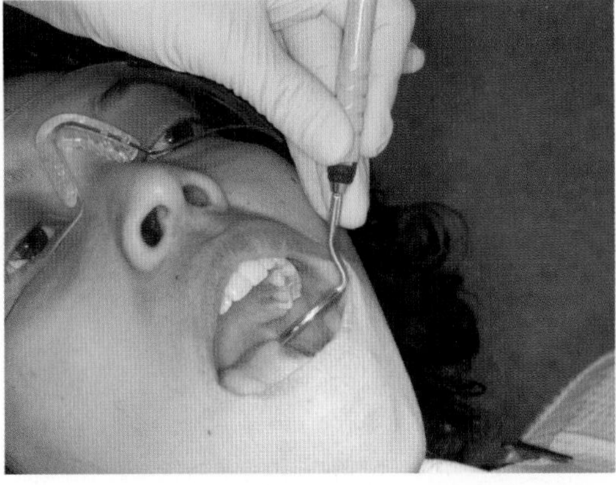

Figure 4-2. Extraoral Finger Rest. The ring finger rests on the patient's chin or cheek to stabilize the mirror. An extraoral finger rest is used most commonly to stabilize the mouth mirror in the oral cavity.

INTRAORAL FULCRUM

Box 4-1. Characteristics of Intraoral Fulcrum

- Provides stable support for the hand.
- Enables the hand and instrument to move as a unit.
- Facilitates precise stroke length and pressure against the tooth surface.
- Decreases the likelihood of injury to the patient or clinician if the patient moves unexpectedly during instrumentation.

TABLE 4-1. Summary Sheet: Technique for Intraoral Fulcrum

	Technique:
Grasp	Hold the instrument in a modified pen grasp.
Fulcrum	Keep ring finger straight, with the tip of the finger supporting the weight of the hand.
Location	Position the finger rest of the dominant hand near the tooth being instrumented. • Depending on the tooth being instrumented and the size of your hand, the finger rest may be 1 to 4 teeth away from the tooth on which you are working. • A finger rest is always established "**out of the line of fire**." The phrase "out of the line of fire" refers to the concept that the finger rest is never established directly above the tooth surface being worked on. If the finger rest is on the tooth being worked on, it is possible that the clinician's finger will be injured by the sharp cutting edge. Staying out of the line of fire lessens the likelihood of instrument sticks.
Rest	Place the finger rest on the same arch as the tooth being instrumented. • Rest the fingertip of the fulcrum finger on an incisal (or occlusal) surface or on the occlusofacial or occlusolingual line angle of a tooth. • The teeth are saliva-covered, so you will be more likely to slip if you establish a finger rest directly on the facial or lingual surface. • Avoid resting on a mobile tooth or one with a large carious lesion.

Section 2
Wrist Position for Instrumentation

NEUTRAL WRIST POSITION

Neutral wrist position is the ideal positioning of the wrist while performing work activities and is associated with decreased risk of musculoskeletal injury (Box 4-2).[6]

Box 4-2. Neutral Hand Position

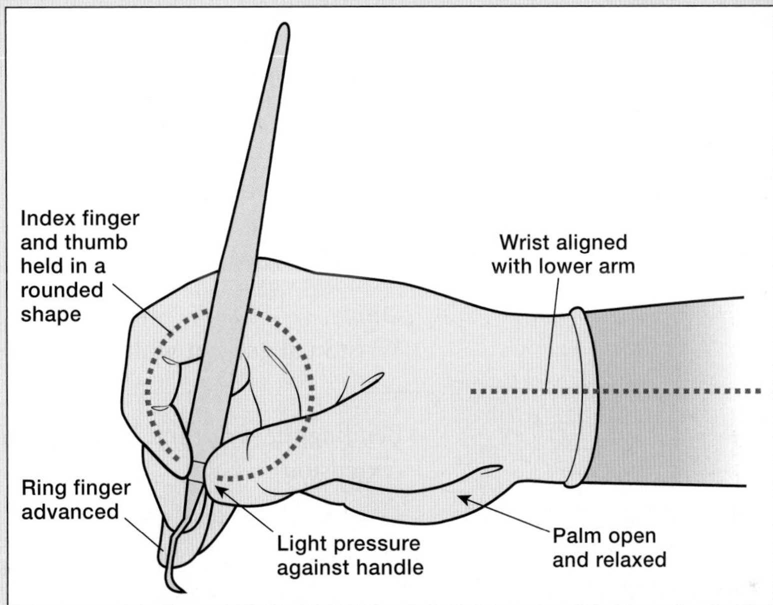

Figure 4-3. Neutral Hand Position for Periodontal Instrumentation

- Wrist aligned with the long axis of the lower arm
- Little finger-side of the palm rotated slightly downward
- Palm open and relaxed
- Thumb, middle, and index fingers held in a rounded shape
- Light finger pressure against the instrument handle
- Ring finger advanced ahead of other fingers in the grasp

GUIDELINES FOR NEUTRAL WRIST POSITION

Keeping the wrist aligned with the long axis of the arm decreases musculoskeletal stresses on the wrist joint. Avoiding fully flexed or fully extended joint positions keeps the muscles used to control hand movements at more ideal muscle lengths for generating motions.[7–9]

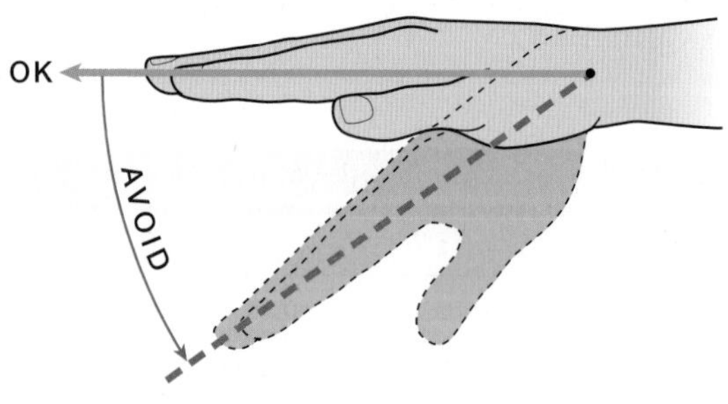

OK:
Wrist aligned with the long axis of the forearm

AVOID:
Bending the wrist and hand down toward the palm (flexion)

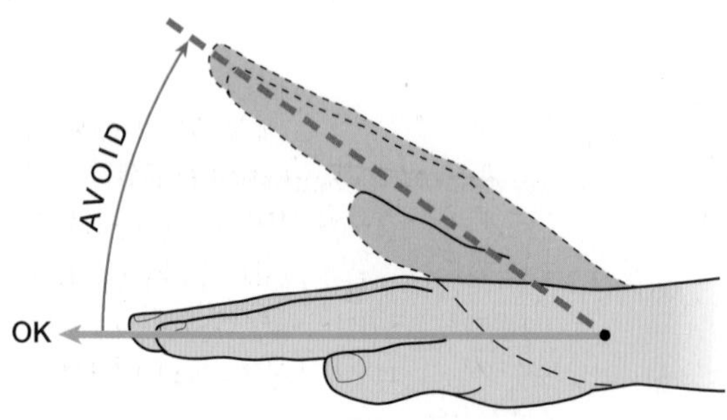

OK:
Wrist in alignment with the forearm

AVOID:
Bending the wrist and hand up and back (extension)

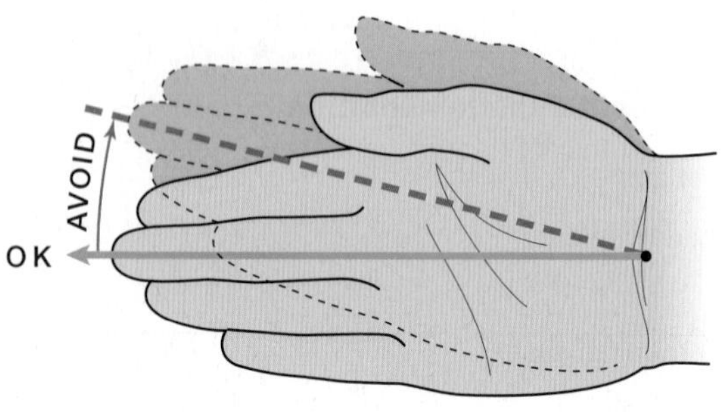

OK:
Wrist aligned with long axis of forearm

AVOID:
Bending the wrist toward the thumb (radial deviation)

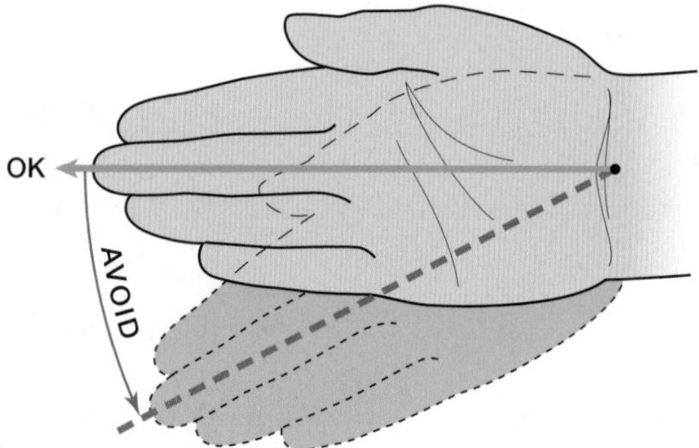

OK:
Wrist in alignment with the long axis of the forearm

AVOID:
Bending the wrist toward the little finger (ulnar deviation)

Section 3
The Dental Mirror

TYPES OF DENTAL MIRRORS

A clinician uses a dental mirror to view tooth surfaces that cannot be seen using direct vision (Fig. 4-4). The three common types of dental mirrors are the front surface mirror, concave mirror, and the plane mirror. The characteristics of each type of dental mirror are listed in Table 4-2.

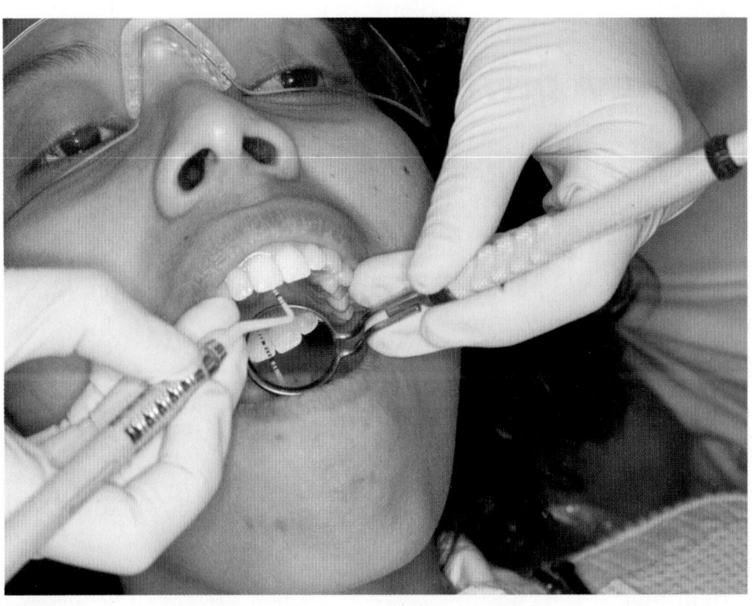

Figure 4-4. Dental Mirror or Mouth Mirror. The working-end of a dental mirror has a reflecting mirrored surface used to view tooth surfaces that cannot be seen directly.

TABLE 4-2. Types of Mirror Surfaces

Type	Characteristics
Front Surface	• Reflecting surface is on the front surface of the glass • Produces a clear mirror image with no distortion • Most commonly used type because of good image quality • Reflecting surface of mirror is easily scratched
Concave	• Reflecting surface is on the front surface of the mirror lens • Produces a magnified image (image is enlarged) • Magnification distorts the image
Plane (Flat Surface)	• Reflecting surface is on the back surface of the mirror lens • Produces a double image (ghost image) • Double image may be distracting

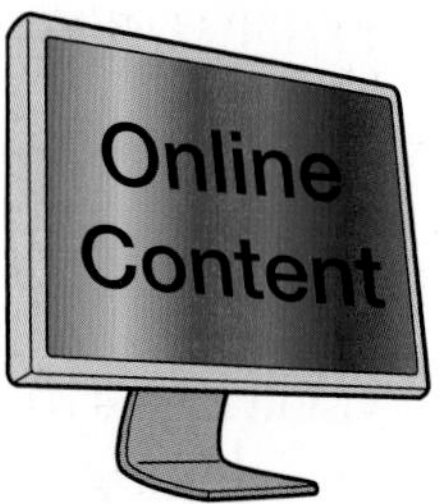

Videos for the topic of mirror use can be viewed online at http://thepoint.lww.com/GehrigFundamentals7e

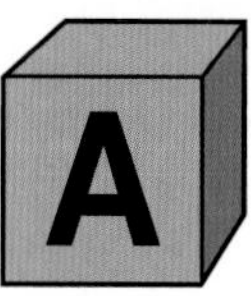

SKILL BUILDING. USING A DENTAL MIRROR

Directions: Watch the online video presentation on mirror use. Practice using a dental mirror in the oral cavity by following the instructions in Figures 4-5 to 4-9.

The dental mirror is used in four ways during periodontal instrumentation: (1) indirect vision, (2) retraction, (3) indirect illumination, and (4) transillumination.

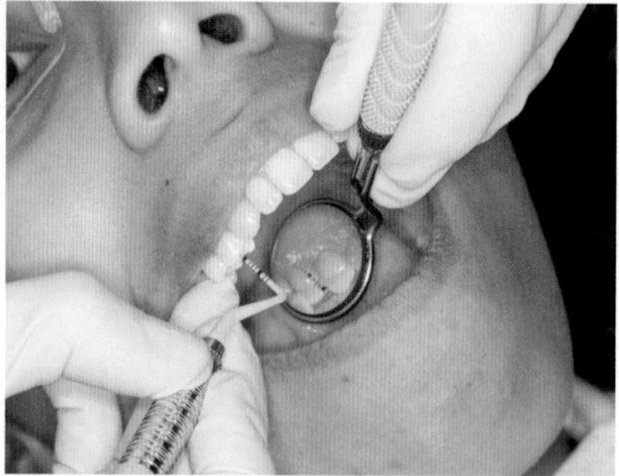

Figure 4-5. Indirect Vision. Indirect vision is the use of a dental mirror to view a tooth surface or intraoral structure that cannot be seen directly.

- Practice using the mirror to indirectly view the lingual surfaces of the maxillary right first premolar.
- Establish an extraoral or intraoral finger rest with your nondominant hand.
- Note that you can see the dental instrument in the mirror.

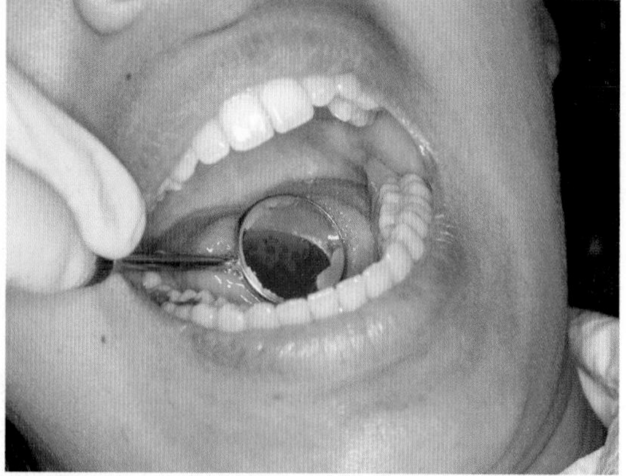

Figure 4-6. Retraction of Tongue. Retraction is the use of the mirror head to hold the patient's cheek, lip, or tongue so that the clinician can view tooth surfaces that are otherwise hidden from view by these soft tissue structures.

- Practice using the back of the mirror to retract the tongue away from the mandibular posterior teeth.
- Use the mirrored side to view the lingual surfaces indirectly.

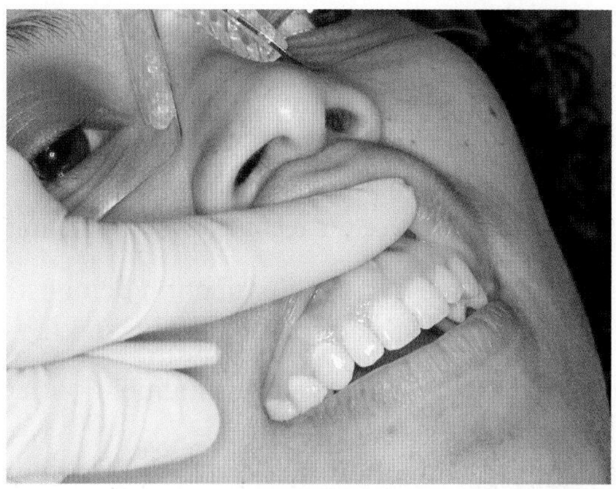

Figure 4-7. Retraction of Lip.

- Practice using the index finger of your nondominant hand to retract the lip away from the facial aspect of anterior teeth. The patient will be more comfortable if a finger rather than the mirror is used for retraction of the lip.
- **Tip:** The mirror may be held in the palm of the hand when retracting with the finger. Palming the mirror avoids having to put down the mirror and pick it up again when moving on to another sextant.

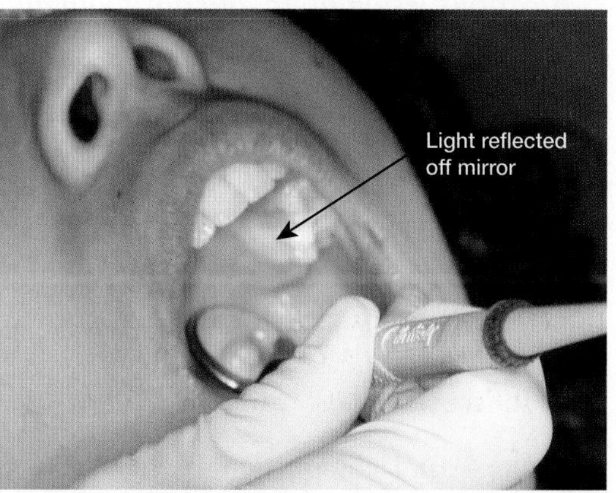

Figure 4-8. Indirect illumination. **Indirect illumination** is the use of the mirror surface to reflect light onto a tooth surface in a dark area of the mouth.

- Practice using the mirrored surface to direct additional light onto the lingual surfaces of the maxillary left molars. (Shine the light from the dental light or dental headlights onto the mirrored surface. The light will reflect off the mirror onto the lingual surfaces.)

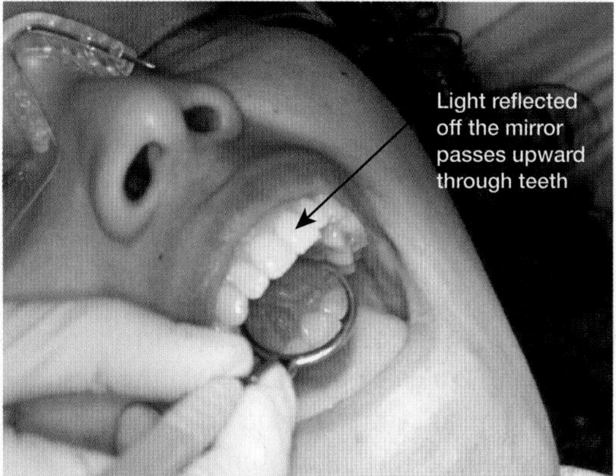

Figure 4-9. Transillumination. **Transillumination** is the technique of directing light off of the mirror surface and through the anterior teeth. (*trans* = through + *illumination* = lighting up.) As light is reflected off the mirror surface, the light beams pass back through the teeth.

- Follow the directions on the next page to practice transillumination of the anterior teeth.

Box 4-3. Techniques to Stop Fogging of Reflecting Surface

Use one of the following techniques to stop fogging of the reflecting surface:

- Warm the reflecting surface against the patient's buccal mucosa
- Ask patient to breathe through the nose
- Wipe the reflecting surface with a commercial defogging solution
- Wipe the reflecting surface with a gauze square moistened with mouthwash

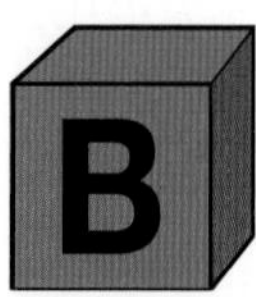

SKILL BUILDING. TRANSILLUMINATION

Directions: Practice the technique for transillumination by following the instructions in Figures 4-10 to 4-12.

The technique of transillumination demonstrates caries as dark regions within the enamel of an interproximal surface of an anterior tooth.

- When employing the transillumination technique, ***the mirror is used to reflect light through anterior teeth.***
- Transillumination is effective only with anterior teeth because they are thin enough to allow light to pass through.
- ***A carious lesion of an anterior tooth appears as a shadow when an anterior tooth is transilluminated.***

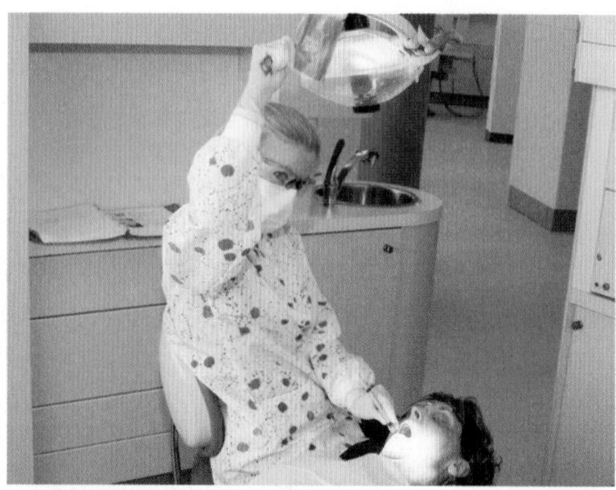

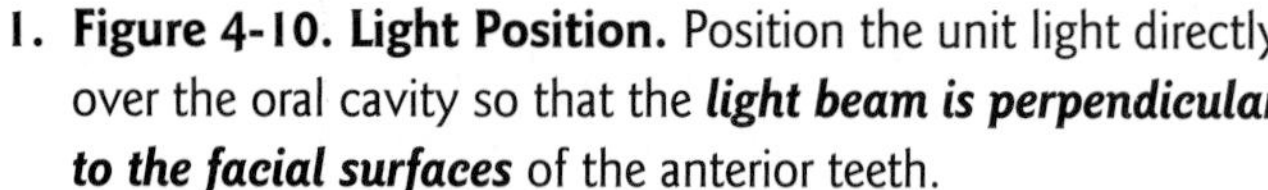

1. **Figure 4-10. Light Position.** Position the unit light directly over the oral cavity so that the ***light beam is perpendicular to the facial surfaces*** of the anterior teeth.

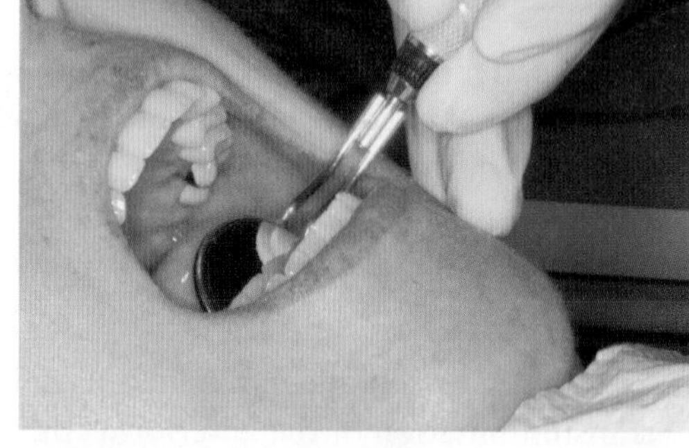

2. **Figure 4-11. Position Mouth Mirror. *Position yourself in the 12 o'clock position.*** Hold the mirror behind the mandibular central incisors so that the reflecting surface is parallel to the lingual surfaces.

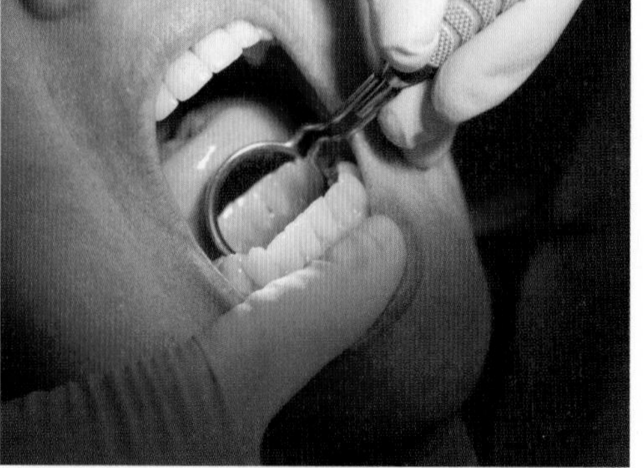

3. **Figure 4-12. View Transilluminated Anterior Teeth.** If you have correctly positioned the light and the mirror, the anterior teeth will appear to "glow." Remember, in this case, you are looking ***directly at the teeth and not in the mirror***.

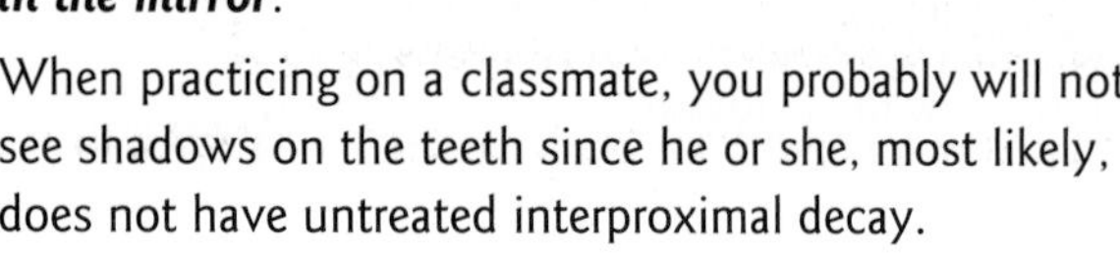

   When practicing on a classmate, you probably will not see shadows on the teeth since he or she, most likely, does not have untreated interproximal decay.

BUILDING BLOCKS FROM POSITION TO FINGER REST

Precise, accurate performance of the building block skills is essential if periodontal instrumentation is to be effective, efficient, safe for the patient, and comfortable for the clinician.

- Research on psychomotor skill acquisition indicates that a high level of mastery in the performance of skill building blocks is essential to successful mastery of periodontal instrumentation.
- The building block skills are the foundation that "supports" successful periodontal instrumentation.
- While practicing finger rests, it is important to complete each of the skills listed in Figure 4-13 in sequence.

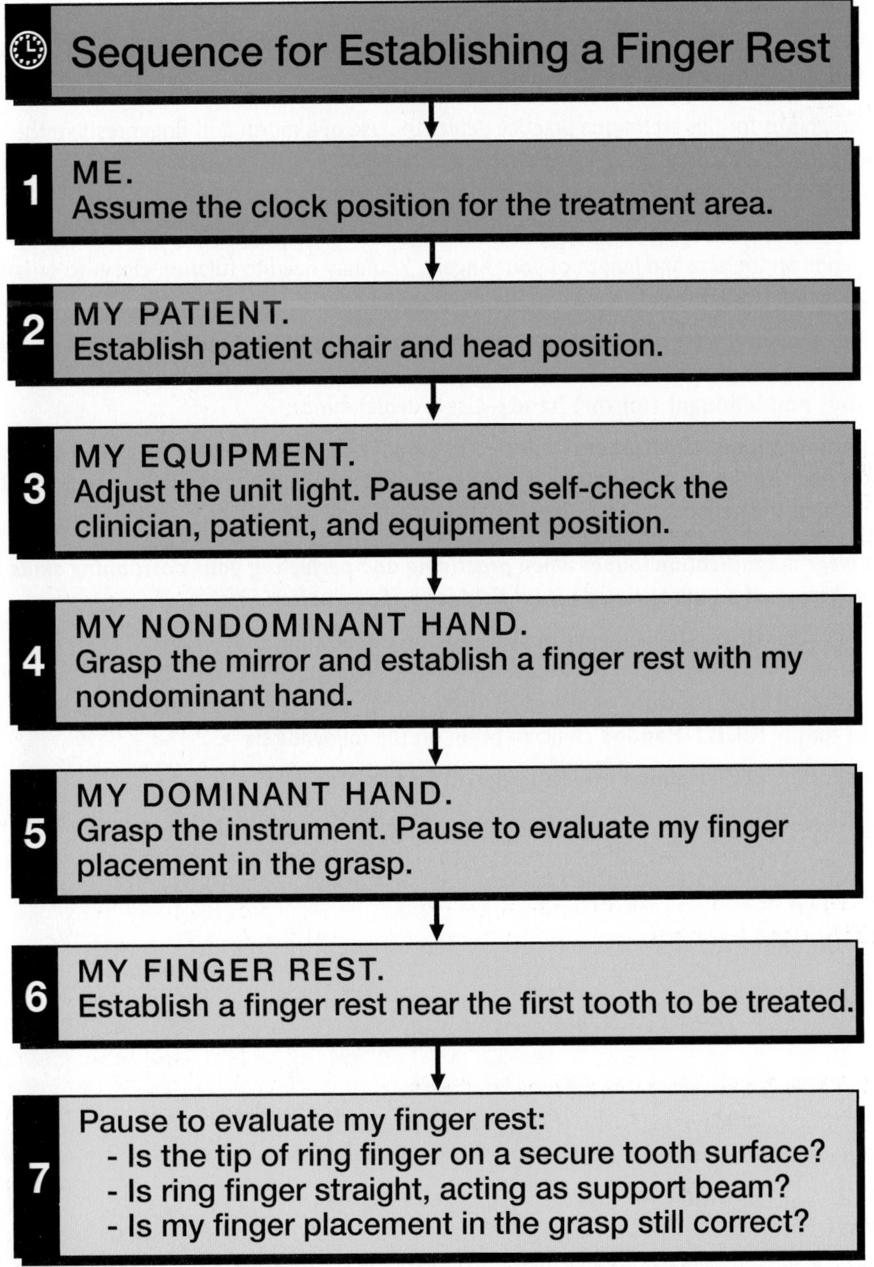
Sequence for Establishing a Finger Rest
1
ME.
Assume the clock position for the treatment area.
2
MY PATIENT.
Establish patient chair and head position.
3
MY EQUIPMENT.
Adjust the unit light. Pause and self-check the clinician, patient, and equipment position.
4
MY NONDOMINANT HAND.
Grasp the mirror and establish a finger rest with my nondominant hand.
5
MY DOMINANT HAND.
Grasp the instrument. Pause to evaluate my finger placement in the grasp.
6
MY FINGER REST.
Establish a finger rest near the first tooth to be treated.
7
Pause to evaluate my finger rest:
- Is the tip of ring finger on a secure tooth surface?
- Is ring finger straight, acting as support beam?
- Is my finger placement in the grasp still correct?

Figure 4-13. Establishing a Finger Rest. When establishing a finger rest, it is important to proceed in the small, explicit steps outlined in this flow chart.[10]

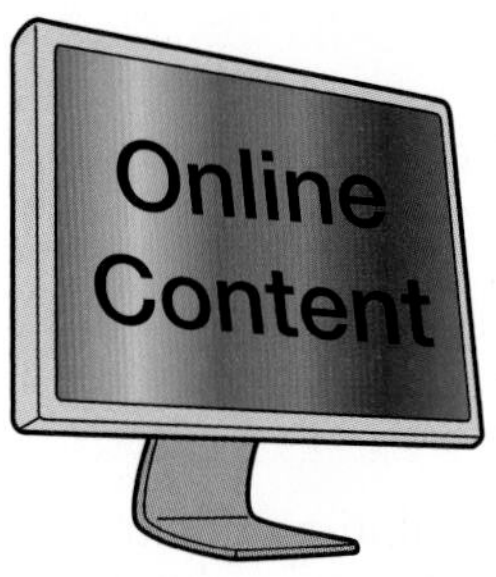

A video on the topic of finger rests can be viewed online at http://thepoint.lww.com/GehrigFundamentals7e

Box 4-4. Directions for Sections 4 and 5 of This Module

1. The next two sections of this module contain instructions for practicing finger rests for each treatment area of the mouth.
2. The photographs for this technique practice depict the use of a mirror and finger rests in the anterior treatment areas. Some photographs were taken on a patient. Others were taken using a manikin and without gloves so that you can easily see the finger placement in the grasp.
3. The photographs provide a *general guideline* for finger rests; however, the location of your own finger rest depends on the size and length of your fingers. You may need to fulcrum closer to or farther from the tooth being treated than is shown in the photograph.
4. Focus your attention on mastering mirror use, wrist position, and the finger rests. Use the following instruments in this module:
    - **For your nondominant (mirror) hand**—Use a dental mirror.
    - **For your dominant (instrument) hand**—(a) Remove the mirror head from one of your dental mirrors and use the mirror handle as if it were a periodontal instrument, or (b) use a periodontal probe to represent the periodontal instrument in this module.
5. ***Do not wear magnification loupes when practicing and perfecting your positioning skills in this module. You need an unrestricted visual field for self-evaluation.***
6. Figure 4-13 summarizes the sequence of skills used in establishing a finger rest.

The remainder of this module is divided into right- and left-handed sections.

- Instructions for the **RIGHT-Handed** clinician begin on the following page.
- Instructions for the **LEFT-Handed** clinician begin in Section 5 on page 112.

Section 4
Technique Practice: RIGHT-Handed Clinician

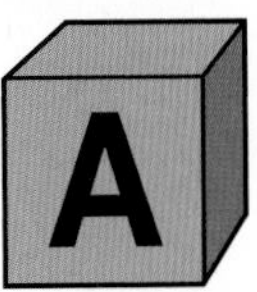

SKILL BUILDING. MANDIBULAR ANTERIOR TEETH, SURFACES TOWARD

Directions: Practice establishing a finger rest for the mandibular anterior teeth, surfaces toward, by referring to Figures 4-14 to 4-21.

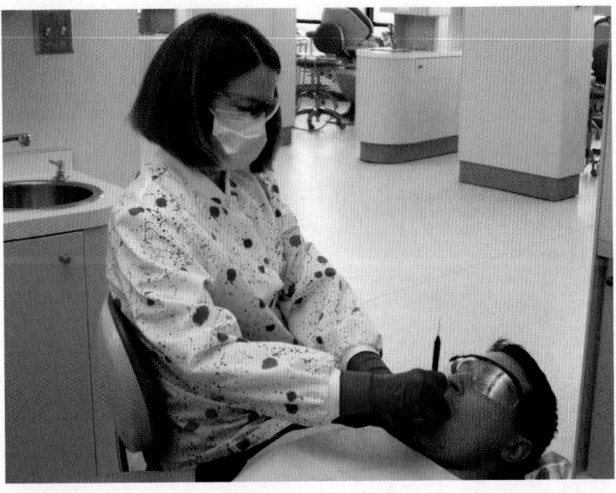

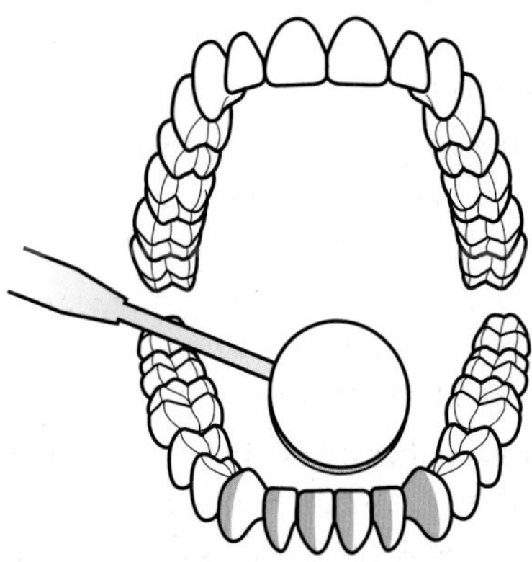

Figure 4-14. Clock Position for Mandibular Anterior Teeth, Surfaces Toward. The clinician's clock position for the mandibular anterior surfaces toward the clinician—facial and lingual aspects—is the 8 to 9 o'clock position. The patient should be in a chin-down head position.

Box 4-5. Handle Positions for Mandibular Anterior Teeth

1. Hold the hand in a palm-down position.
2. Rest the handle against the index finger somewhere in the green shaded area.

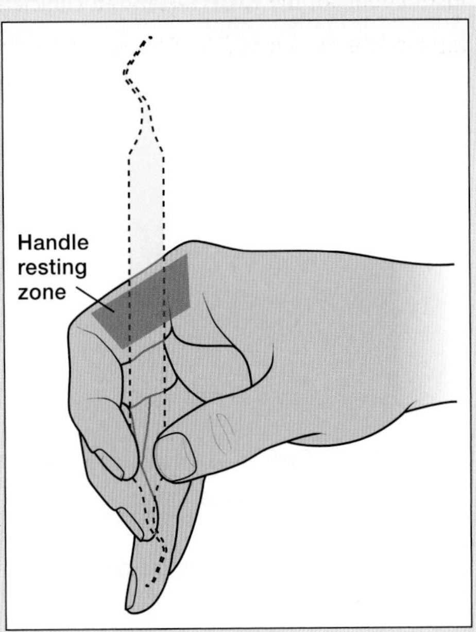

Figure 4-15. Handle Positions for Mandibular Treatment Areas.

RIGHT-Handed Clinician

Mandibular Anteriors, Facial Aspect: Surfaces Toward

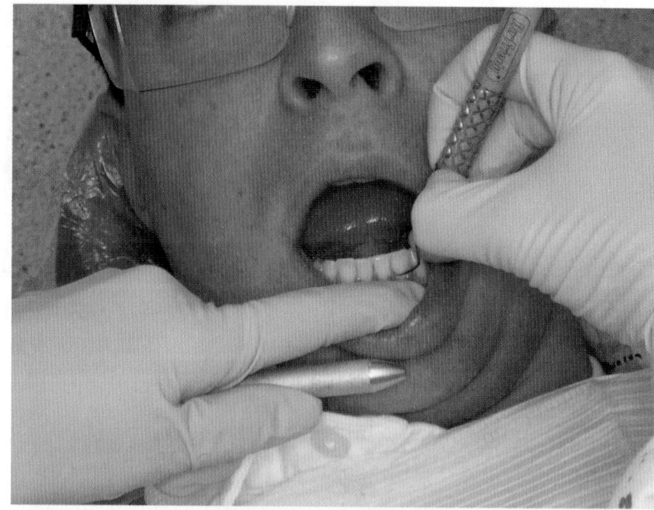

Figure 4-16. Retraction. Retract the lip with the index finger or thumb of your left hand.

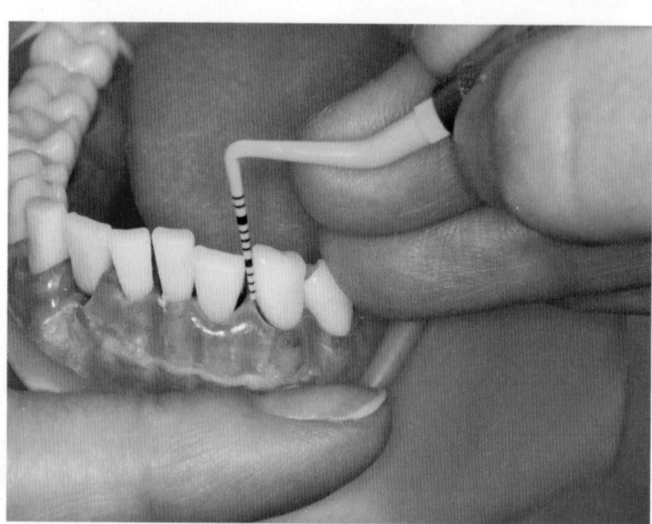

Figure 4-17. Task 1—Mesial Surface of the Left Canine. Finger rest on an occlusofacial line angle.
Place the instrument tip on the mesial surface of the left canine.

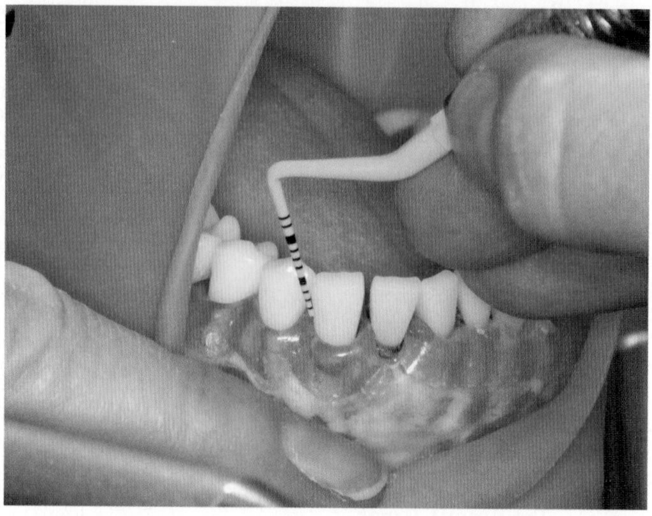

Figure 4-18. Task 2—Distal Surface of Right Canine. Finger rest on an incisal edge.
Place the instrument tip on the distal surface of the right canine.

Mandibular Anteriors, Lingual Aspect: Surfaces Toward

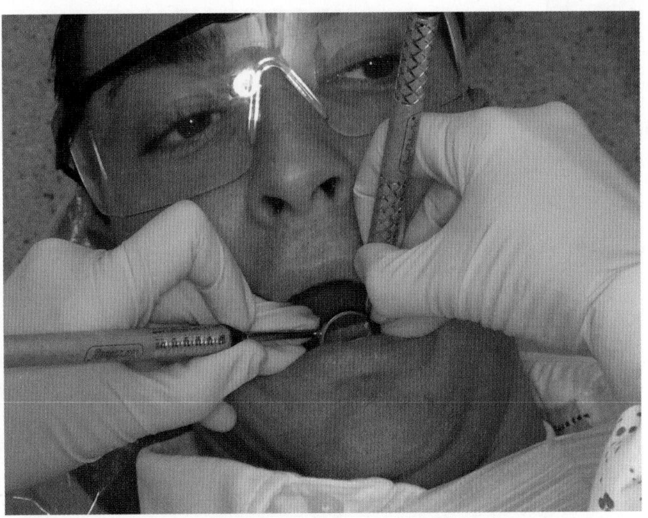

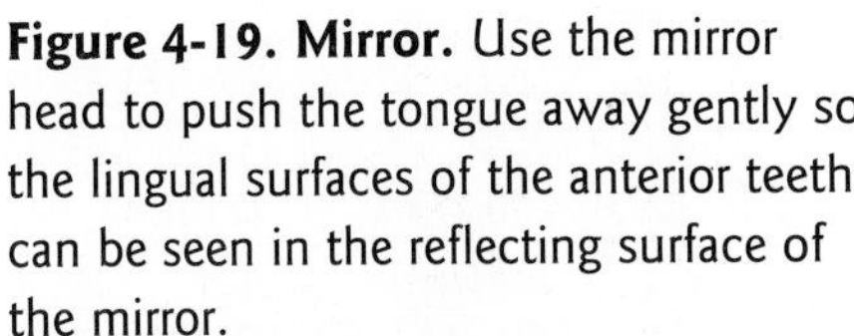

Figure 4-19. Mirror. Use the mirror head to push the tongue away gently so the lingual surfaces of the anterior teeth can be seen in the reflecting surface of the mirror.
Note that the clinician pictured is using an extraoral finger rest for the nondominant "mirror" hand.

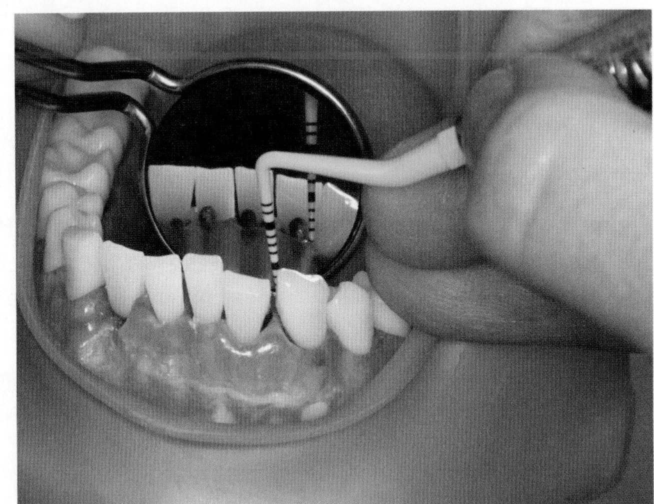

Figure 4-20. Task 1—Mesial Surface of the Left Canine. Finger rest on an occlusofacial line angle.
Place the instrument tip on the mesial surface of the left canine.

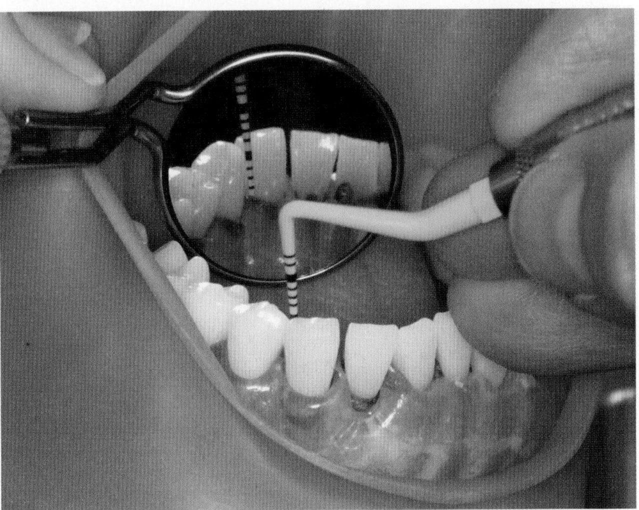

Figure 4-21. Task 2—Distal Surface of the Right Canine. Finger rest on an incisal edge. Place the instrument tip on the distal surface of the right canine.

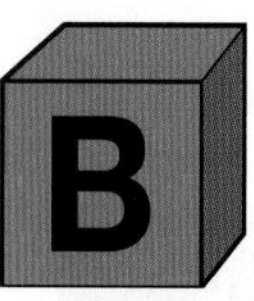

SKILL BUILDING. MANDIBULAR ANTERIOR TEETH, SURFACES AWAY

Directions: Practice establishing a finger rest for the mandibular anterior teeth, surfaces away, by referring to Figures 4-22 to 4-29.

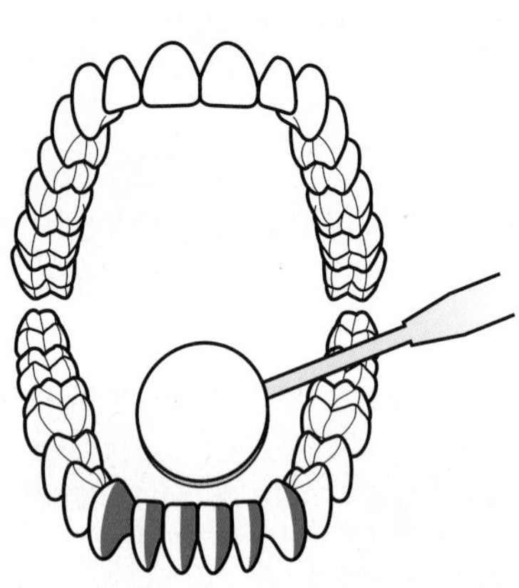

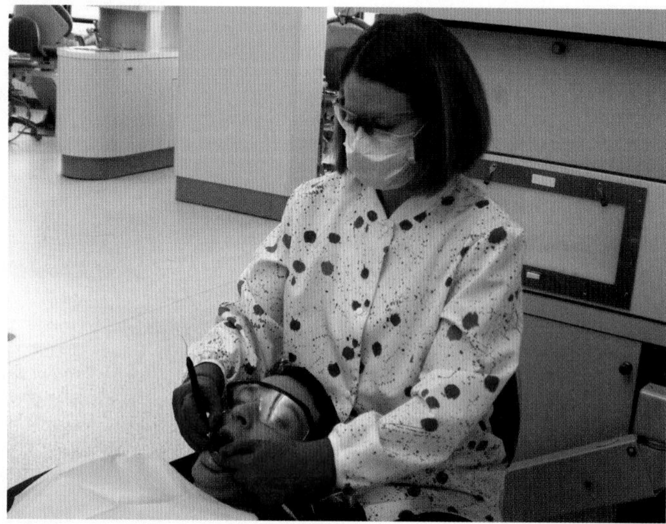

Figure 4-22. Clock Position for Mandibular Anterior Teeth, Surfaces Away. The clinician's clock position for the mandibular anterior surfaces away from the clinician—facial and lingual aspects—is the 11 to 1 o'clock position. The patient is in a chin-down head position.

Box 4-6. Handle Positions for Mandibular Anterior Teeth

1. Hold the hand in a palm-down position.
2. Rest the handle against the index finger somewhere in the green shaded area.

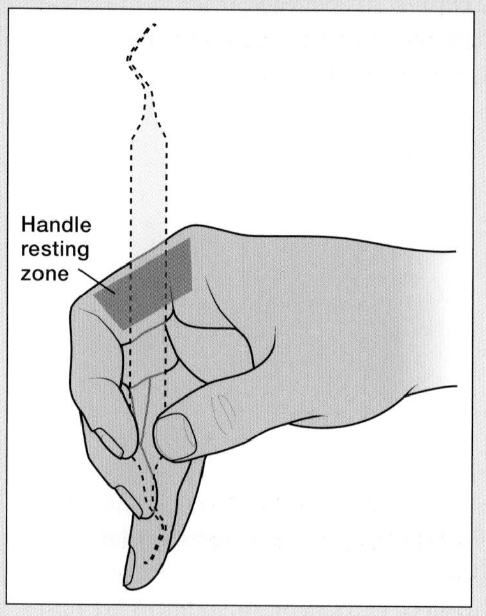

Figure 4-23. Handle Positions for Mandibular Treatment Areas.

Mandibular Anteriors, Facial Aspect: Surfaces Away

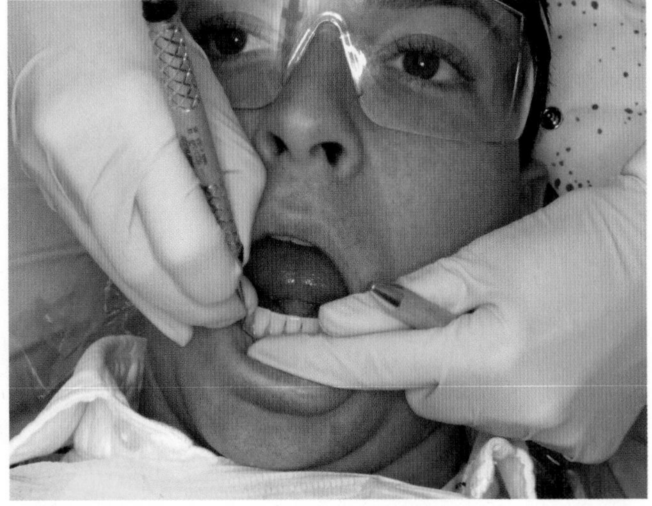

Figure 4-24. Retraction. Retract the lip with your index finger or thumb.
Note that the clinician pictured is holding the mirror in the palm of her hand.

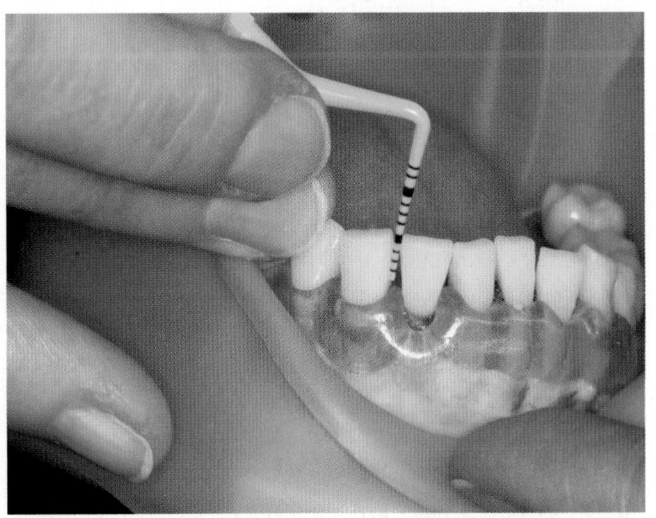

Figure 4-25. Task 1—Mesial Surface of the Right Canine. Finger rest on an occlusofacial line angle.
Place the instrument tip on the mesial surface of the right canine.

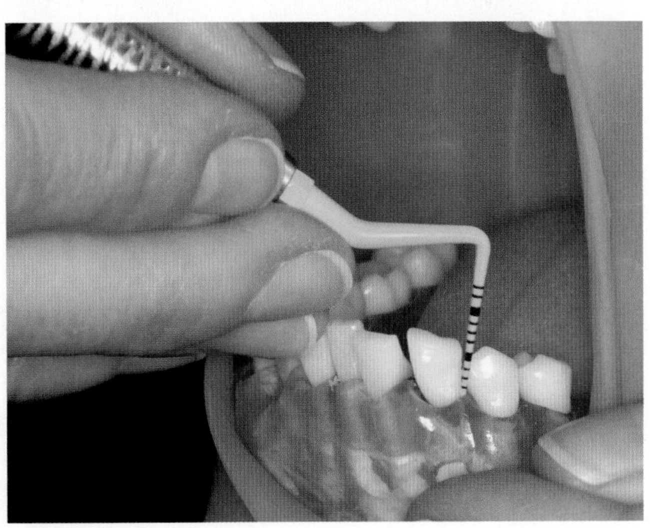

Figure 4-26. Task 2—Distal Surface of the Left Canine. Finger rest on an incisal edge.
Place the instrument tip on the distal surface of the left canine.

Mandibular Anteriors, Lingual Aspect: Surfaces Away

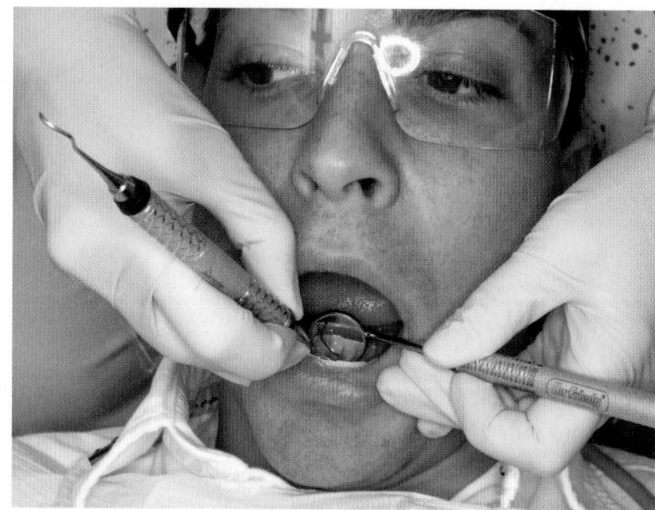

Figure 4-27. Mirror. Use the mirror head to push the tongue back gently so that the lingual surfaces of the teeth can be seen.

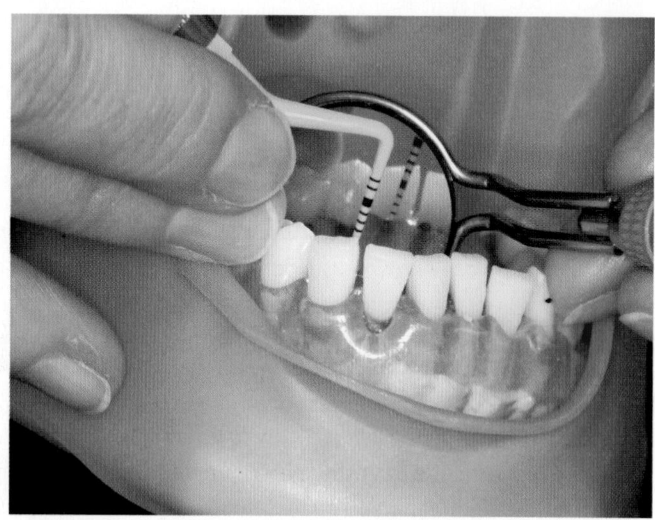

Figure 4-28. Task 1—Mesial Surface of the Right Canine. Finger rest on an occlusofacial line angle. Place the instrument tip on the mesial surface of the right canine.

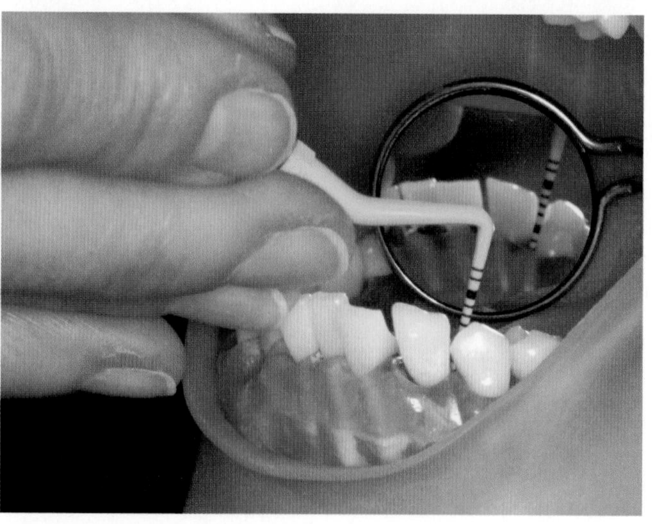

Figure 4-29. Task 2—Distal Surface of the Left Canine. Finger rest on an incisal edge. Place the instrument tip on the distal surface of the left canine.

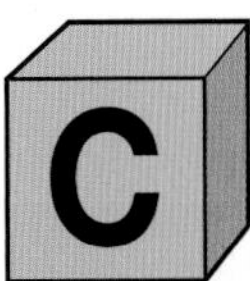

SKILL BUILDING. MAXILLARY ANTERIOR TEETH, SURFACES TOWARD

Directions: Practice establishing a finger rest for the maxillary anterior teeth, surfaces toward, by referring to Figures 4-30 to 4-37.

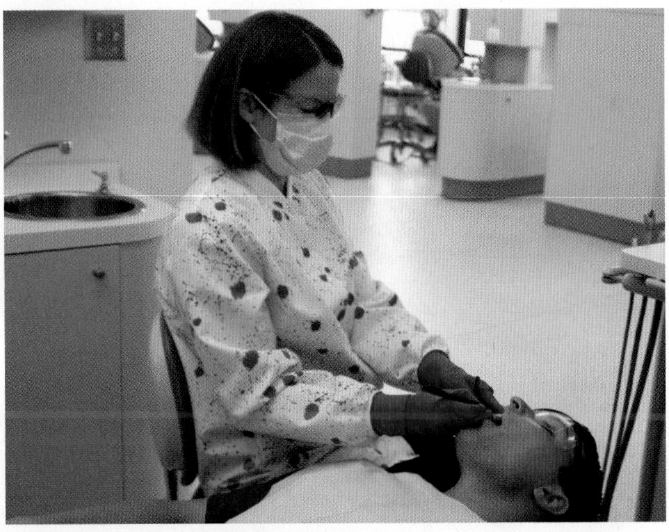

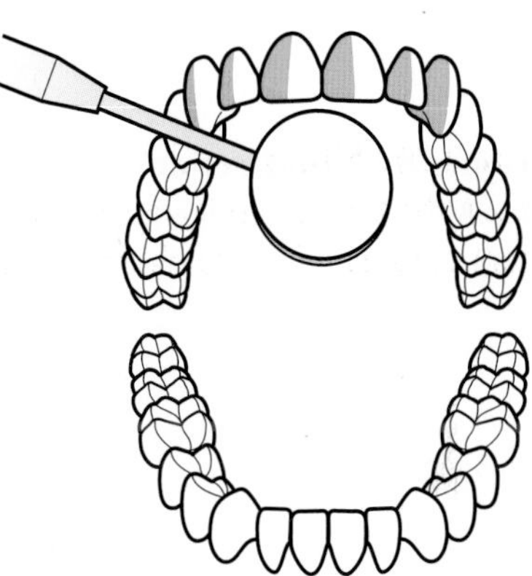

Figure 4-30. Clock Position for Maxillary Anterior Teeth, Surfaces Toward. The clinician's clock position for the maxillary anterior surfaces toward the clinician—facial and lingual aspects—is the 8 to 9 o'clock position. The patient should be in a chin-up head position.

Box 4-7. Handle Positions for Maxillary Anterior Teeth

1. Hold the hand in a palm-up position.
2. Rest the handle against the index finger somewhere in the green shaded area.

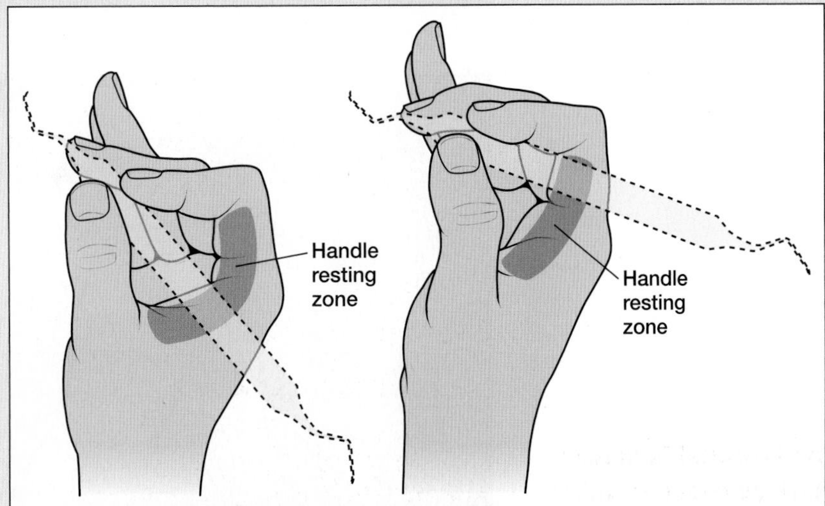

Figure 4-31. Handle Positions for Maxillary Treatment Areas.

Maxillary Anteriors, Facial Aspect: Surfaces Toward

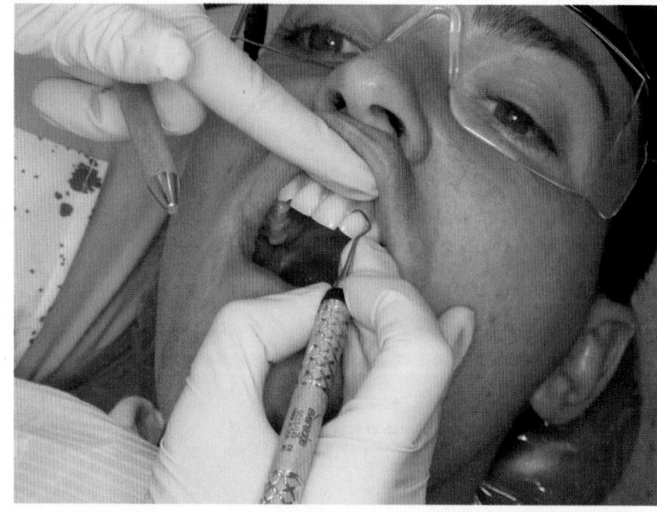

Figure 4-32. Retraction. Retract the lip with the index finger or thumb of your left hand.

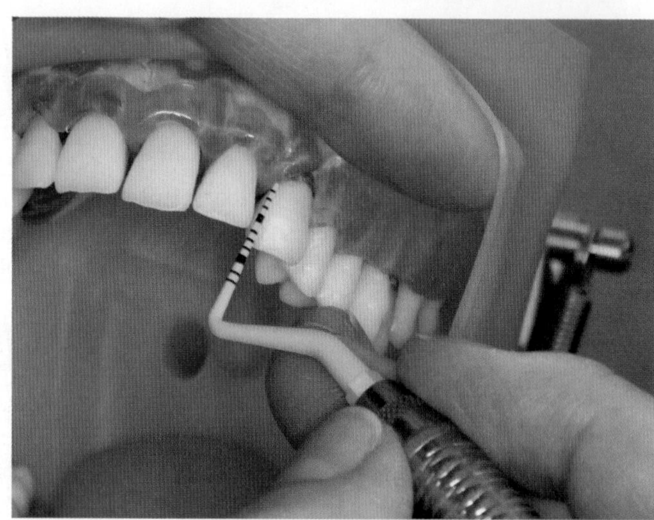

Figure 4-33. Task 1—Mesial Surface of the Left Canine. Finger rest on an occlusofacial line angle.
Place the instrument tip on the mesial surface of the left canine.

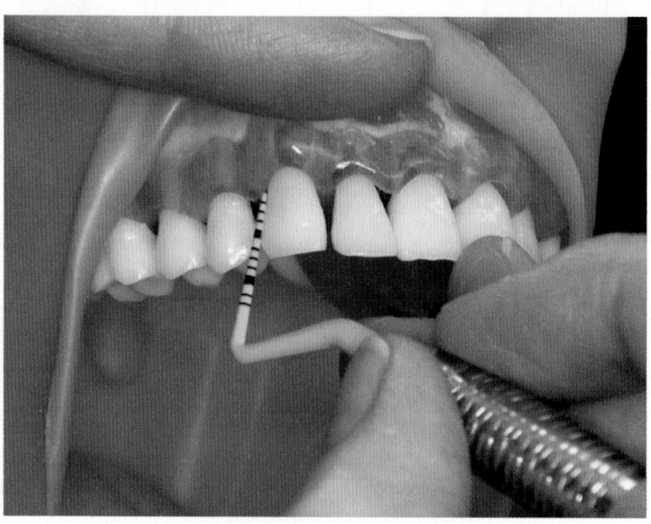

Figure 4-34. Task 2—Distal Surface of Right Canine. Finger rest on an incisal edge. Place the instrument tip on the distal surface of the right canine.

Maxillary Anteriors, Lingual Aspect: Surfaces Toward

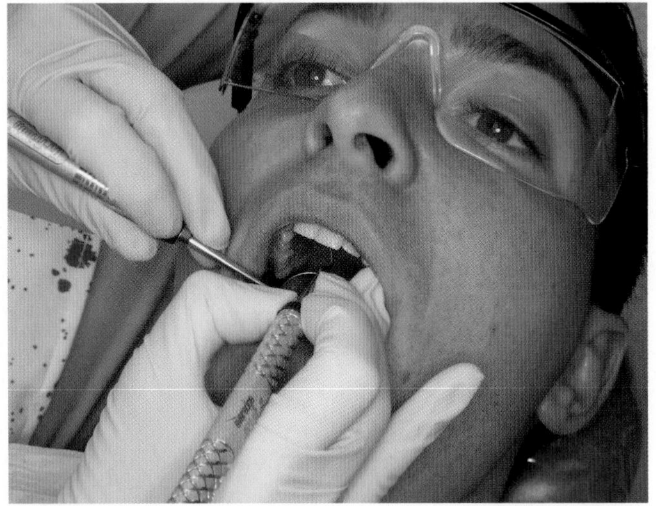

Figure 4-35. Mirror. Position the mirror head so the lingual surfaces of the anterior teeth can be seen in the reflecting surface of the mirror.

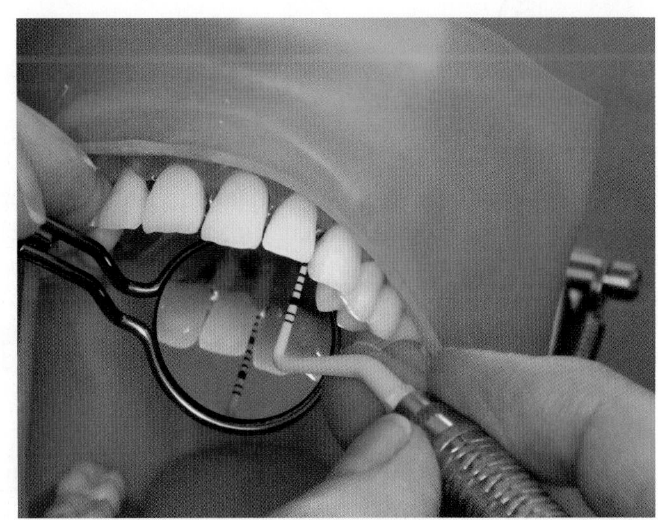

Figure 4-36. Task 1—Mesial Surface of the Left Canine. Finger rest on an occlusofacial line angle.
Place the instrument tip on the mesial surface of the left canine.

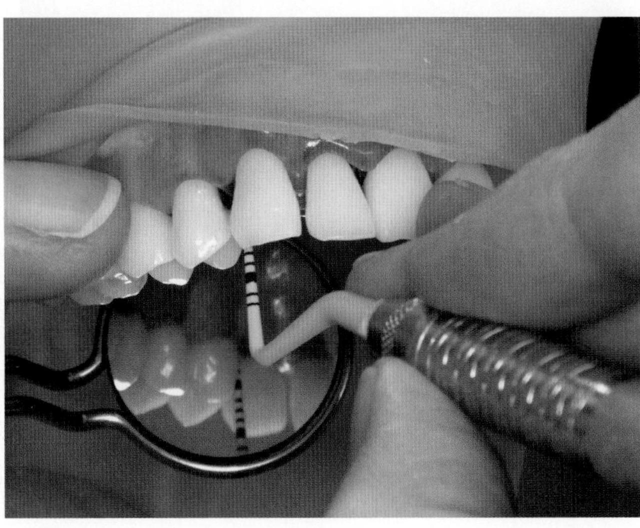

Figure 4-37. Task 2—Distal Surface of the Right Canine. Finger rest on an incisal edge.
Place the instrument tip on the distal surface of the right canine.

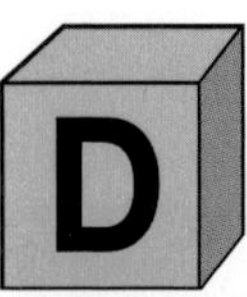

SKILL BUILDING. MAXILLARY ANTERIOR TEETH, SURFACES AWAY

Directions: Practice establishing a finger rest for the maxillary anterior teeth, surfaces away, by referring to Figures 4-38 to 4-45.

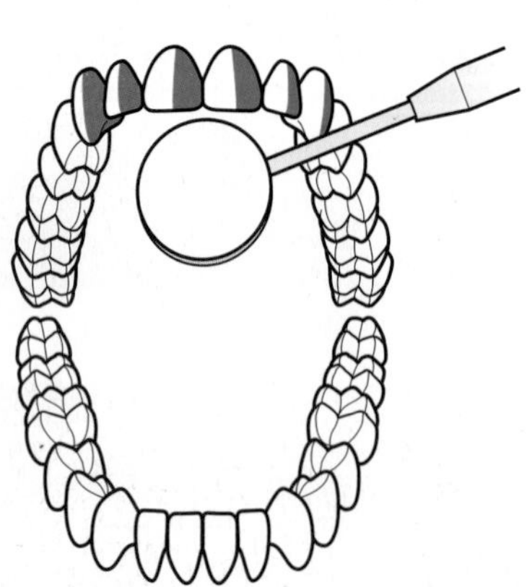

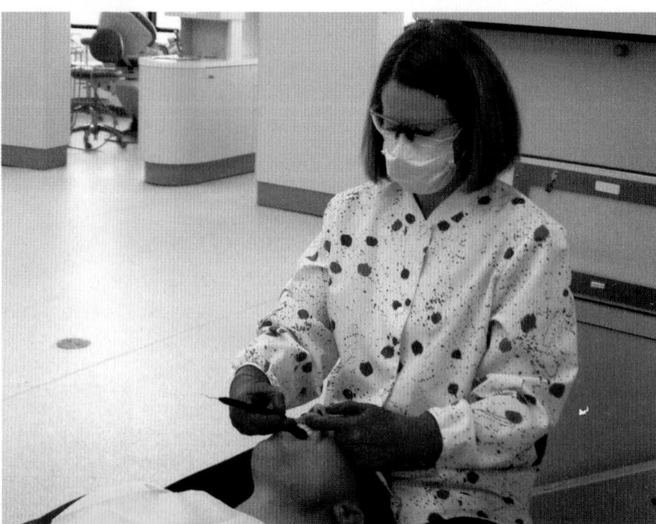

Figure 4-38. Clock Position for Maxillary Anterior Teeth, Surfaces Away. The clinician's clock position for the maxillary anterior surfaces away from the clinician—facial and lingual aspects—is the 11 to 1 o'clock position. The patient is in a chin-up head position.

Box 4-8. Handle Positions for Maxillary Anterior Teeth

1. Hold the hand in a palm-up position.
2. Rest the handle against the index finger somewhere in the green shaded area.

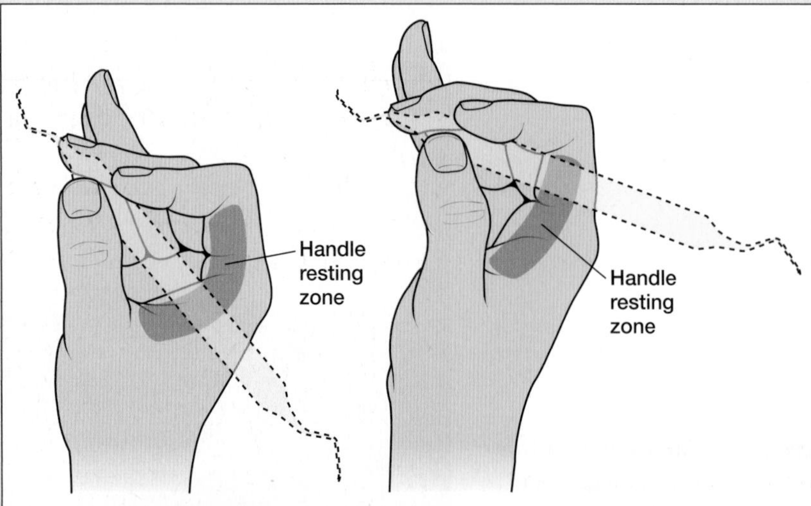

Figure 4-39. Handle Positions for Maxillary Treatment Areas.

Maxillary Anteriors, Facial Aspect: Surfaces Away

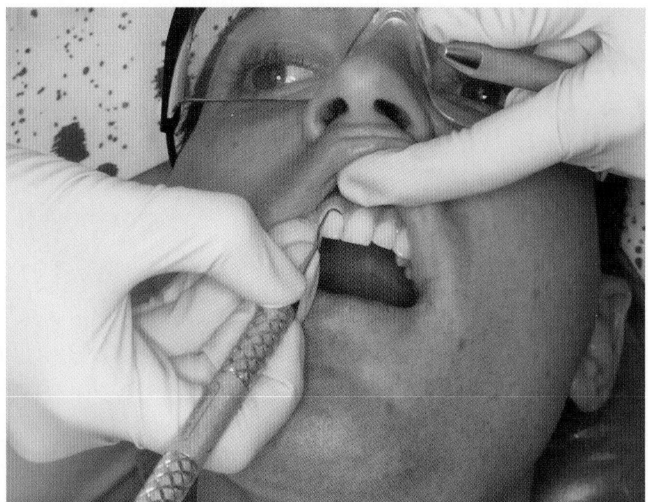

Figure 4-40. Retraction. Retract the lip with your index finger or thumb.
Technique hint: Your dominant hand is positioned correctly if you can see the underside of your middle and ring fingers.

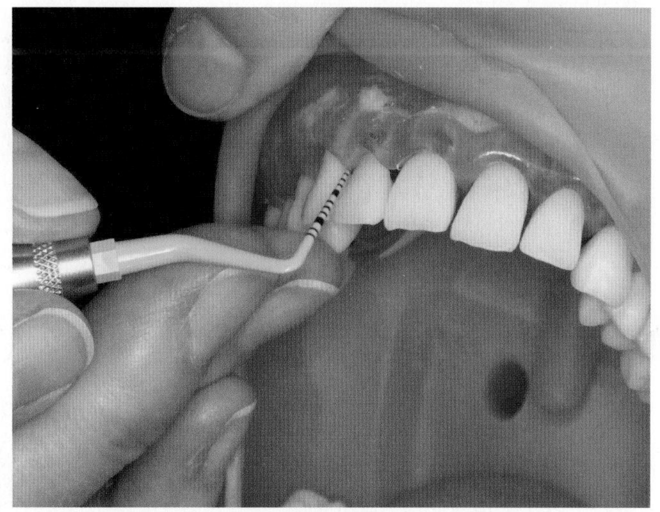

Figure 4-41. Task 1—Mesial Surface of the Right Canine. Finger rest on an occlusal surface.
Place the instrument tip on the mesial surface of the right canine.

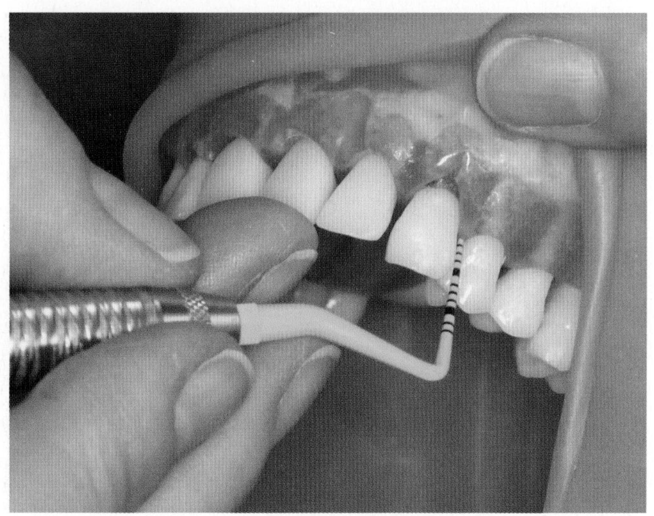

Figure 4-42. Task 2—Distal Surface of the Left Canine. Finger rest on an incisal edge.
Place the instrument tip on the distal surface of the left canine.

Maxillary Anterior Sextant, Lingual Aspect: Surfaces Away

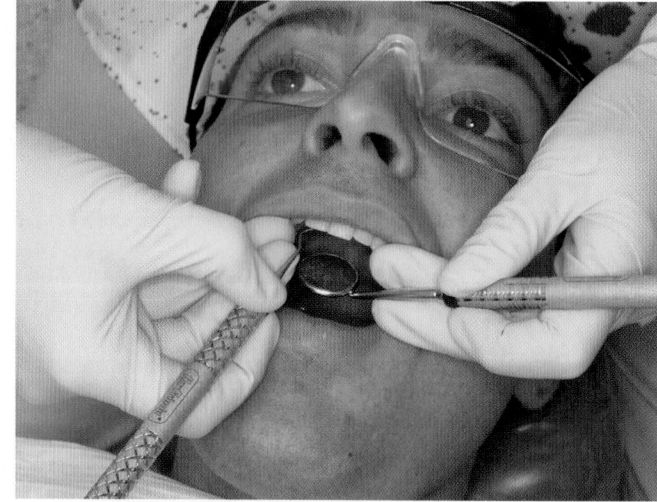

Figure 4-43. Mirror. Position the mirror head so that the lingual surfaces of the teeth can be seen.
Technique hint: Your dominant hand is positioned correctly if you can see the underside of your middle and ring fingers.

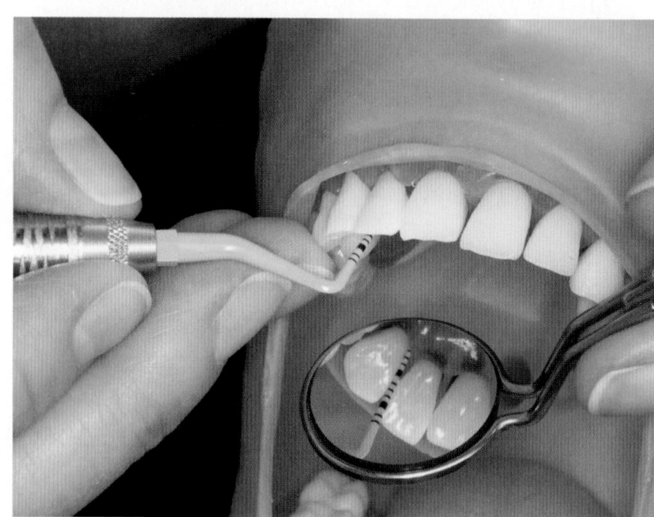

Figure 4-44. Task 1—Mesial Surface of the Right Canine. Finger rest on an occlusal surface.
Place the instrument tip on the mesial surface of the right canine.

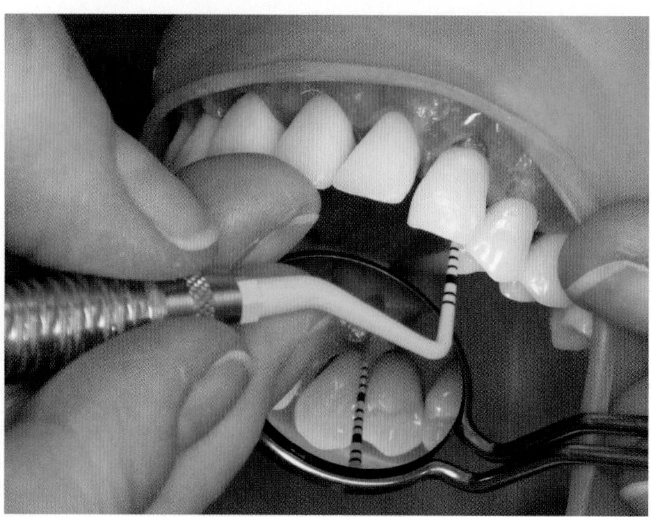

Figure 4-45. Task 2—Distal Surface of the Left Canine. Finger rest on an incisal edge.
Place the instrument tip on the distal surface of the left canine.

REFERENCE SHEET FOR ANTERIOR TREATMENT AREAS FOR THE RIGHT-HANDED CLINICIAN

Photocopy this reference sheet in Table 4-3 and use it for quick reference as you practice your skills. Place the photocopied reference sheet in a plastic page protector for longer use.

TABLE 4-3. Reference Sheet: Anterior Treatment Areas

Treatment Area	Clock Position	Patient's Head
Mandibular Teeth		
Facial Surfaces TOWARD	8:00–9:00	
Lingual Surfaces TOWARD		Slightly toward
		Chin DOWN
Facial Surfaces AWAY	11:00–1:00	
Lingual Surfaces AWAY		
Maxillary Teeth		
Facial Surfaces TOWARD	8:00–9:00	
Lingual Surfaces TOWARD		Slightly toward
		Chin UP
Facial Surfaces AWAY	11:00–1:00	
Lingual Surfaces AWAY		

Note: This ends the section for RIGHT-Handed clinicians. Turn to page 125 for Section 6: Modified Fulcruming Techniques.

Section 5
Technique Practice: LEFT-Handed Clinician

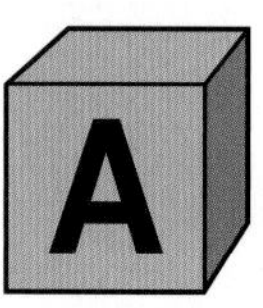

SKILL BUILDING. MANDIBULAR ANTERIOR TEETH, SURFACES TOWARD

Directions: Practice establishing a finger rest for the mandibular anterior teeth, surfaces toward, by referring to Figures 4-46 to 4-53.

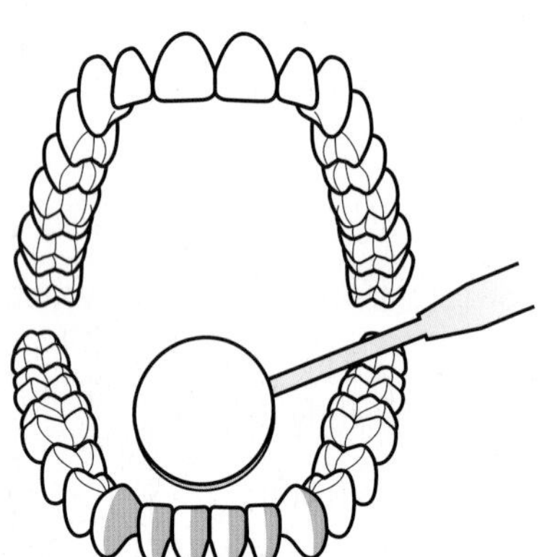

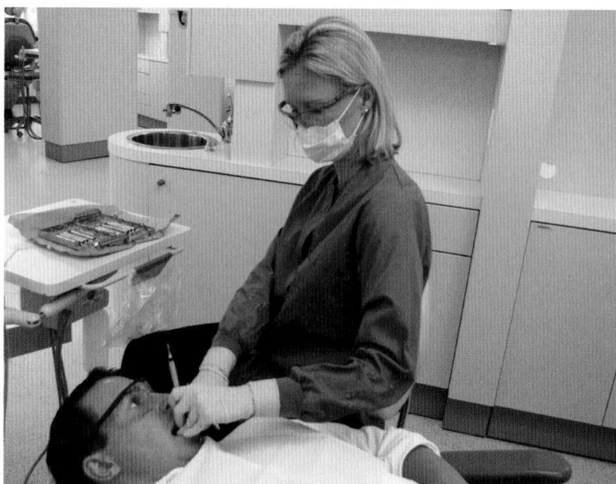

Figure 4-46. Clock Position for Mandibular Anterior Teeth, Surfaces Toward. The clinician's clock position for the mandibular anterior surfaces toward the clinician—facial and lingual aspects—is the 3 to 4 o'clock position. The patient should be in a chin-down head position.

Box 4-9. Handle Positions for Mandibular Anterior Teeth

1. Hold the hand in a palm-down position.
2. Rest the handle against the index finger somewhere in the green shaded area.

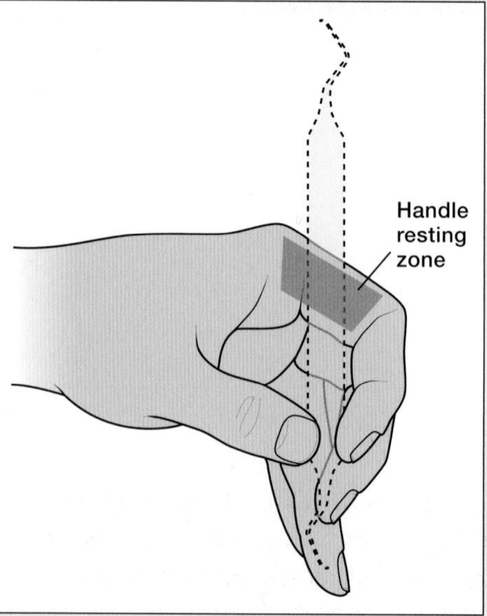

Figure 4-47. Handle Positions for Mandibular Treatment Areas.

Mandibular Anteriors, Facial Aspect: Surfaces Toward

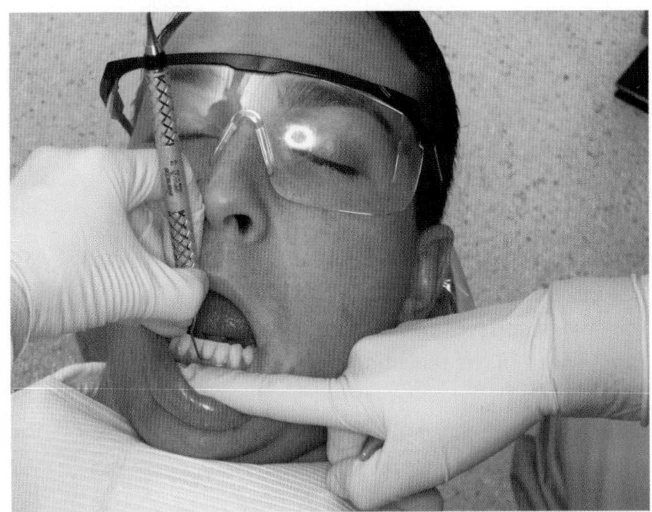

Figure 4-48. Retraction. Retract the lip with the index finger or thumb of your right hand.

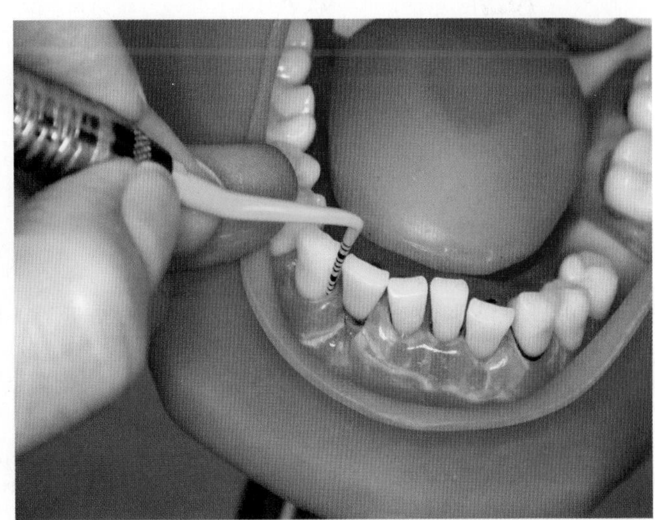

Figure 4-49. Task 1—Mesial Surface of the Right Canine. Finger rest on an occlusofacial line angle.
Place the instrument tip on the mesial surface of the right canine.

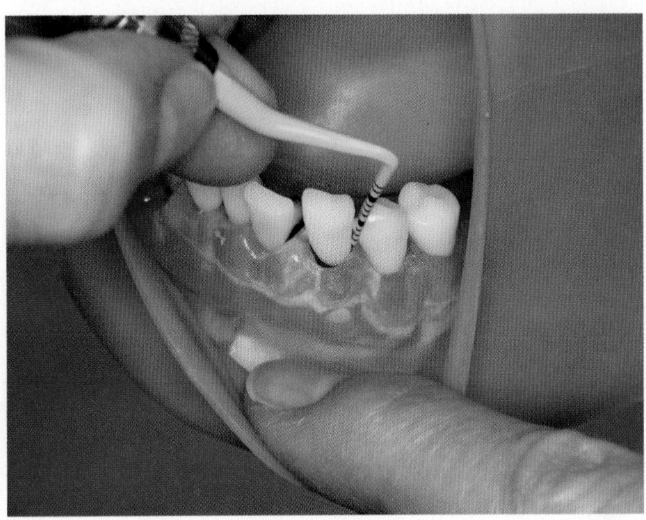

Figure 4-50. Task 2—Distal Surface of Left Canine. Finger rest on an incisal edge. Place the instrument tip on the distal surface of the left canine.

Mandibular Anteriors, Lingual Aspect: Surfaces Toward

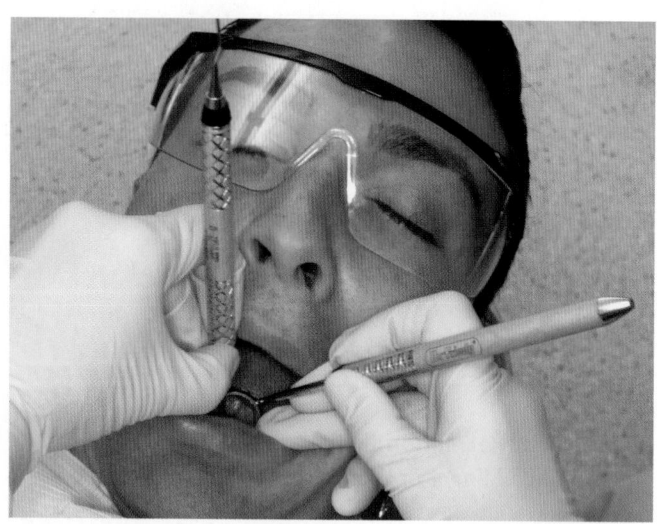

Figure 4-51. Mirror. Use the mirror head to push the tongue away gently so the lingual surfaces of the anterior teeth can be seen in the reflecting surface of the mirror.
Note that the clinician pictured here is using an extraoral fulcrum for her mirror hand.

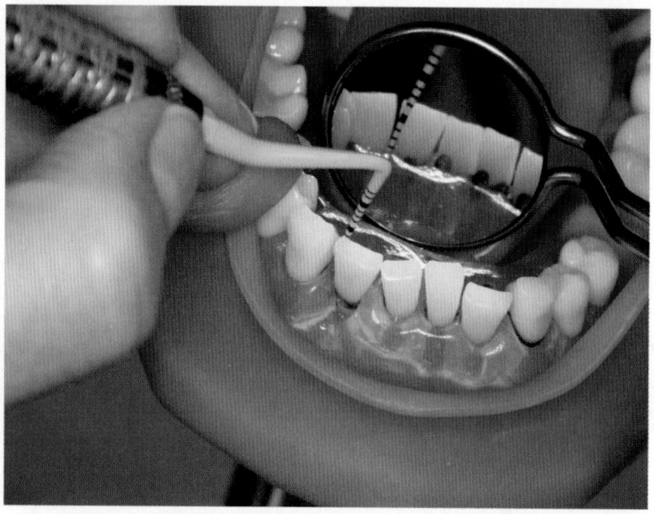

Figure 4-52. Task 1—Mesial Surface of the Right Canine. Finger rest on an occlusofacial line angle.
Place the instrument tip on the mesial surface of the right canine.

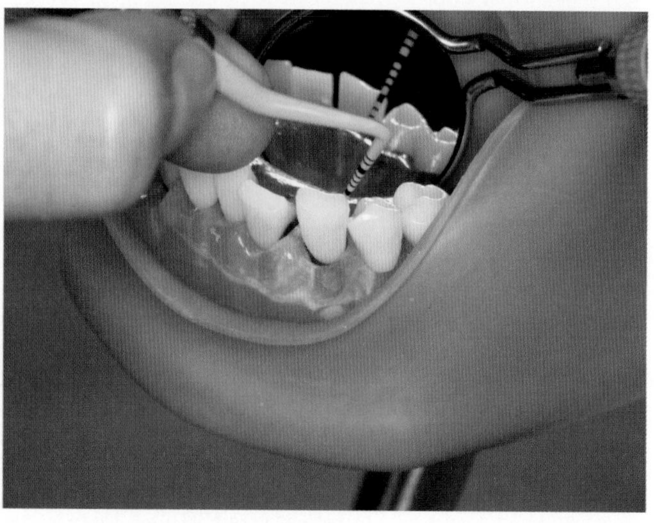

Figure 4-53. Task 2—Distal Surface of the Left Canine. Finger rest on an incisal edge. Place the instrument tip on the distal surface of the left canine.

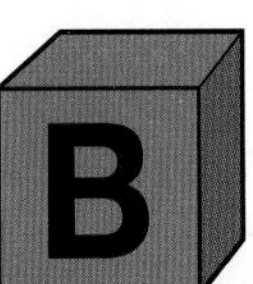

SKILL BUILDING. MANDIBULAR ANTERIOR TEETH, SURFACES AWAY

Directions: Practice establishing a finger rest for the mandibular anterior teeth, surfaces away, by referring to Figures 4-54 to 4-61.

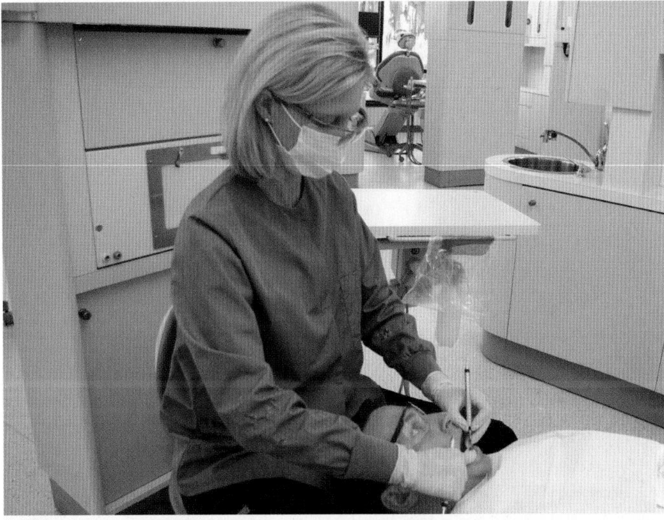

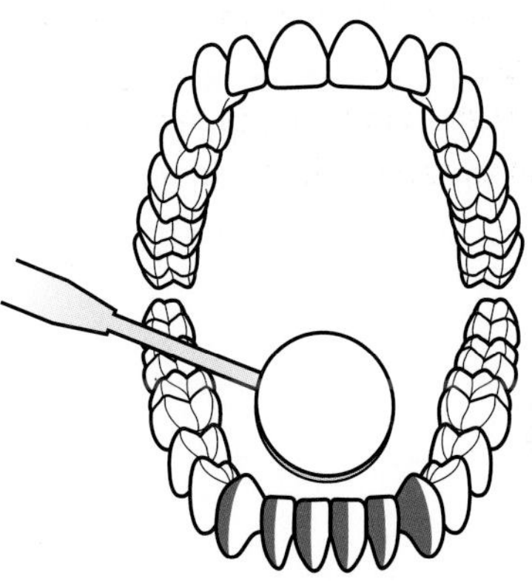

Figure 4-54. Clock Position for Mandibular Anterior Teeth, Surfaces Away. The clinician's clock position for the mandibular anterior surfaces away from the clinician—facial and lingual aspects—is the 11 to 1 o'clock position. The patient is in a chin-down head position.

Box 4-10. Handle Positions for Mandibular Anterior Teeth

1. Hold the hand in a palm-down position.
2. Rest the handle against the index finger somewhere in the green shaded area.

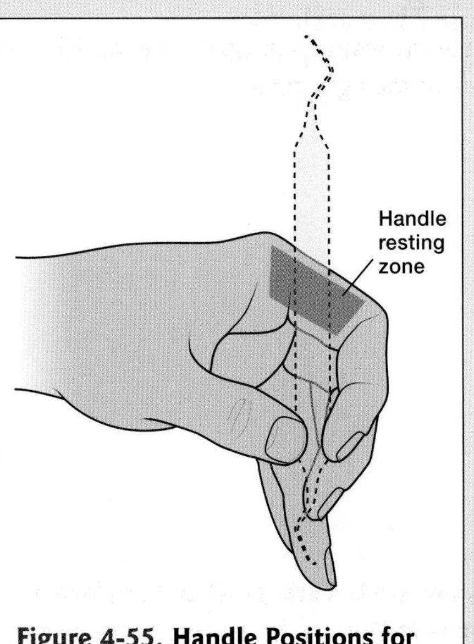

Figure 4-55. Handle Positions for Mandibular Treatment Areas.

Mandibular Anteriors, Facial Aspect: Surfaces Away

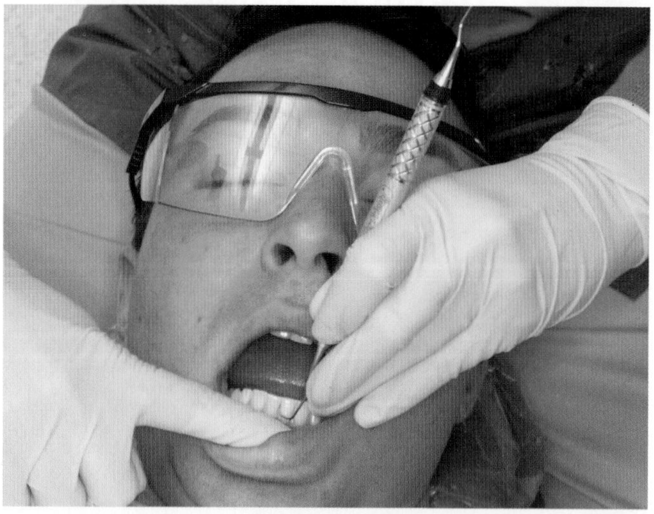

Figure 4-56. Retraction. Retract the lip with your index finger or thumb.
Hold the mirror in your palm until it is needed for another treatment area.

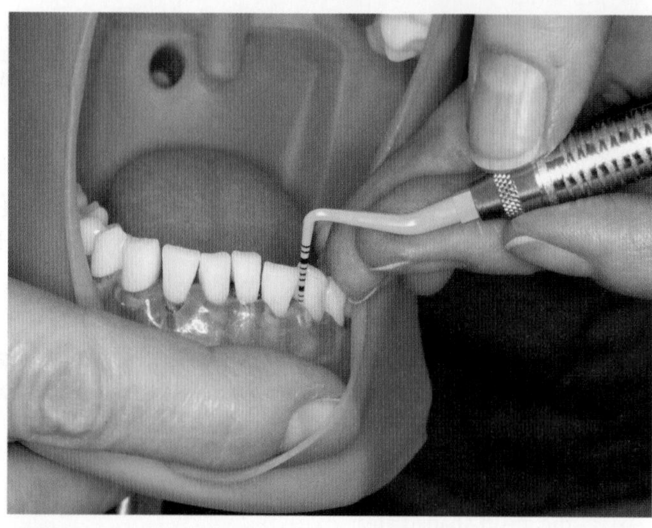

Figure 4-57. Task 1—Mesial Surface of the Left Canine. Finger rest on an occlusofacial line angle.
Place the instrument tip on the mesial surface of the left canine.

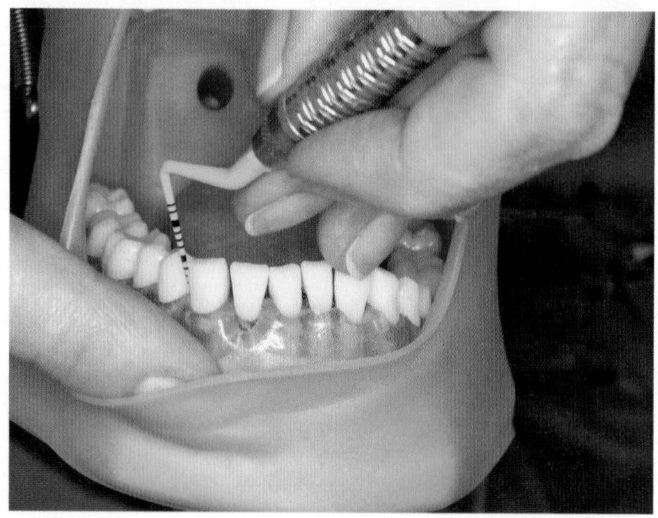

Figure 4-58. Task 2—Distal Surface of the Right Canine. Finger rest on an incisal edge.
Place the instrument tip on the distal surface of the right canine.

Mandibular Anteriors, Lingual Aspect: Surfaces Away

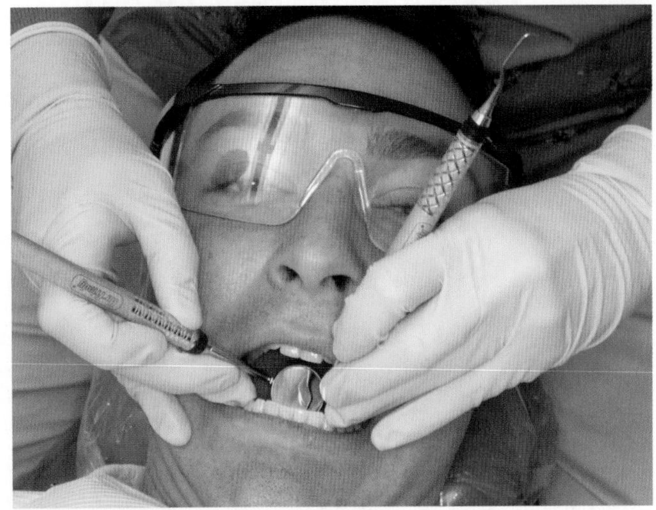

Figure 4-59. Mirror. Use the mirror head to push the tongue back gently so that the lingual surfaces of the teeth can be seen.

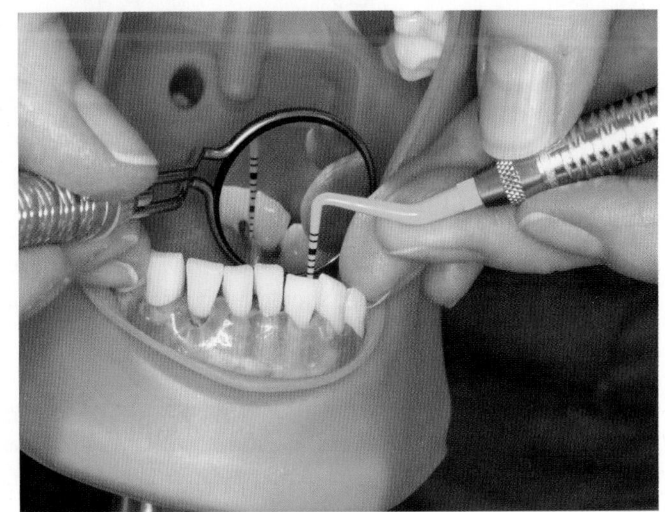

Figure 4-60. Task 1—Mesial Surface of the Left Canine. Finger rest on an occlusofacial line angle.
Place the instrument tip on the mesial surface of the left canine.

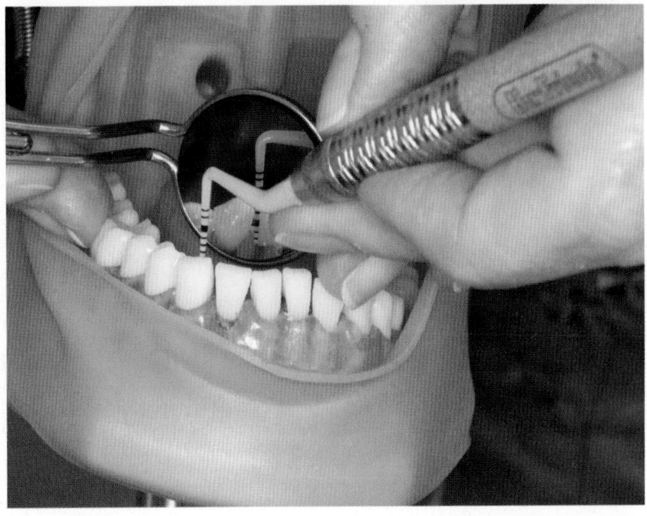

Figure 4-61. Task 2—Distal Surface of the Right Canine. Finger rest on an incisal edge.
Place the instrument tip on the distal surface of the right canine.

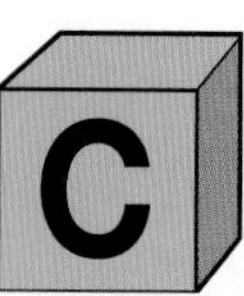

SKILL BUILDING. MAXILLARY ANTERIOR TEETH, SURFACES TOWARD

Directions: Practice establishing a finger rest for the maxillary anterior teeth, surfaces toward, by referring to Figures 4-62 to 4-69.

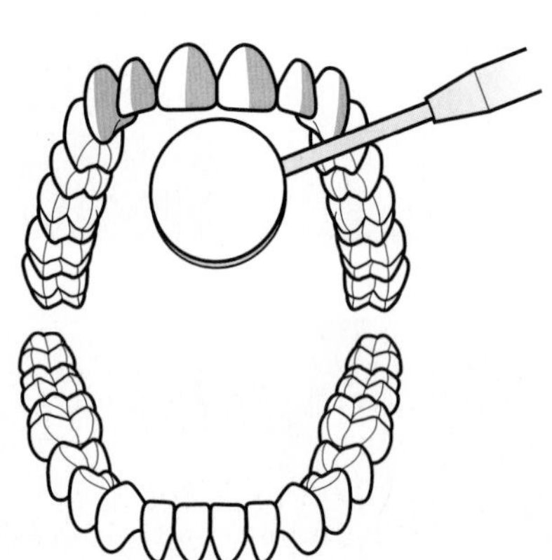

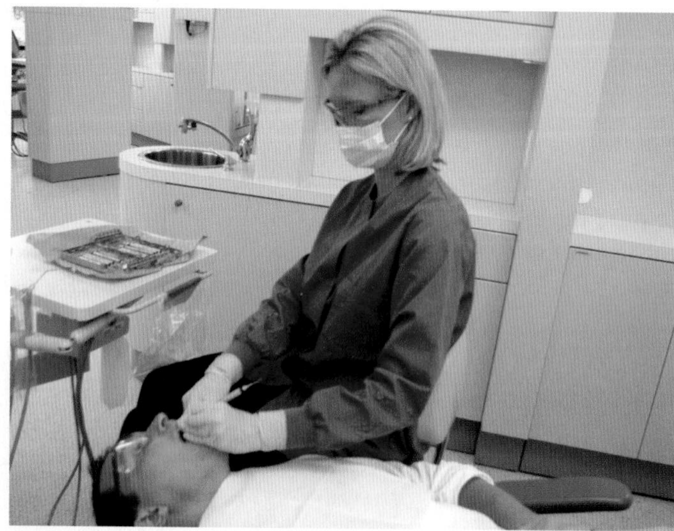

Figure 4-62. Clock Position for Maxillary Anterior Teeth, Surfaces Toward. The clinician's clock position for the maxillary anterior surfaces toward the clinician—facial and lingual aspects—is the 3 to 4 o'clock position. The patient should be in a chin-up head position.

Box 4-11. Handle Positions for Maxillary Anterior Teeth

1. Hold the hand in a palm-up position.
2. Rest the handle against the index finger somewhere in the green shaded area.

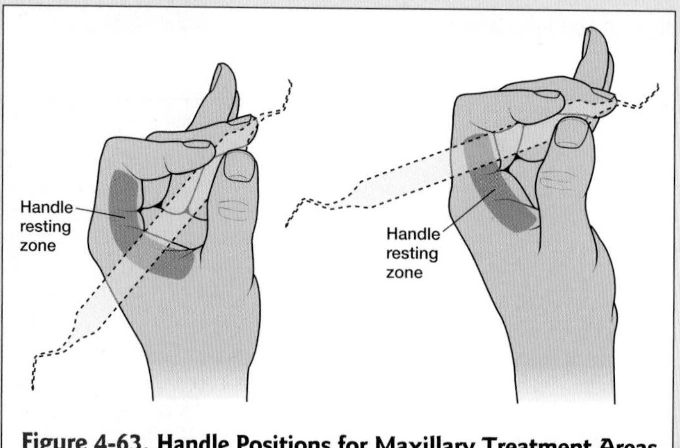

Figure 4-63. Handle Positions for Maxillary Treatment Areas.

Maxillary Anteriors, Facial Aspect: Surfaces Toward

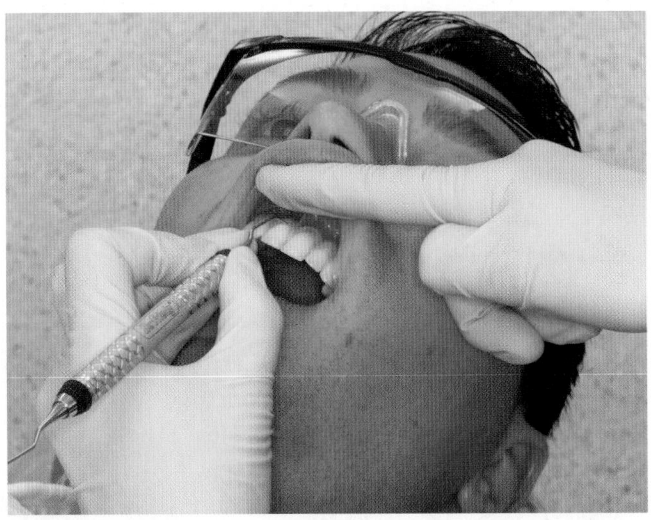

Figure 4-64. Retraction. Retract the lip with the index finger or thumb of your right hand.

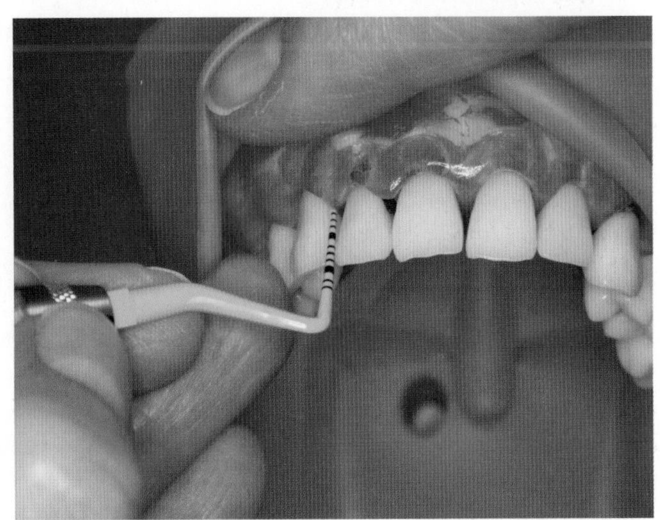

Figure 4-65. Task 1—Mesial Surface of the Right Canine. Finger rest on an occlusofacial line angle.
Place the instrument tip on the mesial surface of the right canine.

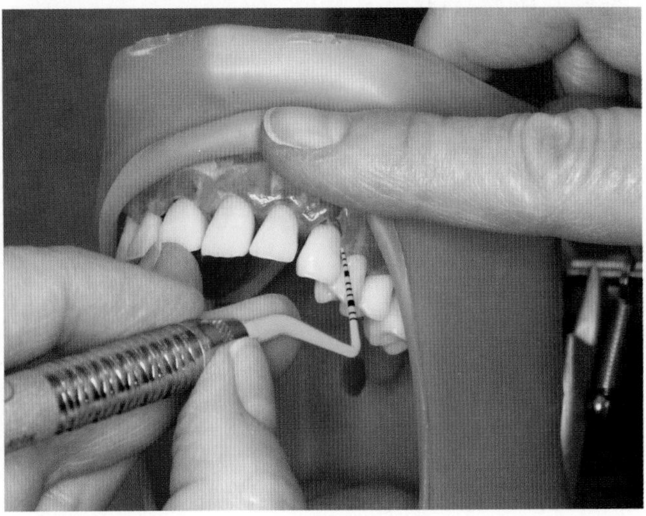

Figure 4-66. Task 2—Distal Surface of Left Canine. Finger rest on an incisal edge.
Place the instrument tip on the distal surface of the left canine.

Maxillary Anteriors, Lingual Aspect: Surfaces Toward

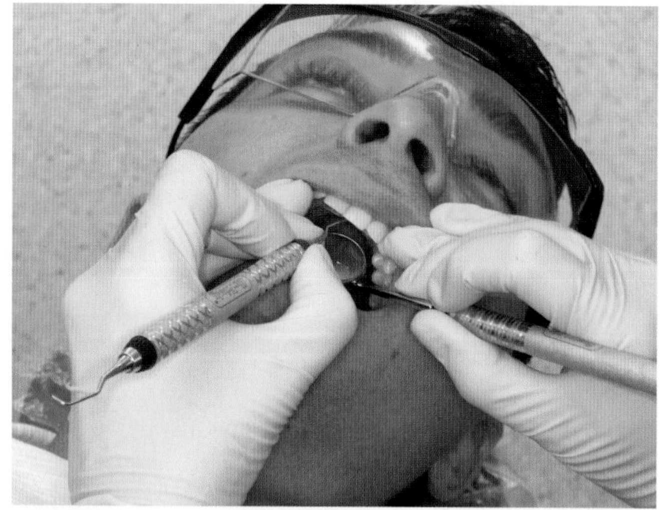

Figure 4-67. Mirror. Position the mirror head so the lingual surfaces of the anterior teeth can be seen in the reflecting surface of the mirror.

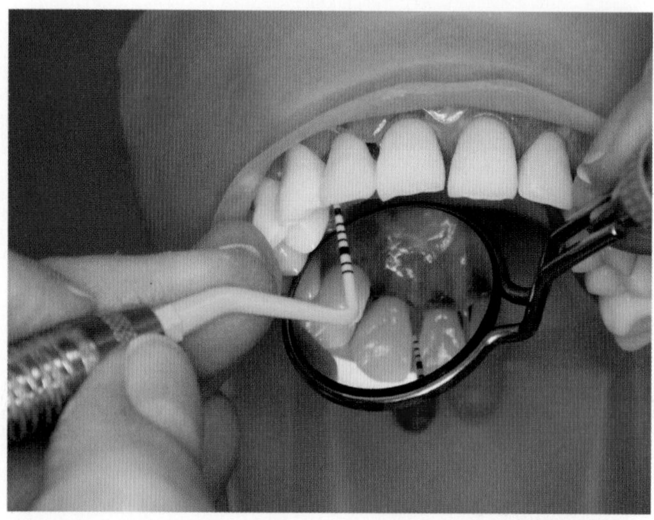

Figure 4-68. Task 1—Mesial Surface of the Right Canine. Finger rest on an occlusofacial line angle.
Place the instrument tip on the mesial surface of the right canine.

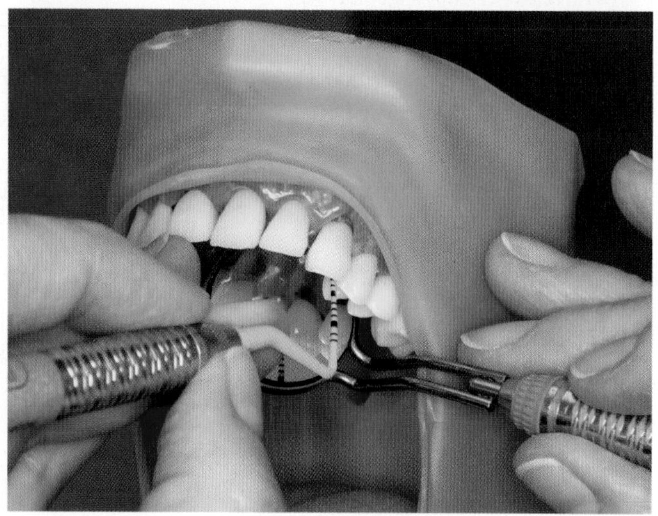

Figure 4-69. Task 2—Distal Surface of the Left Canine. Finger rest on an incisal edge.
Place the instrument tip on the distal surface of the left canine.

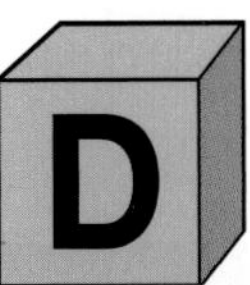

SKILL BUILDING. MAXILLARY ANTERIOR TEETH, SURFACES AWAY

Directions: Practice establishing a finger rest for the maxillary anterior teeth, surfaces away, by referring to Figures 4-70 to 4-77.

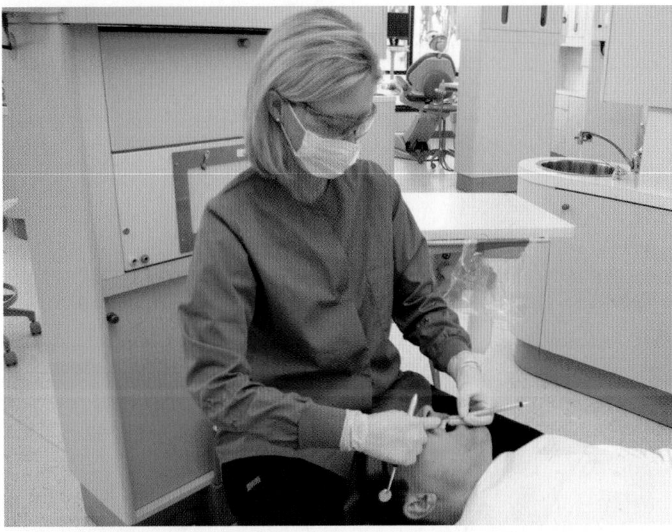

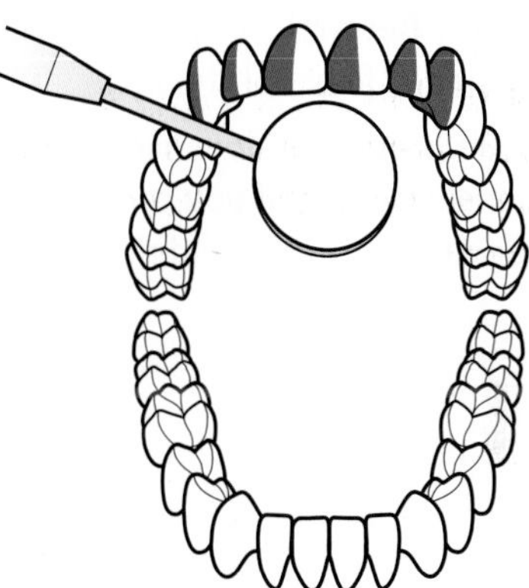

Figure 4-70. Clock Position for Maxillary Anterior Teeth, Surfaces Away. The clinician's clock position for the maxillary anterior surfaces away from the clinician—facial and lingual aspects—is the 11 to 1 o'clock position. The patient is in a chin-up head position.

Box 4-12. Handle Positions for Maxillary Anterior Teeth

1. Hold the hand in a palm-up position.
2. Rest the handle against the index finger somewhere in the green shaded area.

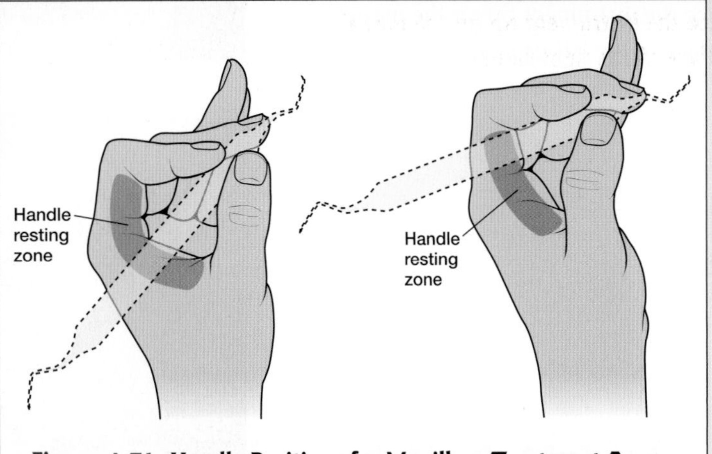

Figure 4-71. Handle Positions for Maxillary Treatment Areas.

Maxillary Anteriors, Facial Aspect: Surfaces Away

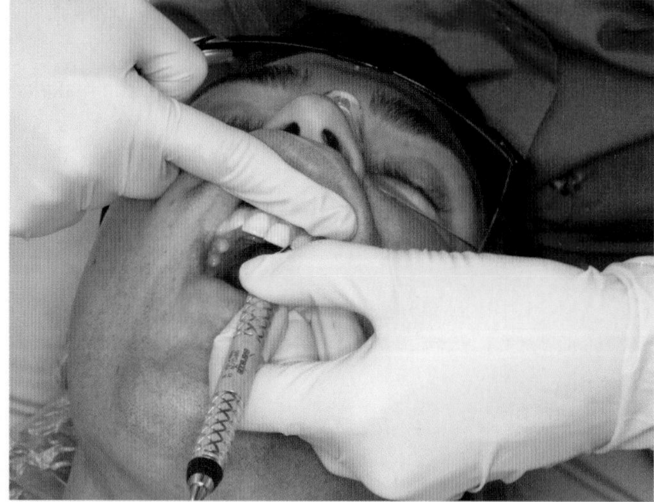

Figure 4-72. Retraction. Retract the lip with your index finger or thumb.

Technique hint: Your dominant hand is positioned correctly if you can see the underside of your middle and ring fingers.

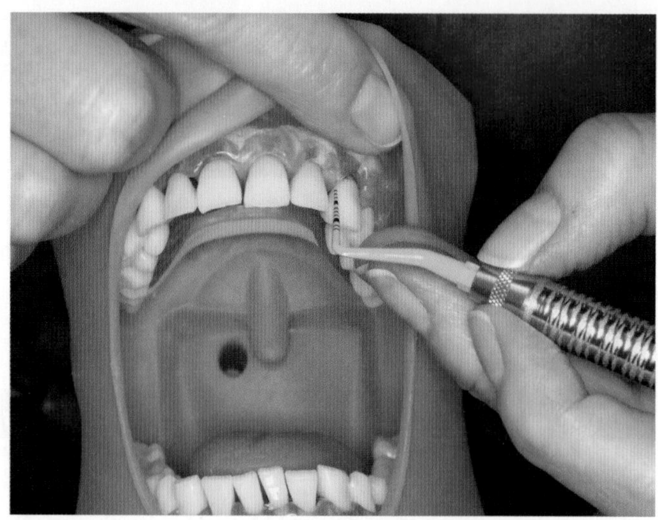

Figure 4-73. Task 1—Mesial Surface of the Left Canine. Finger rest on an occlusal surface.

Place the instrument tip on the mesial surface of the left canine.

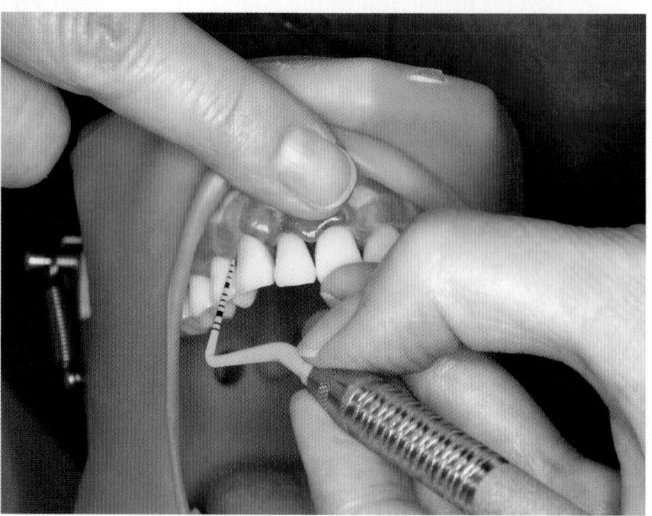

Figure 4-74. Task 2—Distal Surface of the Right Canine. Finger rest on an incisal edge.

Place the instrument tip on the distal surface of the right canine.

Maxillary Anteriors, Lingual Aspect: Surfaces Away

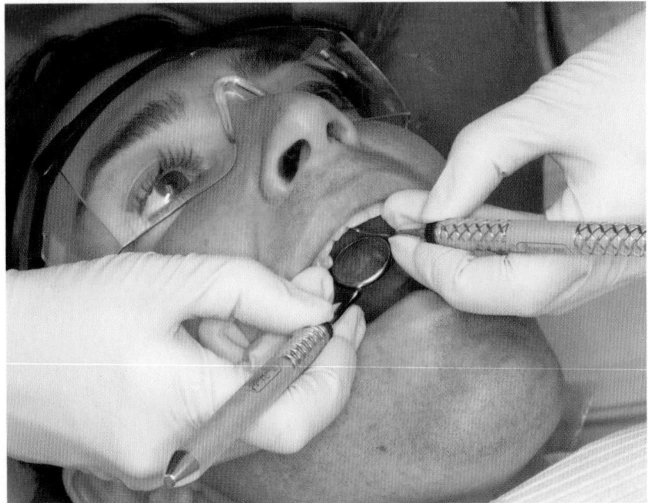

Figure 4-75. Mirror. Position the mirror head so that the lingual surfaces of the teeth can be seen.

Technique hint: Your dominant hand is positioned correctly if you can see the underside of your middle and ring fingers.

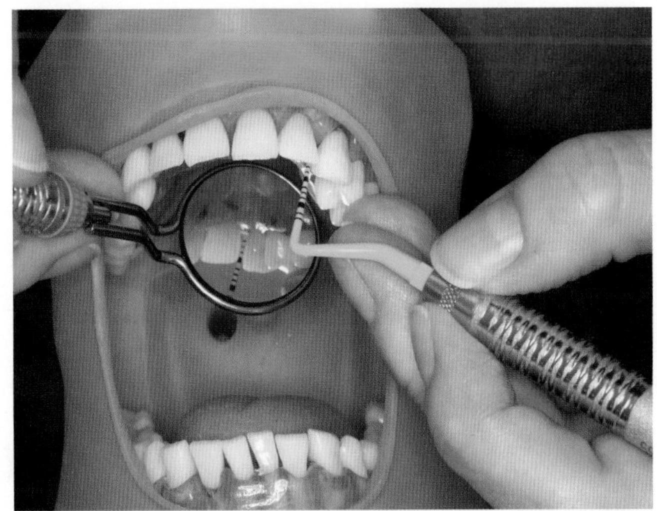

Figure 4-76. Task 1—Mesial Surface of the Left Canine. Finger rest on an occlusal surface.

Place the instrument tip on the mesial surface of the left canine.

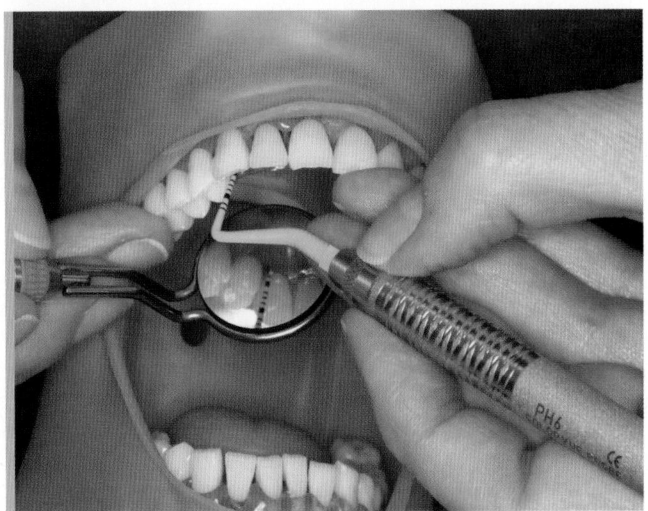

Figure 4-77. Task 2—Distal Surface of the Right Canine. Finger rest on an incisal edge.

Place the instrument tip on the distal surface of the right canine.

REFERENCE SHEET FOR ANTERIOR TREATMENT AREAS FOR THE LEFT-HANDED CLINICIAN

Photocopy this reference sheet in Table 4-4 and use it for quick reference as you practice your skills. Place the photocopied reference sheet in a plastic page protector for longer use.

TABLE 4-4. Reference Sheet: Anterior Treatment Areas

Treatment Area	Clock Position	Patient's Head
Mandibular Teeth		
Facial Surfaces TOWARD Lingual Surfaces TOWARD	3:00–4:00	Slightly toward Chin DOWN
Facial Surfaces AWAY Lingual Surfaces AWAY	11:00–1:00	
Maxillary Teeth		
Facial Surfaces TOWARD Lingual Surfaces TOWARD	3:00–4:00	Slightly toward Chin UP
Facial Surfaces AWAY Lingual Surfaces AWAY	11:00–1:00	

Section 6
Modified Fulcruming Techniques

There are times when it is difficult to obtain parallelism with the lower shank or to adapt the cutting edge when using a standard intraoral fulcrum. In instances when a standard intraoral fulcrum does not seem to work well, a modified fulcruming technique can improve access to the tooth surface. For example, when working within a deep periodontal pocket, sometimes it is difficult to position the lower shank parallel to the root surface being treated. In such instances, modified fulcruming techniques are useful in obtaining parallelism.

- Modified fulcruming techniques require greater clinician skill and are helpful when working in areas of limited access, such as a narrow deep pocket.
- ***Before attempting modified fulcruming techniques, the clinician should have mastered the fundamentals of neutral position and standard intraoral fulcruming techniques.***

FINGER-ON-FINGER FULCRUM

The finger-on-finger fulcrum is accomplished by resting the ***ring finger of the dominant hand*** on the ***index finger of the nondominant hand.***

- This technique allows the clinician to fulcrum in line with the long axis of the tooth to improve parallelism of the lower shank to the tooth surface.
- The nondominant index finger provides a stable rest for the clinician's dominant hand and provides improved access to deep periodontal pockets.

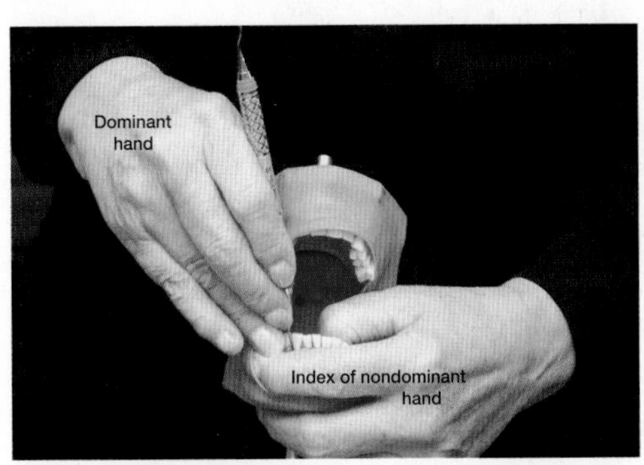

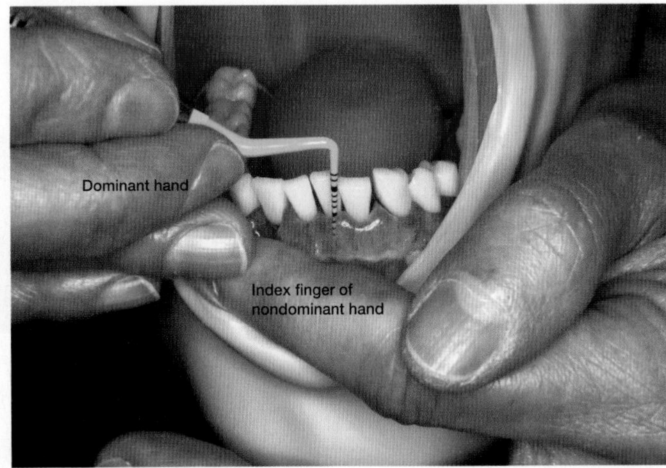

Figure 4-78. Finger-on-Finger Fulcrum on Mandibular Arch. The photo shows a right-handed clinician using a modified finger rest while working on the mandibular anterior teeth, facial aspect.

- The clinician pictured is seated in the 12 o'clock position behind the patient.
- The clinician rests the ring finger of the dominant hand on the index finger of his or her nondominant hand.
- Note that the periodontal probe is inserted in a deep periodontal pocket.

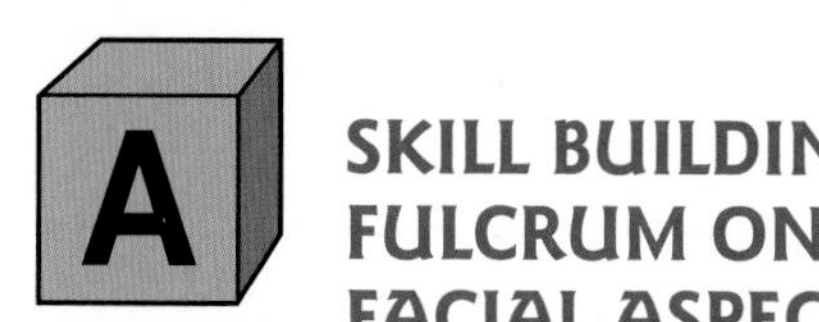

SKILL BUILDING. FINGER-ON-FINGER FULCRUM ON MANDIBULAR ANTERIORS, FACIAL ASPECT

Directions: Practice establishing a modified finger rest for the facial aspect of the mandibular anterior teeth by referring to Figures 4-79 to 4-81.

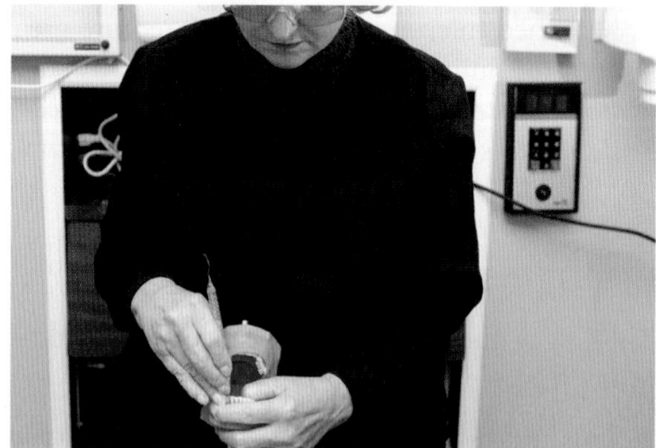

Figure 4-79. Step 1: Clock Position. Sit in the 11 to 1 o'clock position behind the patient.

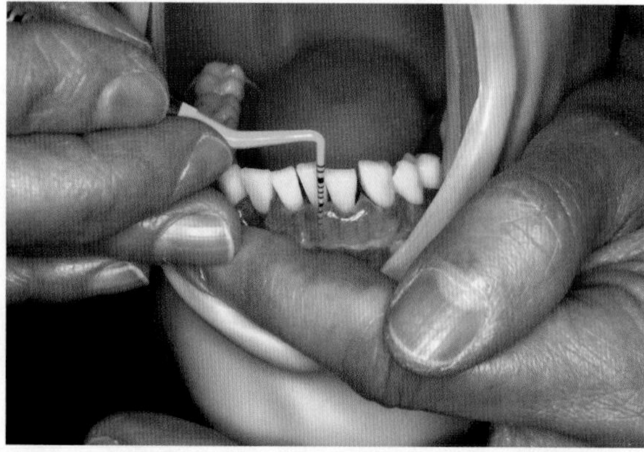

Figure 4-80. Step 2: Establish a Modified Finger Rest.

- Wrap the index finger of your ***nondominant hand*** around the mandibular alveolar mucosa in the mucobuccal fold.
- Rest the ring finger of the ***dominant hand*** on your index finger.

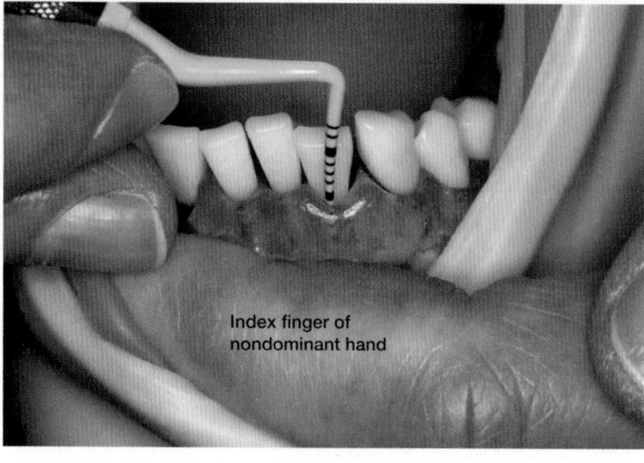

Figure 4-81. Close-up View. This photo shows a close-up view of the finger-on-finger fulcrum with the ring finger resting on the index finger of the non-dominant hand.

B SKILL BUILDING. FINGER-ON-FINGER FULCRUM ON MAXILLARY ANTERIORS, FACIAL ASPECT

Directions: Practice establishing a modified finger rest for the facial aspect of the maxillary anterior teeth by referring to Figures 4-82 to 4-84.

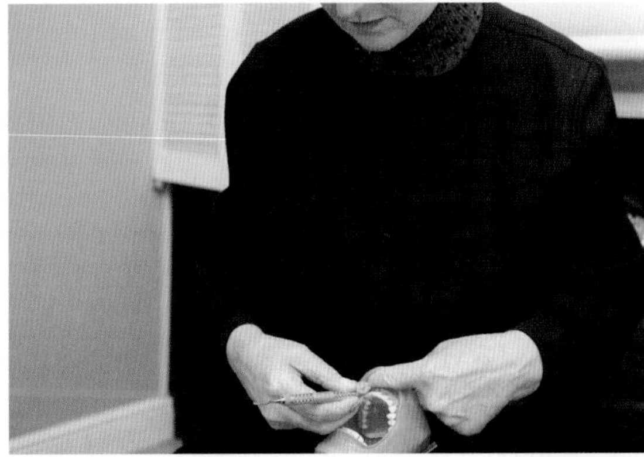

Figure 4-82. Step 1: Clock Position. Sit in the 11 to 1 o'clock position behind the patient.

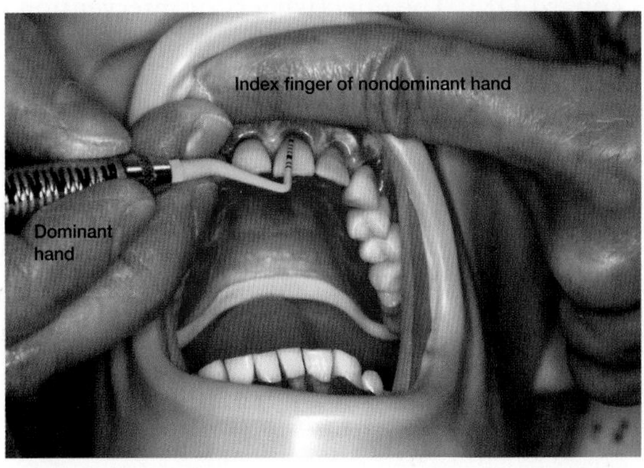

Figure 4-83. Step 2: Establish a Modified Finger Rest.

- Rest the index finger of your ***nondominant hand*** against the maxillary alveolar mucosa in the mucobuccal fold.
- Rest the ring finger of the ***dominant hand*** on your index finger.

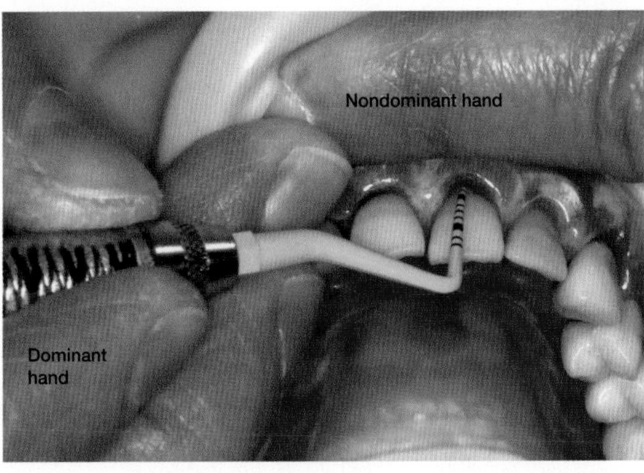

Figure 4-84. Close-up View. This photo shows a close-up view of the finger-on-finger fulcrum with the ring finger resting on the index finger of the nondominant hand.

REFERENCES

1. Dong H, Barr A, Loomer P, Rempel D. The effects of finger rest positions on hand muscle load and pinch force in simulated dental hygiene work. *J Dent Educ*. 2005;69:453–460.
2. Dong H, Loomer P, Villanueva A, Rempel D. Pinch forces and instrument tip forces during periodontal scaling. *J Periodontol*. 2007;78:97–103.
3. Millar D. Reinforced periodontal instrumentation and ergonomics. The best practice to ensure optiminal performance and career longevity. *CDHA*. 2009;24:8–16.
4. Scaramucci M. Getting a grasp. *Dimen Dent Hyg*. 2008;6:24–26.
5. Meador HL. The biocentric technique: a guide to avoiding occupational pain. *J Dent Hyg*. 1993;67:38–51.
6. Sugawara E. The study of wrist postures of musicians using the WristSystem (Greenleaf Medical System). *Work*. 1999;13:217–228.
7. Liskiewicz ST, Kerschbaum WE. Cumulative trauma disorders: an ergonomic approach for prevention. *J Dent Hyg*. 1997;71:162–167.
8. Loren GJ, Shoemaker SD, Burkholder TJ, Jacobson MD, Friden J, Lieber RL. Human wrist motors: biomechanical design and application to tendon transfers. *J Biomech*. 1996;29:331–342.
9. Michalak-Turcotte C. Controlling dental hygiene work-related musculoskeletal disorders: the ergonomic process. *J Dent Hyg*. 2000;74:41–48.
10. Hauser AM, Bowen DM. Primer on preclinical instruction and evaluation. *J Dent Educ*. 2009;73:390–398.

RECOMMENDED READING

Leonard DM. The effectiveness of intervention strategies used to educate clients about prevention of upper extremity cumulative trauma disorders. *Work*. 2000;14:151–157.

Liskiewicz ST, Kerschbaum WE. Cumulative trauma disorders: an ergonomic approach for prevention. *J Dent Hyg*. 1997;71:162–167.

Marcoux BC, Krause V, Nieuwenhuijsen ER. Effectiveness of an educational intervention to increase knowledge and reduce use of risky behaviors associated with cumulative trauma in office workers. *Work*. 2000;14:127–135.

Michalak-Turcotte C. Controlling dental hygiene work-related musculoskeletal disorders: the ergonomic process. *J Dent Hyg*. 2000;74:41–48.

Section 7
Skill Application

PRACTICAL FOCUS

Your course assignment is to visit a local dental office and photograph a clinician at work. Your photographs are shown below in Figures 4-85 to 4-88. (1) Evaluate each photograph for position, grasp, and finger rest. (2) For each incorrect element, describe: (a) how the problem could be corrected and (b) the musculoskeletal problems that could result from each positioning problem.

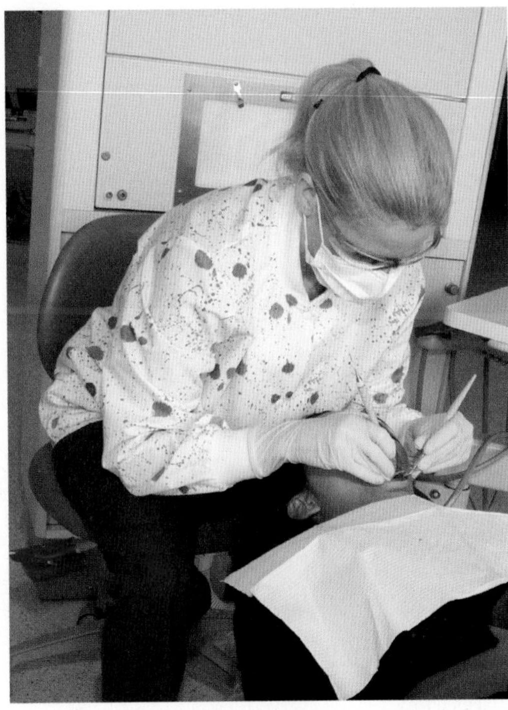

Figure 4-85. Photo 1.

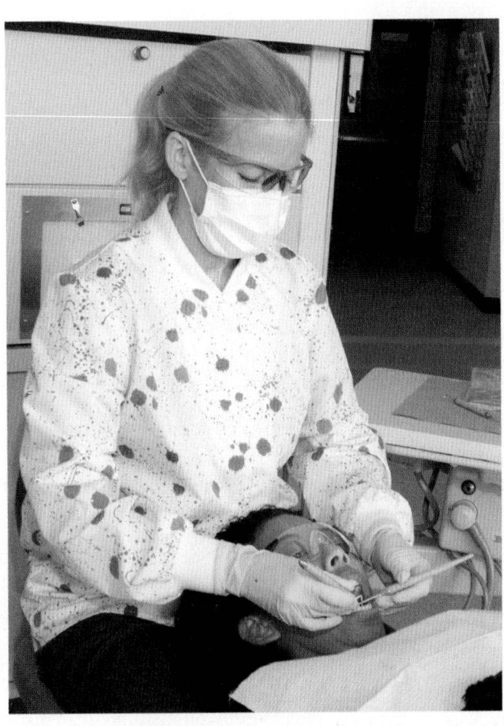

Figure 4-86. Photo 2.

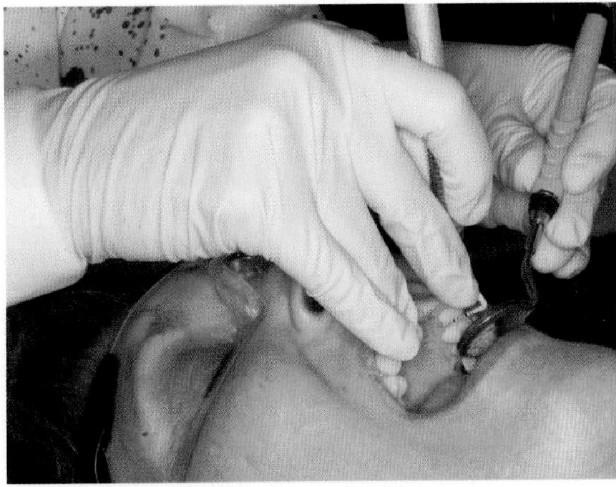

Figure 4-87. Photo 3.

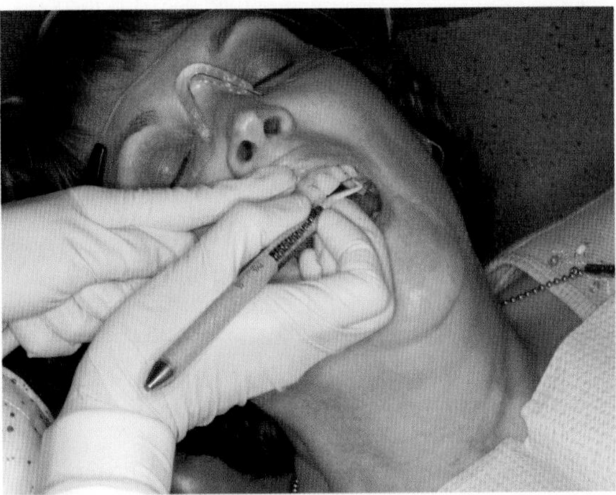

Figure 4-88. Photo 4.

STUDENT SELF-EVALUATION MODULE 4 MIRROR AND FINGER RESTS IN ANTERIOR SEXTANTS

Student: ______________________________
Date: ______________________________

Area 1 = mandibular anteriors, facial aspect
Area 2 = mandibular anteriors, lingual aspect
Area 3 = maxillary anteriors, facial aspect
Area 4 = maxillary anteriors, lingual aspect

DIRECTIONS: Self-evaluate your skill level in each treatment area as: **S** (satisfactory) or **U** (unsatisfactory).

Criteria				
Positioning/Ergonomics	**Area 1**	**Area 2**	**Area 3**	**Area 4**
Adjusts clinician chair correctly				
Reclines patient chair and ensures that patient's head is even with top of headrest				
Positions instrument tray within easy reach for front, side, or rear delivery as appropriate for operatory configuration				
Positions unit light at arm's length or dons dental headlight and adjusts it for use				
Assumes the recommended clock position				
Positions backrest of patient chair for the specified arch and adjusts height of patient chair so that clinician's elbows remain at waist level when accessing the specified treatment area				
Asks patient to assume the head position that facilitates the clinician's view of the specified treatment area				
Maintains neutral position				
Directs light to illuminate the specified treatment area				
Instrument Grasp: Dominant Hand	**Area 1**	**Area 2**	**Area 3**	**Area 4**
Grasps handle with tips of finger pads of index finger and thumb so that these fingers are opposite each other on the handle, but do NOT touch or overlap				
Rests pad of middle finger lightly on instrument shank; middle finger makes contact with ring finger				
Positions the thumb, index, and middle fingers in the "knuckles-up" convex position; hyperextended joint position is avoided				
Holds ring finger straight so that it supports the weight of hand and instrument; ring finger position is "advanced ahead of" the other fingers in the grasp				
Keeps index, middle, ring, and little fingers in contact; "like fingers inside a mitten"				
Maintains a relaxed grasp; fingers are NOT blanched in grasp				
Finger Rest: Dominant Hand	**Area 1**	**Area 2**	**Area 3**	**Area 4**
Establishes secure finger rest that is appropriate for tooth to be treated				
Once finger rest is established, pauses to self-evaluate finger placement in the grasp, verbalizes to evaluator his/her self-assessment of grasp, and corrects finger placement if necessary				

Note to Course Instructors:
To download Module Evaluations for this textbook, go to http://thepoint.lww.com/GehrigFundamentals7e and log on to access the Instructor Resources for *Fundamentals of Periodontal Instrumentation and Advanced Root Instrumentation*.

Module 5

Mirror and Finger Rests in Mandibular Posterior Sextants

Module Overview

This module describes techniques for using a dental mirror and finger rests in the mandibular posterior treatment areas. The fulcrum improves the precision of instrumentation strokes, prevents sudden movements that could injure the patient, and reduces muscle load to the clinician's hand.[1–5]

Module Outline

Key Terms: Review these Key Terms from Chapter 4.

Neutral wrist position
Fulcrum
Support beam
Finger rest
Extraoral fulcrum
Intraoral fulcrum
Finger-on-finger fulcrum

Learning Objectives

1. Position equipment so that it enhances neutral positioning.
2. Maintain neutral positioning when practicing finger rests in the mandibular posterior sextants.
3. While seated in the correct clock position for the treatment area, access the mandibular posterior teeth with optimum vision while maintaining neutral positioning.
4. Demonstrate correct mirror use, grasp, and finger rest in each of the mandibular posterior sextants while maintaining neutral positioning of your wrist.
5. Demonstrate finger rests using precise finger placement on the handle of a periodontal instrument:
   - Finger pads of thumb and index finger are opposite one another on handle.
   - Thumb and index finger do not overlap each other on the handle.
   - Pad of middle finger rests lightly on the shank.
   - Thumb, index, and middle fingers are in a "knuckles-up" position.
   - Ring finger is straight and supports weight of the hand.
6. Recognize incorrect mirror use, grasp, or finger rest and describe how to correct the problem(s).
7. Understand the relationship between proper stabilization of the dominant hand during instrumentation and the prevention of (1) musculoskeletal problems in the clinician's hands and (2) injury to the patient.
8. Understand the relationship between the large motor skills, such as positioning, and small motor skills, such as finger rests. Recognize the importance of initiating these skills in a step-by-step manner.

Section 1
Building Blocks for Posterior Sextants

BUILDING BLOCKS FROM POSITION TO FINGER REST

Precise, accurate performance of the building block skills is essential if periodontal instrumentation is to be effective, efficient, safe for the patient, and comfortable for the clinician.

- Research on psychomotor skill acquisition indicates that a high level of mastery in the performance of skill building blocks is essential to successful mastery of periodontal instrumentation.
- The building block skills are the foundation that "supports" successful periodontal instrumentation.
- While practicing finger rests, it is important to complete each of the skills listed in Figure 5-1 in sequence.

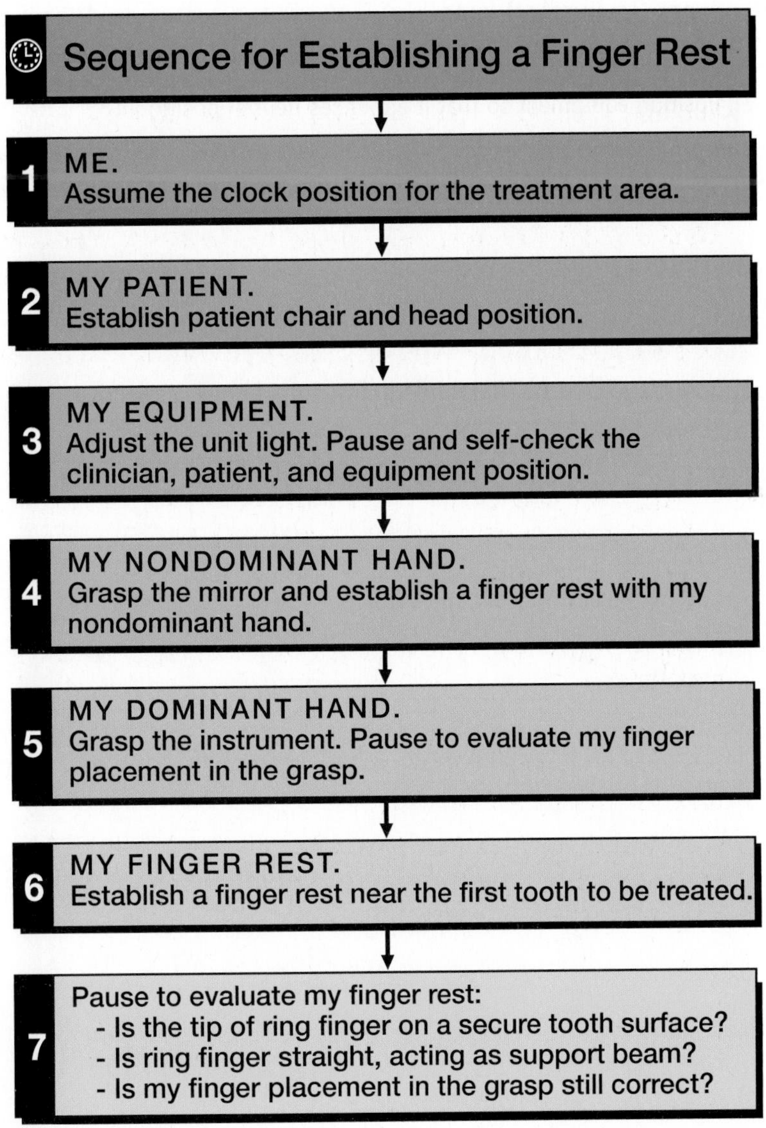
Sequence for Establishing a Finger Rest
1
ME.
Assume the clock position for the treatment area.
2
MY PATIENT.
Establish patient chair and head position.
3
MY EQUIPMENT.
Adjust the unit light. Pause and self-check the clinician, patient, and equipment position.
4
MY NONDOMINANT HAND.
Grasp the mirror and establish a finger rest with my nondominant hand.
5
MY DOMINANT HAND.
Grasp the instrument. Pause to evaluate my finger placement in the grasp.
6
MY FINGER REST.
Establish a finger rest near the first tooth to be treated.
7
Pause to evaluate my finger rest:
- Is the tip of ring finger on a secure tooth surface?
- Is ring finger straight, acting as support beam?
- Is my finger placement in the grasp still correct?

Figure 5-1. Establishing a Finger Rest. When establishing a finger rest, it is important to proceed in the small, explicit steps outlined in this flow chart.[6]

Directions for Technique Practice:

1. The photographs for this technique practice depict the use of a mirror and finger rests in the mandibular posterior treatment areas. Some photographs were taken on a patient. Others were taken using a manikin and without gloves so that you can easily see the finger placement in the grasp.
2. The photographs provide a *general guideline* for finger rests; however, the location of your own finger rest depends on the size and length of your fingers. You may need to fulcrum closer to or farther from the tooth being treated than is shown in the photograph.
3. Focus your attention on mastering mirror use, wrist position, and the finger rests. Use the following instruments in this module:
   - **For your nondominant (mirror) hand**—Use a dental mirror.
   - **For your dominant (instrument) hand**—(a) Remove the mirror head from one of your dental mirrors and use the mirror handle as if it were a periodontal instrument, or (b) use a periodontal probe to represent the periodontal instrument in this module.
4. *Do not wear magnification loupes for this technique practice. It is important to have a view of the patient's head and your hands and wrists when learning finger rests.*

Note: The technique practice for LEFT-Handed clinicians begins in Section 3 on page 143.

Section 2
Technique Practice: RIGHT-Handed Clinician

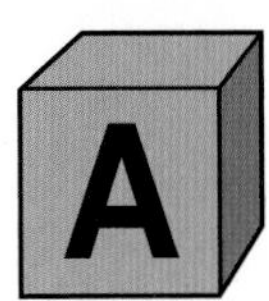

SKILL BUILDING. USING THE MIRROR FOR RETRACTION

Directions: Practice retracting the cheek by referring to Figures 5-2 and 5-3.

Retracting the buccal mucosa away from the facial surfaces of the posterior teeth can be a challenging task, especially if your patient tenses his or her cheek muscles. It is a good idea to practice the retraction technique before attempting the posterior finger rests.

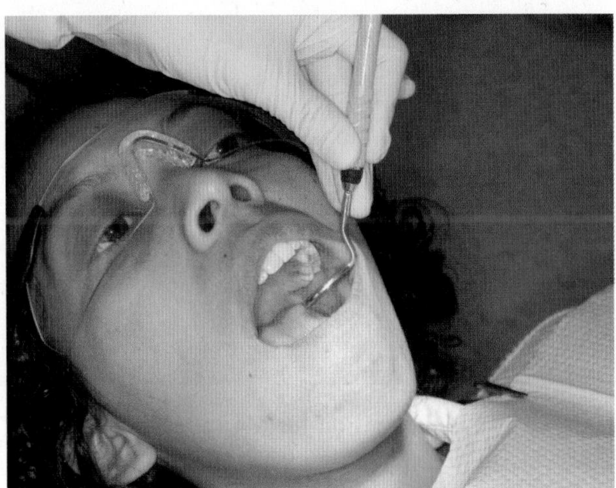

Figure 5-2. Step 1.

1. Assume a 10 to 11 o'clock position for the facial aspect of the mandibular left posteriors.
2. Grasp the mirror in your nondominant hand.
3. Place the mirror head between the dental arches with the reflecting surface parallel to the maxillary occlusal surfaces ("Frisbee-style").
4. Slide the mirror back until it is in line with the second molar.

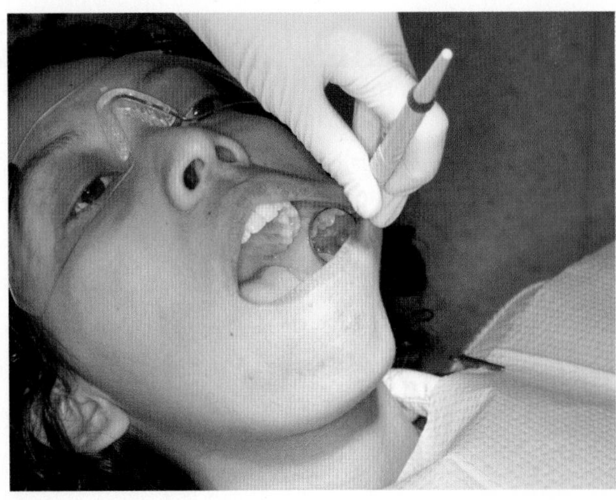

Figure 5-3. Step 2.

5. Position the mirror by turning the mirror handle until the mirror head is parallel to the buccal mucosa. The back of the mirror head rests against the buccal mucosa, and the mirror's reflecting surface is facing the facial surfaces of the teeth.
6. Establish an extraoral finger rest on the side of the patient's cheek.
7. Use your arm muscles for retraction. Pulling with only your finger muscles is a difficult and tiring way to retract the cheek.

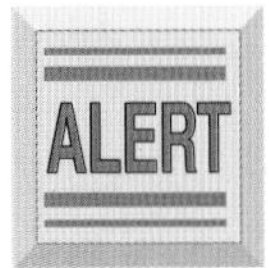

Avoid hitting the mirror head against the patient's teeth or resting the outer rim of the mirror head against the patient's gingival tissues.

Do not use the instrument shank for retraction. Retracting in this manner will be uncomfortable for your patient.

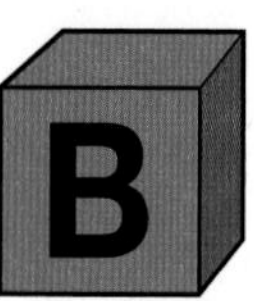

SKILL BUILDING. MANDIBULAR POSTERIOR SEXTANTS, ASPECTS FACING TOWARD

Directions: Practice establishing a finger rest for the mandibular posterior teeth, aspects facing toward, by referring to Figures 5-4 to 5-11.

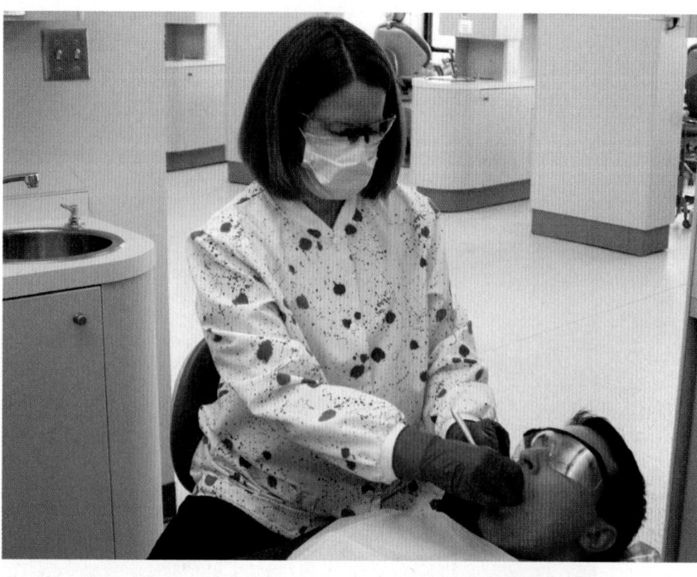

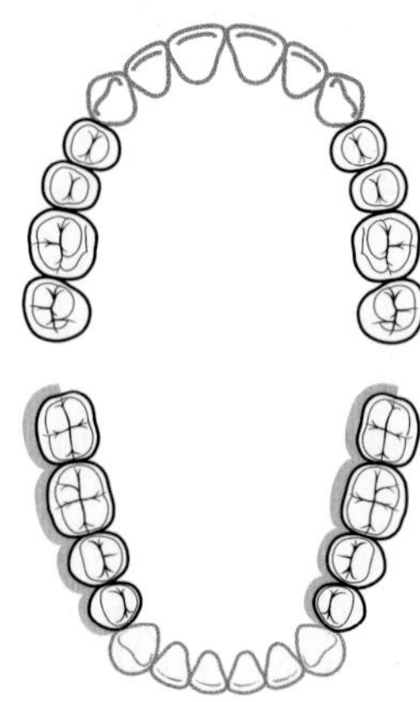

Figure 5-4. Clock Position for Mandibular Posterior Teeth, Aspects Facing Toward the Clinician. The clinician's clock position for the mandibular posterior aspects toward the clinician is the 9 o'clock position. The patient should be in a chin-down head position.

Box 5-1. Handle Positions for Mandibular Posterior Teeth

1. Hold the hand in a palm-down position.
2. Rest the handle against the index finger somewhere in the green shaded area.

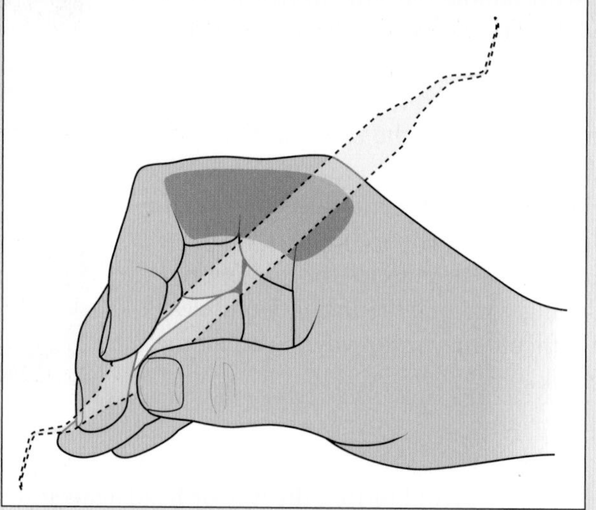

Figure 5-5. Handle Positions for Mandibular Posterior Treatment Areas.

Mandibular Right Posterior Sextant, Facial Aspect

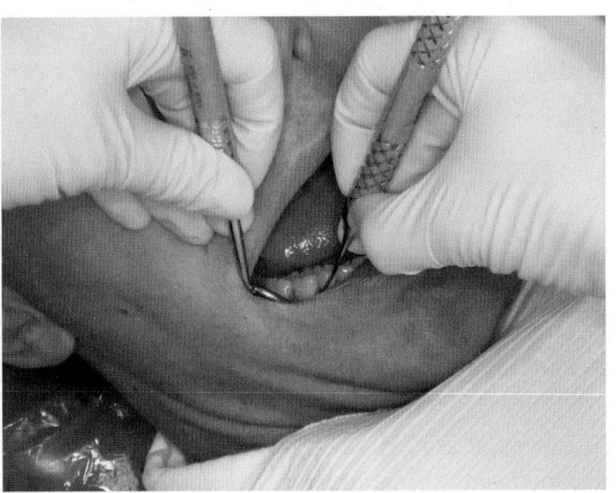

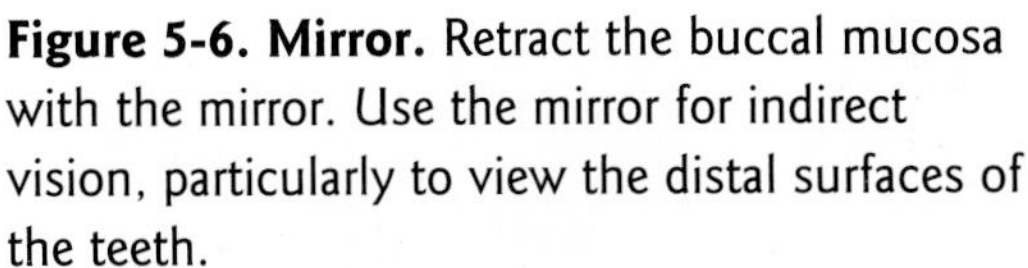

Figure 5-6. Mirror. Retract the buccal mucosa with the mirror. Use the mirror for indirect vision, particularly to view the distal surfaces of the teeth.

Note that the clinician pictured here is using an extraoral finger rest for the mouth mirror.

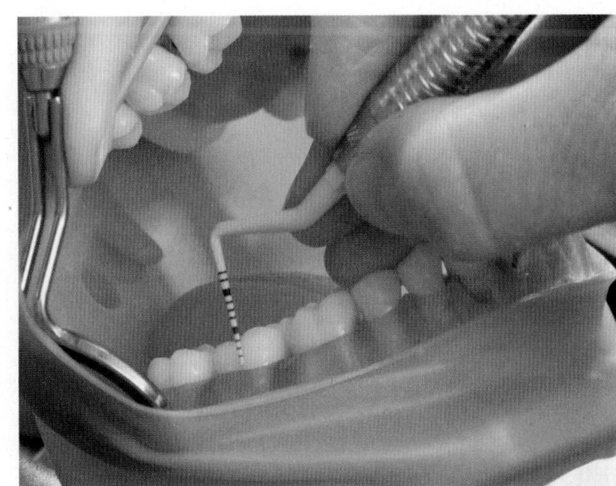

Figure 5-7. Task 1—Second Molar, Facial Aspect. Finger rest on an occlusal surface.

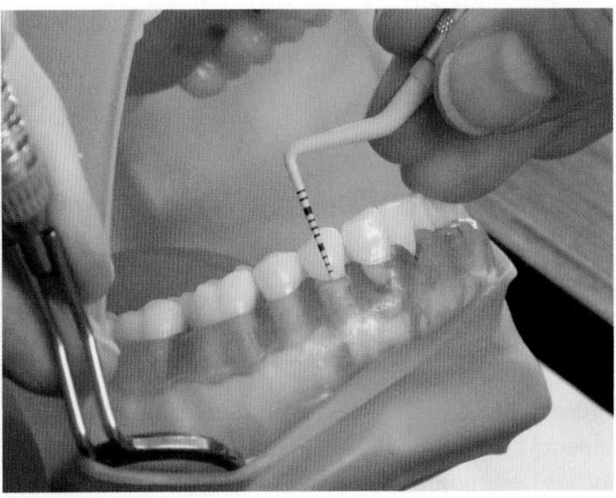

Figure 5-8. Task 2—First Premolar, Facial Aspect. Finger rest on an incisal surface of one of the mandibular anteriors.

Mandibular Left Posterior Sextant, Lingual Aspect

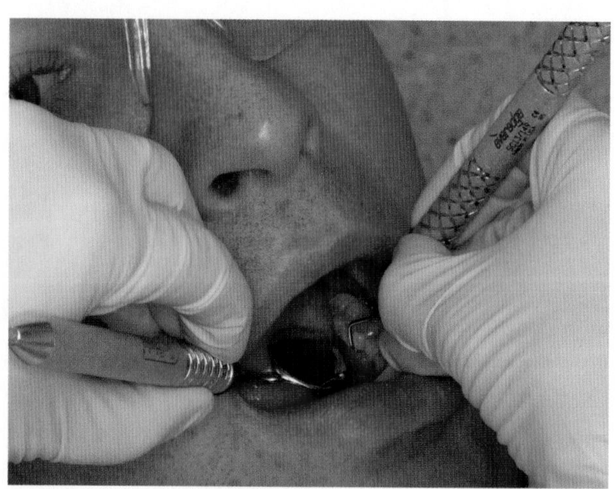

Figure 5-9. Mirror. Use the mirror to gently move the tongue away from the teeth, toward the midline of the mouth. Once in position, the mirror is also used for indirect vision of the tooth surfaces.

Tip: Avoid pressing down against the floor of the mouth with the mirror head.

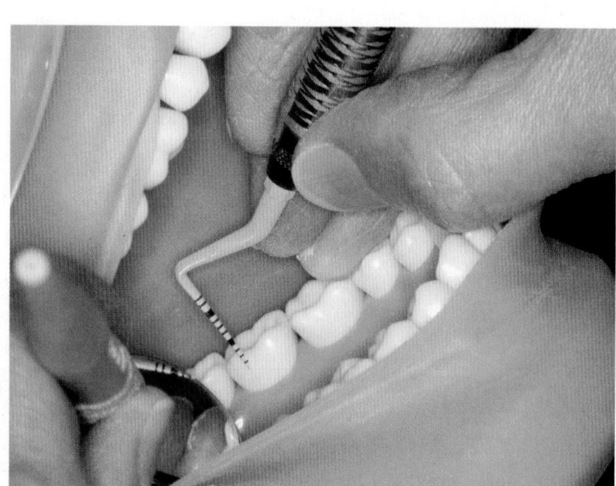

Figure 5-10. Task 1—Second Molar, Lingual Aspect. Finger rest on an occlusofacial line angle.

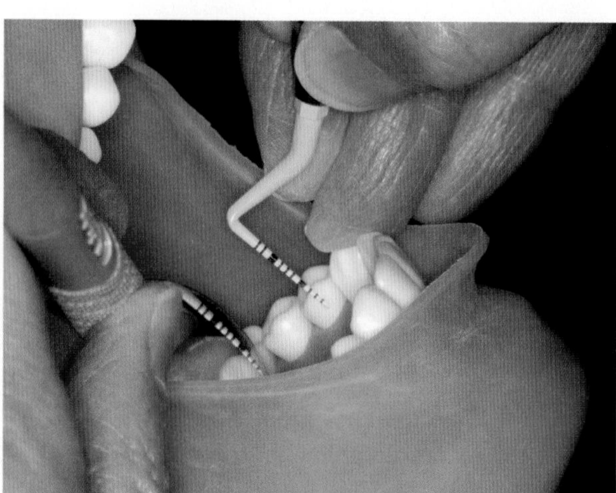

Figure 5-11. Task 2—First Premolar, Lingual Aspect. Finger rest on an incisal edge of one of the mandibular anterior teeth.

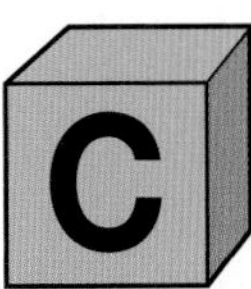

SKILL BUILDING. MANDIBULAR POSTERIOR SEXTANTS, ASPECTS FACING AWAY

Directions: Practice establishing a finger rest for the mandibular posterior teeth, aspects facing away, by referring to Figures 5-12 to 5-19.

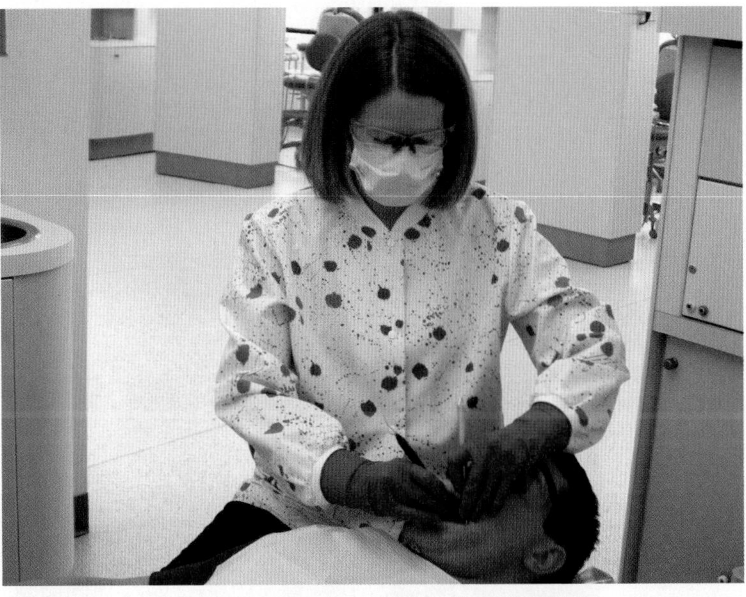

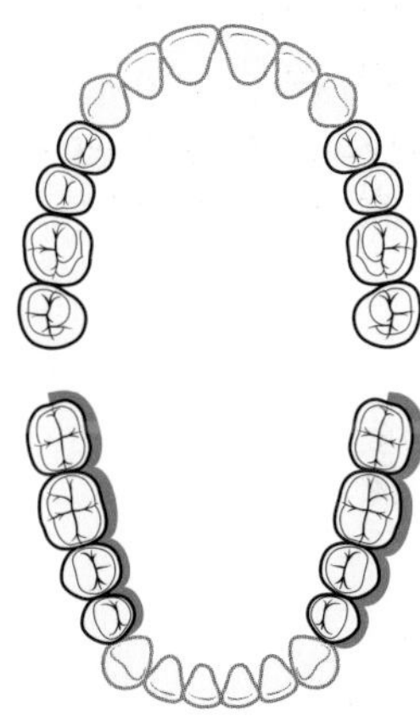

Figure 5-12. Clock Position for Mandibular Posterior Teeth, Aspects Facing Away from the Clinician. The clinician's clock position for the mandibular posterior aspects facing away from the clinician is a 10 to 11 o'clock position. The patient should be in a chin-down head position.

Box 5-2. Handle Positions for Mandibular Posterior Teeth

1. Hold the hand in a palm-down position.
2. Rest the handle against the index finger somewhere in the green shaded area.

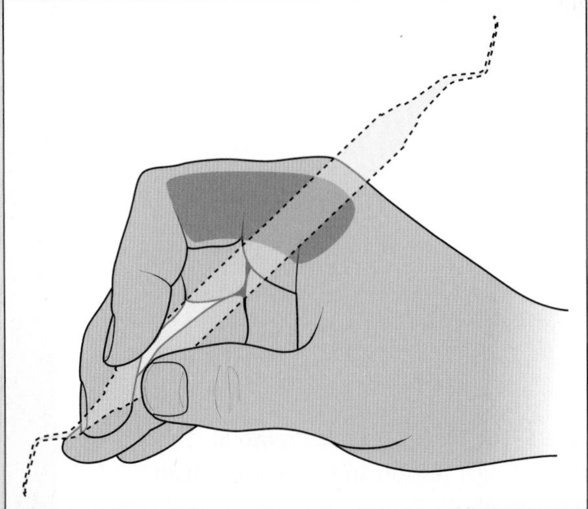

Figure 5-13. Handle Positions for Mandibular Posterior Treatment Areas.

Mandibular Left Posterior Sextant, Facial Aspect

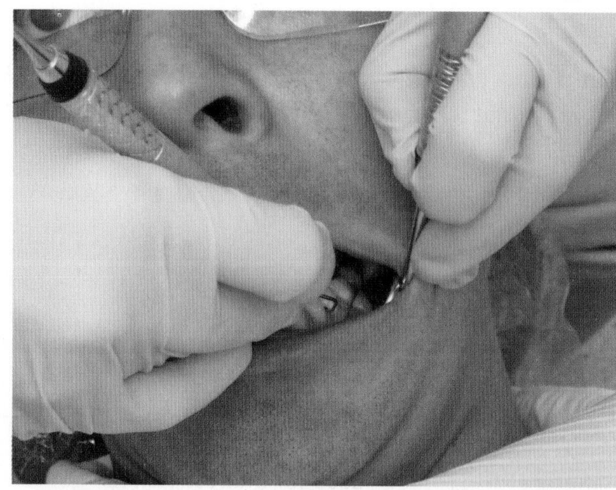

Figure 5-14. Retraction. Use the mirror to retract the buccal mucosa down and away from the teeth.

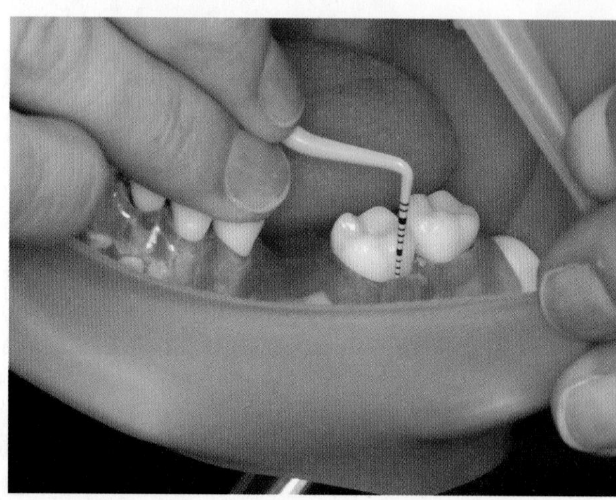

Figure 5-15. Task 1—Second Molar, Facial Aspect. Finger rest on an occlusofacial line angle.

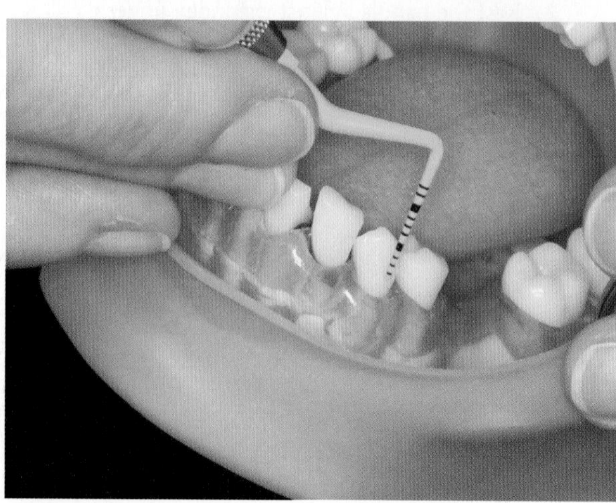

Figure 5-16. Task 2—First Premolar, Facial Aspect. Finger rest on an incisal edge of an anterior tooth.

Mandibular Right Posterior Sextant, Lingual Aspect

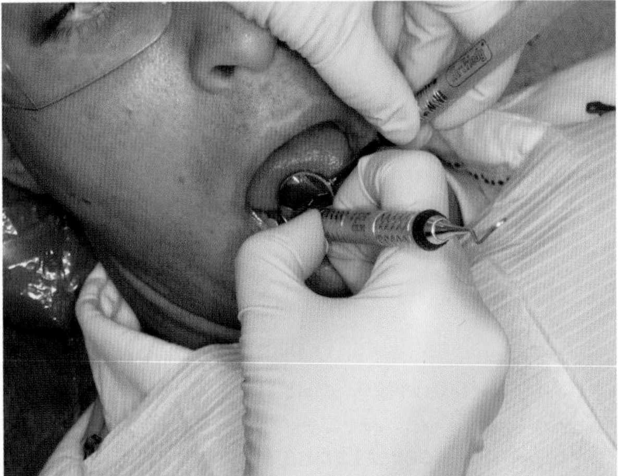

Figure 5-17. Mirror. Use the mirror head to push the tongue back gently so that the lingual surfaces of the teeth can be seen. Once in position, the mirror is also used for indirect vision.

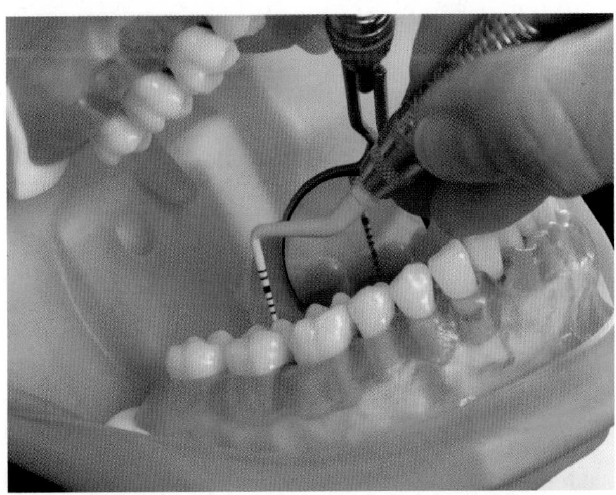

Figure 5-18. Task 1—Second Molar, Lingual Aspect. Finger rest on an occlusal surface.

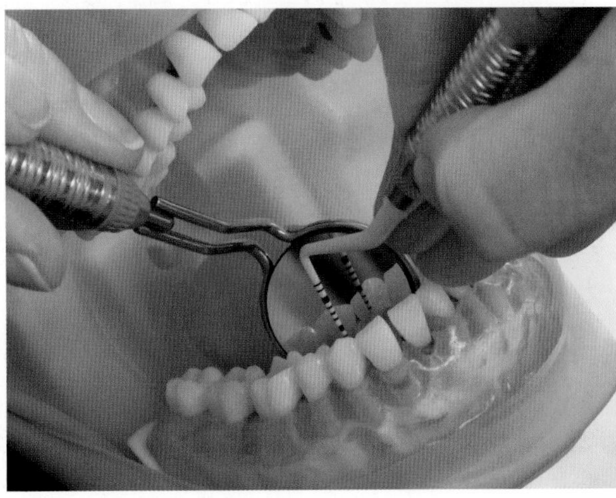

Figure 5-19. Task 2—First Premolar, Lingual Aspect. Finger rest on an incisal edge of an anterior tooth.

REFERENCE SHEET FOR MANDIBULAR POSTERIOR SEXTANTS (RIGHT-HANDED CLINICIANS)

Photocopy this reference sheet and use it for quick reference as you practice your skills. Place the photocopied reference sheet in a plastic page protector for longer use.

TABLE 5-1. Reference Sheet: Mandibular Posterior Sextants

Treatment Area	Clock Position	Patient's Head
Posterior Aspects Facing Toward (Right Posterior, Facial Aspect) (Left Posterior, Lingual Aspect)	9:00	Straight or slightly away Chin DOWN
Posterior Aspects Facing Away (Right Posterior, Lingual Aspect) (Left Posterior, Facial Aspect)	10:00–11:00	Toward Chin DOWN

Note: This ends the section for RIGHT-Handed clinicians. Turn to page 151 for Section 4 of this module.

Section 3
Technique Practice: LEFT-Handed Clinician

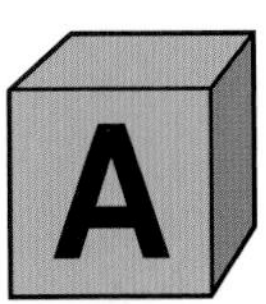

SKILL BUILDING. USING THE MIRROR FOR RETRACTION

Directions: Practice retracting the cheek by referring to Figures 5-20 and 5-21.
Retracting the buccal mucosa away from the facial surfaces of the posterior teeth can be a challenging task, especially if your patient tenses his or her cheek muscles. It is a good idea to practice the retraction technique before attempting the posterior finger rests.

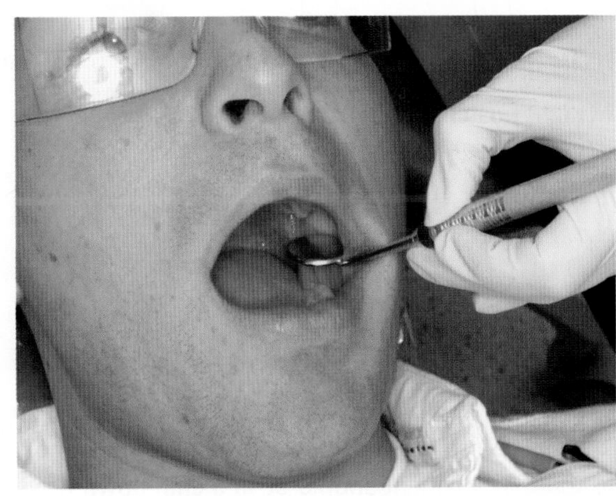

Figure 5-20. Step 1.

1. Assume a 1 to 2 o'clock position for the facial aspect of the mandibular right posteriors.
2. Grasp the mirror in your nondominant hand.
3. Place the mirror head between the dental arches with the reflecting surface parallel to the maxillary occlusal surfaces ("Frisbee-style").
4. Slide the mirror back until it is in line with the second molar.

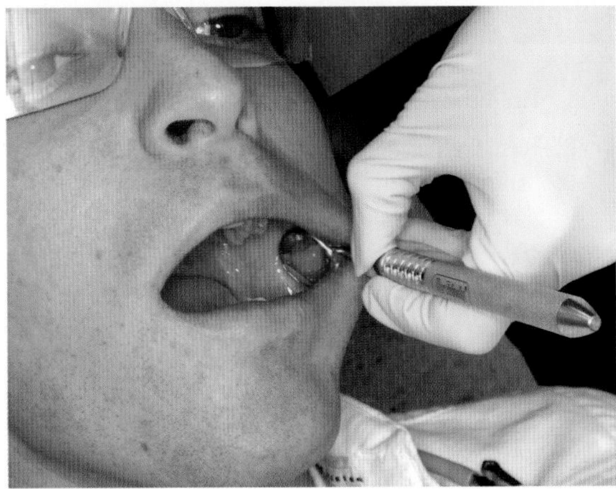

Figure 5-21. Step 2.

5. Position the mirror by turning the mirror handle until the mirror head is parallel to the buccal mucosa. The back of the mirror head is against the buccal mucosa, and the mirror's reflecting surface is facing the facial surfaces of the teeth.
6. Establish an extraoral finger rest on the side of the patient's cheek.
7. Use your arm muscles for retraction. Pulling with only your finger muscles is a difficult and tiring way to retract the cheek.

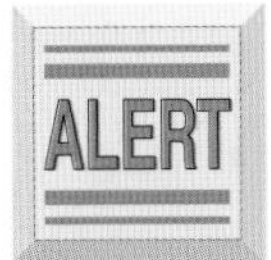

Avoid hitting the mirror head against the patient's teeth or resting the outer rim of the mirror head against the patient's gingival tissues.
Do not use the instrument shank for retraction. Retracting in this manner will be uncomfortable for your patient.

LEFT-Handed Clinician

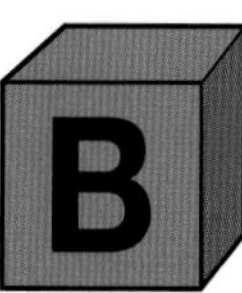

SKILL BUILDING. MANDIBULAR POSTERIOR SEXTANTS, ASPECTS FACING TOWARD

Directions: Practice establishing a finger rest for the mandibular posterior teeth, aspects facing toward, by referring to Figures 5-22 to 5-29.

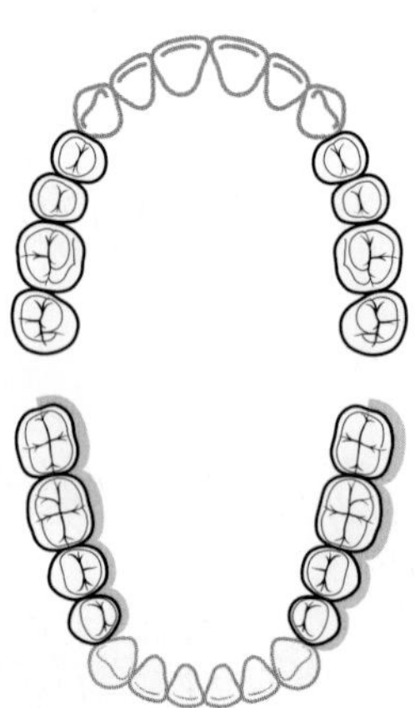

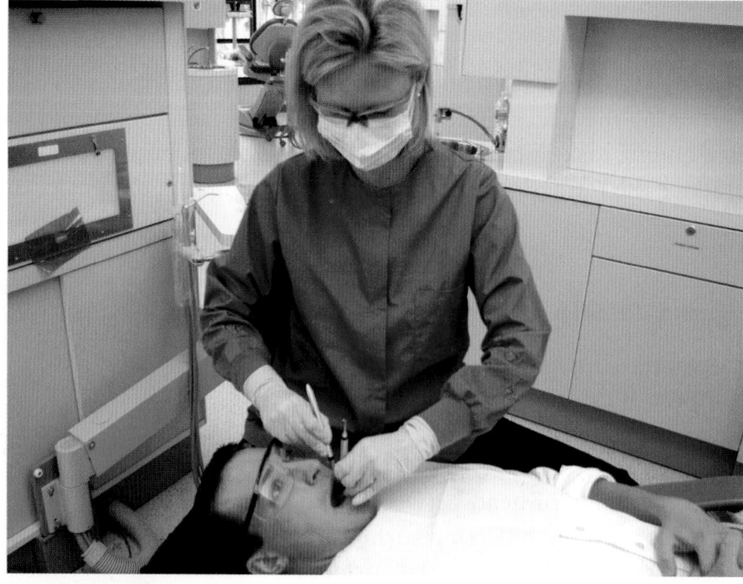

Figure 5-22. Clock Position for Mandibular Posterior Teeth, Aspects Facing Toward the Clinician. The clinician's clock position for the mandibular posterior aspects toward the clinician is the 3 o'clock position. The patient should be in a chin-down head position.

Box 5-3. Handle Positions for Mandibular Posterior Teeth

1. Hold the hand in a palm-down position.
2. Rest the handle against the index finger somewhere in the green shaded area.

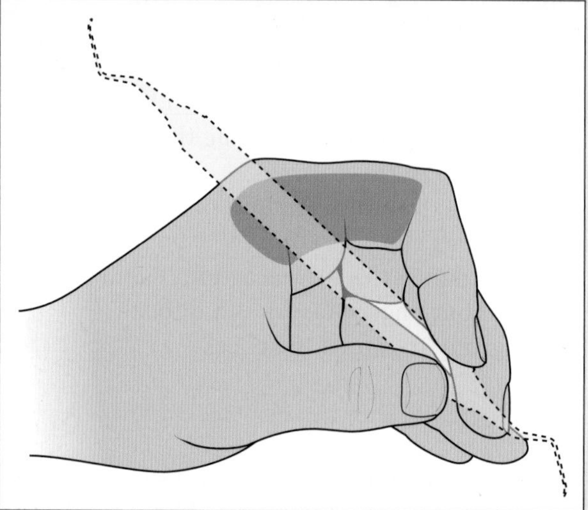

Figure 5-23. Handle Positions for Mandibular Posterior Treatment Areas.

Mandibular Left Posterior Sextant, Facial Aspect

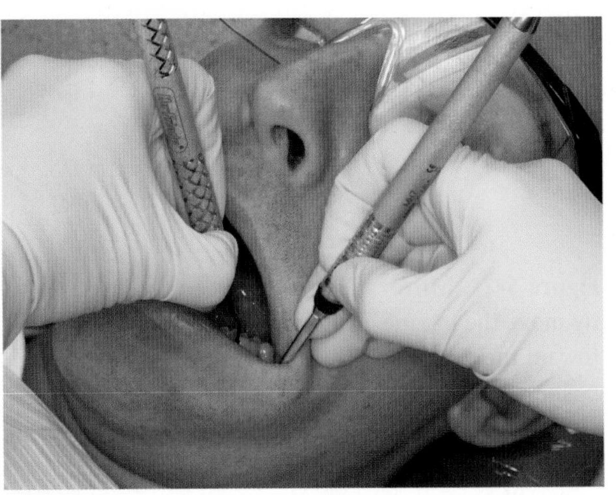

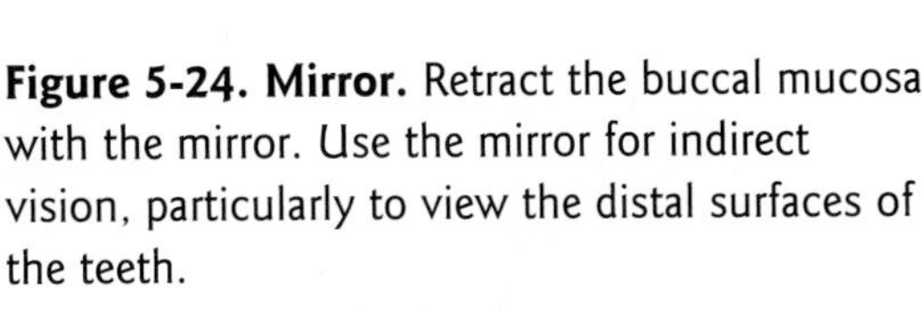

Figure 5-24. Mirror. Retract the buccal mucosa with the mirror. Use the mirror for indirect vision, particularly to view the distal surfaces of the teeth.

Note that the clinician pictured here is using an extraoral finger rest with the mouth mirror.

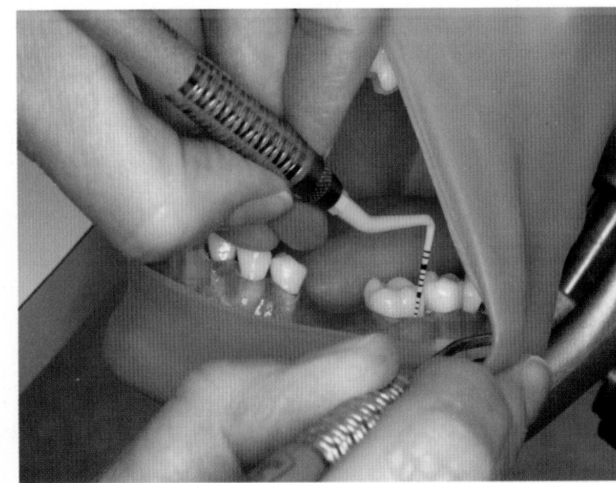

Figure 5-25. Task 1—Second Molar, Facial Aspect. Finger rest on an occlusal surface.

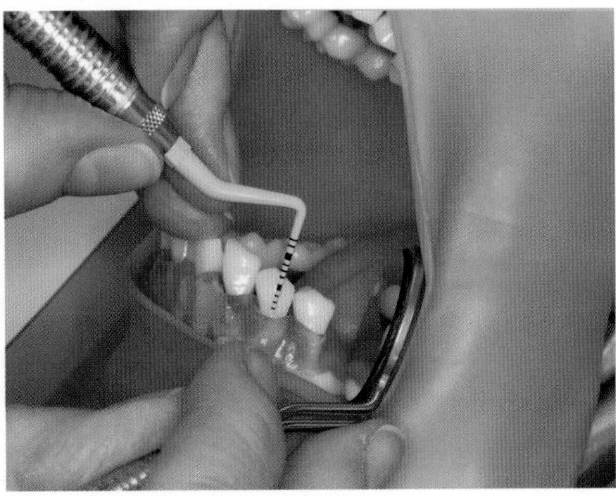

Figure 5-26. Task 2—First Premolar, Facial Aspect. Finger rest on an incisal surface of one of the mandibular anteriors.

Mandibular Right Posterior Sextant, Lingual Aspect

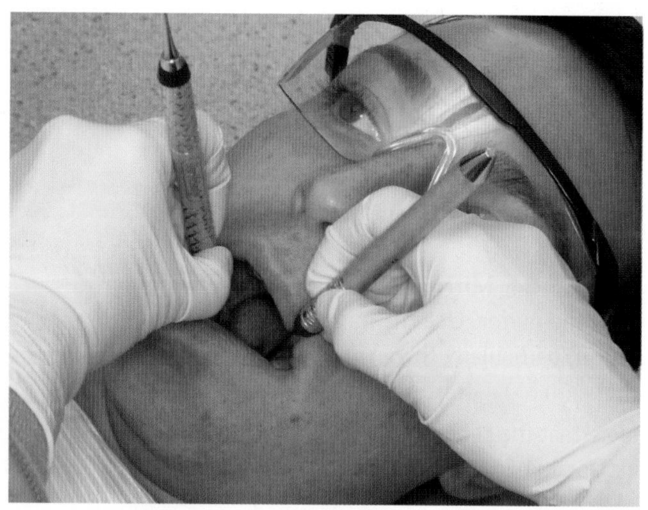

Figure 5-27. Mirror. Use the mirror to gently move the tongue away from the teeth, toward the midline of the mouth. Once in position, the mirror is also used for indirect vision of the tooth surfaces.

Tip: Avoid pressing down against the floor of the mouth with the mirror head.

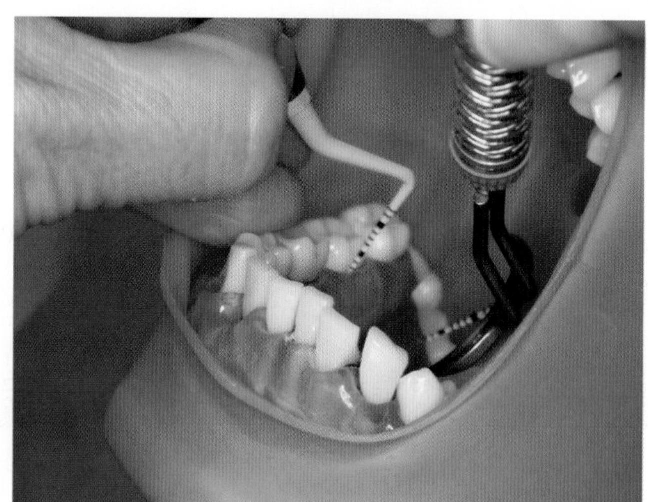

Figure 5-28. Task 1—Second Molar, Lingual Aspect. Finger rest on an occlusofacial line angle.

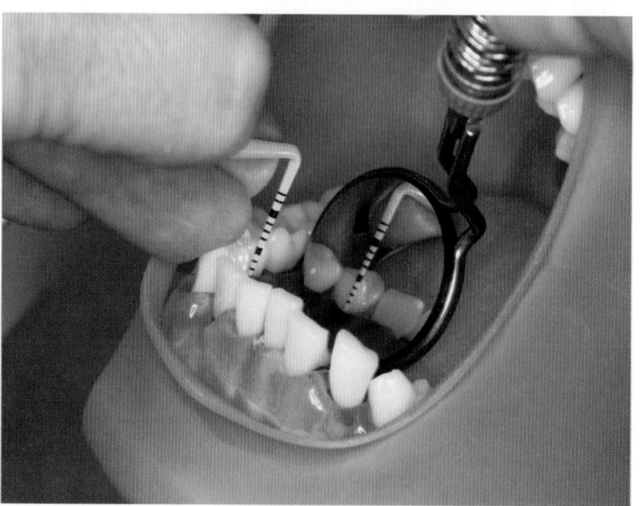

Figure 5-29. Task 2—First Premolar, Lingual Aspect. Finger rest on an incisal edge of one of the mandibular anterior teeth.

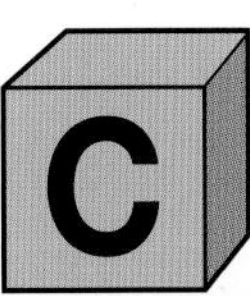

SKILL BUILDING. MANDIBULAR POSTERIOR SEXTANTS, ASPECTS FACING AWAY

Directions: Practice establishing a finger rest for the mandibular posterior teeth, aspects facing away, by referring to Figures 5-30 to 5-37.

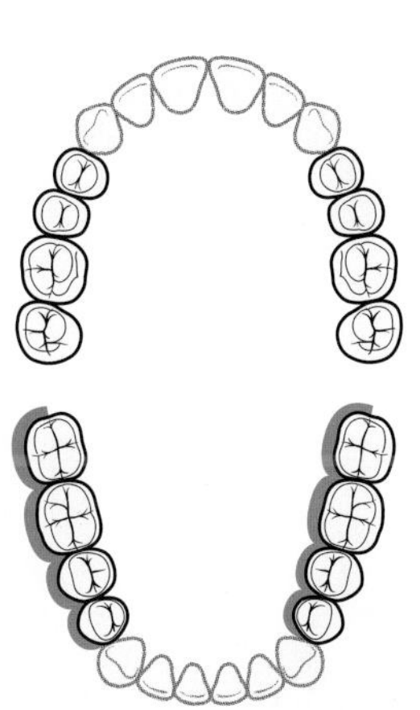

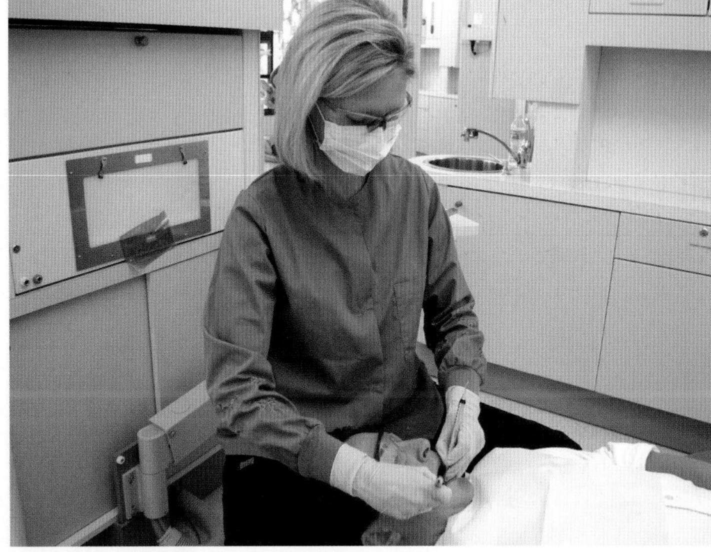

Figure 5-30. Clock Position for Mandibular Posterior Teeth, Aspects Facing Away from the Clinician. The clinician's clock position for the mandibular posterior aspects facing away from the clinician is a 1 to 2 o'clock position. The patient should be in a chin-down head position.

Box 5-4. Handle Positions for Mandibular Posterior Teeth

1. Hold the hand in a palm-down position.
2. Rest the handle against the index finger somewhere in the green shaded area.

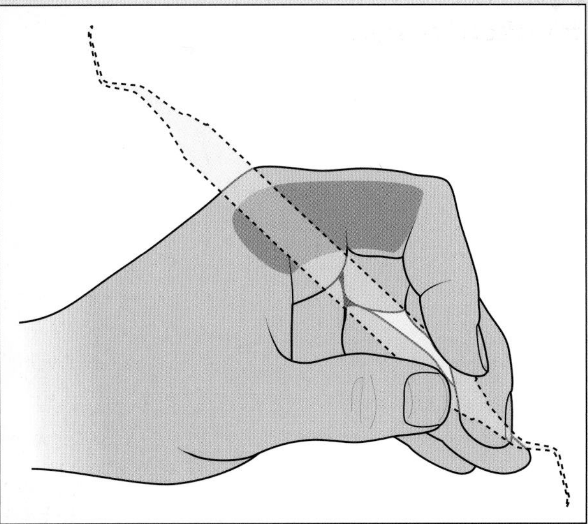

Figure 5-31. Handle Positions for Mandibular Posterior Treatment Areas.

Mandibular Right Posterior Sextant, Facial Aspect

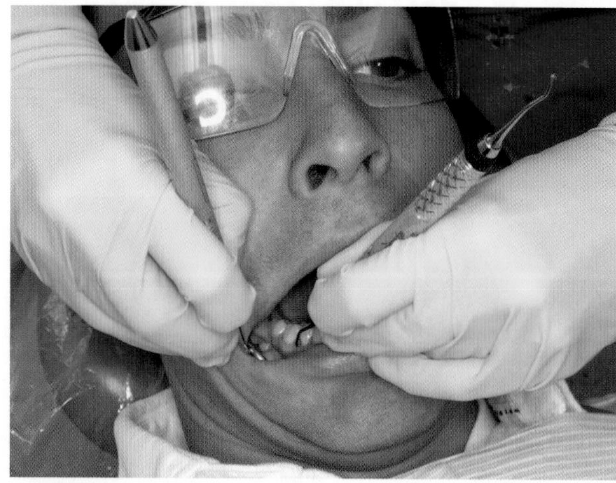

Figure 5-32. Retraction. Use the mirror to retract the buccal mucosa down and away from the teeth.

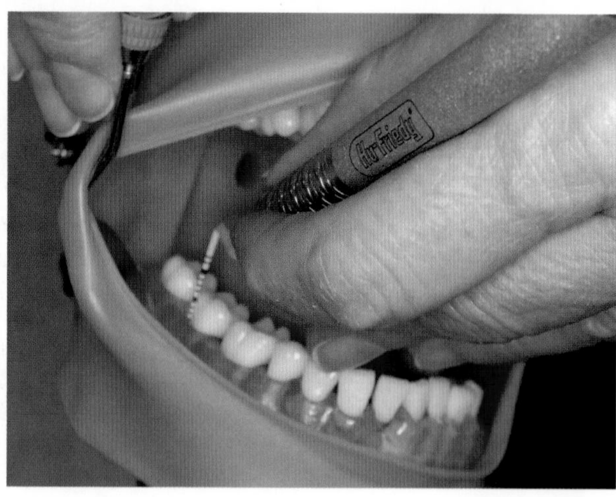

Figure 5-33. Task 1—Second Molar, Facial Aspect. Finger rest on an occlusofacial line angle.

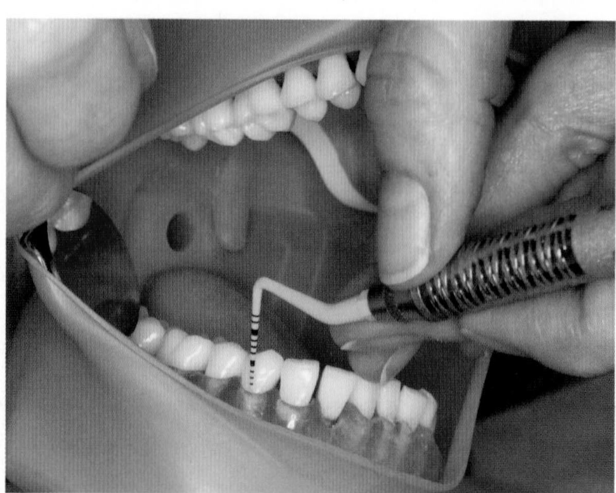

Figure 5-34. Task 2—First Premolar, Facial Aspect. Finger rest on an incisal surface of one of the mandibular anterior teeth.

Mandibular Left Posterior Sextant, Lingual Aspect

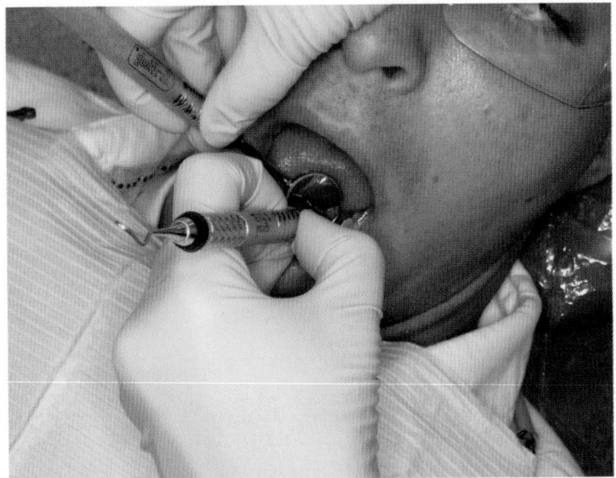

Figure 5-35. Mirror. Use the mirror head to push the tongue back gently so that the lingual surfaces of the teeth can be seen. Once in position, the mirror is also used for indirect vision.

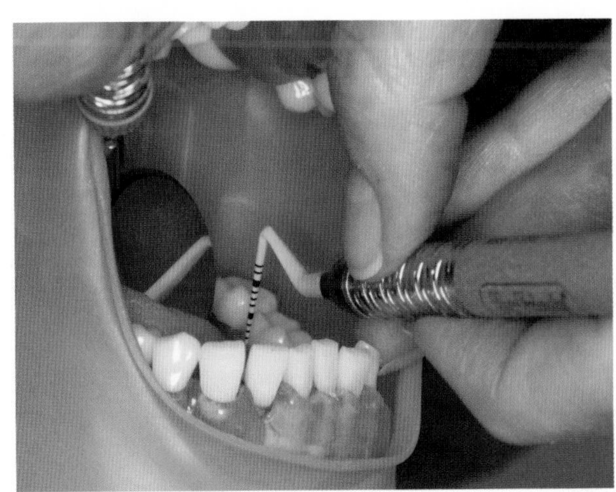

Figure 5-36. Task 1—Second Molar, Lingual Aspect. Finger rest on an occlusal surface.

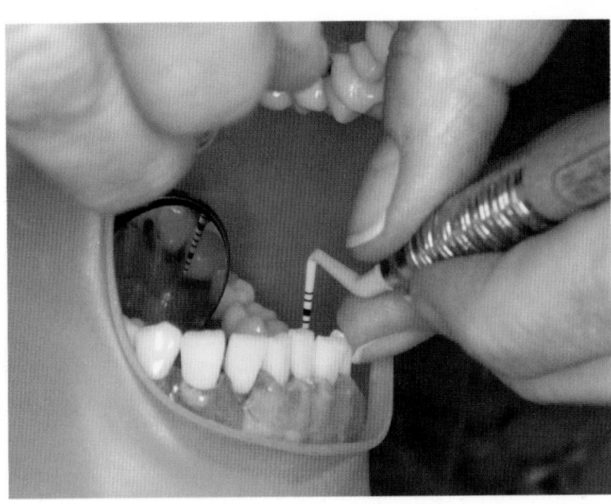

Figure 5-37. Task 2—First Premolar, Lingual Aspect. Finger rest on an incisal edge of an anterior tooth.

REFERENCE SHEET FOR MANDIBULAR POSTERIOR SEXTANTS (LEFT-HANDED CLINICIANS)

Photocopy this reference sheet and use it for quick reference as you practice your skills. Place the photocopied reference sheet in a plastic page protector for longer use.

TABLE 5-2. Reference Sheet: Mandibular Posterior Sextants

Treatment Area	Clock Position	Patient's Head
Posterior Aspects Facing Toward (Left Posterior, Facial Aspect) (Right Posterior, Lingual Aspect)	3:00	Straight or slightly away Chin DOWN
Posterior Aspects Facing Away (Left Posterior, Lingual Aspect) (Right Posterior, Facial Aspect)	1:00–2:00	Toward Chin DOWN

Section 4
Alternate Clock Positions and Finger Rests

After mastering the basic skills of clinician position and fulcruming techniques, variations of these basic skills may be modified for use with treatment areas that are difficult to access.

- When the traditional clock positions for the mandibular arch have been mastered, it is possible to use an alternative seated position in certain circumstances. Alternate clock positions can facilitate access to root surfaces within deep periodontal pockets.
- In instances when a standard intraoral fulcrum does not seem to work well, a modified fulcruming technique can improve access to the tooth surface. For example, when working within a deep periodontal pocket, sometimes it is difficult to position the lower shank parallel to the root surface being treated. In such instances, modified fulcruming techniques are useful in obtaining parallelism.
- ***When employing alternate positioning or fulcruming techniques, the clinician should always maintain a neutral seated position and a neutral wrist position.***

Alternative techniques for the right-handed clinician begin on this page.
Alternate techniques for the left-handed clinician are on page 153.

ALTERNATE TECHNIQUES FOR THE RIGHT-HANDED CLINICIAN

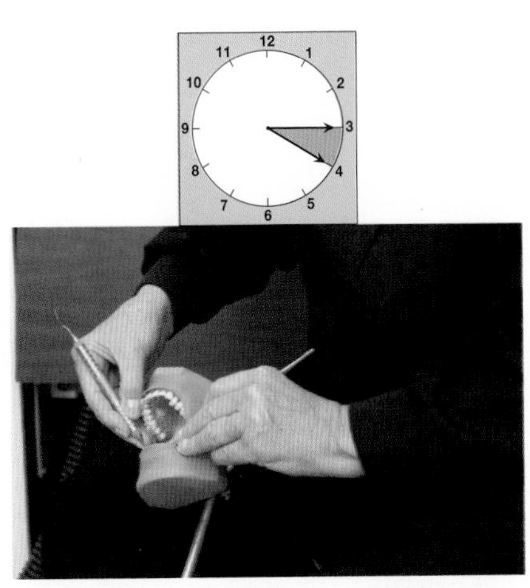

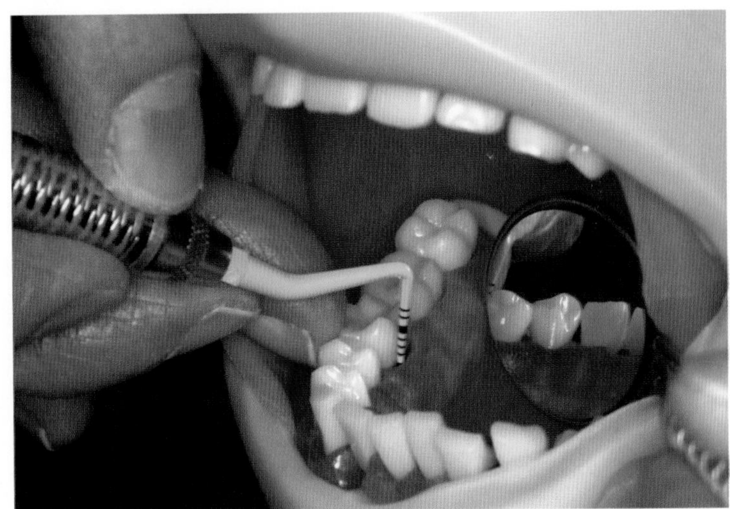

Figure 5-38. Mandibular Right Posteriors, Lingual Aspect.

- Alternate clock position is at 3 to 4 o'clock.
- Finger rest is a standard intraoral fulcrum.

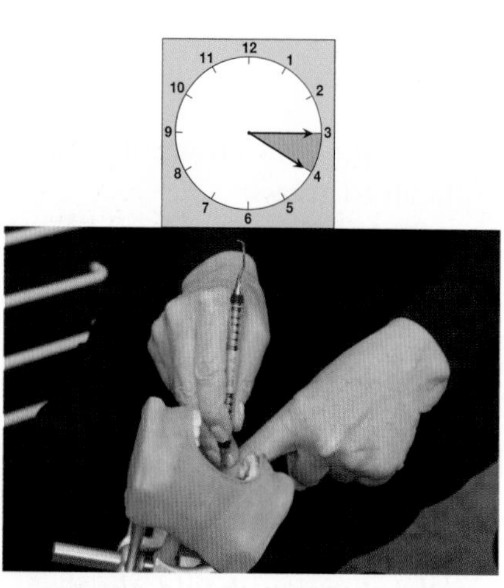

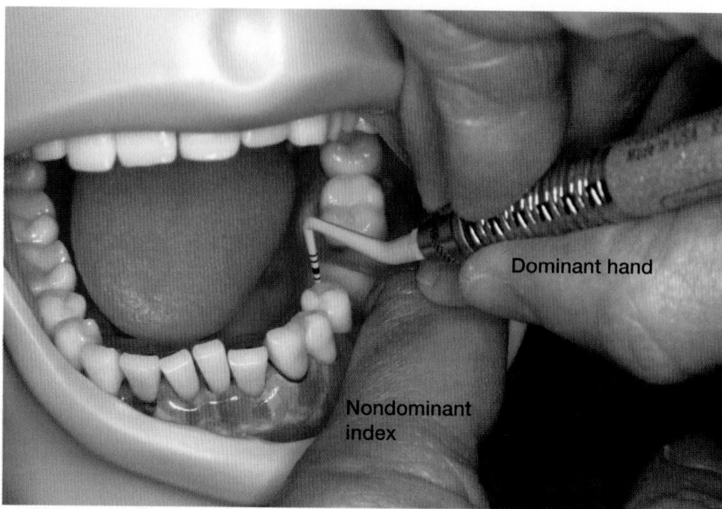

Figure 5-39. Mandibular Left Posteriors, Lingual Aspect.

- Alternate clock position is at 3 to 4 o'clock.
- Modified finger rest is a finger-on-finger fulcrum.

ALTERNATE TECHNIQUES FOR THE LEFT-HANDED CLINICIAN

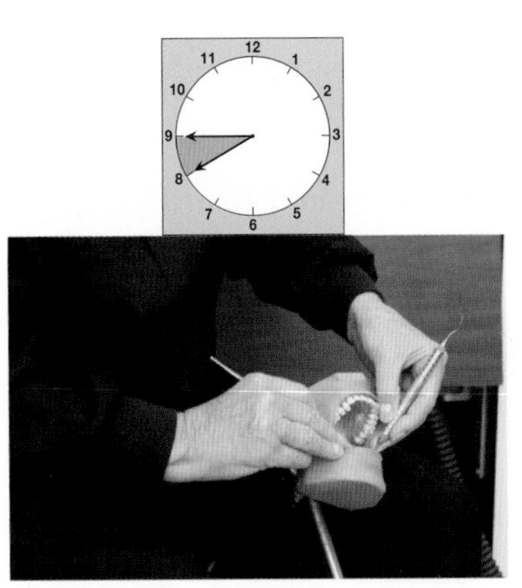

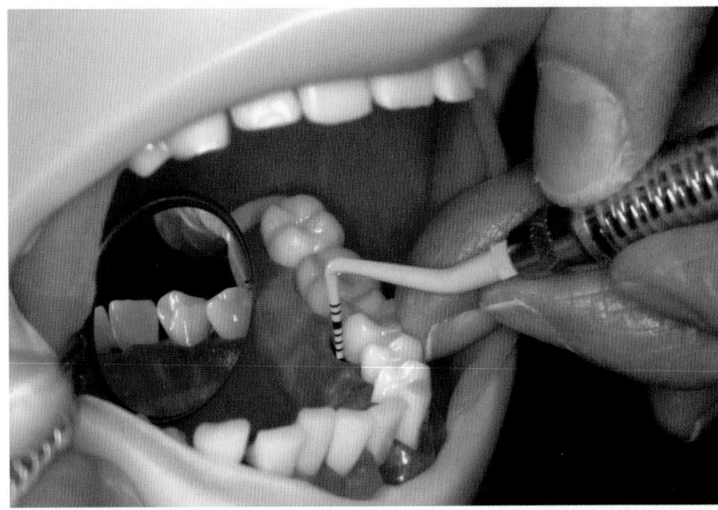

Figure 5-40. Mandibular Left Posteriors, Lingual Aspect.

- Alternate clock position is at 8 to 9 o'clock.
- Finger rest is a standard intraoral fulcrum.

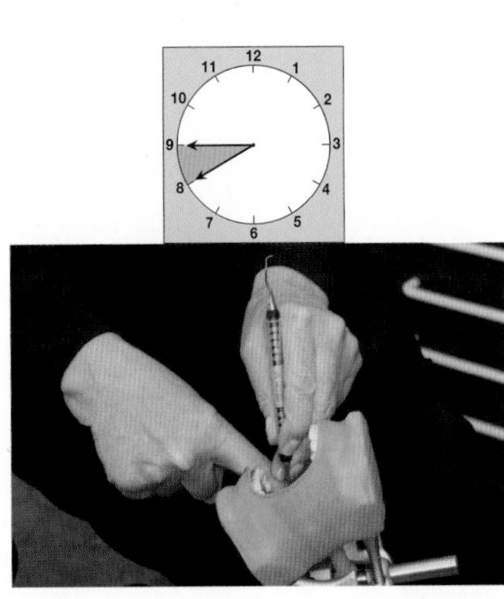

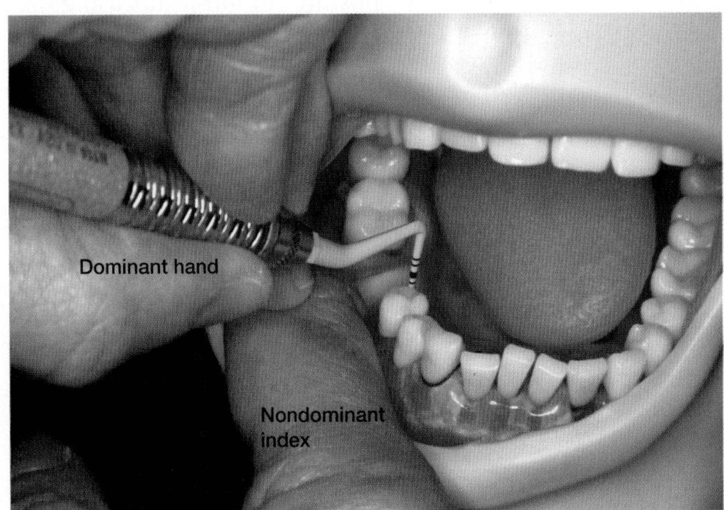

Figure 5-41. Mandibular Right Posteriors, Lingual Aspect.

- Alternate clock position is at 8 to 9 o'clock.
- Modified finger rest is a finger-on-finger fulcrum.

REFERENCES

1. Dong H, Barr A, Loomer P, Rempel D. The effects of finger rest positions on hand muscle load and pinch force in simulated dental hygiene work. *J Dent Educ*. 2005;69:453–460.
2. Dong H, Loomer P, Villanueva A, Rempel D. Pinch forces and instrument tip forces during periodontal scaling. *J Periodontol*. 2007;78:97–103.
3. Millar D. Reinforced periodontal instrumentation and ergonomics. The best practice to ensure optiminal performance and career longevity. *CDHA*. 2009;24:8–16.
4. Scaramucci M. Getting a grasp. *Dimen Dent Hyg*. 2008;6:24–26.
5. Meador HL. The biocentric technique: a guide to avoiding occupational pain. *J Dent Hyg*. 1993;67:38–51.
6. Hauser AM, Bowen DM. Primer on preclinical instruction and evaluation. *J Dent Educ*. 2009;73:390–398.

RECOMMENDED READING

Leonard DM. The effectiveness of intervention strategies used to educate clients about prevention of upper extremity cumulative trauma disorders. *Work*. 2000;14:151–157.

Liskiewicz ST, Kerschbaum WE. Cumulative trauma disorders: an ergonomic approach for prevention. *J Dent Hyg*. 1997;71:162–167.

Marcoux BC, Krause V, Nieuwenhuijsen ER. Effectiveness of an educational intervention to increase knowledge and reduce use of risky behaviors associated with cumulative trauma in office workers. *Work*. 2000;14:127–135.

Michalak-Turcotte C. Controlling dental hygiene work-related musculoskeletal disorders: the ergonomic process. *J Dent Hyg*. 2000;74:41–48.

Sugawara E. The study of wrist postures of musicians using the WristSystem (Greenleaf Medical System). *Work*. 1999;13:217–228.

Section 5
Skill Application

PRACTICAL FOCUS

1. **Musculoskeletal Pain.** A second-year student has been complaining about back and shoulder pain after each clinic period of treating patients. You observe him in clinic and notice that he is positioning his patient too high, so that he must hold his elbows up to reach the patient's mouth. Unfortunately, many clinicians do not self-check their large motor skills (thinking these skills to be unimportant). To experience the importance of large motor skills for yourself, position your patient so that the tip of the patient's mouth is level with the mid-region of your chest (base of your sternum). Establish a finger rest in each of the mandibular treatment areas. What kind of muscle strain do you think you might experience if you were to work for several hours with the patient positioned in this manner?

2. **Photo Analysis.** Your course assignment is to visit a local dental office and photograph a clinician at work on the mandibular posterior teeth. Your photographs are shown below. (1) Evaluate each photograph for position, grasp, and finger rest. (2) For each incorrect element, describe: (a) how the problem could be corrected and (b) the musculoskeletal problems that could result from each positioning problem.

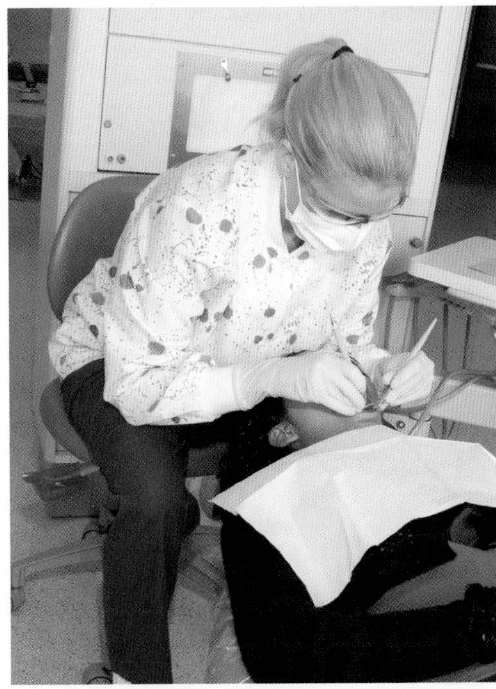

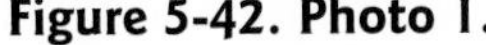

Figure 5-42. Photo 1.

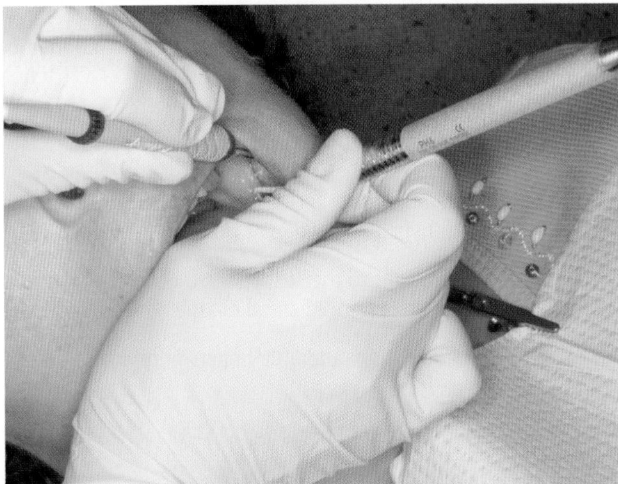

Figure 5-43. Photo 2.

STUDENT SELF-EVALUATION MODULE 5 — MIRROR AND RESTS IN MANDIBULAR POSTERIOR SEXTANTS

Student: ______________________________

Date: ______________________________

Area 1 = right posterior sextant, facial aspect
Area 2 = right posterior sextant, lingual aspect
Area 3 = left posterior sextant, facial aspect
Area 4 = left posterior sextant, lingual aspect

DIRECTIONS: Self-evaluate your skill level in each treatment area as: **S** (satisfactory) or **U** (unsatisfactory).

Criteria				
Positioning/Ergonomics	**Area 1**	**Area 2**	**Area 3**	**Area 4**
Adjusts clinician chair correctly				
Reclines patient chair and ensures that patient's head is even with top of headrest				
Positions instrument tray within easy reach for front, side, or rear delivery as appropriate for operatory configuration				
Positions unit light at arm's length or dons dental headlight and adjusts it for use				
Assumes the recommended clock position				
Positions backrest of patient chair for the specified arch and adjusts height of patient chair so that clinician's elbows remain at waist level when accessing the specified treatment area				
Asks patient to assume the head position that facilitates the clinician's view of the specified treatment area				
Maintains neutral position				
Directs light to illuminate the specified treatment area				
Instrument Grasp: Dominant Hand	**Area 1**	**Area 2**	**Area 3**	**Area 4**
Grasps handle with tips of finger pads of index finger and thumb so that these fingers are opposite each other on the handle, but do NOT touch or overlap				
Rests pad of middle finger lightly on instrument shank; middle finger makes contact with ring finger				
Positions the thumb, index, and middle fingers in the "knuckles-up" convex position; hyperextended joint position is avoided				
Holds ring finger straight so that it supports the weight of hand and instrument; ring finger position is "advanced ahead of" the other fingers in the grasp				
Keeps index, middle, ring, and little fingers in contact—"like fingers inside a mitten"				
Maintains a relaxed grasp; fingers are NOT blanched in grasp				
Finger Rest: Dominant Hand	**Area 1**	**Area 2**	**Area 3**	**Area 4**
Establishes secure finger rest that is appropriate for tooth to be treated				
Once finger rest is established, pauses to self-evaluate finger placement in the grasp, verbalizes to evaluator his or her self-assessment of grasp, and corrects finger placement if necessary				

Module 6

Mirror and Finger Rests in Maxillary Posterior Sextants

Module Overview

This module describes techniques for using a dental mirror and finger rests in the maxillary posterior treatment areas. The fulcrum improves the precision of instrumentation strokes, prevents sudden movements that could injure the patient, and reduces muscle load to the clinician's hand.[1–5]

Module Outline

Key Terms: Review these key terms from Chapter 4.

Neutral wrist position
Fulcrum
Support beam
Finger rest
Extraoral fulcrum
Intraoral fulcrum
Finger-on-finger fulcrum

Learning Objectives

1. Position equipment so that it enhances neutral positioning.
2. Maintain neutral positioning when practicing finger rests in the maxillary posterior sextants.
3. While seated in the correct clock position for the treatment area, access the maxillary posterior teeth with optimum vision while maintaining neutral positioning.
4. Demonstrate correct mirror use, grasp, and finger rest in each of the maxillary posterior sextants while maintaining neutral positioning of your wrist.
5. Demonstrate finger rests using precise finger placement on the handle of a periodontal instrument:
   - Finger pads of thumb and index finger are opposite one another on handle.
   - Thumb and index finger do not overlap each other on the handle.
   - Pad of middle finger rests lightly on the shank.
   - Thumb, index, and middle fingers are in a "knuckles-up" position.
   - Ring finger is straight and supports weight of the hand.
6. Recognize incorrect mirror use, grasp, or finger rest and describe how to correct the problem(s).
7. Understand the relationship between proper stabilization of the dominant hand during instrumentation and the prevention of (1) musculoskeletal problems in the clinician's hands and (2) injury to the patient.
8. Understand the relationship between the large motor skills, such as positioning, and small motor skills, such as finger rests. Recognize the importance of initiating these skills in a step-by-step manner.
9. Demonstrate exercises that lessen muscle imbalances through chairside stretching throughout the workday.

Section 1
Building Blocks for Posterior Sextants

BUILDING BLOCKS FROM POSITION TO FINGER REST

Precise, accurate performance of the building block skills is essential if periodontal instrumentation is to be effective, efficient, safe for the patient, and comfortable for the clinician.

- Research on psychomotor skill acquisition indicates that a high level of mastery in the performance of skill building blocks is essential to successful mastery of periodontal instrumentation.
- The building block skills are the foundation that "supports" successful periodontal instrumentation.
- While practicing finger rests, it is important to complete each of the skills listed in Figure 6-1 in sequence.

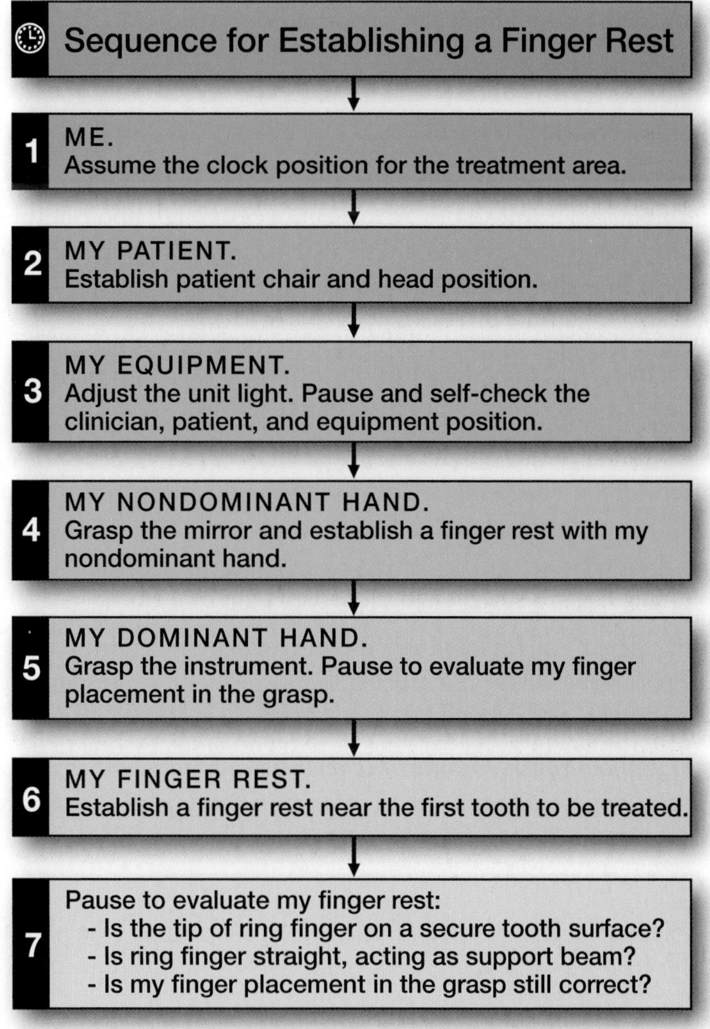
Sequence for Establishing a Finger Rest
1
ME.
Assume the clock position for the treatment area.
2
MY PATIENT.
Establish patient chair and head position.
3
MY EQUIPMENT.
Adjust the unit light. Pause and self-check the clinician, patient, and equipment position.
4
MY NONDOMINANT HAND.
Grasp the mirror and establish a finger rest with my nondominant hand.
5
MY DOMINANT HAND.
Grasp the instrument. Pause to evaluate my finger placement in the grasp.
6
MY FINGER REST.
Establish a finger rest near the first tooth to be treated.
7
Pause to evaluate my finger rest:
- Is the tip of ring finger on a secure tooth surface?
- Is ring finger straight, acting as support beam?
- Is my finger placement in the grasp still correct?

Figure 6-1. Establishing a Finger Rest. When establishing a finger rest, it is important to proceed in the small, explicit steps outlined in this flow chart.[5]

INDIRECT VISION AND PREVENTION OF MUSCULOSKELETAL STRAIN

Dental healthcare providers who routinely use a mirror for indirect vision have less pain in the neck and shoulders and fewer headaches than clinicians who use indirect vision less often.[1] Clinicians who do not use a mirror for indirect vision tend to keep their heads bent to the side and rotated more than 15° during patient treatment.[2]

Experience the Difference for Yourself:

1. Sit in the recommended clock position, and endeavor to view the lingual aspect of the maxillary right posterior sextant.
2. Without using a mirror, view these lingual surfaces. How does your body position change in order to view the lingual surfaces?
3. Now, view the lingual surfaces using indirect vision with a mirror. Compare your body position with and without the use of indirect vision.

Directions for Technique Practice:

1. The photographs for this technique practice depict the use of a mirror and finger rests in the maxillary posterior treatment areas. Some photographs were taken on a patient. Others were taken using a manikin and without gloves so that you can easily see the finger placement in the grasp.
2. The photographs provide a general guideline for finger rests; however, the location of your own finger rest depends on the size and length of your fingers. You may need to fulcrum closer to or farther from the tooth being treated than is shown in the photograph.
3. Focus your attention on mastering mirror use, wrist position, and the finger rests. Use the following instruments in this module:
   - For your nondominant (mirror) hand—Use a dental mirror.
   - For your dominant (instrument) hand—(a) Remove the mirror head from one of your dental mirrors and use the mirror handle as if it were a periodontal instrument, or (b) use a periodontal probe to represent the periodontal instrument in this module.
4. ***Do not wear magnification loupes for this technique practice. It is important to have a view of the patient's head and your hands and wrists when learning finger rests.***

Note: The technique practice for LEFT-Handed clinicians begins in Section 3 on page 168.

Section 2
Technique Practice: RIGHT-Handed Clinician

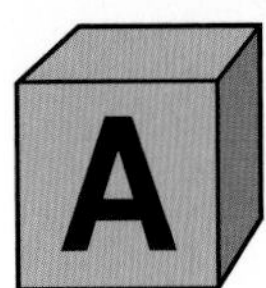

SKILL BUILDING. MAXILLARY POSTERIOR SEXTANTS, ASPECTS FACING TOWARD

Directions: Practice establishing a finger rest for the maxillary posterior teeth, aspects facing toward, by referring to Figures 6-2 to 6-9.

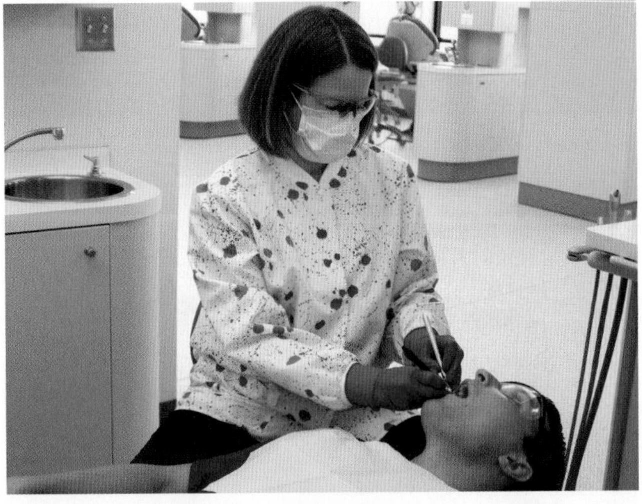

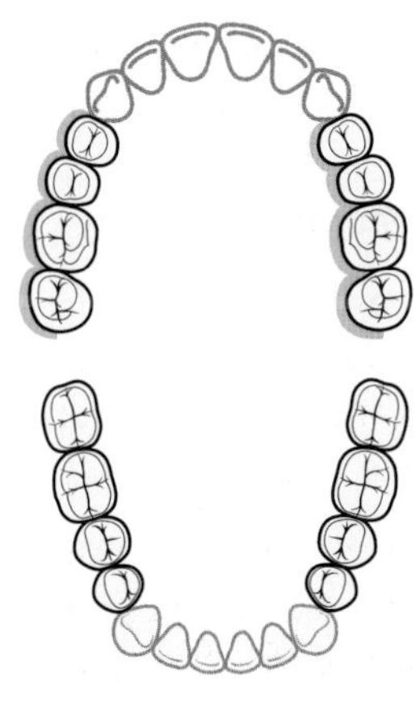

Figure 6-2. Clock Position for Maxillary Posterior Teeth, Aspects Facing Toward the Clinician. The clinician's clock position for the maxillary posterior aspects toward the clinician is the 9 o'clock position. The patient should be in a chin-up head position.

Box 6-1. Handle Positions for Maxillary Posterior Teeth

1. Hold the hand in a palm-up position.
2. Rest the handle against the index finger somewhere in the green shaded area.

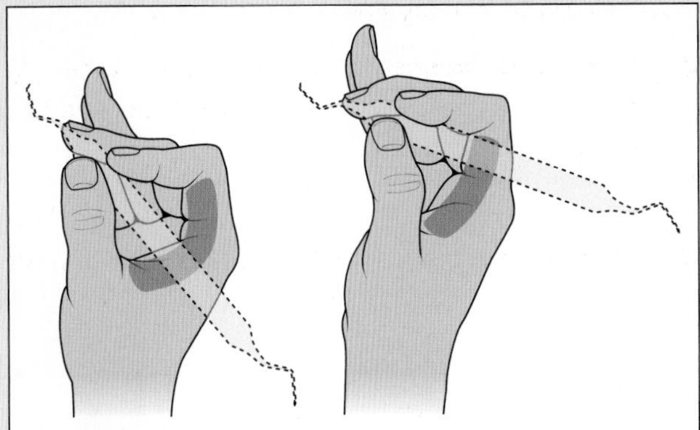

Figure 6-3. Handle Positions for Maxillary Posterior Treatment Areas.

Maxillary Right Posterior Sextant, Facial Aspect

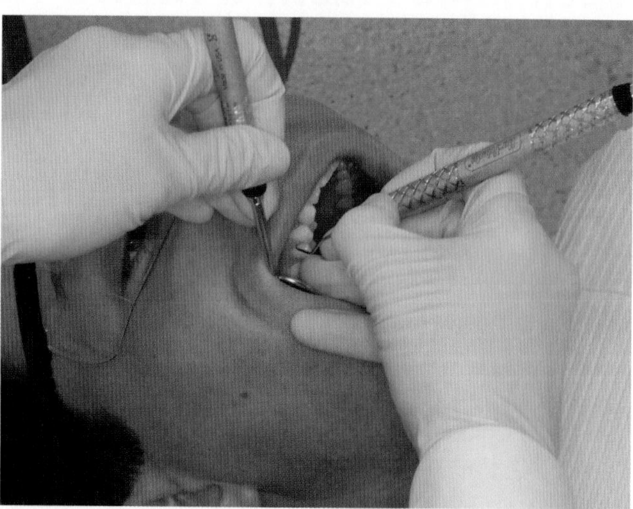

Figure 6-4. Retraction. Retract the buccal mucosa with the mirror. Use the mirror for indirect vision, particularly to view the distal surfaces of the teeth.

Note the clinician pictured here is using an extraoral finger rest with the dental mirror.

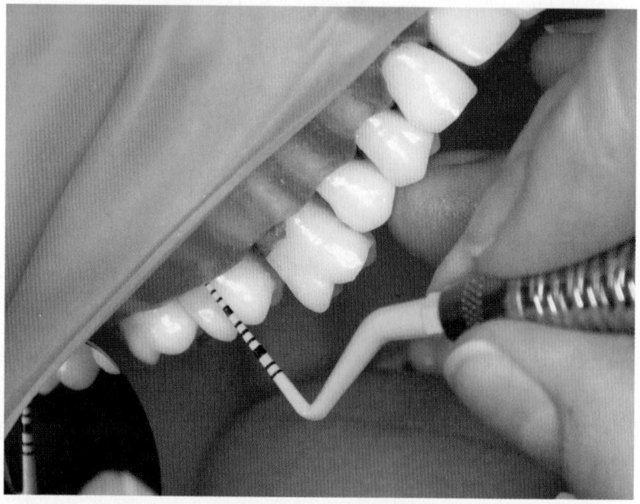

Figure 6-5. Task 1—Second Molar, Facial Aspect. Finger rest on an occlusal surface.

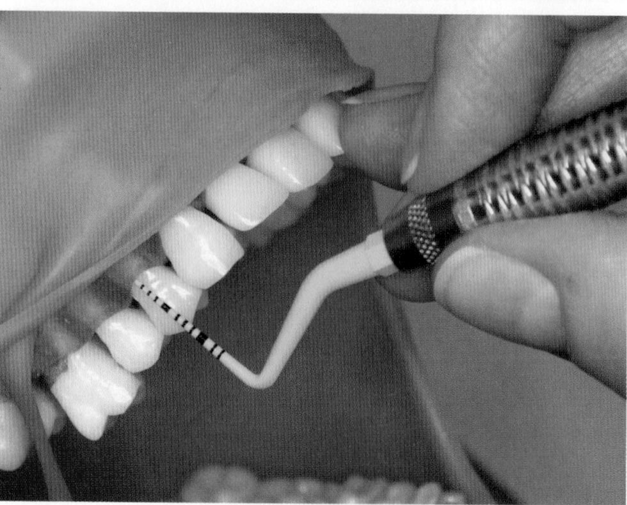

Figure 6-6. Task 2—First Premolar, Facial Aspect. Finger rest on an incisal surface of one of the maxillary anteriors.

Maxillary Left Posterior Sextant, Lingual Aspect

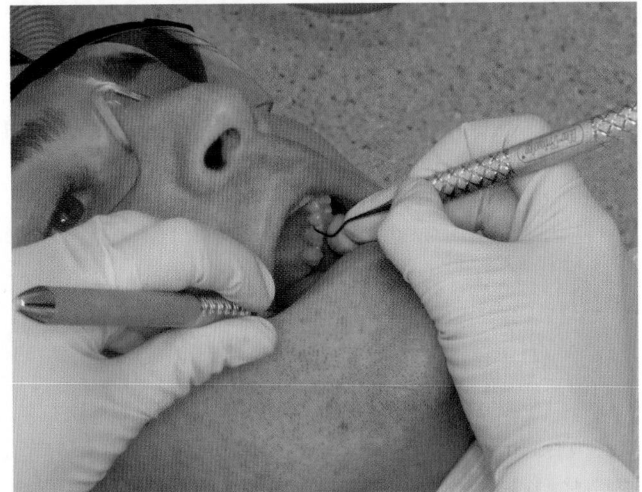

Figure 6-7. Mirror. Use the mirror to view the distal surfaces of the teeth.

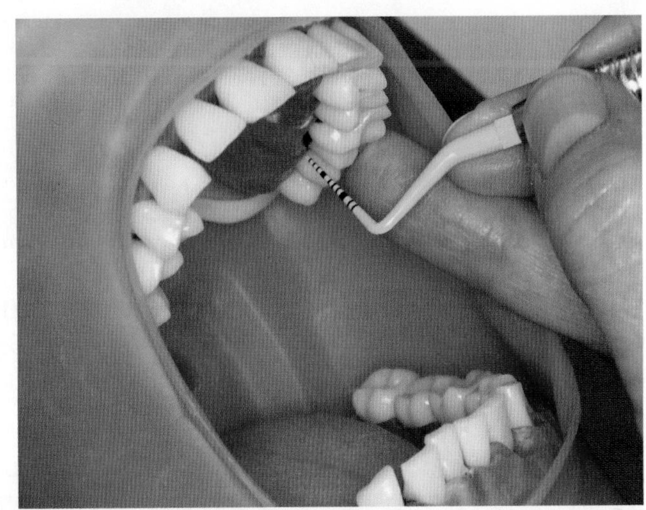

Figure 6-8. Task 1—Second Molar, Lingual Aspect. Finger rest on an occluso-facial line angle.

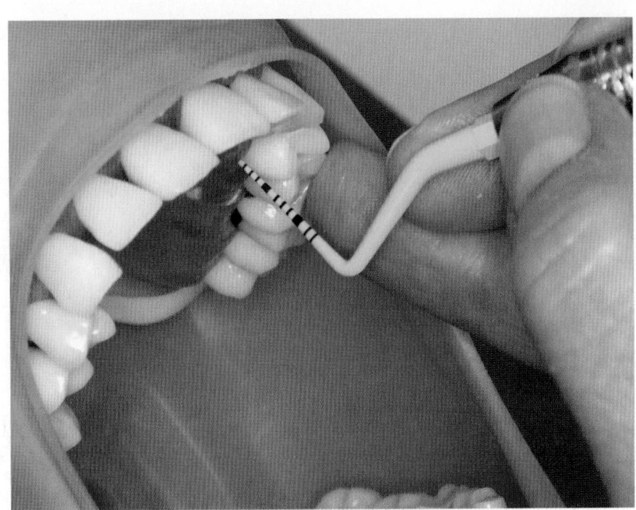

Figure 6-9. Task 2—First Premolar, Lingual Aspect. Finger rest on the occlusofacial line angle or an incisal edge.

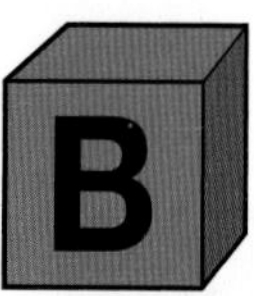

SKILL BUILDING. MAXILLARY POSTERIOR SEXTANTS, ASPECTS FACING AWAY

Directions: Practice establishing a finger rest for the maxillary posterior teeth, aspects facing away, by referring to Figures 6-10 to 6-17.

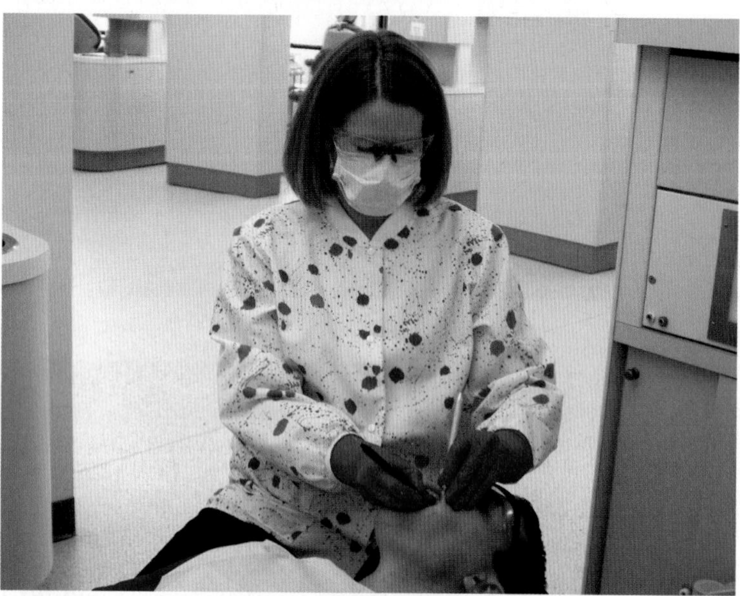

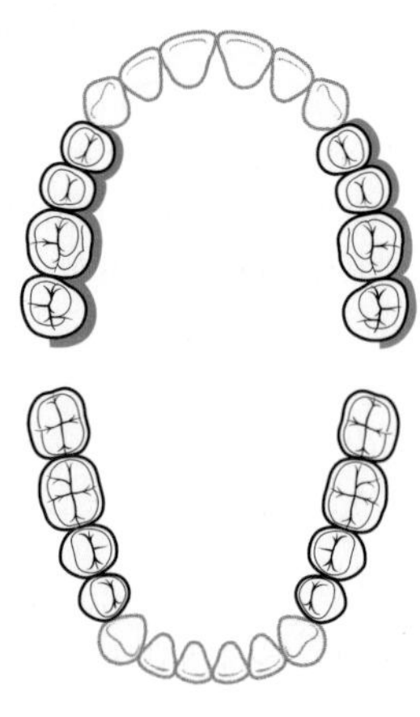

Figure 6-10. Clock Position for Maxillary Posterior Teeth, Aspects Facing Away from the Clinician. The clinician's clock position for the maxillary posterior aspects facing away from the clinician is a 10 to 11 o'clock position. The patient should be in a chin-up head position.

Box 6-2. Handle Positions for Maxillary Posterior Teeth

1. Hold the hand in a palm-up position.
2. Rest the handle against the index finger somewhere in the green shaded area.

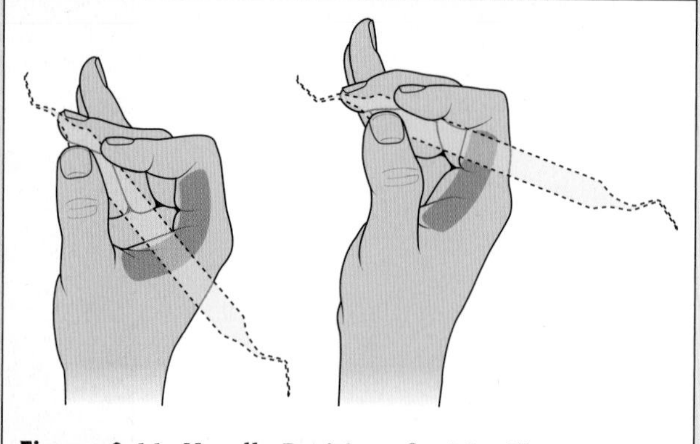

Figure 6-11. Handle Positions for Maxillary Posterior Treatment Areas.

Maxillary Left Posterior Sextant, Facial Aspect

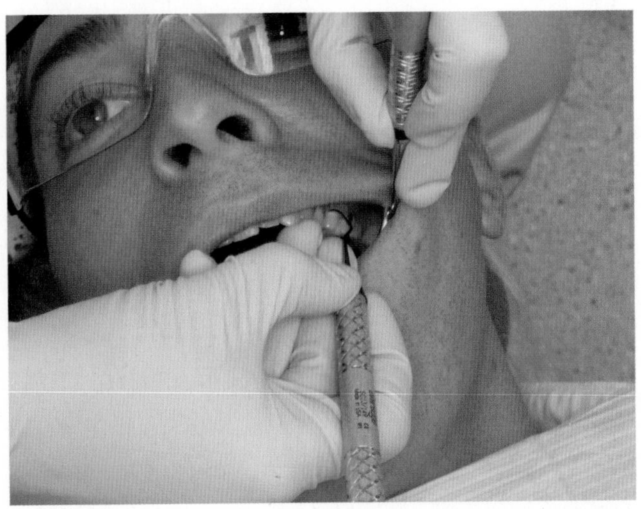

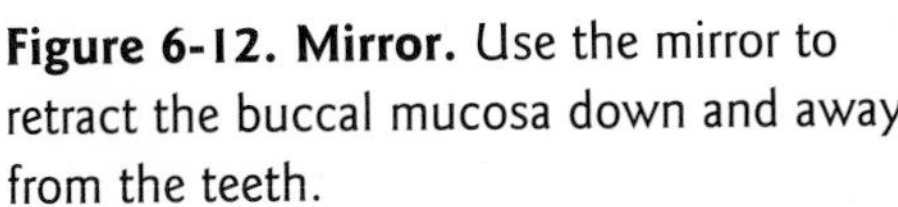

Figure 6-12. Mirror. Use the mirror to retract the buccal mucosa down and away from the teeth.

Technique hint: Your dominant hand is positioned correctly if you can see the underside of your middle and ring fingers.

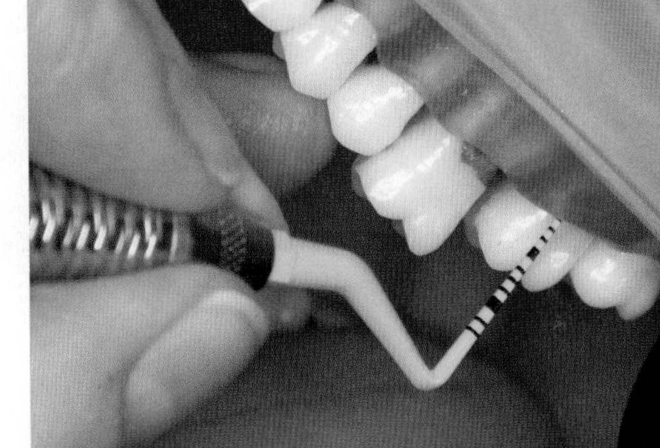

Figure 6-13. Task 1—Second Molar, Facial Aspect. Finger rest on an occlusal surface.

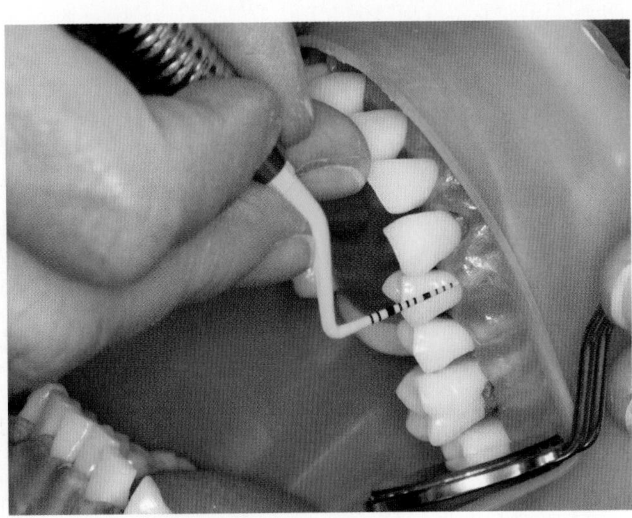

Figure 6-14. Task 2—First Premolar, Facial Aspect. Finger rest on an incisal edge of an anterior tooth.

Maxillary Right Posterior Sextant, Lingual Aspect

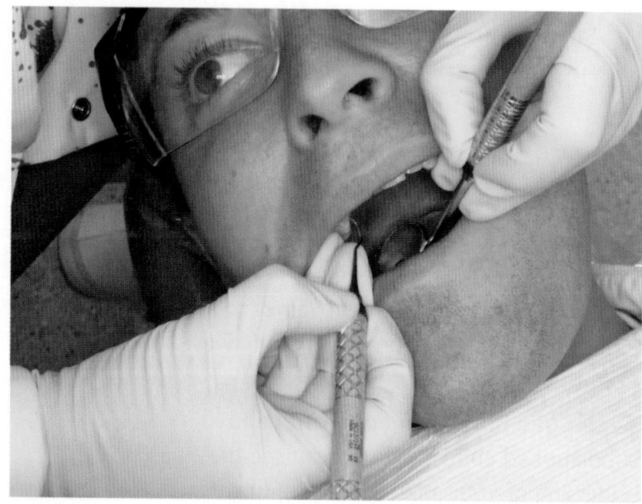

Figure 6-15. Mirror. Use the mirror for indirect vision.

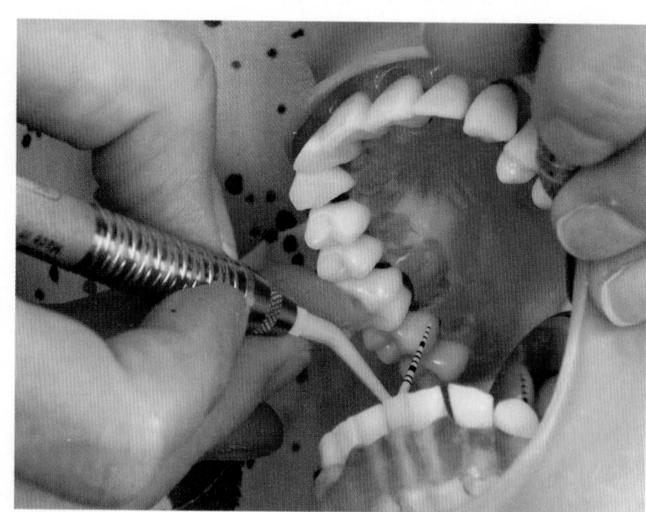

Figure 6-16. Task 1—Second Molar, Lingual Aspect. Finger rest on an occlusal surface.

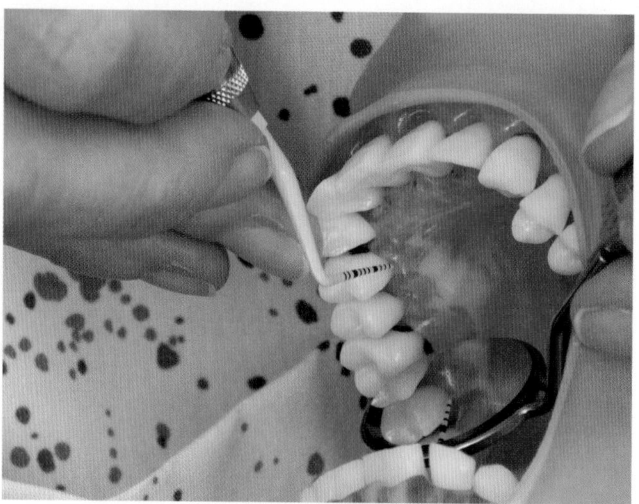

Figure 6-17. Task 2—First Premolar, Lingual Aspect. Finger rest on the occlusal surface or an incisal edge.

REFERENCE SHEET FOR MAXILLARY POSTERIOR SEXTANTS (RIGHT-HANDED CLINICIAN)

Photocopy this reference sheet and use it for quick reference as you practice your skills. Place the photocopied reference sheet in a plastic page protector for longer use.

TABLE 6-1. Reference Sheet: Maxillary Posterior Sextants

Treatment Area	Clock Position	Patient's Head
Posterior Aspects Facing Toward (Right Posterior, Facial Aspect) (Left Posterior, Lingual Aspect)	9:00	Straight or slightly away Chin UP
Posterior Aspects Facing Away (Right Posterior, Lingual Aspect) (Left Posterior, Facial Aspect)	10:00–11:00	Toward Chin UP

Note: This ends the section for RIGHT-Handed clinicians. Turn to page 175 for Section 4: Alternate Clock Positions and Finger Rests.

Section 3
Technique Practice: LEFT-Handed Clinician

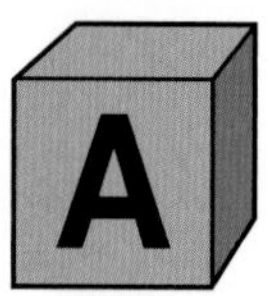

SKILL BUILDING. MAXILLARY POSTERIOR SEXTANTS, ASPECTS FACING TOWARD

Directions: Practice establishing a finger rest for the maxillary posterior teeth, aspects facing toward, by referring to Figures 6-18 to 6-25.

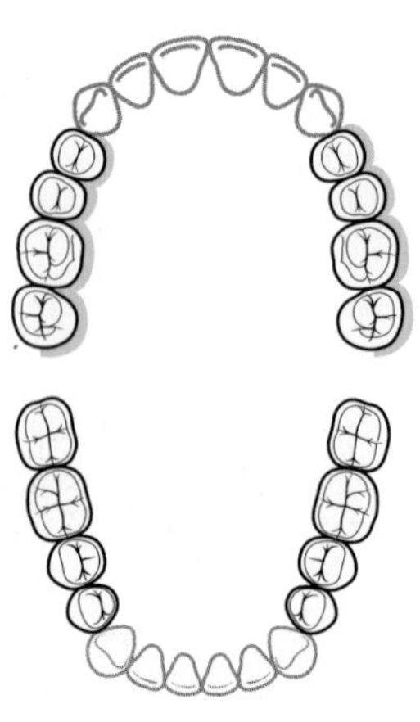

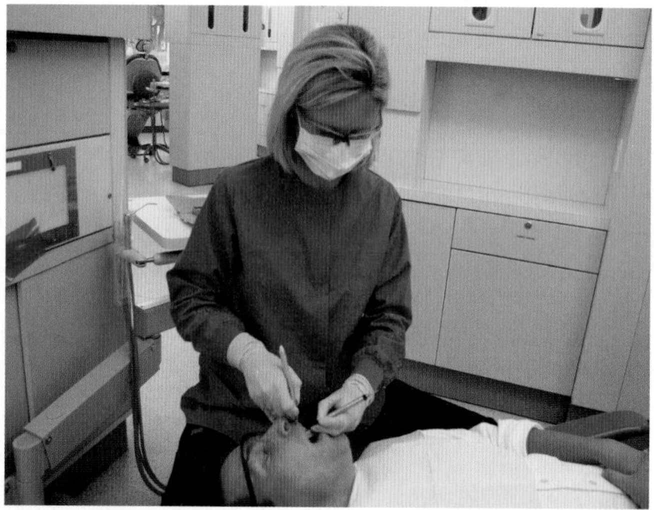

Figure 6-18. Clock Position for Maxillary Posterior Teeth, Aspects Facing Toward the Clinician. The clinician's clock position for the maxillary posterior aspects toward the clinician is the 3 o'clock position. The patient should be in a chin-up head position.

Box 6-3. Handle Positions for Maxillary Posterior Teeth

1. Hold the hand in a palm-up position.
2. Rest the handle against the index finger somewhere in the green shaded area.

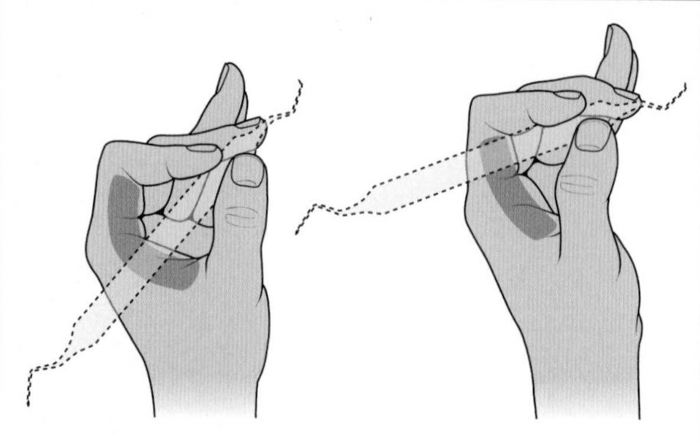

Figure 6-19. Handle Positions for Maxillary Posterior Treatment Areas.

TECHNIQUE PRACTICE: MAXILLARY POSTERIOR SEXTANTS

AQ5

Maxillary Left Posterior Sextant, Facial Aspect

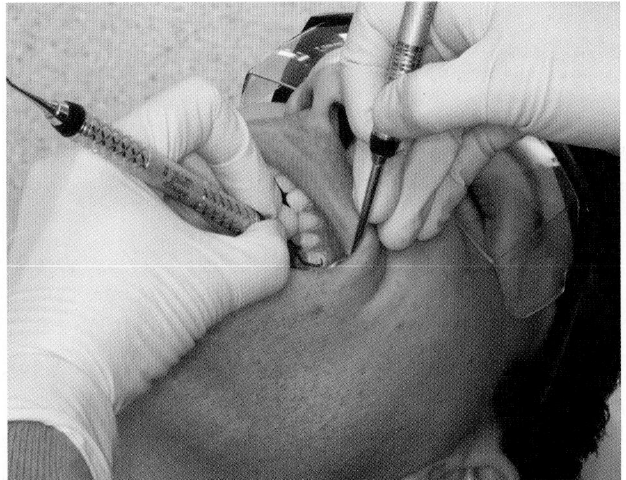

Figure 6-20. Mirror. Retract the buccal mucosa with the mirror. Use the mirror for indirect vision, particularly to view the distal surfaces of the teeth.

Note the clinician pictured here is using an extraoral finger rest with the dental mirror.

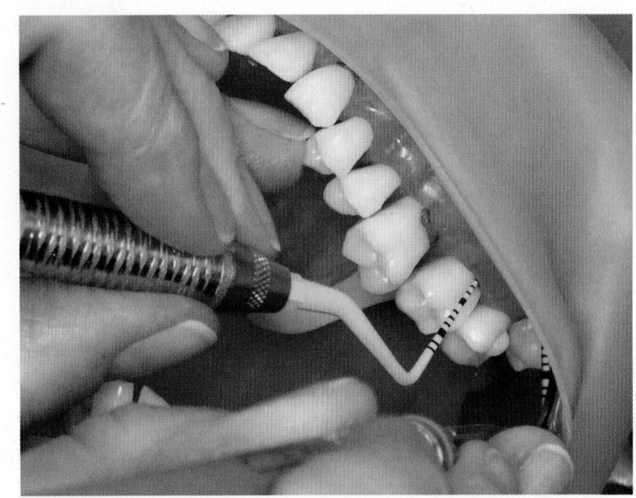

Figure 6-21. Task 1—Second Molar, Facial Aspect. Finger rest on an occlusal surface.

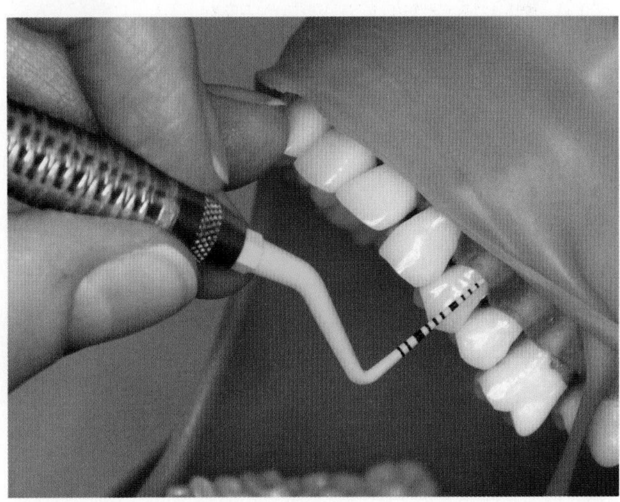

Figure 6-22. Task 2—First Premolar, Facial Aspect. Finger rest on an incisal surface of one of the maxillary anteriors.

Maxillary Right Posterior Sextant, Lingual Aspect

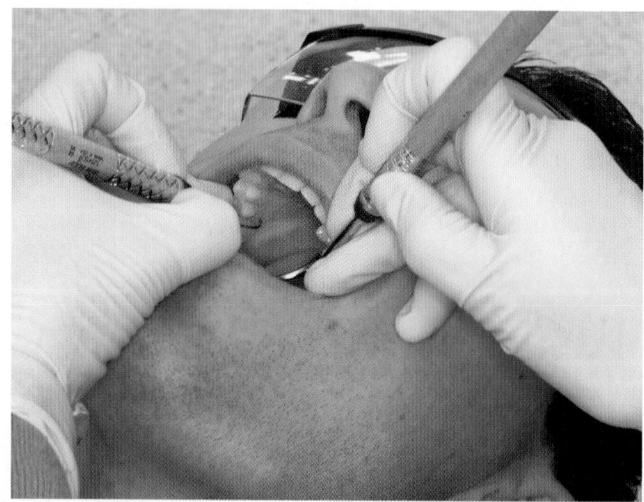

Figure 6-23. Mirror. Use the mirror to view the distal surfaces of the teeth.

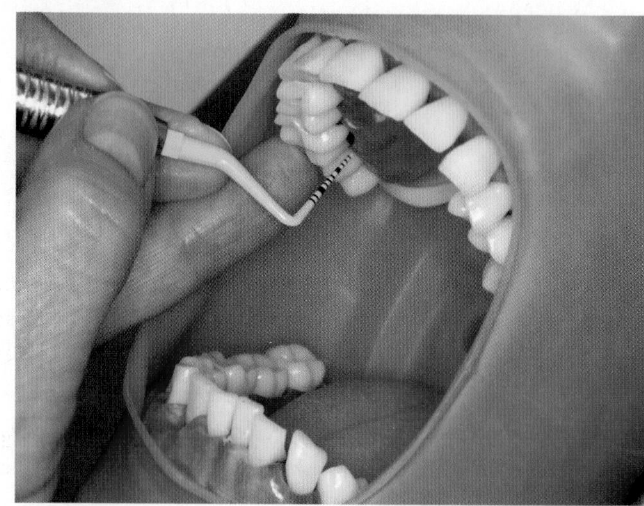

Figure 6-24. Task 1—Second Molar, Lingual Aspect. Finger rest on an occluso-facial line angle.

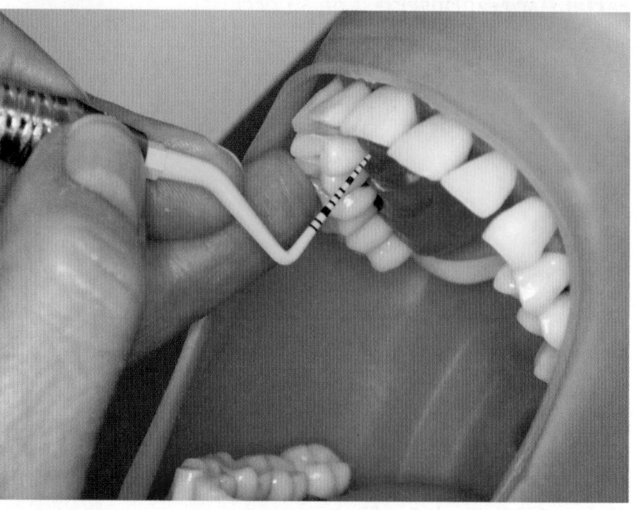

Figure 6-25. Task 2—First Premolar, Lingual Aspect. Finger rest on the occlusofacial line angle or an incisal edge.

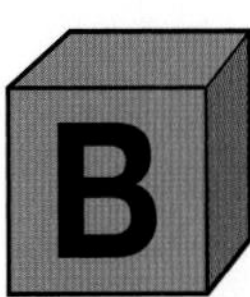

SKILL BUILDING. MAXILLARY POSTERIOR SEXTANTS, ASPECTS FACING AWAY

Directions: Practice establishing a finger rest for the maxillary posterior teeth, aspects facing away, by referring to Figures 6-26 to 6-33.

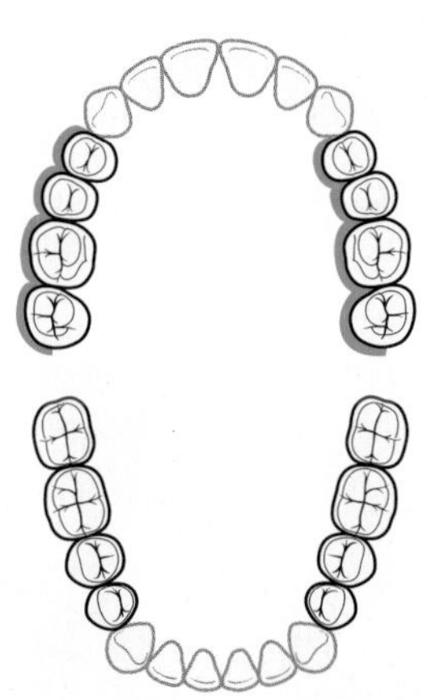

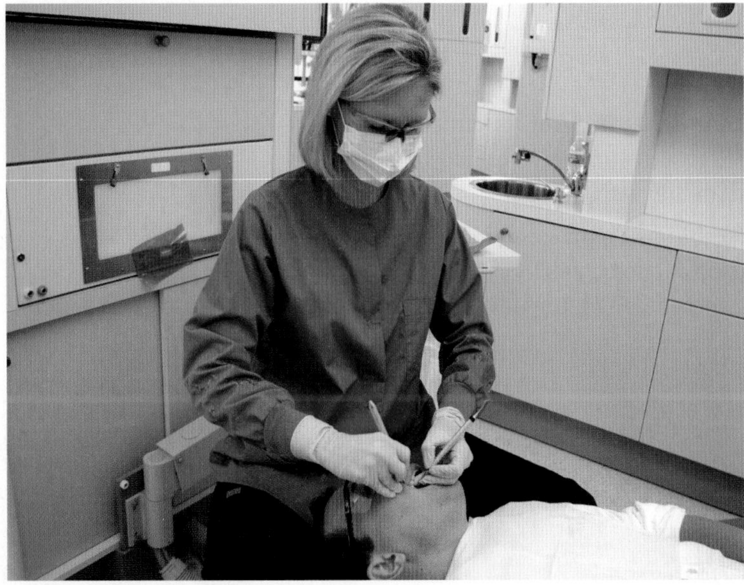

Figure 6-26. Clock Position for Maxillary Posterior Teeth, Aspects Facing Away from the Clinician. The clinician's clock position for the maxillary posterior aspects facing away from the clinician is a 1 to 2 o'clock position. The patient should be in a chin-up head position.

Box 6-4. Handle Positions for Maxillary Posterior Teeth

1. Hold the hand in a palm-up position.
2. Rest the handle against the index finger somewhere in the green shaded area.

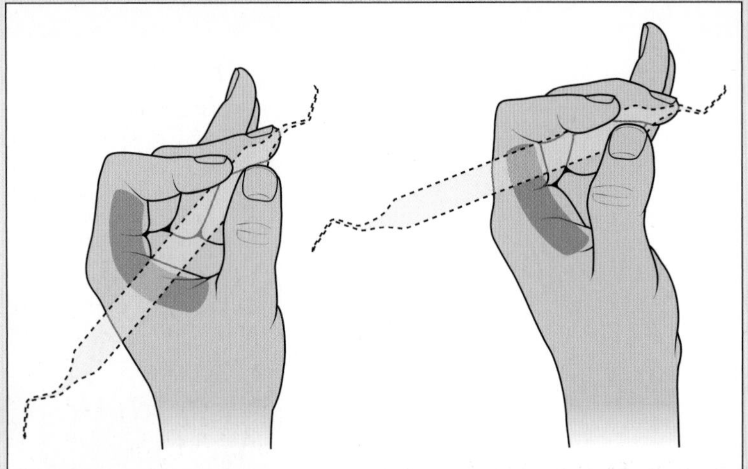

Figure 6-27. Handle Positions for Maxillary Posterior Treatment Areas.

Maxillary Right Posterior Sextant, Facial Aspect

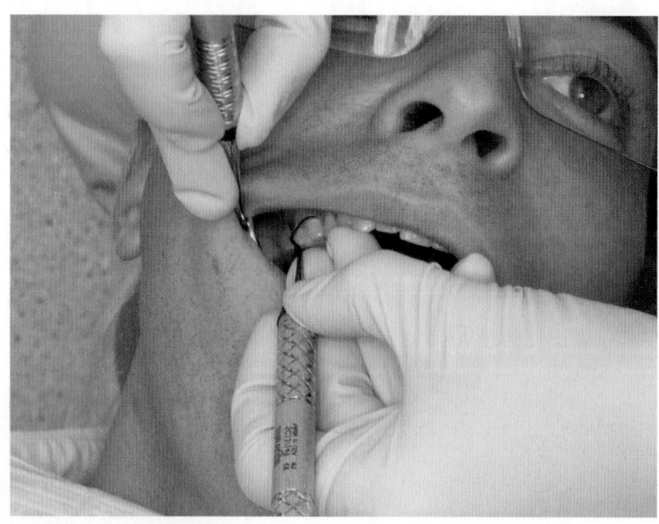

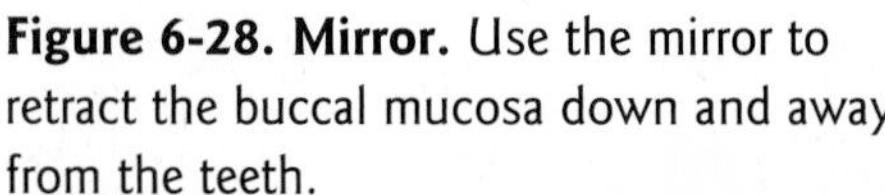

Figure 6-28. Mirror. Use the mirror to retract the buccal mucosa down and away from the teeth.

Technique hint: Your dominant hand is positioned correctly if you can see the underside of your middle and ring fingers.

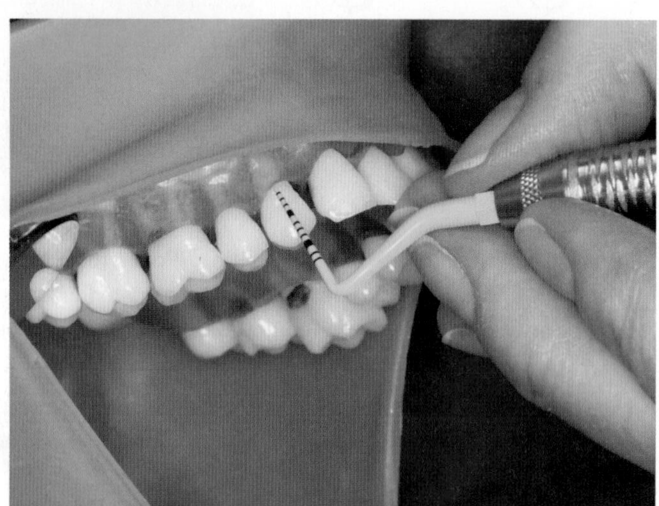

Figure 6-29. Task 1—Second Molar, Facial Aspect. Finger rest on an occlusal surface.

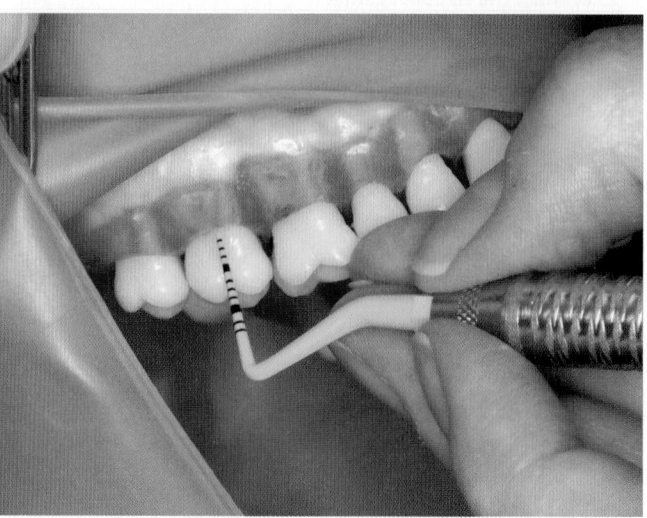

Figure 6-30. Task 2—First Premolar, Facial Aspect. Finger rest on an incisal edge of an anterior tooth.

Maxillary Left Posterior Sextant, Lingual Aspect

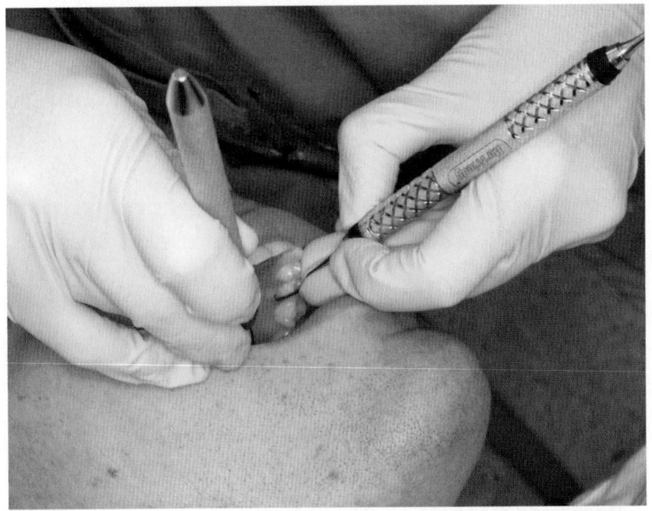

Figure 6-31. Mirror. Use the mirror for indirect vision.

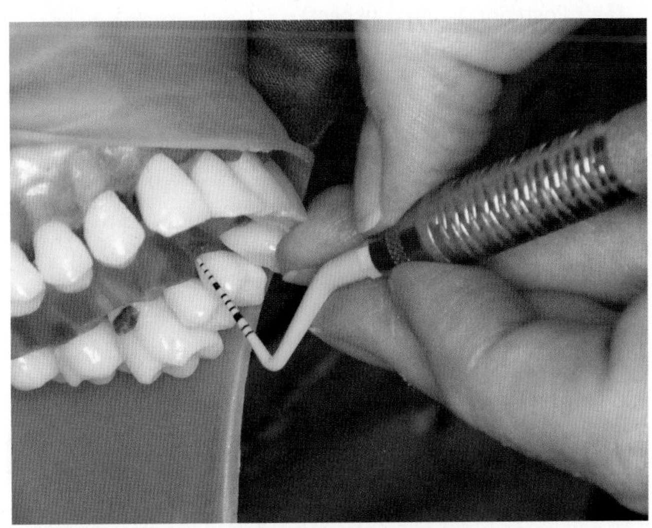

Figure 6-32. Task 1—Second Molar, Lingual Aspect. Finger rest on an occlusal surface.

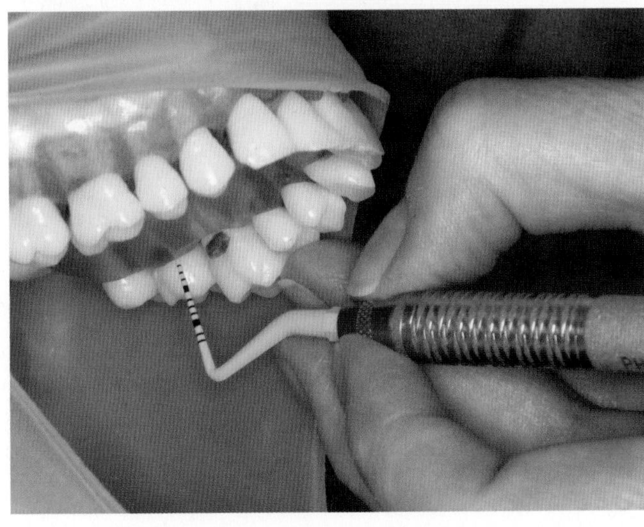

Figure 6-33. Task 2—First Premolar, Lingual Aspect. Finger rest on the occlusal surface or an incisal edge.

REFERENCE SHEET FOR MAXILLARY POSTERIOR SEXTANTS (LEFT-HANDED CLINICIAN)

Photocopy this reference sheet and use it for quick reference as you practice your skills. Place the photocopied reference sheet in a plastic page protector for longer use.

TABLE 6-2. Reference Sheet: Maxillary Posterior Sextants

Treatment Area	Clock Position	Patient's Head
Posterior Aspects Facing Toward (Left Posterior, Facial Aspect) (Right Posterior, Lingual Aspect)	3:00	Straight or slightly away Chin UP
Posterior Aspects Facing Away (Left Posterior, Lingual Aspect) (Right Posterior, Facial Aspect)	1:00–2:00	Toward Chin UP

Section 4
Alternate Finger Rests

- For right-handed clinicians, the facial aspect of the maxillary right posterior sextant sometimes may be difficult to access. Likewise, the facial aspect of the maxillary left posterior sextant may be challenging for left-handed clinicians. Some clinicians find that using a finger-on-finger modified fulcrum assists them in keeping the lower shank parallel to the root surfaces when working in deep periodontal pockets. Figures 6-34 and 6-35 depict this alternate technique. ***Before attempting modified fulcruming techniques, the clinician should have mastered the fundamentals of neutral position and standard intraoral fulcruming techniques.***

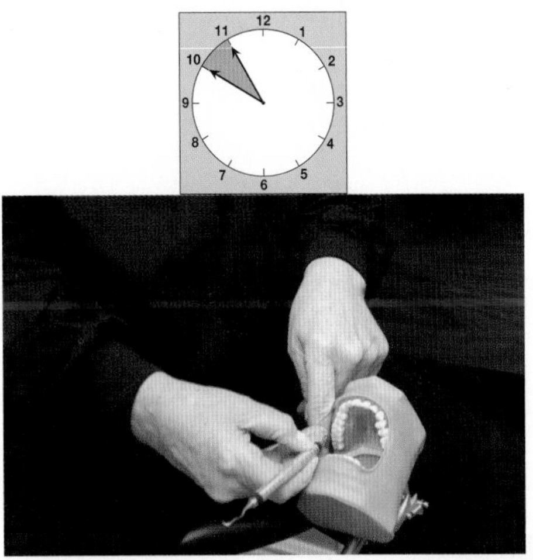

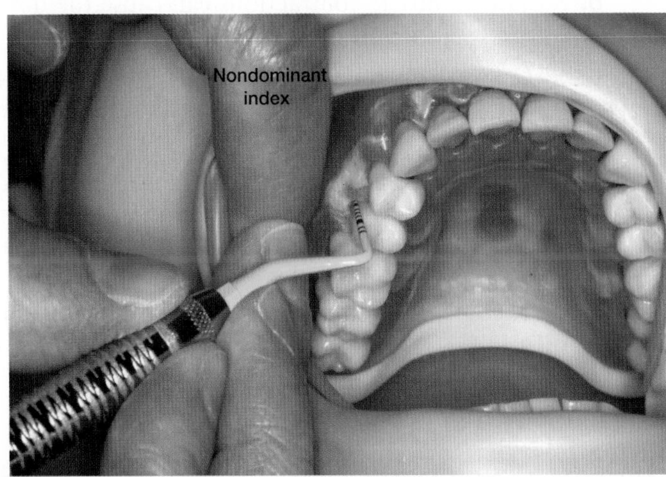

Figure 6-34. RIGHT-Handed Clinician: Maxillary Right Posteriors, Facial Aspect.

- Use traditional clock position of 10 to 11 o'clock.
- Use finger-on-finger fulcrum.

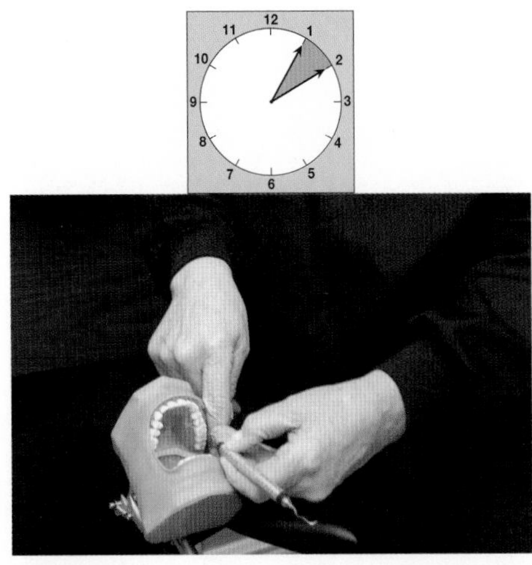

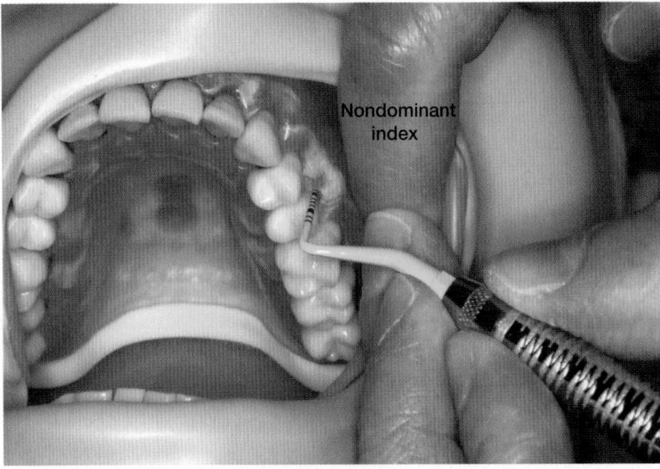

Figure 6-35. LEFT-Handed Clinician: Maxillary Left Posteriors, Facial Aspect.

- Use traditional clock position of 1 to 2 o'clock.
- Use finger-on-finger fulcrum.

Section 5
Preventive Strategies: Stretches

1. Strong postural muscles of the trunk and shoulders stabilize the body in the neutral seated position, allowing the arms and hands to perform the exacting task of periodontal instrumentation.
2. Most dental hygienists sit for sustained periods of time in static positions that can cause muscle tension and stiffness.
   a. Prolonged, static, and unbalanced seated postures are the most common causes of musculoskeletal disorders in dentists and dental hygienists.
   b. Sustained muscle contractions can cause the development of tender spots in muscles and deterioration of the vertebral joints and discs.
   c. Over time, unbalanced seated positions cause muscle imbalances—tightness in one muscle group and weakness in the opposing group—leading to musculoskeletal pain.
3. Performing chairside stretching exercises offers numerous benefits (Box 6-5).
   a. Many authors recommend short work breaks and a routine of chairside stretching throughout the day between patients.[2,4–8]
   b. A schedule of brief, yet frequent rest periods is more beneficial than lengthy infrequent stretching breaks. Chairside stretches should be performed every 30 to 60 minutes throughout the day.

Box 6-5. Benefits of Stretching

- Warms up muscles before beginning to work[7]
- Helps prevent muscle strains and spasms[7,9]
- Decreases muscle soreness and tender spots[7,10]
- Increases production of joint synovial fluid to reduce friction between joints during movement[5]
- Increases range of motion, which promotes increased flexibility[7,11,12]
- Increases coordination, which enhances control of fine motor skills[7,13]
- Increases nutrient supply to the vertebral discs of the spine[7]
- Reduces stress and promotes relaxation[7,14,15]

Box 6-6. How to Stretch Safely

- Assume the starting position for the stretch.
- Breathe in deeply as you begin the stretch.
- Hold the stretch for about 6 seconds.
- Slowly release the stretch as you return to the starting position. Repeat the stretch if time allows.
- Never stretch in a painful range. If stretching increases your pain, stop immediately.

MINI-BREAK CHAIRSIDE STRETCHES

Lydia T. Pierce, LPT, demonstrates chairside stretches in Figures 6-36 to 6-43. It is beneficial to perform stretches in short mini-breaks every 30 to 60 minutes throughout the day. Refer to Box 6-6 for guidelines for stretching safely.

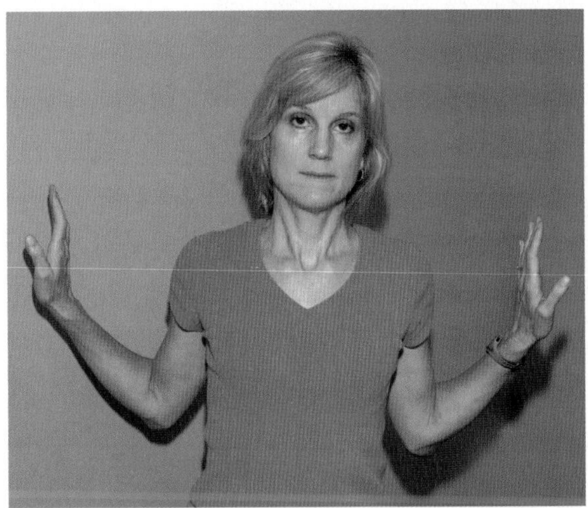

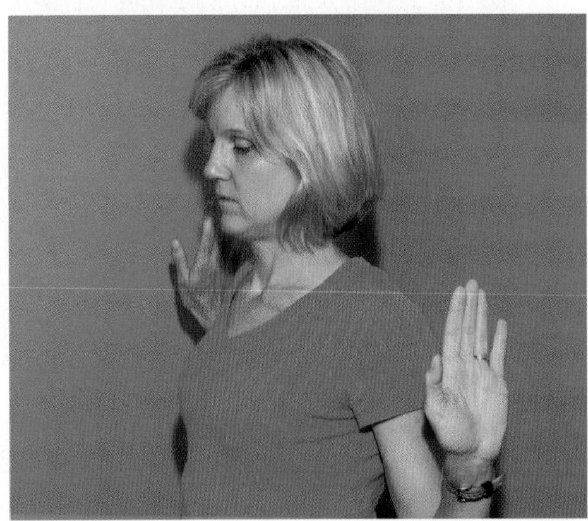

Figure 6-36. The Butterfly Stretch.

- Stand or sit with your hands positioned at about chest height.
- Lift your sternum and relax your neck.
- Lead with your little fingers as you move your elbows and palms to the side of your torso. Squeeze your shoulder blades together while keeping your neck relaxed.
- Hold for 6 seconds. Repeat 6 times.

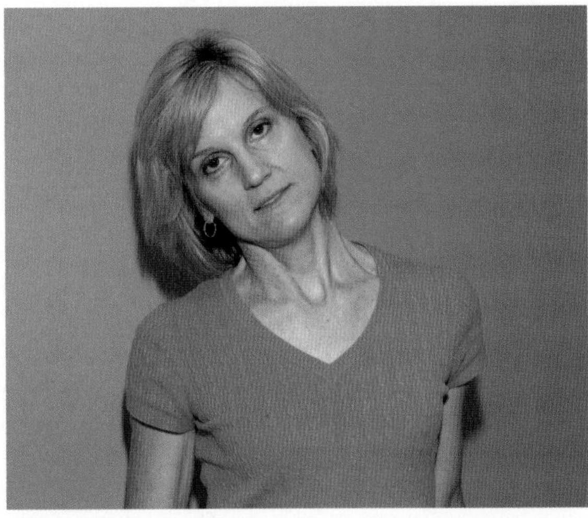

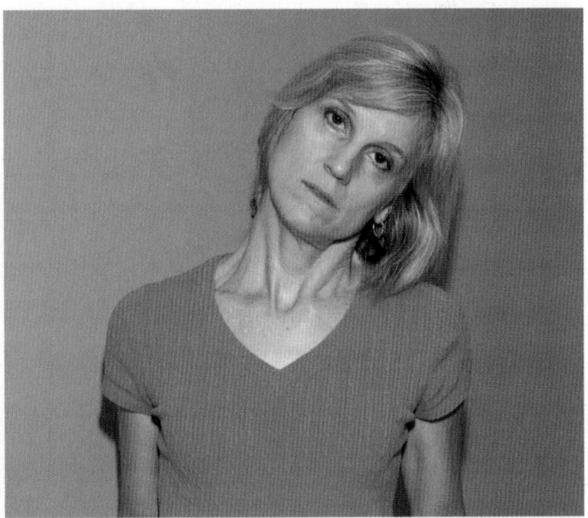

Figure 6-37. The Head Tilt.

- In a seated position, relax your neck and hold your shoulders down and back.
- Move your right ear to the right shoulder and hold for 6 seconds.
- Repeat the same sequence to the left.
- Repeat 6 times.

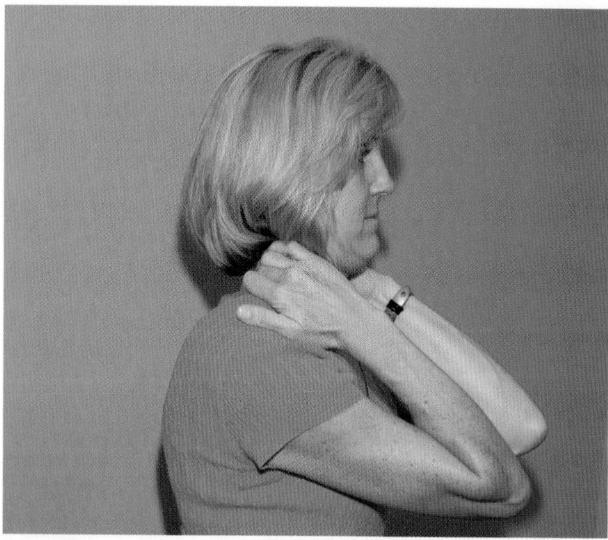

Figure 6-38. The Chin Tuck.

- In a seated position, relax your neck and hold your shoulders down and back.
- Place your hands against the back of your neck as you pull your chin straight back (chin tuck). Hold for 6 seconds.
- Repeat 6 times.

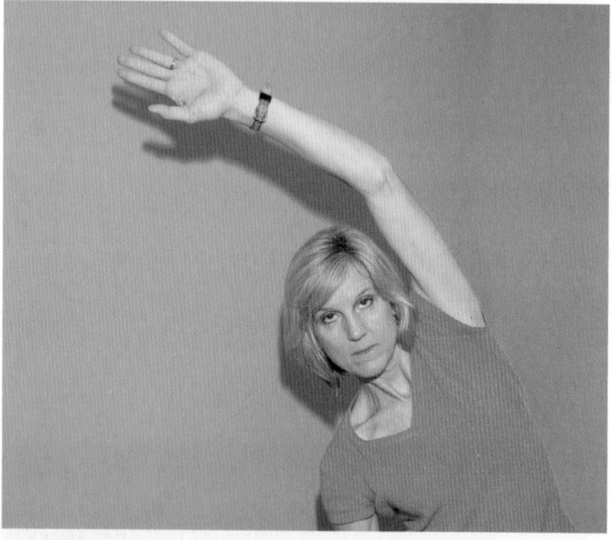

Figure 6-39. The Arm-Torso Stretch.

- In a seated position, relax your neck and hold your shoulders down and back.
- Maintain your feet in a tripod position as you stretch your right arm overhead while bending your torso to the right. Hold for 6 seconds.
- Repeat the same sequence to the left.
- Repeat 6 times.

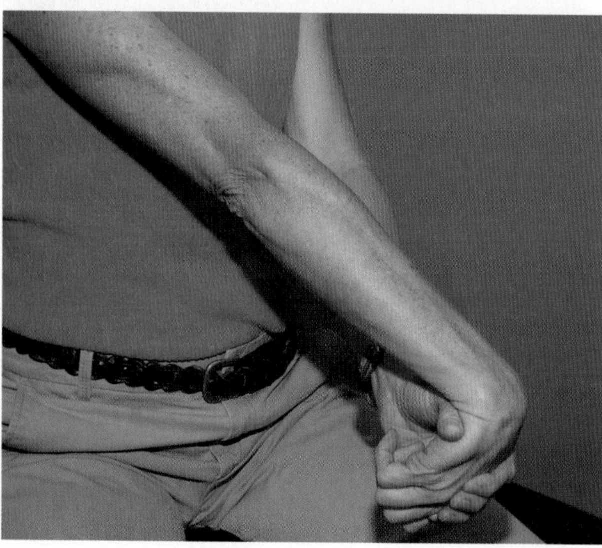

Figure 6-40. The Extensor Stretch.

- In a seated position, relax your neck and hold your shoulders down and back.
- Hold your right arm straight with palm down.
- Use your left hand to gently pull the right wrist downward. Hold stretch for 6 seconds.
- Repeat the same sequence for the left wrist.
- Repeat 6 times.

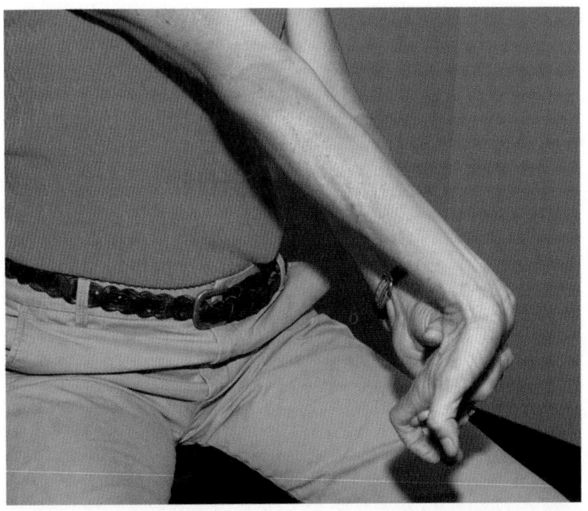

Figure 6-41. The Flexor Stretch.

- In a seated position, relax your neck and hold your shoulders down and back.
- Hold right arm straight with palm up.
- Use your left hand to gently pull the right wrist backward. Hold stretch for 6 seconds.
- Repeat the same sequence for the left wrist.
- Repeat 6 times.

HIP-HINGE TECHNIQUE PRACTICE

To maintain neutral seated position, the clinician should hinge from the hips—rather than round the back—to move closer to the patient. A common positioning error is rounding the back in order to get closer to the treatment area (Fig. 6-42A). Instead of rounding the back, the clinician should hinge at the hips to move closer to the treatment area (Fig. 6-42B).

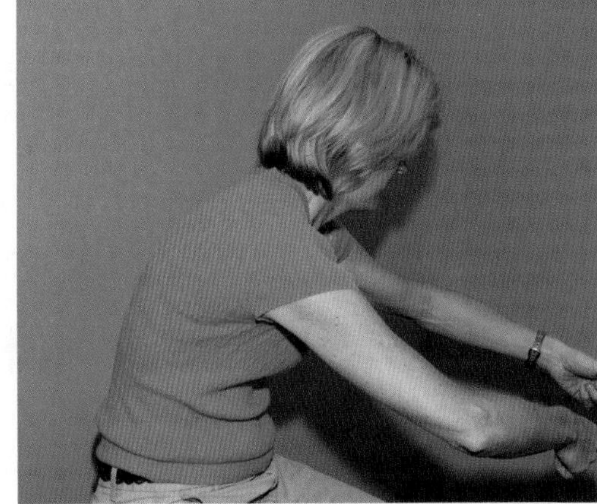

Figure 6-42A. Incorrect Technique. Rounding the back is a common positioning error used by clinicians in an attempt to move closer to the treatment area.

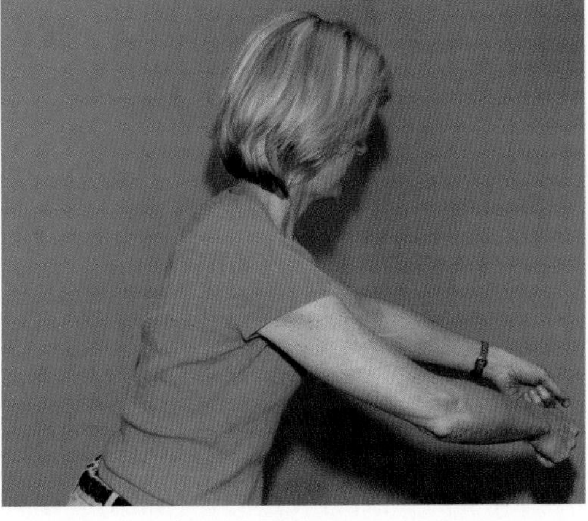

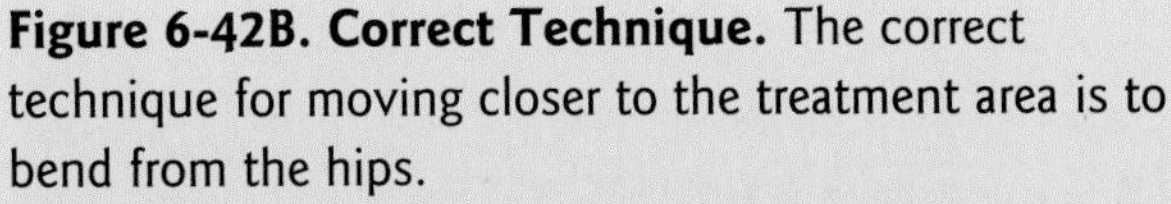

Figure 6-42B. Correct Technique. The correct technique for moving closer to the treatment area is to bend from the hips.

Practice the hip hinge by following these steps:

- In a seated position, relax your neck and hold your shoulders down and back, with chest up.
- Practice the correct technique for leaning toward the patient by hinging at the hips instead of at the mid-back.
- Repeat 6 times.

AFTER A LONG DAY: AT-HOME STRETCH

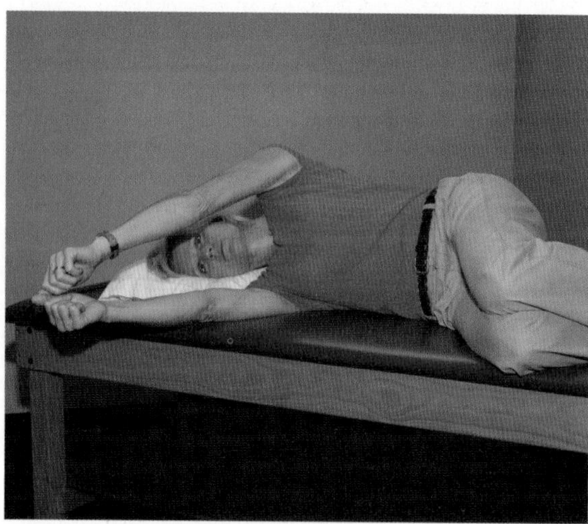

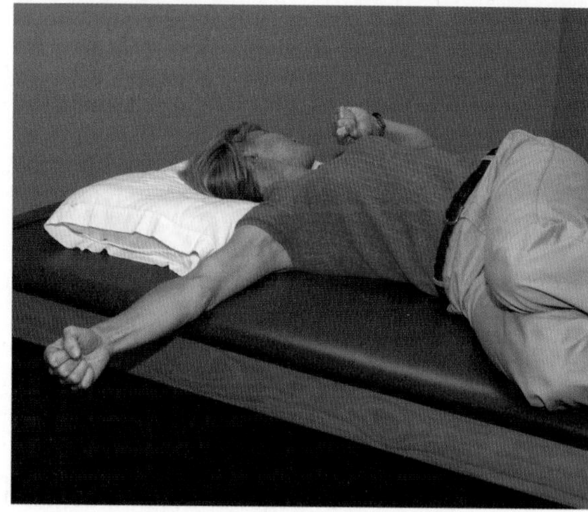

Figure 6-43. The Bow and Arrow.

- Lie on your right side in bed with your head and neck supported by a pillow.
- Hold the lower arm straight.
- Pull the top arm back as if pulling an arrow in a bow. As you pull the top arm back, follow your moving arm with your head and torso.
- Hold for 6 seconds. Repeat 6 times.
- Repeat the same sequence lying on your left side.

REFERENCES

1. Rundcrantz BL, Johnsson B, Moritz U. Cervical pain and discomfort among dentists. Epidemiological, clinical and therapeutic aspects. Part 1. A survey of pain and discomfort. *Swed Dent J*. 1990;14:71–80.
2. Rundcrantz BL, Johnsson B, Moritz U. Occupational cervico-brachial disorders among dentists. Analysis of ergonomics and locomotor functions. *Swed Dent J*. 1991;15:105–115.
3. Andrews N, Vigoren G. Ergonomics: muscle fatigue, posture, magnification, and illumination. *Compend Contin Educ Dent*. 2002;23:261–266, 268, 270.
4. Dylla J, Forrest J. Stretching and strengthening for balance and stability: part 1. *Access*. 2006;11:38–43.
5. Hauser AM, Bowen DM. Primer on preclinical instruction and evaluation. *J Dent Educ*. 2009;73:390–398.
6. Tovoc T, Gutmann M. Making the principles of ergonomics work for you. *Dimen Dent Hyg*. 2005;3:16–18, 20–21.
7. Valachi B. *Practice Dentistry Pain-Free: Evidence-Based Strategies to Prevent Pain and Extend Your Career*. Portland, OR: Posturedontics Press; 2008.
8. Wann O, Canull B. Ergonomics and dental hygienists. *Comtemp Oral Hyg*. 2003;3:16–22.
9. Coppin RJ, Wicke DM, Little PS. Managing nocturnal leg cramps–calf-stretching exercises and cessation of quinine treatment: a factorial randomised controlled trial. *Br J Gen Pract*. 2005;55:186–191.
10. Rahnama N, Rahmani-Nia F, Ebrahim K. The isolated and combined effects of selected physical activity and ibuprofen on delayed-onset muscle soreness. *J Sports Sci*. 2005;23:843–850.
11. Decicco PV, Fisher MM. The effects of proprioceptive neuromuscular facilitation stretching on shoulder range of motion in overhand athletes. *J Sports Med Phys Fitness*. 2005;45:183–187.
12. Decoster LC, Cleland J, Altieri C, Russell P. The effects of hamstring stretching on range of motion: a systematic literature review. *J Orthop Sports Phys Ther*. 2005;35:377–387.
13. Lane JM, Nydick M. Osteoporosis: current modes of prevention and treatment. *J Am Acad Orthop Surg*. 1999;7:19–31.
14. Khasky AD, Smith JC. Stress, relaxation states, and creativity. *Percept Mot Skills*. 1999;88:409–416.
15. Parshad O. Role of yoga in stress management. *West Indian Med J*. 2004;53:191–194.

RECOMMENDED READING

Leonard DM. The effectiveness of intervention strategies used to educate clients about prevention of upper extremity cumulative trauma disorders. *Work*. 2000;14:151–157.

Liskiewicz ST, Kerschbaum WE. Cumulative trauma disorders: an ergonomic approach for prevention. *J Dent Hyg*. 1997;71:162–167.

Marcoux BC, Krause V, Nieuwenhuijsen ER. Effectiveness of an educational intervention to increase knowledge and reduce use of risky behaviors associated with cumulative trauma in office workers. *Work*. 2000;14:127–135.

Michalak-Turcotte C. Controlling dental hygiene work-related musculoskeletal disorders: the ergonomic process. *J Dent Hyg*. 2000;74:41–48.

Sugawara E. The study of wrist postures of musicians using the WristSystem (Greenleaf Medical System). *Work*. 1999;13:217–228.

Section 6
Skill Application

MUSCULOSKELETAL RISK ASSESSMENT

Do you sometimes forget about neutral body position as you concentrate on the finger rests? Use this checklist to assess your habits. ***A "YES" answer means that changes are indicated.***

TABLE 6-3. Body Breakers Risk Assessment Checklist

Structure	Incorrect Body Mechanics	YES	NO
Head	Tilted to one side?	☐	☐
	Tipped too far forward?	☐	☐
Shoulders	Lifted up toward ears?	☐	☐
	Tense?	☐	☐
	Hunched forward?	☐	☐
Upper Arms	Held more than 20° away from body?	☐	☐
Elbows	Held above waist level?	☐	☐
Wrists	Hand bent up? Down?	☐	☐
	Hand angled toward thumb? Toward little finger?	☐	☐
	Thumb-side of palm tipped down?	☐	☐
Hands	Gloves too tight?	☐	☐
	Fingers blanched in grasp?	☐	☐
	Fingers tense?	☐	☐
Back	Rounded back?	☐	☐
Hips	Perched forward on seat?	☐	☐
	All weight on one hip?	☐	☐
Legs	Under back of patient's chair?	☐	☐
	Thighs "cut" by edge of chair seat?	☐	☐
	Legs crossed?	☐	☐
Feet	Dangling?	☐	☐
	Ankles crossed?	☐	☐

PRACTICAL FOCUS

1. **Evaluate Fundamental Skills.** Your course assignment is to visit a local dental office and photograph a clinician at work on the maxillary teeth. Your photographs are shown below.
   a. Evaluate each photograph for clinician and patient position, grasp, and finger rest.
   b. For each incorrect element, describe: (a) how the problem could be corrected and (b) the musculoskeletal problems that could result from each positioning problem.

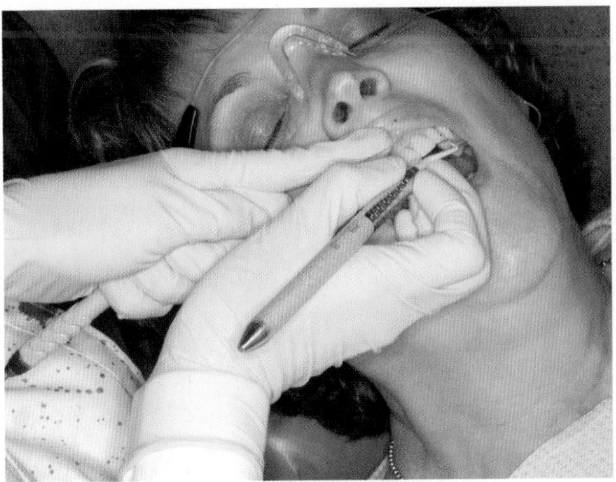

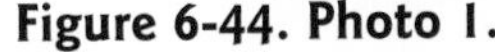

Figure 6-44. Photo 1.

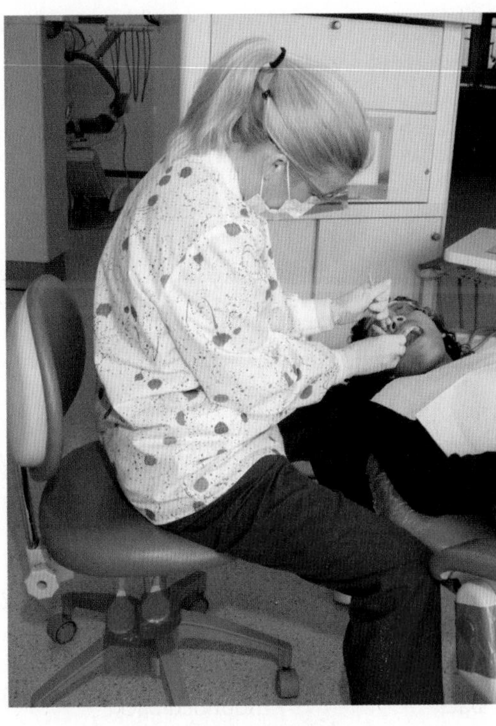

Figure 6-45. Photo 2.

2. **Precise Instrument Control.** This activity simulates the skills you will need to use when placing the instrument's working-end on the various tooth surfaces while using indirect vision. Margaret Starr designed this activity when she was a dental hygiene student learning to use indirect vision for periodontal instrumentation.

   Materials and Equipment: Printed page from a textbook or magazine, a dental mirror, and a sharpened pencil.

   a. Lay the printed page flat on a desk or tabletop. Hold a dental mirror in your non-dominant hand and position it on the page. Angle the mirror head so that you are able to see several letters reflected in the mirror. How do the letters appear?
   b. Still looking in the mirror, locate a letter "e" in one of the words. Grasp the pencil in a modified pen grasp and touch the pencil point to the "e" *on the paper*.
   c. Move the mirror to a different location on the paper. Looking in the mirror, select a letter and touch it with the pencil point.

STUDENT SELF-EVALUATION MODULE 6 MIRROR AND RESTS IN MAXILLARY POSTERIOR SEXTANTS

Student: ______________________

Date: ______________________

Area 1 = right posterior sextant, facial aspect
Area 2 = right posterior sextant, lingual aspect
Area 3 = left posterior sextant, facial aspect
Area 4 = left posterior sextant, lingual aspect

DIRECTIONS: Self-evaluate your skill level in each treatment area as: **S** (satisfactory) or **U** (unsatisfactory).

Criteria				
Positioning/Ergonomics	**Area 1**	**Area 2**	**Area 3**	**Area 4**
Adjusts clinician chair correctly				
Reclines patient chair and ensures that patient's head is even with top of headrest				
Positions instrument tray within easy reach for front, side, or rear delivery as appropriate for operatory configuration				
Positions unit light at arm's length or dons dental headlight and adjusts it for use				
Assumes the recommended clock position				
Positions backrest of patient chair for the specified arch and adjusts height of patient chair so that clinician's elbows remain at waist level when accessing the specified treatment area				
Asks patient to assume the head position that facilitates the clinician's view of the specified treatment area				
Maintains neutral position				
Directs light to illuminate the specified treatment area				
Instrument Grasp: Dominant Hand	**Area 1**	**Area 2**	**Area 3**	**Area 4**
Grasps handle with tips of finger pads of index finger and thumb so that these fingers are opposite each other on the handle, but do NOT touch or overlap				
Rests pad of middle finger lightly on instrument shank; middle finger makes contact with ring finger				
Positions the thumb, index, and middle fingers in the "knuckles-up" convex position; hyperextended joint position is avoided				
Holds ring finger straight so that it supports the weight of hand and instrument; ring finger position is "advanced ahead of" the other fingers in the grasp				
Keeps index, middle, ring, and little fingers in contact; "like fingers inside a mitten"				
Maintains a relaxed grasp; fingers are NOT blanched in grasp				
Finger Rest: Dominant Hand	**Area 1**	**Area 2**	**Area 3**	**Area 4**
Establishes secure finger rest that is appropriate for tooth to be treated				
Once finger rest is established, pauses to self-evaluate finger placement in the grasp, verbalizes to evaluator his/her self-assessment of grasp, and corrects finger placement if necessary				

Module 7

Instrument Design and Classification

Module Overview

Module 7 introduces the various design characteristics of periodontal instruments. To select an appropriate instrument for a particular instrumentation task, the clinician must have a thorough understanding of the design features of the handles, shanks, and working-ends of periodontal instruments. With so many instruments currently on the market and new designs introduced regularly, it is impossible for anyone clinician to recognize each instrument by name. Fortunately, a clinician who understands the principles of design and classification can easily determine the intended use of any unfamiliar instrument.

Module Outline

Key Terms

Knurling pattern
Balanced instrument
Simple shank design
Complex shank design
Rigid shank
Flexible shank
Visual information
Tactile sensitivity
Vibrations
Functional shank
Lower shank
Terminal shank
Extended lower shank
Unpaired working-ends
Paired working-ends
Design name
Design number
Face
Back
Lateral surfaces
Cutting edge
Toe of working-end
Tip of working-end
Cross section
Classifications
Periodontal probe
Explorer
Sickle scaler
Curet
Periodontal file

Learning Objectives

1. Identify each working-end of a periodontal instrument by its design name and number.
2. Recognize the design features of instrument handles and shanks, and discuss how these design features relate to the instrument's use.
3. Describe the advantages and limitations of the various design features available for instrument handles and shanks.
4. Given a variety of periodontal instruments, demonstrate the ability to select instruments with handle design characteristics that will reduce the pinch force required to grasp the instrument.
5. Given a variety of periodontal instruments, sort the instruments into those with simple shank design and those with complex shank design.
6. Given a variety of sickle scalers and curets, identify the face, back, lateral surfaces, cutting edges, and toe or tip on each working-end.
7. Given a variety of periodontal instruments, determine the intended use of each instrument by evaluating its design features and classification.
8. Given any instrument, identify where and how it may be used on the dentition (i.e., assessment or calculus removal, anterior/posterior teeth, supragingival or subgingival use).

Section I
Design Characteristics of Instrument Handle

The design characteristics of periodontal instruments vary widely from manufacturer to manufacturer. Selecting instruments with ergonomic design is important in the prevention of musculoskeletal injury during instrumentation. The design characteristics of the handle, shank, and working-end should be considered when selecting instruments for periodontal instrumentation. Identification of the parts of a periodontal instrument is reviewed in Figure 7-1.

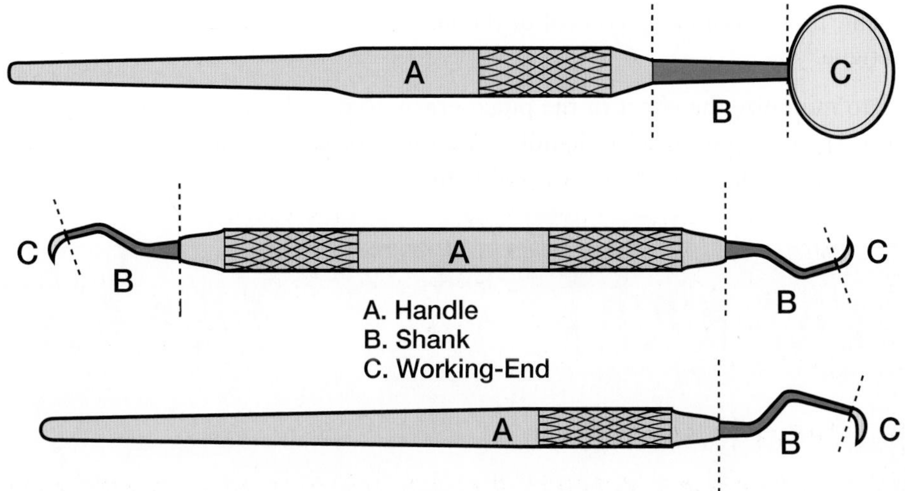

Figure 7-1. Parts of a Periodontal Instrument. The parts of a periodontal instrument are **(A)** the handle, **(B)** the shank, and **(C)** the working-end.

VARIATION IN HANDLE DESIGN

1. Instrument handles are available in a wide variety of diameters and textures.
   a. Handle design is an important component in the prevention of musculoskeletal injury during instrumentation. Hand injuries are a significant cause of pain among dental hygienists and may be related to the pinch force used to grasp the handle during periodontal instrumentation.[1]
   b. Figure 7-2 shows examples of different handle diameters and texture. Tables 7-1 and 7-2 present examples of commonly used periodontal instruments and mouth mirrors.
2. In selecting an instrument handle, there are three characteristics to consider: (1) weight, (2) diameter, and (3) texture.[2–6] Table 7-3 summarizes criteria for selecting instruments with ergonomic handle design.
   a. **Instrument Weight**
      1. The literature suggests that the optimal weight of a periodontal instrument is 15 g or less.[5,7]
      2. Lightweight instruments place less stress on the muscles of the hand and require less pinch force during periodontal instrumentation.[7]
   b. **Handle Diameter.** The literature suggests that the optimal handle diameter for periodontal instruments and mirrors is 10 mm.[1,5,7]
      1. Small diameter handles (7 mm) require more pinch force to hold and tend to cause muscle cramping.[7]

2. Large diameter handles (10 mm) and padded handles require the least pinch force when performing periodontal instrumentation.[7]
3. Lightweight instruments (15 g) with larger diameter handles (10 mm) require the least amount of pinch force.[7]

c. **Handle Texture.** Another term for texturing is a knurling pattern. Texturing increases the static friction between the fingers and handle, resulting in reduced pinch force in the grasp.[8–11]

1. Handles with no texturing decrease control of the instrument in the wet environment of the oral cavity and increase muscle fatigue.
2. Handles with raised texturing are easier to hold in the wet oral environment, thus maximizing control of the instrument and reducing muscle fatigue.[11]

3. In order to minimize the effect of the pinch grasp used with the modified pen grasp, it may be helpful to select handles in a range of larger diameters, thus providing some variety for the muscles of your fingers.[2–4,6]

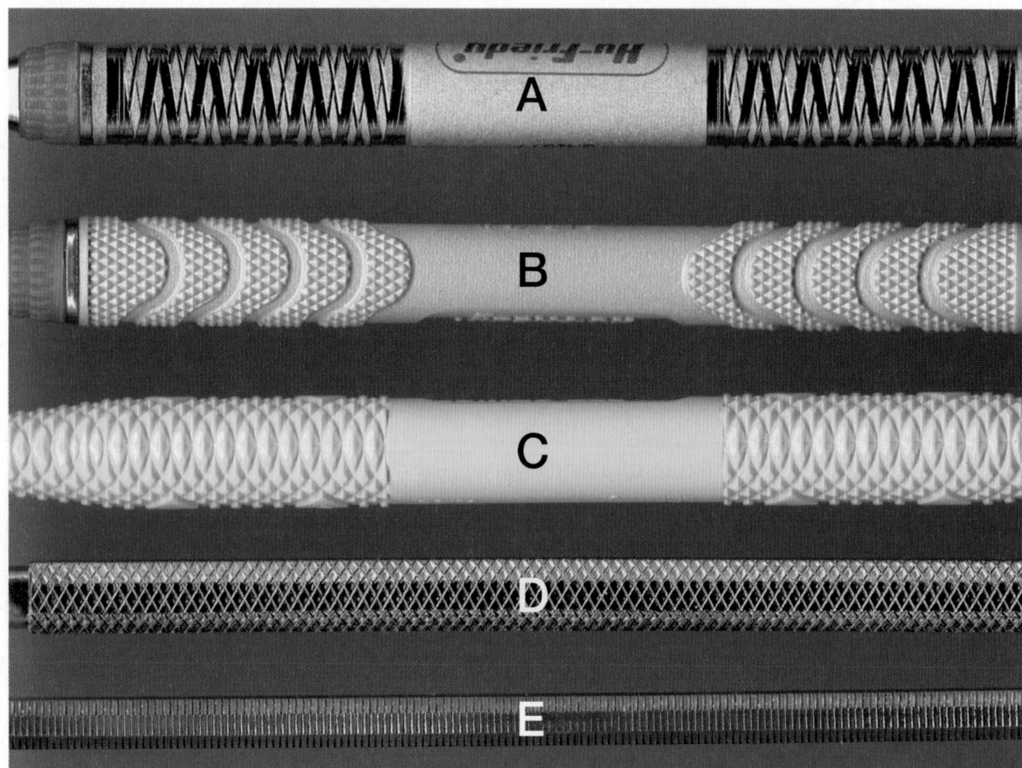

Figure 7-2. Handle Diameter and Texturing. The diameter and texturing of a handle varies greatly from manufacturer to manufacturer. Shown here are examples of the variations in design characteristics of instrument handles.

- Instruments A, B, and C with large diameter handles and bumpy texturing would be easy to hold and reduce muscle fatigue.
- Instruments A, B, and C have additional texturing on the tapered portion of the handle. This feature reduces muscle strain for short-fingered clinicians who must grip the tapered portion of the handle.
- Instrument D has a smaller diameter handle and less pronounced texturing.
- Instrument E has a small diameter handle and very limited texturing.

TABLE 7-1. Summary of Handle Designs for Periodontal Instruments*

Manufacturer	Design	Diameter (mm)	Weight (g)	Padding
American Eagle	EagleLite Resin	9.5	15	No
Brasseler USA	#2 handle (standard)	6	25	No
Brasseler USA	#4 handle	8	15	No
Brasseler USA	#6 handle	9.5	20	No
Brasseler USA	Elite handle	11	20	No
G. Hartzell & Son	A-Grip handle	9	15	No
Hu-Friedy	Standard handle	6.5	20	No
Hu-Friedy	#4 handle	8	20	No
Hu-Friedy	#7 handle	9.5	20	No
Hu-Friedy	#8 handle	9.5	20	No
Miltex	GripLite Size 6 resin handle	10	15	No
Nordent	DuraLite HEXagonal handle	9.5	15	No
Nordent	DuraLite ROUND handle with ControlRing grip	9.5	15	No
Premier	Big Easy Ultralight	11	15	Yes
Premier	Big Easy Stainless Steel	10	25	Yes
Premier	LightTouch Round handle	8	20	No

TABLE 7-2. Summary of Handle Designs for Dental Mirrors*

Manufacturer	Design	Diameter (mm)	Weight (g)	Padding
American Eagle	Standard handle	6.5	35	No
American Eagle	Resin handle	10	16	No
American Eagle	Stainless steel handle	10	30	No
Brasseler USA	#2 handle (standard)	6	35	No
Brasseler USA	#6 handle	9	20	No
Brasseler USA	Elite handle	10	30	No
Clive Craig Co.	Autoclavable plastic mirror	7	5	No
Hu-Friedy	Standard handle	6	25	No
Hu-Friedy	#6 handle	9.5	30	No
Hu-Friedy	#7 handle	9.5	30	No
Hu-Friedy	#8 handle	10	15	No
Miltex	GripLite Size 6 resin handle	10	15	No
Nordent	DuraLite ROUND handle with ControlRing grip	9.5	20	No
PDT-Cruise	Standard handle	10	15	No
Premier	Big Easy Stainless Steel	10	30	Yes
Premier	LightTouch Round handle	6	25	No

* Tables 7-1 and 7-2 reprinted from Simmer-Beck M, Branson BG. An evidence-based review of ergonomic features of dental hygiene instruments. *Work*. 2010;35:477–485, with permission from IOS Press.

TABLE 7-3. Handle Selection Criteria

Recommended:	Avoid:
• Large handle diameter (10 mm)	• Small handle diameter (7 mm)
• Lightweight hollow handle (15 g)	• Heavy, solid metal handle
• Raised texturing	• No texturing or nonraised texturing

BALANCE OF THE HANDLE AND WORKING-END

A periodontal instrument is said to be balanced when its working-ends are aligned with an imaginary line that runs vertically through the center of the handle lengthwise (the long axis of the handle). Figure 7-3 compares an instrument that is not balanced with a balanced instrument.

1. During instrumentation, balance ensures that finger pressure applied against the handle is transferred to the working-end, resulting in pressure against the tooth.
2. An instrument that is not balanced is more difficult to use and stresses the muscles of the hand and arm.
3. An easy method for determining whether an instrument is balanced is to place the instrument on a line of a lined writing tablet. Align the midline of the handle with a line on the paper; the instrument is balanced if the working-ends are centered on the line.

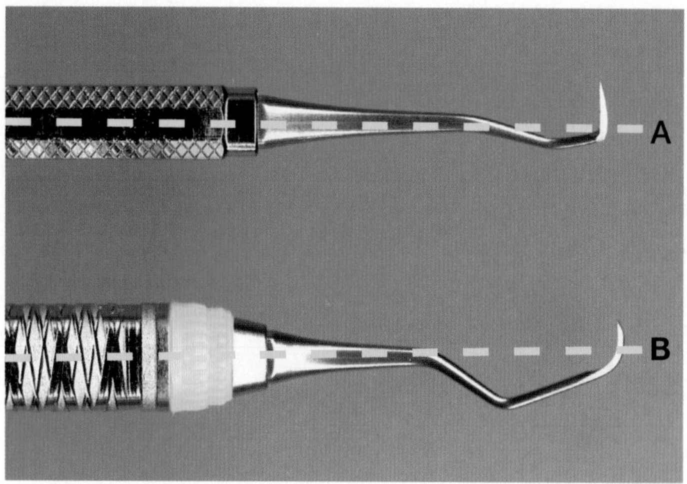

Figure 7-3. Instrument Balance. An instrument in which the working-end is aligned with the long axis of the handle is termed *balanced*. A balanced instrument ensures that pressure applied with the fingers against the handle is transferred to the working-end. In the photograph above, instrument **A** is not balanced. Instrument **B** is balanced because the working-end is centered on a line running through the long axis of the handle.

Section 2
Design Characteristics of Instrument Shank

SIMPLE AND COMPLEX SHANK DESIGN

The shanks of most periodontal instruments are bent in one or more places to facilitate placement of the working-end against the tooth surface.

1. Simple shank design—a shank that is bent in one plane (front-to-back). Figure 7-4A shows a curet with a simple shank design. Application of an instrument with a simple shank is shown in Figure 7-5.
   a. Another term for a simple shank is a straight shank.
   b. Instruments with simple shanks are used primarily on anterior teeth.
2. Complex shank design—a shank that is bent in two planes (front-to-back and side-to-side) to facilitate instrumentation of posterior teeth. Figure 7-4B shows a curet with a complex shank design. Application of an instrument with a complex shank is illustrated in Figures 7-6 and 7-7.
   a. Another term for a complex shank is an angled or curved shank.
   b. The crowns of posterior teeth are rounded and overhang their roots. An instrument with a complex shank is needed to reach around a posterior crown and onto the root surface.

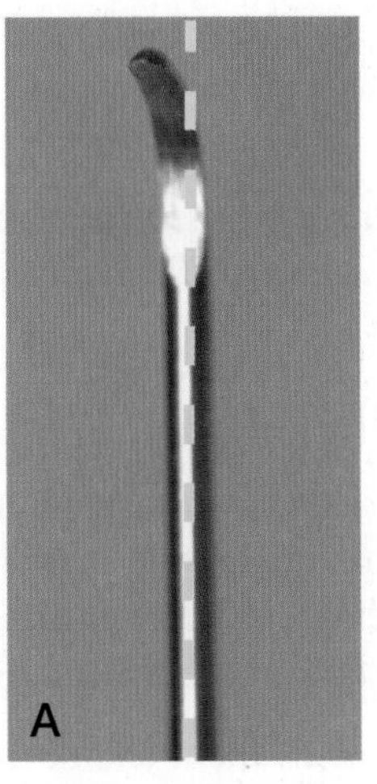

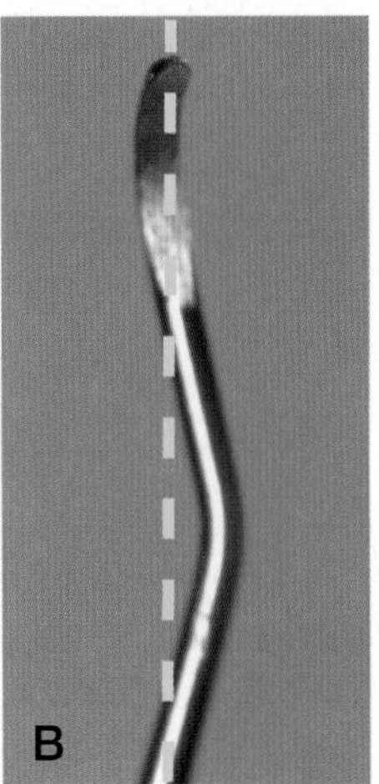

Figure 7-4. Simple and Complex Shank Design.

To determine whether the shank is simple or complex, hold the instrument so that the working-end tip or toe is facing you.

- Instrument **A** has a simple shank design.
- Instrument **B** has a complex shank design.

APPLICATION OF SIMPLE AND COMPLEX SHANKS

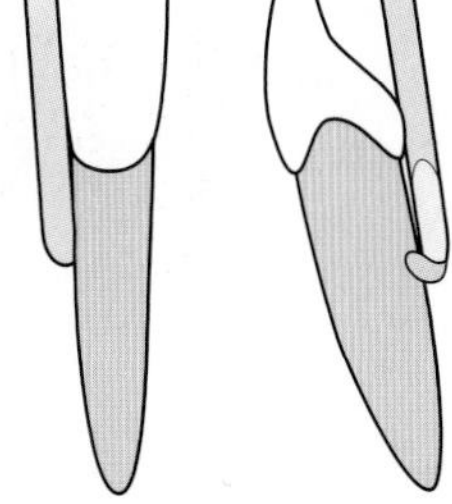

Figure 7-5. Simple Shank on an Anterior Tooth. The crowns of anterior teeth are wedge-shaped. A simple straight shank design is adequate to reach along the crown and onto the root surface.

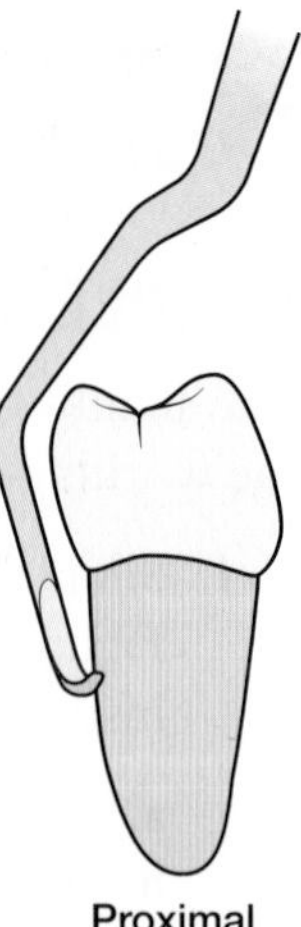

Figure 7-6. Complex Shank on a Lingual Surface. The illustration shows a mandibular molar when viewed from the mesial aspect. The drawing depicts the shank bends that allow the working-end to be placed on the lingual surface of the tooth root.

Front-to-back shank bends enable the working-end to reach around the crown and onto the lingual and facial surfaces of the root.

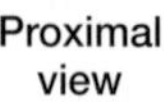

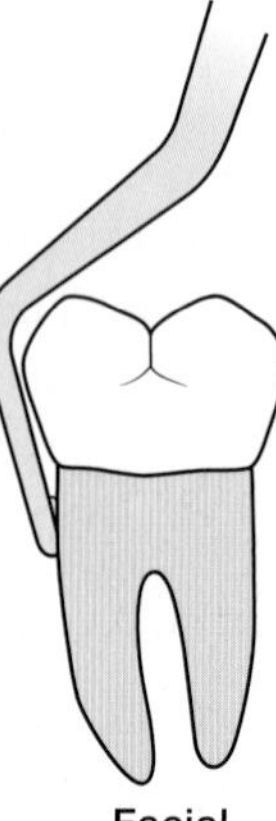

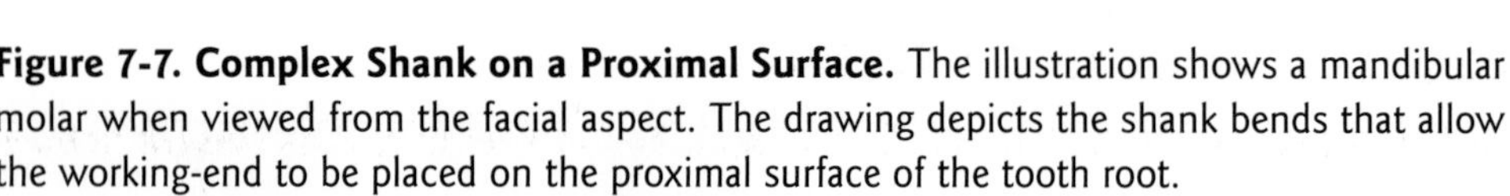

Figure 7-7. Complex Shank on a Proximal Surface. The illustration shows a mandibular molar when viewed from the facial aspect. The drawing depicts the shank bends that allow the working-end to be placed on the proximal surface of the tooth root.

Side-to-side shank bends enable the working-end to reach around the crown and onto proximal (mesial and distal) surfaces of the tooth.

SHANK FLEXIBILITY

An important characteristic of an instrument shank is its strength. To remove calculus deposits, the clinician applies pressure against the handle and shank to press the working-end against the tooth surface. The type and diameter of metal used in a shank determines its strength. Instrument shanks are classified as either rigid or flexible in design.

1. Rigid shank—an instrument shank that will withstand the pressure needed to remove heavy calculus deposits. A large calculus deposit can be removed more quickly and with less effort if the instrument has a rigid shank.
2. Flexible shank—an instrument shank that will not withstand the pressure needed to remove heavy calculus deposits but works well to remove small and medium-size calculus deposits.
    a. When used against a heavy calculus deposit, a flexible shank will bend or flex as pressure is applied against the deposit.

b. Flexible shanks enhance the amount of tactile information transmitted to the clinician's fingers. For this reason, a flexible shank design is desirable for instruments—such as explorers—that are used to locate calculus deposits hidden beneath the gingival margin.
   1. Visual information is of limited use when using instruments beneath the gingival margin since the clinician cannot see the working-end hidden subgingivally.
   2. *Instead of using visual information, the clinician must rely on his or her sense of touch to locate the calculus deposits hidden beneath the gingival margin.*[12]
   3. Tactile sensitivity is the clinician's ability to feel vibrations transmitted from the instrument working-end with his or her fingers as they rest on the shank and handle.
   4. Vibrations are created when the working-end quivers slightly as it moves over irregularities on the surface of the tooth.
      a) These vibrations are transmitted from the working-end through the shank and into the handle.
      b) The ability to feel vibrations through the instrument handle is similar in nature to the ability to feel sensations in the soles of the feet when rollerblading over a gravel surface. The rollers encounter the gravel and transmit vibrations to the soles of the feet.

THE FUNCTIONAL AND LOWER SHANK

The instrument shank extends from below the working-end to the junction of the instrument handle.

1. The portion of the shank that allows the working-end to be adapted to the tooth surface is called the functional shank. The dotted line in Figure 7-8 indicates the functional shank of a periodontal instrument.
   a. The functional shank begins below the working-end and extends to the last bend in the shank nearest the handle.
   b. Instruments with short functional shanks are used on the crowns of the teeth. For example, an instrument with a short functional shank might be used to remove supragingival calculus deposits from a tooth crown.
   c. Instruments with long functional shanks are used on both the crowns and roots of the teeth (Table 7-4). Instruments with long functional shanks might be used to detect calculus deposits beneath the gingival margin on the roots of the teeth.
2. The section of the functional shank that is nearest to the working-end is termed the lower shank. Another term for the lower shank is the terminal shank. In Figure 7-8, the blue shading indicates the lower shank of the instrument.
   a. *The ability to identify the lower shank is important because the lower shank provides an important visual clue for the clinician in selecting the correct working-end for the particular tooth surface to be instrumented.*
   b. A general rule for working-end selection is that the lower shank should be parallel to the tooth surface—distal, mesial, facial, or lingual—of the crown or root surface to be instrumented.
   c. The lower shank may be standard or extended in length (Fig. 7-9). An extended lower shank has a shank length that is 3 mm longer than that of a standard lower shank. Instruments designed for use in deep periodontal pockets have extended lower shanks.

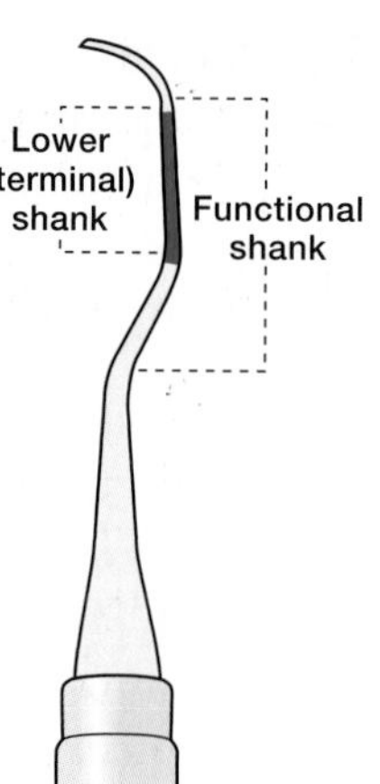

Figure 7-8. Functional and Lower Shanks.

- The functional shank, indicated by the dotted line, begins below the working-end and extends to the last bend in the shank nearest the handle.
- The lower shank, indicated by the blue shading, is the portion of the functional shank nearest to the working-end. The lower shank is important in selecting the correct working-end of an instrument.

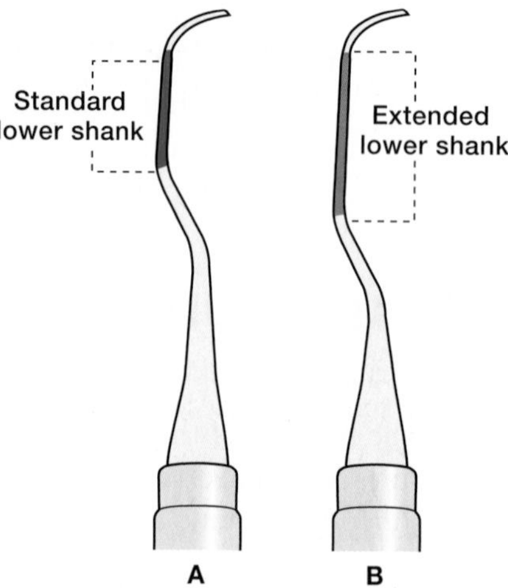

Figure 7-9. Standard and Extended Lower Shank Designs. Some instruments, such as the Gracey curets, are available with either a standard or extended lower shank design.

- In the illustration, **A** represents a curet with a standard lower shank length.
- Illustration **B** shows the same instrument, but with an extended lower shank.
- The instrument with the extended shank is ideal for use in deep periodontal pockets or when using advanced fulcruming techniques.

TABLE 7-4. Shank Design Related to Instrument Use

Shank Design	Use
Simple shank with short functional length	***Supra***gingival use on anterior teeth
Simple shank with long functional length	***Sub***gingival use on anterior teeth
Complex shank with short functional length	***Supra***gingival use on posterior teeth
Complex shank with long functional length	***Sub***gingival use on posterior teeth

Section 3

Design Characteristics of Instrument Working-End

SINGLE- AND DOUBLE-ENDED INSTRUMENTS

1. Periodontal instruments are available in single-ended and double-ended configurations. Figures 7-10 and 7-11 show examples of single-ended and double-ended instruments. Dental mirrors are usually single-ended instruments. Curets frequently are found on double-ended instruments.
2. Some double-ended instruments have unpaired working-ends that are dissimilar. An example of a double-ended instrument with unpaired working-ends is an explorer and a probe combination. Figure 7-11A shows a double-ended instrument with unpaired, dissimilar working-ends; one end is a curet, and the other is a sickle scaler.
3. Many double-ended instruments have paired working-ends that are exact mirror images. An example of an instrument with paired working-ends is a Gracey 11/12 curet. Figure 7-11B shows a double-ended instrument with paired working-ends; these curets are mirror images.

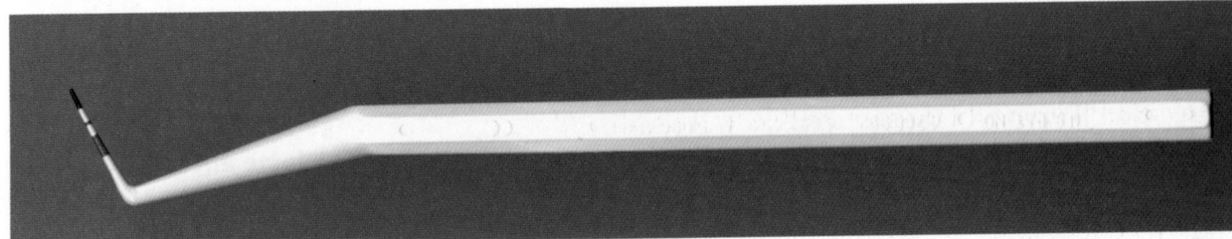

Figure 7-10. Single-Ended Instrument. This photo shows an example of a single-ended instrument. The single working-end is a periodontal probe.

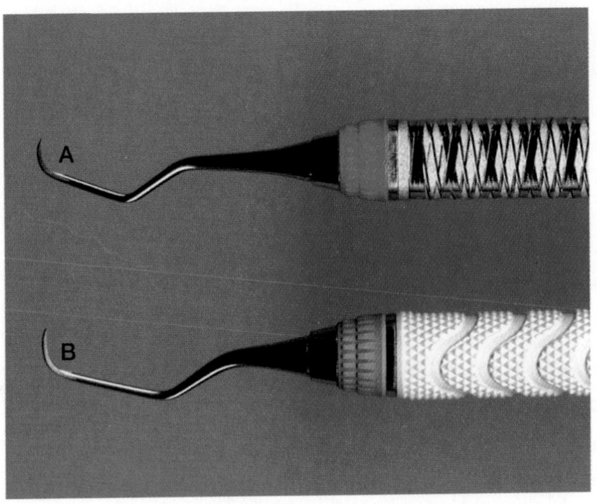

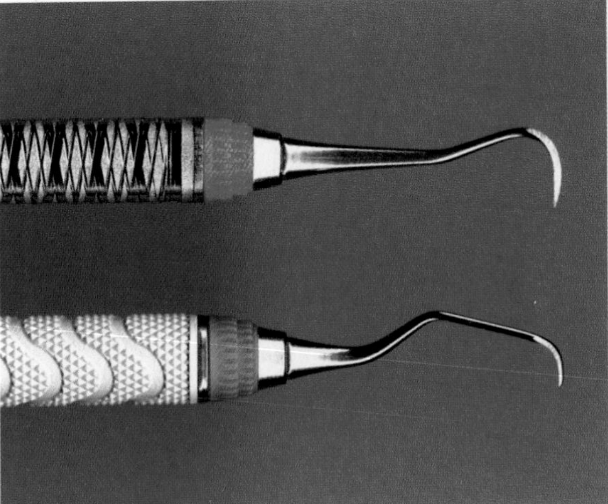

Figure 7-11. Double-Ended Instruments. Instrument A has unpaired, dissimilar working-ends. **Instrument B** has paired, mirror-image working-ends.

DESIGN NAME AND NUMBER

A unique design name and number(s) identifies each individual periodontal instrument.

1. The design name identifies the school or individual originally responsible for the design or development of an instrument or group of instruments.
   - Instruments are often named after the designer or an academic institution.
   - A well-known example is the design name "Gracey." In the late 1930s, Dr. Clayton H. Gracey designed the 14 original single-ended instruments in this series that bears his name.
2. The design number is a number designation that, when combined with the design name, provides an exact identification of the working-end.
   - Using an instrument from the Gracey series of periodontal curets as an example—Gracey 11—"Gracey" is the design name and "11" is the design number that identifies a specific instrument in this instrument series.

WORKING-END IDENTIFICATION

The design name and number are usually stamped on the handle of a periodontal instrument. A double-ended instrument will have two design numbers; each number identifies a working-end of the instrument. For example, the original Gracey series of instruments includes seven double-ended instruments, such as the Gracey 3/4, Gracey 5/6, Gracey 11/12, and Gracey 13/14. Figures 7-12 and 7-13 explain how to determine the correct design number on a double-ended instrument.

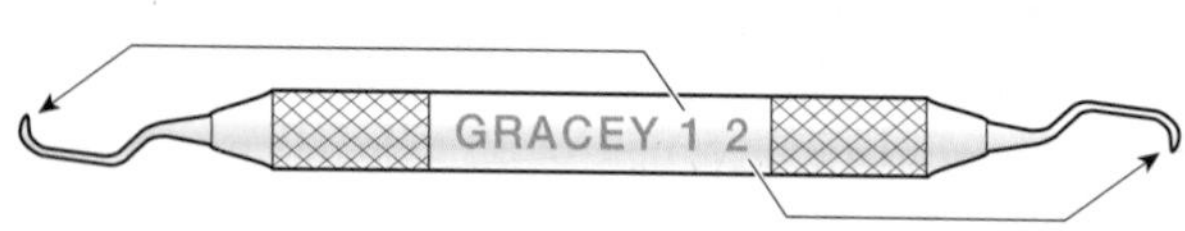

Figure 7-12. Design Name and Number Marked Along the Handle. In this example, the name and numbers are marked across the long axis of the handle; each working-end is identified by the number closest to it.

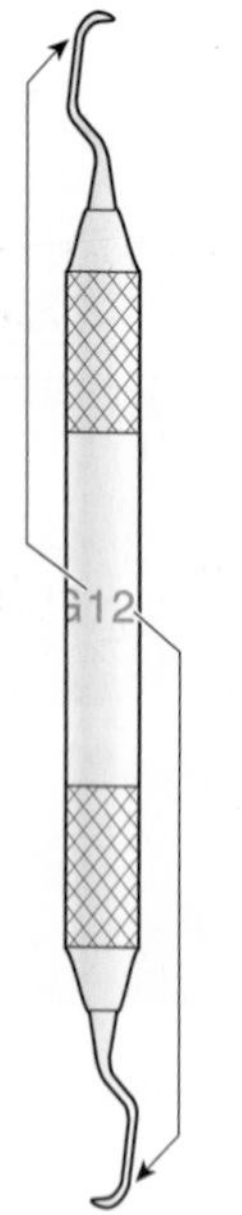

Figure 7-13. Design Name and Number Marked Around the Handle. In this example, the name and numbers are marked around the handle; the first number (on the left) identifies the working-end at the top end of the handle, and the second number identifies the working-end at the lower end of the handle.

PARTS OF THE WORKING-END

An instrument's function is determined primarily by the design of its working-end. Some instruments are used to assess the teeth or soft tissues; others are used to remove calculus deposits. To determine an instrument's use, it is necessary to be able to identify the face, back, lateral surfaces, cutting edges, and toe or tip of the working-end (Figs. 7-14 to 7-17).

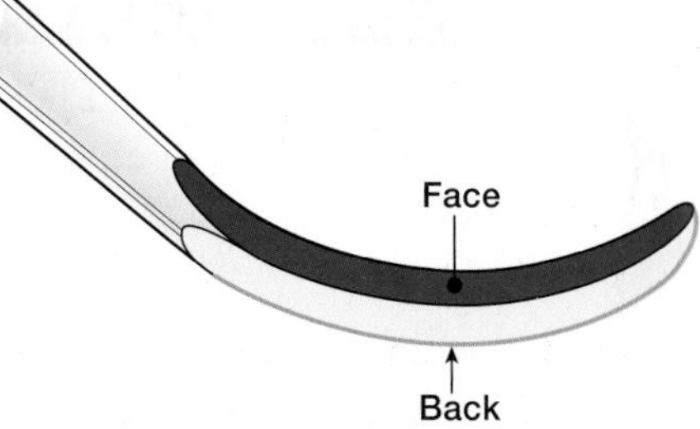

Figure 7-14. Face and Back of the Working-End. The surface shaded in purple on this illustration is the instrument **face**. The surface opposite the face—indicated by a gold line—is the instrument **back**.

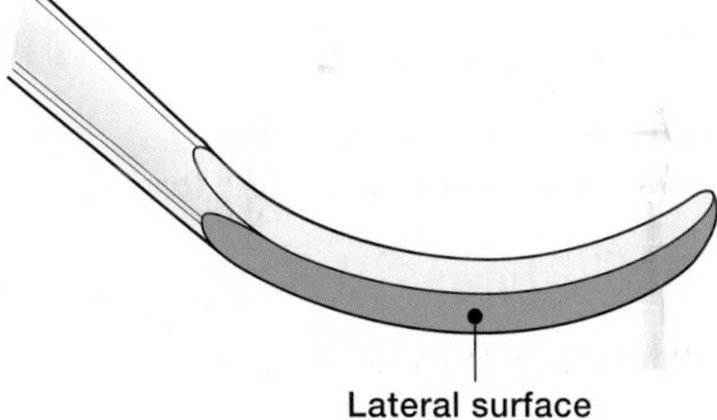

Figure 7-15. Lateral Surfaces of the Working-End. The surfaces of the working-end on either side of the face are called the **lateral surfaces** of the instrument. The green shading on this illustration indicates one lateral surface of the working-end.

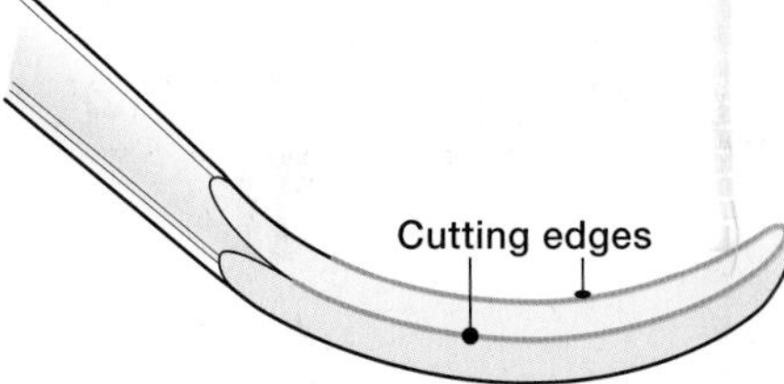

Figure 7-16. Cutting Edge of the Working-End. The **cutting edge** is a sharp area of the working-end formed where the face and lateral surfaces meet. The orange lines on this illustration indicate the cutting edges of the working-end.

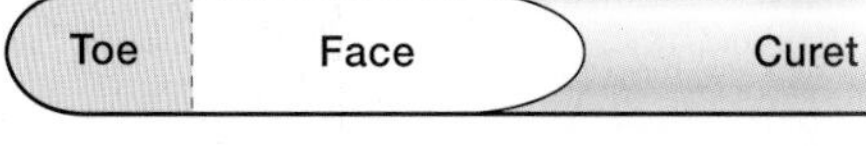

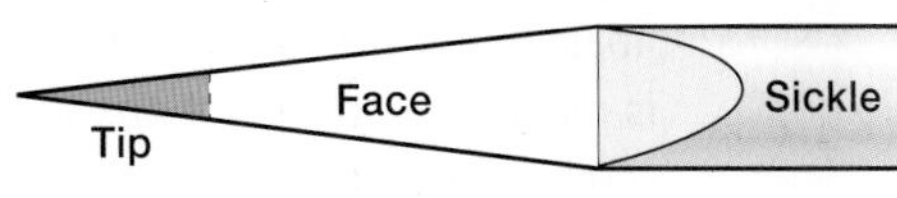

Figure 7-17. Toe or Tip of the Working-End. These illustrations show a curet and a sickle scaler from a bird's-eye view, looking directly down on the instrument face.

The cutting edges of a curet meet to form a rounded surface called a toe. The cutting edges of a sickle scaler meet in a point called a tip.

THE WORKING-END IN CROSS SECTION

A cross section is a cut through something at an angle perpendicular to its long axis in order to view its interior structure. A well-known example is a cross section of a tree that shows its growth rings and tells its age.

- The cross section of a working-end determines whether it can be used subgingivally beneath the gingival margin or is restricted to supragingival use.
- At first, understanding cross sections may seem difficult, but looking at an everyday object pictured in Figure 7-18 should help to clarify this concept. Figures 7-19 to 7-21 illustrate periodontal instruments in cross section.

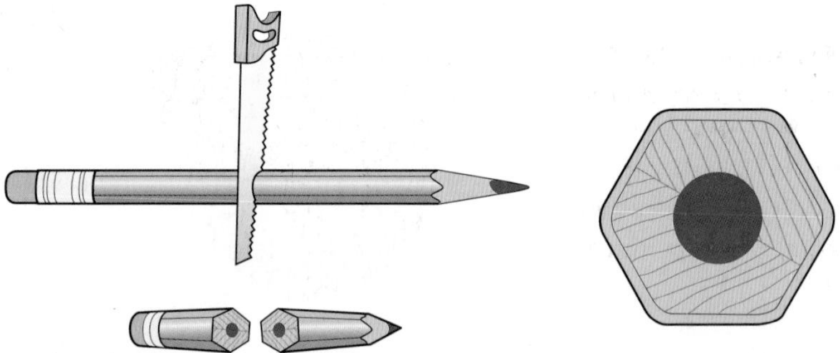

Figure 7-18. Creating a Cross Section of a Pencil. Imagine sawing a lead pencil into two parts by cutting it in the middle perpendicular to the long axis of the pencil. When the pencil has been cut, it is possible to view its shape in cross section. The pencil is hexagonal (six-sided) in cross section.

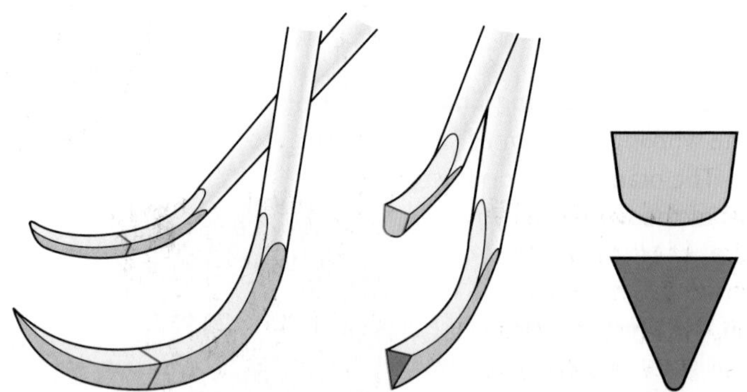

Figure 7-19. Instrument Working-Ends in Cross Section. In a similar manner, imagine cutting the working-ends of periodontal instruments in half. After the cut is made, the cross sections of the working-ends are visible. The top instrument is semi-circular in cross section. The lower instrument is triangular in cross section.

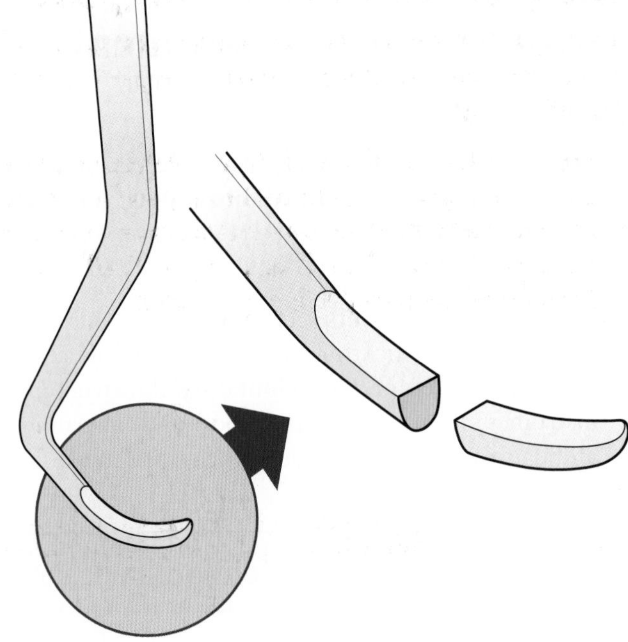

Figure 7-20. Cross Section of a Curet. The semi-circular cross section of a periodontal instrument is shown in yellow on this illustration. Curets are calculus removal instruments that are semi-circular in cross section. The working-end of a curet has a rounded back and toe.

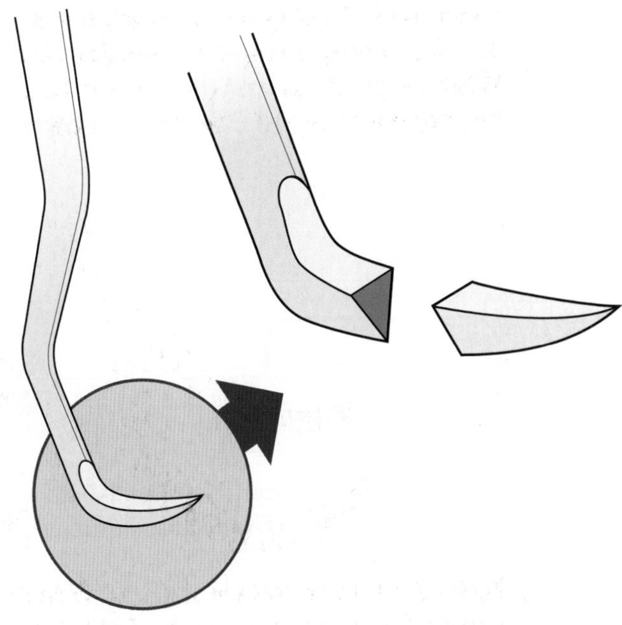

Figure 7-21. Cross Section of a Sickle Scaler. The triangular cross section of a periodontal instrument is shown in green on this illustration. Sickle scalers are calculus removal instruments that are triangular in cross section. The working-end of a sickle scaler has a pointed back and pointed tip.

Section 4
Introduction to Instrument Classification

Periodontal instruments are divided into types, or classifications, based on the specific design characteristics of the working-ends (Fig. 7-22). This section presents a basic introduction to instrument classification; detailed information about each of the different instrumentation classifications is presented in later modules.

- Nonsurgical, hand-activated periodontal instruments are classified as periodontal probes, explorers, sickle scalers, periodontal files, curets, hoes, or chisels. These commonly used instrument classifications are pictured in Figures 7-23 to 7-27.
- Hoes and chisels are periodontal hand instruments that are rarely used in modern periodontal instrumentation. Mechanized (powered) instruments have largely replaced the function of hoes and chisels for removing large, heavy calculus deposits.

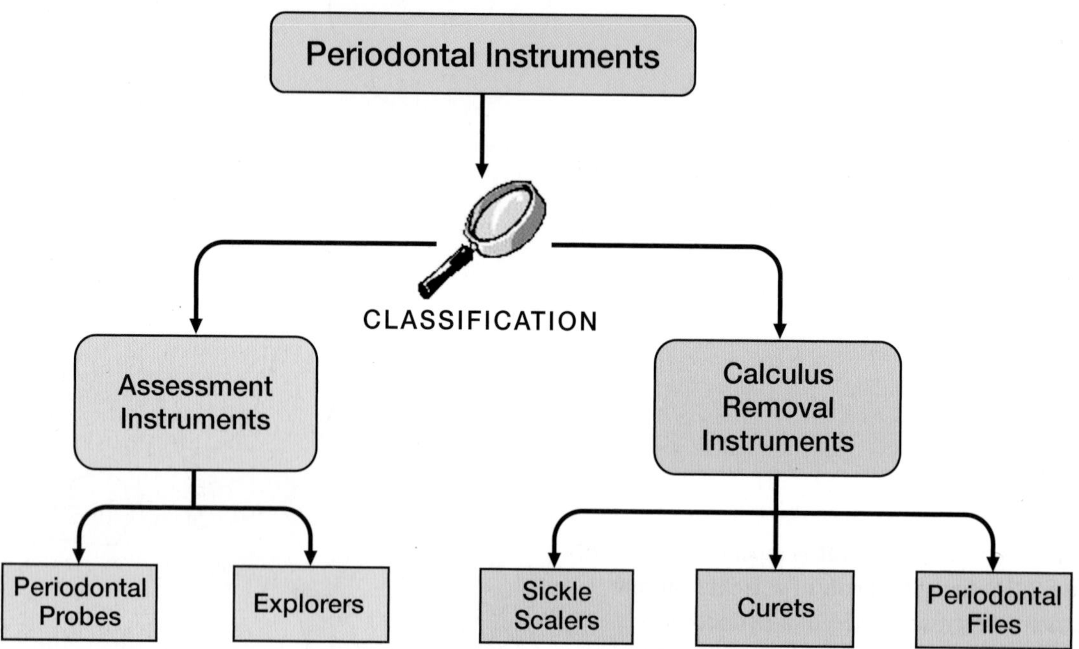

Figure 7-22. Classification of Hand-Activated Periodontal Instruments. Two major classifications of periodontal instruments are assessment instruments and calculus removal instruments.

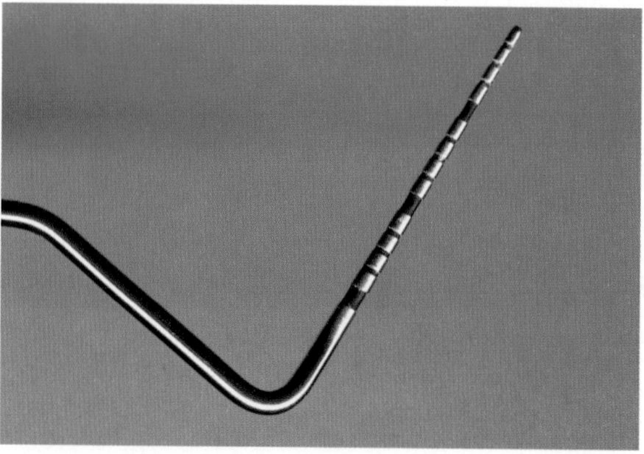

Figure 7-23. Periodontal Probe. The periodontal probe is a slender assessment instrument used to evaluate the health of the periodontal tissues. Probes have blunt, rod-shaped working-ends that are circular or rectangular in cross section.

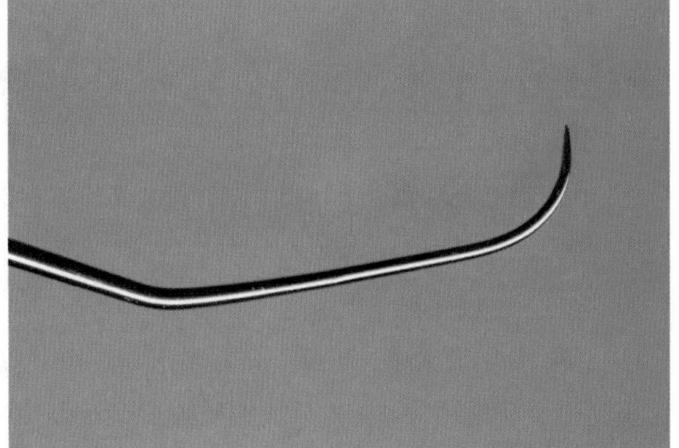

Figure 7-24. Explorer. An explorer is an assessment instrument used to locate calculus deposits, tooth surface irregularities, and defective margins on restorations. Explorers have flexible shanks and are circular in cross section.

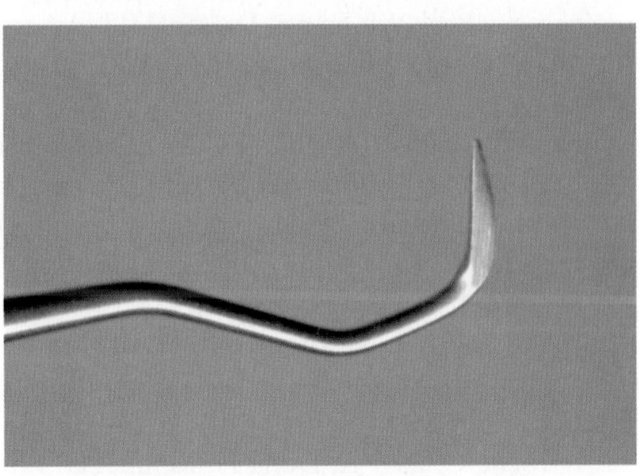

Figure 7-25. Sickle Scaler. A sickle scaler is a periodontal instrument used to remove calculus deposits from the crowns of the teeth. The working-end of a sickle scaler has a pointed back and pointed tip and is triangular in cross section.

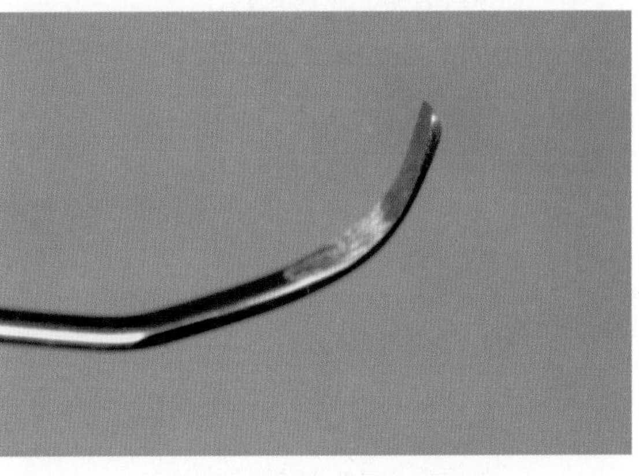

Figure 7-26. Curet. A curet is a periodontal instrument used to remove calculus deposits from the crowns and roots of the teeth. The working-end of a curet has a rounded back and rounded toe and is semi-circular in cross section. Two curet subtypes are the universal curet and area-specific curet.

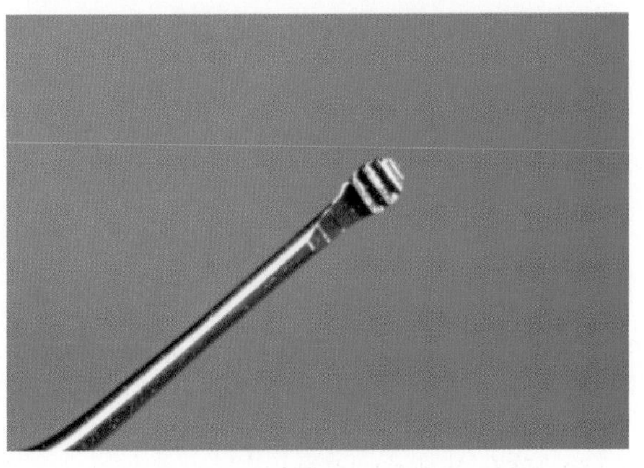

Figure 7-27. A Periodontal File. A periodontal file is an instrument used to crush large calculus deposits. Each working-end of a periodontal file has several cutting edges.

REFERENCES

1. Dong H, Loomer P, Barr A, Laroche C, Young E, Rempel D. The effect of tool handle shape on hand muscle load and pinch force in a simulated dental scaling task. *Appl Ergon*. 2007;38: 525–531.
2. Horstman SW, Horstman BC, Horstman FS. Ergonomic risk factors associated with the practice of dental hygiene: a preliminary study. *Prof Safety*. 1997;42:49–53.
3. Liskiewicz ST, Kerschbaum WE. Cumulative trauma disorders: an ergonomic approach for prevention. *J Dent Hyg*. 1997;71:162–167.
4. Michalak-Turcotte C. Controlling dental hygiene work-related musculoskeletal disorders: the ergonomic process. *J Dent Hyg*. 2000;74:41–48.
5. Simmer-Beck M, Branson BG. An evidence-based review of ergonomic features of dental hygiene instruments. *Work*. 2010;35:477–485.
6. van der Beek AJ, Frings-Dresen MH. Assessment of mechanical exposure in ergonomic epidemiology. *Occup Environ Med*. 1998;55:291–299.
7. Dong H, Barr A, Loomer P, Laroche C, Young E, Rempel D. The effects of periodontal instrument handle design on hand muscle load and pinch force. *J Am Dent Assoc*. 2006;137:1123–1130.
8. Bobjer O, Johansson SE, Piguet S. Friction between hand and handle. Effects of oil and lard on textured and non-textured surfaces; perception of discomfort. *Appl Ergon*. 1993;24:190–202.
9. Fredrick L, Armstrong T. Effect of friction and load on pinch force in hand transfer task. *Ergonomics*. 1995;38:2447–2454.
10. Johansson RS, Westling G. Roles of glabrous skin receptors and sensorimotor memory in automatic control of precision grip when lifting rougher or more slippery objects. *Exp Brain Res*. 1984;56:550–564.
11. Laroche C, Barr A, Dong H, Rempel D. Effect of dental tool surface texture and material on static friction with a wet gloved fingertip. *J Biomech*. 2007;40:697–701.
12. Rucker LM, Gibson G, McGregor C. Getting the "feel" of it: the non-visual component of dimensional accuracy during operative tooth preparation. *J Can Dent Assoc*. 1990;56:937–941.

Section 5
Skill Application

PRACTICAL FOCUS

1. **Working-End Design.** Use nail polish to identify the design elements of several periodontal instruments as illustrated in Figure 7-28 below.

   Equipment: Ask your instructor to help you assemble the following instruments—a sickle scaler, a universal curet, and an area-specific curet.

   Materials: Four bottles of nail polish in different colors and nail polish remover or orange solvent (to remove nail polish from your instruments at the completion of this activity).

   a. Paint the lateral surfaces of each working-end with one color of nail polish.
   b. Use a contrasting color of polish to paint the face of each instrument.
   c. Paint the back of each instrument.
   d. Paint the functional shank on each instrument. Compare the functional shank lengths on the various instruments.
   e. Use a contrasting color of polish to paint the lower shank on each instrument.
   f. Ask an instructor to check your work.

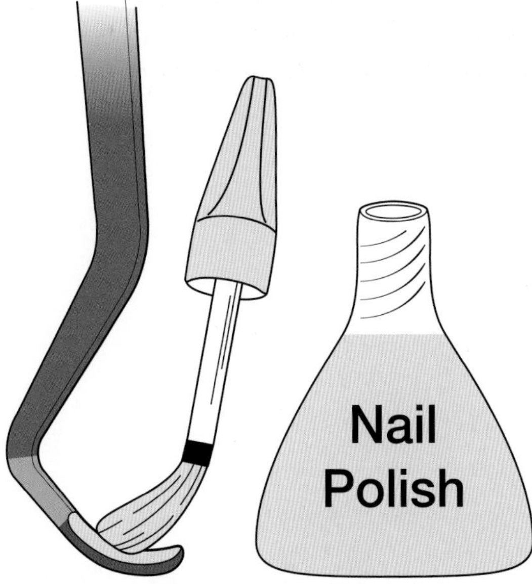

Figure 7-28. Identify Parts of Instrument with Nail Polish. Use different shades of nail polish to mark the following areas of a periodontal instrument: face, back, lateral surfaces, functional shank, and lower shank.

The Practical Focus activities continue on the next page.

2. **The World of Periodontal Instruments.** The periodontal instruments in your school's kit are only a small sample of the many instrument designs on the market.

    - Select one of the instrument manufacturers' websites listed below.
    - Go to the website and explore the variety of periodontal instruments available on the site. Select one instrument that is NOT part of your school's instrument kit.
    - Identify the design characteristics of the instrument.
    - Post the following information in your course instructor's drop box:
        - Website that you accessed online
        - Instrument selected by item number, product number, or design name and number
        - Description of the design characteristics of the working-ends

Manufacturer Sites:

- http://www.am-eagle.com
- http://www.dentalez.com/stardental/hygiene
- http://www.jjinstruments.com (click on dental and then select periodontal curettes)
- http://www.hu-friedy.com
- http://www.nordent.com
- http://www.pdtdental.com/products.php
- http://www.premusa.com/dental/instruments.asp
- http://www.smartpractice.com (enter hygiene instruments in the product search box)

3. **Evaluation of Design Characteristics: Instrument Kit.** Assemble a variety of periodontal instruments from your instrument kit, including assessment and calculus removal instruments. For each instrument, determine its classification and intended use by evaluating the design features of the shank and working-end. Enter the information in Table 7-5.

TABLE 7-5. Evaluation of Instrument Design and Classification

Instrument	Shank Simple or complex? Short or long?	Working-End Pointed tip? Rounded toe?	Classification	Instrument Use Assessment? Calculus removal?
A				
B				
C				
D				
E				
F				
G				
H				
I				
J				
K				
L				
M				
N				

STUDENT SELF-EVALUATION MODULE 7 INSTRUMENT DESIGN AND CLASSIFICATION

Student: ______________________

Date: ______________________

Instrument 1 = ______________________

Instrument 2 = ______________________

Instrument 3 = ______________________

Instrument 4 = ______________________

DIRECTIONS: Self-evaluate your skill level as: **S** (satisfactory) or **U** (unsatisfactory).

Criteria				
Instrument	1	2	3	4
Identifies each working-end by its design name and number				
Determines if the instrument is balanced				
Working-End	1	2	3	4
Identifies the classification of each working-end				
Identifies the parts of the working-end (face, back, lateral surfaces, tip or toe, and cutting edges)				
States the shape of the working-end in cross section				
Shank	1	2	3	4
Identifies the functional shank				
Identifies the lower (terminal) shank				
Identifies the shank as simple or complex				

Module 8

Technique Essentials: Movement and Orientation to Tooth Surface

Module Overview

This module introduces two techniques that are essential to effective periodontal instrumentation: (1) the manner in which the instrument is moved during periodontal instrumentation and (2) the orientation of the instrument to the various tooth surfaces in the dentition during periodontal instrumentation.

- Movement of the instrument involves (a) using the muscles of the fingers, hand, and arm to move the working-end across the tooth surface, (b) pivoting on the fulcrum finger, and (c) rolling the instrument handle as the working-end moves around the tooth.
- Orientation involves alignment of the instrument to the tooth surface to be instrumented.

Module Outline

Key Terms

- Motion activation
- Wrist motion activation
- Digital motion activation
- Rolling the instrument handle
- Drive finger
- Pivot
- Tooth surface being instrumented

Learning Objectives

1. Define motion activation as it relates to periodontal instrumentation.
2. Name two types of motion activation commonly used in periodontal instrumentation.
3. Define and explain the uses of wrist motion activation during periodontal instrumentation.
4. Using a pencil or periodontal probe, demonstrate the correct technique for wrist motion activation.
5. When demonstrating wrist motion activation, use correct instrumentation technique such as: using the fulcrum finger as a support beam, maintaining correct grasp, and maintaining neutral wrist position.
6. Define and explain the uses of digital motion activation during periodontal instrumentation.
7. Using a pencil or periodontal probe, demonstrate the correct technique for digital motion activation.
8. When demonstrating digital motion activation, use correct instrumentation technique such as: using the fulcrum finger as a support beam, maintaining correct grasp, and maintaining neutral wrist position.
9. Define and explain the use of the handle roll during periodontal instrumentation.
10. Using a pen or pencil, demonstrate the handle roll using correct technique including: correct modified pen grasp, knuckles-up position, fulcrum finger as a support beam, and neutral wrist position.
11. Using a pen or pencil and Figure 8-8A or 8-8B, demonstrate how to pivot on the fulcrum finger.
12. Explain how the teeth are positioned in the dental arches.
13. Using a periodontal probe and a typodont or tooth model, correctly orient the working-end of a probe to the various tooth surfaces of the dentition.

Section I
Moving the Working-End

Motion activation is the muscle action used to move the working-end of a periodontal instrument across a tooth surface.

1. Two types of motion activation commonly used in periodontal instrumentation are wrist motion activation and digital motion activation.
   a. Wrist motion activation is the most commonly used type of movement used for periodontal instrumentation.
      1. This type of activation employs the hand, wrist, and arm—moving as a unit—to produce a rotating motion used to move the working-end across a tooth surface.
      2. A clinician experiences less fatigue with wrist activation than if finger movements are used to move the instrument during periodontal instrumentation.
      3. Wrist motion activation is recommended for calculus removal with hand-activated instruments.
   b. Digital motion activation is a less commonly used type of movement for periodontal instrumentation.
      1. This type of activation moves the instrument by making push-pull movements with the thumb, index, and middle fingers. For example, on mandibular teeth, the fingers are used to pull the working-end up the tooth, and then a push movement returns the working-end back to its starting position.
      2. Digital motion activation is used whenever physical strength is not required during instrumentation. It is used most commonly with powered instruments such as ultrasonic and sonic instruments. With powered instruments, the machine, rather than the clinician, provides the force necessary for calculus removal.
      3. Digital motion activation also may be used to instrument areas where movement is very restricted, such as when instrumenting furcation areas.
2. It is important to remember that instrumentation strokes are tiny movements. The working-end is moved only a few millimeters with each stroke.

WRIST MOTION ACTIVATION

Wrist motion activation is the act of rotating the hand and wrist as a unit to provide the power for an instrumentation stroke.

1. This movement is a rotating motion similar to the action of turning a doorknob.
2. The way the fulcrum finger is used is an important element in the controlled movement of the working-end across a tooth surface.
   a. During motion activation, the fulcrum finger supports the weight of the hand and assists in controlling the movement of the working-end.
   b. Throughout the production of an instrument stroke, the fulcrum finger should remain pressed against the tooth.
   c. The slight pressure of the finger against the tooth allows the fulcrum to act like a "brake" to stop the movement at the end of each stroke. If the instrument tip flies off of the tooth at the end of a stroke, the clinician did not stop the stroke by pressing down with the fulcrum against the tooth.

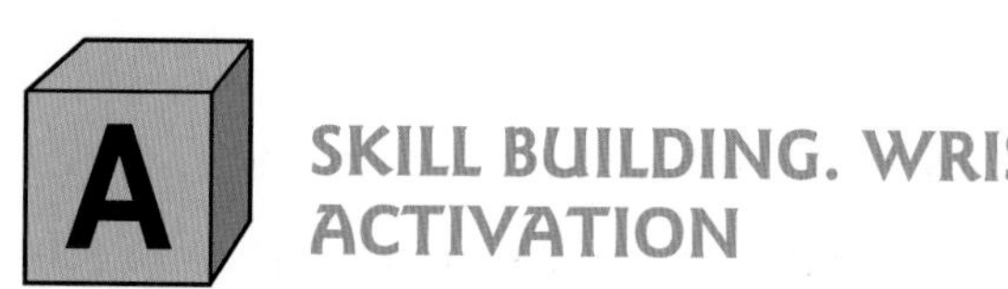

SKILL BUILDING. WRIST MOTION ACTIVATION

Directions: This skill building activity is designed to help you experience wrist motion activation. Keep in mind that the movements in this practice are broad, large movements when compared with the tiny, precise movements used to instrument a tooth.

1. **Get Ready.** Grasp a periodontal probe or pencil with a modified pen grasp in your *dominant hand*. The photographs below show a right-handed clinician.
2. **Get Set: Starting Position**
   - Establish a finger rest with your ring finger on a countertop. Your thumb, middle, and index fingers should be in a curved, knuckles-out position and relaxed. Your ring finger is advanced ahead of the other fingers in the grasp and held straight to act as a support beam for your hand.
   - The photograph below shows the starting position, **Position A.**
   - The end of the periodontal probe or pencil should be touching the countertop, and the long axis of the periodontal probe or pencil should be perpendicular ($\perp$) to the countertop.
   - Your wrist should be in neutral position so that the back of your hand and wrist are in straight alignment and your arm is parallel (=) to the countertop.
3. **Activate Motion**
   - Press your ring finger downward against the counter in preparation for motion.
   - Using a similar motion to turning a doorknob, rotate your hand and wrist as a unit away from your body into **Position B** shown below. As you make this movement, the end of the periodontal probe or pencil lifts off of the countertop.
   - Throughout the motion, your ring finger continues to press down against the countertop and does not lift off the counter.
4. **Reposition for Next Movement.** Return the periodontal probe or pencil to **Position A** by rotating your hand and wrist back toward your body.

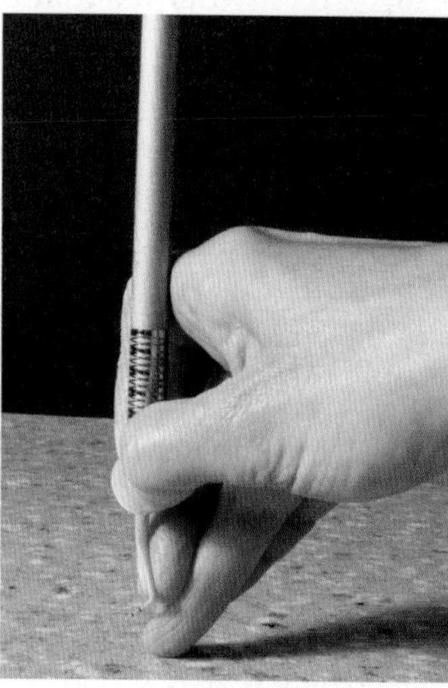

Figure 8-1A. Wrist Motion Activation. Position A at start of activation.

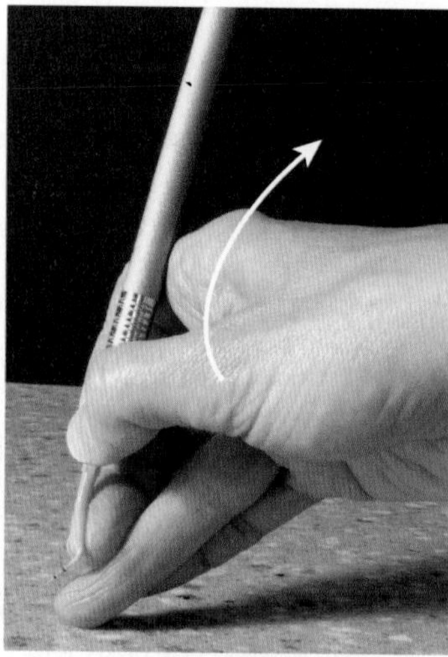

Figure 8-1B. Wrist Motion Activation. Position B at end of activation.

DIGITAL MOTION ACTIVATION

Digital motion activation is moving the instrument by flexing the thumb, index, and middle fingers.

1. Digital motion activation is used whenever physical strength is not required during instrumentation.
2. It may be used with periodontal probes, explorers, and ultrasonic instruments. With ultrasonic (automated, powered) instruments, the machine, rather than the clinician, provides the force necessary for calculus removal.
3. Digital motion activation also may be used to instrument areas where movement is very restricted, such as when instrumenting the furcation areas of multirooted teeth.

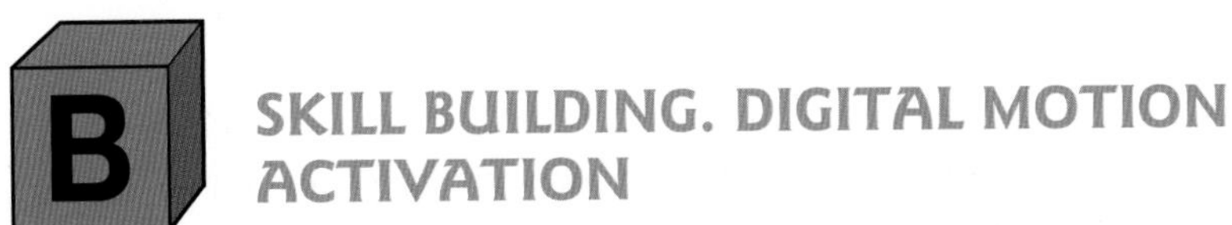

SKILL BUILDING. DIGITAL MOTION ACTIVATION

Directions: Follow these steps to practice digital motion activation.

1. **Get Ready.** Grasp a periodontal probe or pencil with a modified pen grasp in your *dominant hand*. The photographs below show a right-handed clinician.
2. **Get Set: Starting Position**
   - Establish a finger rest with your ring finger on the edge of a textbook so that the working-end of the probe extends over the side of the book. Your thumb, middle, and index fingers should be in a curved, knuckles-out position and relaxed. Your ring finger is advanced ahead of the other fingers in the grasp and held straight to act as a support beam for your hand. The photograph below shows the starting position, **Position A.**
   - Your wrist should be in neutral position so that the back of your hand and wrist are in straight alignment and your arm is parallel (=) to the countertop.
3. **Activate Motion**
   - Press your ring finger downward against the textbook in preparation for motion.
   - Use digital motion activation to pull the tip of the periodontal probe or pencil upward by pulling your thumb, index, and middle fingers toward the palm of your hand into **Position B.**
   - Your ring finger should remain motionless pressing down against the textbook.
4. **Reposition for Next Movement.** Return the periodontal probe or pencil to **Position A** by pushing downward with your thumb, index, and middle fingers. Note that you have little strength and your fingers would fatigue quickly when using this type of motion activation.

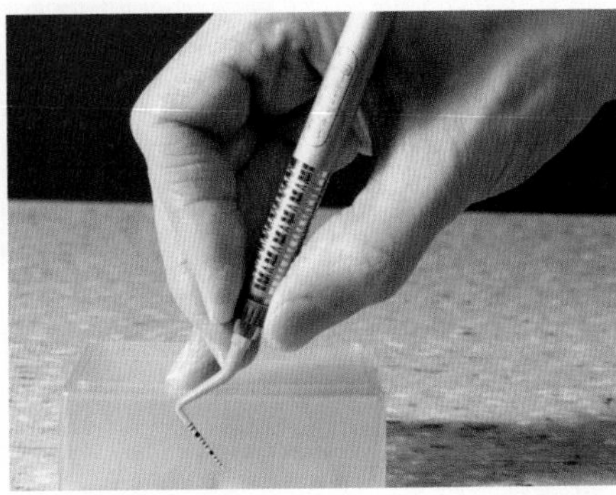

Figure 8-2A. Digital Activation, Position A.

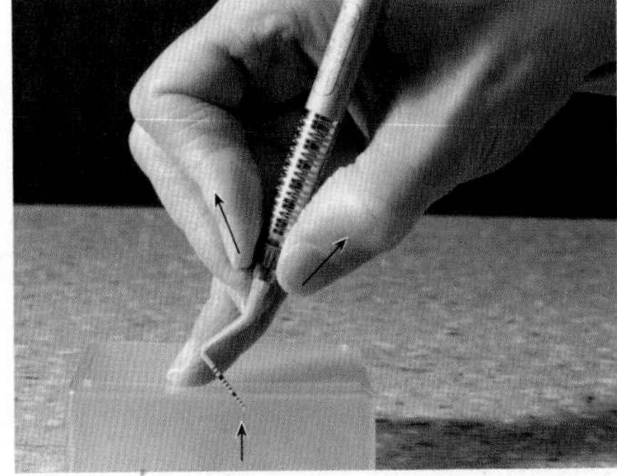

Figure 8-2B. Digital Activation, Position B.

Section 2
Rolling the Instrument Handle

Rolling the instrument handle is the act of turning the handle between the thumb and index finger. The purpose is to maintain precise contact of the working-end to the tooth surface as it moves around the tooth. Either the index finger *or* the thumb acts as the drive finger used to turn the instrument. The finger used to roll the handle determines the direction in which the working-end will turn.

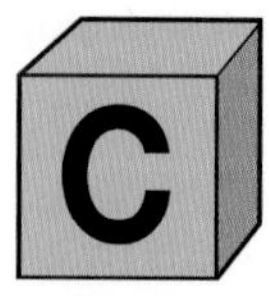

SKILL BUILDING. THE HANDLE ROLL

Directions: This skill building activity is designed to help you learn how to use your thumb and index finger to roll an instrument. Use a pen with lettering running along its length. The lettering on the pen provides a visual reference point as the pen turns between your fingers.

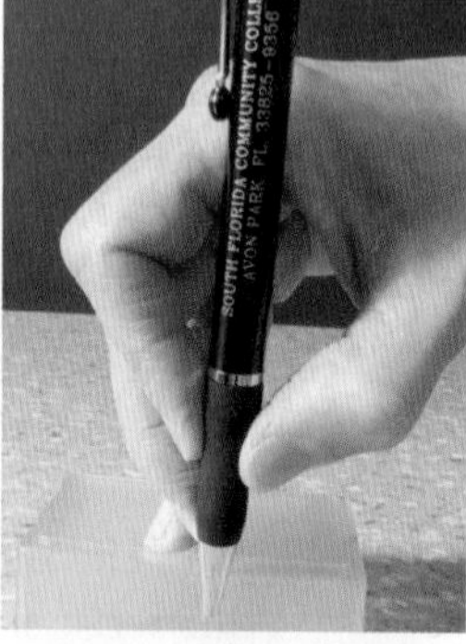

Figure 8-3. Get Ready. Establish a finger rest on a textbook and allow the tip of the pen to extend over the side of the book.

- Grasp the pen so that the lettering is visible between your index finger and thumb.
- *Space your thumb and index finger slightly apart on the pen shaft. Touching or overlapping the fingers makes it more difficult to roll the pen.*

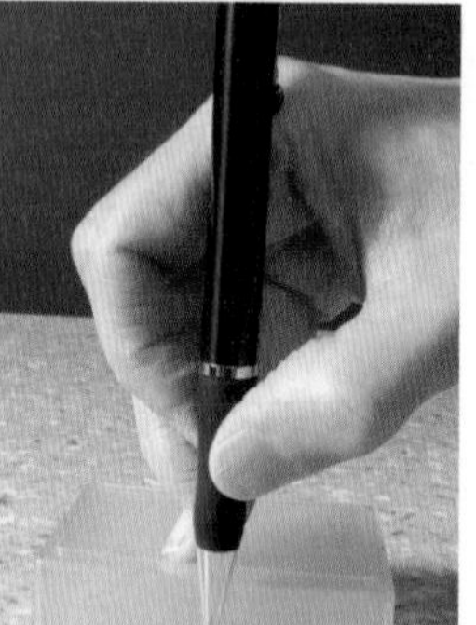

Figure 8-4. Roll in a Clockwise Direction. Roll the pen between your index finger and thumb in a clockwise direction until the lettering is no longer visible. Does your index finger or your thumb act as the drive finger to turn the instrument in a clockwise direction?

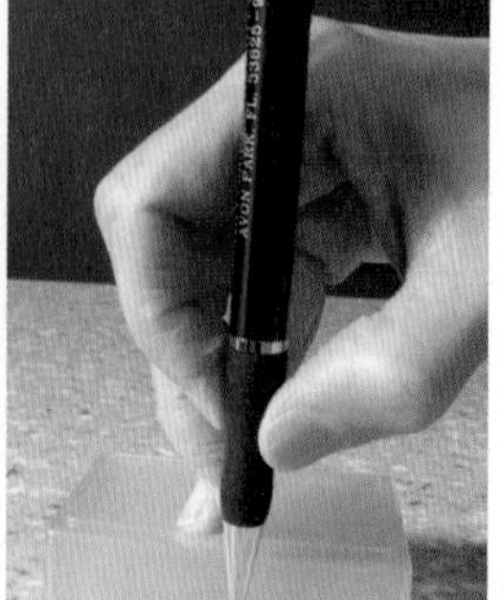

Figure 8-5. Roll in a Counter-Clockwise Direction. Finally, turn the pen in a counter-clockwise direction, back toward the starting position. Continue rolling until the pen has returned to the original starting position.
Does your index finger or your thumb act as the drive finger to turn the instrument in a counter-clockwise direction?

Section 3
Pivoting on the Fulcrum

THE HAND PIVOT

A pivot is something, such as a rod, that supports an object as it turns or rotates—for example, spinning around while balanced on one foot like a ballerina. In this example, a foot and leg act as the pivot that supports the rest of the body as it turns. In periodontal instrumentation, the fulcrum finger acts as the pivot that supports the hand as it turns.

- Pivoting the hand and arm assists the clinician in keeping the working-end against the tooth as it moves around the tooth.
- Pivoting is used principally when moving around a line angle and onto the proximal surface of a tooth. For example, moving the working-end from the facial surface—around the mesiofacial line angle—and onto the mesial surface of a molar tooth.

EXAMPLE OF PIVOTING ON FULCRUM

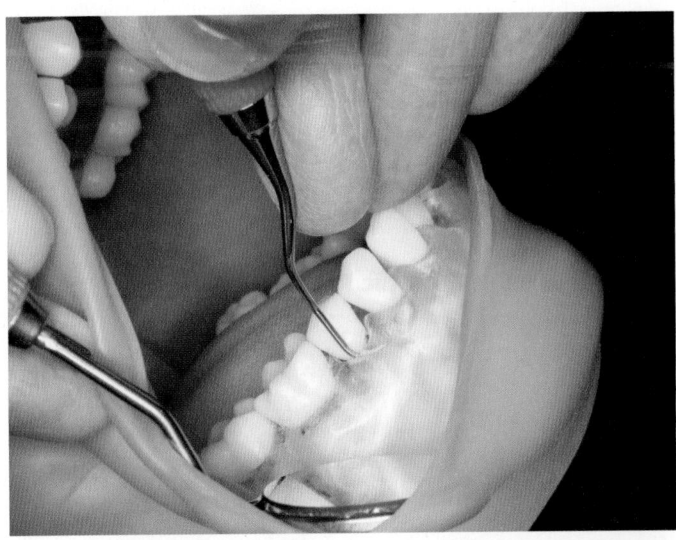

Figure 8-6. Prior to Pivot on Facial Surface.

- The clinician pictured here is moving the working-end across the facial surface of the second premolar.
- Note that while working on the facial surface, only the ***underside*** of the middle finger is visible in this photo.

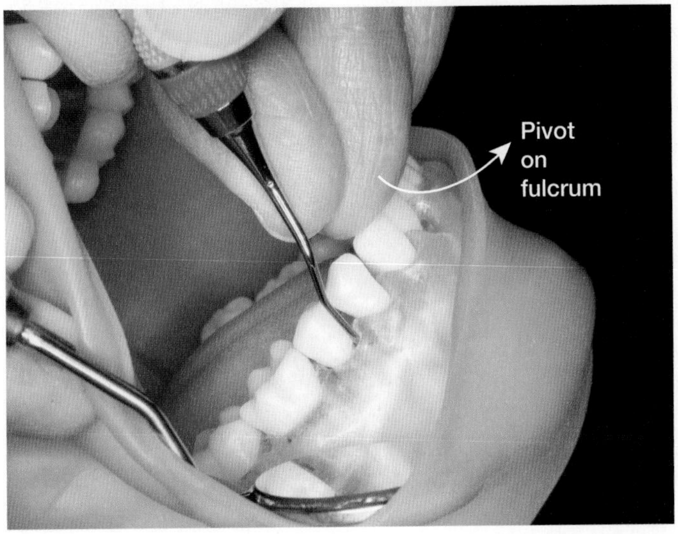

Pivot
on
fulcrum

Figure 8-7. After Pivot.

- As the clinician reaches the mesiofacial line angle, he or she pivots on the fulcrum finger to rotate the hand slightly.
- With a slight pivot of the hand, the clinician has moved the working-end from the facial surface onto the mesial surface of the premolar.
- Note that the ***side*** of the middle finger is visible after the hand pivot.

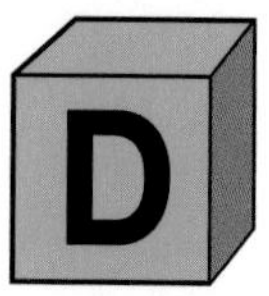

SKILL BUILDING. THE HAND PIVOT

Directions: This skill building activity will assist you in learning to pivot on your fulcrum finger. As with all movements when working in the oral cavity, the pivot is a tiny movement used to reposition your hand.

1. **Get Ready.**
   - *RIGHT-handed clinicians* use Figure 8-8A. *LEFT-handed clinicians* use Figure 8-8B.
   - Grasp a pencil in a modified pen grasp and establish a fulcrum in the circle on the illustration.
   - Touch the pencil point to the "X" on the illustration.
   - Begin with the midline of your hand and arm aligned with dotted **Line A.**
2. **Pivot.** Push down lightly and pivot on your fulcrum finger as you swing the midline of your hand and arm as a unit to align with dotted **Line B.** Be sure to maintain neutral wrist position.

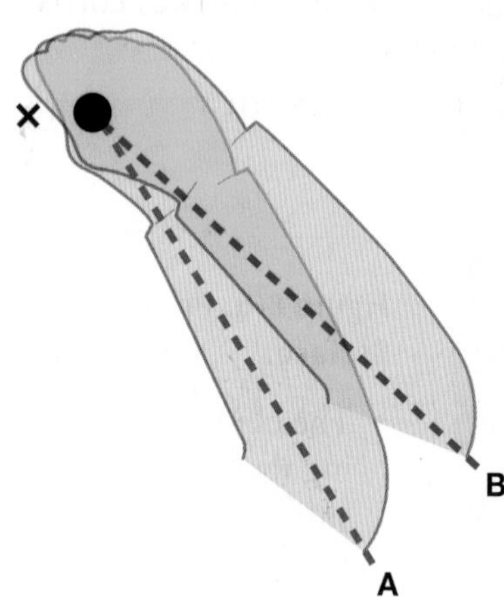

Figure 8-8A. For the Right-Handed Clinician.

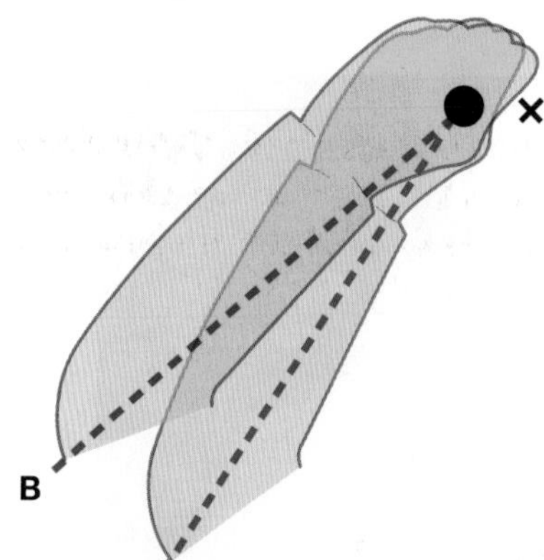

Figure 8-8B. For the Left-Handed Clinician.

Section 4
Orientation of Instrument to Tooth Surface

ANGULATION OF TEETH IN DENTAL ARCHES

The placement of the working-end in relation to the tooth surface being instrumented is a critical element in periodontal instrumentation.

1. Much periodontal instrumentation occurs on the root surfaces of the teeth.
2. Correct placement of the working-end to the ***root surface being instrumented*** is facilitated if the clinician has a clear visual picture of the angulation of the teeth in the dental arches.
   a. As illustrated in Figure 8-9A, a common misconception is that most teeth are positioned vertically in the dental arches. The teeth, however, do not sit like fence posts sticking straight down into the soil. This incorrect visual picture of the teeth in the dental arches results in positioning the lower shank incorrectly in relation to the root surface being instrumented.
   b. As illustrated in Figure 8-9B, the teeth usually are tilted in the dental arches. This correct visual picture of the teeth in the dental arches facilitates correct alignment of the lower shank with the root surface being instrumented.
3. Figures 8-10 and 8-11 illustrate the true angulation of the maxillary and mandibular teeth in the dental arches.

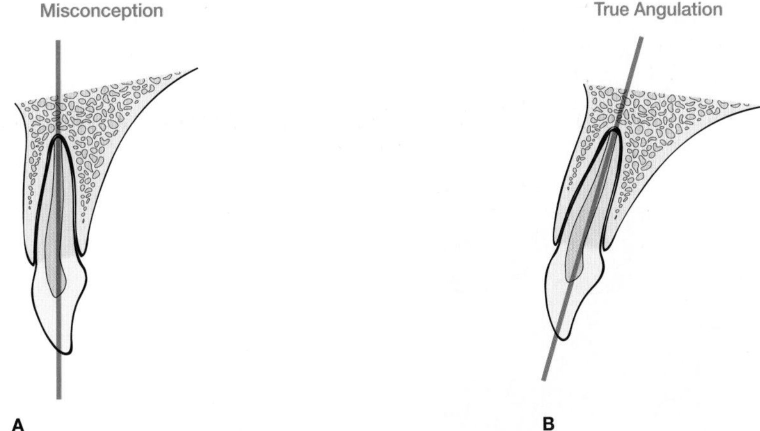

Figure 8-9. Angulation of the Teeth in the Dental Arches. A. Incorrect Visual Picture. A common misconception is that most teeth are positioned vertically in the dental arches. **B. True Angulation.** Most teeth are tilted in the dental arch.

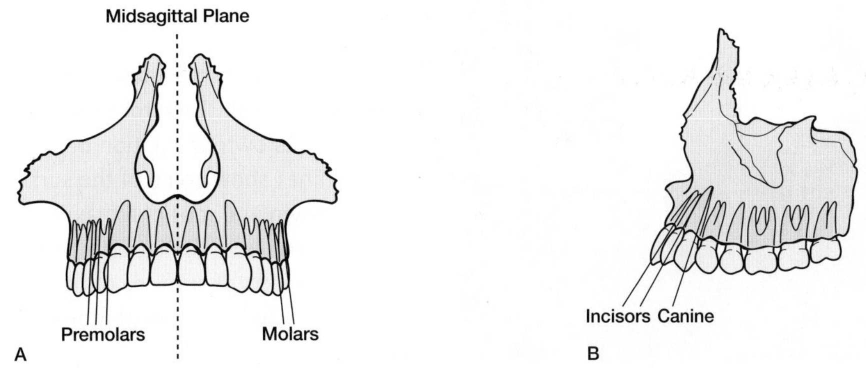

Figure 8-10. Maxillary Teeth Angulation. The roots of all the maxillary teeth incline inward.

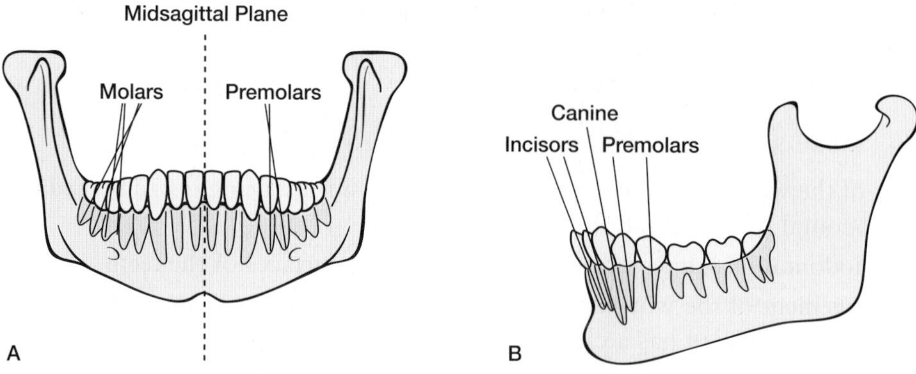

Figure 8-11. Mandibular Teeth Angulation. The roots of the mandibular anterior teeth usually tilt inward. The roots of the mandibular premolars usually are positioned more nearly vertical. The roots of the mandibular molars tilt slightly outward.

ORIENTATION TO TOOTH SURFACE

Initial placement of the working-end against the tooth surface begins by orienting the lower shank with the tooth surface to be instrumented.

1. Orienting the instrument with the tooth surface to be instrumented requires some thought on the part of the clinician.
2. A single tooth has many surfaces, each with its own orientation including the convex, rounded posterior tooth crowns, tapering root surfaces, divergent roots, and root concavities. Figure 8-12 illustrates the many surface orientations of a maxillary first molar when viewed from the facial aspect.

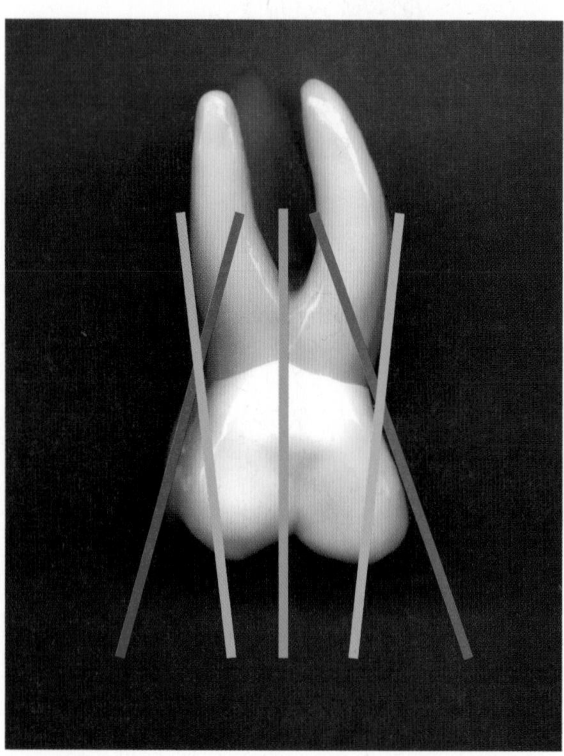

Figure 8-12. Tooth Surface Planes for Instrumentation. Each tooth has many surfaces each with its own orientation or surface plane. The colored lines show some of the surface orientations on the crown and root of a maxillary first molar when viewed from the facial aspect. Note that the orientations of surfaces of the crown differ significantly from the orientations of the surfaces of the root.

Figures 8-13 to 8-18 illustrate incorrect and correct orientation to various tooth surfaces in the dentition.

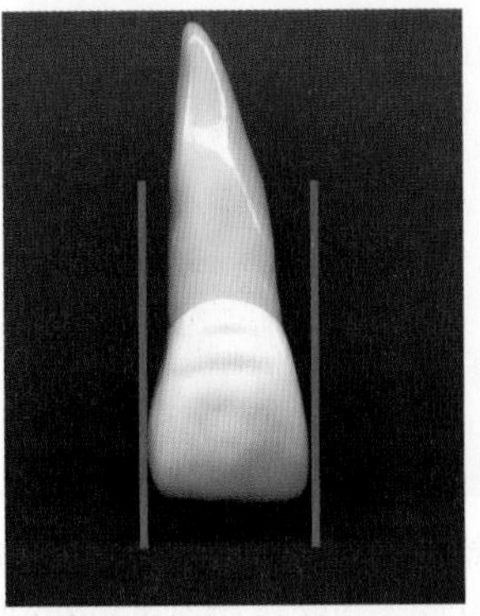

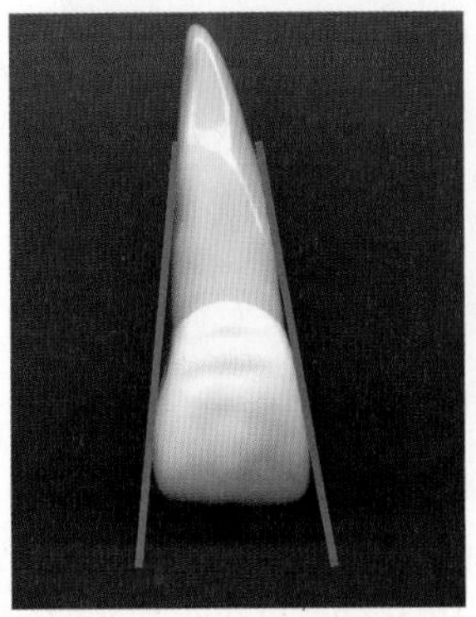

Figure 8-13. Orientation to Proximal Surfaces. A. Incorrect. The red lines indicate incorrect alignment to the distal and mesial surfaces of a maxillary central incisor. **B. Correct.** The green lines indicate correct alignment to the distal and mesial proximal surfaces of a maxillary central incisor.

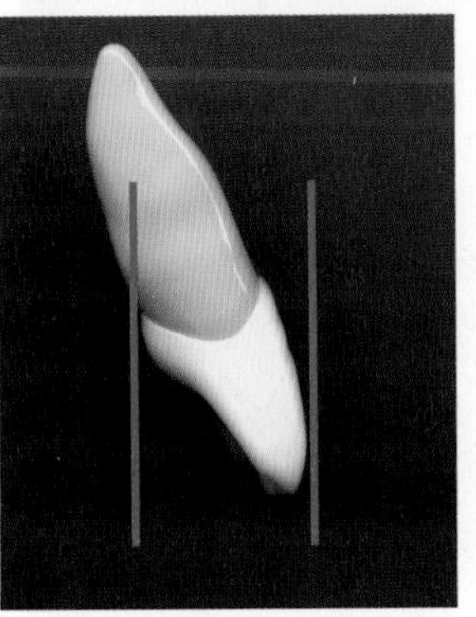

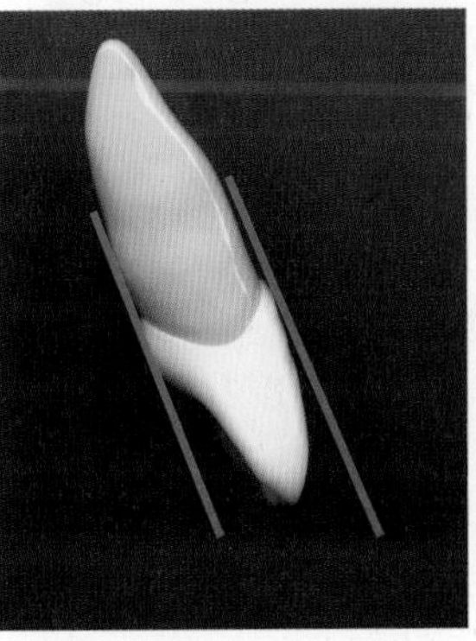

Figure 8-14. Orientation to Facial and Lingual Surfaces. A. Incorrect. The red lines indicate incorrect alignment to the lingual and facial surfaces of a maxillary central incisor. **B. Correct.** The green lines indicate correct alignment to the lingual and facial surfaces of a maxillary central incisor.

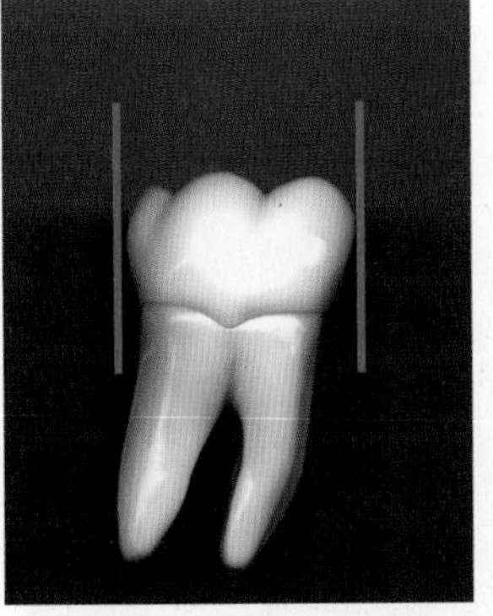

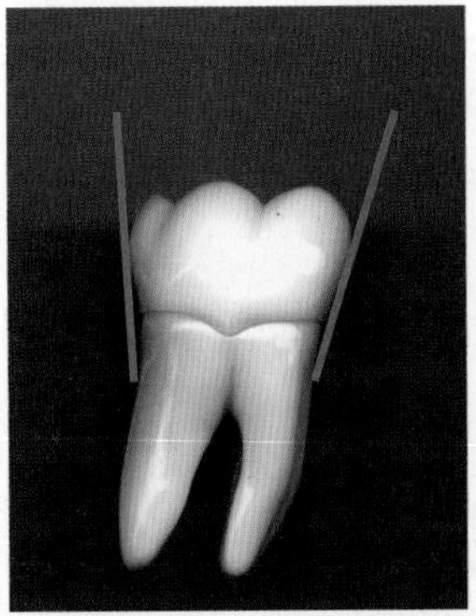

Figure 8-15. Orientation to Proximal Surfaces. A. Incorrect. The red lines indicate incorrect alignment to the distal and mesial surfaces of a mandibular molar. **B. Correct.** The green lines indicate correct alignment to the distal and mesial proximal surfaces of a mandibular molar.

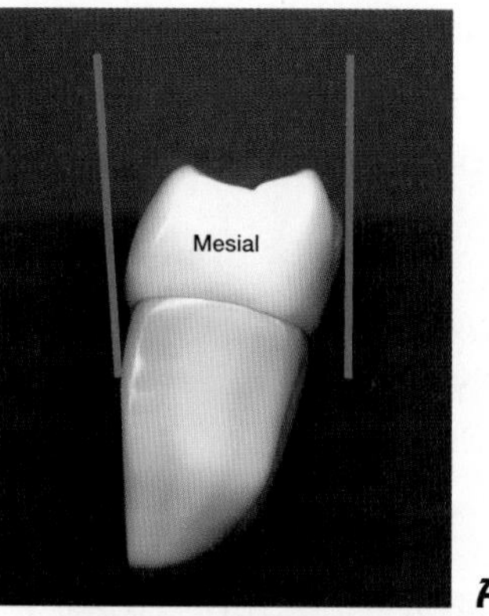

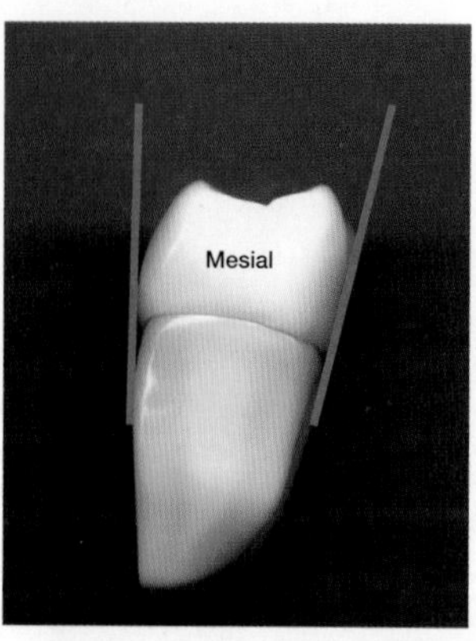

Figure 8-16. Orientation to Facial and Lingual Surfaces. **A. Incorrect.** The red lines indicate incorrect alignment to the lingual and facial surfaces of a mandibular molar. **B. Correct.** The green lines indicate correct alignment to the lingual and facial surfaces of a mandibular molar.

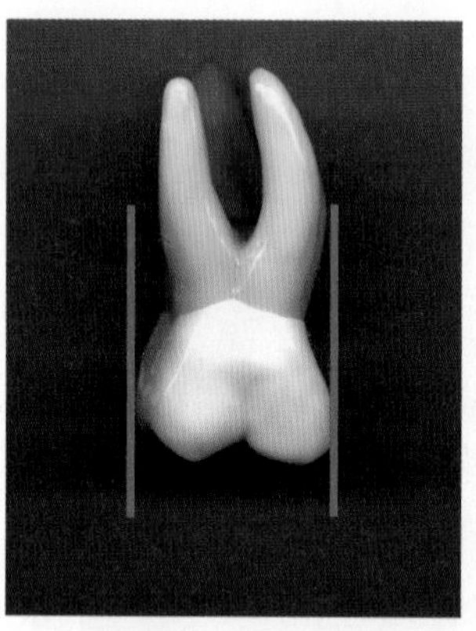

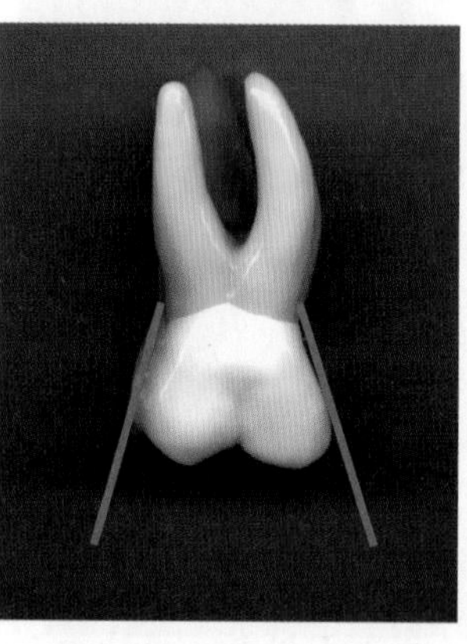

Figure 8-17. Orientation to Proximal Surfaces. **A. Incorrect.** The red lines indicate incorrect alignment to the distal and mesial surfaces of a maxillary molar. **B. Correct.** The green lines indicate correct alignment to the distal and mesial proximal surfaces of a maxillary molar.

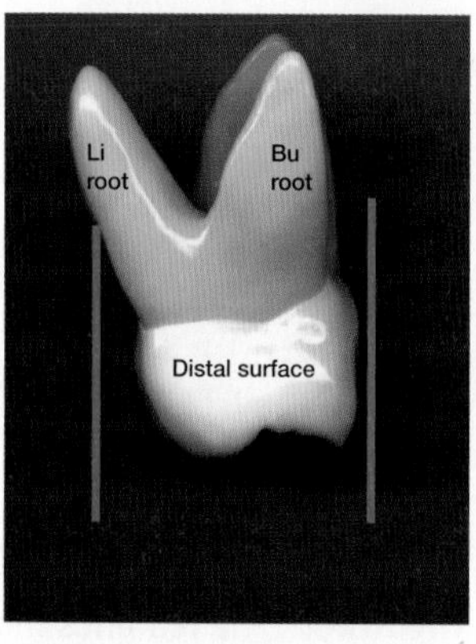

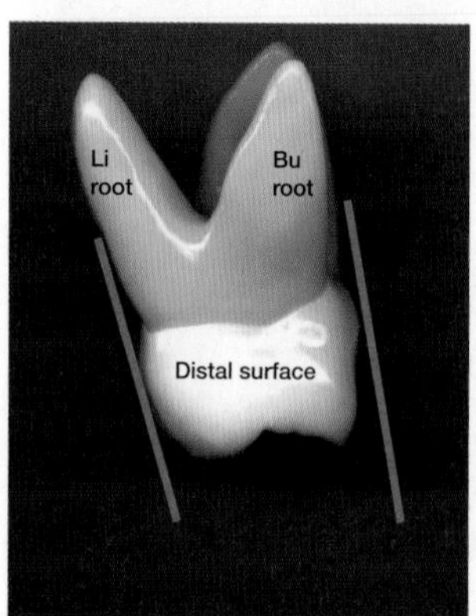

Figure 8-18. Orientation to Facial and Lingual Surfaces. **A. Incorrect.** The red lines indicate incorrect alignment to the lingual and facial surfaces of a maxillary molar. **B. Correct.** The green lines indicate correct alignment to the lingual and facial surfaces of a maxillary molar.

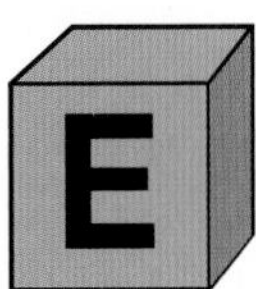

SKILL BUILDING. ALIGNMENT TO TOOTH SURFACE

Directions: This skill building activity is designed to assist you in learning to align the working-end of a periodontal probe to various tooth surfaces in the dentition. The working-end of a periodontal probe should be positioned parallel to the tooth surface being instrumented.

Directions:

- Equipment: A periodontal typodont with flexible or removable gingiva and a periodontal probe
- Practice orienting a periodontal probe to the facial, lingual, mesial, and distal aspects of the first molar in the four posterior sextants and a central incisor tooth in both anterior sextants of the mouth. A few examples are shown below in Figures 8-19 to 8-21.

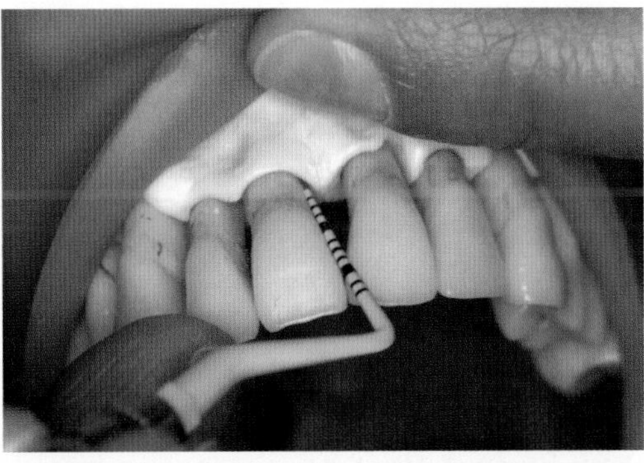

Figure 8-19. Orientation to Mesial Surface of Maxillary Central Incisor.

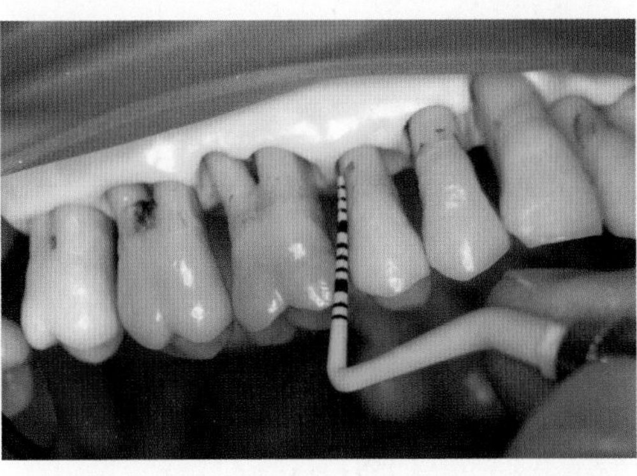

Figure 8-20. Orientation to Distal Surface of Maxillary Second Premolar.

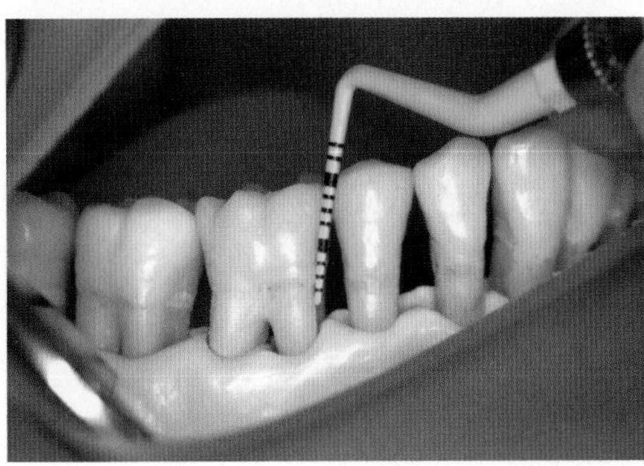

Figure 8-21. Orientation to Mesial Surface of Mandibular Molar.

RECOMMENDED READING

Canakci V, Orbak R, Tezel A, Canakci CF. Influence of different periodontal curette grips on the outcome of mechanical non-surgical therapy. *Int Dent J*. 2003;53:153–158.

Dong H, Barr A, Loomer P, Rempel D. The effects of finger rest positions on hand muscle load and pinch force in simulated dental hygiene work. *J Dent Educ*. 2005;69:453–460.

Dufour LA, Bissell HS. Periodontal attachment loss induced by mechanical subgingival instrumentation in shallow sulci. *J Dent Hyg*. 2002;76:207–212.

Hauser AM, Bowen DM. Primer on preclinical instruction and evaluation. *J Dent Educ*. 2009;73:390–398.

Ruhling A, Konig J, Rolf H, Kocher T, Schwahn C, Plagmann HC. Learning root debridement with curettes and power-driven instruments. Part II: clinical results following mechanical, nonsurgical therapy. *J Clin Periodontol*. 2003;30:611–615.

Section 5
Skill Application

STUDENT SELF-EVALUATION MODULE 8 | **MOVEMENT AND ORIENTATION TO TOOTH SURFACE**

Student: ______________________ Date: ______________________

DIRECTIONS: Self-evaluate your skill level as: **S** (satisfactory) or **U** (unsatisfactory).

Criteria	
Wrist Motion: Uses a pencil to demonstrate wrist motion activation	**Eval.**
Uses modified pen grasp with precise finger placement on the pencil	
Uses ring finger as a support beam	
Maintains neutral wrist position throughout activation	
Digital Motion: Uses a pencil to demonstrate digital motion activation	**Eval.**
Uses modified pen grasp with precise finger placement on the pencil	
Uses ring finger as a support beam	
Maintains neutral wrist position throughout activation	
Pivot: Uses pencil and Figure 8-8A or 8-8B to demonstrate pivoting on the fulcrum finger	**Eval.**
Uses modified pen grasp with precise finger placement on the pencil	
Uses ring finger as a support beam	
Maintains neutral wrist position during pivot	
Handle Roll: Demonstrates rolling a pencil in a clockwise and counter-clockwise direction	**Eval.**
Uses modified pen grasp with precise finger placement on the pencil	
Uses ring finger as a support beam	
Maintains neutral wrist position	
Orientation to Tooth Surfaces: Uses a typodont or tooth models and a periodontal probe	**Eval.**
Demonstrates how to correctly orient the probe tip to the anterior teeth in the dentition, including facial, lingual, and proximal surfaces	
Demonstrates how to correctly orient the probe tip to the mandibular posterior teeth	
Demonstrates how to correctly orient the probe tip to the maxillary posterior teeth	

Module 9

Technique Essentials: Adaptation

Module Overview

An instrumentation stroke is the act of moving the working-end of a periodontal instrument across a tooth surface. The production of an instrumentation stroke involves several precise techniques. These include (1) motion activation, (2) orientation to the tooth surface, (3) adaptation, and (4) angulation. This module discusses adaptation of the working-end to the tooth surface. Motion activation and orientation to the tooth surface were discussed in Module 8. Module 13 covers the topic of angulation of the working-end.

Adaptation refers to the positioning of the first 1 or 2 mm of the working-end's lateral surface in contact with the tooth. For successful instrumentation, correct adaptation must be maintained as the working-end is moved over a tooth surface.

Module Outline

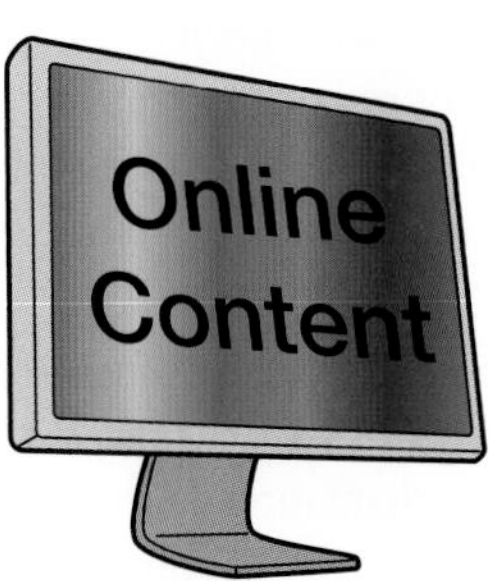

A video on the topic of adaptation can be viewed at http://thepoint.lww.com/GehrigFundamentals7e

Key Terms

Adaptation

Leading-third of working-end

Toe-third (curet)

Tip-third (sickle scaler)

Learning Objectives

1. Define the term adaptation as it relates to periodontal instrumentation.
2. Identify the leading-, middle-, and heel-third of the working-end of a sickle scaler and a curet.
3. Using a typodont and an anterior sickle scaler, describe and demonstrate correct adaptation of the working-end to the midline and line angle of a mandibular anterior tooth.
4. Explain problems associated with incorrect adaptation during periodontal instrumentation.
5. Using Figure 9-9 and a pencil, demonstrate how to maintain adaptation to curved surfaces while using correct modified pen grasp and wrist motion activation.
6. Given a universal curet and a typodont, explain how to use visual clues to select the correct working-end for use on the distal surface of a mandibular premolar tooth.
7. Use precise finger placement on the handle of a periodontal instrument while demonstrating adaptation and selection of the correct working-end for a treatment area:
   - Finger pads of thumb and index finger are opposite one another on handle.
   - Thumb and index finger do not overlap each other on the handle.
   - Pad of middle finger rests lightly on the shank.
   - Thumb, index, and middle fingers are in a "knuckles-up" position.
   - Ring finger is straight and supports weight of the hand.

Note to Course Instructor: Typodonts for Technique Practice

One excellent source of periodontal typodonts with flexible gingiva for technique practice is Kilgore International, Inc.: 800-892-9999 or online at http://www.kilgoreinternational.com. These typodonts are an excellent addition to student instrument kits to be used when learning instrumentation technique and for patient instruction in self-care (home care) techniques in clinic.

Typodonts allow students to practice techniques such as insertion without danger of injury to the sulcular or junctional epithelium of a partner.[1] Also, there is the advantage that students can see for themselves the results of improper adaptation on the synthetic gingival tissue. In later modules, students can use typodonts to practice instrumentation on root surfaces—the most important and difficult areas of the tooth on which to master instrumentation.[2]

Section I
Adaptation of the Working-End

ADAPTATION OF THE LEADING-THIRD OF THE WORKING-END

Adaptation is the act of placing the first 1 or 2 mm of the working-end's lateral surface in contact with the tooth.

1. The three sections of a working-end are the (1) leading-third, (2) middle-third, and (3) heel-third. Figure 9-1 presents a bird's-eye view—looking down on the face—of a curet and a sickle scaler showing the three sections of each working-end. The leading-third is the anterior portion of the working-end.
2. **Correct adaptation of the working-end to the tooth surface requires positioning the working-end so that the *leading-third of the working-end* is in contact with the tooth surface.** Figures 9-2 and 9-3 show examples of correct and incorrect adaptation.

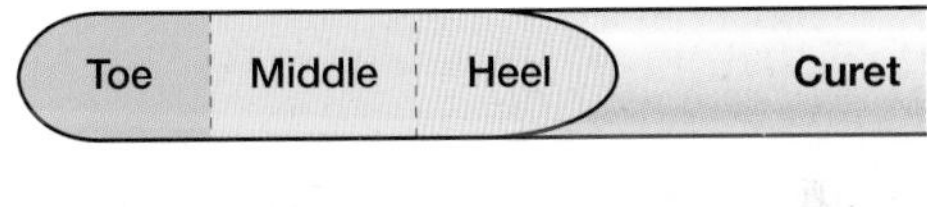

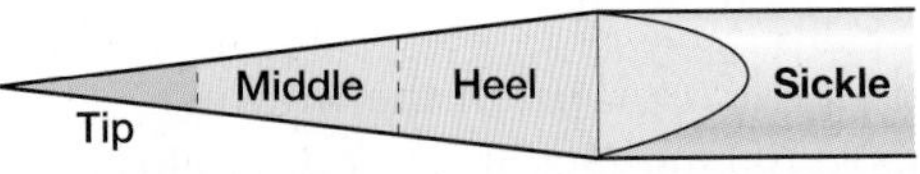

Figure 9-1. Leading-Third.

- *On curets*, the leading-third is termed the toe-third of the working-end.
- *On sickle scalers*, the leading-third is termed the tip-third of the working-end.

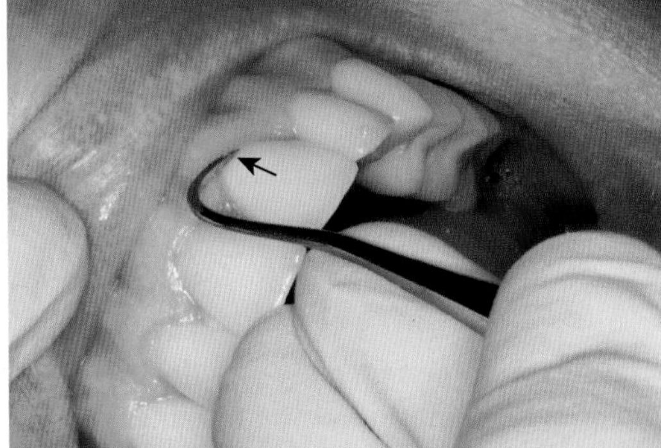

Figure 9-2. Correct Adaptation. The tip-third of this sickle scaler is **correctly** adapted to the facial surface of the incisor tooth.

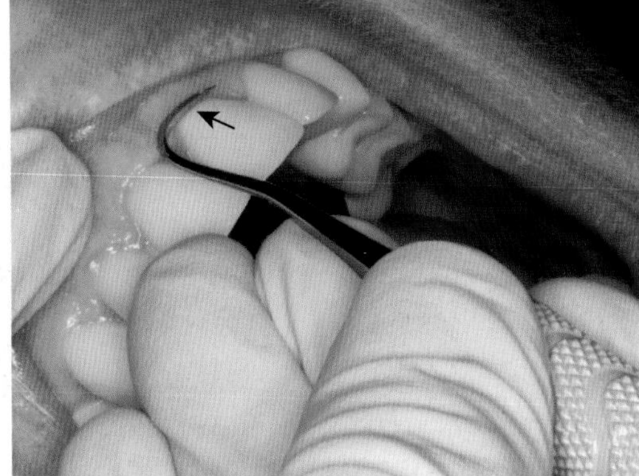

Figure 9-3. Incorrect Adaptation. Here, the middle-third of the working-end is **incorrectly** adapted to the tooth. Note how the instrument tip is sticking out and could injure the soft tissue (ouch!).

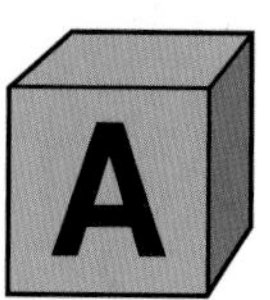

SKILL BUILDING. ADAPTATION TO THE TOOTH CROWN

Directions:

1. Assemble the following equipment: anterior sickle scaler and a dental typodont. Follow the steps illustrated on this and the following page as demonstrated in Figures 9-4 to 9-7.
2. Treatment Area: **RIGHT-Handed clinician:** Mandibular anteriors, facial surfaces TOWARD your nondominant hand; **LEFT-Handed clinician:** Mandibular anteriors, facial surfaces AWAY FROM your nondominant hand

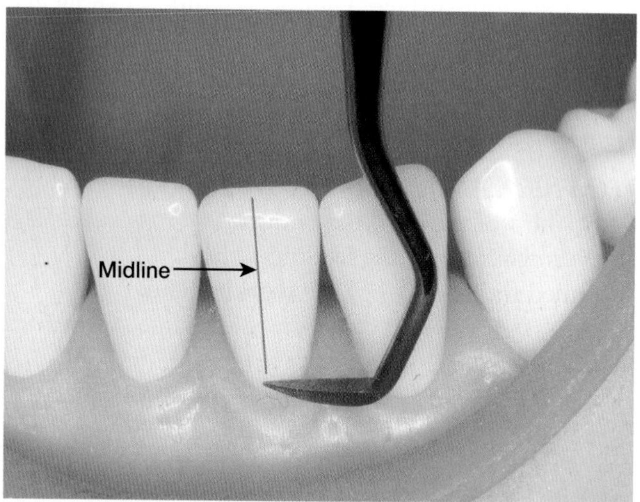

Figure 9-4. Practice Correct Adaptation on the Facial Surface.

- Adapt the ***tip-third*** of the working-end to the midline of the tooth. **This is the correct way to adapt the working-end to the midline.**
- Note that the ***middle- and heel-thirds*** of the working-end are NOT in contact with the tooth surface.

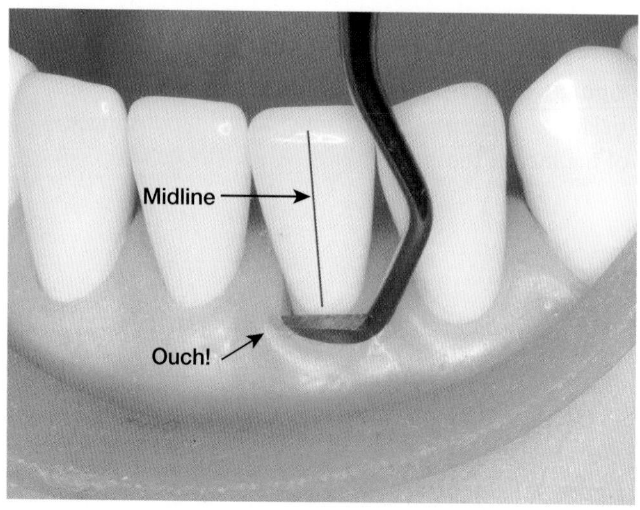

Figure 9-5. Experience the Results of Incorrect Adaptation at the Midline.

- Adapt the middle-third of the working-end to the midline the tooth.
- Look carefully at the instrument. Note that the tip-third of the working-end is NOT adapted to the tooth. **In fact, it is sticking out. This is the incorrect technique.**
- What could happen to the soft tissue if the working-end were incorrectly adapted in this manner?

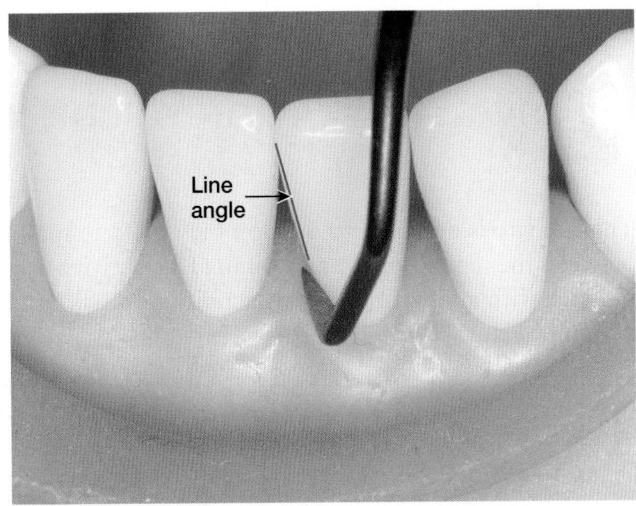

Figure 9-6. Practice Correct Adaptation on the Line Angle.

- Adapt the tip-third of a sickle scaler to the line angle of the tooth. **This is the correct way to adapt the working-end to a line angle.**
- Note that the middle- and heel-thirds of the working-end are not adapted to the tooth.

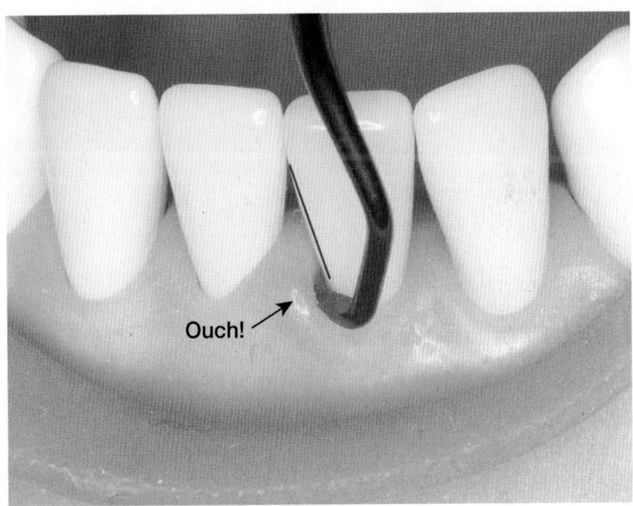

Figure 9-7. Experience the Results of Incorrect Adaptation at the Line Angle.

- Adapt the middle-third of the working-end to the line angle.
- **This incorrect adaptation is a mistake commonly made by beginning clinicians when moving from the facial surface onto the distal surface.**
- Can you see why this is not the correct technique for adaptation? OUCH!

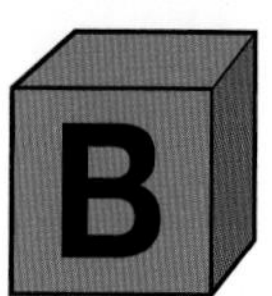

SKILL BUILDING. MAINTAINING ADAPTATION TO CURVED SURFACES

This activity is designed to develop the ability to maintain adaptation by rolling an instrument between the index finger and thumb. This activity uses a pencil and an abstract line to provide practice with adaptation. **In this activity, you will practice adapting a *vertical mark* to the abstract design in Figure 9-9.**

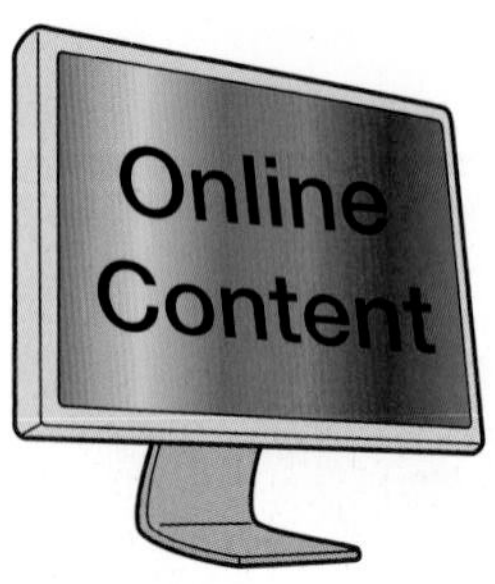

A video for this topic can be viewed at http://thepoint.lww.com/GehrigFundamentals7e

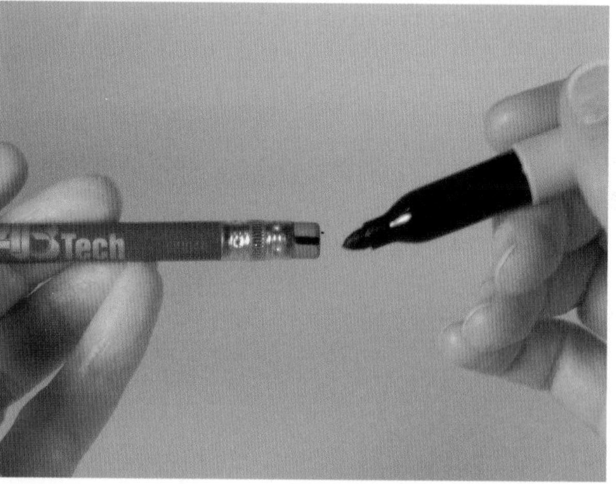

Figure 9-8A. Prepare a Pencil.

- Use a pen to make a vertical mark on the pencil eraser. The line should extend from the base of the eraser to the top of the eraser.
- In this activity, you will try to adapt the **vertical mark** to the abstract design on the next page.

INSTRUCTIONS: Follow Steps 1 to 5 to practice adapting the vertical mark to the abstract line in Figure 9-9.

1. Hold the pencil in a modified pen grasp. Imagine that the **vertical mark** on the eraser is the leading-third of the working-end.
2. **Right-handed clinicians:** Begin near the letter **R**. Imagine that you are working on the anterior surfaces toward you.
   Left-handed clinicians: Begin near the letter L. Imagine that you are working on the anterior surfaces toward you.
3. Establish a fulcrum near the end of the abstract line in Figure 9-9. Figure 9-8B depicts this step.
   - Touch the **vertical mark** on the eraser to the first dot on Figure 9-9.
     - If you are right-handed, this will be the first dot beside the letter **R**.
     - If you are left-handed, this will be the first dot beside the letter L.
   - The **vertical mark** is now adapted to the first dot.

4. Adapt to the second dot by following these steps:
   - Keep your finger rest on the book, and use wrist motion activation to lift the eraser off of the paper away from the first dot.
   - Still holding the eraser off the paper, slide your finger rest closer to the second dot.
   - Roll the pencil until the **vertical mark** is directly above the second dot on the abstract line. Use wrist motion activation to return the eraser to the paper so that the mark is adapted to the second dot.
5. Continue to slide your finger rest as you move along the design (Fig. 9-8C), rolling the pencil to adapt the **vertical mark** to each dot until you reach the opposite end of the line (Fig. 9-8D).

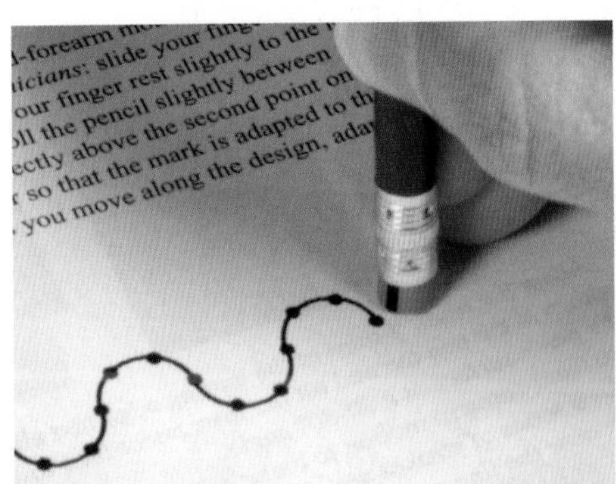

Figure 9-8B. Step 1. Establish a fulcrum near the end of the abstract line (Fig. 9-9). Touch the vertical mark on the eraser to the first dot.

- If you are right-handed, this will be the first dot beside the letter **R**.
- If you are left-handed, this will be the first dot beside the letter **L**.

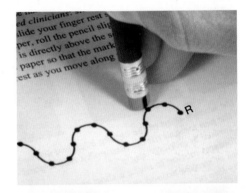

Figure 9-8C. Adapt to the Second and Third Dots, Proceeding Along the Line.

- Maintain your finger rest and use wrist motion activation to lift the eraser off of the paper.
- Slide your finger rest closer to the second dot.
- Roll the pencil until the vertical mark is above the second dot. Use wrist motion activation to return the eraser to the paper so that the mark is adapted to the second dot.
- Repeat this process for the third dot.

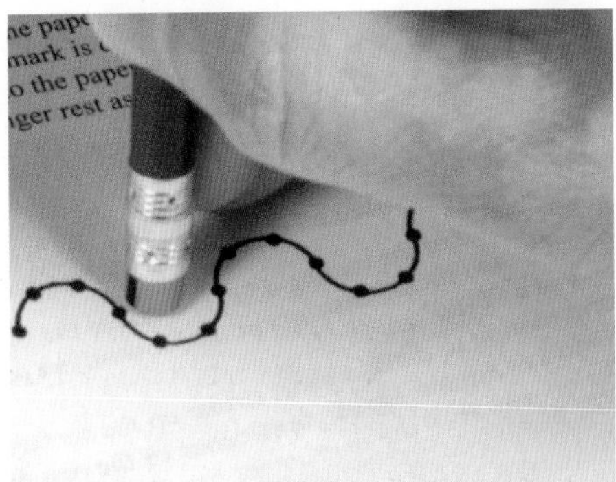

Figure 9-8D. Continue. Continue to slide your finger rest as you move along the design (Fig. 9-8C), rolling the pencil to adapt the vertical mark to each dot until you reach the opposite end of the line.

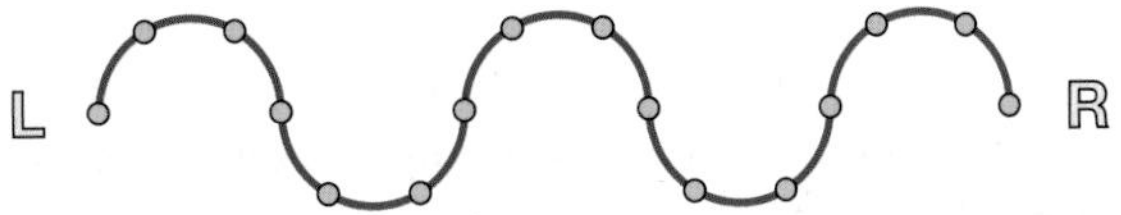

Figure 9-9. Abstract Line. Use this abstract line to develop your skills of adaptation.

Section 2
Selecting the Correct Working-End

Before using a double-ended instrument on a posterior tooth, the clinician first must determine which working-end to use. To select the correct working-end, the clinician observes the relationship of the lower shank to the distal surface of the tooth. The position of the lower shank provides a visual clue to the correct working-end. ***It is helpful to use a premolar tooth for working-end selection, because a premolar is more easily viewed than a molar tooth.***

- *Visual Clue for the Correct Working-End:* The lower shank is parallel to the distal surface, and the functional shank goes *"up and over the tooth."* Figure 9-10 shows the correct working-end for the facial aspect of the mandibular right posterior sextant.
- *Visual Clue for the Incorrect Working-End:* The lower shank is NOT parallel to the distal surface, and the functional shank is *"down and around the tooth."* Figure 9-11 shows the incorrect working-end for the facial aspect of the mandibular right posterior sextant.

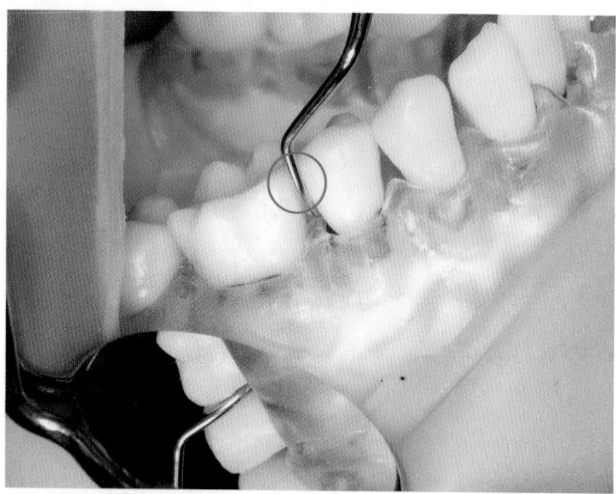

Figure 9-10. Correct Working-End. This photograph shows working-end **A** of the instrument adapted to the distal surface of a mandibular premolar tooth.

This is the **CORRECT working-end** because the *lower shank is parallel to the distal surface.*

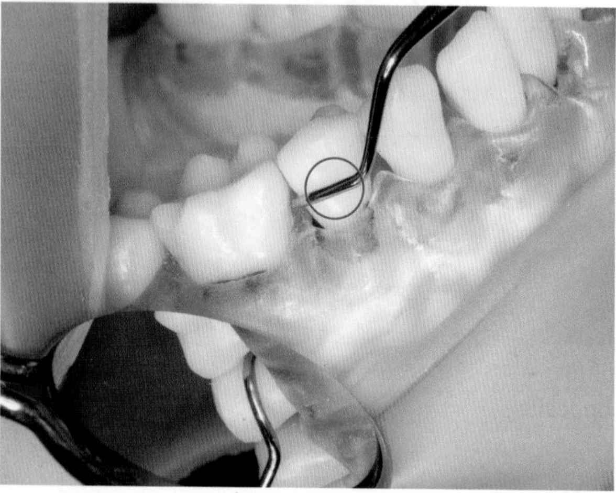

Figure 9-11. Incorrect Working-End. This photograph shows working-end **B** of the instrument adapted to the distal surface of a mandibular premolar tooth.

This is the **INCORRECT working-end** because the *lower shank is NOT parallel to the distal surface.*

Complete the Skill Building exercise on the following page to gain experience in selecting the correct end of a double-ended instrument.

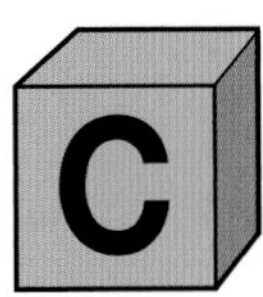

SKILL BUILDING. WORKING-END SELECTION, POSTERIOR TEETH

Materials: Ask your instructor to help you pick an instrument for this Skill Building exercise. Use a universal curet, such as a Barnhart 1/2 or a Columbia 13/14. If you do not have a universal curet in your instrument kit, you can use a Langer 1/2 or a posterior sickle. Use a typodont to practice working-end selection.

1. **Right-Handed clinician:** Mandibular right posterior sextant, facial aspect. **Left-Handed clinician:** Mandibular left posterior sextant, facial aspect.
2. Remember: "Me, My patient, My light, My dominant hand, My nondominant hand."
3. Grasp the curet in your dominant hand and establish a finger rest to work on the distal surface of the first premolar.
4. Maintain your finger rest as you randomly select one working-end of the instrument and place it on the distal surface of the first premolar tooth.
5. Assess the visual clues for this working-end.
   - Is the lower shank parallel to the distal surface?
   - Does the functional shank go "up and over the tooth" or "down and around the tooth"?
6. Repeat the process with the other working-end of the instrument.
7. Based on the visual clues, which is the correct working-end?
8. Ask your instructor to check your results.

REFERENCES

1. Dufour LA, Bissell HS. Periodontal attachment loss induced by mechanical subgingival instrumentation in shallow sulci. *J Dent Hyg*. 2002;76:207–212.
2. Ruhling A, Konig J, Rolf H, Kocher T, Schwahn C, Plagmann HC. Learning root debridement with curettes and power-driven instruments. Part II: clinical results following mechanical, non-surgical therapy. *J Clin Periodontol*. 2003;30:611–615.

Section 3
Skill Application

PRACTICAL FOCUS: OBSERVATION OF CLINICIAN TECHNIQUE

Directions: Analyze the photos for Case 1 and Case 2 on this and the following page.

Case 1. Your friend, Marybeth, has difficulty removing calculus on the mandibular teeth. In addition, she frequently lacerates the papillae when working on the mandibular anteriors. Marybeth simply does not know what she is doing wrong! She asks you to observe her in clinic and give her feedback about the problems she is encountering. The three photos below are typical of your observations as Marybeth worked on the mandibular anteriors, facial, and lingual aspects. What problems, if any, did your observe? How might Marybeth correct these problems?

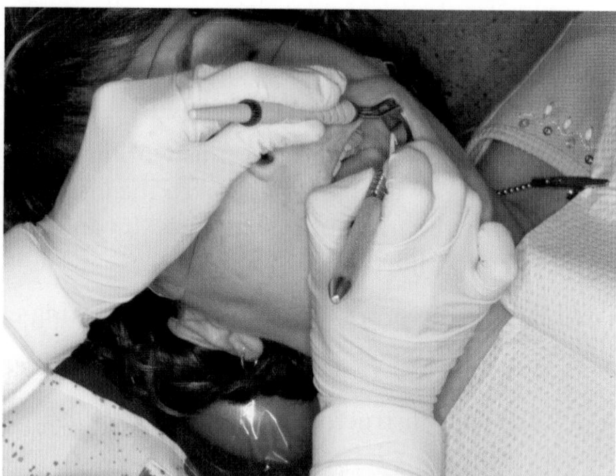

B

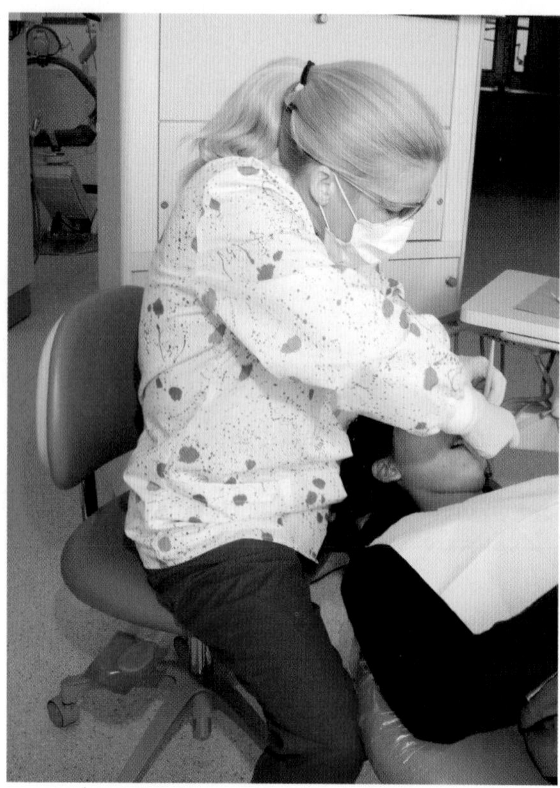

A

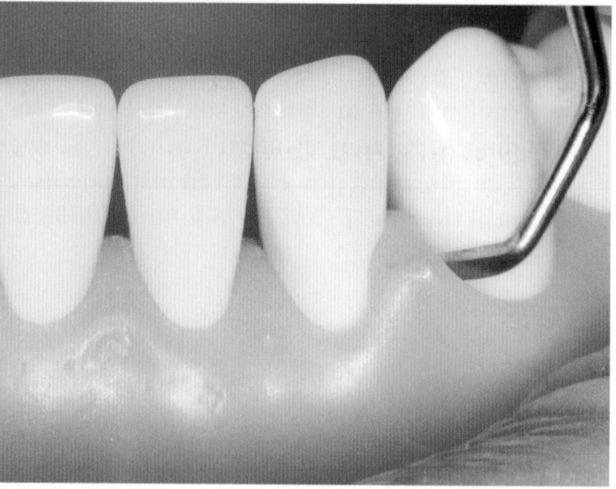

C

Figures 9-12, A–C. Case 1.

Case 2. Observe your classmate, Marybeth, as she practices determining the correct working-end of an explorer. The three photos below are typical of your observations as Marybeth worked on the mandibular posterior sextant. (1) Evaluate each photograph. (2) If you find any problems, explain how each problem could be corrected.

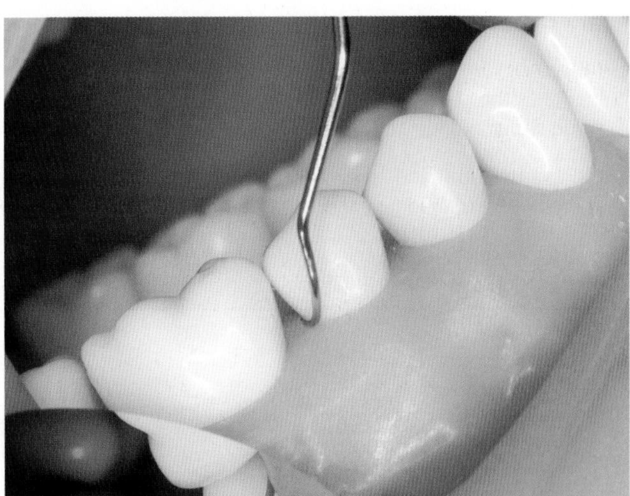

B

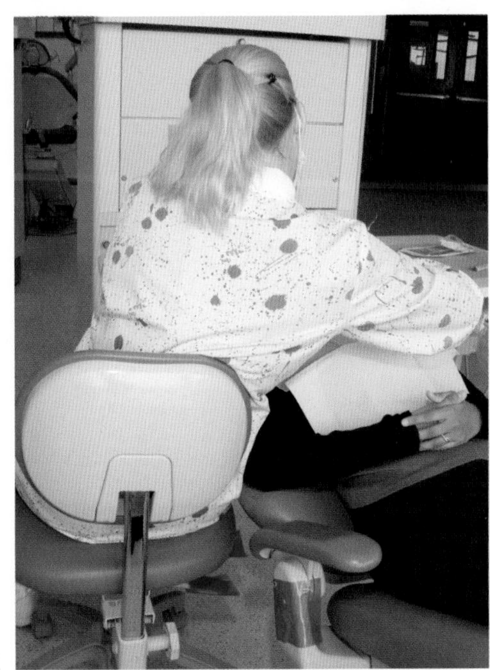

A

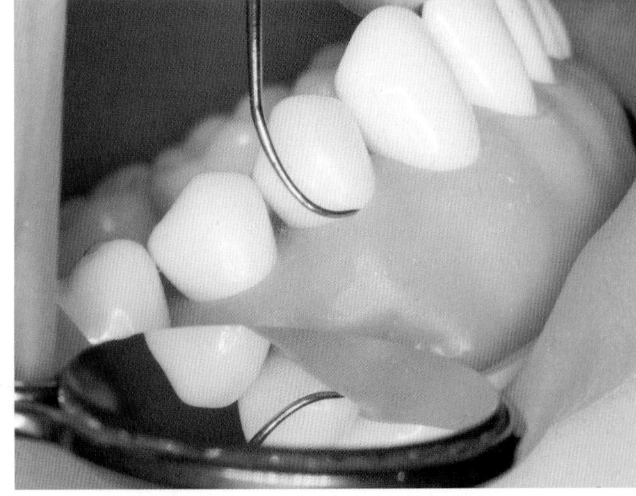

C

Figures 9-13, A–C. Case 2.

STUDENT SELF-EVALUATION MODULE 9 ADAPTATION

Student: ______________________ Date: ______________________

DIRECTIONS: Self-evaluate your skill level as: **S** (satisfactory) or **U** (unsatisfactory).

Criteria	
	Eval.
Identifies the (1) tip-third or toe-third, (2) middle-third, and (3) heel-third of the cutting edge on a sickle scaler and a curet	
Using a typodont and an anterior sickle scaler, adapts the tip-third of the cutting edge to the (1) midline and (2) line angle of a canine tooth while maintaining a correct grasp and finger rest	
Given a universal curet, selects the correct working-end for use on the distal surface of a mandibular premolar tooth while maintaining a correct grasp and finger rest	

Module 10

Technique Essentials: Instrumentation Strokes

Module Overview

An instrumentation stroke is the act of moving the working-end of a periodontal instrument over the tooth surface. The three basic directions employed with an instrumentation stroke are vertical, oblique, and horizontal. The three types of instrumentation stroke—assessment, calculus removal, and root debridement—each have unique characteristics and functions during periodontal instrumentation.

Module Outline

Key Terms

Instrumentation stroke
Junctional epithelium
Vertical stroke direction
Oblique stroke direction
Horizontal stroke direction
Assessment stroke
Calculus removal stroke
Root debridement stroke
Residual calculus deposit
"Out of the line of fire"

Learning Objectives

1. Using a sickle scaler and a periodontal typodont, demonstrate the three basic stroke directions: vertical, oblique, and horizontal.
2. Compare and contrast the functions and characteristics of three types of instrumentation strokes: assessment, calculus removal, and root debridement.
3. Demonstrate how to stabilize the hand and instrument to perform an instrumentation stroke by using an appropriate intraoral fulcrum and the ring finger as a "support beam" for the hand.
4. Demonstrate the elements of an assessment stroke in a step-by-step manner.
5. Use precise finger placement on the handle of a periodontal instrument while demonstrating assessment strokes:
   - Finger pads of thumb and index finger are opposite one another on handle.
   - Thumb and index finger do not overlap each other on the handle.
   - Pad of middle finger rests lightly on the shank.
   - Thumb, index, and middle fingers are in a "knuckles-up" position.
   - Ring finger is straight and supports weight of the hand.

Section 1
Characteristics of Instrumentation Strokes

The act of moving the working-end of a periodontal instrument against the tooth surface is termed the instrumentation stroke. Instrumentation strokes are used to assess the character of the tooth surface (such as to locate calculus deposits hidden beneath the gingival tissue) and to remove calculus deposits from the tooth surfaces.

1. One example of an instrumentation stroke occurs when the working-end of a curet is positioned apical to—beneath—a calculus deposit in preparation for a calculus removal stroke. The instrument stroke occurs as the working-end is moved coronally against the calculus deposit to dislodge it from the tooth surface.
2. The working-end of an explorer is used to make a series of light, flowing instrumentation strokes over the root surface for the purpose of detecting calculus deposits scattered over the root surface of the tooth.
3. An important principle regarding movement of the working-end over a tooth surface relates to the working-end and the junctional epithelium.
   - The junctional epithelium is the soft epithelial tissue that forms the base of a gingival sulcus or periodontal pocket.
   - The cutting edge of a curet or sharp point of an explorer would injure the junctional epithelium and thus should not come in contact with the soft tissue base of a sulcus or periodontal pocket.

STROKE DIRECTION

An instrumentation stroke may be made in one of three directions. The stroke direction varies depending on the tooth surface being instrumented, with the clinician selecting the best stroke direction to access the particular area of the tooth. Figure 10-1 illustrates the three basic stroke directions: vertical, oblique, and horizontal strokes. Table 10-1 summarizes the uses of these strokes. Figures 10-2 to 10-5 show these three strokes in use.

1. ***Vertical and oblique instrumentation strokes always should be made in a coronal direction away from the soft tissue base of the sulcus or periodontal pocket.***
2. Horizontal instrumentation strokes are most useful when working around the line angles of a posterior tooth or at the midline of an anterior tooth. This type of stroke is discussed in more detail in later modules of this book. ***It is important to note that the working-end does not come in contact with the junctional epithelium when using a horizontal stroke.***

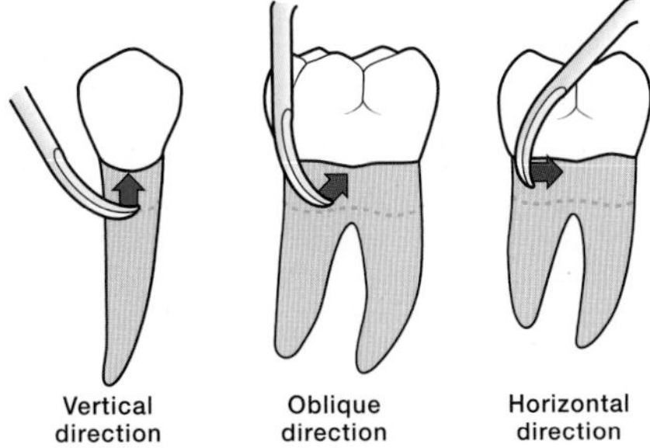

Figure 10-1. Stroke Directions for Instrumentation. Three stroke directions can be used for assessment and calculus removal with a periodontal instrument: vertical, oblique, or horizontal.

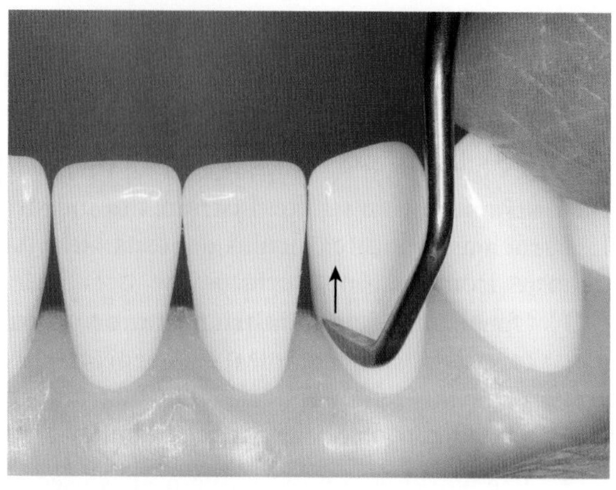

Figure 10-2. Vertical Stroke.

- On *anterior teeth*, vertical strokes are used on the facial, lingual, and proximal surfaces.
- On *posterior teeth*, vertical strokes are used primarily on the mesial and distal surfaces.

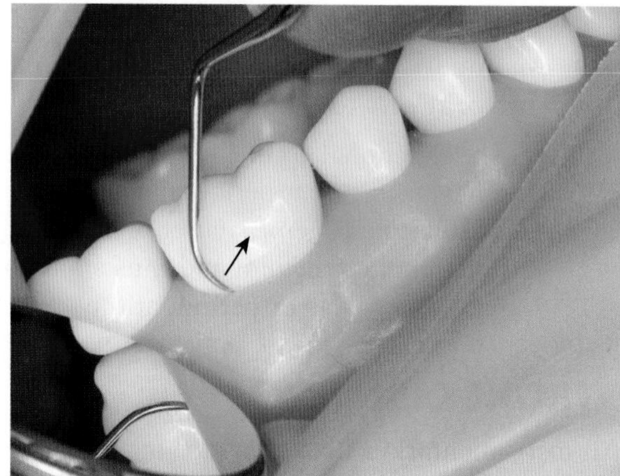

Figure 10-3. Oblique Stroke. Oblique strokes are used most commonly on the *facial and lingual surfaces* of posterior teeth.

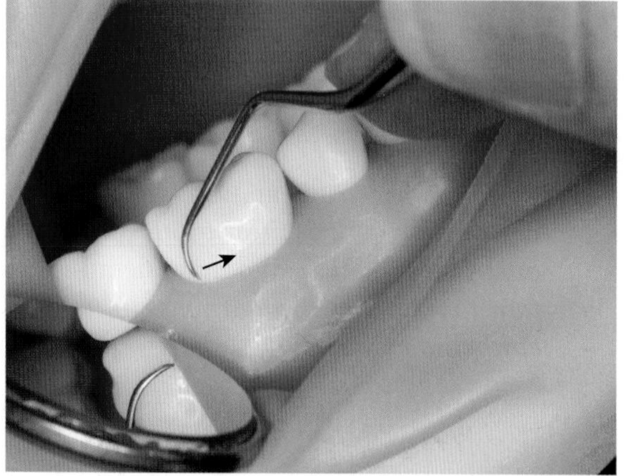

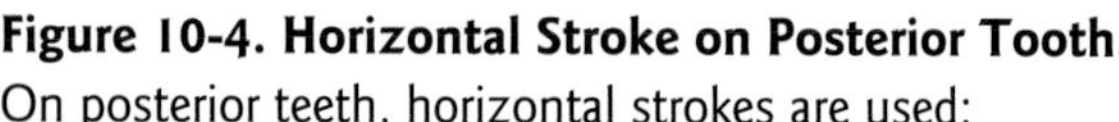

Figure 10-4. Horizontal Stroke on Posterior Tooth. On posterior teeth, horizontal strokes are used:

- Around line angles
- In furcation areas
- In deep pockets that are too narrow to allow vertical or oblique strokes

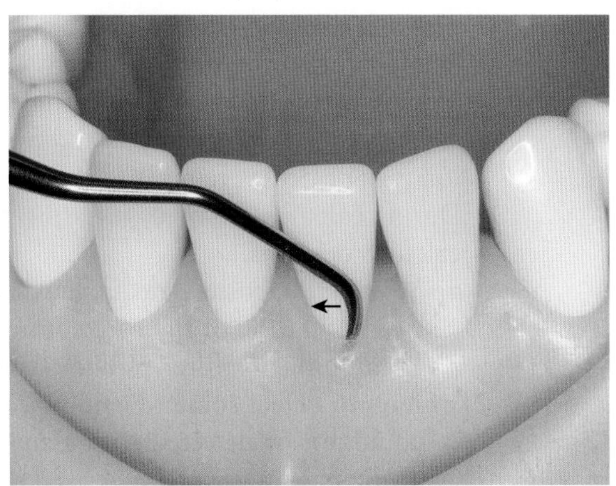

Figure 10-5. Horizontal Stroke on Anterior Tooth.

- The *facial and lingual surfaces* of anterior teeth are difficult to instrument because these teeth have a narrow mesial–distal width. Horizontal strokes are very effective in removing calculus from these narrow root surfaces.
- The working-end is used in a toe-down position. A short, controlled horizontal stroke is made on the tooth surface.

TABLE 10-1. Stroke Directions on Anterior and Posterior Teeth

Tooth Surfaces	Primary	Secondary
Facial or lingual surfaces of anterior teeth	Vertical	
Facial or lingual surfaces of posterior teeth	Oblique	Vertical
Mesial and distal tooth surfaces	Vertical	Horizontal, oblique
Midlines of root surfaces of anterior teeth	Horizontal	Vertical
Line angles of posterior teeth	Horizontal	Oblique, vertical
Furcation areas of multirooted teeth	Horizontal	Vertical
Narrow, deep pockets	Horizontal	Vertical

TYPES OF INSTRUMENTATION STROKES

The characteristics of an instrumentation stroke change depending on the purpose of the stroke. Periodontal instruments are used to assess characteristics of the root surface, remove calculus deposits, and refine root surfaces to facilitate soft tissue healing. Each of these functions requires an instrumentation stroke with unique properties. The three types of instrumentation strokes are the assessment stroke, calculus removal stroke, and root debridement stroke.

1. Assessment Stroke: Evaluation of the Characteristics of the Root Surface

A. Also known as an exploratory stroke.

B. An assessment stroke is a type of instrumentation stroke used to locate calculus deposits or other tooth surface irregularities hidden beneath the gingival margin.

1. The fine working-end and flexible shank of an explorer are used to enhance tactile information to the clinician's fingers. The superior tactile conduction of an explorer makes it the instrument of choice for (1) *initially locating subgingival calculus deposits* and for (2) *re-evaluating tooth surfaces* following calculus removal.
2. During calculus removal, assessment strokes are used with curets to locate calculus deposits.
   a. When all deposits detectable with a curet have been removed, a definitive evaluation of the root surface should be made using an explorer.
   b. Because the explorer provides superior tactile information, it is common to detect some remaining calculus deposits with an explorer that could not be detected with a curet.

C. Assessment strokes are characterized by:
1. Fingers relaxed in the modified pen grasp
2. Feather-light strokes against the tooth surface

2. Calculus Removal Stroke: Remove Supragingival and Subgingival Calculus

A. A calculus removal stroke is a type of instrumentation stroke used with sickle scalers and universal and area-specific curets to remove calculus deposits from the tooth.
1. A calculus removal stroke is characterized by a very short, controlled, biting stroke made with moderate pressure of the cutting edge against the tooth surface.
2. The fulcrum finger supports the hand and instrument during a stroke. At the initiation (start) of a stroke, the clinician presses down against the tooth.
3. Each stroke is a tiny movement of the working-end; the working-end only moves a few millimeters. After each calculus removal stroke, the clinician pauses and then uses a feather-light assessment stroke to determine if the deposit has been completely removed.

B. Calculus removal strokes are not used on tooth surfaces that are free of calculus deposits.
1. ***Instrumentation practice on student partners who have healthy shallow sulci is not recommended since instrumentation practice may result in periodontal attachment loss.***[1]
2. ***Periodontal typodonts with flexible "gingiva" are recommended for students learning instrumentation. Periodontal typodonts allow students to practice insertion into periodontal pockets. Instrumentation practice on periodontal typodonts is ideal since skilled instrumentation of root surfaces is vital to successful dental hygiene therapy.***[2–4]

3. Root Debridement Stroke: Refine Root Surface to Facilitate Tissue Healing

A. The root debridement stroke is a type of instrumentation stroke used to remove residual calculus deposits, bacterial plaque, and by-products from root surfaces exposed due to gingival recession or within deep periodontal pockets. Residual calculus deposits are very tiny deposits remaining on the root surface that can be removed using the lighter pressure of a root debridement stroke.

B. A root debridement stroke is characterized by:
1. A shaving stroke made with light pressure with the cutting edge against the tooth cementum.
2. A stroke that is slightly longer than a calculus removal stroke.

C. ***Conservation of cementum is an important goal of instrumentation.***

1. It is currently believed that conservation of cementum enhances healing of the soft tissues after instrumentation. In periodontal health, an important function of cementum is to attach the periodontal ligament fibers to the root surface. During the healing process after disease, cementum is thought to contribute to repair of the periodontium.[5–9]
2. In addition, research studies indicate that complete removal of cementum from the root surface, exposing the ends of dentinal tubules, may allow bacteria to travel from the periodontal pocket into the pulp in some instances.[10]
3. Over the course of many years, overzealous instrumentation can result in removal of all cementum and exposure of the underlying dentin. Within deep periodontal pockets, a plastic "implant" curet or a slim-tipped ultrasonic instrument may be used for plaque removal when no residual calculus deposits are present.

D. The root debridement stroke should not be confused with root planing. As traditionally defined, the term root planing involves the routine, intentional removal of cementum and the instrumenting of all root surfaces to a glassy smooth texture.

1. Until relatively recently, it was thought that intentional removal of most cementum was always needed to ensure the removal of all calculus as well as all bacterial products from the root surfaces.
2. It is now understood that vigorous root planing is not universally needed to reestablish periodontal health in all sites of periodontitis. Rather than vigorous root planing and removal of most or all of the cementum, bacterial products can be removed from the root surfaces with a minimal loss of cementum.

TABLE 10-2. Stroke Characteristics with Hand-Activated Instruments

	Assessment Stroke	**Calculus Removal Stroke**	**Root Debridement Stroke**
Purpose	To assess tooth anatomy and detect calculus and other plaque-retentive factors	To lift calculus deposits off of the tooth surface	To remove residual calculus and disrupt bacterial plaque from root surfaces within deep periodontal pockets
Used with	Probes, explorers, curets	Sickle scalers, curets	Curets
Lateral pressure	Contact with tooth surface, but no pressure	Moderate pressure against tooth surface	Light pressure against tooth surface
Character	Flowing, feather-light stroke of moderate length	Brief, tiny biting stroke	Lighter shaving stroke of moderate length
Number	Many, to evaluate the entire root surface	Limited to areas with calculus deposits	Many, covering entire subgingival root surface

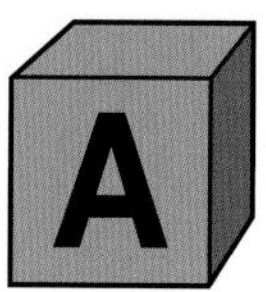

SKILL BUILDING. ASSESSMENT STROKE WITH AN EXPLORER

Directions:

- **Right-Handed clinicians** work on the mandibular right first molar, facial aspect.
- **Left-Handed clinicians** work on the mandibular left first molar, facial aspect.
- Use a periodontal typodont with removable or flexible "gingiva" so that you can practice as if working in a deep periodontal pocket. Use an explorer such as an 11/12-type explorer for this technique practice.
- **Establish a Finger Rest.** Establish an intraoral finger rest near but not directly over the surface to be instrumented. The finger rest should not be positioned in line with the working-end of the instrument to prevent sticking the ring finger when making a stroke. Position the finger rest **"out of the line of fire"** near to the tooth surface to be instrumented.

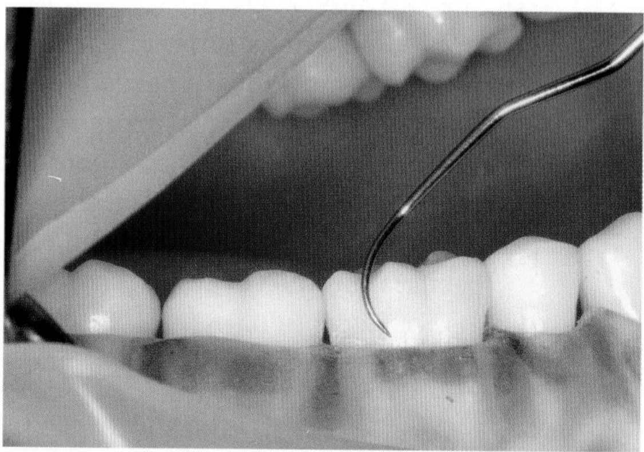

1. Figure 10-6. Get Ready. Prepare to assess the facial aspect of the molar. Establish a finger rest and place the working-end of the explorer in the middle-third of the crown. *Place the leading-third of the side of the explorer—**not the point**—against the tooth surface.* The explorer tip should "hug" the tooth surface.

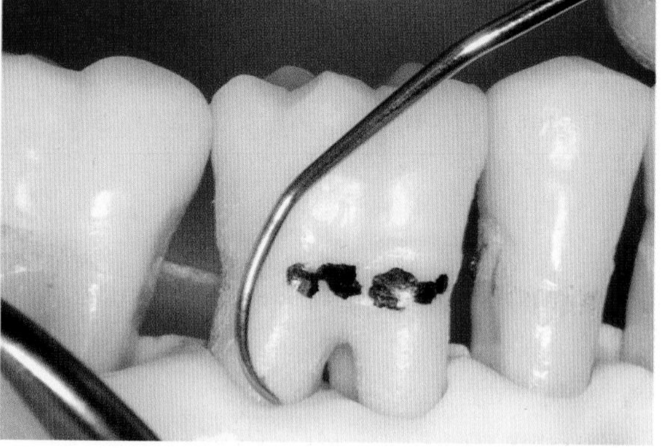

2. Figure 10-7. Insert. Gently slide the tip of the explorer beneath the gingival margin keeping the tip against the tooth surface.

- When working on a periodontal typodont, insert the tip of the explorer well into the "periodontal pocket."
- *In a real mouth, the explorer is inserted until the back of the working-end touches the junctional epithelium at the base of the pocket.*

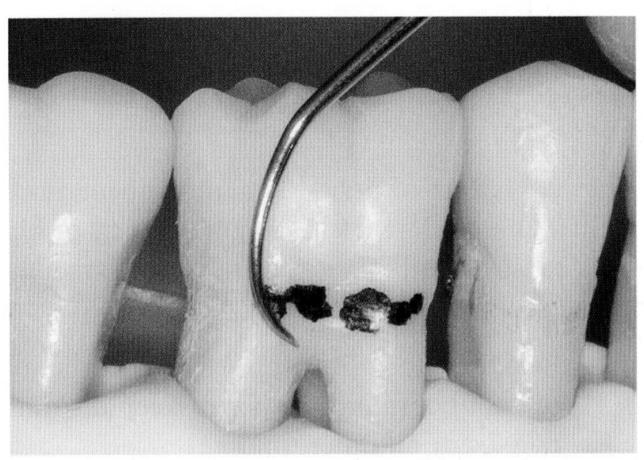

3. Figure 10-8. Make an Assessment Stroke.

- Use wrist activation to make an instrumentation stroke, away from the soft tissue at the base of the pocket.
- As you make the *feather-light* assessment stroke, you will encounter a calculus deposit.
- As the explorer tip moves over the calculus deposit, you will feel tiny vibrations with your fingertips on the shank and handle.

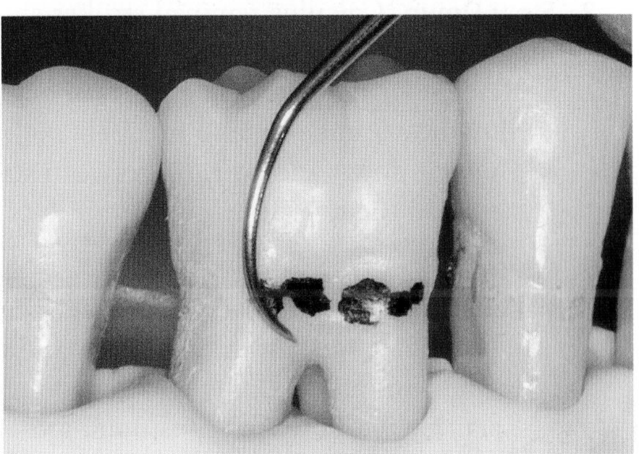

4. Figure 10-9. Employ Recommended Technique.

- *Assessment strokes are **feather-light** strokes.*
- Keep the fingers in your grasp very relaxed when making assessment strokes.
- A tight grasp will prevent you from feeling calculus deposits. (Tip: If your fingers are blanched, your grasp is too tight.)

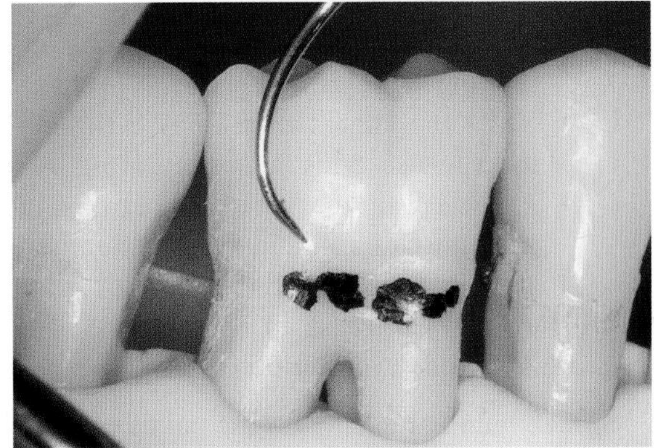

5. Figure 10-10. Stop the Assessment Stroke.

- Stop each stroke just beneath the gingival margin. (Tip: Your fulcrum finger should NOT lift off of the tooth at the end of a stroke.)
- At the gingival margin, do not remove the explorer tip from the pocket. Removing and reinserting with each stroke will traumatize the gingival tissue.

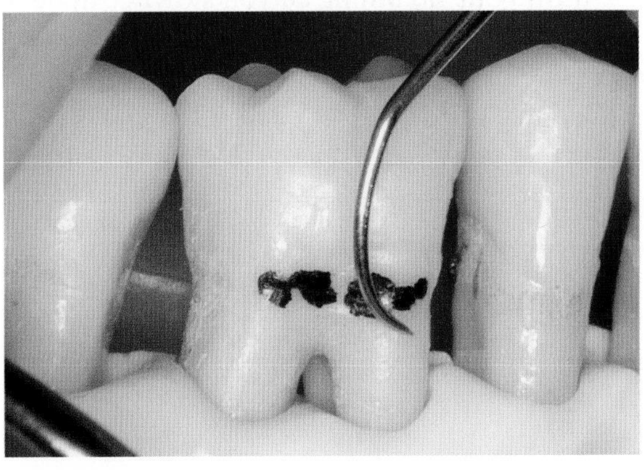

6. Figure 10-11. Make a Series of Assessment Strokes.

- Practice making a series of feather-light strokes across the facial surface.
- With each stroke, glide to the base of the pocket, make an assessment stroke, stop near the gingival margin, and repeat.
- Remember to *keep your fingers very relaxed in the grasp*.
- Keep your touch *feather-light against the tooth surface*.

Section 2
Strategies for Avoiding Injury during Instrumentation

The very nature of periodontal instrumentation means that the clinician engages in repetitive movements. One of the most damaging aspects of repetitive movements is maintaining the hand, arm, and back muscles in the same positions for extended time periods. Some suggestions for reducing muscle stain are listed below.

1. **Relax.** Only apply pressure against the tooth surface ***during*** a calculus removal or root debridement stroke. Keep the muscles of the fingers, hand, and wrist relaxed at all other times.

2. **Slow Down.** Calculus removal strokes should **not** be made in a rapid, nonstop manner as if keeping time to a beat.
   - Remember that the faster the pace of the strokes, the more difficult it is to control them.
   - Slow down; take time to precisely make each individual stroke and pause between strokes.
   - Slowing down and pausing between strokes makes each stroke more accurate and lessens stress on the muscles.
3. **Pause**
   - Pause at the end of each calculus removal stroke to relax the muscles. This does not mean taking the hand out of the mouth and laying the instrument down after each stroke. Rather, simply relax the muscles to lightly grasp the instrument handle.
   - Relax the hand when repositioning the working-end in preparation for the next stroke. In terms of avoiding musculoskeletal injury, this step is the most important.
4. **During Instrumentation**
   - Approximately every 20 minutes, stop and return the instrument to the tray setup. Stretch the fingers apart and hold the stretch for a few seconds.
   - Relax the fingers and slowly curl them inward without clenching. Keep the fingers curled for a few seconds before repeating. Repeat several times.
   - Allow a little recovery time between instrumentation-intensive activities to cool and lubricate muscles and tendons. A 10-minute break each hour from instrumentation provides sufficient recovery time. Without short breaks, the need for recovery builds and the threat of injury increases.
   - Rest your eyes periodically by pausing and focusing on distant objects.
5. **Between Patients.** Rub the palms of your hands together until they feel warm. Close your eyes and cup your warmed hands over them. Relax and concentrate on your breathing as you slowly exhale and inhale for 5 to 10 seconds.

REFERENCES

1. Dufour LA, Bissell HS. Periodontal attachment loss induced by mechanical subgingival instrumentation in shallow sulci. *J Dent Hyg*. 2002;76:207–212.
2. Rucker LM, Gibson G, McGregor C. Getting the "feel" of it: the non-visual component of dimensional accuracy during operative tooth preparation. *J Can Dent Assoc*. 1990;56:937–941.
3. Ruhling A, Konig J, Rolf H, Kocher T, Schwahn C, Plagmann HC. Learning root debridement with curettes and power-driven instruments. Part II: clinical results following mechanical, nonsurgical therapy. *J Clin Periodontol*. 2003;30:611–615.
4. Ruhling A, Schlemme H, Konig J, Kocher T, Schwahn C, Plagmann HC. Learning root debridement with curettes and power-driven instruments. Part I: a training program to increase effectivity. *J Clin Periodontol*. 2002;29:622–629.
5. Goncalves PF, Gurgel BC, Pimentel SP, Sallum EA, Sallum AW, Casati MZ, et al. Effect of two different approaches for root decontamination on new cementum formation following guided tissue regeneration: a histomorphometric study in dogs. *J Periodontal Res*. 2006;41:535–540.
6. Goncalves PF, Gurgel BC, Pimentel SP, Sallum EA, Sallum AW, Casati MZ, et al. Root cementum modulates periodontal regeneration in class III furcation defects treated by the guided tissue regeneration technique: a histometric study in dogs. *J Periodontol*. 2006;77:976–982.
7. Goncalves PF, Lima LL, Sallum EA, Casati MZ, Nociti FH Jr. Root cementum may modulate gene expression during periodontal regeneration: a preliminary study in humans. *J Periodontol*. 2008;79:323–331.
8. Nyman S, Westfelt E, Sarhed G, Karring T. Role of "diseased" root cementum in healing following treatment of periodontal disease. A clinical study. *J Clin Periodontol*. 1988;15:464–468.
9. Zaman KU, Sugaya T, Hongo O, Kato H. A study of attached and oriented human periodontal ligament cells to periodontally diseased cementum and dentin after demineralizing with neutral and low pH etching solution. *J Periodontol*. 2000;71:1094–1099.
10. Berutti E. Microleakage of human saliva through dentinal tubules exposed at the cervical level in teeth treated endodontically. *J Endod*. 1996;22:579–582.

Section 3
Skill Application

STUDENT SELF-EVALUATION MODULE 10 INSTRUMENTATION STROKE

Student: ______________________ Date: ______________________

DIRECTIONS: Self-evaluate your skill level as: **S** (satisfactory) or **U** (unsatisfactory).

- **Right-Handed Clinician:** demonstrate on facial surface of the mandibular right first molar facial
- **Left-Handed Clinician:** demonstrate on facial surface of the mandibular left first molar facial

Criteria	
Assessment Stroke on Facial Surface of a Mandibular First Molar	**Eval.**
Establishes a correct finger rest and selects the correct working-end of the explorer	
Places explorer working-end in the middle-third of the crown in preparation for insertion	
Pauses to assess finger placement in the modified pen grasp; corrects finger position, if necessary	
Gently inserts the working-end beneath the gingival margin keeping the tip-third against the tooth surface	
Using a relaxed grasp, keeps the tip-third in contact with the tooth surface and slides the working-end to the base of the pocket	
Maintaining a relaxed grasp, makes a feather-light assessment stroke away from the junctional epithelium	
Stops the assessment stroke just beneath the gingival margin (fulcrum finger does not lift off of the tooth at the end of a stroke)	
Makes a series of feather-light strokes across the facial surface of the tooth	
Maintains a relaxed grasp with no finger blanching during the entire assessment process of the facial surface	

Module 11

Periodontal Probes and Basic Probing Technique

MODULE OVERVIEW

The periodontal probe is a periodontal instrument that is calibrated in millimeter increments and used to evaluate the health of the periodontal tissues. Findings from an examination with a calibrated probe are an important part of a comprehensive periodontal assessment to determine the health of the periodontal tissues. This module presents the design characteristics of calibrated periodontal probes and step-by-step instructions for use of a calibrated periodontal probe.

Module Outline

Key Terms

Periodontal probe
Gingiva
Free gingiva
Gingival margin
Gingival sulcus
Attached gingiva
Sulcus
Junctional epithelium
Periodontitis
Periodontal pocket
Gingival pocket
Apical migration
Pseudo-pocket
Probing depth
Periodontal chart
Probing
Walking stroke

Learning Objectives

1. Identify the design characteristics of a calibrated periodontal probe.
2. Identify the millimeter markings on several calibrated periodontal probes including some probe designs that are not in your school instrument kit.
3. Describe the rationale and technique for periodontal probing.
4. Identify factors that can affect the accuracy of periodontal probing.
5. Discuss the characteristics of effective probing technique in terms of adaptation and angulation of the tip, amount of pressure needed, instrumentation stroke, and number and location of probe readings for each tooth.
6. Using a calibrated periodontal probe, demonstrate correct adaptation on facial, lingual, and proximal surfaces and beneath the contact area of two adjacent teeth.
7. Activate a calibrated periodontal probe using a walking stroke and correct probing technique.
8. While using correct positioning, mirror, grasp, and finger rests, demonstrate correct probing technique in all sextants of the dentition.
9. Determine probing depths accurately to within 1 mm of an instructor's reading.
10. Define the term junctional epithelium.
11. Differentiate between a normal sulcus and a periodontal pocket and describe the position of the probe in each.

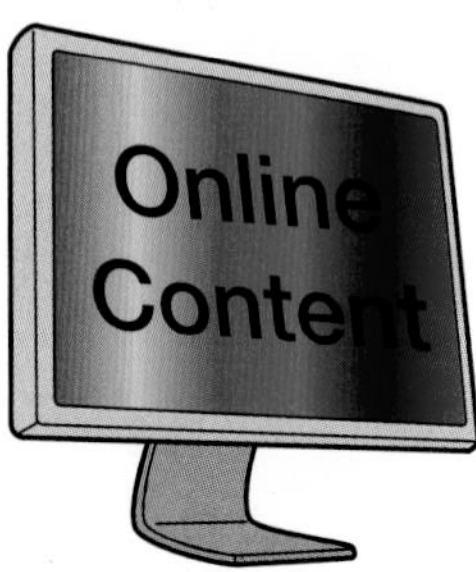

Videos for this topic can be viewed online at http://thepoint.lww.com/GehrigFundamentals7e

Section 1
The Periodontal Probe

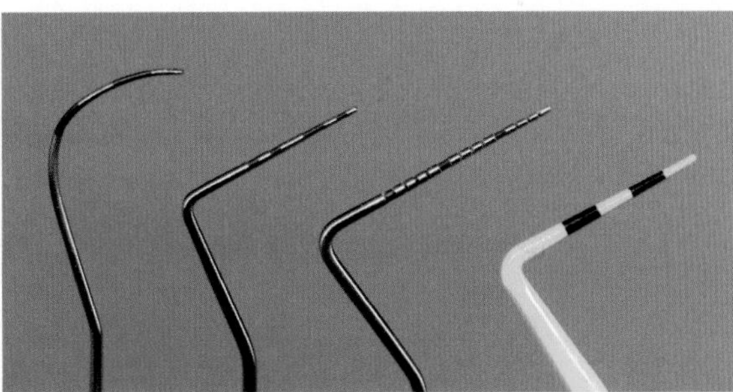

Figure 11-1. Calibrated Periodontal Probes. The **periodontal probe** is a periodontal instrument that is calibrated in millimeter increments and used to evaluate the health of the periodontal tissues.

DESIGN CHARACTERISTICS AND FUNCTIONS

1. **Design of Periodontal Probes**
   - **a.** A periodontal probe has a blunt, rod-shaped working-end that may be circular or rectangular in cross section and is calibrated with millimeter markings (Fig. 11-1).
   - **b.** The working-end and the shank meet in a defined angle that is usually greater than 90°.
2. **Function of Periodontal Probes**
   - **a. Primary Function. Detect periodontal pockets to determine the health status of the periodontium.**
     1. The most convenient and reliable way of detecting and measuring periodontal pockets is through the use of a periodontal probe. A periodontal probe is used to obtain a physical measurement of the distance between the gingival margin and the base of a periodontal pocket.
     2. In 1958, the eminent periodontist, B.J. Orban described the periodontal probe as the "eye of the clinician beneath the gingival margin," an essential part of a complete periodontal examination.[1]
     3. The periodontal probe is the most important clinical tool for obtaining information about the health status of the periodontium. In other words, is the tissue healthy or diseased?[2–4]
   - **b. Other Functions.** In addition to measuring periodontal pocket depths, the periodontal probe has numerous other uses in the periodontal assessment.[2–4] These other uses of the periodontal probe are explained in the module on advanced probing techniques.
     - Measure clinical attachment loss
     - Measure extent of recession of the gingival margin
     - Measure the width of the attached gingiva
     - Measure the size of intraoral lesions
     - Assess bleeding on probing
     - Determine mucogingival relationships
     - Monitoring the longitudinal response of the periodontium to treatment

PROBE DESIGNS

Different probes, such as Michigan, Williams, Marquis, Goldman-Fox, and Nabers probes, have different dimensions and a different diameter at the tip (Table 11-1). The tip diameters range from 0.28 mm for the Michigan "O" probe to 0.7 mm for the Williams probe.[2] Most periodontal probes are made of stainless steel, but some are made of titanium and plastic.

TABLE 11-1. Examples of Probe Designs

Probe	Design Characteristics
Williams Probe 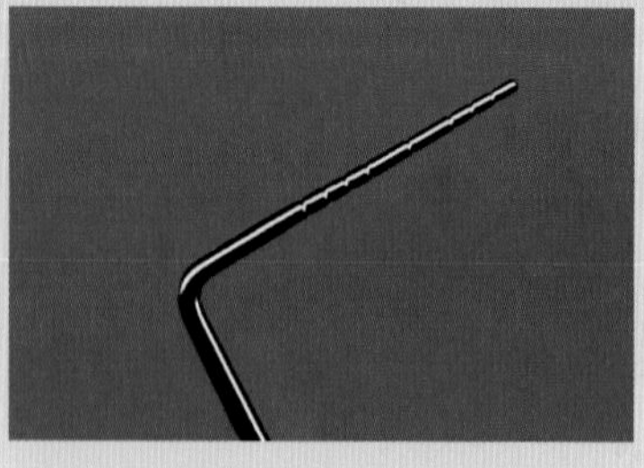 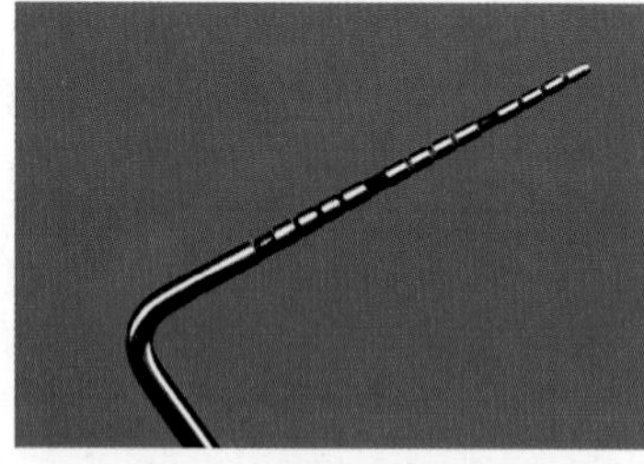	• Prototype for most subsequent probe designs (standard on which later probe designs are based) • Williams was a periodontist who specialized in the study of the relationship between pocket formation and local infection.[5] • Thin, round working-end • Millimeter grooves at 1, 2, 3, 5, 7, 8, 9, and 10 mm (markings at 4 and 6 mm are missing to avoid confusion in reading the markings)
University of North Carolina (UNC-12 and UNC-15) Probe 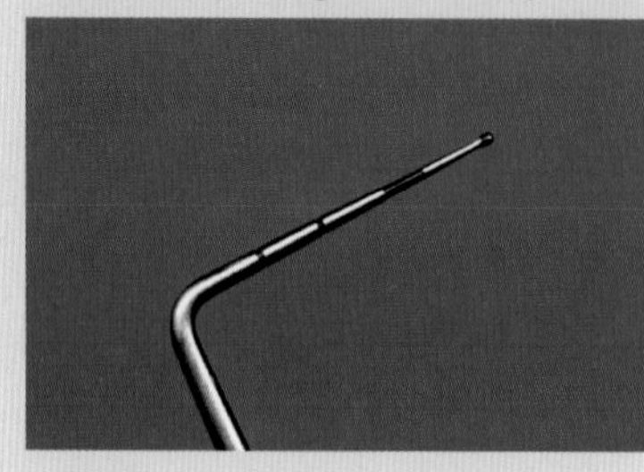	• Preferred probe for use in clinical research • Millimeter markings at each millimeter • UNC-12 color-coded at 4 and 9 mm • UNC-15 color-coded at 4, 9, and 14 mm • Thin, round working-end
World Health Organization (WHO) 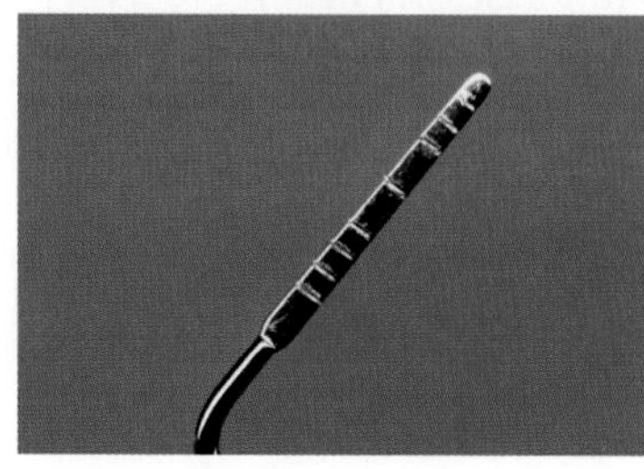	• Has a unique ball-end of 0.5 mm in diameter, which is attached to a 16-mm-long working-end • Markings at 3.5, 5.5, 8.5, and 11.5 mm • Advocated for use in epidemiology and routine periodontal screening in general dental practice • Thin, round working-end
Goldman Fox Probe	• Millimeter grooves at 1, 2, 3, 5, 7, 8, 9, and 10 mm (markings at 4 and 6 mm are missing) • Flat working-end

(continues)

TABLE 11-1. Examples of Probe Designs *(continued)*

Probe	Design Characteristics
Novatech Probe 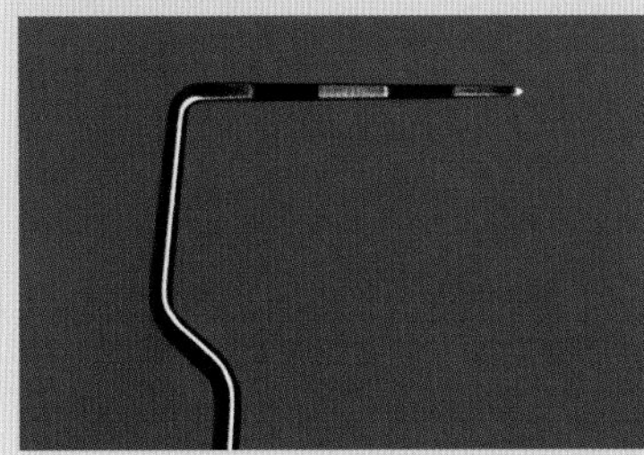	• Unique shank design with upward and right-angled bend to facilitate access to the distal surfaces of molars • Novatech probe pictured has millimeter markings at 3, 6, 9, and 12 mm. • Available in a variety of millimeter calibrations
Plastic Probe 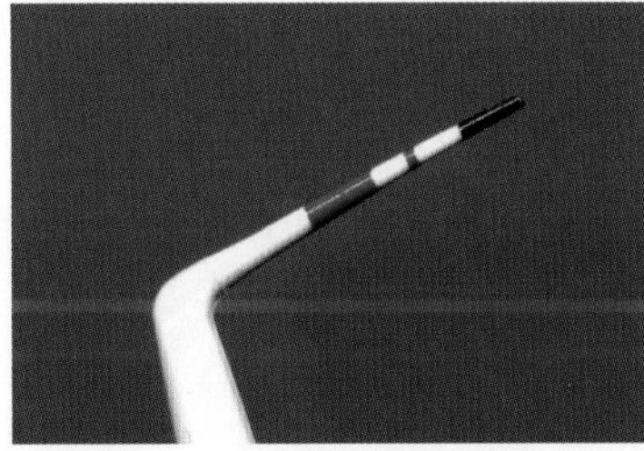	• Color-coded in a variety of millimeter calibrations • PerioWise probe pictured has millimeter markings at 3, 5, 7, and 10 mm. • Round, tapered working-end • Color-coding facilitates reading • Recommended if probing dental implants • Sterilizable for reuse
Florida Probe 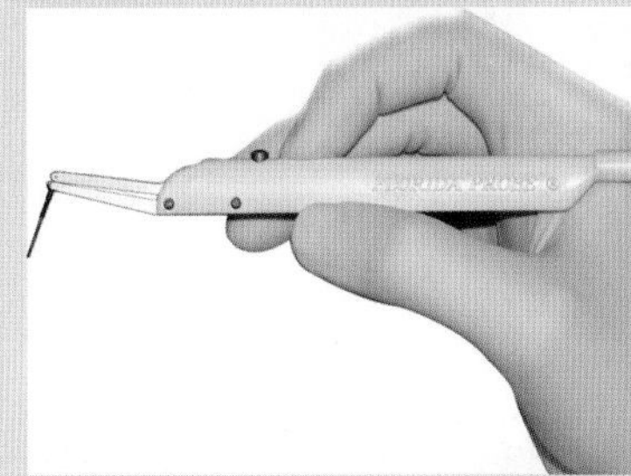 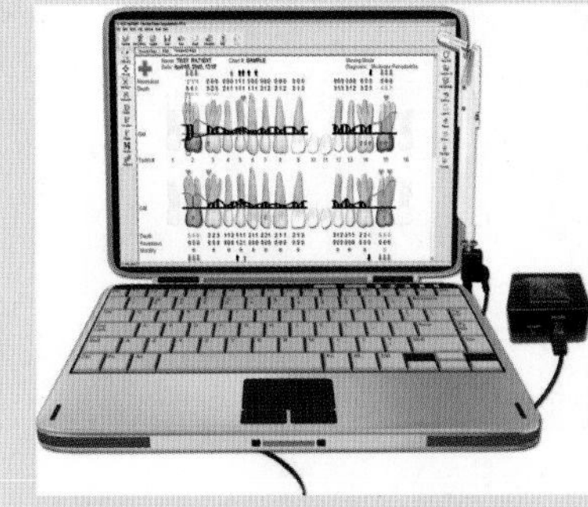	• Computer-assisted probe with digital readouts and computer storage of data • Constant probing pressure of 15 g is provided by coil springs inside the handpiece. • Consists of a probe handpiece and sleeve; a displacement transducer; a foot switch; and a computer interface[6] • Measurement of the probe depth is made electronically and transferred automatically to the computer when the foot switch is pressed. • Can also record missing teeth, recession, pocket depth, bleeding, suppuration, furcation involvement, mobility, and plaque assessment[7] (Photographs of Florida Probe courtesy of Florida Probe Corporation.)

MILLIMETER MARKINGS

Calibrated probes are marked in millimeter increments and are used like miniature rulers for making intraoral measurements.

1. **Millimeter Markings**
   a. Grooves, colored indentations, or colored bands may be used to indicate the millimeter markings on the working-end of a periodontal probe.
   b. Each millimeter may be indicated on the probe, or only certain millimeter increments may be marked (Figs. 11-2 and 11-3).
   c. If uncertain how a probe is calibrated, a millimeter ruler may be used to determine the millimeter markings.
2. **Color-Coding.** Color-coded probes are marked in bands (often black in color) with each band being several millimeters in width.

EXAMPLES OF PROBE CALIBRATIONS

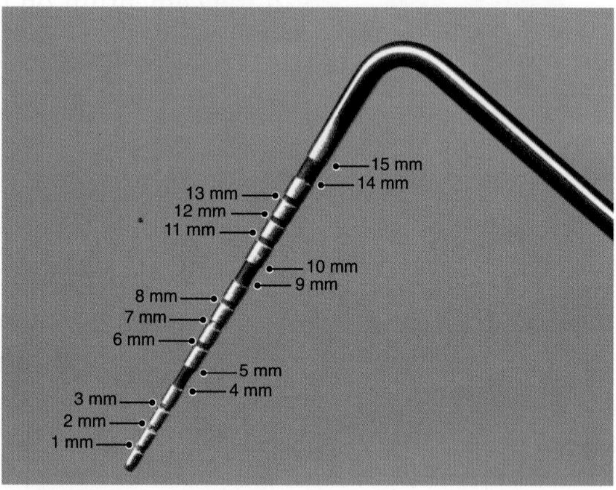

Figure 11-2. Markings at Each Millimeter. The UNC-15 probe has millimeter markings at 1, 2, 3, 4, 5, 6, 7, 8, 9, 10, 11, 12, 13, 14, and 15 mm. Colored bands between 4 and 5 mm, 9 and 10 mm, and 14 and 15 mm facilitate reading of the markings.

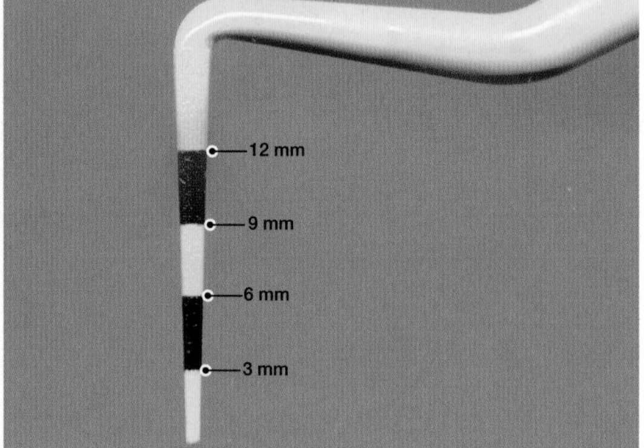

Figure 11-3. Color-Coded Probe. This probe is marked in alternating black and yellow bands; each band is 3 mm in length. The millimeter markings are at 3, 6, 9, and 12 mm on this particular probe.

Section 2
Assessing Tissue Health

REVIEW OF PERIODONTAL ANATOMY IN HEALTH

The gingiva is the tissue that covers the cervical portions of the teeth and the alveolar processes of the jaws (Fig. 11-4).

1. **The Free Gingiva.** The free gingiva is the unattached portion of the gingiva that surrounds the tooth in the region of the cementoenamel junction (CEJ).
   a. The tissue of the free gingiva fits closely around the tooth—in a turtleneck manner—but is not directly attached to it. This tissue, because it is unattached, may be moved gently away from the tooth surface with a periodontal probe.
   b. The free gingiva meets the tooth in a thin rounded edge called the gingival margin.
2. **The Gingival Sulcus.** The gingival sulcus is a shallow, V-shaped *space* between the free gingiva and the tooth surface.
3. **The Attached Gingiva.** The attached gingiva is the part of the gingiva that is tightly connected to the cementum on the cervical-third of the root and to the periosteum (connective tissue cover) of the alveolar bone.

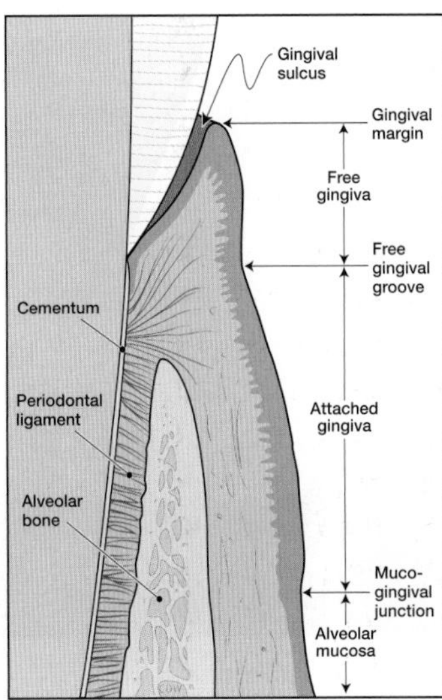

Figure 11-4. The Gingival Tissues in Cross Section. The structures of the healthy periodontium in cross section. The sulcus is a V-shaped, shallow space around the tooth. The base of the sulcus is formed by the junctional epithelium.

IDENTIFICATION OF PERIODONTAL POCKETS

The periodontal probe is the most important clinical tool for obtaining information about the health status of the periodontium.

1. **The Healthy Sulcus**
   a. In health, the tooth is surrounded by a sulcus. The junctional epithelium is the tissue that forms the base of the sulcus by attaching to the enamel of the crown near the CEJ.
   b. ***Anatomically, the gingival sulcus is defined as the distance from the gingival margin to the coronal-most part of the junctional epithelium.***[8] The true anatomic determination of the bottom of the pocket can be obtained solely through a histologic examination.[9]

c. The depth of a clinically normal gingival sulcus is from 1 to 3 mm, as measured using a periodontal probe (Fig. 11-5).
d. Probing depths on the mesial and distal surfaces are slightly deeper than depths on lingual surfaces. Probing depths on facial surfaces exhibit the least depth.[3,10]

2. **The Periodontal Pocket**

a. Periodontitis is a bacterial infection of all parts of the periodontium including the gingiva, periodontal ligament, alveolar bone, and cementum.
   1. Clinically, periodontitis is identified by the presence of a periodontal pocket—a sulcus that is greater than 3 mm.[11]
   2. Therefore, the correct identification of periodontal pockets is fundamental in the recognition of periodontitis.
b. A periodontal pocket is a gingival sulcus that has been deepened by disease. In a periodontal pocket, the junctional epithelium forms the base of the pocket by attaching to the root surface somewhere apical to (below) the CEJ. A periodontal pocket results from destruction of alveolar bone and the periodontal ligament fibers that surround the tooth.
c. The depth of a periodontal pocket, as measured by a periodontal probe, will be greater than 3 mm (Fig. 11-6). It is common to have pockets measuring 5 to 6 mm in depth.

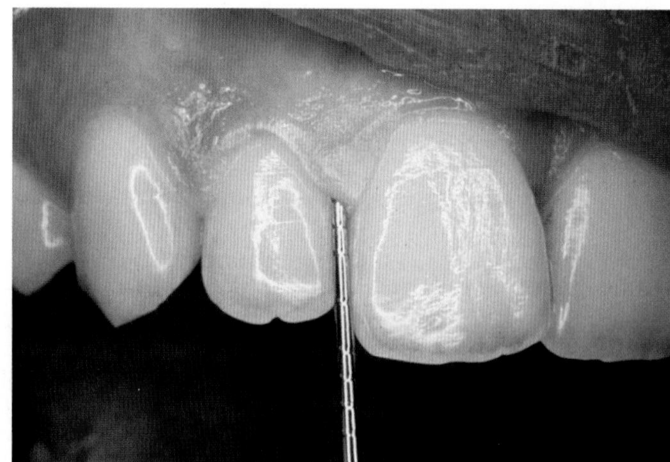

Figure 11-5. Probe in a Healthy Sulcus. The photograph shows a periodontal probe inserted into a healthy gingival sulcus, the space between the free gingiva and the tooth. A healthy sulcus is 1 to 3 mm deep, as measured with a periodontal probe.

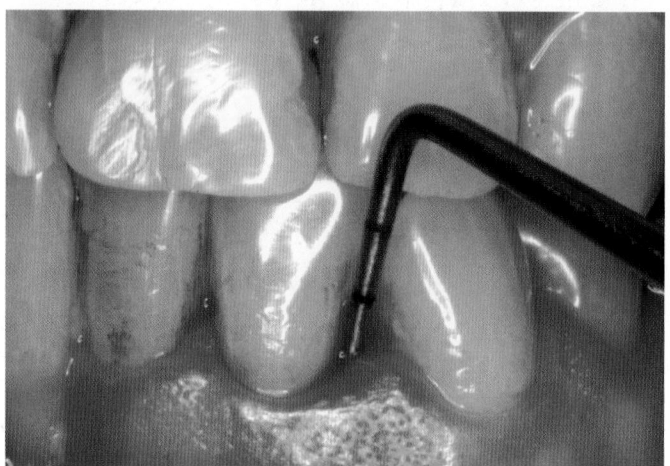

Figure 11-6. Probe in a Periodontal Pocket. The photograph shows a periodontal probe inserted into a periodontal pocket. In a periodontal pocket, the junctional epithelium is located on the root somewhere below the CEJ. The depth of a periodontal pocket, as measured by a periodontal probe, will be greater than 3 mm.

POCKET FORMATION

1. **Gingival Sulcus.** In health, the junctional epithelial cells attach to the enamel of the tooth crown (Fig. 11-7).
2. **Gingival Pocket.** A gingival pocket is a deepening of the gingival sulcus. The increased probing depth seen in a gingival pocket is due to (1) detachment of the coronal portion of the junctional epithelium from the tooth and (2) increased tissue size due to swelling of the tissue (Fig. 11-8).
3. **Periodontal Pocket.** A periodontal pocket forms as the result of the (1) apical migration of the junctional epithelium and (2) destruction of the periodontal ligament fibers and alveolar bone (Fig. 11-9). Apical migration is the movement of the cells of the junctional epithelium from their normal position—coronal to the CEJ—to a position apical to the CEJ. In periodontitis, the junctional epithelial cells attach to the cementum of the tooth root.

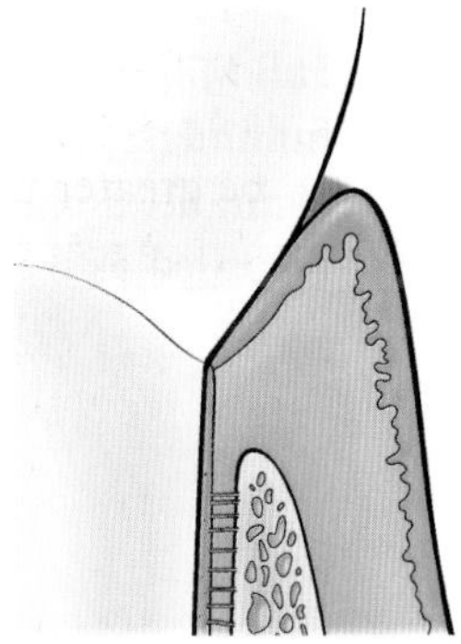

Figure 11-7. Gingival Sulcus.

- In health, the junctional epithelium is located slightly apical to—above—the CEJ.
- The junctional epithelium (JE) attaches along its entire length to the enamel of the crown.

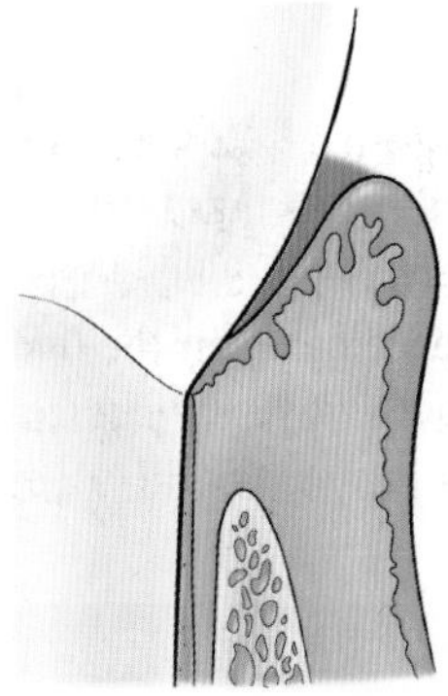

Figure 11-8. Gingival Pocket.

- In gingivitis, the coronal-most portion of the junctional epithelium detaches from the tooth, resulting in an increased probing depth.
- Compare the sulcus depth in this illustration with that shown in Figure 11-7.
- In some cases of gingivitis, the gingival tissue swells, resulting in an increased probing depth known as a pseudo-pocket.

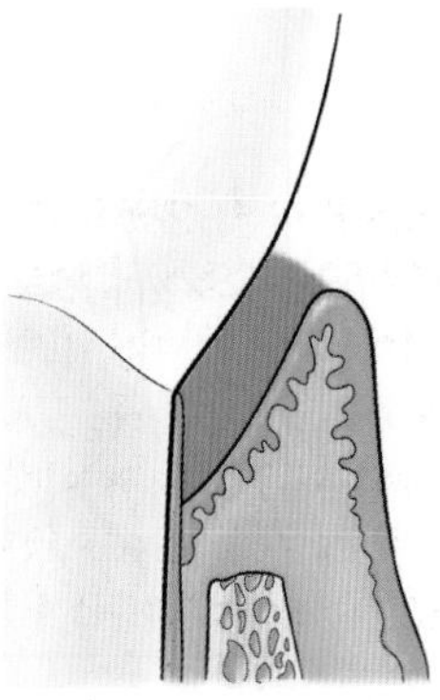

Figure 11-9. Periodontal Pocket.

- In a periodontal pocket, the junctional epithelium is located on the root somewhere below the CEJ.
- The deeper probing depth of a periodontal pocket is due to the apical migration of the junctional epithelium.

Section 3
Reading and Recording Depth Measurements

CLINICAL PROBING DEPTH MEASUREMENT

A probing depth is a measurement of the depth of a sulcus or periodontal pocket (Fig. 11-10). It is determined by measuring the distance from the gingival margin to the base of the sulcus or pocket with a calibrated periodontal probe.

1. **Six Areas per Tooth.** Probing depth measurements are recorded for six specific areas on each tooth: (1) distofacial, (2) facial, (3) mesiofacial, (4) distolingual, (5) lingual, and (6) mesiolingual (Box 11-1).
2. **One Reading per Area.** Only one reading per area is recorded. If the probing depths vary within an area, the deepest reading obtained in that area is recorded. For example, if the probing depths in the facial surface ranged from 3 to 6 mm, only the 6-mm reading would be entered on the chart for the facial area (Fig. 11-11).
3. **Full Millimeter Measurements.** Probing depths are recorded to the nearest full millimeter. Round up measurements to the next higher whole number; for example, a reading of 3.5 mm is recorded as 4 mm or a reading of 5.5 mm is recorded as 6 mm.

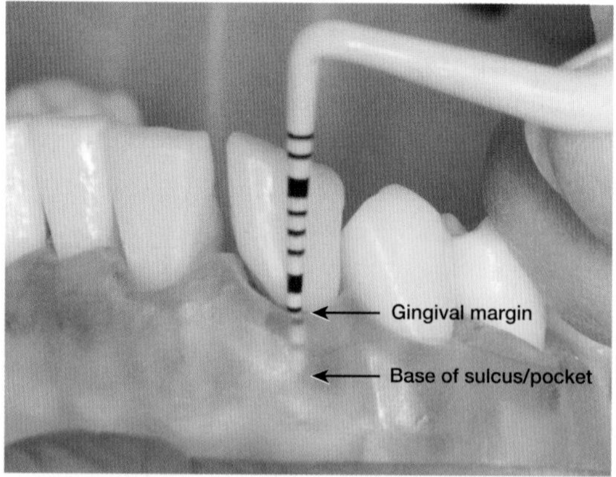

Figure 11-10. Probing Depth. A probing depth is the distance in millimeters from the *gingival margin* to the base of the sulcus or periodontal pocket as measured with a calibrated probe.

Box 11-1. Record Measurements for Six Areas per Tooth

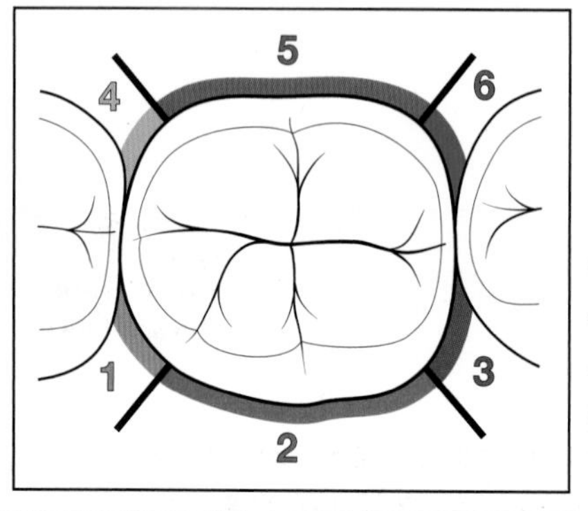

Probing depth measurements are recorded for 6 specific sites on each tooth:

1 - distofacial line angle to the midline of distal surface
2 - facial surface
3 - mesiofacial line angle to the midline of mesial surface
4 - distolingual line angle to the midline of distal surface
5 - lingual surface
6 - mesiolingual line angle to the midline of mesial surface

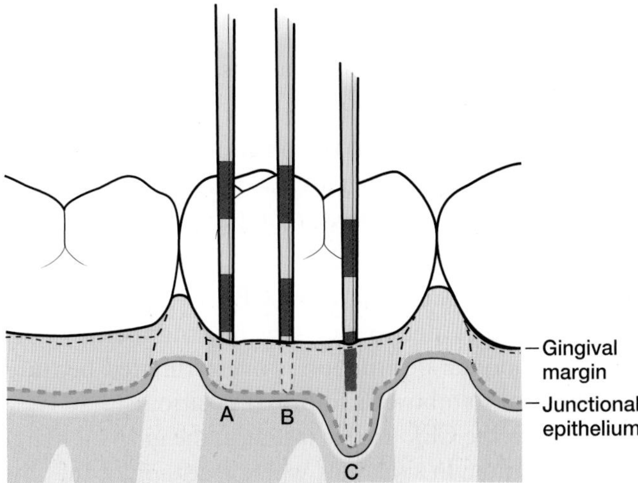

Figure 11-11. Record the Deepest Reading per Area. In the illustration shown here, the depth of the pocket base varies considerably at points **A**, **B**, and **C** in the facial surface.

- Points A and B on the facial surface measure 3 mm.
- Point C on the facial surface is a 6-mm reading. Because only a single reading can be recorded for the facial surface, the deepest reading at point C is recorded for the facial surface.

PERIODONTAL CHART

Probing depth measurements are recorded on a periodontal chart. Most periodontal charts include rows of boxes that are used to record the probing depths on the facial and lingual aspects of the teeth (Fig. 11-12).

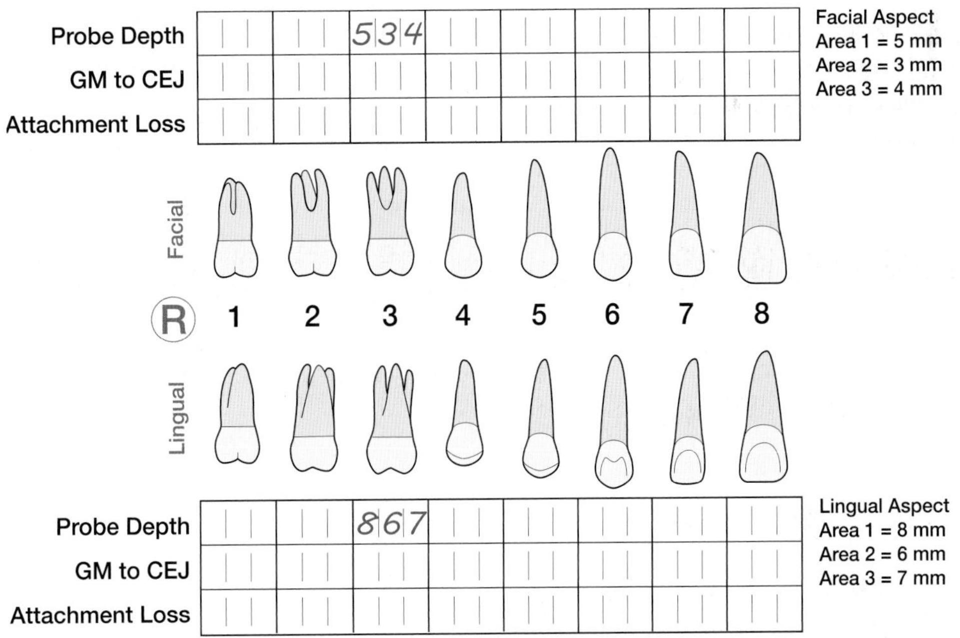

Figure 11-12. Recording Probing Depths. Probing depths for the facial and lingual aspects of the maxillary right first molar are recorded on the periodontal chart shown here. (Key: GM = gingival margin; CEJ = cementoenamel junction.)

LIMITATIONS OF PROBING MEASUREMENTS

Probing depth measurements have their limitations. Various factors can affect how accurately probing depths reflect the extent of periodontal destruction.[2,3,9,12–14]

1. **Position of the Gingival Margin.** In health, the position of the gingival margin is slightly coronal to (above) the CEJ. ***If the gingival margin is not in its normal location—slightly coronal to the CEJ—probing depths will NOT accurately reflect the health of periodontium.***
   a. **Gingival Margin Significantly Coronal to the CEJ.** Frequently, the gingival tissue is swollen or overgrown due to gingivitis or drug therapy.[15] In such cases, the extent of periodontal destruction is overestimated because the gingival margin is coronal to (above) its normal position.
   b. **Gingival Margin Apical to the CEJ.** In this instance, the gingival margin is apical to (below) its normal location. In situations where recession of the gingival margin is present, probing depth readings can substantially underestimate the true extent of periodontal destruction.
2. **Reading Errors due to Naturally Occurring States**
   a. Reading errors may result from naturally occurring states, such as interference from calculus deposits on the tooth surface, the presence of an overhanging restoration, or the crown's contour.[14] Figure 11-13 depicts two states that can interfere with probing.
   b. When a calculus deposit is encountered, the probe is gently teased out and around the deposit or the calculus deposit is removed so that the probe can be inserted to the base of the pocket.
3. **Reading Errors due to Probing Technique and Equipment**
   a. Technique errors include incorrect angulation and positioning of the probe, incorrect amount of pressure applied to the probe, misreading the probe calibrations, and recording the measurements incorrectly.[14]
   b. Other variables that influence measurements include the diameter and shape of the probe, calibration scale of the probe, and the degree of inflammation in the periodontal tissues.
   c. Manufacturing errors can result in the widths of probe markings differing by as much as 0.7 mm between probes.[13]
   d. A research study by van Weringh et al.[16] suggests that the diameter of the instrument handle of a probe has an effect on the force exerted with a periodontal probe.

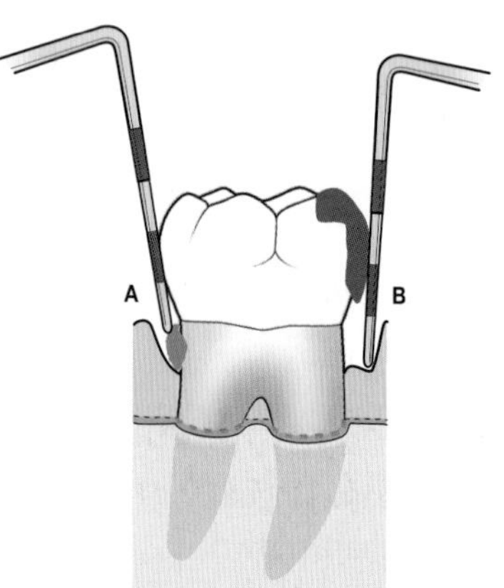

Figure 11-13. Interference with Probe Insertion. Reading errors may result from interference of **(A)** a large calculus deposit or **(B)** overhanging restoration.

Section 4
Probing Technique

ALIGNMENT AND ADAPTATION

1. **Insertion and Adaptation.** Once a probe is inserted into a periodontal pocket, ***the working-end is kept parallel to the root surface.*** Figure 11-14 depicts correct and incorrect alignment of a probe to the root surface.
   a. The tip should be kept as flat against the root surface as possible as the working-end is inserted to the base of the pocket.
   b. Even though the probing involves contact of the working-end with the root surface, no pressure should be used with a probing stroke.
2. **Obtaining Alignment on Distal Surfaces of Maxillary Molars.** Often, it is difficult to align the probe's working-end to the distal surfaces of the maxillary molars because the mandible is in the way. This problem can be overcome by repositioning the instrument handle to the side of the patient's face. This solution is depicted in Figure 11-15.

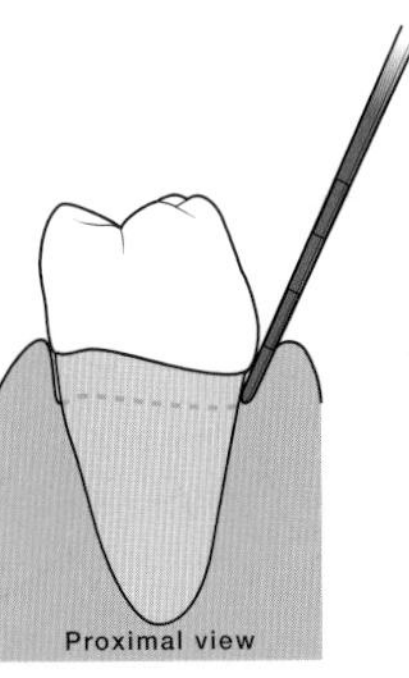

Figure 11-14A. Correct Adaptation to Proximal Surface. This illustration shows correct adaptation of the probe with the working-end parallel to the root surface.

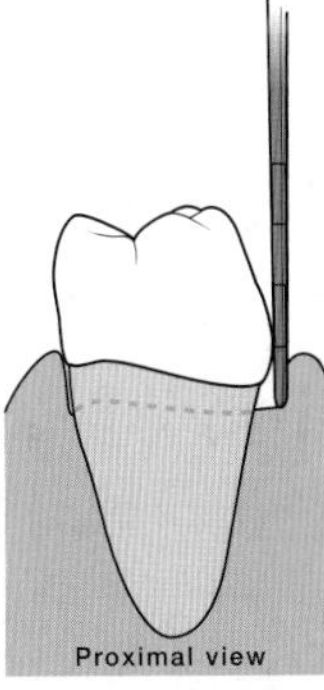

Figure 11-14B. Incorrect Adaptation to Proximal Surface. In this example, the probe is not parallel to the root surface, resulting in an underestimation of the measurement.

PROBING MAXILLARY MOLARS

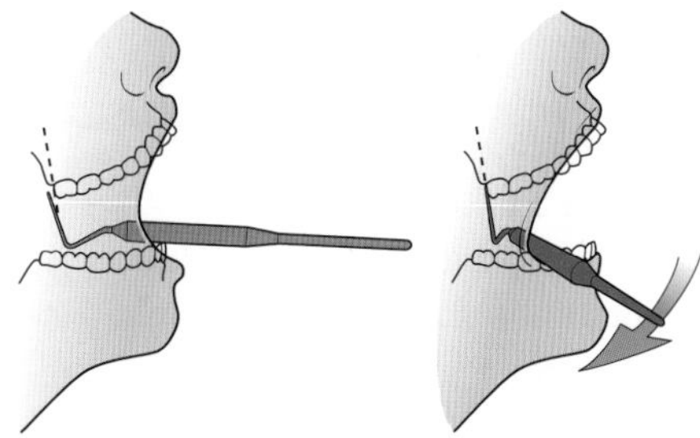

Figure 11-15. Technique for Distal Surfaces of the Maxillary Molars. Often, it is difficult to probe the distal surfaces of the maxillary molars because the mandible is in the way. This problem can be overcome by repositioning the instrument handle to the side of the patient's face.

PROBING PROXIMAL ROOT SURFACES

1. **Periodontal Pocketing on Proximal Root Surfaces**
   - **a.** It is important to assess the proximal surfaces of a tooth because periodontal pockets are common on the mesial and distal surfaces.
   - **b.** *The proximal surfaces should be probed from both the facial and lingual aspects to assure that the entire circumference of the junctional epithelium is assessed* (Fig. 11-16).
2. **Technique for Probing Proximal Root Surfaces.** *When two adjacent teeth are in contact, a special technique is used to probe the depth of the junctional epithelium directly beneath the contact area.* The two-step technique used on a proximal—mesial or distal—surface is depicted in Figure 11-17.
   1. **Step 1:** Keeping the working-end of the probe in contact with the proximal root surface, walk the probe across the proximal surface until it touches the contact area (Fig. 11-17A). The area beneath the contact area cannot be probed directly because the probe will not fit between the adjacent teeth.
   2. **Step 2:** Slant the probe slightly so that the tip reaches under the contact area. The tip of the probe extends under the contact area while the upper portion touches the contact area (Fig. 11-17B). With the probe in this position, *gently press downward to touch the junctional epithelium.*

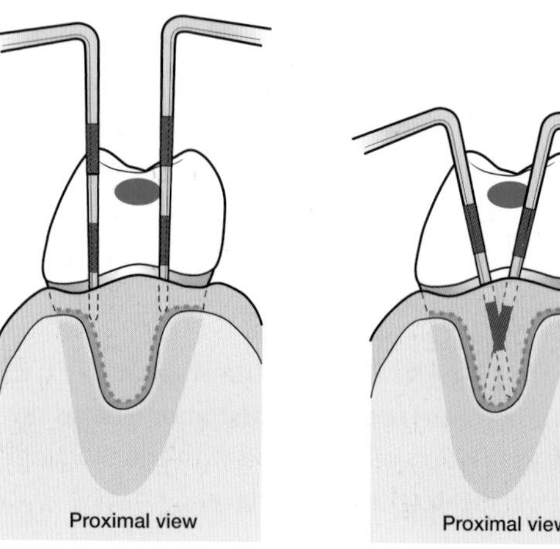

Figure 11-16. Assessing the Proximal Surface. The proximal surface of a tooth is assessed from both the facial and lingual aspects of the dental arch.

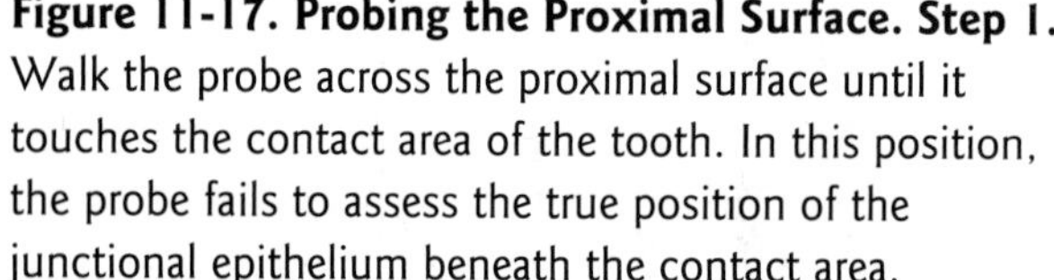

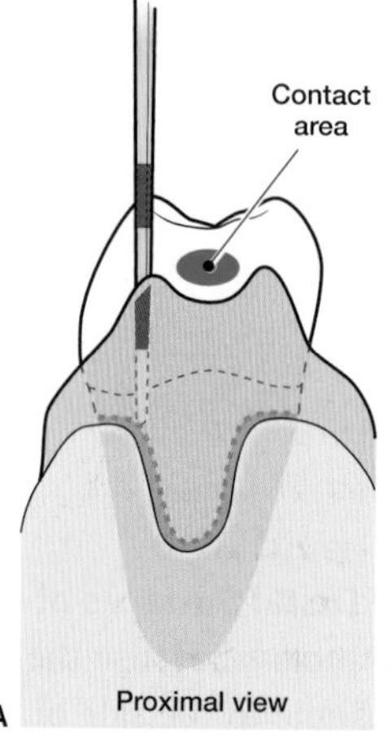

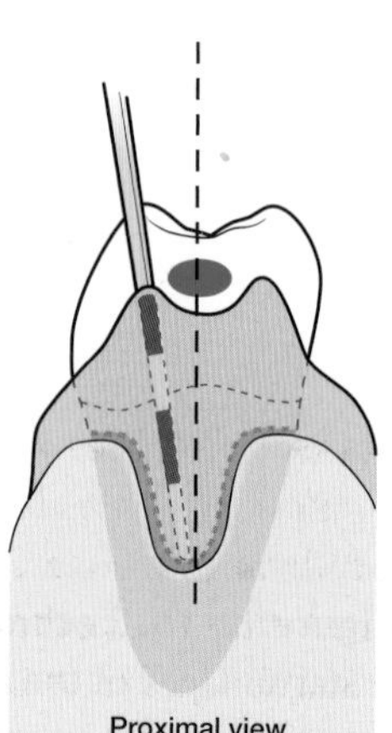

Figure 11-17. Probing the Proximal Surface. Step 1. Walk the probe across the proximal surface until it touches the contact area of the tooth. In this position, the probe fails to assess the true position of the junctional epithelium beneath the contact area.

Step 2. Slant the working-end of the probe so that the tip extends under the contact area to reach the midline of the proximal surface. With the probe in this position, gently press downward to touch the junctional epithelium.

THE WALKING STROKE

Probing is the act of walking the tip of a probe along the junctional epithelium within the sulcus or pocket for the purpose of assessing the health status of the periodontal tissues. Careful probing technique is essential if the information obtained with a periodontal probe is to be accurate.

1. **Description of Walking Stroke**
   a. The walking stroke is the movement of a calibrated probe around the perimeter of the base of a sulcus or pocket.
   b. Walking strokes are used to cover the entire circumference of the sulcus or pocket base. ***It is essential to evaluate the entire circumference of the pocket base—all the way around the entire tooth—because the junctional epithelium is not necessarily at a uniform depth from the gingival margin. In fact, differences in the depths of two neighboring sites along the pocket base are common.***
2. **Production of the Walking Stroke**
   a. Walking strokes are a series of bobbing strokes made within the sulcus or pocket. The stroke begins when the probe is inserted into the sulcus or periodontal pocket while *keeping the probe tip against and in alignment with the root surface.*
   b. The probe is inserted until the tip encounters the resistance of the junctional epithelium that forms the base of the sulcus or periodontal pocket. The junctional epithelium feels soft and resilient when touched by the probe.
   c. The walking stroke is created by moving the probe up and down (↕) in short bobbing strokes and forward in 1-mm increments (↔). With each down stroke, the probe returns to touch the junctional epithelium (Fig. 11-18).
   d. The probe is not removed from the sulcus or periodontal pocket with each upward stroke. Removing and reinserting the probe repeatedly can traumatize the tissue at the gingival margin.
   e. The pressure exerted with the probe tip against the junctional epithelium should be between 10 and 20 g. A sensitive scale that measures weight in grams can be used to standardize the probing pressure.
   f. Either wrist or digital (finger) activation may be used with the probe because only light pressure is used when probing.

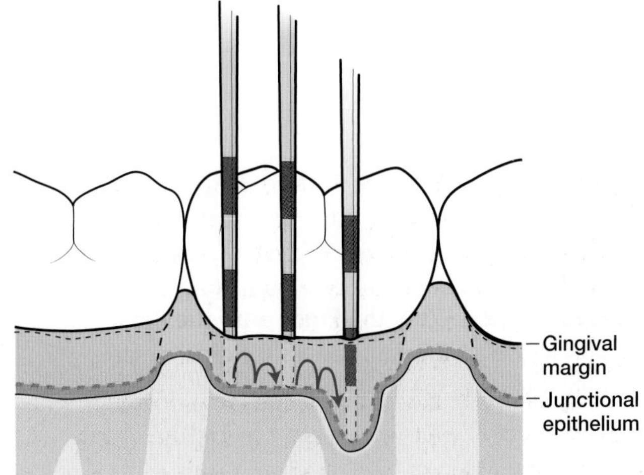

Figure 11-18. The Walking Stroke. The walking stroke is a series of bobbing strokes along the junctional epithelium (JE). Each up-and-down stroke should be approximately 1 to 2 mm in length (↕). The strokes must be very close together, about 1 mm apart (↔).

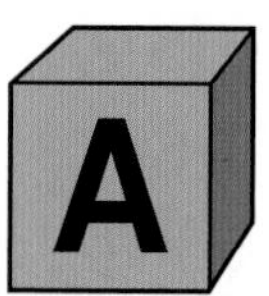

SKILL BUILDING. PROBING TECHNIQUE ON POSTERIOR TEETH

Directions:

- Follow steps 1 to 11 to practice probing the facial aspect of a mandibular first molar (Figs. 11-19 to 11-29). **Right-Handed clinicians:** Begin your practice session with the mandibular right posterior sextant, facial aspect. **Left-Handed clinicians:** Begin your practice session with the mandibular left posterior sextant, facial aspect.
- Remember: *"Me, My patient, My light, My dominant hand, My nondominant hand, My finger rest, My adaptation."*

1. **Figure 11-19. Area 1.** First, assess from the distofacial line angle to the midline of the distal surface. Insert the probe near the distofacial line angle of the *first molar*.

   Keep the side of the working-end in contact with the root surface as you gently slide the probe to touch the pocket base.

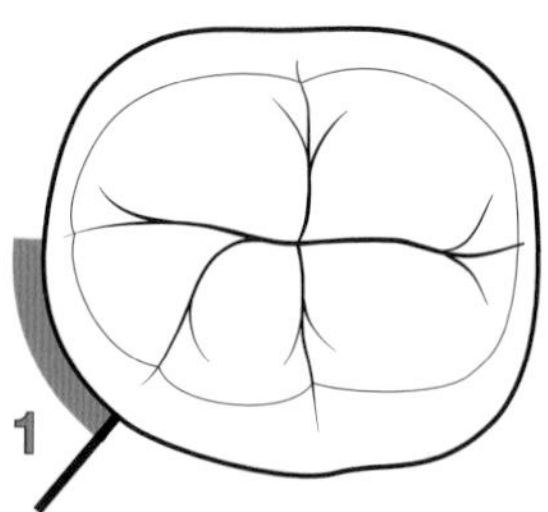

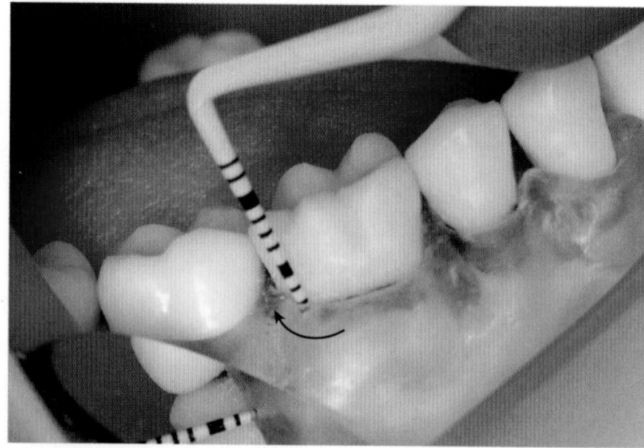

2. **Figure 11-20. Begin to Probe Area 1.** Keeping the working-end in contact with the tooth, initiate a series of short, bobbing strokes ***toward the distal surface***. Use a walking stroke, keeping your strokes close together. Gently touch the junctional epithelium at the base of the sulcus or pocket with each downward stroke of the probe.

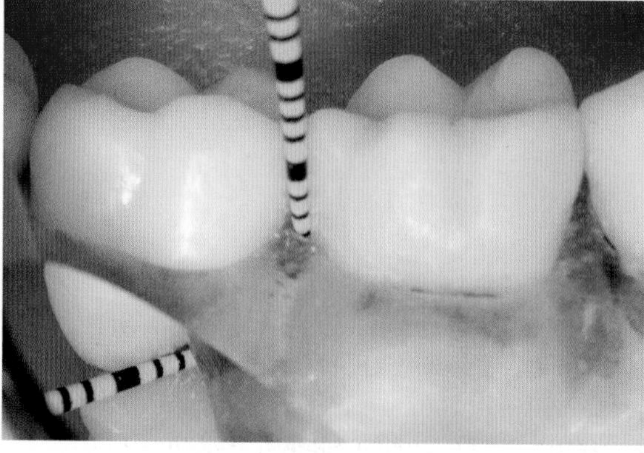

3. **Figure 11-21. Walk the Probe onto the Proximal Surface.** Walk the probe across the distal surface until it touches the contact area.

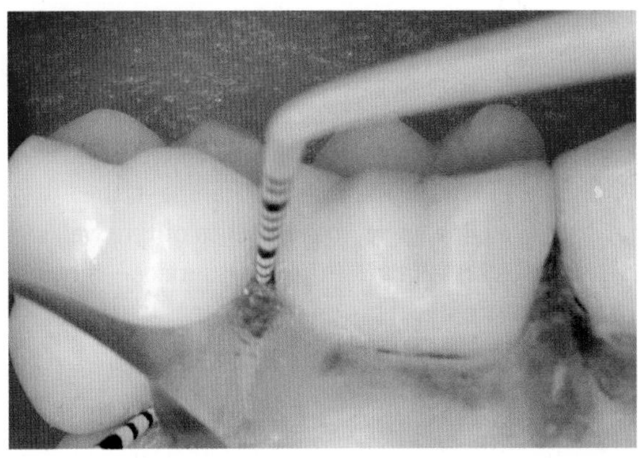

4. **Figure 11-22. Assess beneath the Contact Area.** Tilt the probe so that the tip reaches beneath the contact area (the upper portion of the probe touches the contact area).

   Gently press downward to touch the junctional epithelium.

   Enter the deepest reading encountered for Area 1 on the periodontal chart.

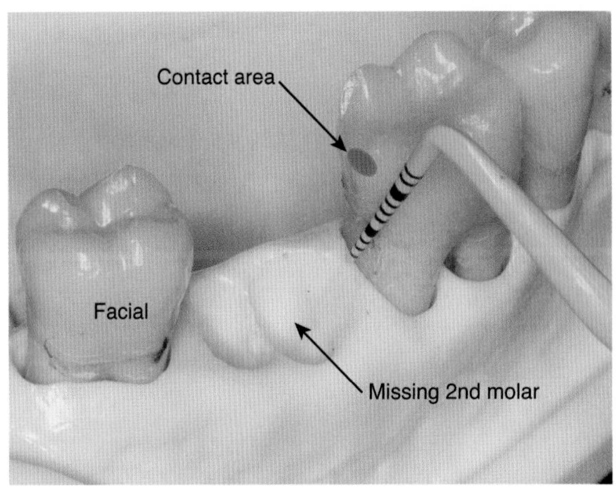

5. **Figure 11-23. Technique Check: Distal View.** *In this photo, the adjacent tooth has been removed* to provide a view of the correct probe position for assessing the tissue beneath the contact area from the facial aspect. Tilt your probe in a similar manner.

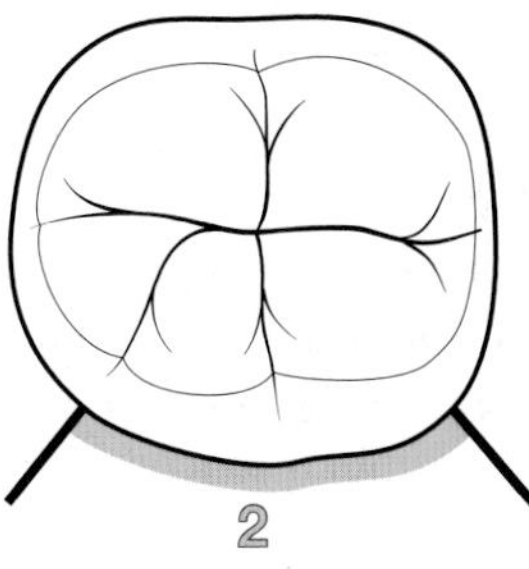

6. **Figure 11-24. Area 2.** Prepare to assess Area 2, the facial surface from the distofacial line angle to the mesiofacial line angle.

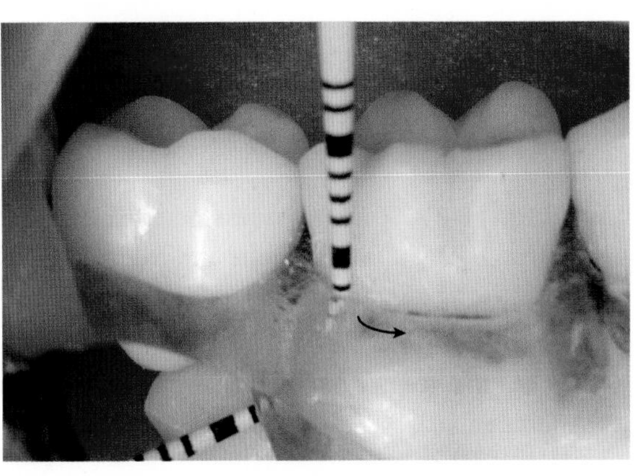

7. **Figure 11-25. Probe Area 2.** Reposition the probe at the distofacial line angle in preparation for assessing Area 2, the facial surface.

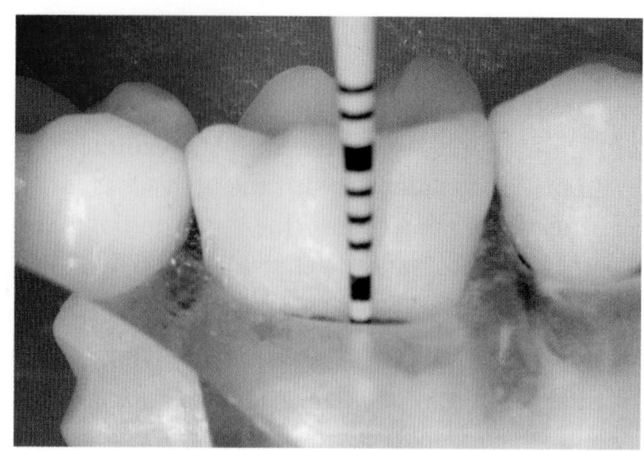

8. **Figure 11-26. Probe Area 2.** Starting at the distofacial line angle, make a series of tiny walking strokes across Area 2—the facial surface—moving in a forward direction toward the mesiofacial line angle.

   Record the deepest measurement in Area 2 on the periodontal chart.

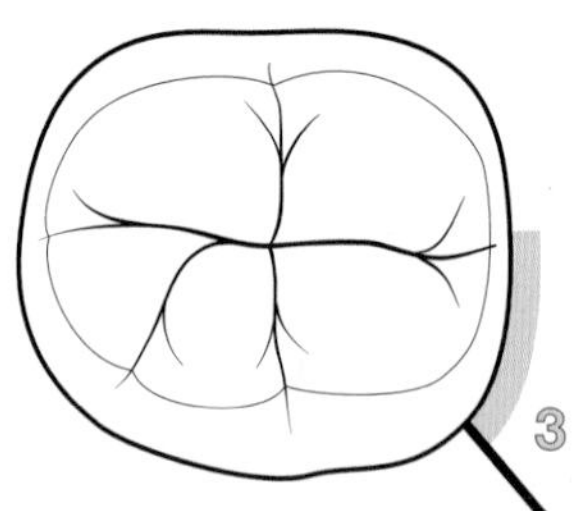

9. **Figure 11-27. Area 3.** Finally, probe Area 3 from the mesiofacial line angle to the midline of the mesial surface.

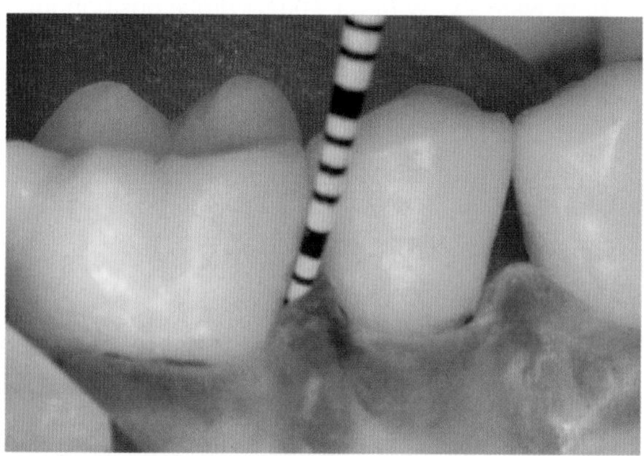

10. **Figure 11-28. Probe Area 3.** Starting at the mesiofacial line angle, walk the probe across the mesial surface until it touches the contact area.

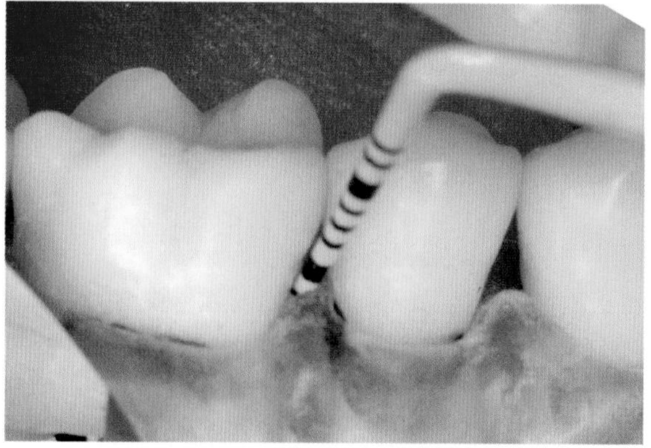

11. **Figure 11-29. Area 3. Assess beneath the Contact Area.** Tilt the probe and extend the tip beneath the contact area. Press down gently to touch the junctional epithelium.

    Record the deepest reading for Area 3 on the periodontal chart.

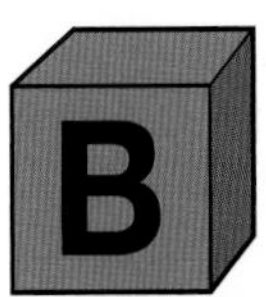

SKILL BUILDING. PROBING TECHNIQUE ON ANTERIOR TEETH

Directions:

- Follow steps 1 to 11 below to practice probing the facial aspect of a maxillary canine (Figs. 11-30 to 11-40). **Divide the facial aspect of each tooth into three sections.** For an anterior tooth, a probing depth measurement is recorded for the following three areas of the facial aspect: (1) distofacial area, (2) facial surface, and (3) mesiofacial area.
    - Begin by probing the distofacial area and record the deepest measurement for this area.
    - Next, probe the facial surface and record the deepest measurement.
    - Finally, probe the mesiofacial area and record the deepest measurement on a periodontal chart.
- ***Right-handed clinicians:*** Begin this practice session with the maxillary right canine, facial aspect. ***Left-handed clinicians:*** Begin this practice session with the maxillary left canine, facial aspect.

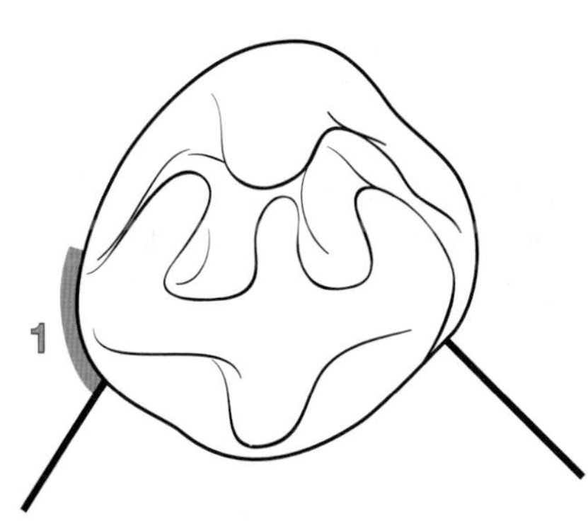

1. **Figure 11-30. Area 1.** Begin with Area 1 from the distofacial line angle to the midline of the distal surface of the canine. (This drawing shows the incisal view of a canine.)

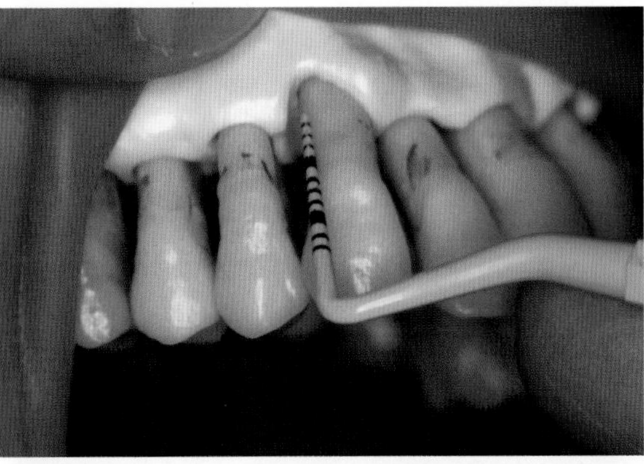

2. **Figure 11-31. Area 1. Insert at the Distofacial Line Angle.** Begin by inserting the probe at the distofacial line angle of the canine. You are now in position to assess the distal area of the facial aspect.

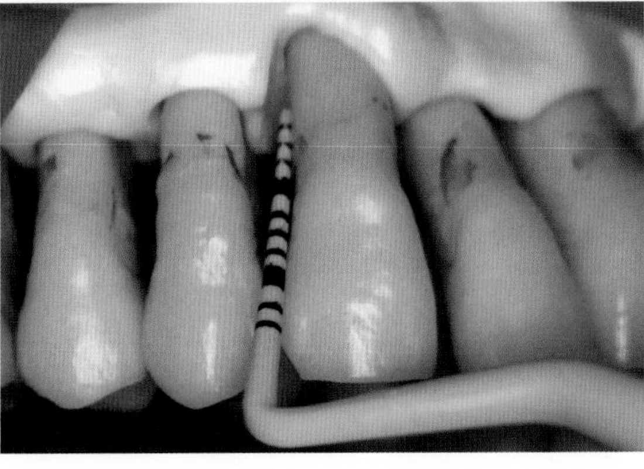

3. **Figure 11-32. Area 1. Walk toward the Distal Surface.** Walk the probe across the distal surface until it touches the contact area. Gently touch the junctional epithelium at the base of the sulcus or pocket with each downward stroke of the probe.

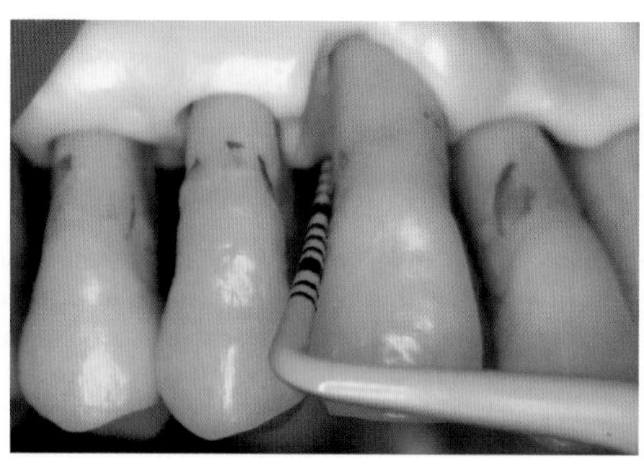

4. **Figure 11-33. Area 1. Assess beneath the Contact Area.** Tilt the probe and extend the tip beneath the contact area. Press down gently to touch the junctional epithelium.

   Record the deepest measurement for Area 1 on the periodontal chart as the distofacial reading.

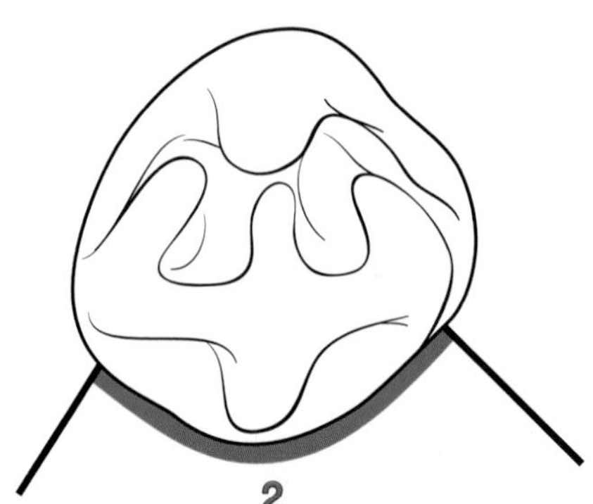

5. **Figure 11-34. Area 2.** The second area is the facial surface, extending from the distofacial line angle to the mesiofacial line angle. (This drawing shows the incisal view of a canine.)

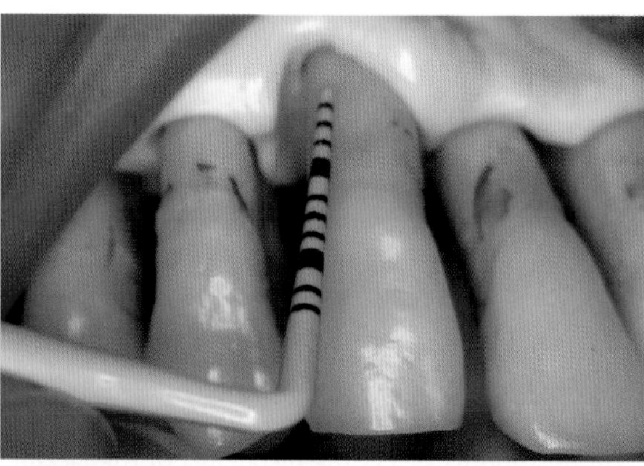

6. **Figure 11-35. Area 2. Reposition the Probe at the Distofacial Line Angle.** Remove the probe from the sulcus and reinsert it at the distofacial line angle. You are now in position to probe the facial surface of the canine.

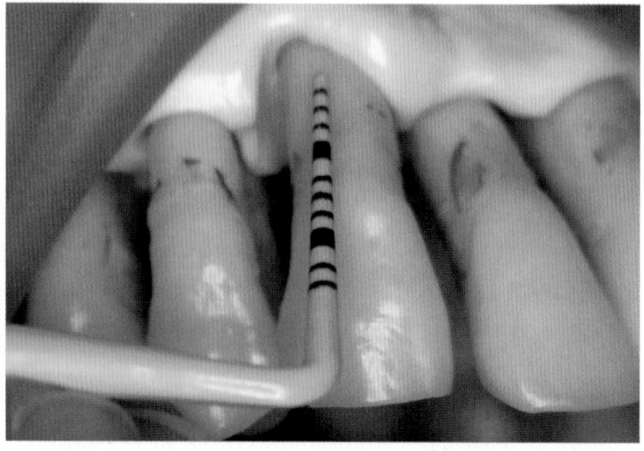

7. **Figure 11-36. Area 2. Assess the Facial Surface.** Make a series of walking strokes across the facial surface.

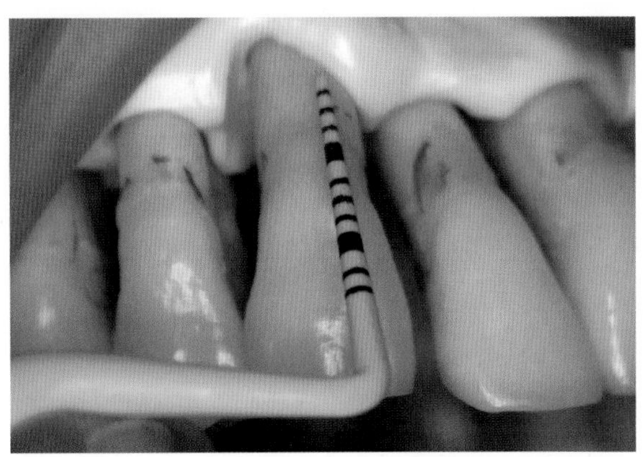

8. **Figure 11-37. Area 2. Walk toward the Mesial Surface.** Walk across the facial surface, stopping at the mesiofacial line angle.

   Record the deepest reading in Area 2 on the periodontal chart.

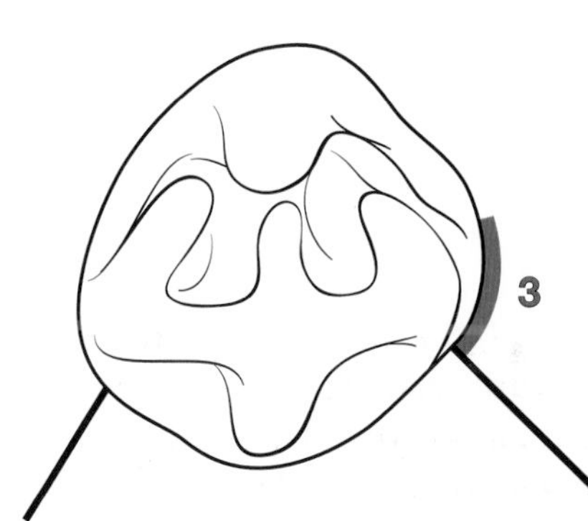

9. **Figure 11-38. Area 3.** Finally, assess Area 3 from the mesiofacial line angle to the midline of the mesial surface. (This drawing shows the incisal view of a canine.)

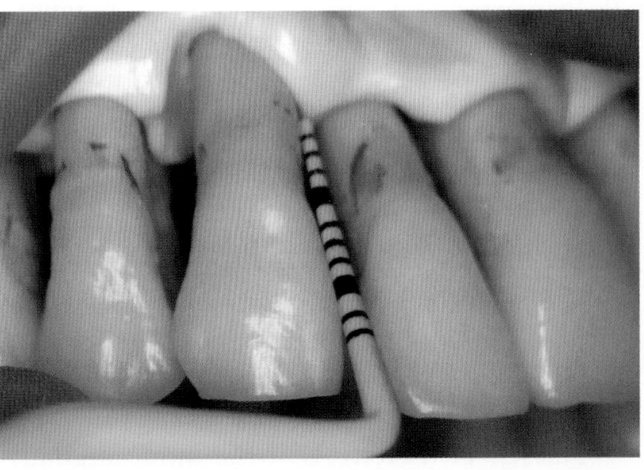

10. **Figure 11-39. Area 3.** Begin with the probe positioned at the mesiofacial line angle. Walk the probe onto the mesial surface until it touches the contact area.

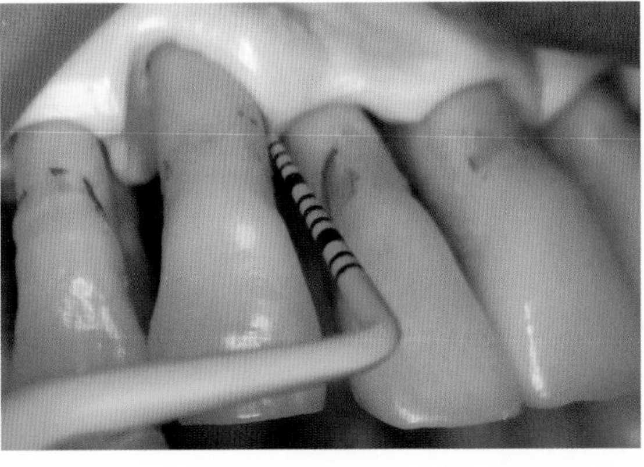

11. **Figure 11-40. Area 3. Assess beneath the Contact Area.** On adjacent *anterior teeth*, only a slight tilt is needed to probe the col area. Gently probe the col area.

    Record the deepest reading for Area 3 on the periodontal chart.

Note to Course Instructors: Please refer to the module on Advanced Probing Techniques for content on advanced assessments with periodontal probes: (1) gingival recession, (2) tooth mobility, (3) oral deviations, (4) width of attached gingiva, (5) clinical attachment level, and (6) furcation involvement.

REFERENCES

1. Orban BJ. *Periodontics: A Concept–Theory and Practice*. St. Louis, MO: Mosby; 1958.
2. Khan S, Cabanilla LL. Periodontal probing depth measurement: a review. *Compend Contin Educ Dent*. 2009;30:12–14, 16, 18–21.
3. Hefti AF. Periodontal probing. *Crit Rev Oral Biol Med*. 1997;8:336–356.
4. Wilkins EM. *Clinical Practice of the Dental Hygienist*. Baltimore, MD: Lippincott Williams & Wilkins; 2005.
5. Williams CHM. Some newer periodontal findings of practical importance to the general practitioner. *J Can Dent Assoc*. 1936;2:333–340.
6. Gibbs CH, Hirschfeld JW, Lee JG, Low SB, Magnusson I, Thousand RR, et al. Description and clinical evaluation of a new computerized periodontal probe—the Florida probe. *J Clin Periodontol*. 1988;15:137–144.
7. Osborn JB, Stoltenberg JL, Huso BA, Aeppli DM, Pihlstrom BL. Comparison of measurement variability in subjects with moderate periodontitis using a conventional and constant force periodontal probe. *J Periodontol*. 1992;63:283–289.
8. Listgarten M. Ultrastructure of the dento-gingival junction after gingivectomy. *J Periodontal Res*. 1972;7:151–160.
9. Listgarten MA. Periodontal probing: what does it mean? *J Clin Periodontol*. 1980;7:165–176.
10. Persson GR. Effects of line-angle versus midproximal periodontal probing measurements on prevalence estimates of periodontal disease. *J Periodontal Res*. 1991;26:527–529.
11. American Academy of Periodontology. *The American Academy of Periodontology Glossary of Periodontal Terms*. Chicago, IL: The American Academy of Periodontology; 1992.
12. Chamberlain AD, Renvert S, Garrett S, Nilvéus R, Egelberg J. Significance of probing force for evaluation of healing following periodontal therapy. *J Clin Periodontol*. 1985;12:306–311.
13. van der Zee E, Davies EH, Newman HN. Marking width, calibration from tip and tine diameter of periodontal probes. *J Clin Periodontol*. 1991;18:516–520.
14. Badersten A, Nilveus R, Egelberg J. Reproducibility of probing attachment level measurements. *J Clin Periodontol*. 1984;11:475–485.
15. Hassell TM, Hefti AF. Drug-induced gingival overgrowth: old problem, new problem. *Crit Rev Oral Biol Med*. 1991;2:103–137.
16. van Weringh M, Barendregt DS, Rosema NA, Timmerman MF, van der Weijden GA. A thin or thick probe handle: does it make a difference? *Int J Dent Hyg*. 2006;4:140–144.

Section 5
Skill Application

PRACTICAL FOCUS

1. **Probing Depths.** Using the color-coded probe shown in Figure 11-41, measure and record the probing depths for the three teeth illustrated in Figures 11-42 to 11-44 below.

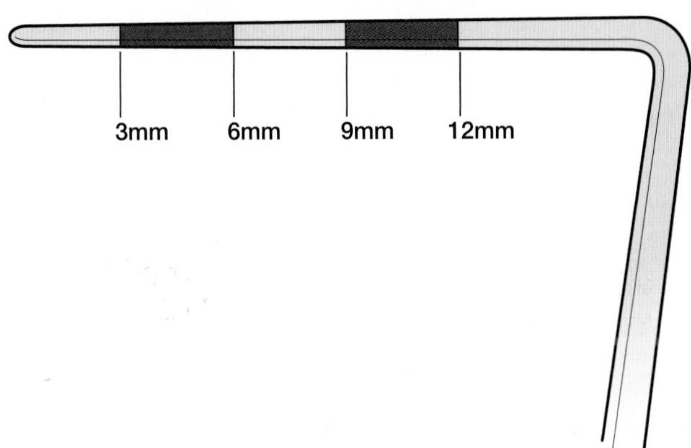

Figure 11-41. Probe Millimeter Markings.

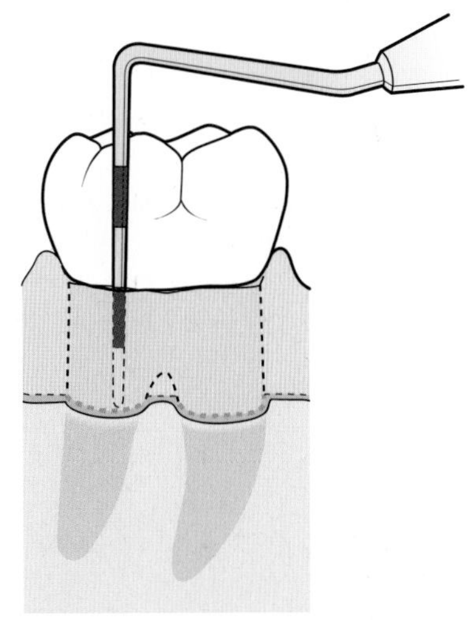

Figure 11-42. Tooth A.
Probing Depth = ___ mm

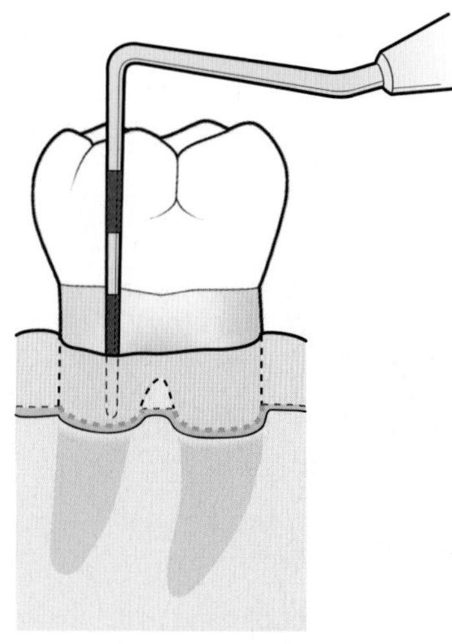

Figure 11-43. Tooth B.
Probing Depth = ___ mm

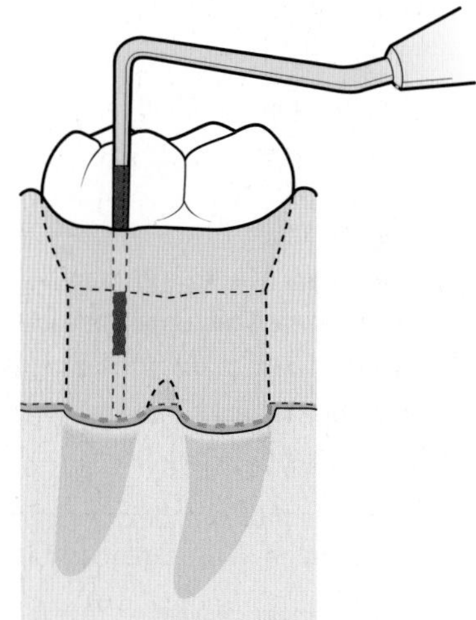

Figure 11-44. Tooth C.
Probing Depth = ___ mm

Assess the Probing Depths. Look closely at teeth **A**, **B**, and **C** above.

1. Compare the bone level on these three teeth? Is the level of bone the same or different for these teeth?
2. Compare the probing depths. Do the probing depths provide you with an accurate picture of the amount of bone lost from around each of the teeth?

STUDENT SELF-EVALUATION MODULE 11 BASIC PROBING TECHNIQUE

Student: ______________________________

Date: ______________________________

Anterior Area 1 = ______________________

Anterior Area 2 = ______________________

Posterior Area 3 = ______________________

Posterior Area 4 = ______________________

DIRECTIONS: Self-evaluate your skill level in each treatment area as: **S** (satisfactory) or **U** (unsatisfactory).

Criteria				
Positioning/Ergonomics	**Area 1**	**Area 2**	**Area 3**	**Area 4**
Adjusts clinician chair correctly				
Reclines patient chair and assures that patient's head is even with top of headrest				
Positions instrument tray within easy reach for front, side, or rear delivery as appropriate for operatory configuration				
Positions unit light at arm's length or dons dental headlight and adjusts it for use				
Assumes the recommended clock position				
Positions backrest of patient chair for the specified arch and adjusts height of patient chair so that clinician's elbows remain at waist level when accessing the specified treatment area				
Asks patient to assume the head position that facilitates the clinician's view of the specified treatment area				
Maintains neutral position				
Directs light to illuminate the specified treatment area				
Instrument Grasp: Dominant Hand	**Area 1**	**Area 2**	**Area 3**	**Area 4**
Grasps handle with tips of finger pads of index finger and thumb so that these fingers are opposite each other on the handle, but do NOT touch or overlap				
Rests pad of middle finger lightly on instrument shank; middle finger makes contact with ring finger				
Positions the thumb, index, and middle fingers in the "knuckles-up" convex position; hyperextended joint position is avoided				
Holds ring finger straight so that it supports the weight of hand and instrument; ring finger position is "advanced ahead of" the other fingers in the grasp				
Keeps index, middle, ring, and little fingers in contact; "like fingers inside a mitten"				
Maintains a relaxed grasp; fingers are NOT blanched in grasp				
Finger Rest: Dominant Hand	**Area 1**	**Area 2**	**Area 3**	**Area 4**
Establishes secure finger rest that is appropriate for tooth to be treated				
Once finger rest is established, pauses to self-evaluate finger placement in the grasp, verbalizes to evaluator his/her self-assessment of grasp, and corrects finger placement if necessary				

(Note student self-evaluation continues on the next page)

STUDENT SELF-EVALUATION MODULE 11 BASIC PROBING TECHNIQUE (continued)

Criteria				
Insertion	**Area 1**	**Area 2**	**Area 3**	**Area 4**
Establishes 0° angulation in preparation for insertion				
Gently inserts explorer tip beneath the gingival margin to base of sulcus or pocket				
Probing Technique	**Area 1**	**Area 2**	**Area 3**	**Area 4**
Orients probe working-end parallel to the root surface being probed				
Keeps tip in contact with the root surface				
Uses small walking strokes within the sulcus or periodontal pocket; maintains the probe beneath the gingival margin with each stroke				
Tilts probe and extends tip beneath contact area to assess interproximal area (col area)				
Covers entire circumference of the junctional epithelium with walking strokes				
Maintains neutral wrist position throughout motion activation				
Obtains measurement readings that are within 1 mm of the evaluator's measurements				

Module 12

Explorers

Module Overview

Explorers have flexible wire-like working-ends used to detect subgingival calculus deposits for the purpose of assessing the progress and completeness of periodontal instrumentation. This module presents the design characteristics of explorers and step-by-step instructions for their use in the detection of root surface irregularities and calculus deposits.

Module Outline

Key Terms

Assessment instruments
Explorers
Explorer tip
Lower shank
Supragingival instrumentation
Subgingival instrumentation
Assessment stroke
Exploratory stroke
Tactile sensitivity
Calculus
Plaque retentive
Supragingival calculus deposits
Subgingival calculus deposits
Residual calculus deposits
Spicule of calculus
Nodule of calculus
Calculus ledge
Calculus ring
Veneer of calculus
Finger-like calculus formation
Carious lesion

Learning Objectives

1. Given a variety of explorer designs, identify the design characteristics of each explorer.
2. Given a variety of explorer designs, identify the explorer tip.
3. Identify and describe the advantages and limitations of various explorer designs.
4. Describe how the clinician can use visual clues to select the correct working-end of a double-ended explorer.
5. Demonstrate correct adaptation of the explorer tip.
6. Describe and demonstrate an assessment stroke with an explorer.
7. Demonstrate detection of supragingival calculus deposits using compressed air.
8. Demonstrate correct use of an Orban-type explorer in the anterior sextants while maintaining correct position, correct finger rests, and precise finger placement in the grasp.
9. Demonstrate correct use of an 11/12-type explorer in the anterior sextants while maintaining correct position, correct finger rests, and precise finger placement in the grasp.
10. Demonstrate correct use of an 11/12-type explorer in the posterior sextants while maintaining correct position, correct finger rests, and precise finger placement in the grasp.
11. Name and describe several common types of calculus deposit formations.
12. Explain why the forceful application of an explorer tip into a carious pit or fissure could be potentially harmful.

Section 1
Explorers

FUNCTIONS AND DESIGN CHARACTERISTICS

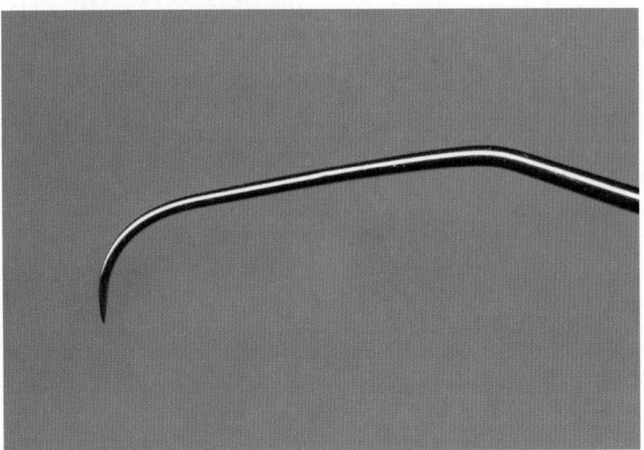

Figure 12-1. Explorer. An explorer is an assessment instrument with a flexible wire-like working-end.

1. Functions of Explorers

a. Assessment instruments—such as periodontal probes and explorers—are used to determine the health of the periodontal tissues, tooth anatomy, and the texture of tooth surfaces.

b. Explorers are used to detect, by tactile means, the texture and character of tooth surfaces before, during, and after periodontal instrumentation to assess the progress and completeness of instrumentation.

   1. The explorer's flexible working-end quivers as it is moved over tooth surface irregularities such as dental calculus (tartar).
   2. Dental calculus deposits frequently are located subgingivally below the gingival margin where they cannot be detected visually. Since these subgingival calculus deposits cannot be seen, the clinician must rely on his or her sense of touch to find and remove these hidden deposits. The explorer with its highly flexible working-end is the instrument of choice for detection of subgingival calculus deposits.
   3. Explorers also are used to examine tooth surfaces for dental anomalies and anatomic features such as grooves, curvatures, or root furcations and to assess dental restorations and sealants.

2. Design of Explorers

a. Explorers are made of flexible metal that conducts vibrations from the working-end to the clinician's fingers resting on the instrument shank and handle.

b. Explorers are circular in cross section and may have unpaired (dissimilar) or paired working-ends.

c. The working-end is 1 to 2 mm in length and is referred to as the explorer tip.

d. ***The actual point of the explorer is not used to detect dental calculus; rather, the side of explorer tip is applied to the tooth surface.***

EXPLORER TIP AND LOWER SHANK

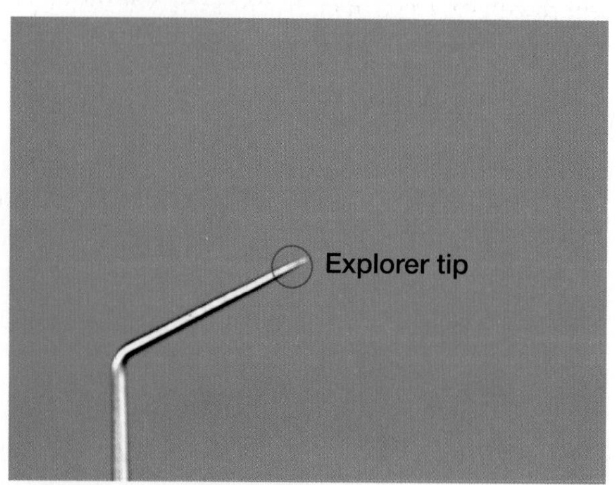

Figure 12-2. The Explorer Tip. For periodontal instrumentation, the explorer tip is defined as 1 to 2 mm of the *side* of the explorer. The tip is adapted to the tooth for detection of dental calculus or root surface irregularities. **The actual *point* of the explorer is never used for detection of calculus.**

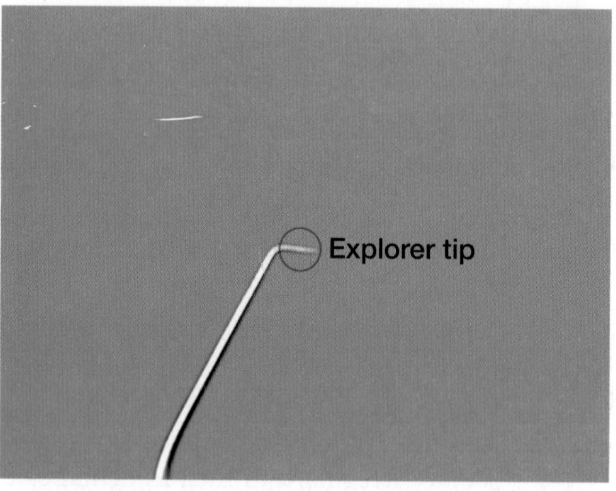

Figure 12-3. Explorer Tip Design. Explorers are available in a variety of different designs. On this explorer, the tip is bent at a 90° angle to the lower shank. Such an explorer design is ideal for subgingival instrumentation.

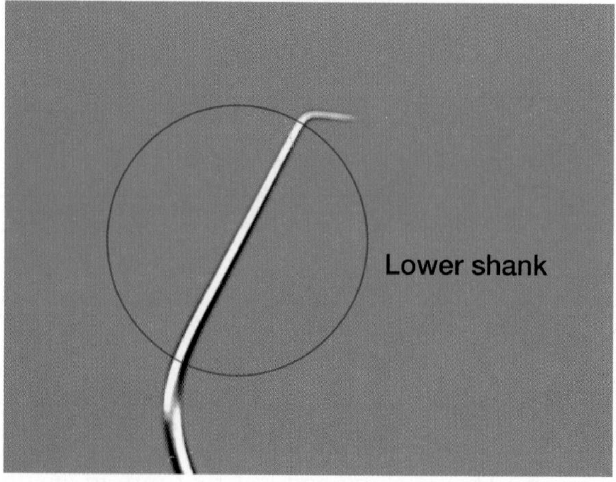

Figure 12-4. Lower Shank. The lower shank is the section of the shank nearest to the explorer tip. The lower shank provides an important visual clue for the clinician when positioning the instrument. In posterior sextants, the lower shank should be parallel to the tooth surface being instrumented.

EXPLORER DESIGN TYPES

Explorers are available in a variety of design types. All design types are not well suited to subgingival use; therefore, the clinician should be knowledgeable about the recommended use of each design type.

1. Supragingival instrumentation—use of an instrument coronal to (above) the gingival margin. For example, use of an explorer to examine the margins of restorations or dental sealants.
2. Subgingival instrumentation—use of an instrument apical to (below) the gingival margin. For example, use of an explorer to detect calculus deposits hidden beneath the gingival margin.

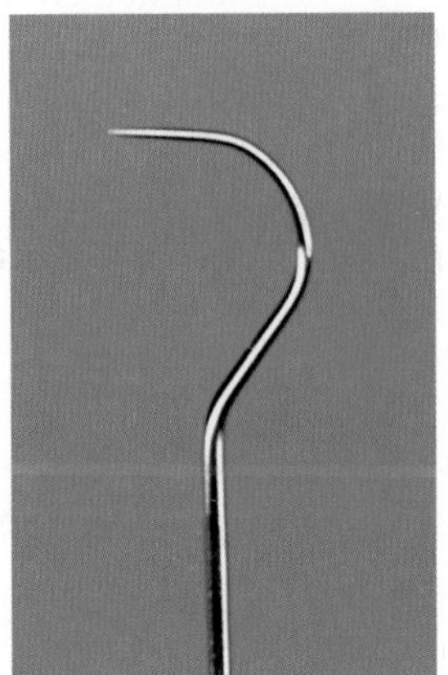

Figure 12-5. Shepherd Hook Explorer—gets its name because it resembles the long stick with a curved end that was used by ancient shepherds to catch sheep.

Use:

- *Supragingival* examination of the margins of restorations or to assess for sealant retention.
- NOT recommended for subgingival use because the point could injure the soft tissue at the base of the sulcus or pocket.

Examples: 23 and 54 explorers.

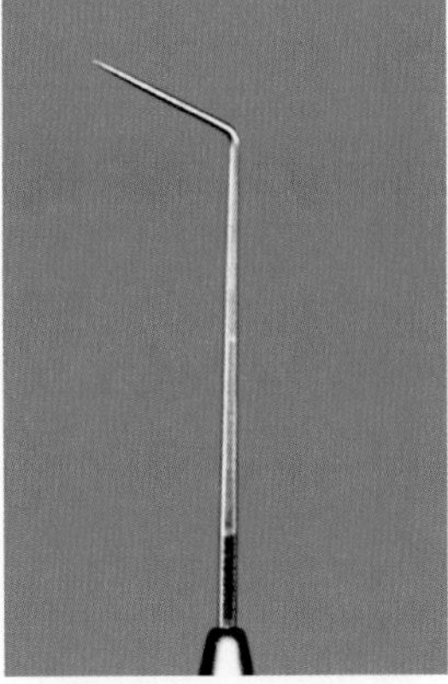

Figure 12-6. Straight Explorer.

Use:

- *Supragingival* examination of the margins of restorations or to assess for sealant retention.
- NOT recommended for subgingival use because the point could injure the soft tissue at the base of the sulcus or pocket.

Examples: 6, 6A, 6L, and 6XL explorers.

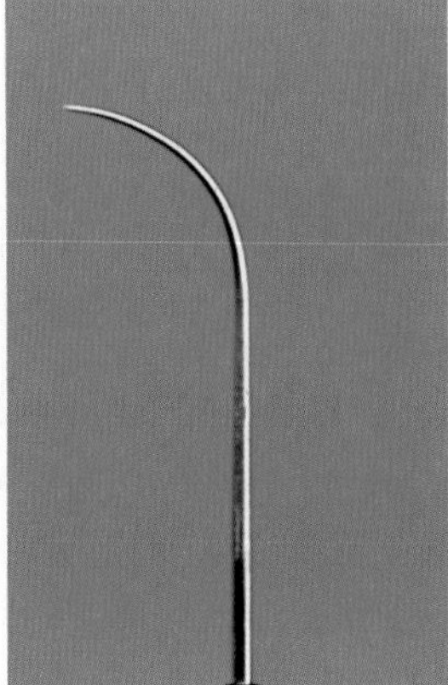

Figure 12-7. Curved Explorer.

Use:

- Calculus detection in normal sulci or shallow pockets.
- Care must be taken not to injure the soft tissue base of the sulcus or pocket if the working-end is used subgingivally.

Examples: 3 and 3A explorers.

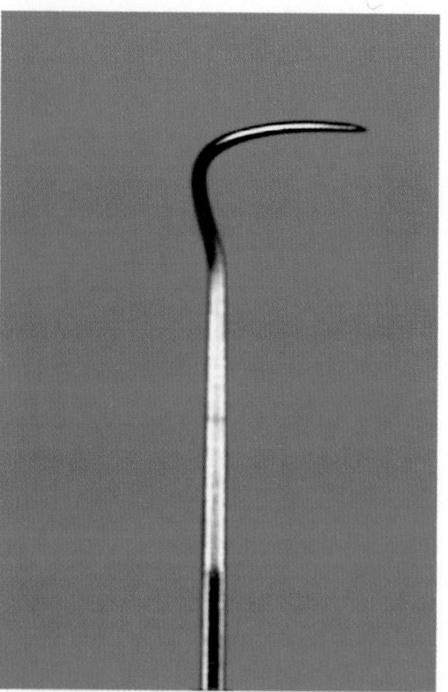

Figure 12-8. Pigtail and Cowhorn Explorers—get their names because they resemble a pig's tail or a bull's horns.

Use:

- Calculus detection in normal sulci or shallow pockets extending no deeper than the cervical-third of the root.
- The curved lower shank causes considerable stretching of the tissue away from the root surface.

Examples: 3ML, 3CH, and 2A explorers.

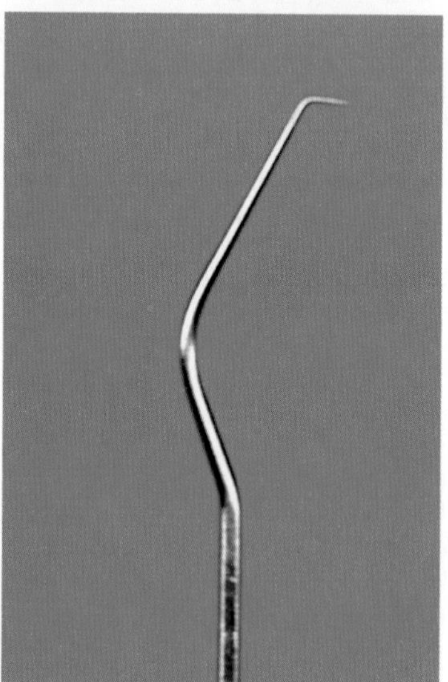

Figure 12-9. Orban-Type Explorer.

Design Characteristics:

- The tip is bent at a 90° angle to the lower shank; this feature allows the *back of the tip* (instead of the point) to be directed against the soft tissue at the base of the sulcus or pocket.
- The straight lower shank allows insertion in narrow pockets with only slight stretching of the tissue away from the root surface.

Use: Assessment of anterior root surfaces and the facial and lingual surfaces of posterior teeth. Difficult to adapt to the line angles and proximal surfaces of the posterior teeth.

Examples: 17, 20F, and TU17 explorers.

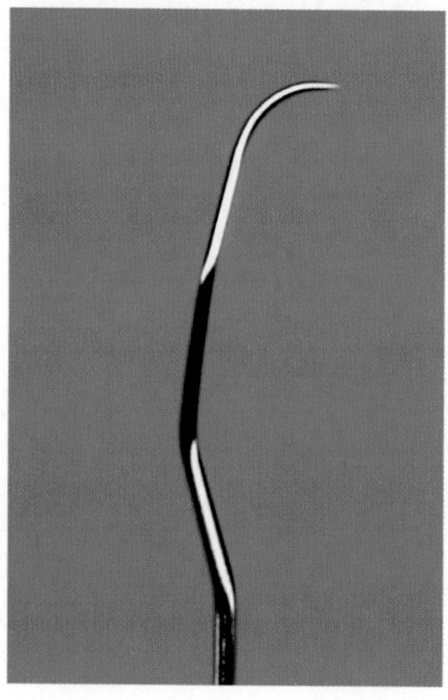

Figure 12-10. 11/12-Type Explorer—an explorer with several advantageous design characteristics.

Design Characteristics:

- Like the Orban-type explorers, the tip is at a 90° angle to the lower shank.
- The long complex shank design makes it equally useful when working on anterior and posterior teeth with normal sulci or deep periodontal pockets.

Use: Assessment of root surfaces on anterior and posterior teeth.

Examples: ODU 11/12 and 11/12AF explorers.

THE ASSESSMENT STROKE

An assessment stroke, also called an exploratory stroke, is used to detect calculus deposits or other tooth surface irregularities. Assessment strokes require a high degree of precision. The proper use of an explorer requires light, controlled strokes.

1. During subgingival instrumentation, the clinician relies on his or her sense of touch to locate calculus deposits hidden beneath the gingival margin.
2. Tactile sensitivity is the ability to detect tooth irregularities by feeling vibrations transferred from the explorer tip to the handle.
   - For example, the explorer tip quivers slightly as it travels over rough calculus deposits on the tooth surface. These vibrations are transmitted from the tip, through the shank, and into the handle.
   - The clinician feels the vibrations with his or her fingertips resting on the handle and instrument shank.
3. The fine working-end and flexible shank of an explorer are used to enhance tactile information to the clinician's fingers.
   - The superior tactile conduction of an explorer makes it the instrument of choice for (1) *initially locating subgingival calculus deposits* and for (2) *re-evaluating tooth surfaces* following calculus removal.
4. *During calculus removal*, the curet is used for calculus detection.
   - When all deposits detectable with a curet have been removed, a definitive evaluation of the root surface should be made using an explorer.
   - Because the explorer provides superior tactile information, it is common to detect some remaining calculus deposits with an explorer that could not be detected with a curet.

TABLE 12-1. Assessment Stroke with an Explorer

Grasp	Relaxed grasp; middle finger rests lightly on shank
Adaptation	1–2 mm of the side of the tip are adapted
Lateral pressure	Light pressure with working-end against tooth
Activation	Wrist activation is usually recommended; however, digital activation is acceptable with an explorer because physical strength is not required for assessment strokes
Stroke characteristics	Fluid, sweeping strokes
Stroke number	Many overlapping strokes are used to cover every square millimeter of the root surface
Common errors	AVOID a tight, tense "death grip" on handle AVOID applying pressure with the middle finger against the instrument shank as this will reduce tactile information to the finger

SUBGINGIVAL ASSESSMENT WITH AN EXPLORER

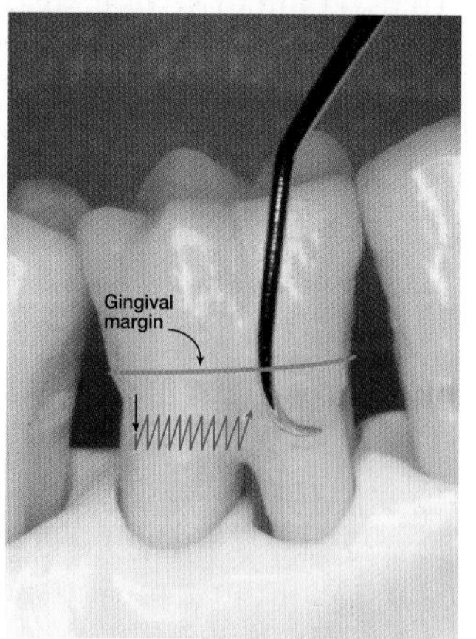

Figure 12-11. Subgingival Exploring. Subgingival assessment strokes should be short in length and involve many overlapping strokes covering every square millimeter of the root surface.

Steps for Subgingival Exploration:

1. **Get Ready and Insert.** Adapt the explorer tip to the tooth surface above the gingival margin in the middle-third of the crown. Gently slide the tip under the gingival margin.
2. **Insert to Base of Pocket.** Keep the tip constantly in contact with the root surface. Gently slide the explorer in an apical direction until the back of the tip touches the soft tissue base of the sulcus or pocket. The attached tissue will have a soft, elastic feel.
3. **Initiate Assessment Stroke in Coronal Direction.** Move the tip forward slightly and use a vertical or oblique stroke to move the explorer up the surface of the root. Keep the tip in contact with the root surface as you move the tip up toward the gingival margin. Concentrate as the tip moves over the tooth surface; be alert for quivers of the tip that indicate a calculus deposit.
4. **Control Stroke Length.** Do not remove the explorer tip from the sulcus or pocket as you make an upward stroke. Removing and reinserting the tip repeatedly can traumatize the tissue at the gingival margin. Bring the explorer tip to a point just beneath the gingival margin and move the tip forward slightly.
5. **Reposition at Base of Pocket.** Maintaining the tip in contact with the tooth surface, return the tip to the base of the sulcus or pocket. As you move the tip, remain alert for tactile information transmitted through the instrument shank.
6. **Divide Root into Apical, Middle, and Cervical Sections.** Keep your assessment strokes short, approximately 2 to 3 mm in length.
   - If you are working within a normal sulcus, your strokes will extend from the base of the sulcus to a point just beneath the gingival margin.
   - Within a pocket, first, explore the portion of the root next to the base of the pocket. Then, move the tip up and explore the midsection on the root. Finally, assess the section near the gingival margin. The depth of the pocket will determine how many sections—3 mm in height—are needed to cover the entire root surface.
7. **Considerations for Proximal Surfaces.** On the distal and mesial proximal surfaces, lead with the point of the explorer tip. Do not "back" into the proximal surface. Your strokes should reach under the contact area, so that half of the proximal surface is explored from the facial aspect and half from the lingual aspect of the tooth.

Section 2
Technique Practice—Anterior Teeth

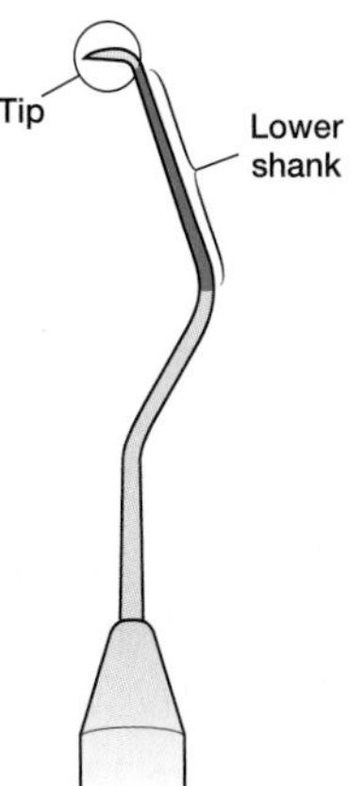

Figure 12-12. The Orban-Type Explorer. An Orban-type explorer, such as a TU17, is an excellent choice for subgingival assessment of the anterior teeth. The straight lower shank allows insertion in narrow pockets with only slight tissue stretching away from the root surface. The tip design allows the back of the tip—rather than the sharp point—to be directed against the junctional epithelium.

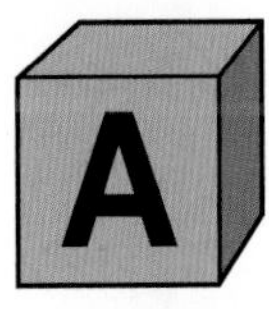

SKILL BUILDING. STEP-BY-STEP TECHNIQUE ON FACIAL AND LINGUAL SURFACES

- Follow steps 1 to 8 to practice exploring the mandibular anterior teeth with an Orban-type explorer (Figs. 12-13 to 12-20).
- Remember: "Me, My patient, My light, My dominant hand, My nondominant hand, My finger rest, My adaptation."

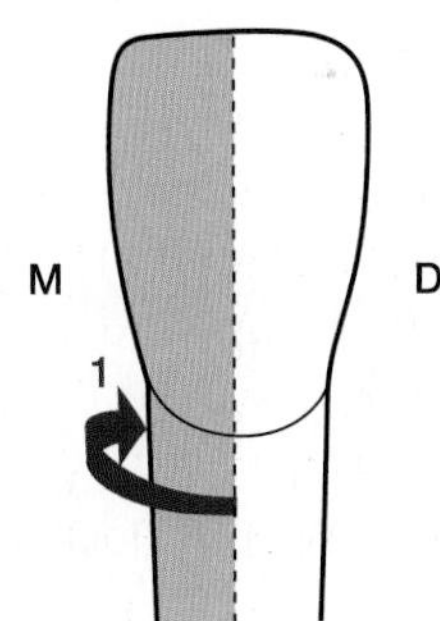

1. **Figure 12-13. Tooth Surface.** First, practice on the mandibular left central incisor, facial aspect.
   - **Right-Handed** clinicians—*surface toward.*
   - **Left-Handed** clinicians—*surface away.*

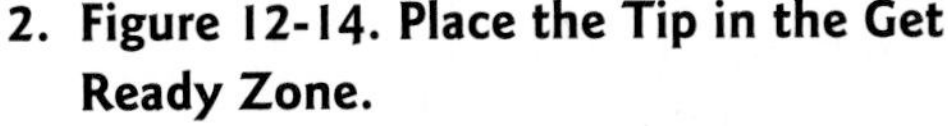

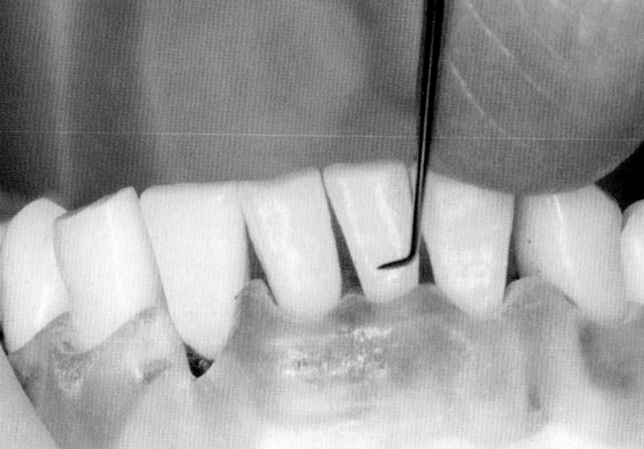

2. **Figure 12-14. Place the Tip in the Get Ready Zone.**
   - Place the tip on the middle-third of the crown near the midline of the facial surface.
   - The point of the explorer should face in the direction of the mesial surface.

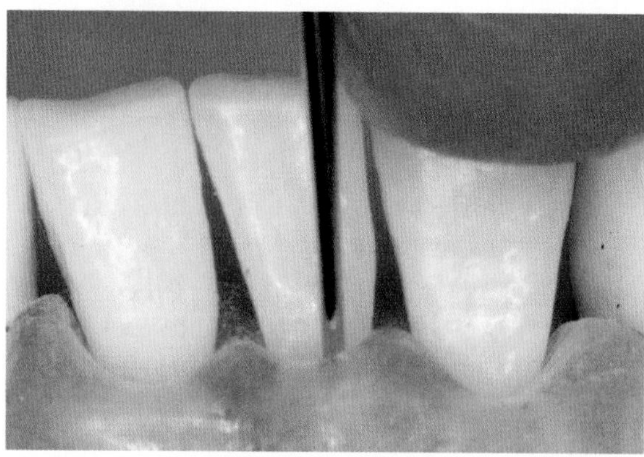

3. **Figure 12-15. Insert.** Gently insert the working-end beneath the gingival margin keeping the tip in contact with the tooth surface.

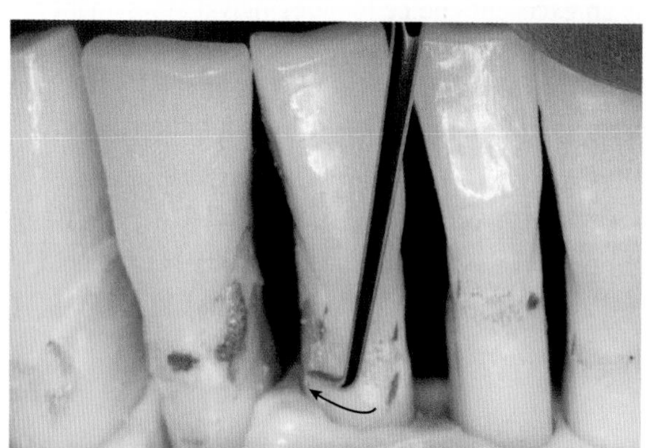

4. **Figure 12-16. Work across the Facial Surface.**
    - Make assessment strokes across the facial surface working toward the mesial surface.
    - It may be helpful to remove the gingival tissue from the typodont to facilitate practice on the root surfaces.
    - As you approach the mesiofacial line angle, roll the instrument handle to maintain adaptation.

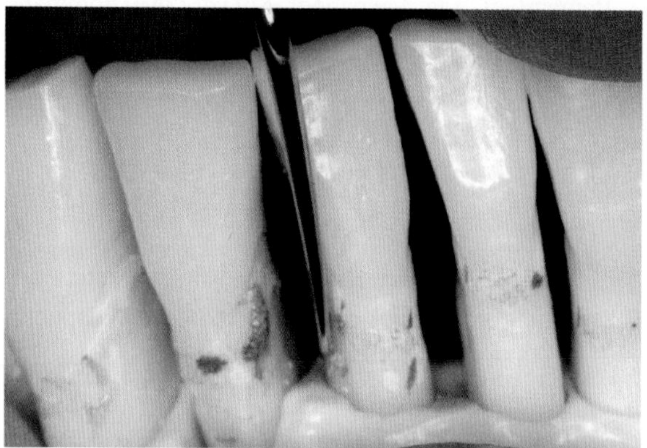

5. **Figure 12-17. Explore the Mesial Surface.** Continue making strokes under the contact area until you have explored at least halfway across the mesial proximal surface. (The other half of the mesial surface is assessed from the lingual aspect of the tooth.)

6. **Figure 12-18. Technique Check.** This photograph shows a dental typodont with the gingiva removed. Note the position of the explorer tip on the mesial surface of this canine tooth. Correct technique demands that the explorer reach at least the halfway point of the proximal surface under the contact area.

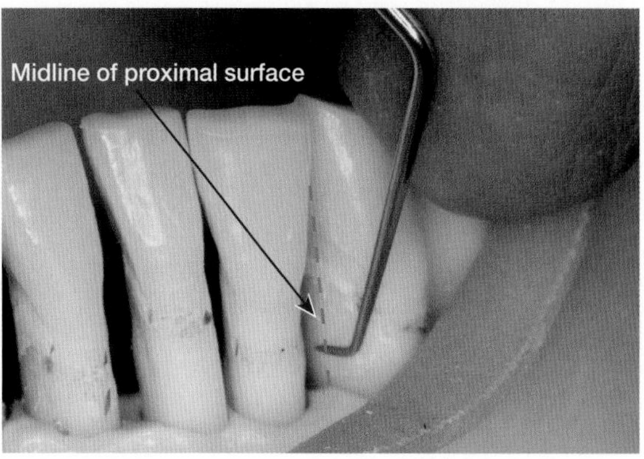

7. **Figure 12-19. Sequence 1.** Next, use the sequence shown in this illustration to explore the colored tooth surfaces of the facial aspect. Begin with the left canine and end with the right canine.

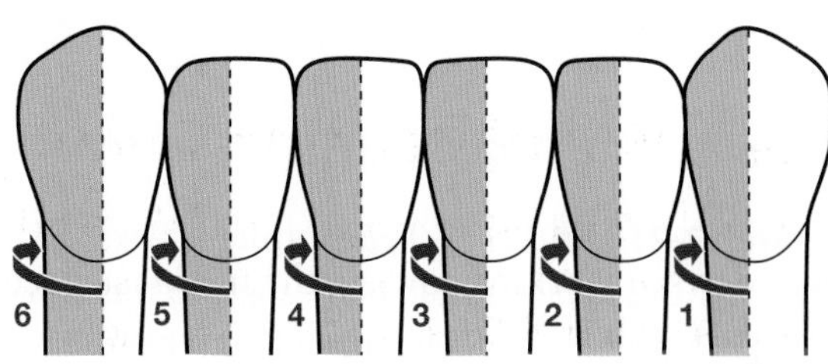

8. **Figure 12-20. Sequence 2.** Change your clock position and complete the remaining facial surfaces, beginning with the right canine and ending with the left canine.

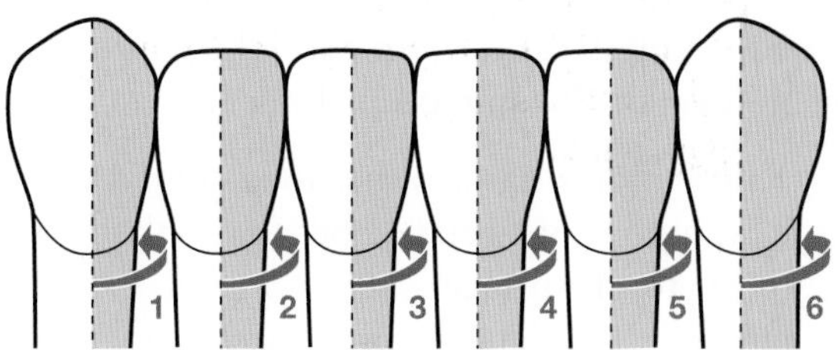

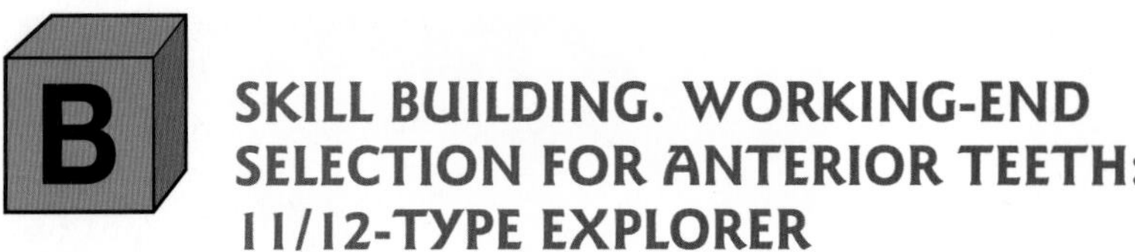

SKILL BUILDING. WORKING-END SELECTION FOR ANTERIOR TEETH: 11/12-TYPE EXPLORER

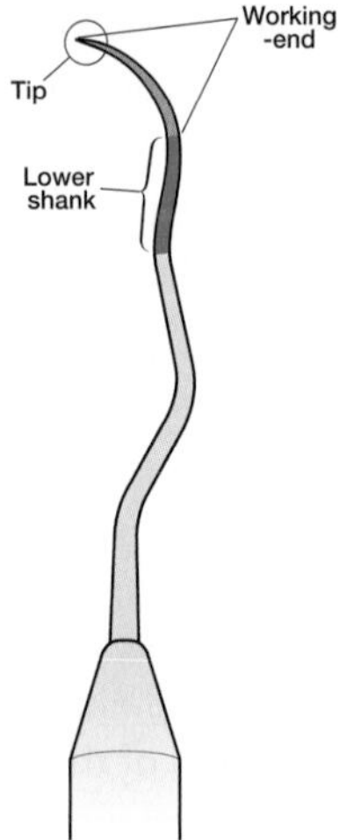

Figure 12-21. An 11/12-Type Explorer. Like the Orban-type explorer, the tip of this explorer is at a 90° angle to the lower shank. The ODU 11/12 is a double-ended instrument with mirror image working-ends.

The working-end design of an 11/12-type explorer makes it more challenging to adapt to the anterior teeth than an Orban-type explorer.

- This explorer has a rather long curved working-end.
- It is important to remember that only the terminal 2 mm of the side of tip are actually adapted to the tooth surface.
- Figure 12-22 depicts correct working-end selection. Incorrect working-end selection is shown in Figure 12-23.

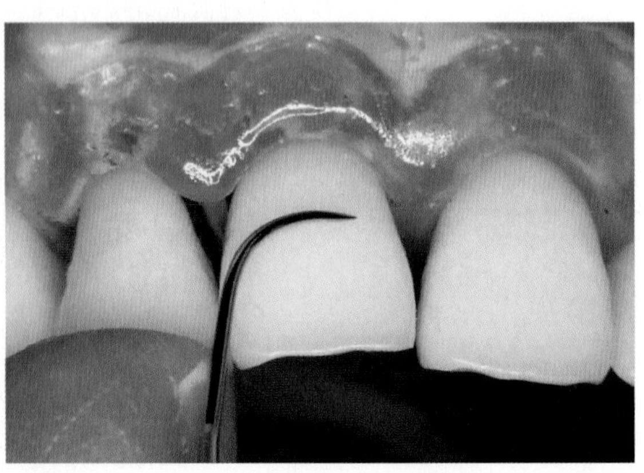

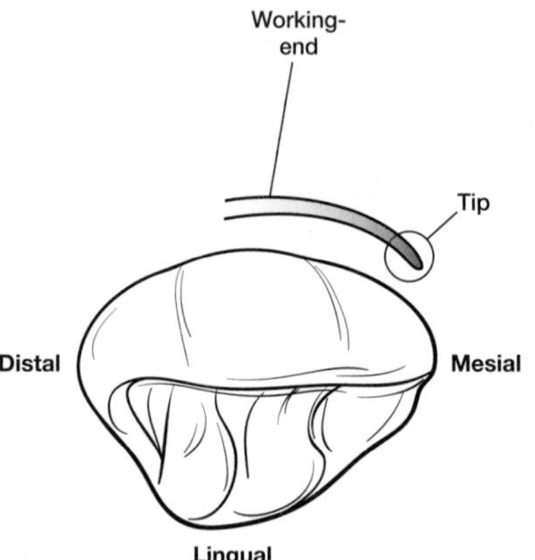

Figure 12-22. Correct Working-End.

- The photo and illustration show the correct working-end for use on the midline of the facial surface to the midline of the mesial surface. (This is the surface away from the right-handed clinician and the surface toward the left-handed clinician.)
- *The correct working-end is 12.* The correct working-end curves inward toward—"wraps around"—the facial surface.

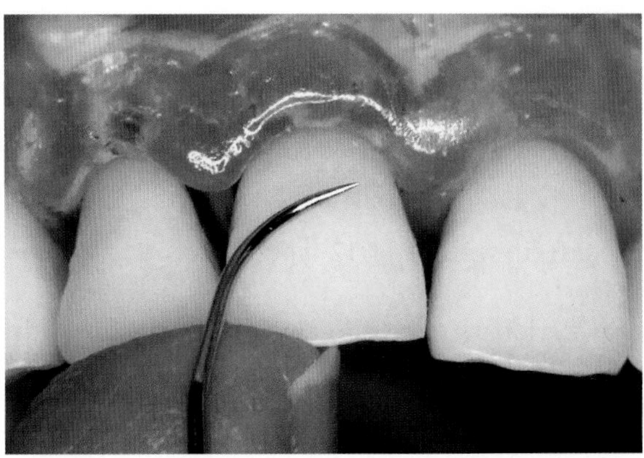

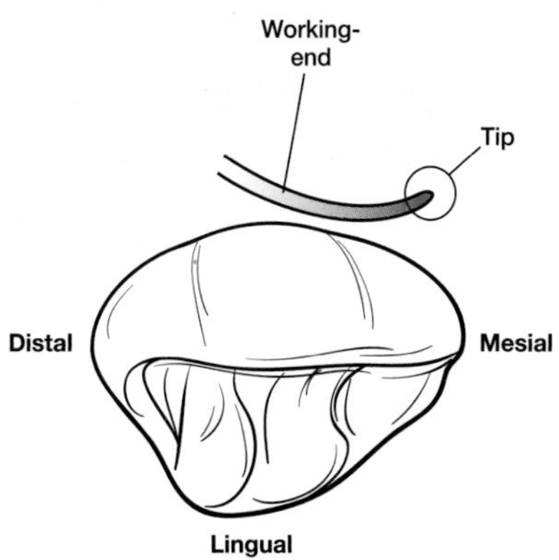

Figure 12-23. Incorrect Working-End.

- The photo and illustration show the incorrect working-end for use on the midline of the facial surface to the midline of the mesial surface. (This is the surface away from the right-handed clinician and the surface toward the left-handed clinician.)
- *The incorrect working-end is 11.* The incorrect working-end curves outward, away from the facial surface.

Box 12-1. Visual Clue Anterior Teeth: "Wrapping" the Working-End

1. A useful visual clue in selecting the correct working-end of an 11/12-type explorer is to select the working-end that "wraps around" or "curves toward" the tooth surface.
   - ***When using this visual clue, it is vital to understand that the entire working-end does not wrap around the tooth during an assessment stroke. During an assessment stroke, only the tip of the working-end is adapted to the tooth surface.***
   - "Wrapping" the working-end is simply a useful verbal description when explaining working-end selection.
2. Selecting the working-end that curves inward toward the tooth surface facilitates adaptation of the explorer tip to the curved surfaces of the anterior teeth.
3. Using the explorer in this manner is very similar to the way that a universal curet is adapted to the anterior teeth. Thus, this method aids in transfer of the technique from the explorer to the universal curet.

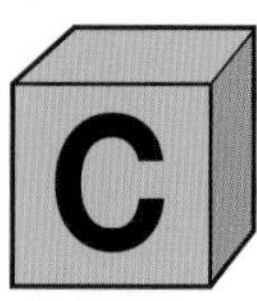

SKILL BUILDING. ANTERIOR TEETH WITH 11/12-TYPE EXPLORER

- Follow steps 1 to 6 to practice exploring the maxillary anterior teeth with an 11/12-type explorer (Figs. 12-24 to 12-29).
- **Right-handed clinicians** begin practice with the surfaces away; **left-handed clinicians** begin practice with the surfaces toward.
- Remember: "Me, My patient, My light, My dominant hand, My nondominant hand, My finger rest, My adaptation."

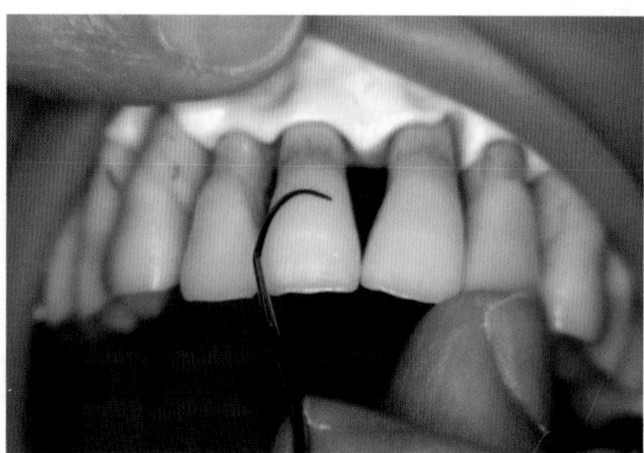

1. **Figure 12-24. Select the Correct Working-End.**
    - Select the correct working-end for use on the midline of the facial surface to the midline of the mesial surface (right-handed clinician: surface away; left-handed clinician: surface toward).
    - The correct working-end is the **12**.

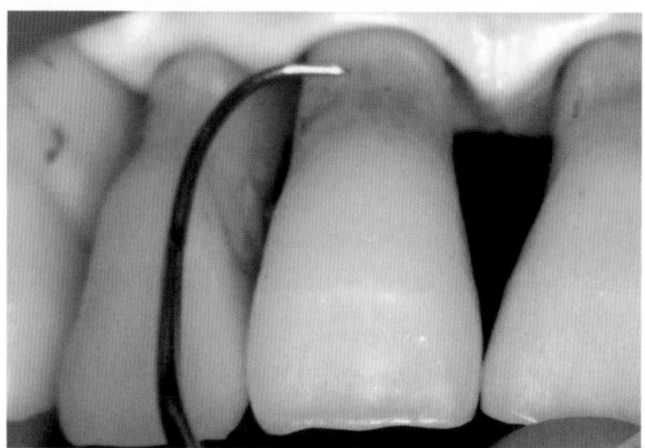

2. **Figure 12-25. Insert and Position for Instrumentation.**
    - Gently insert the #12 working-end to the base of the pocket.
    - Position the tip slightly to the right of the midline with the tip facing toward the mesial surface.
    - Make a series of assessment strokes in the direction of the mesial surface.

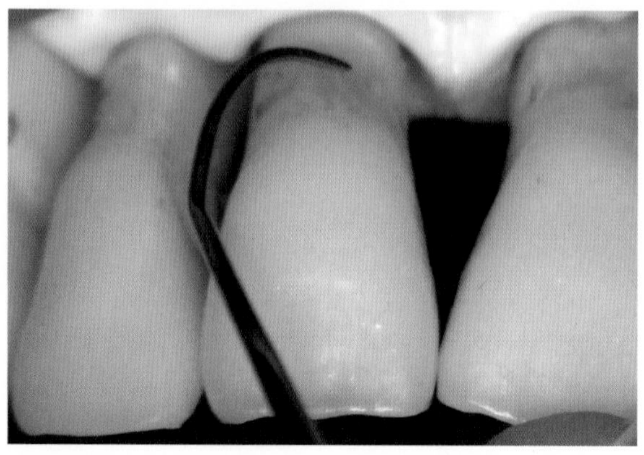

3. **Figure 12-26. Work across the Facial Surface.**
    - Make assessment strokes across the facial surface.
    - Roll the instrument handle to keep just the tip of the working-end adapted to the root surface.

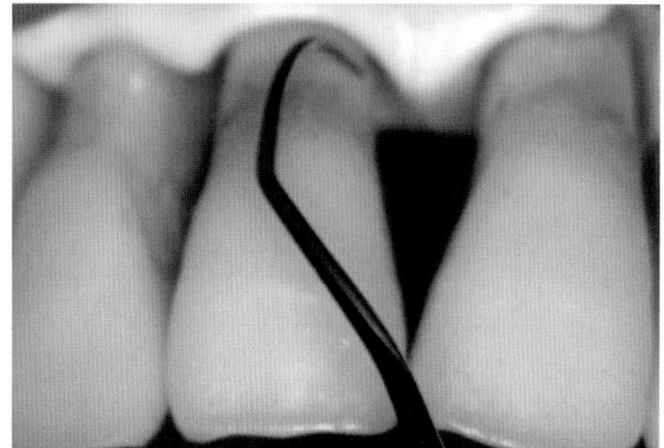

4. **Figure 12-27. Move around the Line Angle.** Roll the instrument handle to move the tip around the mesiofacial line angle.

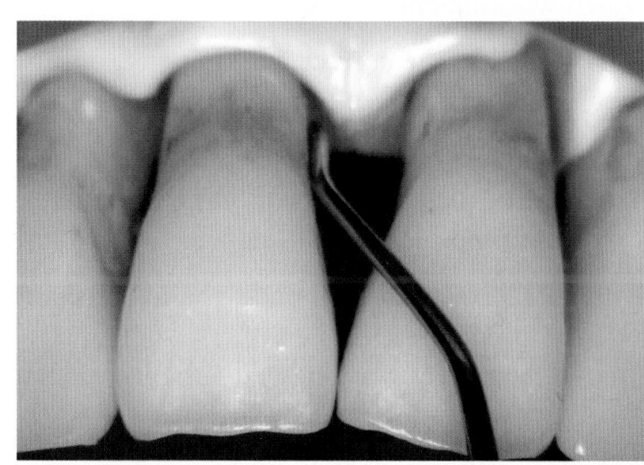

5. **Figure 12-28. Assess the Mesial Surface.** Assess at least halfway across the mesial surface from the facial aspect.

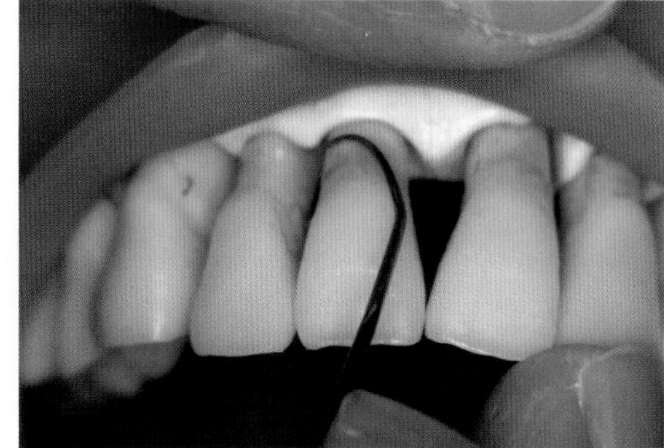

6. **Figure 12-29. Assess the Other Half of the Tooth.**
   - Select the correct working-end to instrument the surface toward if you are right-handed (or the surface away if you are left-handed).
   - The correct working-end is the **11**.

Section 3

Technique Practice—Posterior Teeth

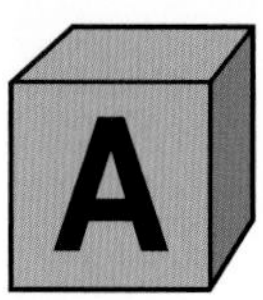

SKILL BUILDING. WORKING-END SELECTION FOR POSTERIOR TEETH: 11/12-TYPE EXPLORER

Before using a double-ended explorer on the posterior sextants, the clinician must first determine which working-end to use.

1. To select the correct working-end, observe the relationship of the lower shank to the distal surface of the tooth.
2. Pick a tooth that is easily seen, such as the first premolar tooth. Randomly select one of the explorer working-ends and adapt the tip to the distal surface of the first premolar.
   a. Correct working-end—the lower shank is parallel to the distal surface of the premolar (Fig. 12-30).
   b. Incorrect working-end—the lower shank extends across the facial surface of the premolar (Fig. 12-31).
3. Using the mandibular right posterior sextant as an example, one working-end of the explorer adapts to the facial aspect, and the other working-end adapts to the lingual aspect of the sextant.

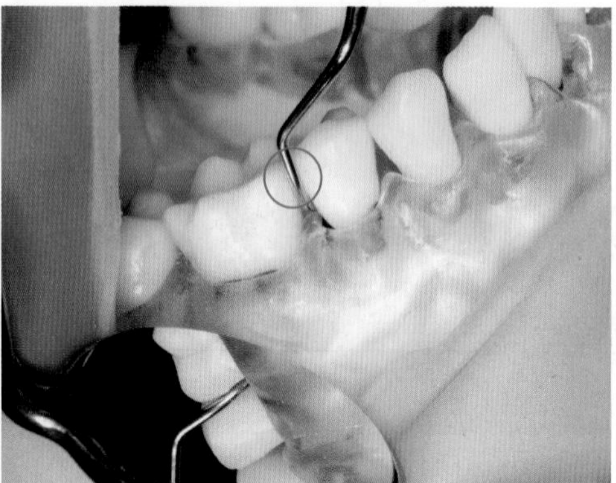

Figure 12-30. Correct Working-End.

Visual Clue to Correct Working-End:

- *Lower shank* is parallel to the distal surface of the premolar.
- *Functional shank* goes "up and over the premolar tooth."

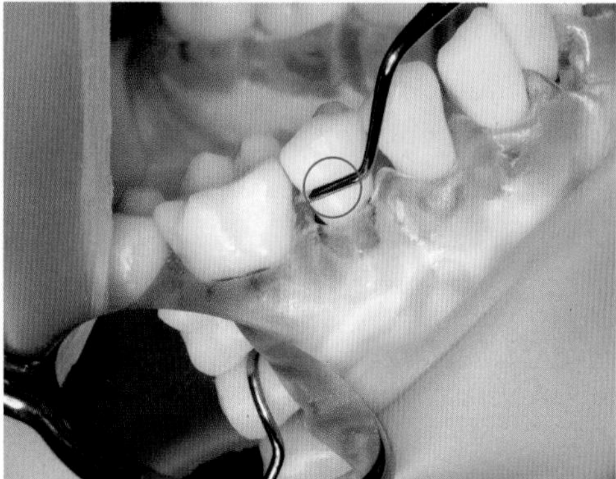

Figure 12-31. Incorrect Working-End.

Visual Clue to Incorrect Working-End:

- *Lower shank* is not parallel to distal surface of the premolar.
- *Functional shank* is "down and around the premolar tooth."

Box 12-2. Working-End Selection on Posterior Teeth

When the working-end is adapted to a distal surface of a posterior tooth, the correct working-end has the following relationship between the shank and the tooth:

- Lower shank is parallel to the distal surface.
- Functional shank goes up and over the tooth.

Think: **"Posterior = Parallel. Functional shank up and over!"**

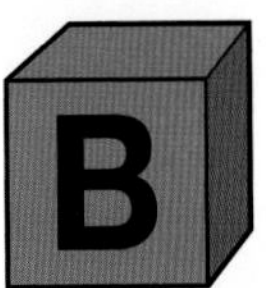

SKILL BUILDING. MANDIBULAR POSTERIOR TEETH WITH 11/12-TYPE EXPLORER

Directions:

- Follow steps 1 to 13 to practice exploring the mandibular right posterior sextant, facial aspect with an 11/12-type explorer (Figs. 12-32 to 12-44).
- Remember: "Me, My patient, My light, My dominant hand, My nondominant hand, My finger rest, My adaptation."

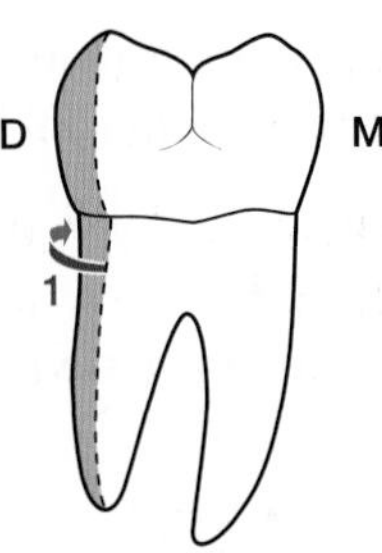

1. **Figure 12-32. Begin with Mandibular First Molar.** As an introduction to exploring the posterior teeth, first, practice on the *mandibular right first molar*. The distal surface is completed first, beginning at the distofacial line angle and working onto the distal surface.

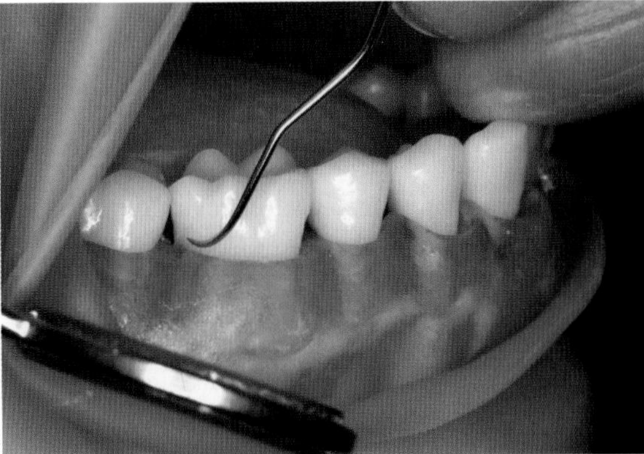

2. **Figure 12-33. Position the Tip Near the Distofacial Line Angle in the Get Ready Zone.**
   - Place the tip in the middle-third of the crown just forward of the distofacial line angle.
   - The tip should aim toward the back of the mouth because this is the direction in which you are working.

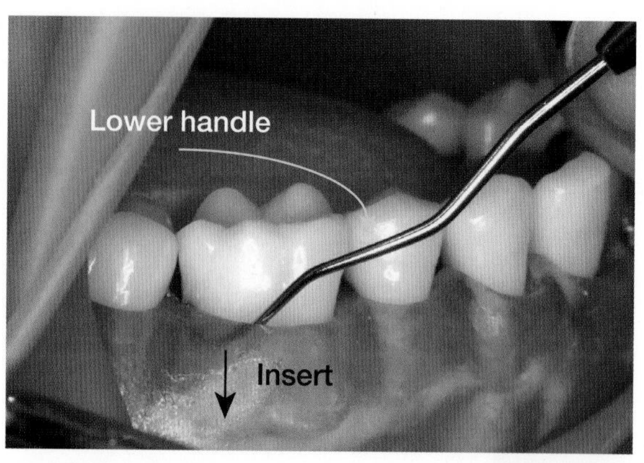

3. **Figure 12-34. Insert.**
   - Lower the instrument handle and adapt the "face" of the explorer tip to the tooth surface.
   - Slide the tip beneath the gingival margin.

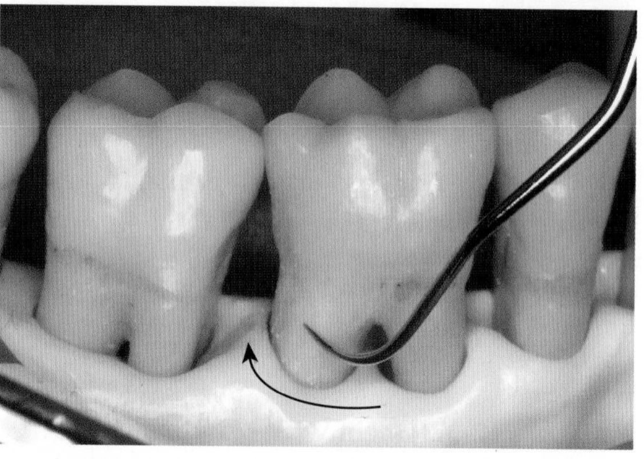

4. **Figure 12-35. Explore Distal Surface.**
   - Return the handle to its normal position.
   - Beginning at the distofacial line angle, make feather-light strokes toward the distal surface.

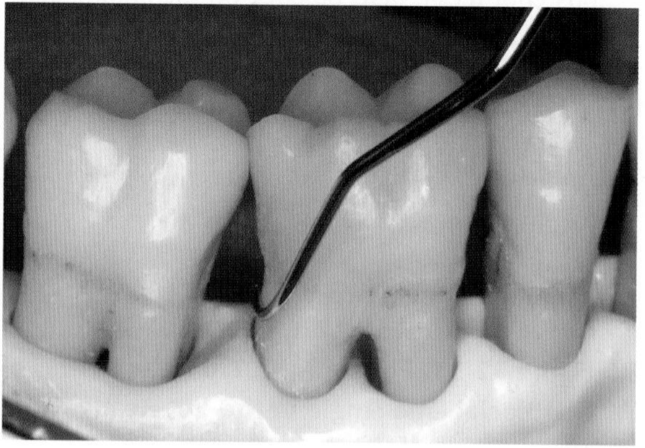

5. **Figure 12-36. Roll the Instrument Handle.**
   - Roll the instrument handle slightly to adapt to the distal surface.
   - Explore at least halfway across the distal surface from the facial aspect. Keep the tip adapted to the tooth surface at all times.

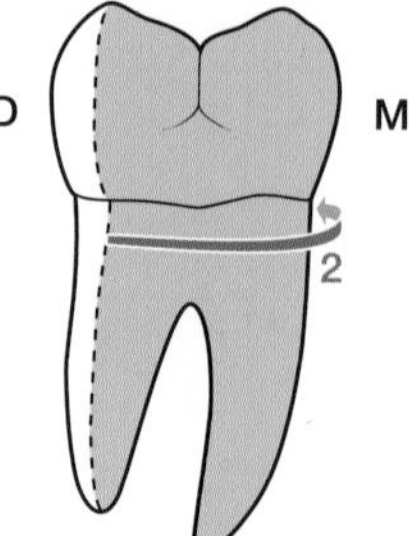

6. **Figure 12-37. Explore the Facial Surface.** You are now ready to explore the facial and mesial surfaces of the tooth, beginning at the distofacial line angle.

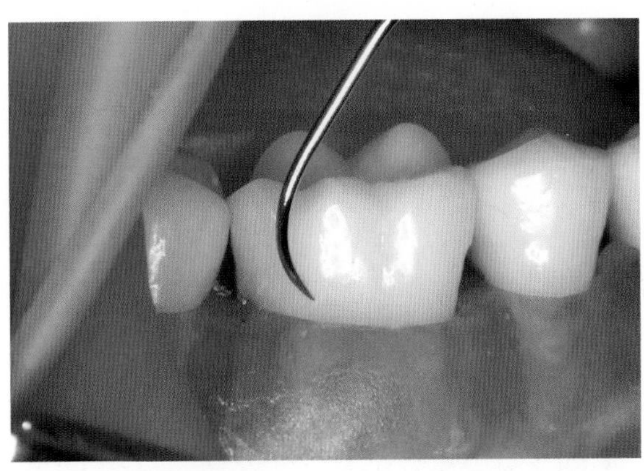

7. **Figure 12-38. Reposition the Tip for Facial Surface.**
    - While maintaining your fulcrum, remove the tip from the sulcus and turn it so that it aims toward the front of the mouth.
    - Place the tip in the middle-third of the facial surface with the point facing forward.

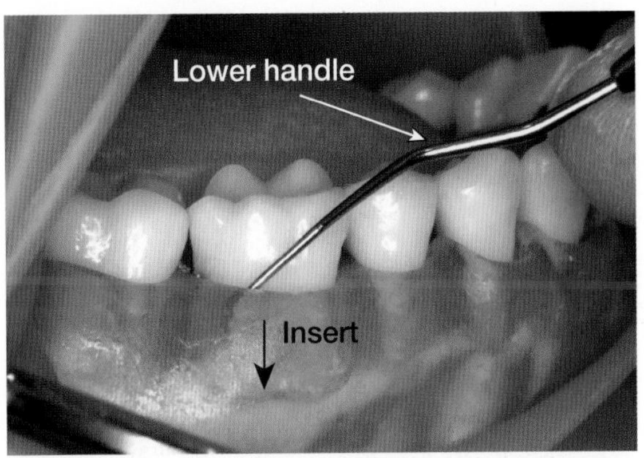

8. **Figure 12-39. Insert.**
    - Lower the instrument handle and place the "face" of the explorer against the facial surface in preparation for insertion.
    - Reinsert the tip and reposition it just to the left of the distofacial line angle.

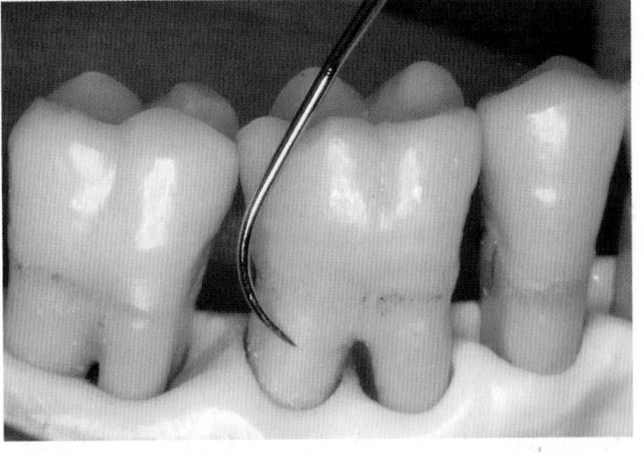

9. **Figure 12-40. Explore the Facial Surface.**
    - Return the handle to its normal position.
    - Beginning at the distofacial line angle, initiate feather-light strokes.

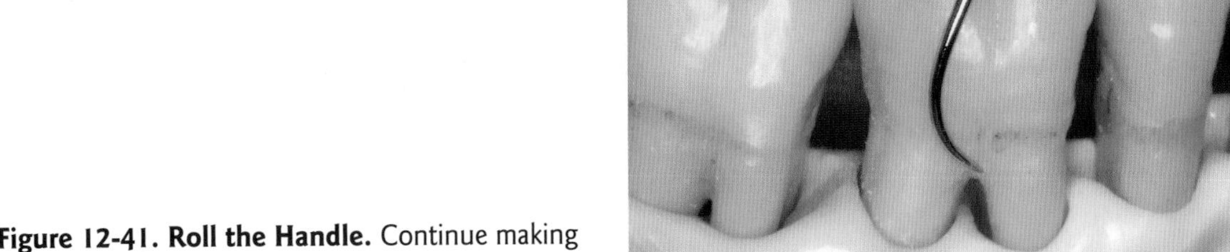

10. **Figure 12-41. Roll the Handle.** Continue making feather-light strokes across the facial surface.

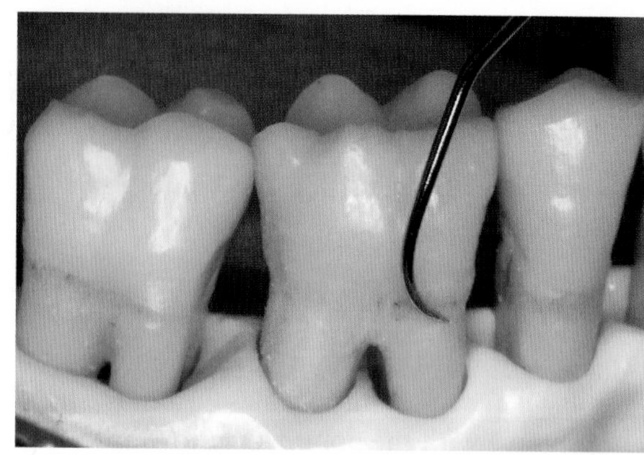

11. **Figure 12-42. Roll the Handle.** As you approach the mesiofacial line angle, roll the handle slightly to maintain adaptation.

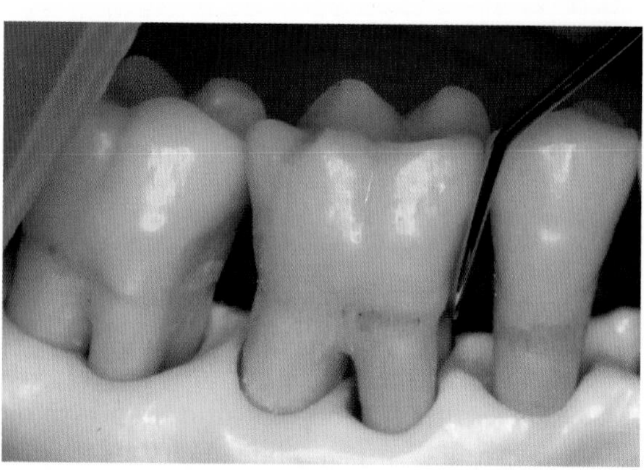

12. **Figure 12-43. Continue Strokes.** Explore at least halfway across the mesial surface from the facial aspect. (The other half of the mesial surface is explored from the lingual aspect.)

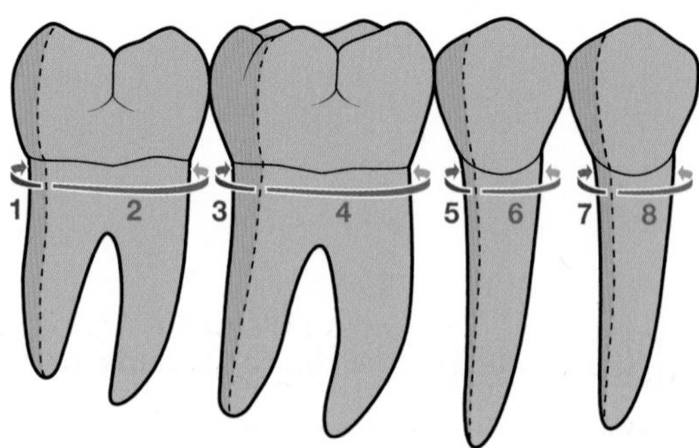

13. **Figure 12-44. Sequence for Sextant.** Next, use the sequence shown in this illustration to explore the facial aspect of the entire sextant, beginning with the posterior-most molar.

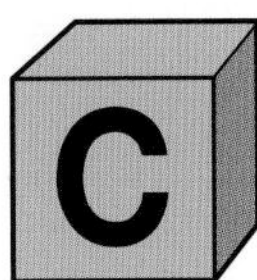

SKILL BUILDING. MAXILLARY POSTERIOR TEETH WITH 11/12-TYPE EXPLORER

Directions:

- Follow steps 1 to 6 to practice exploring the maxillary left posterior sextant, lingual aspect with an 11/12-type explorer (Figs. 12-45 to 12-50).
- Remember: "Me, My patient, My light, My dominant hand, My nondominant hand, My finger rest, My adaptation."

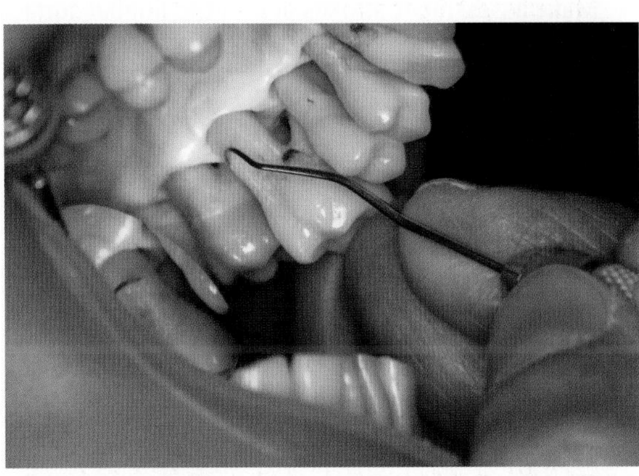

1. **Figure 12-45. Begin at the Distolingual Line Angle.** Position the explorer tip at the distolingual line angle in preparation for assessing the distal surface.

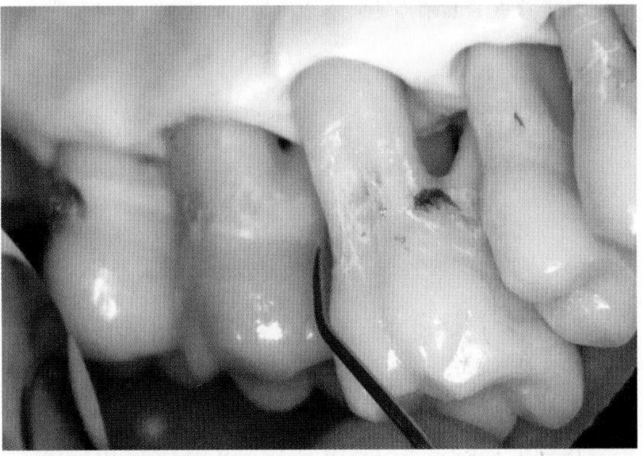

2. **Figure 12-46. Assess the Distal Surface.** Make assessment strokes from the distolingual line angle to the midline of the distal surface.

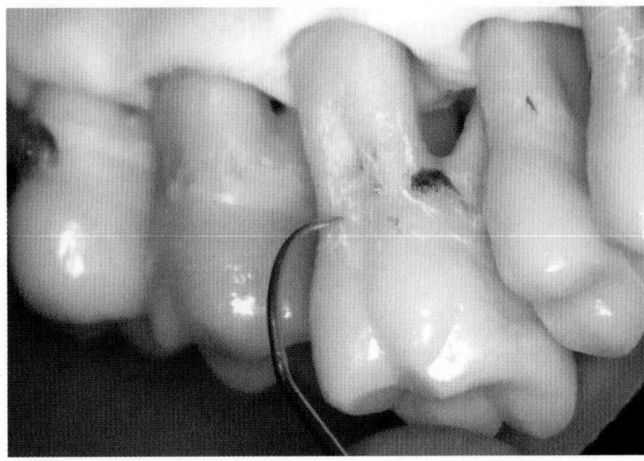

3. **Figure 12-47. Prepare to Assess the Lingual Surface.** Reposition the explorer tip at the distolingual line angle in preparation for assessing the lingual surface.

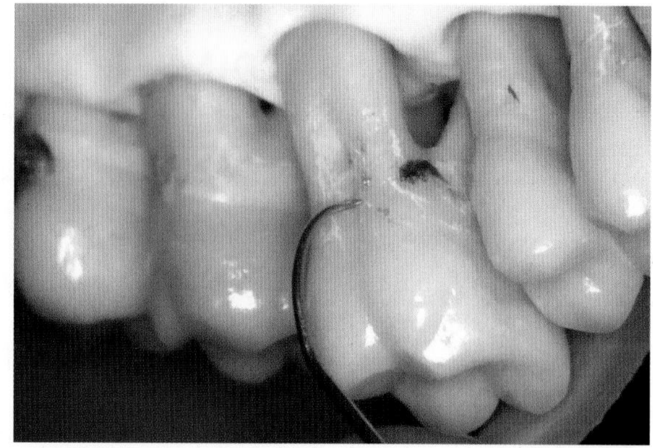

4. **Figure 12-48. Assess the Lingual Surface.** Make assessment strokes across the lingual surface.

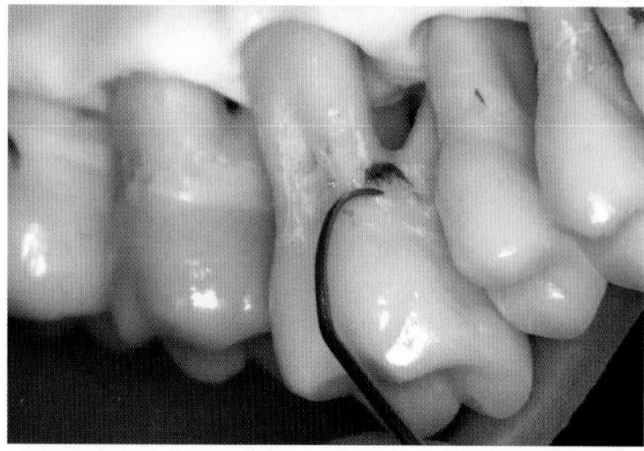

5. **Figure 12-49. Assess the Mesial Surface.** Roll the instrument handle to keep the tip adapted as you work around the mesiolingual line angle. Continue making assessment strokes across the mesial surface.

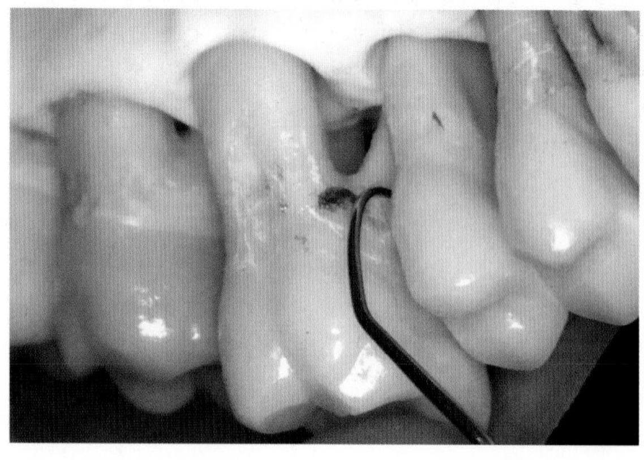

6. **Figure 12-50. Extend Strokes across Mesial Surface.** Continue assessment strokes at least halfway across the mesial surface.

Note to Course Instructor: Exploration of root furcations is covered in Module 20, Advanced Techniques for Root Surface Debridement.

Section 4
Technique Alerts

New clinicians often fail to detect calculus deposits that are located (1) near the distofacial or distolingual line angle of posterior teeth and (2) at the midline of the facial or lingual surfaces of anterior teeth. Undetected calculus deposits may result from not overlapping the assessment strokes sufficiently at the line angles and midlines of teeth. Horizontal strokes are extremely useful for calculus detection in these areas.

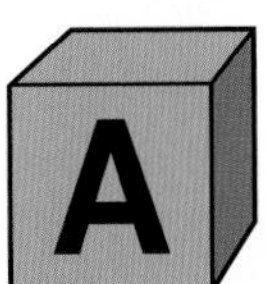

SKILL BUILDING. USE OF HORIZONTAL STROKES FOR CALCULUS DETECTION AT LINE ANGLES OF POSTERIOR TEETH

Follow the steps below to practice horizontal strokes at the distofacial line angle of a molar tooth (Figs. 12-51 and 12-52).

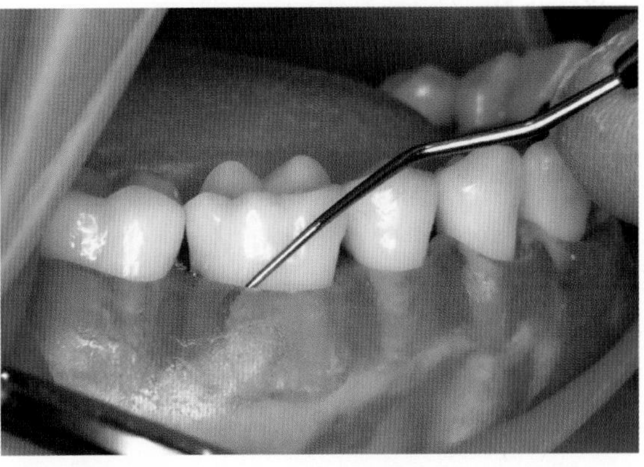

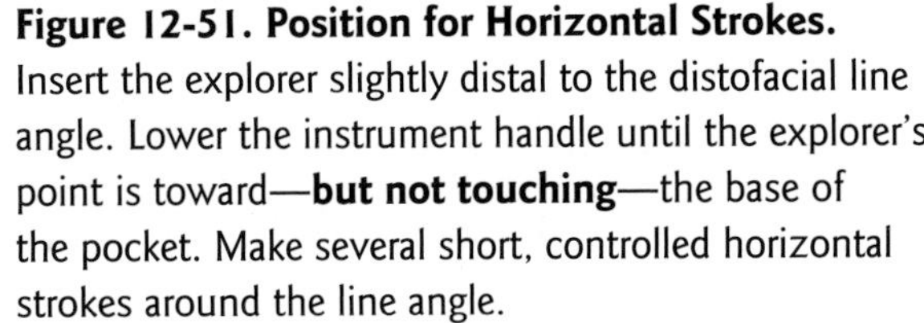
Figure 12-51. Position for Horizontal Strokes. Insert the explorer slightly distal to the distofacial line angle. Lower the instrument handle until the explorer's point is toward—**but not touching**—the base of the pocket. Make several short, controlled horizontal strokes around the line angle.

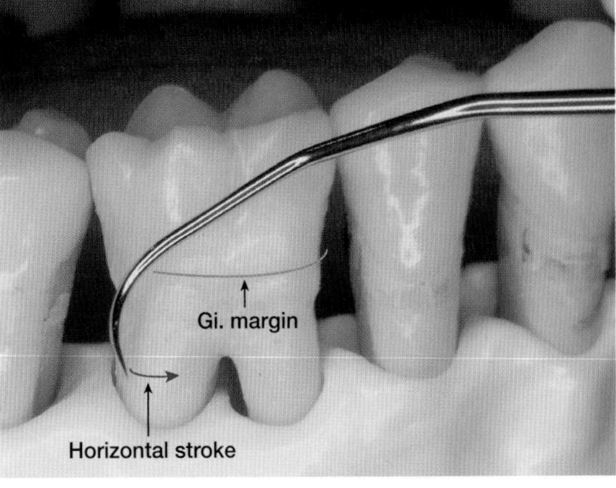

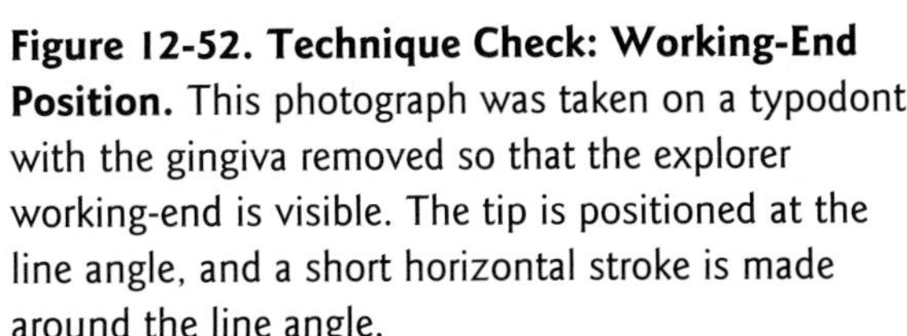
Figure 12-52. Technique Check: Working-End Position. This photograph was taken on a typodont with the gingiva removed so that the explorer working-end is visible. The tip is positioned at the line angle, and a short horizontal stroke is made around the line angle.

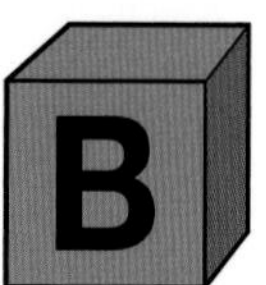

SKILL BUILDING. USE OF HORIZONTAL STROKES FOR CALCULUS DETECTION AT MIDLINES OF ANTERIOR TEETH

Technique Practice: Horizontal Strokes at the Midlines of Anterior Teeth

Follow the directions below to practice making horizontal strokes at the midline of the facial surface of a central incisor (Fig. 12-53). Horizontal strokes are useful for detection of calculus deposits located at the midline of facial or lingual surfaces on anterior teeth.

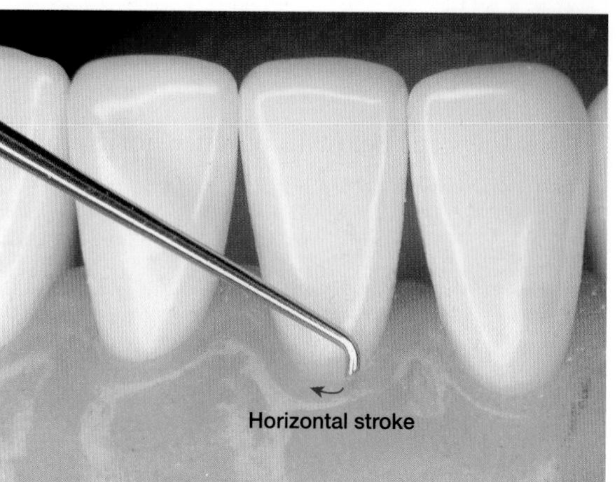

Figure 12-53. Horizontal Strokes: Midline of Anterior Tooth. Insert the explorer tip just distal to the midline.

- Lower the handle until the explorer's point is toward—**but not touching**—the base of the pocket.
- Make several short, controlled horizontal strokes across the midline.

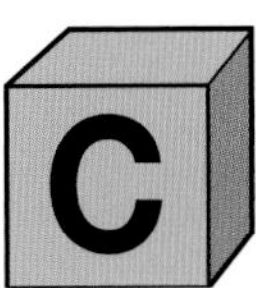

SKILL BUILDING. NEUTRAL WRIST POSITION

The most common positioning error when working on the maxillary posterior treatment areas is failing to maintain a neutral wrist position. A failure to maintain neutral wrist position occurs when the clinician bends the wrist rather than (1) assuming the correct clock position (Fig. 12-54) or (2) adjusting the handle position in the grasp. Correct neutral wrist position is shown in Figure 12-55.

Directions: This technique practice allows you to experience the difference in wrist positions that result from using two different handle positions in the grasp.

1. Equipment: an ODU 11/12-type explorer.
2. **Right-Handed clinicians:** maxillary right central incisor, surface away; facial aspect; **Left-Handed clinicians:** maxillary right central incisor, surface toward.

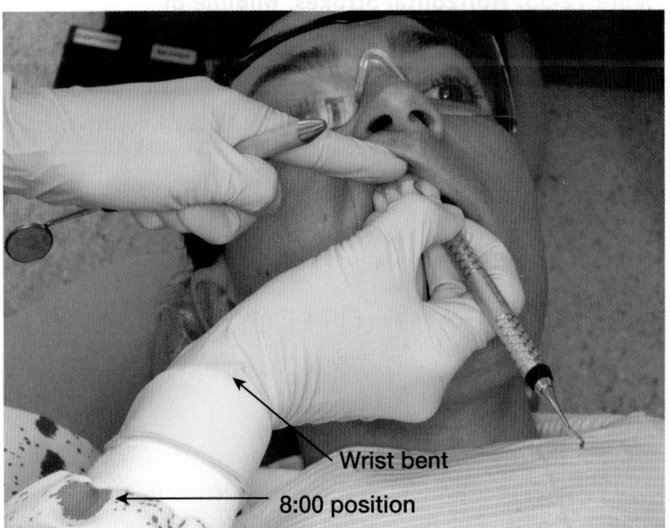

Figure 12-54. Incorrect Wrist Position.

Here the clinician is instrumenting the maxillary anterior surfaces away from the clinician.

- Note that the clinician is incorrectly seated in the 8:00 position.
- In this position, the clinician must bend his or her wrist in order to position the lower shank parallel to the distal surface of the tooth.

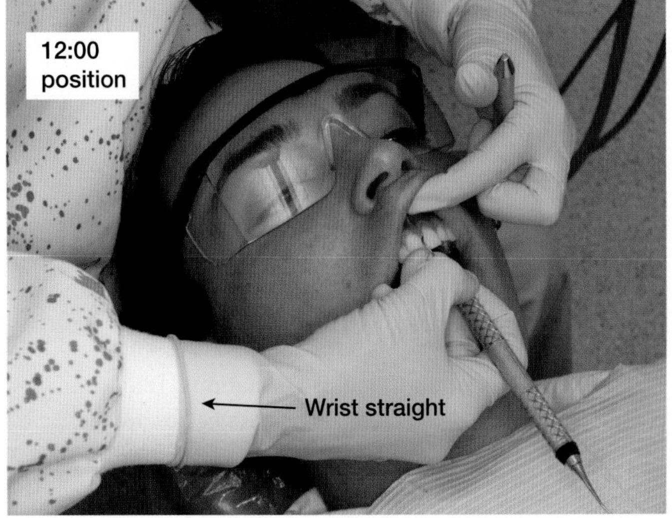

Figure 12-55. Correct Wrist Position.

Here the clinician is correctly seated in the 11 to 12 o'clock position for surfaces away.

- Note that the wrist is in neutral position.
- The instrument handle rests securely against the index finger in the "handle-down" orientation.

Section 5
Detection of Dental Calculus and Caries

TYPES AND CHARACTERISTICS OF CALCULUS DEPOSITS

Calculus is calcified bacterial plaque that forms as a hard tenacious mass on tooth surfaces and dental prostheses. It is commonly known as tartar. Calculus deposits are plaque retentive, meaning that the outer surface of a calculus deposit is covered with a layer of dental plaque biofilm.

1. *Supra*gingival calculus deposits are located coronal to the gingival margin (above the gingival margin).
   - When dried with a stream of compressed air, supragingival calculus has a rough, chalky appearance that contrasts visually with the smooth enamel surfaces.
   - Wet supragingival calculus is difficult to detect because the wet surface reflects light and blends in with the shiny tooth enamel.
2. *Sub*gingival calculus deposits are hidden beneath the gingival margin within the gingival sulcus or periodontal pocket. (Think "***sub***marines travel beneath the surface of the water.") Subgingival calculus deposits often are flattened in shape due to the pressure of the pocket wall against the tooth.
3. Residual calculus deposits are tiny remnants of calculus located on the surface of a tooth root.

THE NATURE OF CALCULUS FORMATION

When attempting to imagine the nature of subgingival deposits, remember that the deposits are built up layer by layer slowly over time.

- Calculus deposits are heavier more often near the cementoenamel junction (CEJ) rather than near the junctional epithelium, as deposits near the CEJ have been forming longer than those near the base of the pocket.
- The most common types of calculus formations are spicules, nodules, ledges, rings, veneers, and finger-like formations.[1] These formations are described in Box 12-3 and depicted in Figure 12-56.

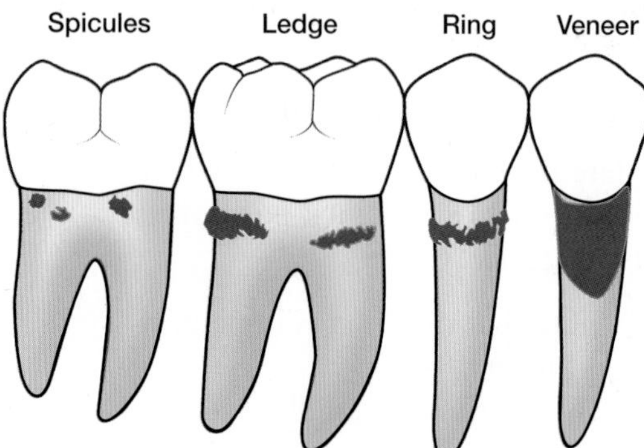

Figure 12-56. Common Calculus Formations. Four common types of calculus formations are spicules, ledges, rings, and veneers.

Box 12-3. Common Calculus Formations

Spicule—an isolated, minute particle or speck of calculus. Commonly found under contact areas, at line angles, and at the midline of a tooth.

Nodule—larger spicule-type formations with a crusty or spiny surface.

Ledge—a long ridge of calculus running parallel to the gingival margin. Common on all tooth surfaces.

Ring—a ridge of calculus running parallel to the gingival margin that encircles the tooth.

Veneer—a thin, smooth coating of calculus with a "shield-like shape" located on a portion of the root surface.

Finger-like formation—a long, narrow deposit running parallel or oblique to the long axis of the root.

INTERPRETATION OF SUBGINGIVAL CONDITIONS

The ability to recognize what you are feeling beneath the gingival margin is a skill that takes time and concentration to develop. The illustrations and descriptions in Figures 12-57 to 12-62 should aid you in interpreting what you feel. (Figures from Trott JR. The cross-subgingival calculus explorer. *Dental Digest*. 1961;67:481–483.)

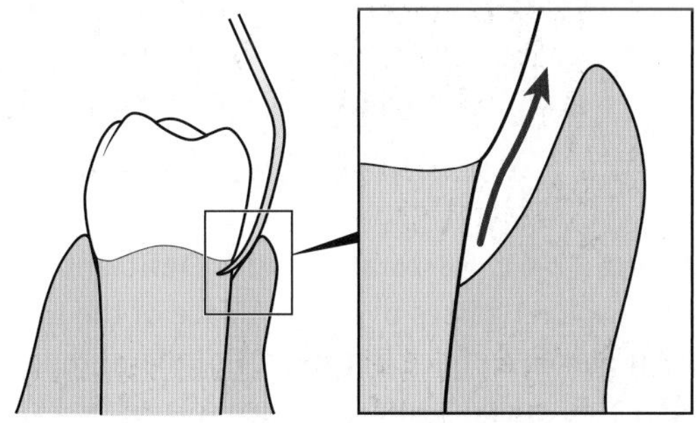

Figure 12-57. Normal Conditions. Your fingers do not feel any interruptions in the path of the explorer as it moves from the junctional epithelium to the gingival margin.

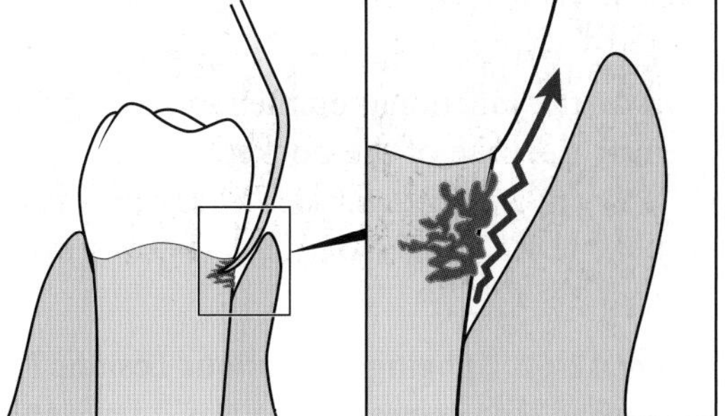

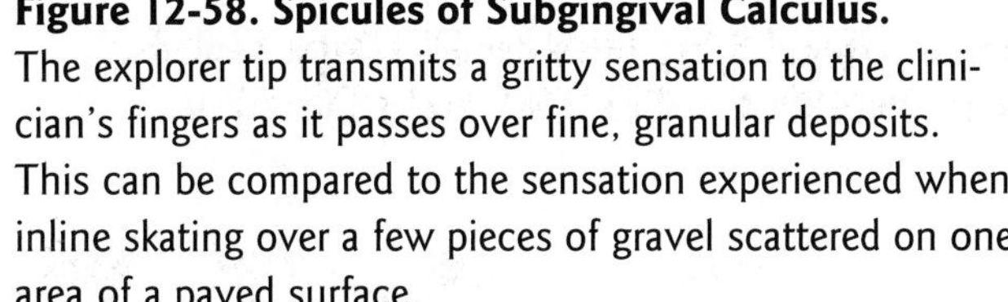

Figure 12-58. Spicules of Subgingival Calculus. The explorer tip transmits a gritty sensation to the clinician's fingers as it passes over fine, granular deposits. This can be compared to the sensation experienced when inline skating over a few pieces of gravel scattered on one area of a paved surface.

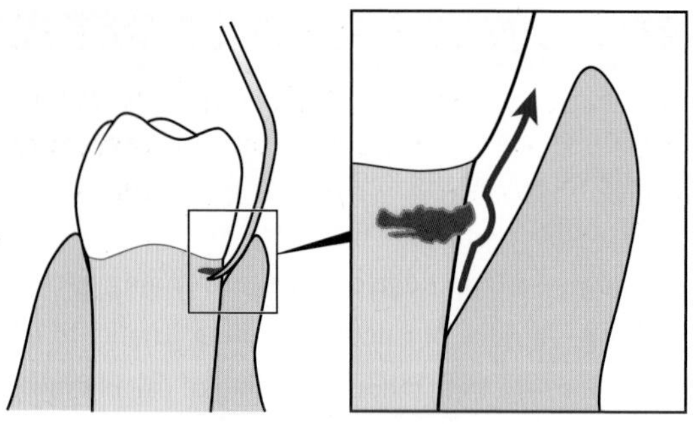

Figure 12-59. Ledge of Subgingival Calculus. As the explorer tip moves along the tooth surface, it moves out and around the raised bump, and returns back to the tooth surface. This is similar to the sensation of skating over speed bumps in a parking lot or over a cobblestone surface.

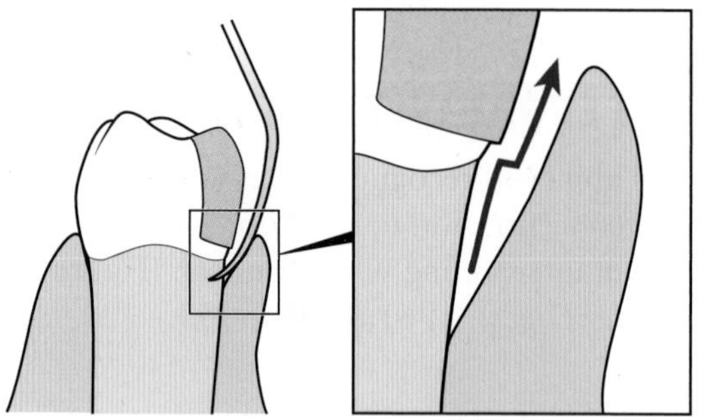

Figure 12-60. Restoration with Overhanging Margin. The explorer's path is blocked by the overhang and must move away from the tooth surface and over the restoration. This is similar to encountering the edge of a section of pavement that is higher than the surrounding pavement. Your skates must move up and over the higher section of pavement.

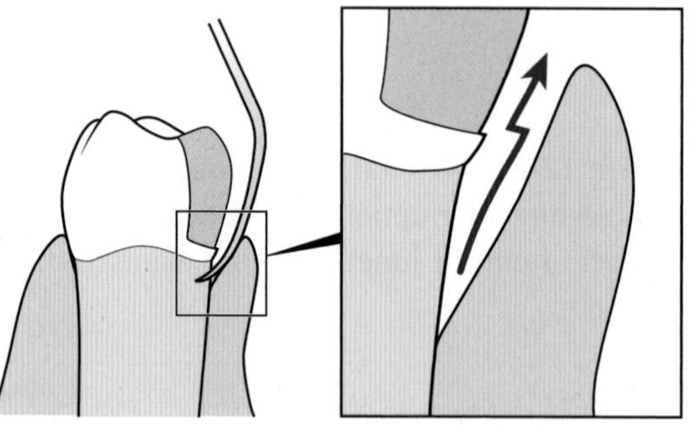

Figure 12-61. Restoration with Deficient Margin. The explorer passes over the surface of the tooth and then dips in to trace the surface of the restoration. This is similar to encountering the edge of a section of pavement that is lower than the surrounding pavement. Your skates must move down onto this section of pavement.

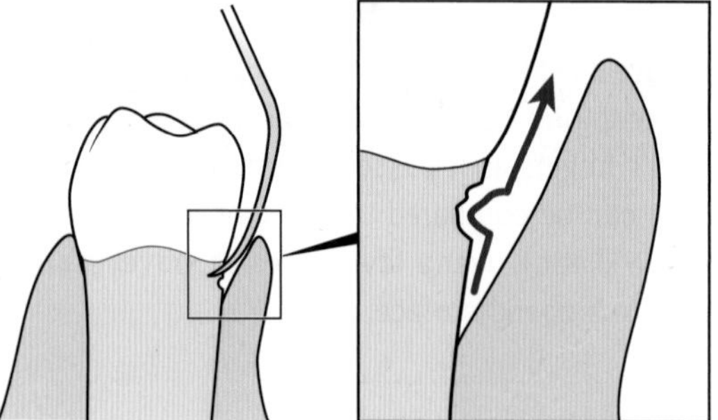

Figure 12-62. Subgingival Carious Lesion. The explorer dips in and then comes out again as it travels along the tooth surface. This would be like skating into a pothole, across the pothole, and then back onto the pavement.

REFERENCE SHEET: UNDETECTED CALCULUS

Errors in exploring technique are the most common cause of a failure to detect subgingival calculus deposits. As this reference sheet shows, often a small change in technique makes a big difference in the ability to detect calculus deposits.

TABLE 12-2. Causes of Undetected Calculus Deposits

Location	Technique Error
No particular pattern of undetected deposits	• Use of inappropriate explorer for task • "Death-grip" on instrument handle • Middle finger not on shank (fewer vibrations can be felt through handle than through the shank) • Middle finger applying pressure against shank, reducing tactile information • Strokes too far apart (not overlapping)
Undetected deposits at midlines of anteriors or line angles of posteriors	• Failure to overlap strokes in these areas • Failure to maintain constant adaptation to surface • Not using horizontal strokes in these areas
Undetected deposits on mesial or distal surfaces	• Strokes not extended apical to contact area so that at least one-half of surface is explored from both the facial and lingual aspects
Undetected *supra*gingival deposits	• Failure to use compressed air for a visual inspection of the teeth, especially facial surfaces of maxillary molars and lingual surfaces of mandibular anterior teeth (Fig. 12-63)
Undetected deposits at base of sulcus or pocket	• Failure to insert explorer to junctional epithelium before initiating stroke

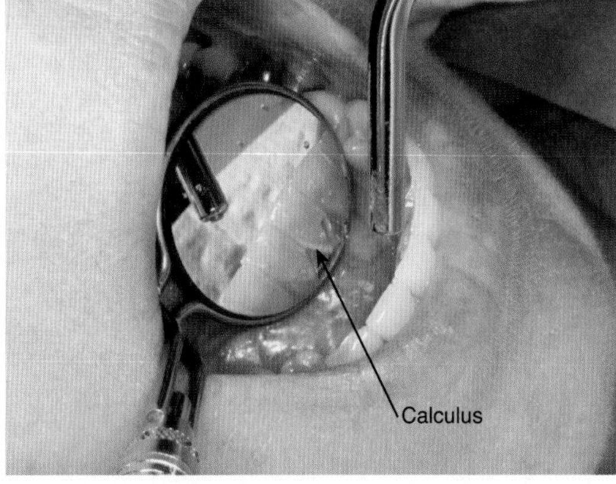

Figure 12-63. Use of Compressed Air for Detection of Supragingival Calculus Deposits. Examine the tooth surfaces visually while applying a continuous stream of air with the air syringe.

DETECTION OF DENTAL CARIES

A carious lesion is a decayed area on the tooth crown or root (Fig. 12-64). Enamel caries often can be detected visually by changes in the appearance of the enamel. An enamel lesion may appear chalky-white, gray, brown, or black in color. Root caries are common in older adults and periodontal patients.

1. **Historic Use of Tactile Methods for Caries Detection.** Historically, the use of the sharp tip of an explorer—gently forced into a pit or fissure—was a commonly used carious lesion detection method.
   - **a.** Research has shown this technique to be unreliable for carious lesion detection and to be potentially harmful.[2–11]
   - **b.** Firm application of a sharp explorer tip into a carious pit or fissure on a tooth surface may actually cause additional damage to the tooth surface that can interfere with subsequent attempts at remineralization of the caries lesion.
     1. Dental lesions initially develop as a subsurface lesion. Early lesions may be reversed—with meticulous patient self-care and application of fluoride—as long as the thin surface layer over the lesion remains intact.[12]
     2. The use of a dental explorer with firm pressure to probe suspicious areas may result in the rupture of the surface layer covering early lesions.[12]
2. **New Detection Aids**
   - **a.** To date, no one form of diagnosis is reliable in detecting all carious lesions or determining if a lesion is active or arrested.[13,14]
   - **b.** Noninvasive detection aids currently available include visual detection, radiographs, laser fluorescence, quantitative light-induced fluorescence, subtraction radiography, and electrical caries measurements.[15] The ideal caries detection method has yet to be identified, but it is likely that dental hygienists will see new developments in the future.

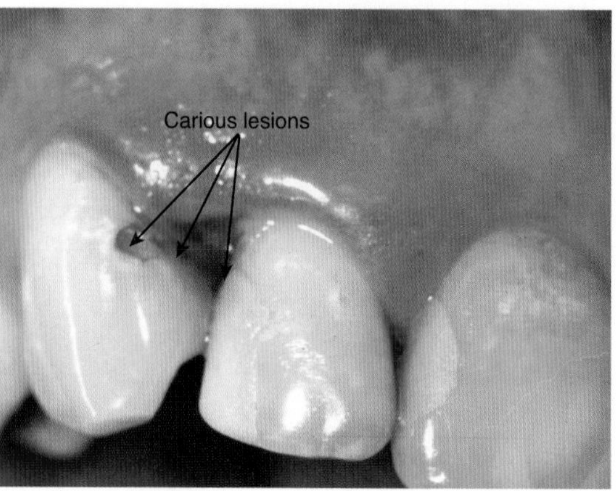

Figure 12-64. Dental Decay. Smooth surface caries on the canine and lateral incisor. Clinically visible carious lesions should NOT be explored.

INTERNATIONAL CARIES DETECTION AND ASSESSMENT SYSTEM (ICDAS)

The International Caries Detection and Assessment System (ICDAS) developed guidelines for the diagnosis of carious lesions on all tooth surfaces at all stages of severity.[10,11,16]

1. The ICDAS detection codes for coronal caries range from 0 to 6 depending on the severity of the lesion. Table 12-3 presents a brief description of the codes.

2. The ICDAS includes codes for the detection and classification of carious lesions on the root surfaces. One score is assigned per root surface. The facial, mesial, distal, and lingual root surfaces are classified based on the codes shown in Table 12-4.

TABLE 12-3. ICDAS Coronal Primary Caries Codes

Code	Description
0	Sound tooth surface, no change after 5 seconds of air drying
1	First visual change in enamel (seen only after prolonged air drying or restricted to within the confines of a pit or fissure)
2	Distinct visual change in enamel; tooth must be viewed wet. When wet, there is a (a) white spot lesion and/or (b) brown carious discoloration that is wider than the natural fissure/fossa that is not consistent with the clinical appearance of sound enamel.
3	Localized enamel breakdown without clinical visual signs of dentinal involvement; once dried for approximately 5 seconds, there is visible loss of tooth structure at the entrance to, or within, the pit or fissure/fossa
4	Underlying dark shadow from dentin; lesion appears as a shadow of discolored dentin visible through an apparently intact enamel surface
5	Distinct cavity with visible dentin; once dried for approximately 5 seconds, there is visible evidence of demineralization (opaque/white, brown, or dark brown walls) at the entrance to or within the pit or fissure, and dentin is exposed
6	Extensive distinct cavity with visible dentin; obvious loss of tooth structure, and dentin is clearly visible on the walls and at the base in a cavity that involves at least half of the tooth surface

TABLE 12-4. ICDAS Codes for Carious Lesions on Root Surfaces

Code	Description
E	Excluded; the root surface cannot be visualized directly because it is covered by gingiva or calculus deposits
0	No unusual discoloration or surface defect OR definite loss of surface continuity that is NOT consistent with the dental caries process; such loss of continuity is commonly associated with abrasion or erosion
1	Clearly demarcated area on the root surface or at the CEJ that is discolored (light/dark brown, black), but there is NO loss of anatomical contour (cavitation) present
2	Clearly demarcated area on the root surface or at the CEJ that is discolored (light/dark brown, black), and there IS loss of anatomical contour (cavitation) present

REFERENCES

1. Gurgan CA, Bilgin E. Distribution of different morphologic types of subgingival calculus on proximal root surfaces. *Quintessence Int.* 2005;36:202–208.
2. Aleksejuniene J, Gorovenko M. Caries detection techniques and clinical practice. *Pract Proced Aesthet Dent.* 2009;21:26–28.
3. Berg JH, Swift EJ Jr. Critical appraisal: current caries detection devices. *J Esthet Restor Dent.* 2010;22:464–470.
4. Braga MM, Mendes FM, Ekstrand KR. Detection activity assessment and diagnosis of dental caries lesions. *Dent Clin North Am.* 2010;54:479–493.
5. Selwitz RH, Ismail AI, Pitts NB. Dental caries. *Lancet.* 2007;369:51–59.
6. Ekstrand K, Qvist V, Thylstrup A. Light microscope study of the effect of probing in occlusal surfaces. *Caries Res.* 1987;21:368–374.
7. Pitts N. *Detection, Assessment, Diagnosis and Monitoring of Caries.* Basel, Switzerland: Karger; 2009.
8. Pitts NB. Implementation. Improving caries detection, assessment, diagnosis and monitoring. *Monogr Oral Sci.* 2009;21:199–208.
9. Pitts NB. How the detection, assessment, diagnosis and monitoring of caries integrate with personalized caries management. *Monogr Oral Sci.* 2009;21:1–14.
10. Shivakumar K, Prasad S, Chandu G. International Caries Detection and Assessment System: a new paradigm in detection of dental caries. *J Conserv Dent.* 2009;12:10–16.
11. Topping GV, Pitts NB. Clinical visual caries detection. *Monogr Oral Sci.* 2009;21:15–41.
12. Stookey G. The evolution of caries detection. *Dimen Dent Hyg.* 2003;October:12–15.
13. NIH Consensus Development Conference on Diagnosis and Management of Dental Caries Throughout Life. Bethesda, MD, March 26–28, 2001. Conference Papers. *J Dent Educ.* 2001;65:935–1179.
14. Ekstrand KR, Zero DT, Martignon S, Pitts NB. Lesion activity assessment. *Monogr Oral Sci.* 2009;21:63–90.
15. Neuhaus KW, Longbottom C, Ellwood R, Lussi A. Novel lesion detection aids. *Monogr Oral Sci.* 2009;21:52–62.
16. Zero DT, Fontana M, Martínez-Mier EA, Ferreira-Zandoná A, Ando M, González-Cabezas C. The biology, prevention, diagnosis and treatment of dental caries: scientific advances in the United States. *J Am Dent Assoc.* 2009;140(suppl 1):25S-34S.

Section 6
Skill Application

PRACTICAL FOCUS

Diagramming Calculus Deposits. This activity will help you to develop tactile detection skills and the ability to form a mental picture of the deposits you detect.

Directions:

1. Begin by creating some objects that will represent tooth roots with calculus deposits.
   - If possible, locate some discarded pieces of old copper or PVC plumbing pipes. The maintenance department at your college or university might be able to supply some.
   - Use synthetic calculus to create "ledges and spicules of calculus" on the surface of the copper tubes.
   - The "calculus deposits" should have a random pattern, and each copper tube should have a unique pattern of "deposits."
   - Allow the "calculus" to dry overnight. Obtain a small *opaque* trash bag.
2. Put an explorer, a copper tube, and both of your hands inside the trash bag.
   - Use your mirror hand to hold the copper tube. Grasp the explorer in your other hand and establish a finger rest on the side of the copper tube.
   - Initiate assessment strokes along the surface of the tube.
   - As you form a mental picture of the "calculus deposits," diagram them on a piece of paper on which you have drawn a rectangle representing the copper tube.
   - Indicate the location and relative size of the "calculus deposits" on the tube.
3. Finally, remove the copper tube from the bag.
   - Compare the actual "calculus deposits" to your drawing (Fig. 12-65). How did you do? Repeat this activity with different copper tubes to improve your detection and visualization skills.

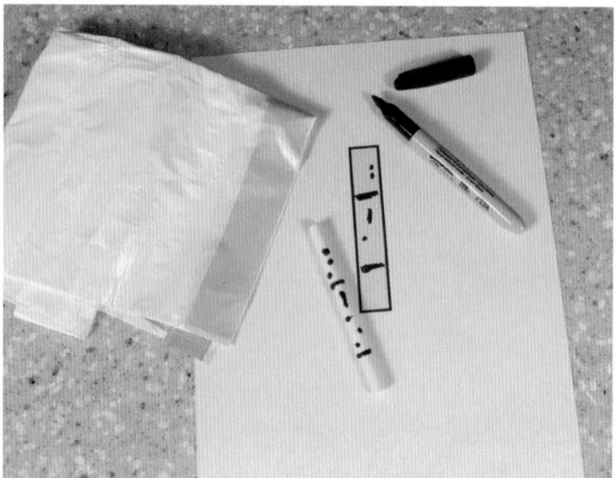

Figure 12-65. Check Your Diagram. Compare the actual deposits on the copper tube with your diagram.

Box 12-4. Reference Sheet for Explorers

General Technique for Calculus Detection:

- Use a relaxed grasp, resting your middle finger lightly on the shank.
- Use the side of the explorer tip, not the actual point.
- Cover every millimeter of the root surface with light, flowing strokes.

Anterior Teeth:

1. **Working-End Selection:** Working-end "wraps" around the tooth, curving toward the tooth surface.
2. **Sequence:** Begin with the surfaces toward you. Start on the canine on the opposite side of the mouth and work toward yourself. (Right-handed: left canine, mesial surface; Left-handed: right canine, mesial surface)

Posterior Teeth:

1. **Working-End Selection:** Lower shank is parallel to tooth surface ("posterior parallel").
2. **Sequence:** Begin with the posterior-most tooth in the sextant. On each tooth, do the distal surface first, followed by facial and mesial (or lingual and mesial) surfaces.

STUDENT SELF-EVALUATION MODULE 12 EXPLORERS

Student: ______________________ Date: ______________________

DIRECTIONS: Self-evaluate your skill level in each treatment area as: **S** (satisfactory) or **U** (unsatisfactory).

Criteria				
Positioning/Ergonomics	**Area 1**	**Area 2**	**Area 3**	**Area 4**
Adjusts clinician chair correctly				
Reclines patient chair and assures that patient's head is even with top of headrest				
Positions instrument tray within easy reach				
Assumes the recommended clock position				
Positions backrest of patient chair for the specified arch and adjusts height of patient chair so that clinician's elbows remain at waist level when accessing the specified treatment area				
Asks patient to assume the head position that facilitates the clinician's view of the specified treatment area				
Directs light to illuminate the specified treatment area				
Instrument Grasp: Dominant Hand	**Area 1**	**Area 2**	**Area 3**	**Area 4**
Grasps handle with tips of finger pads of index finger and thumb				
Rests pad of middle finger lightly on instrument shank				
Positions the thumb, index, and middle fingers in the "knuckles-up" convex position; hyperextended joint position is avoided				
Holds ring finger straight so that it supports the weight of hand and instrument; ring finger position is "advanced ahead of" the other fingers in the grasp				
Keeps index, middle, ring, and little fingers in contact; "like fingers inside a mitten"				
Maintains a relaxed grasp; fingers are NOT blanched in grasp				
Finger Rest: Dominant Hand				
Establishes secure finger rest that is appropriate for tooth to be treated				
Once finger rest is established, pauses to self-evaluate finger placement in the grasp, verbalizes to evaluator his/her self-assessment of grasp, and corrects finger placement if necessary				
Prepare for Instrumentation ("Get Ready")				
Selects correct working-end for tooth surface to be instrumented				
Places the working-end in the "Get Ready Zone" while using a correct finger rest for the treatment area				
Exploring Technique	**Area 1**	**Area 2**	**Area 3**	**Area 4**
Maintains a relaxed grasp to make feather-light, overlapping strokes of an appropriate length				
Stops each assessment stroke beneath the gingival margin (to avoid trauma to the gingival margin); does NOT remove tip from sulcus/pocket with each stroke				
Maintains adaptation of tip; pivots and rolls handle as needed to maintain adaptation				
Covers entire root surface with assessment strokes				
Uses appropriate sequence in the sextant				
Uses overlapping strokes at midlines of anterior teeth, under the contact area, and at line angles of posterior teeth				
Maintains neutral wrist position throughout motion activation				
Ethics and Professionalism				
Punctuality, appearance, demeanor, attitude, composure, honesty				

Module 13

Technique Essentials: Angulation and Calculus Removal

Module Overview

Moving the instrument working-end over the tooth surface to produce an instrumentation stroke involves several small motor skills. Before moving the working-end, it should be positioned correctly against the tooth surface. The two skills used in positioning the working-end are termed adaptation and angulation.

As previously discussed in Module 9, ***adaptation*** refers to the positioning of the first 1 or 2 mm of the working-end's lateral surface in contact with the tooth. ***Angulation*** refers to the relationship between the face of a calculus removal instrument and the tooth surface to which it is applied. For successful instrumentation, correct adaptation and angulation of the working-end must be maintained throughout the entire instrumentation stroke.

This module discusses the elements of an instrumentation stroke including preparation for a stroke, stabilization, insertion, angulation, and stroke production.

Module Outline

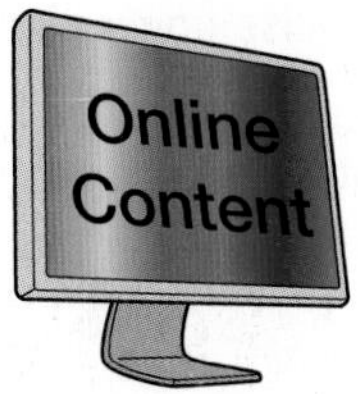

A video on the topic of the calculus removal stroke may be viewed at http://thepoint.lww.com/GehrigFundamentals7e

Key Terms

Angulation	Insertion	"Out of the line of fire"	Burnished calculus deposit
Periodontium	Closed angle	Stabilization	Instrumentation zones
Get Ready Zone		Lateral pressure	

Learning Objectives

1. Define the term angulation as it relates to the use of a curet and sickle scaler for periodontal instrumentation.
2. Explain the problems associated with using an angulation greater than 40° when inserting the working-end beneath the gingival margin and to the base of the sulcus or periodontal pocket.
3. Explain the problems associated with using an angulation greater than 90° for calculus removal.
4. Explain the problems associated with using an angulation less than 45° for calculus removal.
5. Describe how a deposit of calculus is removed from a tooth surface and differentiate that from burnishing.
6. Define the term insertion as it relates to periodontal instrumentation.
7. Using a typodont, describe and demonstrate correct angulation for calculus removal.
8. Define the phrase "Get Ready Zone" as it applies to periodontal instrumentation.
9. List from memory the sequence of steps used for calculus removal strokes as outlined in Figure 13-21.
10. On a periodontal typodont, demonstrate the elements of a calculus removal stroke in a step-by-step manner while maintaining precise finger placement in the grasp and correct fulcruming technique.
11. On a periodontal typodont, demonstrate the elements of a root debridement stroke in a step-by-step manner while maintaining precise finger placement in the grasp and correct fulcruming technique.

Section 1
Relationship of the Instrument Face to the Tooth Surface

Angulation refers to the relationship between the face of a calculus removal instrument and the tooth surface to which it is applied.

1. **Visualizing the Unseen.** *Much periodontal instrumentation takes place beneath the gingival margin. With the working-end hidden beneath the gingival tissue, the dental hygienist needs to be able to visualize the position of the working-end in his or her mind's eye.*[1]
2. **Visualizing in Cross Section.**
   a. To picture the placement of the working-end against the root surface, the hygienist must mentally picture the cross section of the tooth, periodontium, and the instrument working-end.[1] The tissues that surround and support a tooth in the dental arch are known as the periodontium. The components of the periodontium are the gingiva, periodontal ligament, cementum, and alveolar bone.
   b. Figure 13-1 shows a tooth and the periodontium in cross section. Figure 13-2 shows a cross section of a curet.

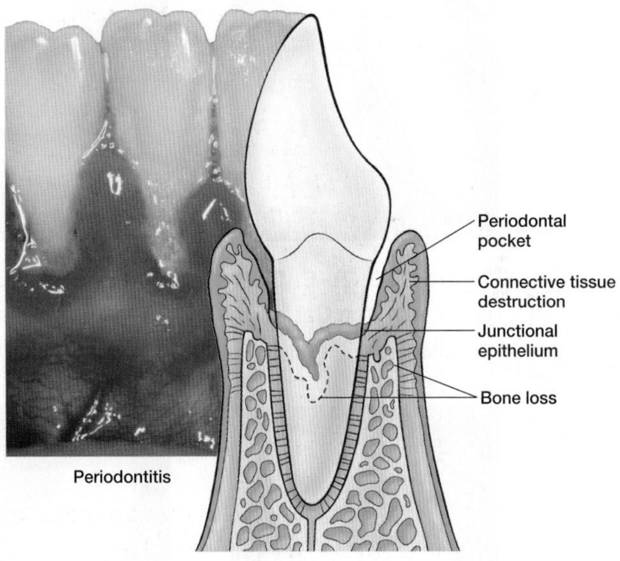

Figure 13-1. The Periodontium in Cross Section. Much of the calculus removal during periodontal instrumentation takes place beneath the gingival margin. An understanding of the periodontium in cross section assists the clinician in visualizing periodontal instrumentation beneath the gingival margin.

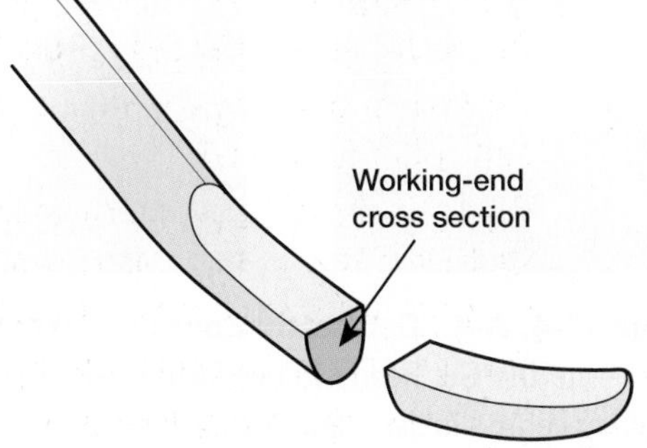

Figure 13-2. Instrument Working-End in Cross Section. A curet is semi-circular in cross section.

Section 2
Insertion beneath the Gingival Margin

PREPARATION FOR INSERTION: THE GET READY ZONE

There are several important steps in preparing for insertion beneath the gingival margin.

- Establishing a secure finger rest near the tooth to be instrumented.
- Selecting the correct working-end of a double-ended instrument.
- Preparing for inserting by placing the working-end on the crown of the tooth in the "*Get Ready Zone.*"

The Get Ready Zone is an area of the crown where the working-end is positioned prior to insertion. ***The Get Ready Zone is located in the middle-third of the crown of the tooth.*** Figures 13-3 and 13-4 show the Get Ready Zones for three teeth on the facial and proximal surfaces.

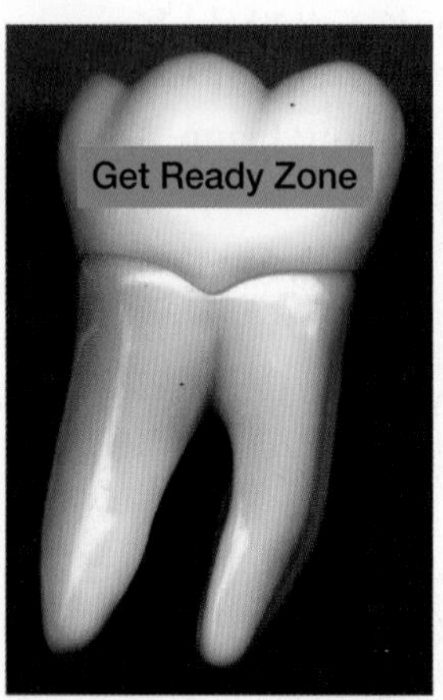

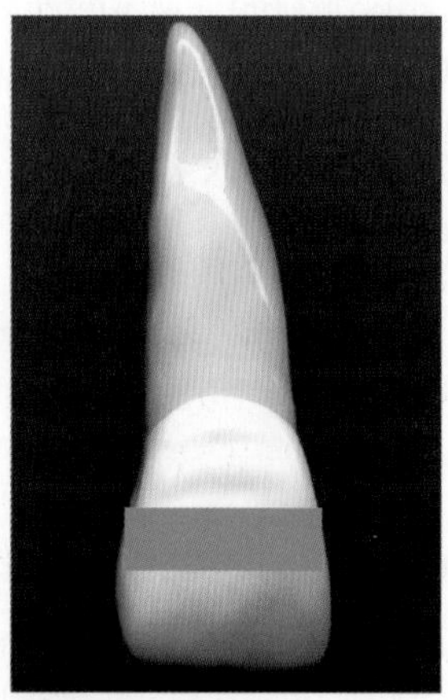
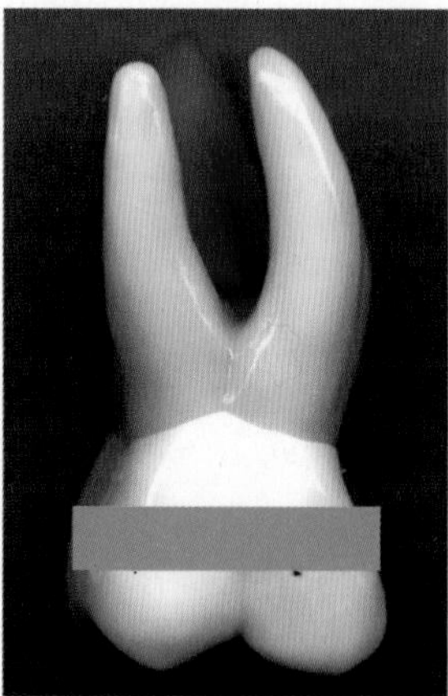

Figure 13-3, A–C. Get Ready Zones on Facial Surfaces. Shown here—shaded in green—are the Get Ready Zones for the facial surfaces of a mandibular first molar, maxillary central incisor, and maxillary first molar.

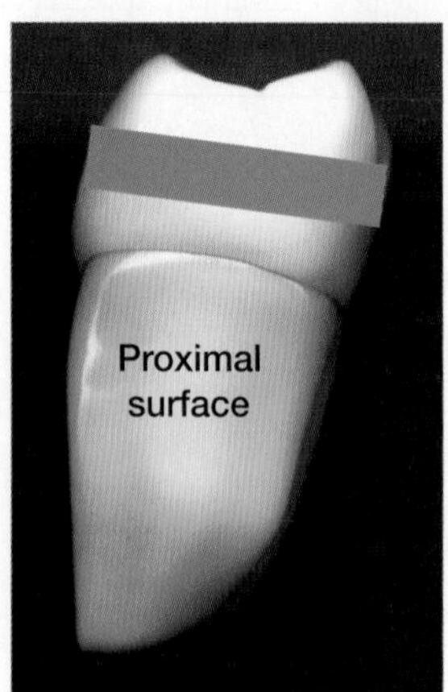

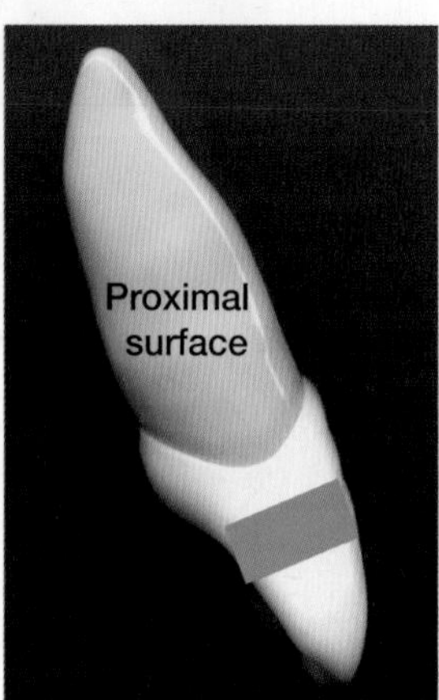

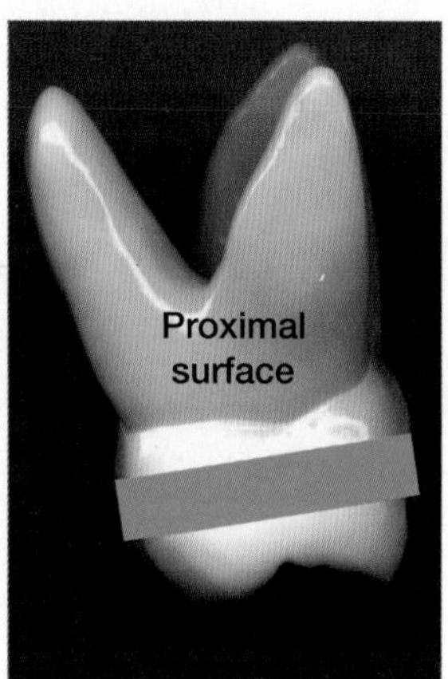

Figure 13-4, A–C. Get Ready Zones on Proximal Surfaces. Shown here—shaded in green—are the Get Ready Zones for the proximal surfaces of a mandibular first molar, maxillary central incisor, and maxillary first molar.

FACE-TO-TOOTH SURFACE ANGULATION FOR INSERTION

Correct face-to-tooth surface angulation of the working-end must be maintained throughout the instrumentation stroke. Each phase of instrumentation requires a precise angulation of the working-end to the tooth surface.

- First, angulation is established to allow the working-end to slide gently beneath the gingival margin.
- Second, an assessment stroke is used to locate a calculus deposit. Once located, the working-end is positioned just apical to the deposit so that the instrument face cups the calculus deposit.
- Third, the angulation of the face-to-tooth surface is established at the proper angulation for calculus removal.
- Finally, angulation is established for root debridement strokes of the root surface.

Angulation during Insertion beneath the Gingival Margin

1. Insertion is the act of gently sliding the working-end beneath the gingival margin into the gingival sulcus or periodontal pocket.
   a. Care must be used during insertion to prevent injury to the soft tissue. The working-end should be kept in contact with the tooth surface during insertion.
   b. Curets are the primary calculus removal instruments for ***sub***gingival instrumentation.
2. ***During insertion, the face-to-tooth surface angulation is an angle between 0° and 40°.*** Figures 13-5 illustrates the proper angulation for insertion.
   a. During insertion, the face of a curet is held against the tooth surface as closely as possible. It should hug the tooth surface throughout the entire process of insertion.
   b. The 0° to 40° angle used for insertion also is referred to as a closed angle because the face is closed against the tooth surface.

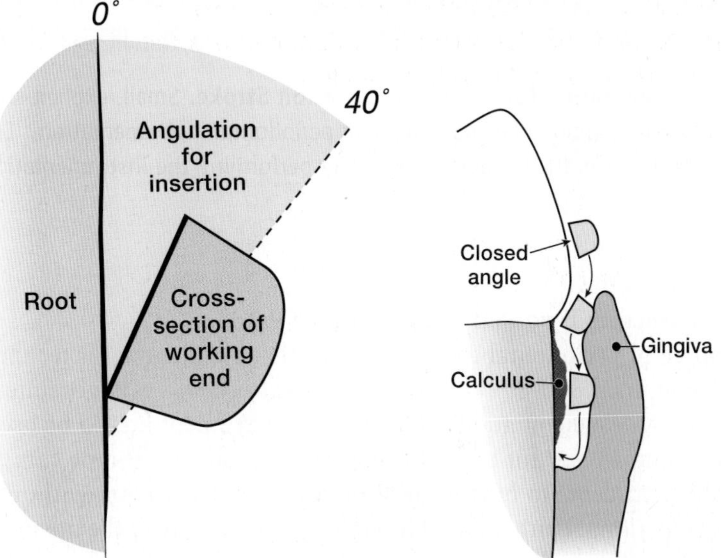

Figure 13-5. Angulation of the Working-End for Insertion. During insertion, the face-to-tooth surface angulation should be an angle between 0° and 40°. The face of the working-end hugs the tooth surface as it slides gently to the base of a periodontal pocket.

FLOW CHART: PREPARATION FOR INSTRUMENTATION

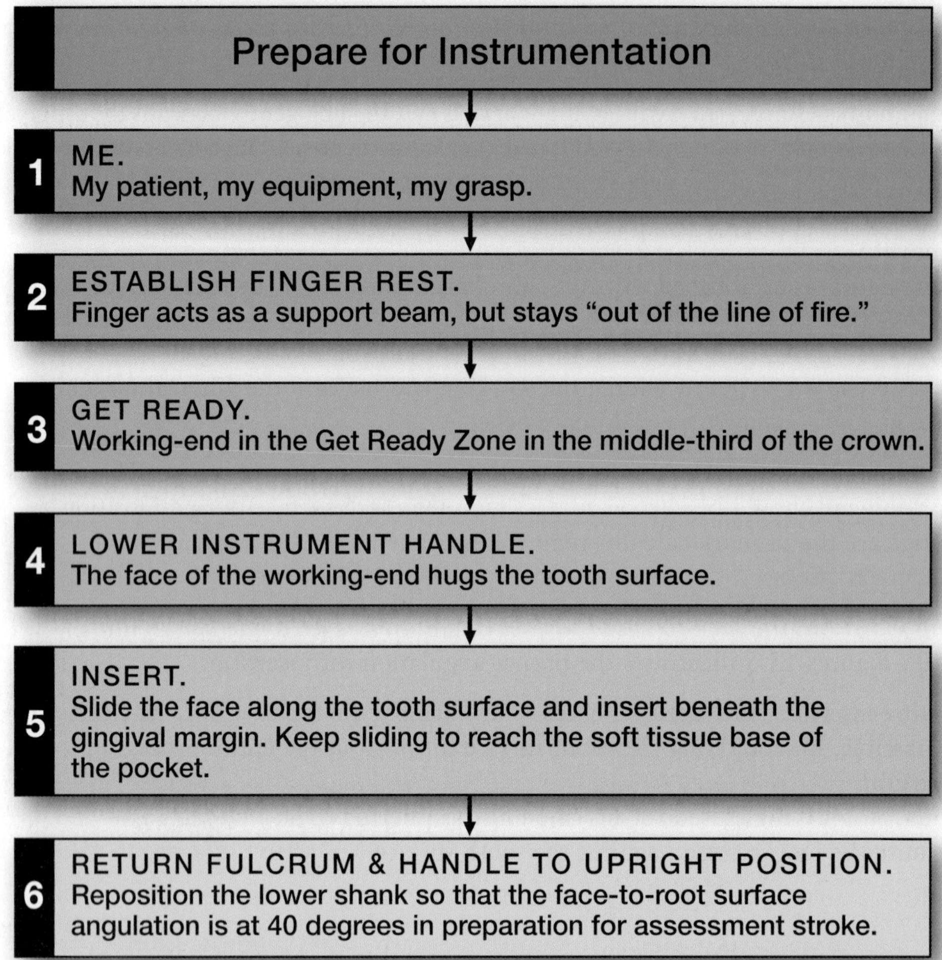

Prepare for Instrumentation
1
ME.
My patient, my equipment, my grasp.
2
ESTABLISH FINGER REST.
Finger acts as a support beam, but stays "out of the line of fire."
3
GET READY.
Working-end in the Get Ready Zone in the middle-third of the crown.
4
LOWER INSTRUMENT HANDLE.
The face of the working-end hugs the tooth surface.
5
INSERT.
Slide the face along the tooth surface and insert beneath the gingival margin. Keep sliding to reach the soft tissue base of the pocket.
6
RETURN FULCRUM & HANDLE TO UPRIGHT POSITION.
Reposition the lower shank so that the face-to-root surface angulation is at 40 degrees in preparation for assessment stroke.

Figure 13-6. Steps in Preparation for an Instrumentation Stroke. Small, explicit steps that clearly define the instrumentation technique facilitate learning periodontal instrumentation.[2] Envisioning the steps prior to attempting a skill assists the learner in accurately performing the instrumentation skill.

Note to Course Instructor: Typodonts for Technique Practice

One excellent source of periodontal typodonts with flexible gingiva for technique practice is Kilgore International, Inc.: 800-892-9999 or online at http://www.kilgoreinternational.com. These typodonts are an excellent addition to student instrument kits to be used when learning instrumentation technique and for patient instruction in self-care (home care) techniques.

Typodonts allow students to practice techniques such as insertion without danger of injury to the sulcular or junctional epithelium of a partner.[3] Also, there is the advantage that students can see for themselves the results of improper adaptation. Periodontal typodonts with flexible or removable gingiva allow students to practice instrumentation on root surfaces—the most important and difficult areas of the tooth on which to master instrumentation.[4]

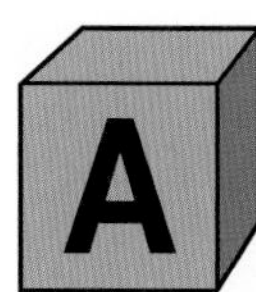

SKILL BUILDING. INSERTION OF A CURET BENEATH THE GINGIVAL MARGIN

Equipment: Periodontal typodont[4] and a universal curet. *If the typodont has removable gingiva, first, practice insertion and then, remove the gingiva so that you can see the working-end of the instrument on the root.*

- Follow steps 1 to 8 to practice insertion on the distal and facial tooth surfaces of a mandibular first molar (Figs. 13-7 to 13-14). **Right-Handed clinician:** Mandibular right posterior sextant, facial aspect. **Left-Handed clinician:** Mandibular left posterior sextant, facial aspect.
- Remember: "Me, My patient, My light, My dominant hand, My nondominant hand."
- The finger rest should not be positioned directly in line with the working-end to prevent cutting the ring finger when making a stroke. ***Position the finger rest "out of the line of fire" near to the tooth surface to be instrumented.***

1. Figure 13-7. Get Ready for Insertion on Distal Surface.

- Turn the toe of working-end toward the distal surface.
- In preparation for insertion, the working-end is placed in the *Get Ready Zone* in the middle-third of the crown.
- In this case, the Get Ready Zone is at the distofacial line angle in the middle-third of the crown.

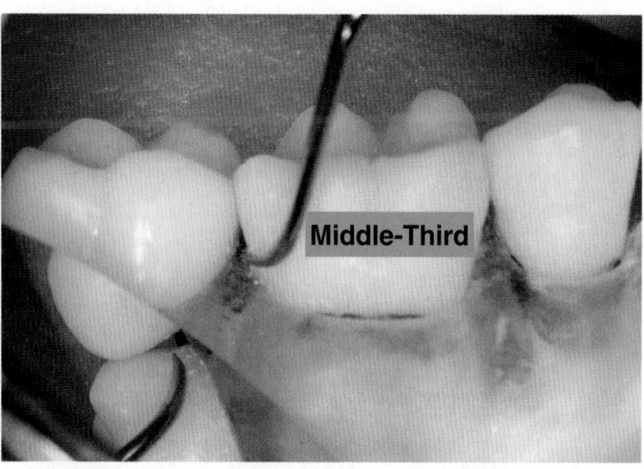

2. Figure 13-8. Prepare for Insertion on Distal Surface.

- Lower your hand and the instrument handle *until the face-to-tooth surface angulation is near to 0°*. (For insertion, it may be necessary to fulcrum briefly on the facial surface.)
- The face of the instrument should hug the distal surface.

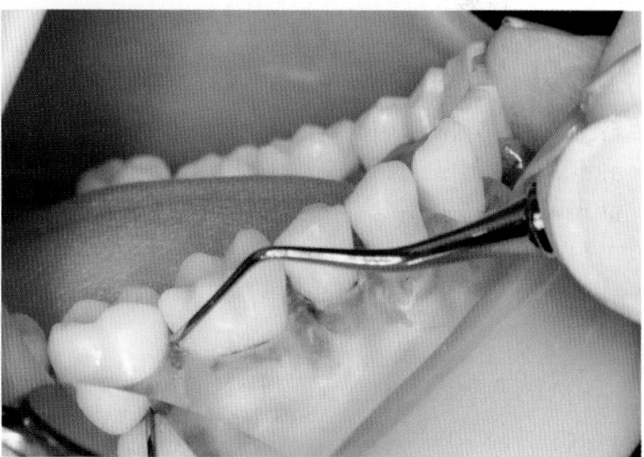

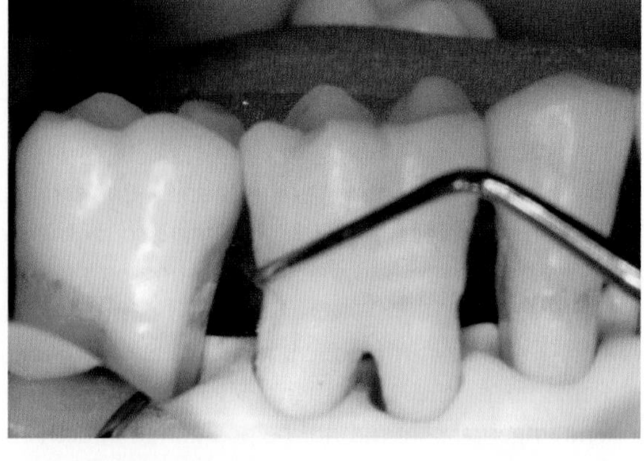

3. Figure 13-9. Insert on Distal Surface.

- Maintaining your hand position, gently slide the working-end beneath the gingival margin and onto the distal surface of the root.
- *Imagine the face of the working-end sliding along the distal surface, all the way to the base of the pocket.*[4]

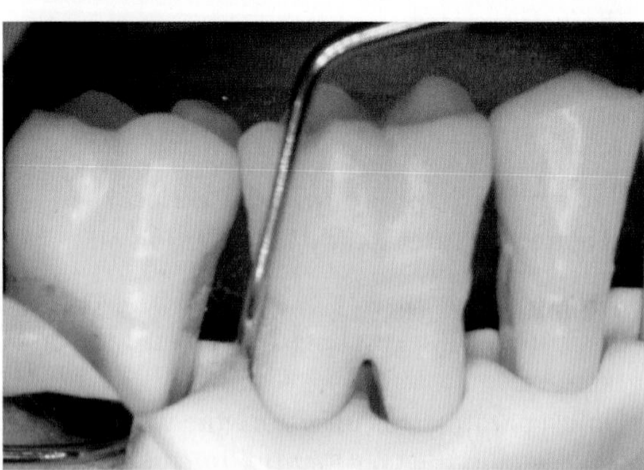

4. Figure 13-10. Return Fulcrum Finger and Handle to Upright Position.

- Return your fulcrum to the occlusofacial line angle of a nearby tooth as you reposition the handle to an upright position.[5]
- Reposition the lower shank so that the face-to-root surface angulation is about 40° in preparation for an assessment stroke.

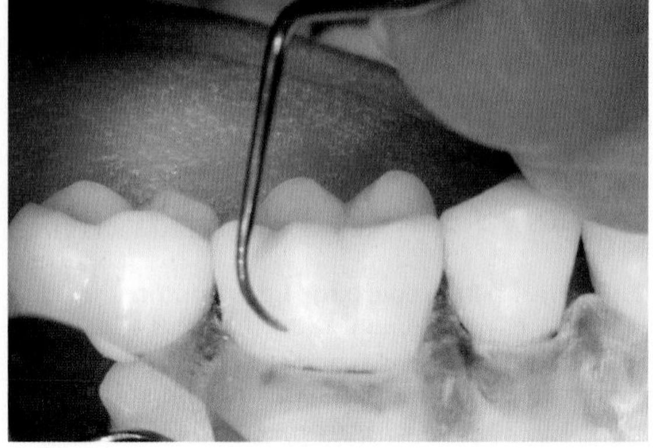

5. Figure 13-11. Get Ready for Insertion on Facial Surface.

- Turn the working-end so that the toe of the curet is "pointing toward" the front of the mouth.
- Place the working-end in the **Get Ready Zone** on the middle-third of the facial surface.

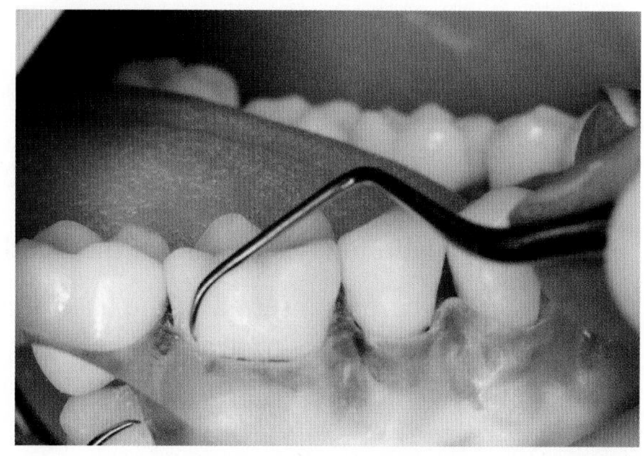

6. Figure 13-12. Prepare for Insertion on Facial Surface.

- Lower your hand and the instrument handle until the curet toe is pointing toward the gingival margin. (For insertion, it may be necessary to fulcrum briefly on the facial surface.)
- Insert at a 0° angulation with the lower shank close to the tooth.
- *The face of the instrument should hug the facial surface.*

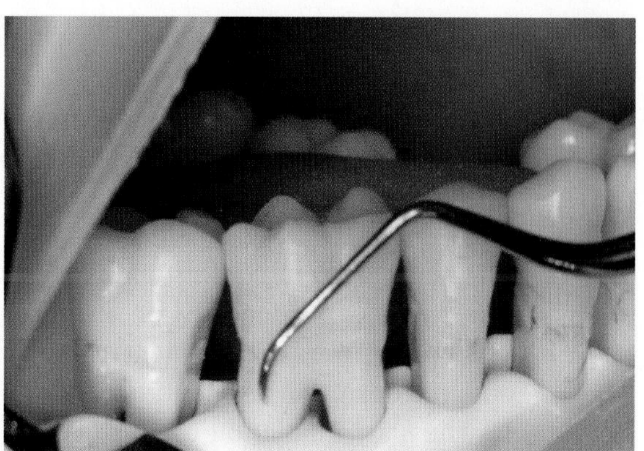

7. Figure 13-13. Insert on Facial Surface.

- Maintaining your hand position, gently slide the working-end beneath the gingival margin and onto the facial surface of the root.
- *Imagine the face of the working-end sliding along the facial surface, all the way to the base of the pocket.*[4]

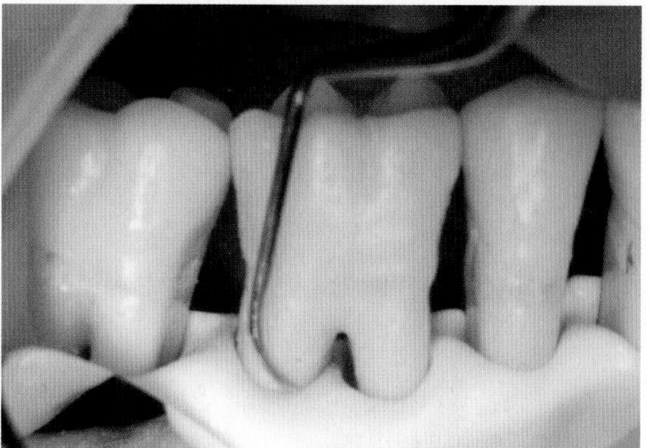

8. Figure 13-14. Return Fulcrum Finger and Handle to Upright Position.

- Return your fulcrum to the occlusofacial line angle of a nearby tooth as you reposition the handle to an upright position.[5]
- Reposition the lower shank so that the face-to-root surface angulation is about 40° in preparation for an assessment stroke.

Section 3

Production of a Calculus Removal Stroke

ANGULATION FOR CALCULUS REMOVAL

1. Angulation during Assessment of the Tooth Surface

a. Once a curet is inserted to the base of a periodontal pocket, it is used with an assessment stroke to detect calculus deposits on the root surface. Assessment strokes are made in a direction that is away from the junctional epithelium.

b. For assessment strokes, the face-to-tooth surface angulation is approximately 40°.

2. Angulation for Calculus Removal

a. *For calculus removal, the face-to-tooth surface angulation is an angle between 45° and 90°.*

b. The ideal angulation for calculus removal is between 70° and 80°. Figure 13-15 depicts the correct angulation for calculus removal.

3. Angulation for Root Debridement

a. Root debridement strokes are used to remove subgingival plaque biofilm, residual calculus deposits, or surface irregularities from the root surface.

b. The goal of root debridement strokes is to preserve as much cementum as possible during instrumentation.
   1. Thus, an angulation used is designed to produce a less aggressive stroke than that used for calculus removal.
   2. *The face-to-root surface angulation for root debridement is an angle between 60° and 70°.*

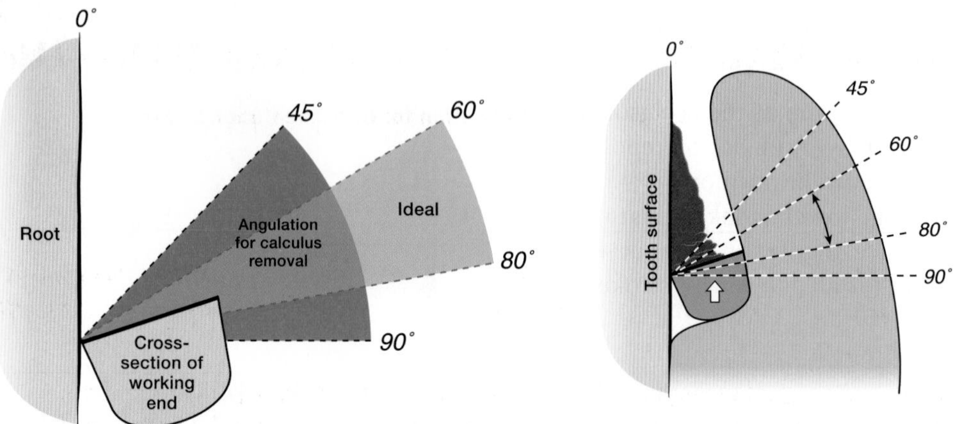

Figure 13-15. Angulation of the Working-End for Calculus Removal. For calculus removal, the face-to-tooth surface angulation should be an angle between 45° and 90°.

- The **correct** *face-to-tooth surface angulation* is greater than 45° and less than 90°.
- Correct angulation allows the cutting edge to bite into the calculus deposit and fracture it from the tooth surface without injuring the soft tissue lining of the periodontal pocket.
- Note that the working-end is positioned apical to (beneath) the calculus deposit.

STABILIZATION AND LATERAL PRESSURE FOR CALCULUS REMOVAL

Two elements used during the production of an instrumentation stroke are stabilization and lateral pressure.

1. Stabilization is the act of preparing for an instrumentation stroke by locking the joints of the ring finger and pressing the fingertip against a tooth surface to provide control for the instrumentation stroke.
    - **a.** Stabilization allows the hand and instrument to function as a unit.
    - **b.** Stabilization provides the control necessary for an effective instrumentation stroke.
2. Lateral pressure is the act of applying equal pressure with the index finger and thumb inward against the instrument handle to press the working-end against a calculus deposit or tooth surface prior to and throughout an instrumentation stroke.

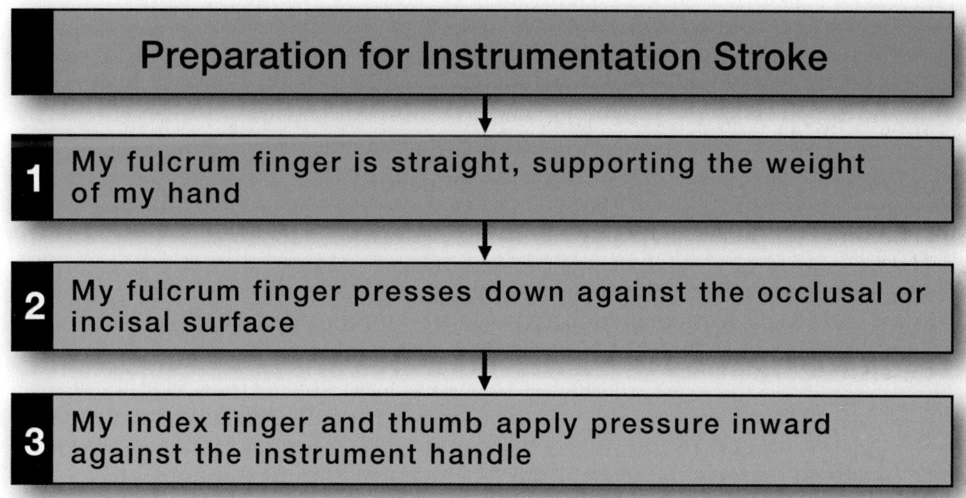

Preparation for Instrumentation Stroke
1 My fulcrum finger is straight, supporting the weight of my hand
2 My fulcrum finger presses down against the occlusal or incisal surface
3 My index finger and thumb apply pressure inward against the instrument handle

Figure 13-16. Flow Chart: Preparation for Instrumentation Stroke.

PREPARATION FOR AN INSTRUMENTATION STROKE

A combination of stabilization and lateral pressure is used to produce a stroke that is at once effective and controlled, yet comfortable for the patient (Fig. 13-16). This combination is accomplished by using these steps:

1. **Stabilizing the Fulcrum Finger.** This is accomplished by locking the joints of the fulcrum finger so that the finger can function as a "support beam" for the hand during the instrumentation stroke.
2. **Stabilizing the Hand and Instrument**
    - **a.** This is accomplished by pressing the tip of the fulcrum finger against the tooth surface.
    - **b.** The extent of the pressure against the tooth ranges from light to firm depending on the type of stroke used.
    - **c.** If the working-end flies off the tooth at the end of a stroke, the clinician is not pressing down against the tooth with the fulcrum finger as the stroke is completed.

3. **Lateral Pressure against the Tooth Surface**
   a. Lateral pressure against the tooth surface is created by applying pressure with the *index finger and thumb* inward against the instrument handle prior to and throughout the instrumentation stroke.
   b. Both fingers must apply pressure equally against the handle or the instrument will be difficult to control.

LATERAL PRESSURE

1. **The Task Determines the Amount of Lateral Pressure**
   a. The instrument classification and instrumentation task determine the amount of lateral pressure needed during instrumentation.
      1. Assessment—requires a feather-light touch against the tooth surface.
      2. Calculus removal—requires firm lateral pressure against the tooth surface.
      3. Root debridement—requires less lateral pressure than a calculus removal stroke.
   b. More pressure applied against the handle and by the fulcrum finger against the tooth results in more pressure against the tooth surface or calculus deposit. Lateral pressure against the tooth surface will range from light to firm; however, heavy pressure is never recommended.
2. **Lateral Pressure and Adaptation during Calculus Removal**
   a. Effective calculus removal depends on a combination of (1) firm lateral pressure and (2) correct angulation. With ideal lateral pressure and angulation, a calculus deposit is fractured from the tooth surface.
   b. Inadequate lateral pressure and/or incorrect angulation result in incomplete calculus removal.
3. **Absence of Lateral Pressure between Strokes.** The techniques of stabilization and lateral pressure are used only (1) immediately prior to beginning a calculus removal stroke and (2) during the production of a calculus removal stroke.
   a. *The finger muscles should be relaxed between strokes and when returning the working-end to the base of the sulcus or pocket after completing a stroke.*
   b. Maintaining constant pressure with the fulcrum finger or when grasping the handle is very stressful to the muscles of the hand and wrist.

STEPS FOR A CALCULUS REMOVAL STROKE

Many fine psychomotor skills are involved in the production of a calculus removal stroke. Figures 13-17 to 13-21 detail the process of initiating, making, and finishing a calculus removal stroke.

A calculus removal stroke involves these steps:

1. **Assess.** Employ an assessment stroke away from the junctional epithelium until a calculus deposit is encountered.
2. **Cup.** Cup the calculus deposit with the face of the curet (Fig. 13-17).
3. **Stroke.** Create a calculus removal stroke by: (a) locking the toe-third against the tooth surface, (b) opening the face to the correct 70° to 80° angulation, while (c) making a short, biting stroke away from the base of the pocket (Fig. 13-18).

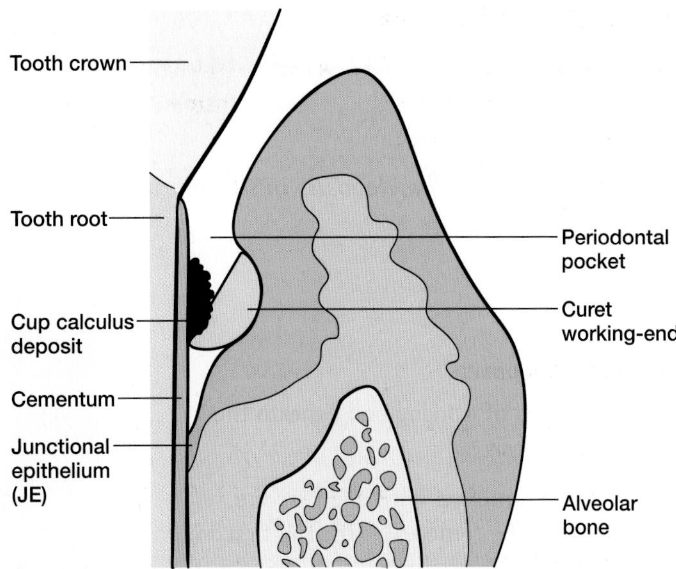

Figure 13-17. Step 1: Assess and Cup the Deposit.

- After inserting a curet to the base of the pocket, employ a light assessment stroke over the root surface until encountering a calculus deposit.
- Size up the calculus deposit with an assessment stroke to determine its size and dimensions.
- Position the curet working-end apical to (beneath) the deposit.
- Cup the deposit with the face of the curet.

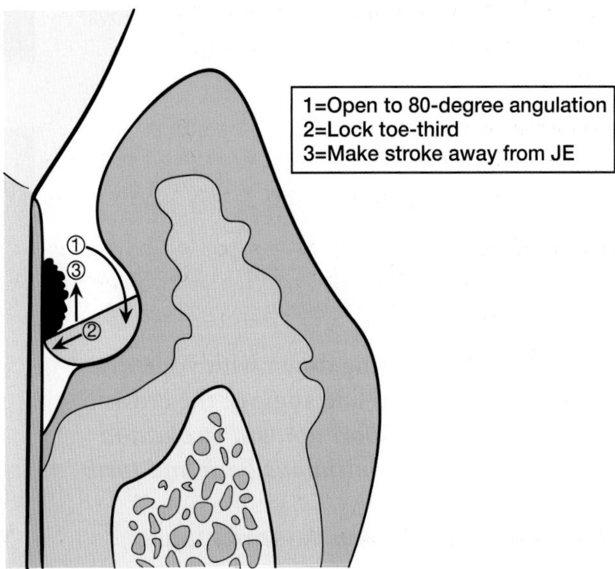

Figure 13-18. Step 2: Stroke.

Reassess your grasp to assure that your fingers are precisely positioned in the grasp and that the fulcrum is straight, supporting your hand.
(1) Prepare for a calculus removal stroke by locking the toe-third against the tooth surface. (2) Activate a stroke by opening the face to a 70° to 80° angulation (3) while making a short, biting stroke away from the base of the pocket. JE, junctional epithelium.

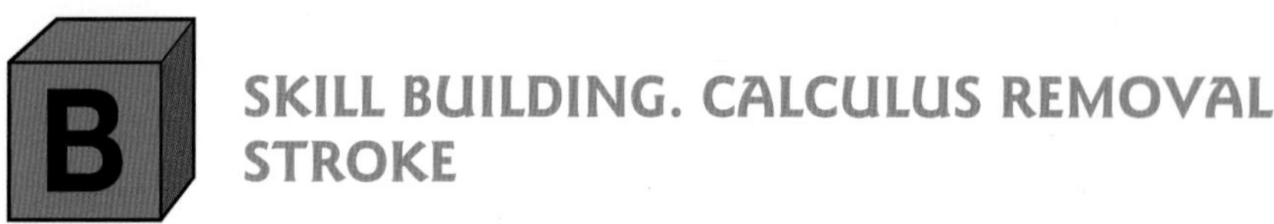

SKILL BUILDING. CALCULUS REMOVAL STROKE

A series of colored dots represent the calculus deposits in the photos below (Figs. 13-19 and 13-20.)

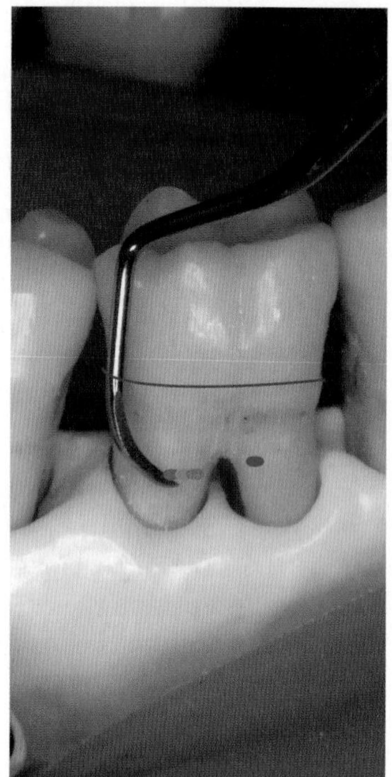

Figure 13-19. Remove a Calculus Deposit.

Step 1: Position. Position the toe-third of working-end beneath the distal-most portion of the calculus deposit.

- Only a portion of the deposit is removed with each stroke.
- In this case, the magenta dot will be removed with the first stroke. Cup the deposit with the working-end.

Step 2: Lock On and Activate.

- "Lock" the toe-third of the working-end against the facial surface of the root.
- *Activate a stroke by opening the face to a 70° to 80° angulation while making a short, biting stroke away from the base of the pocket.*
- Keep the toe-third locked against the facial surface throughout the short, biting stroke.

Step 3: Make a Single Calculus Removal Stroke. Each calculus removal stroke should be a short, biting stroke to lift the deposit from the tooth.

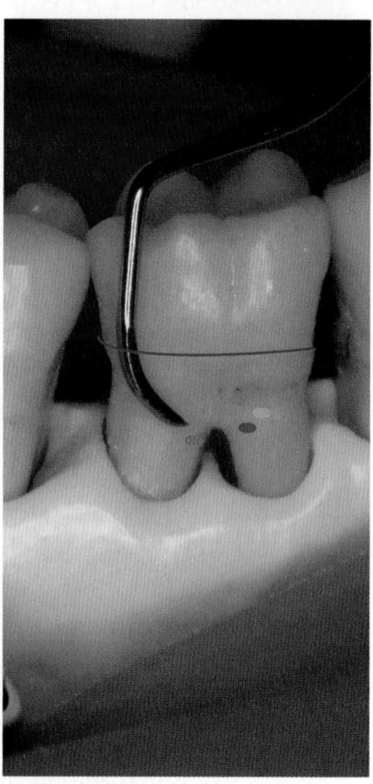

Figure 13-20. End Stroke and Relax.

- End each stroke with precision, by pressing down with your fulcrum finger against the occlusolingual line angle of the crown.
- *Each stroke is distinct; make only one short upward stroke and then pause. Do NOT make a series of continuous back and forth strokes.*
- *Make a single calculus removal stroke, stop the stroke, and immediately relax your fingers in the grasp.*
- Pause for at least 3 seconds after each stroke to prevent strain to the muscles of your hand. To assure that you take time to relax between strokes, stop and silently think: "1-one thousand, 2-one thousand, 3-one thousand."
- The next step is to position the toe-third of the working-end beneath the green dot. Remove the green "deposit" and continue with the blue dot.

FLOW CHART: SEQUENCE FOR CALCULUS REMOVAL STROKE

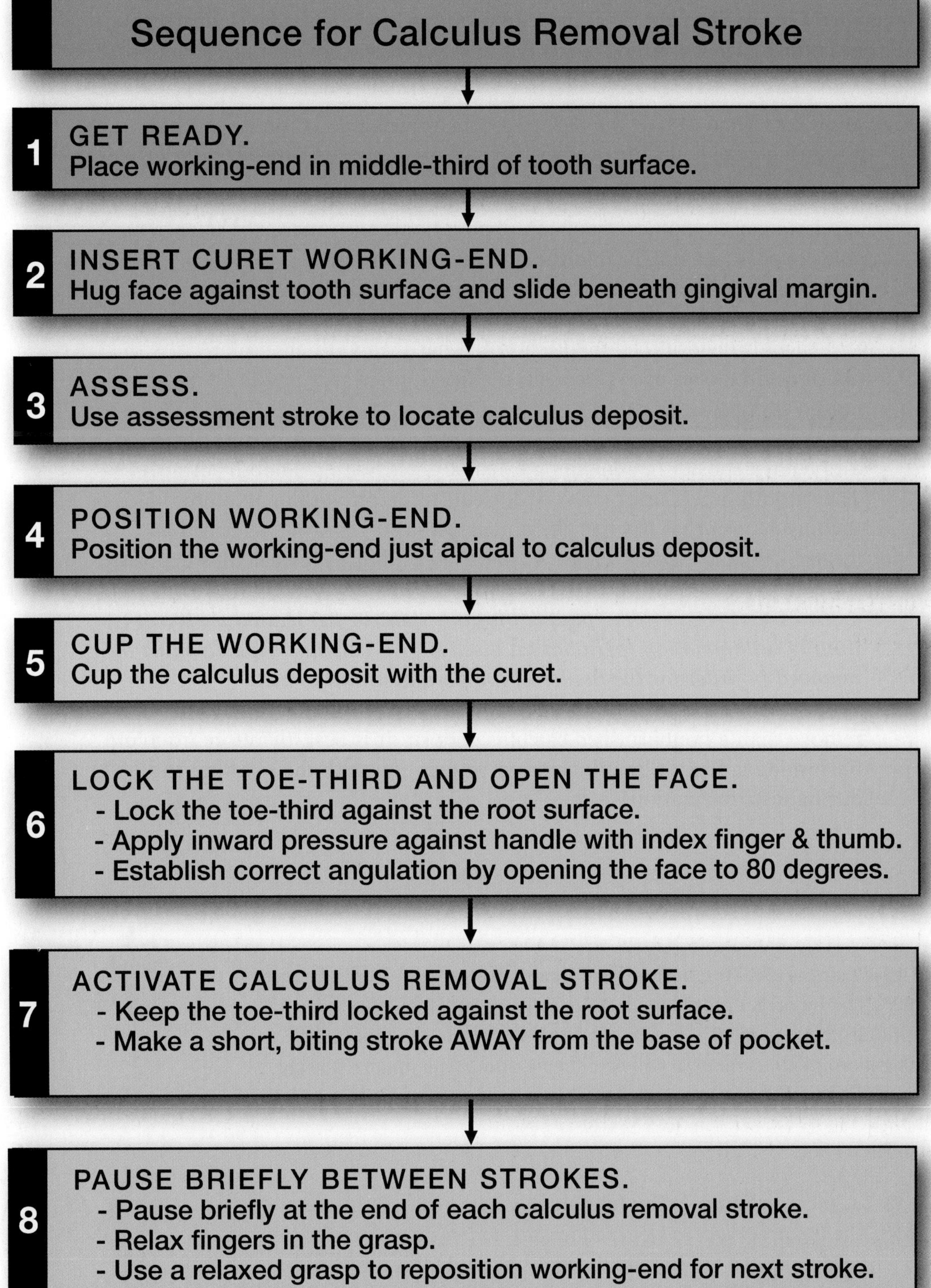

Sequence for Calculus Removal Stroke
1
GET READY.
Place working-end in middle-third of tooth surface.
2
INSERT CURET WORKING-END.
Hug face against tooth surface and slide beneath gingival margin.
3
ASSESS.
Use assessment stroke to locate calculus deposit.
4
POSITION WORKING-END.
Position the working-end just apical to calculus deposit.
5
CUP THE WORKING-END.
Cup the calculus deposit with the curet.
6
LOCK THE TOE-THIRD AND OPEN THE FACE.
- Lock the toe-third against the root surface.
- Apply inward pressure against handle with index finger & thumb.
- Establish correct angulation by opening the face to 80 degrees.
7
ACTIVATE CALCULUS REMOVAL STROKE.
- Keep the toe-third locked against the root surface.
- Make a short, biting stroke AWAY from the base of pocket.
8
PAUSE BRIEFLY BETWEEN STROKES.
- Pause briefly at the end of each calculus removal stroke.
- Relax fingers in the grasp.
- Use a relaxed grasp to reposition working-end for next stroke.

Figure 13-21. Flow Chart Showing Sequence for Calculus Removal.

ANGULATION ERRORS THAT RESULT IN TISSUE INJURY OR BURNISHING

Incorrect angulation of the working-end to the tooth surface is a technique error that results in negative consequences during patient treatment.

1. **Angulation Greater Than 90°.** If the face-to-tooth surface angulation is greater than 90°, one cutting edge will be in contact with the soft tissue lining of the periodontal pocket, injuring the tissue. Figure 13-22 illustrates this technique error.
2. **Angulation Less Than 45°.** If the face-to-tooth surface angulation is less than 45°, the cutting edge will slide over the surface of a calculus deposit, rather than biting into it. This technique error is shown in Figure 13-23.
   a. Incorrect angulation of less than 45° removes only the outermost layer of a calculus deposit, leaving behind the bulk of the deposit.
      1. Calculus deposits form over time in irregular layers, so ordinarily, the outermost layer is rough and jagged. It is the rough characteristic of the calculus deposit that enables it to be detected with an explorer. As the explorer tip moves over a deposit, the tip vibrates as it passes across the jagged surface.
      2. When incorrect technique results in the removal of the outermost layer of a calculus deposit, the remaining calculus is left with a smooth surface. The smooth outer surface is very difficult to detect with an explorer.

   b. A calculus deposit that has had the outermost layer removed is termed a burnished calculus deposit. Figure 13-24 shows a burnished calculus deposit.
      1. ***All calculus deposits, including burnished deposits, are highly porous formations that retain living plaque biofilms that are associated with continuing inflammation (periodontal disease). All calculus deposits must be removed in order for the tissues of the periodontium to heal.***[6,7]
      2. A burnished deposit, with its smooth outer layer, is much more difficult to remove than a nonburnished calculus deposit. It is best, therefore, to avoid burnishing a deposit by using correct angulation with the working-end during instrumentation.

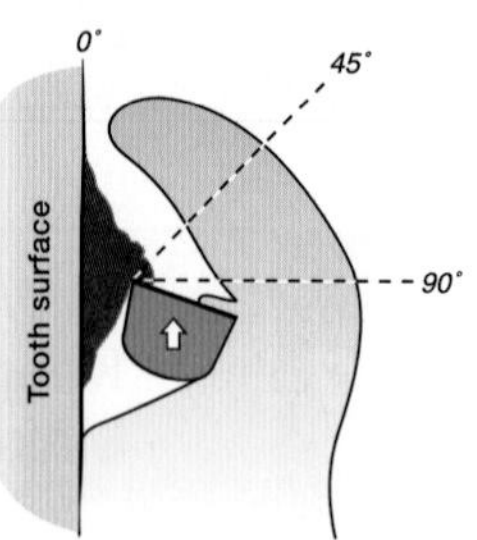

Figure 13-22. Incorrect Angulation for Calculus Removal—Angle Greater Than 90°. The **incorrect** *face-to-tooth surface angulation* shown in this illustration is greater than 90°. The face is tilted away from the root surface. In this position, calculus removal will be difficult, and tissue trauma is likely.

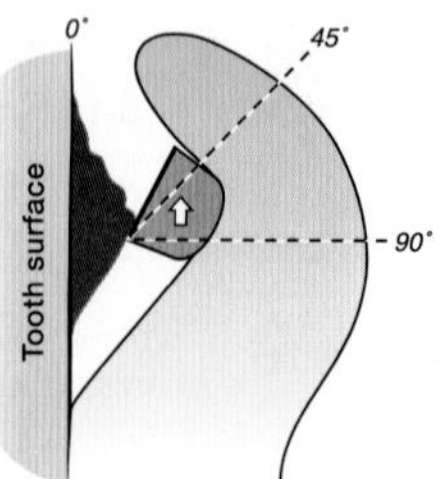

Figure 13-23. Incorrect Angulation for Calculus Removal—Angle Less Than 45°. The **incorrect** *face-to-tooth surface angulation* shown here is less than 45°. The face is tilted too close to the root surface. In this position, the cutting edge cannot bite into the deposit; instead, the face slips over the calculus deposit.

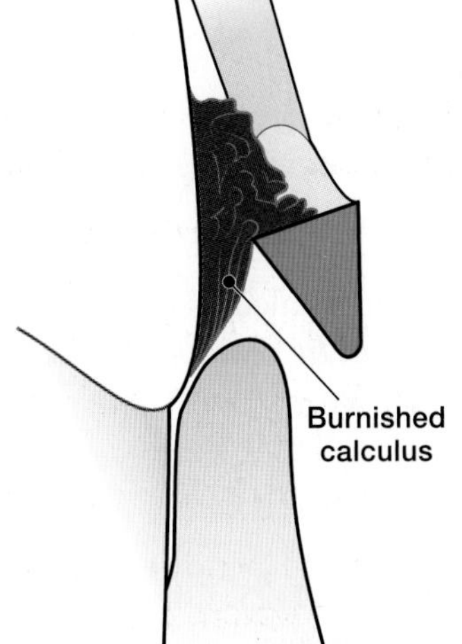

Figure 13-24. Incorrect Technique: Remove Outer Layer.

- The deposit *should not be removed in layers* since removing the outermost layer will leave the deposit with a smooth surface.
- A calculus deposit that has had the outermost layer removed is referred to as a burnished deposit.
- Burnished calculus is difficult to remove because the cutting edge tends to slip over the smooth surface of the deposit.

TABLE 13-1. Reference Sheet: Angulation with Hand-Activated Instruments

	Assessment Stroke	Calculus Removal Stroke	Root Debridement Stroke
Purpose	To assess tooth anatomy; to detect calculus and other plaque-retentive factors	To lift calculus deposits off of the tooth surface	To remove residual calculus; to disrupt bacterial plaque from root surfaces within deep periodontal pockets
Used with	Probes, explorers, curets	Sickle scalers, curets, files	Curets
Face-to-tooth surface angulation	Approximately 40°	70°–80°	60°–70°

Section 4
Stroke Pattern for Calculus Removal

PATTERN FOR REMOVING LARGE SUPRAGINGIVAL DEPOSITS

Often a calculus deposit will be too large to be removed as a single piece. ***Large calculus deposits should be removed in sections using a series of short, firm instrumentation strokes*** (Fig. 13-25).

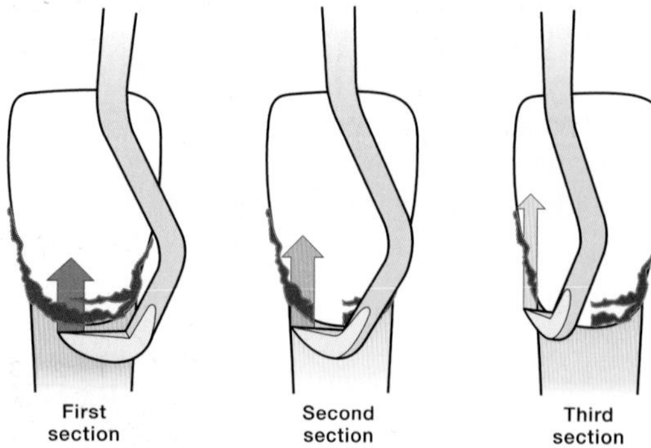

Figure 13-25. Correct Technique: Remove Deposit in Sections.

- Large calculus deposits should be removed in sections.
- Use a series of calculus removal strokes to remove the deposit one section at a time.

PATTERN FOR LOCATING AND REMOVING SUBGINGIVAL DEPOSITS

Locating and removing subgingival calculus deposits is a challenging task because the clinician is working beneath the gingival margin and cannot see the calculus deposits or root surface. For this reason, the clinician must adopt a very systematic pattern of instrumentation strokes. A haphazard stroke pattern will result in missed calculus deposits and unsuccessful treatment of the root surface.

1. **Use Systematic Approach**
   - **a.** It is helpful to think of the root surface as being divided into a series of long narrow instrumentation zones.
   - **b.** ***Each instrumentation zone is only as wide as the toe-third of the instrument's cutting edge.***
2. **Use of Instrumentation Zones for Calculus Removal.** The surface of the root is divided into a pattern of instrumentation zones for the systematic removal of calculus deposits (Fig. 13-26). The steps in employing calculus removal strokes in a series of narrow tracts are as follows:
   - **a.** Begin in "instrumentation zone 1."
     1. Use an assessment stroke with a curet to locate the calculus deposit closest to the soft tissue base of the periodontal pocket.
     2. Calculus deposits adjacent to the junctional epithelium are removed first; those near the gingival margin are removed last.
   - **b.** Place the curet working-end beneath a deposit in zone 1.
     1. Use a tiny calculus removal stroke to snap the entire deposit or a section of a deposit from the root surface.
     2. Reassess the area with the curet using a relaxed assessment stroke.
   - **c.** Continue working in a coronal direction until all deposits in zone 1 have been removed. Figure 13-26 depicts the technique of using instrumentation zones for subgingival calculus removal.

d. Once you have completed zone 1, repeat the process in zone 2. Continue instrumenting each narrow zone in a similar manner until all zones on this aspect of the tooth have been completed.

3. Planning a Calculus Removal Appointment

In planning a calculus removal appointment, the clinician should plan to treat only those tooth surfaces from which the calculus deposits can be completely removed. ***All calculus deposits should be definitely removed from one tooth before starting instrumentation on a second tooth.*** As many calculus removal appointments as needed should be scheduled to treat the entire dentition. Partial calculus removal from a tooth is not recommended. Planning for calculus removal is discussed in detail in Module 21, Calculus Removal: Concepts, Planning, and Patient Cases.

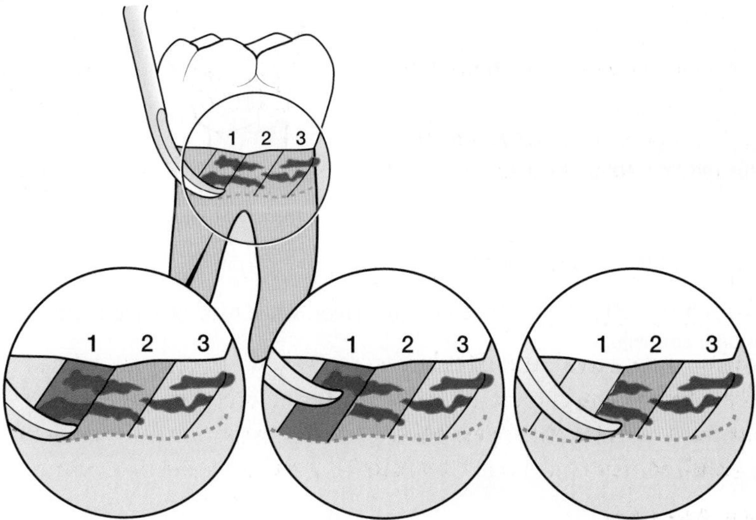

Figure 13-26. Instrumentation Zones for Subgingival Calculus Removal. The root surface is divided into a pattern of instrumentation zones or tracts for the systematic removal of calculus deposits located beneath the gingival tissues. First, all deposits are removed from zone 1, then zone 2, and so on, until all zones are completed.

REFERENCES

1. Rucker LM, Gibson G, McGregor C. Getting the "feel" of it: the non-visual component of dimensional accuracy during operative tooth preparation. *J Can Dent Assoc.* 1990;56:937–941.
2. Hauser AM, Bowen DM. Primer on preclinical instruction and evaluation. *J Dent Educ.* 2009;73:390–398.
3. Dufour LA, Bissell HS. Periodontal attachment loss induced by mechanical subgingival instrumentation in shallow sulci. *J Dent Hyg.* 2002;76:207–212.
4. Ruhling A, Konig J, Rolf H, Kocher T, Schwahn C, Plagmann HC. Learning root debridement with curettes and power-driven instruments. Part II: clinical results following mechanical, non-surgical therapy. *J Clin Periodontol.* 2003;30:611–615.
5. Dong H, Barr A, Loomer P, Rempel D. The effects of finger rest positions on hand muscle load and pinch force in simulated dental hygiene work. *J Dent Educ.* 2005;69:453–460.
6. Stambaugh R. Perioscopy—the new paradigm. *Dimen Dent Hyg.* 2003;1:12–15.
7. Stambaugh RV. A clinician's 3-year experience with perioscopy. *Compend Contin Educ Dent.* 2002;23:1061–1070.

Section 5
Skill Application

STUDENT SELF-EVALUATION MODULE 13 ANGULATION AND CALCULUS REMOVAL

Student: ______________________

Date: ______________________

DIRECTIONS: Self-evaluate your skill level in each treatment area as: **S** (satisfactory) or **U** (unsatisfactory).

Criteria	
Insertion and Calculus Removal Stroke with a Universal Curet	**Area 1**
Positions the working-end in the "Get Ready Zone"	
Inserts the working-end beneath the gingival margin to the soft tissue base of the pocket	
Positions the working-end beneath a calculus deposit with the face cupping the deposit	
Self-assesses grasp for precise finger placement and that fulcrum finger is straight, supporting hand	
Locks the toe-third of the cutting edge against the root surface	
Activates a stroke by opening the face to a 70° to 80° angulation while making a short, biting stroke away from the junctional epithelium	
Precisely stops the stroke and pauses for 3 seconds to relax grasp between strokes	
Insertion and Root Debridement Stroke with an Area-Specific Curet	**Area 1**
Positions the working-end in the "Get Ready Zone"	
Inserts the working-end beneath the gingival margin to the soft tissue base of the pocket	
Self-assesses grasp for precise finger placement and that fulcrum finger is straight, supporting hand	
Activates a stroke by opening the face to a 60° angulation while making a light, shaving stroke away from the junctional epithelium	
Precisely stops the stroke and pauses for 3 seconds to relax grasp between strokes	

Note to Course Instructors: Following this module, there are separate modules devoted to each instrument design classification. Each of these modules provides step-by-step instructions for instrument use and does not rely on the content from any previous instrument module. ***This module structure means that the instrument modules can be covered in any order that you prefer.*** In addition, it is not necessary to include all modules. For example, if sickle scalers are not part of your school's instrument kit, this module does not need to be included in the course.

Module 14

Sickle Scalers

Module Overvie

This module presents [illegible] r sickle scalers and step-by-ste[illegible] nedium-sized or heavy calculus depo[illegible] e 13—Technique Essentials: A[illegible] npleted prior to beginning this n[illegible]

Module Outline

Online Content

A video on the use of a sickle scaler can be viewed at http://thepoint.lww.com/GehrigFundamentals7e

Key Terms

Sickle scaler
Anterior sickle scaler
Posterior sickle scaler
Outer cutting edge
Inner cutting edge

Learning Objectives

1. Given a variety of sickle scaler instruments, identify the design characteristics.
2. List the uses and limitations of sickle scalers.
3. List characteristics of a calculus removal stroke.
4. List from memory the sequence of steps used for calculus removal as outlined in Figure 14-3.
5. Given a posterior sickle scaler, demonstrate how to use visual clues to identify the correct working-end.
6. Demonstrate correct adaptation and angulation of a sickle scaler.
7. Explain why the lower shank of a sickle scaler should be tilted slightly toward the tooth surface being instrumented to obtain correct angulation.
8. Demonstrate correct use of a sickle scaler in the anterior sextants while maintaining correct position, correct finger rests, and precise finger placement in the grasp.

Note to Course Instructor: There is a separate module devoted to each design classification (sickle scalers, universal curets, area-specific curets, periodontal files) and modules covering advanced probing techniques and advanced root instrumentation. Each module provides step-by-step instructions for instrument use and does not rely on the content from any previous instrument module. ***This module structure means that the instrument modules can be covered in any order that you prefer.*** In addition, it is not necessary to include all modules. For example, if sickle scalers are not part of your school's instrument kit, this module does not need to be included in the course.

Section 1
Sickle Scalers

GENERAL DESIGN CHARACTERISTICS

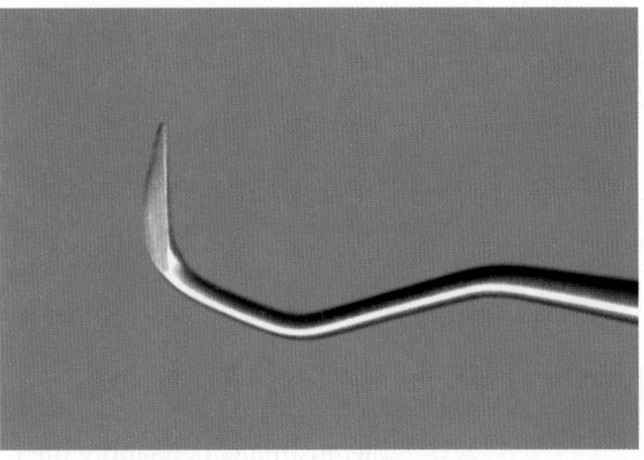

Figure 14-1. Sickle Scaler. The working-end of a sickle scaler.

1. Functions of Sickle Scalers

a. A sickle scaler is a periodontal instrument used to remove calculus deposits from the crowns of the teeth (Figs. 14-1 and 14-2).
b. Sickle scalers are limited to use on enamel surfaces and should NOT be used on root surfaces.

2. Design Characteristics of Sickle Scalers

a. Working-End Design. The working-end of a sickle scaler has several unique design characteristics (Table 14-1).
1. A **pointed back**; some newer sickle scaler designs have working-ends with rounded backs
2. A **pointed tip**
3. A **triangular cross section**
4. **Two cutting edges** per working-end
5. The **face is perpendicular** to the lower shank

b. Anterior and Posterior Instrument Designs
1. Anterior sickle scalers are limited to use on anterior treatment sextants.
   a) Often, they are single-ended instruments because only one working-end is needed to instrument the crowns of the anterior teeth.
   b) It is common, however, to combine two different anterior sickles on a double-ended instrument.
2. Posterior sickle scalers are designed for use on posterior sextants, but they also may be used on anterior teeth.
   a) Usually, two posterior sickles are paired on a double-ended instrument (the working-ends are mirror images of one another).
   b) For example, the Jacquette 34 is paired with the Jacquette 35 (the working-end of the Jacquette 34 is a mirror image of the working-end of the Jacquette 35).

3. Examples of Sickle Scaler Instruments

- **a.** Anterior sickle scalers—OD-1, Jacquette 30, Jacquette 33, Nevi 1, Whiteside-2, USC-128, Towner-U15, Goldman-H6, and Goldman-H7
- **b.** Posterior sickle scalers—Jacquette 34/35, Jacquette 14/15, Jacquette 31/32, Nevi 2, Ball 2/3, Mecca 11/12, and the Catatonia 107/108

WORKING-END DESIGN

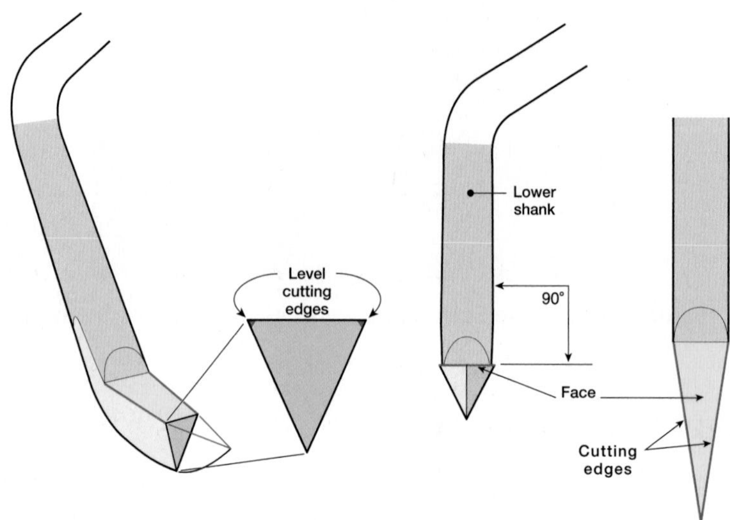

Figure 14-2. Design Characteristics of Sickle Scalers.

TABLE 14-1. Design Characteristics of the Sickle Scaler	
Cross section	Triangular cross section; this design limits use to above the gingival margin because the pointed tip and back could cause tissue trauma
Working-end	Pointed back and tip Two cutting edges per working-end
Face	Face is perpendicular to the lower shank so that cutting edges are level with one another; ***level cutting edges mean that the lower shank must be tilted slightly toward the tooth surface to establish correct angulation***
Application	Anterior teeth—only one single-ended instrument is needed Posterior teeth—one double-ended instrument is needed
Primary functions	Removal of medium- to large-sized calculus deposits Excellent for calculus removal on the (1) proximal surfaces of anterior crowns and (2) enamel surfaces apical to the contact areas of posterior teeth ***Debridement of enamel surfaces; NOT recommended for use on root surfaces***

INNOVATIONS IN SICKLE SCALER DESIGN

Instrument manufacturers are continuously striving to introduce instruments that are more ergonomic in design and efficient at calculus removal. One of the most recent innovations in sickle scaler design is the Nevi series of instruments (Table 14-2).

TABLE 14-2. Nevi Series of Sickle Scalers

Instrument	Characteristics
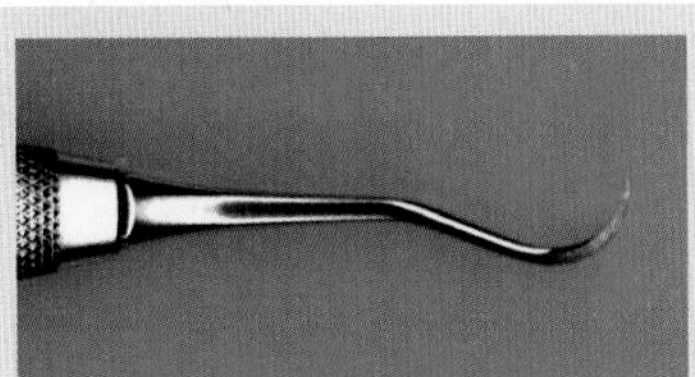 **Nevi 1: Sickle End**	• Sickle-end of the Nevi 1 instrument • Rigid shank • Small, thin sickle • Use on coronal surfaces of anterior teeth
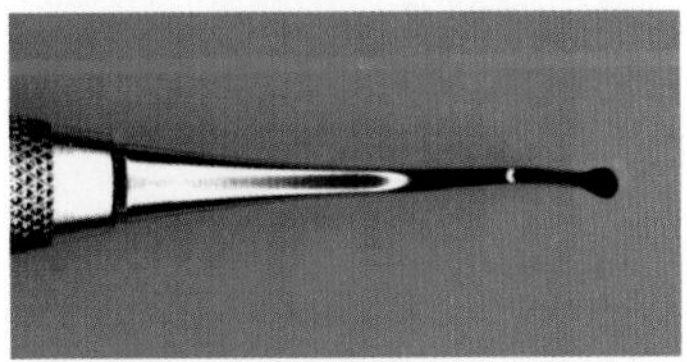 **Nevi 1: Disk End**	• Disk-end of the Nevi 1 instrument • All surfaces are sharp on the disk-end • ***Supra***gingival use on lingual surfaces of anterior teeth
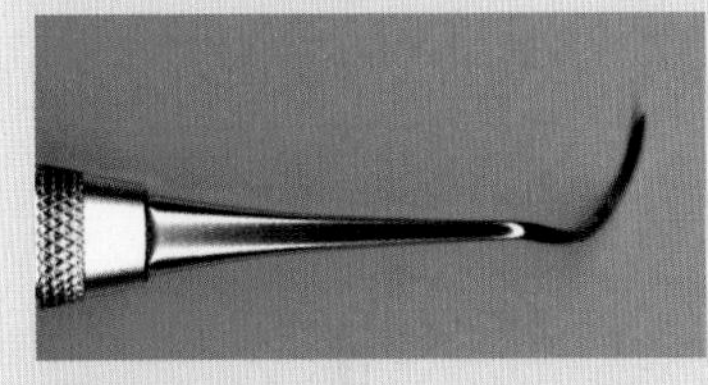 **Nevi 2**	• Paired, mirror-image working-ends • Thin, curved sickles for use on posterior teeth • Long cutting edge facilitates access to proximal tooth surfaces • Use on coronal surfaces of posterior teeth
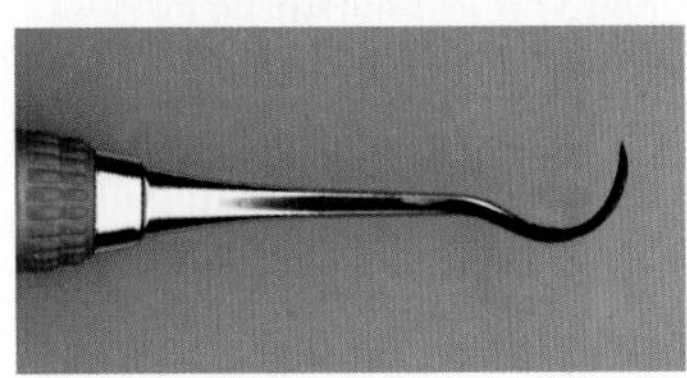 **Nevi 3**	• Paired, mirror-image working-ends • Thin, curved sickles for use on posterior teeth • Long cutting edge facilitates access to proximal tooth surfaces • Use on coronal surfaces of posterior teeth • Excellent for use on pediatric patients
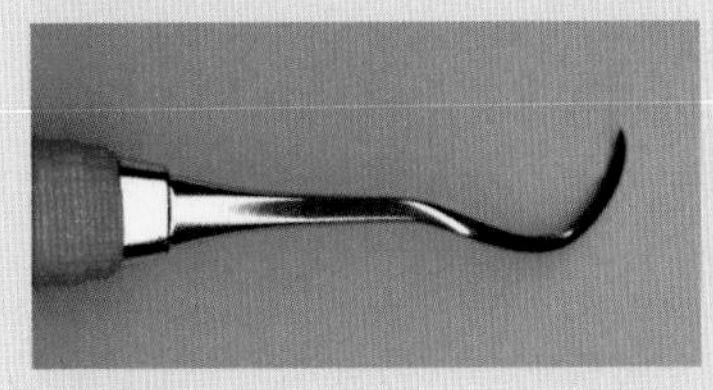 **Nevi 4**	• Paired, mirror-image working-ends • Strong, curved sickles for use on posterior teeth • Rigid working-end and shank • Removal of medium- or large-size deposits

Section 2
Calculus Removal Concepts

CHARACTERISTICS OF THE CALCULUS REMOVAL STROKE

Before beginning the step-by-step technique practice with sickle scalers, review the (1) characteristics of the calculus removal stroke and (2) steps for calculus removal. These concepts are the same for use of sickle scalers and universal curets, and area-specific curet (Table 14-3 and Fig. 14-3).

TABLE 14-3. The Calculus Removal Stroke with Sickle Scaler

Stabilization	Apply pressure with the index finger and thumb inward against the instrument handle and press the tip of the fulcrum finger against the tooth surface
Adaptation	Tip-third of cutting edge is adapted
Angulation	70°–80°; for sickle scalers, the lower shank must be tilted slightly toward the tooth surface to achieve correct angulation
Lateral pressure for calculus removal	Moderate to firm pressure against the tooth surface is maintained during the short, controlled calculus removal stroke made ***away from the soft tissue***
Characteristics	Controlled strokes, short in length
Stroke direction	Vertical strokes are most commonly used on anterior teeth and on the mesial and distal surfaces of posterior teeth Oblique strokes are most commonly used on the facial and lingual surfaces of posterior teeth Horizontal strokes are used at the line angles of posterior teeth and the midlines of the facial or lingual surfaces of anterior teeth
Stroke number	Strokes should be limited to areas where calculus is present; use the minimum number of strokes needed to remove calculus deposits

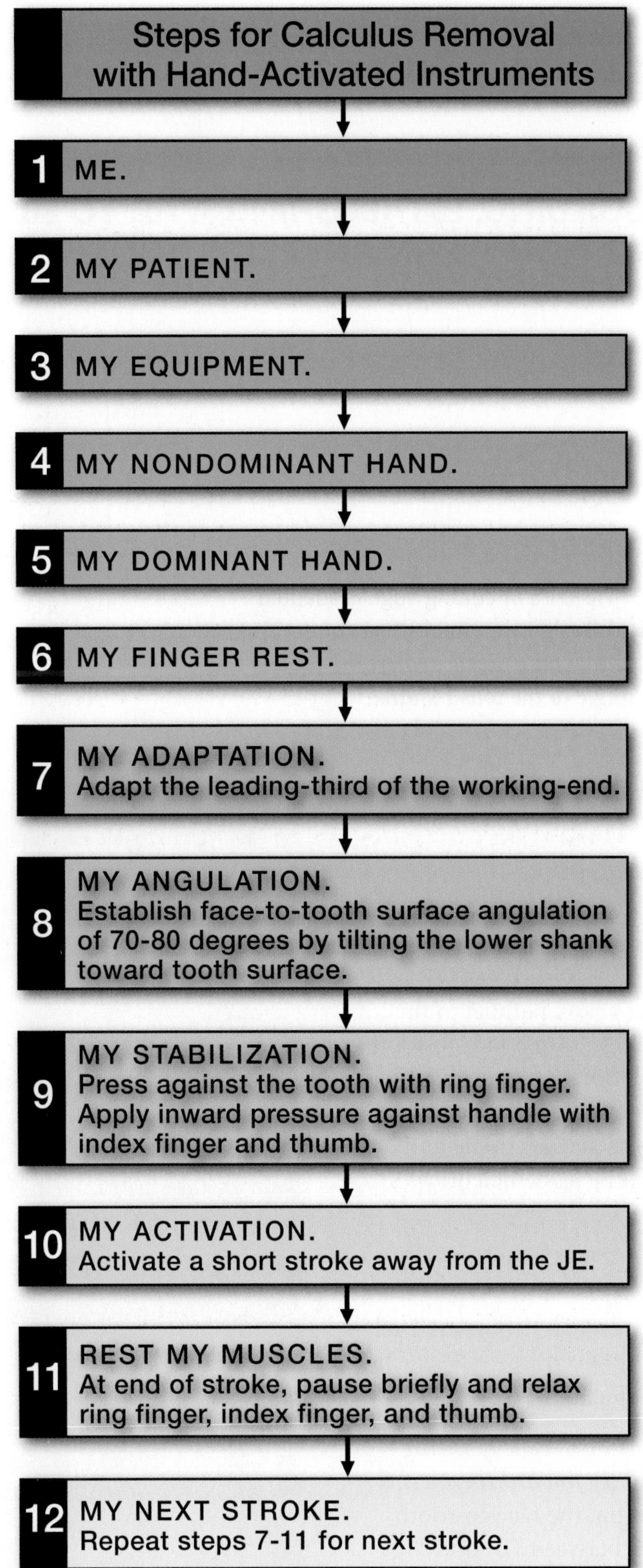

Figure 14-3. Flow Chart for Calculus Removal. (Key: JE = junctional epithelium.)

Section 3
Technique Practice—Anterior Teeth

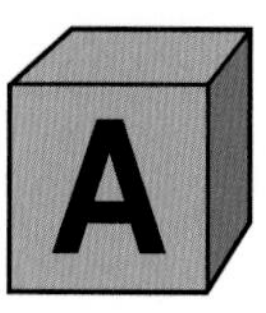

SKILL BUILDING. ESTABLISHING A 70° TO 80° ANGULATION TO AN ANTERIOR TOOTH

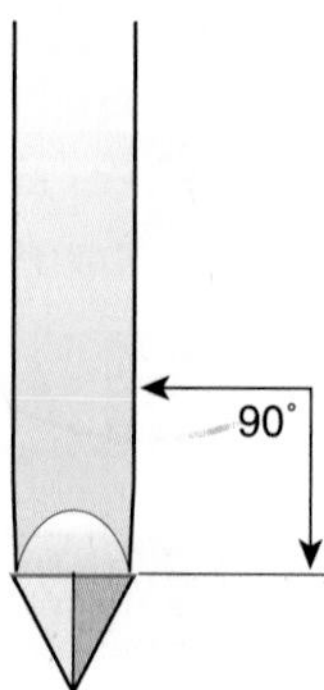

Figure 14-4. Working-End Design. In establishing correct angulation, it is important to remember that ***on a sickle scaler, the face of the working-end is at a 90° angle to the lower shank.***

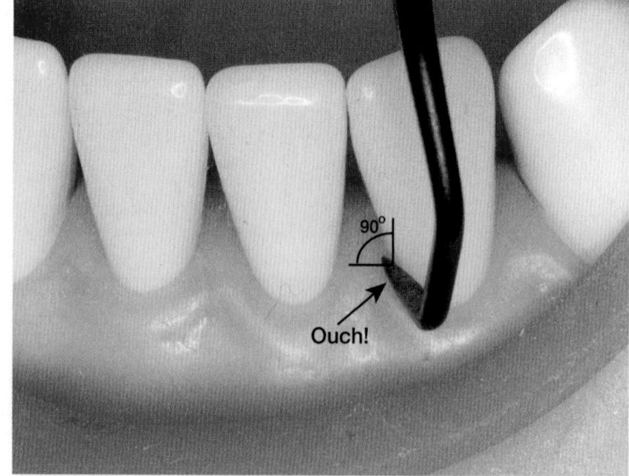

Figure 14-5. Incorrect Angulation.

- Positioning the lower shank parallel to the mesial tooth surface results in a face-to-tooth surface angulation of 90°.
- This angulation means that the other cutting edge could traumatize the soft tissue and calculus removal will be less efficient.

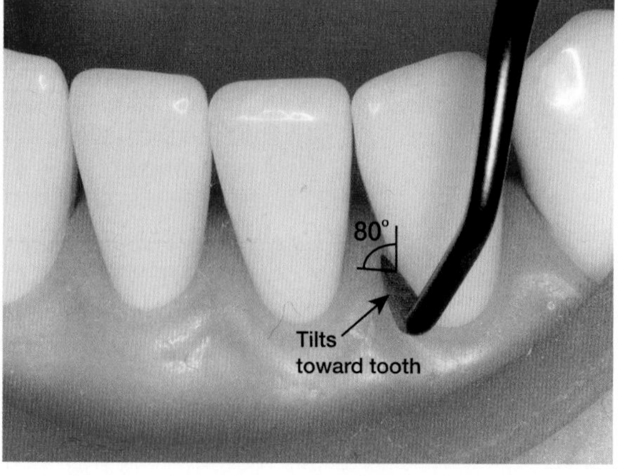

Figure 14-6. Correct Angulation.

- *Correct angulation is achieved by tilting the lower shank slightly toward the mesial surface.* In this position, the face-to-tooth surface angulation is between 70° and 80°.
- With this angulation, the other cutting edge tilts toward the mesial surface and away from the soft tissue.

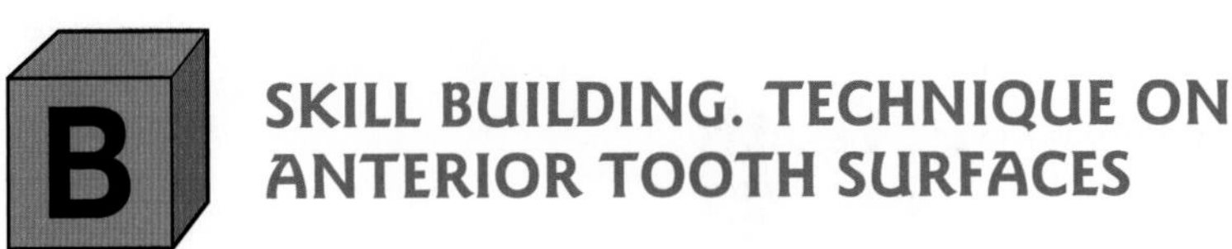

SKILL BUILDING. TECHNIQUE ON ANTERIOR TOOTH SURFACES

APPLICATION OF THE CUTTING EDGES

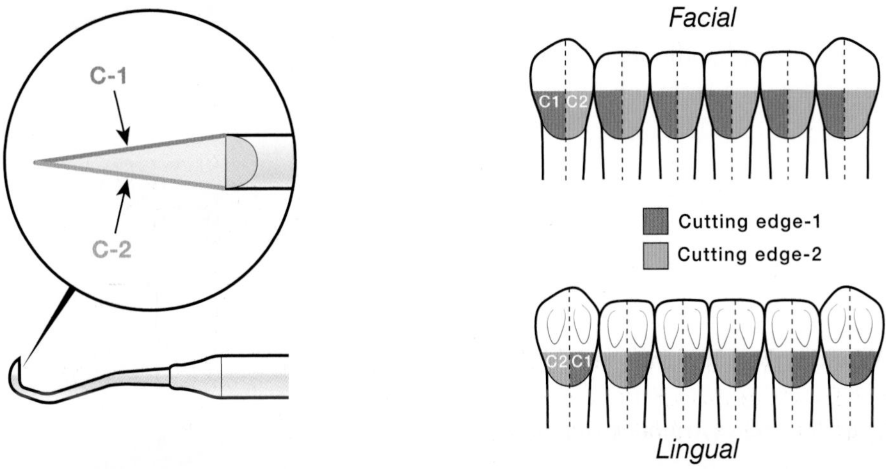

Figure 14-7. Application to Anterior Surfaces. The working-end of an anterior sickle has two cutting edges (C1 and C2). The illustration on the right indicates how the two cutting edges are applied to the tooth surfaces of the anterior teeth.

- Follow steps 1 to 9 to practice use of an anterior sickle scaler on the mandibular anterior teeth (Figs. 14-8 to 14-16).
- Remember: "Me, My patient, My light, My dominant hand, My nondominant hand, My finger rest, My adaptation."

1. **Figure 14-8. Tooth.** As an introduction to using a sickle scaler on the anterior teeth, first, practice on the ***mandibular left canine, facial aspect.***

   Right-Handed clinicians—*surface toward.*
   Left-Handed clinicians—*surface away.*

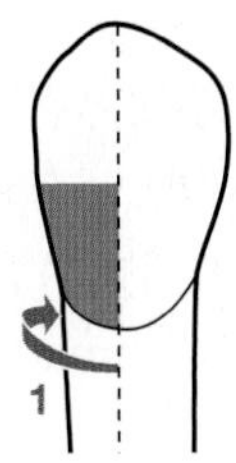

2. **Figure 14-9. Position Working-End Near the Midline.**
   - Establish a 70° to 80° instrument face-to-tooth surface angulation.
   - Aim the tip toward the mesial surface of the tooth.

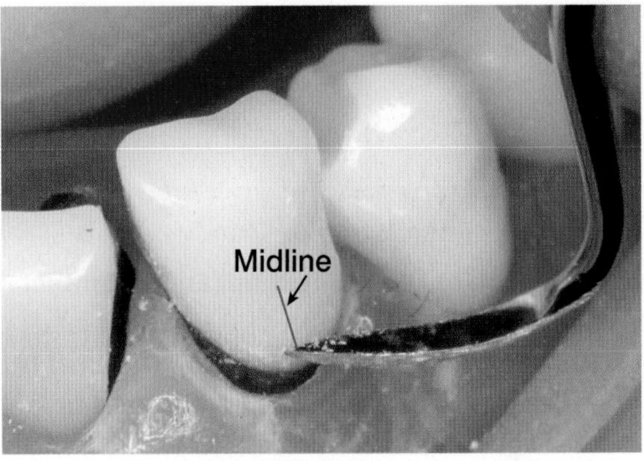

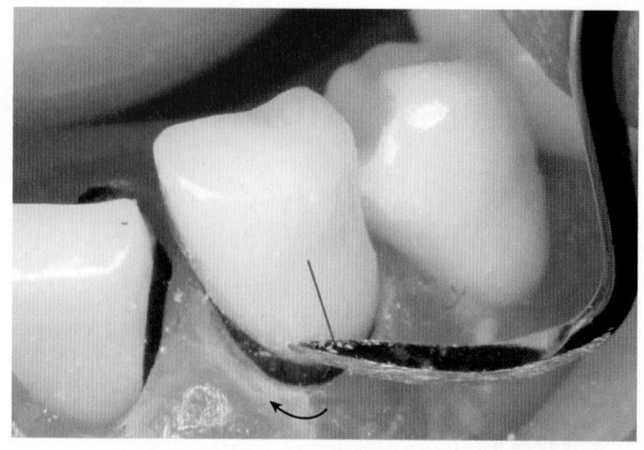

3. **Figure 14-10. Continue across the Facial Surface.**
   - Use overlapping strokes as you work across the facial surface in the direction of the mesial surface.
   - Roll the instrument handle slightly between strokes to maintain adaptation.

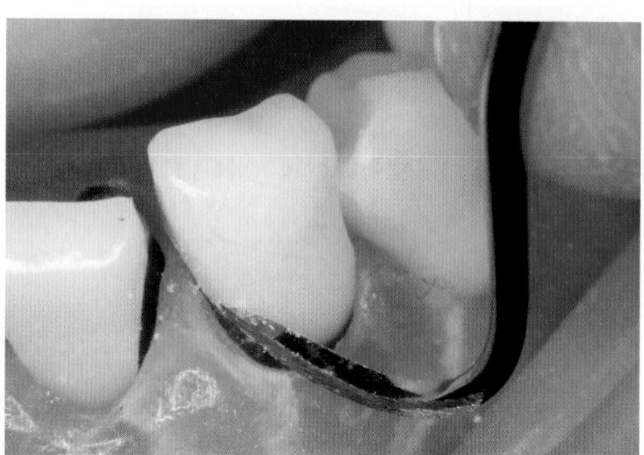

4. **Figure 14-11. Roll the Instrument Handle.** As you approach the mesiofacial line angle, roll the instrument handle to maintain adaptation of the tip-third of the working-end.

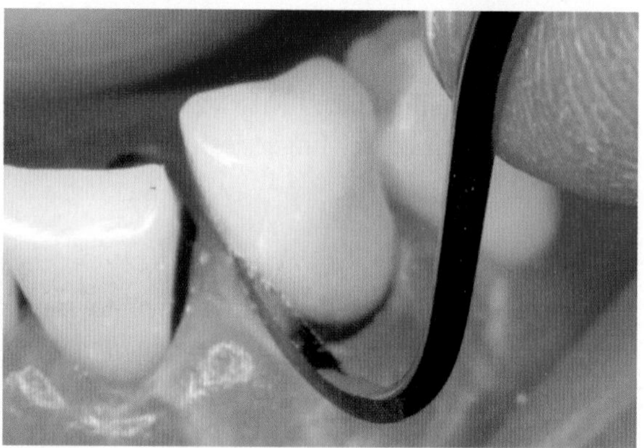

5. **Figure 14-12. Instrument the Mesial Surface.**
   - Check to make sure that you have maintained an angulation of 70° to 80°.
   - Technique check: Keep the tip-third of the cutting edge adapted to the mesial surface. Using the middle-third of the cutting edge might result in trauma to the tissue of the interdental papilla.

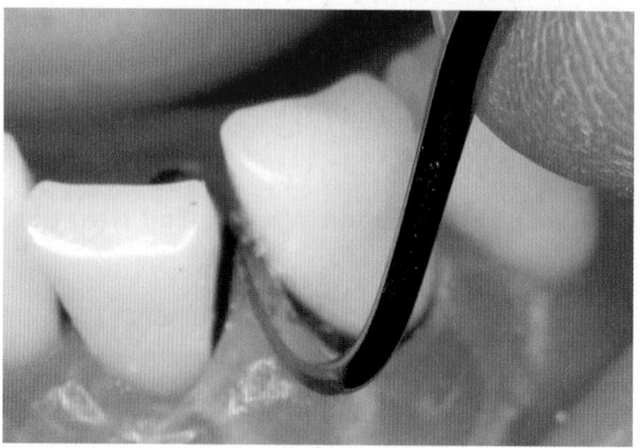

6. **Figure 14-13. Instrument under the Contact Area.** Continue strokes until you work at least halfway across the mesial surface. (The other half of the mesial surface will be instrumented from the lingual aspect of the tooth.)

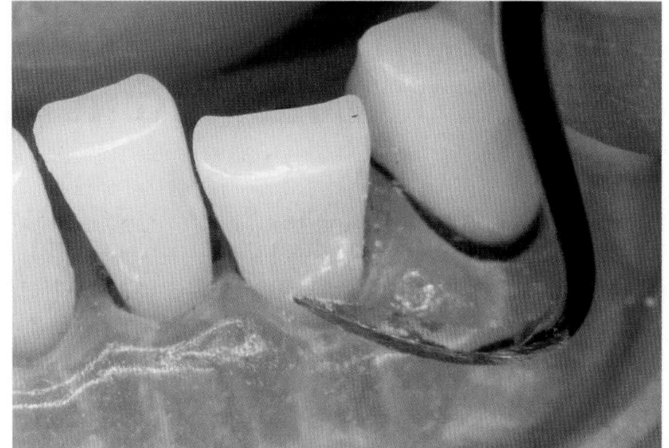

7. **Figure 14-14. Continue with Lateral Incisor.** Move the working-end to the midline of the lateral incisor and proceed in a similar manner with this tooth.

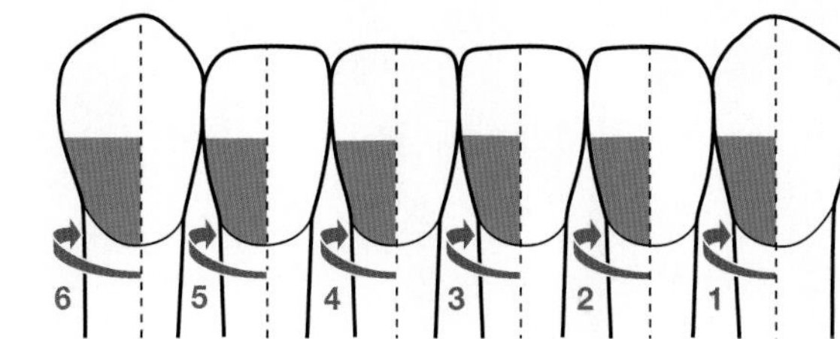

8. **Figure 14-15. Sequence.** Next, use the sequence shown in this illustration to instrument the colored tooth surfaces of the facial aspect. Begin with the left canine and end with the right canine.

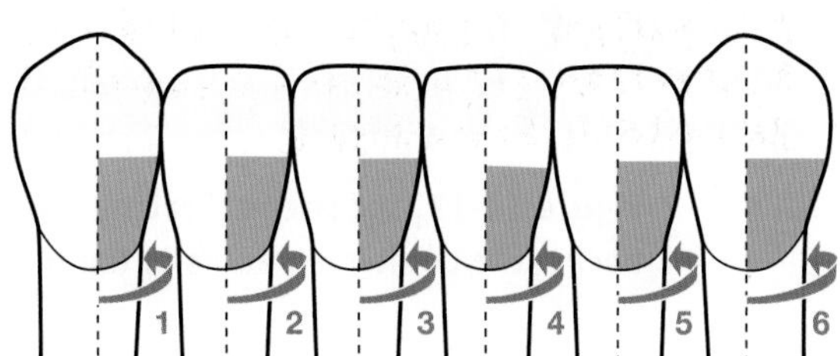

9. **Figure 14-16. Sequence.** Change your clock position and complete the remaining facial surfaces, beginning with the right canine and ending with the left canine.

Box 14-1. Recipe for Artificial Dental Calculus

Create realistic artificial dental calculus for use on typodonts using the following ingredients:

- Plaster of Paris
- Oil-based paint (to give the artificial calculus material color)
- Texture additive for paint
- Shellac

Combine 1 teaspoon of each ingredient to create enough artificial calculus for one typodont. Apply immediately and allow to dry.

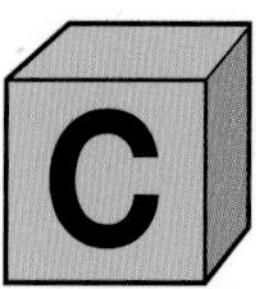

SKILL BUILDING. ADAPTATION ADJACENT TO PAPILLARY GINGIVA

Instrumentation of proximal tooth surfaces adjacent to the papillary gingiva may be challenging to new clinicians. There is a tendency for a new clinician to "trace the pointed contours of the papilla" with the working-end. Instead, correct technique involves positioning the cutting edge against the proximal surface with the working-end between the tooth surface and the pointed projection of the papillary gingiva.

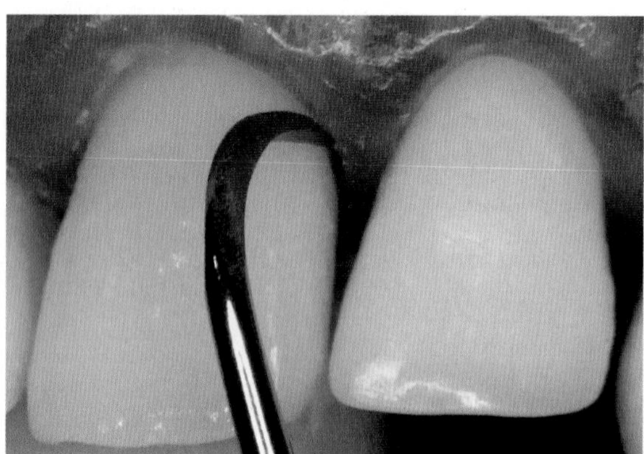

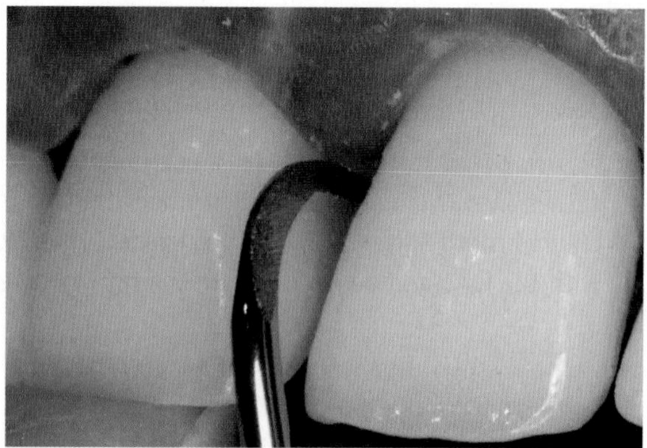

Figure 14-17. Incorrect: Tracing Papillary Contour. Incorrect technique entails tracing the pointed contours of the papilla with the working-end.

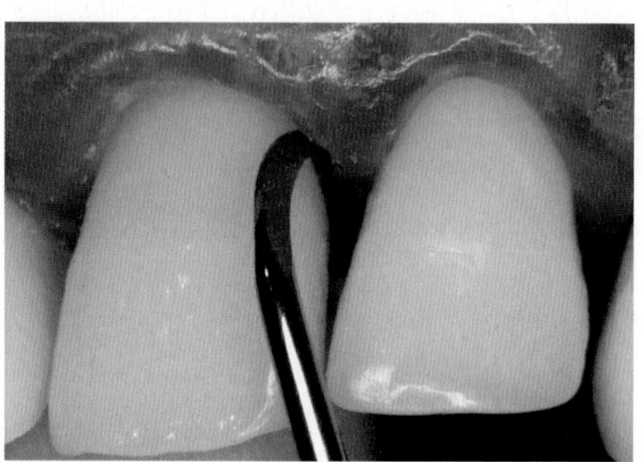

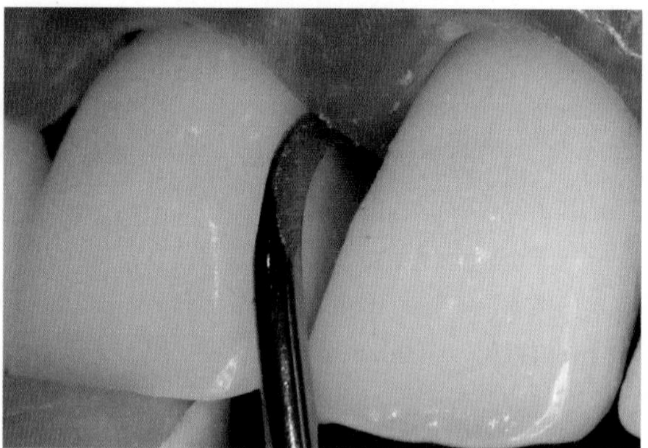

Figure 14-18. Correct Technique. Correct technique involves placing the cutting edge against the proximal surface with the working-end positioned between the tooth and the papillary gingiva. In this position, the cutting edge of the sickle scaler is still adapted to the enamel surface of the tooth crown.

Section 4
Technique Practice—Posterior Teeth

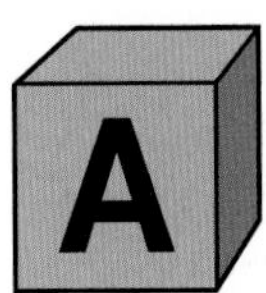

SKILL BUILDING. CHOOSING THE CORRECT WORKING-END OF A POSTERIOR SICKLE SCALER

Method 1: The Lower Shank as a Visual Clue

When a working-end of a posterior sickle scaler is adapted to a distal surface, the correct working-end has the following relationship between the shank and the tooth:

- Lower shank is parallel to the distal surface.
- Functional shank goes up and over the tooth.
- *Think: "Posterior = Parallel. Functional shank up and over!"*

Correct working-end selection of a posterior sickle scaler is shown in Figure 14-19. Figure 14-20 shows the incorrect working-end for the distal surface of the mandibular right second molar, facial aspect.

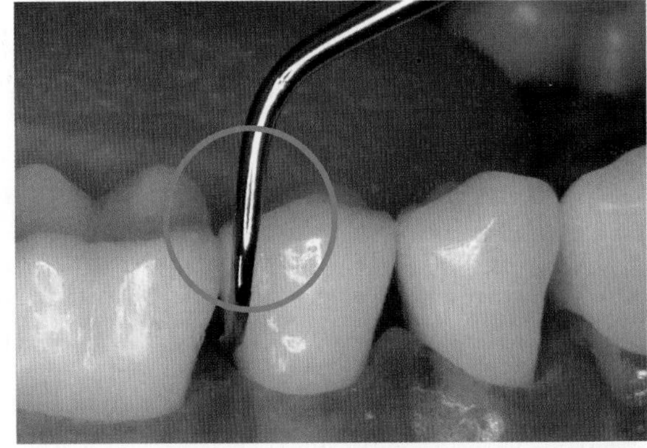

Figure 14-19. Visual Clue for the Correct Working-End.

- The correct working-end is selected when the *lower shank is parallel* to the distal surface.
- The *functional shank goes "up and over the tooth."*

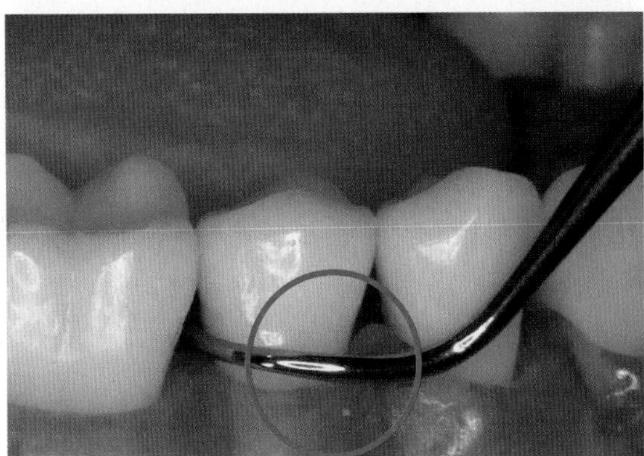

Figure 14-20. Visual Clue for the Incorrect Working-End.

- The incorrect working-end is selected if the *lower shank is not parallel* to the distal surface.
- The *functional shank is "down and around the tooth."*

Method 2: The Inner and Outer Cutting Edges as a Visual Clue

There is a second method for choosing the correct working-end of a posterior sickle scaler. For this method, the cutting edges provide the visual clue (Fig. 14-21). It is not important whether a clinician uses method 1 or method 2 to select the working-end. Each clinician should use the method that is easiest for him or her.

Method 2: *The bends in the functional shank of a posterior sickle scaler cause one of the cutting edges to be nearer to the handle than the other.* Each working-end has two cutting edges, an inner and outer cutting edge (Fig. 14-21).

1. The outer cutting edge is the one that is *farther* from the instrument handle.
2. The inner cutting edge is the one that is *closer* to the instrument handle.

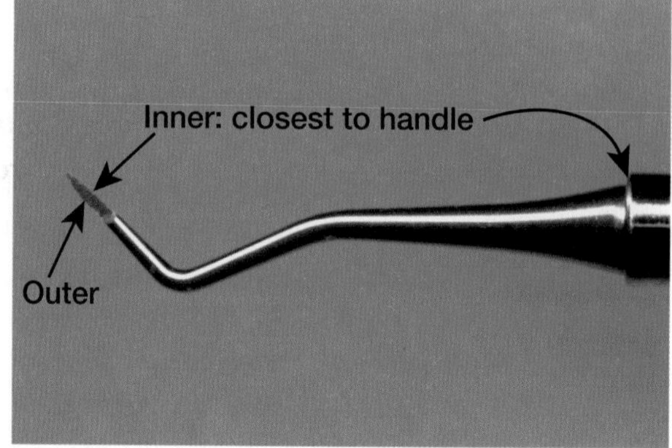

Figure 14-21. Inner and Outer Cutting Edges. To identify the cutting edges, ***hold the instrument so that you are looking down on the face of the working-end.*** One of the cutting edges will be nearer to the instrument handle than the other.

Box 14-2. The Inner and Outer Cutting Edges as a Visual Clue

The ***inner cutting edge*** is used to instrument the ***distal surfaces***.

The ***outer cutting edge*** is used to instrument the ***facial, lingual, and mesial surfaces***.

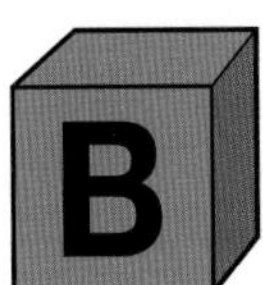

SKILL BUILDING. ESTABLISHING A 70° TO 80° ANGULATION TO A POSTERIOR TOOTH

The relationship of a posterior sickle scaler's face to the lower shank should be kept in mind when establishing angulation of the working-end to the tooth surface (Figs. 14-22 to 14-24). Ideally, the cutting edge-to-tooth angulation is between 70° and 80°.

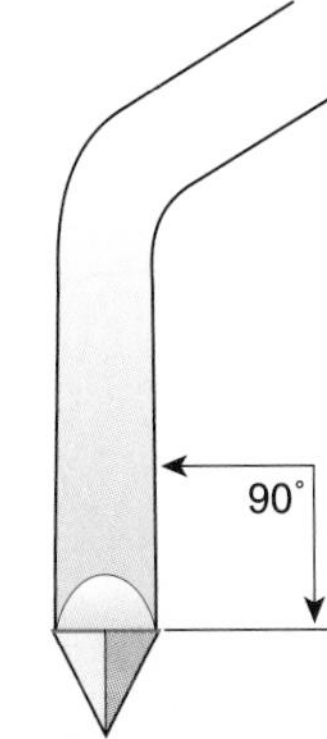

Figure 14-22. Working-End Design of a Posterior Sickle Scaler. In establishing correct angulation, it is important to remember that on a posterior sickle scaler, ***the face of the working-end is at a 90° angle to the lower shank***.

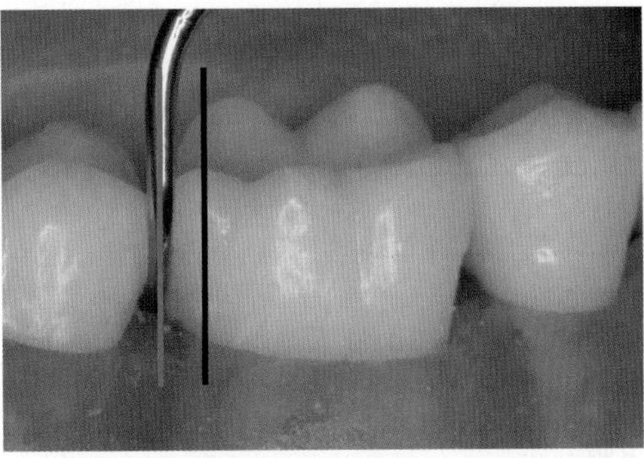

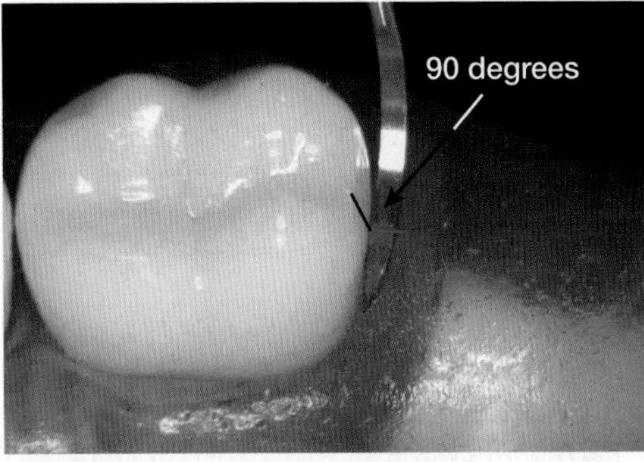

Figure 14-23. Incorrect Angulation. Because the lower shank of a posterior sickle scaler is at a 90° angle to face, positioning the lower shank parallel to the tooth surface results in an incorrect angulation of 90°.

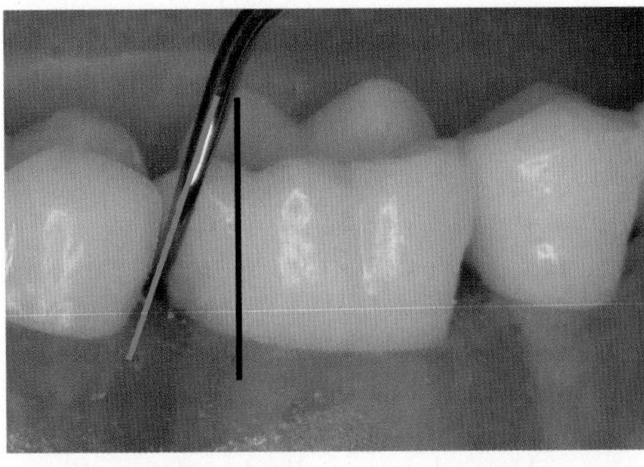

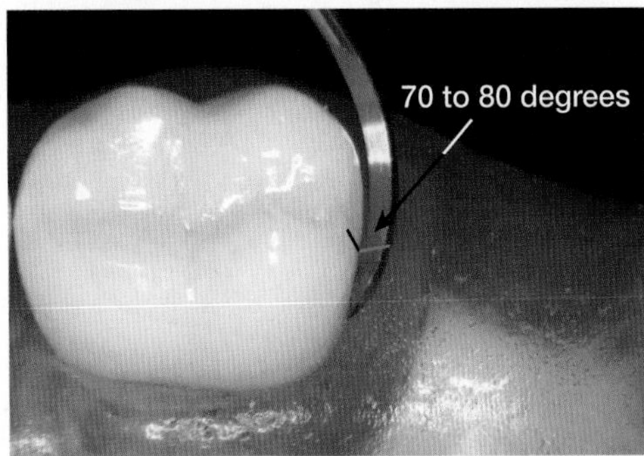

Figure 14-24. Correct Angulation. Correct angulation is achieved by tilting the lower shank slightly toward the tooth surface to be instrumented. In this position, the face-to-tooth surface angulation is correct, between 70° and 80°.

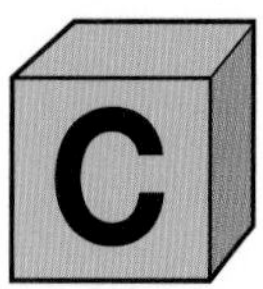

SKILL BUILDING. APPLICATION OF THE CUTTING EDGES TO THE POSTERIOR TEETH

APPLICATION OF THE CUTTING EDGES

All four cutting edges of a posterior sickle scaler are used for calculus removal on the posterior sextants. Figures 14-25 and 14-26 depict application of the cutting edges to the mandibular right posterior sextant. Note that both cutting edges of one working-end—Working-end A—are used on the facial aspect of a tooth, while the cutting edges of the other working-end—Working-end B—are used on the lingual aspect of the same tooth.

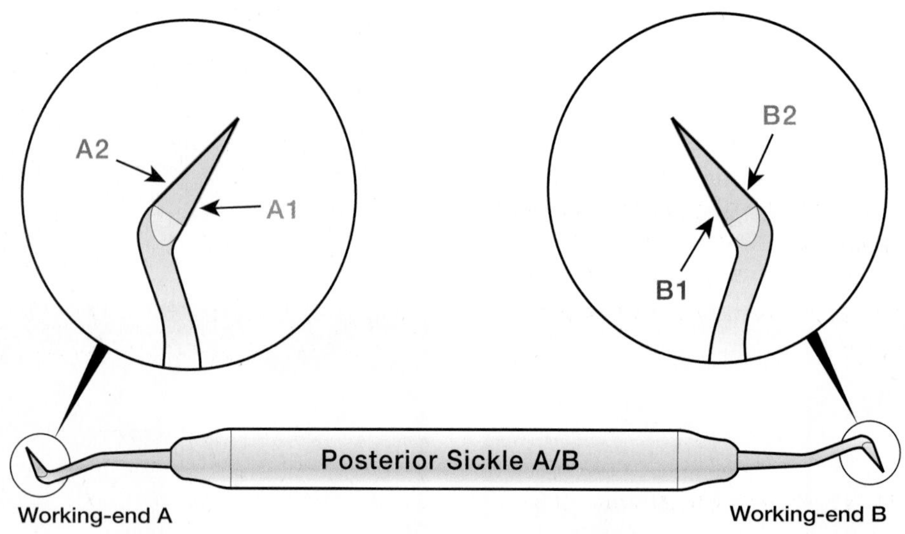

Figure 14-25. Four Cutting Edges of a Posterior Sickle Scaler. A posterior sickle scaler has two working-ends. Working-end A has two cutting edges (A1 and A2). Working-end B has two cutting edges (B1 and B2).

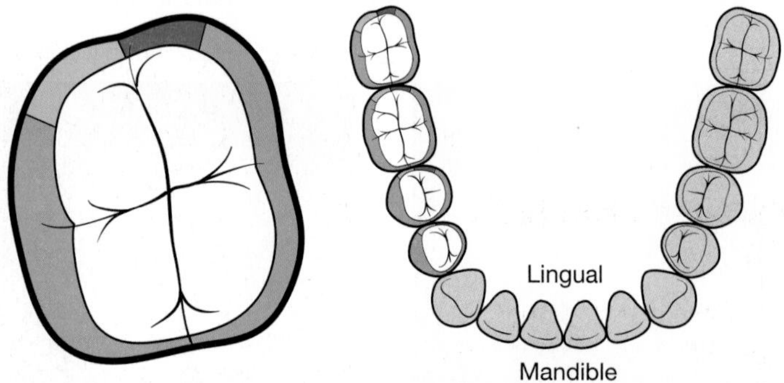

Figure 14-26. Application of Cutting Edges to Posterior Surfaces. These illustrations indicate how the cutting edges of a posterior sickle scaler are applied to the tooth surfaces of the mandibular right first molar and the mandibular right posterior sextant.

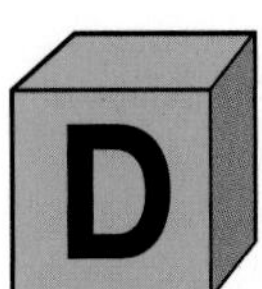

SKILL BUILDING. TECHNIQUE FOR POSTERIOR TEETH

Directions:

- Follow steps 1 to 11 to practice use of a posterior sickle scaler on the mandibular right posterior sextant (Figs. 14-27 to 14-37).
- Remember: "Me, My patient, My light, My dominant hand, My nondominant hand, My finger rest, My adaptation."

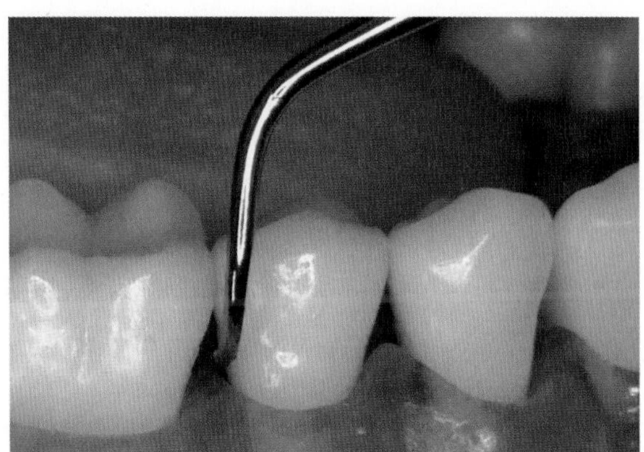

1. **Figure 14-27. Select the Correct Working-End.** When using the lower shank as a visual clue, use a tooth that is easily seen, such as the distal surface of the second premolar, to select the correct working-end.

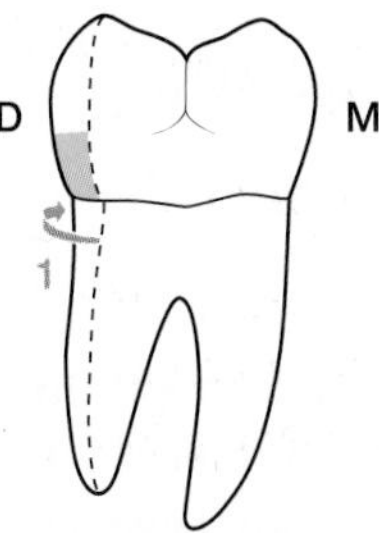

2. **Figure 14-28. Begin with Mandibular First Molar.** As an introduction to the posterior sickle, first practice on the *mandibular right first molar*. The distal surface is completed first, beginning at the distofacial line angle and working onto the distal surface.

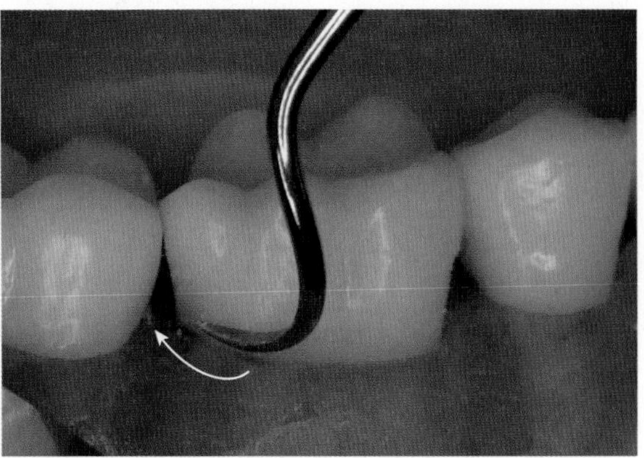

3. **Figure 14-29. Position the Working-End Near the Distofacial Line Angle.**
   - Establish a face-to-tooth surface angulation of between 70° and 80°.
   - The tip should aim toward the back of the mouth because this is the direction in which you are working.

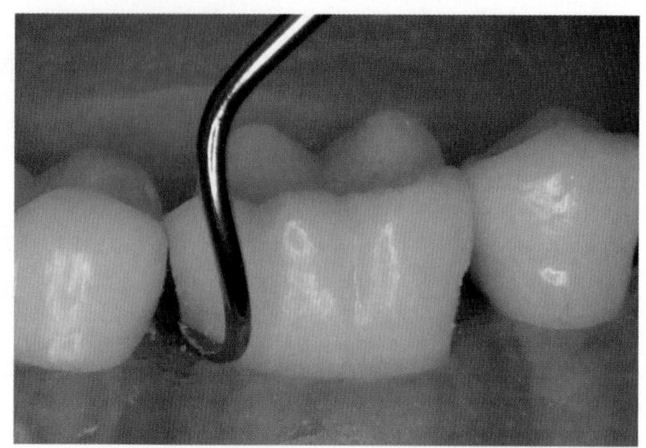

4. **Figure 14-30. Continue Strokes.**
    - Continue making a series of short, precise calculus removal strokes.
    - Remember to roll the instrument handle when working around the distofacial line angle and onto the distal surface.

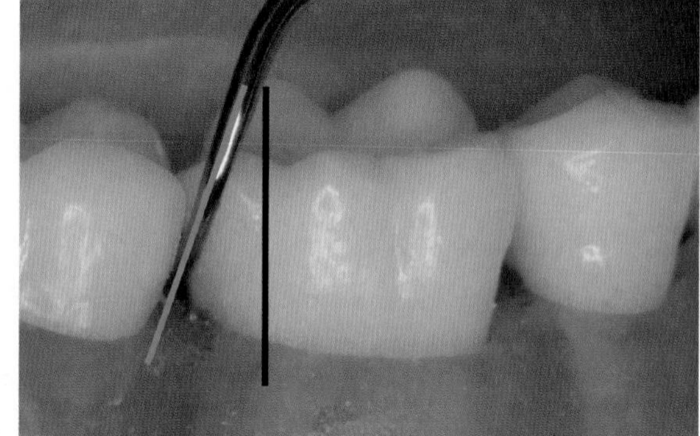

5. **Figure 14-31. Technique Check: Distal Surface.**
    - The sickle's face should be at a 70° to 80° angulation to the distal surface.
    - ***To obtain this angulation, the lower shank will be tilted toward the distal surface.***

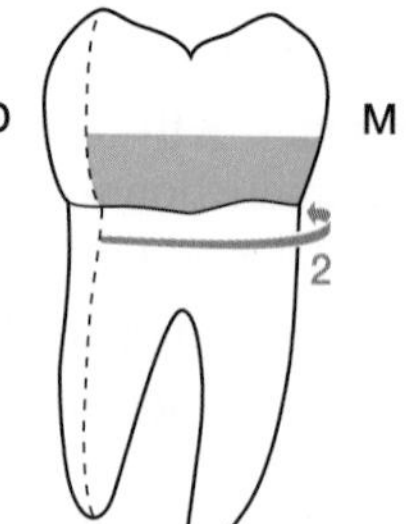

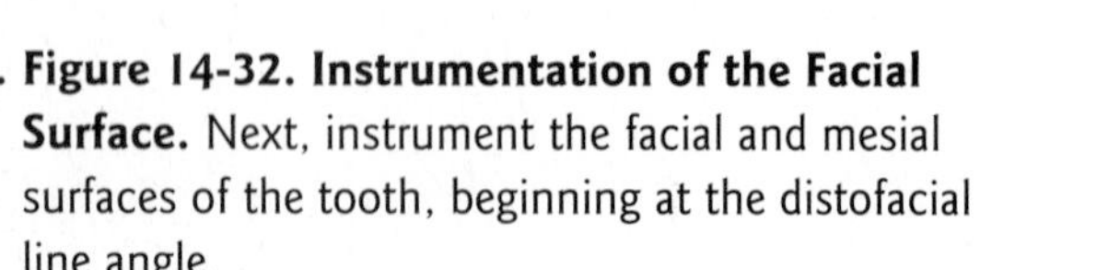

6. **Figure 14-32. Instrumentation of the Facial Surface.** Next, instrument the facial and mesial surfaces of the tooth, beginning at the distofacial line angle.

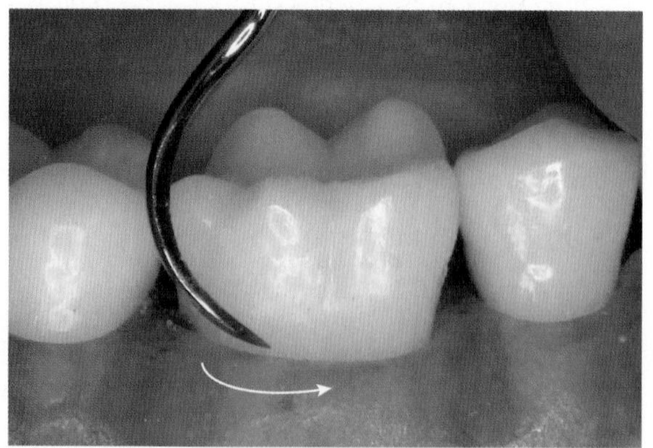

7. **Figure 14-33. Reposition the Working-End at the Line Angle.**
    - While maintaining your fulcrum, lift the working-end away from the tooth and turn it so that it aims toward the front of the mouth.
    - Reposition the working-end at the distofacial line angle.

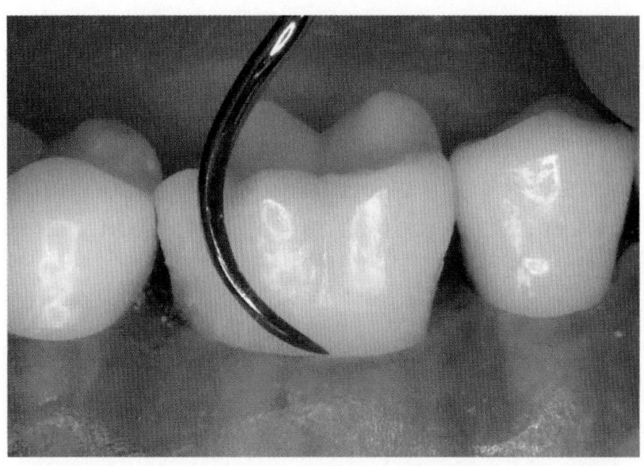

8. Figure 14-34. Work across Facial Surface.

- Continue working across the facial surface. Remember to maintain adaptation at all times.
- As you approach the mesiofacial line angle, roll the handle slightly to maintain adaptation.

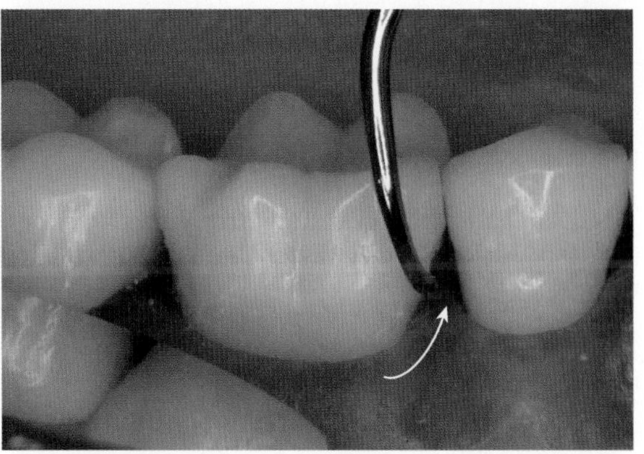

9. Figure 14-35. Instrument the Mesial Surface.

- Tilt the lower shank slightly toward the mesial surface to maintain correct angulation.
- Check the shank position to assure that you have maintained a 70° to 80° face-to-tooth surface angulation.

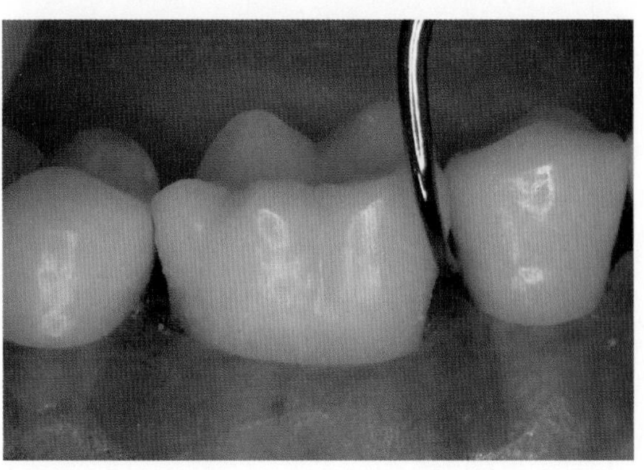

10. Figure 14-36. Continue Strokes. Work at least halfway across the mesial surface from the facial aspect. (The other half will be instrumented from the lingual aspect.)

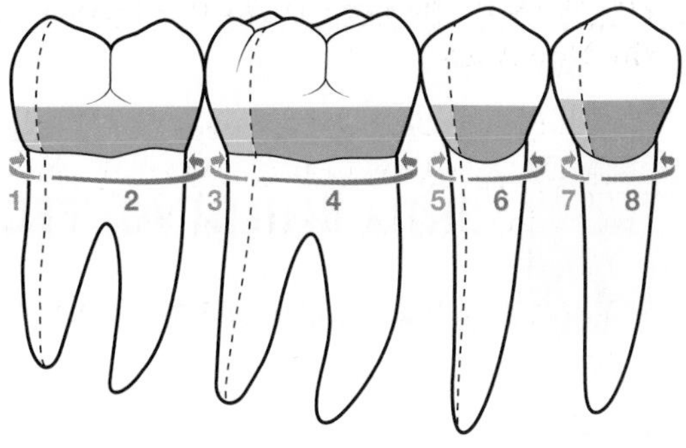

11. Figure 14-37. Sequence for Sextant. Next, use the sequence shown in this illustration to instrument the facial aspect of the entire sextant, beginning with the posterior-most molar. This sequence allows you to instrument the sextant in an efficient manner.

Section 5
Primary Teeth

Instrumentation of primary teeth presents some unique challenges. These include the smaller size of the primary crowns as well as the rougher enamel surfaces and cementoenamel junctions on primary teeth.

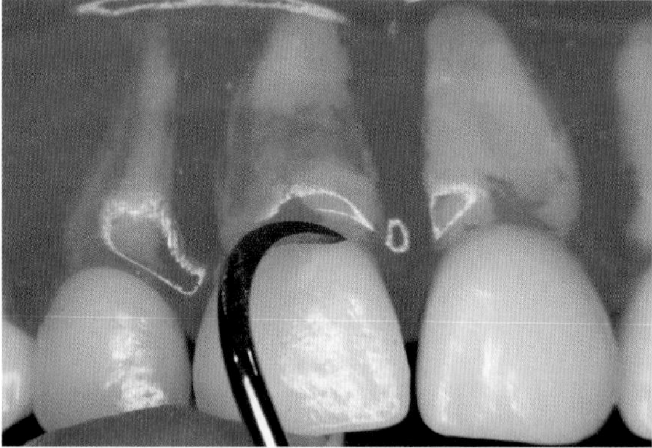

Figure 14-38. Primary Anteriors. The Nevi 1 is a small, thin anterior sickle scaler that works well for the tiny crowns of primary anterior teeth.

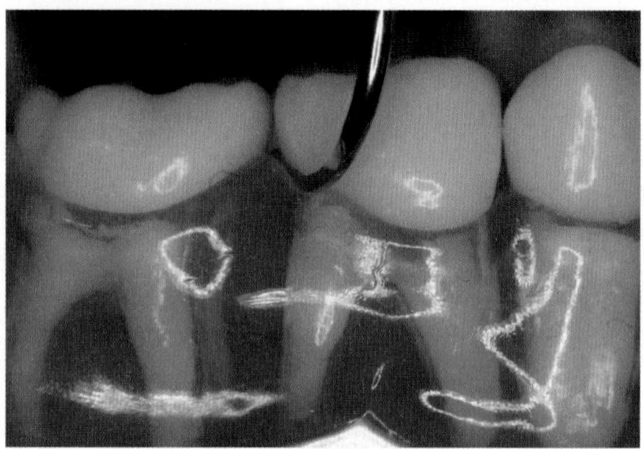

Figure 14-39. Primary Molars. The Nevi 3 posterior sickle scaler has a thin curved working-end that adapts well to primary molars.

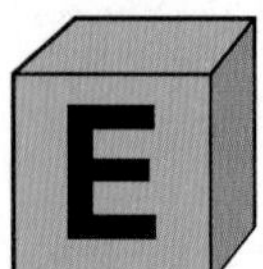

SKILL BUILDING. TECHNIQUE FOR PRIMARY TEETH

Equipment: Typodont with primary or mixed dentition and anterior and posterior sickle scalers.
Directions: Practice using a posterior sickle scaler on primary molar teeth as shown in Figures 14-40 to 14-43.

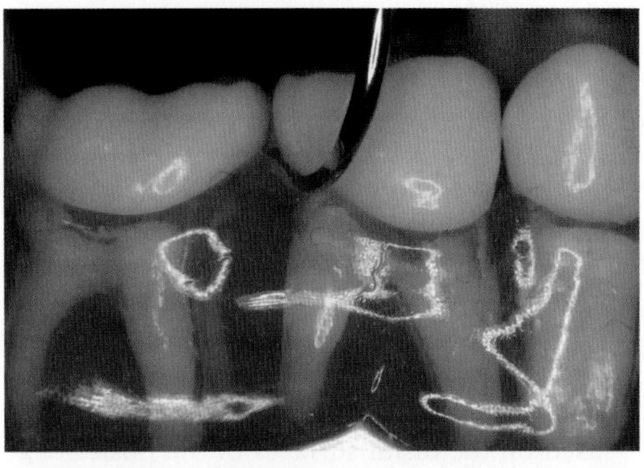

1. Figure 14-40. Get Ready.

- Select the correct working-end and begin instrumentation at the distofacial line angle.
- Work from the distofacial line angle to halfway across the distal surface.

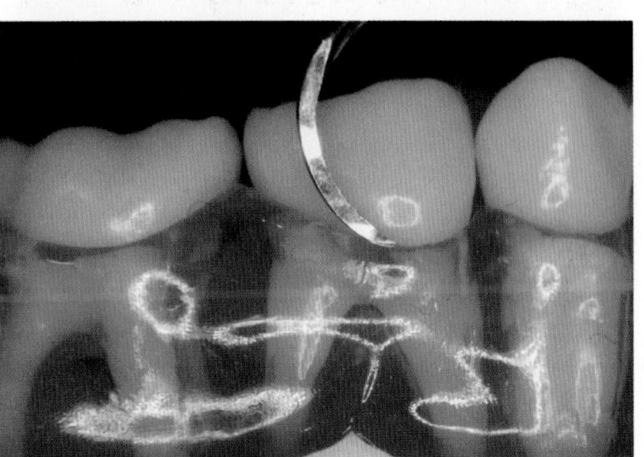

2. Figure 14-41. Instrument the Facial Surface.

- After completing the distal surface, reposition the working-end at the distofacial line angle.
- Make short, precise strokes across the facial surface.

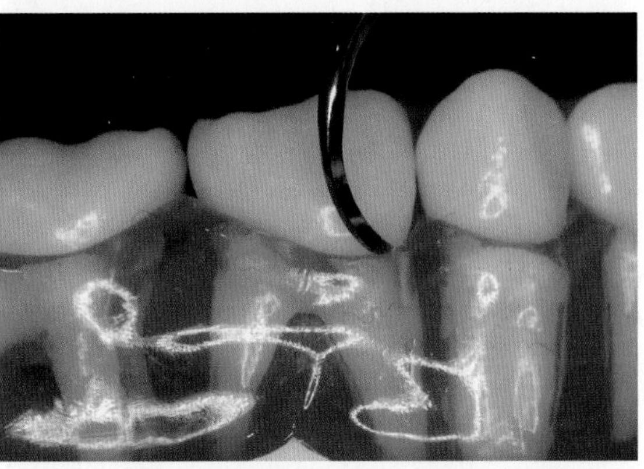

3. Figure 14-42. Roll Instrument Handle at the Mesiofacial Line Angle. At the mesiofacial line angle, roll the instrument handle to maintain adaptation as the working-end moves on to the mesial surface.

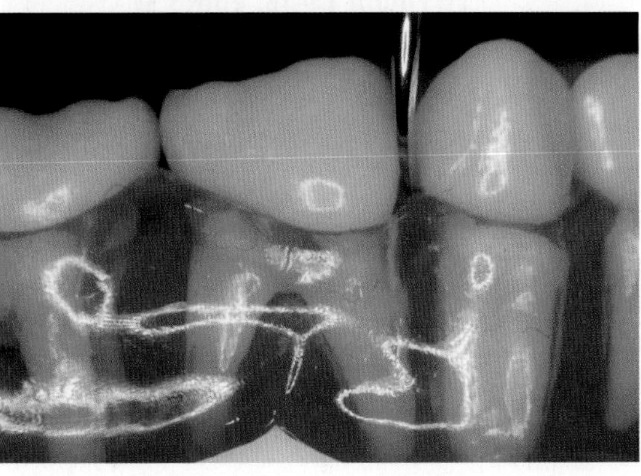

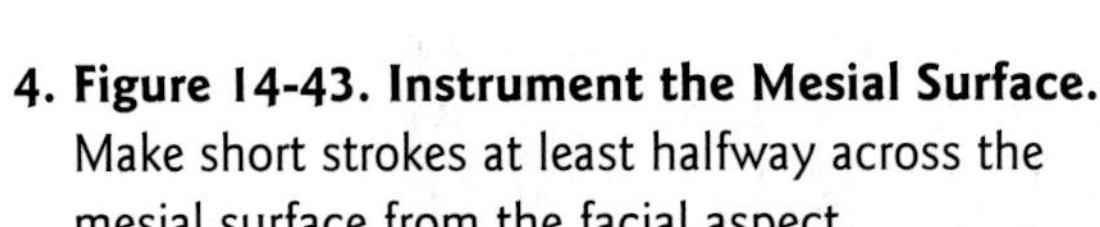

4. Figure 14-43. Instrument the Mesial Surface. Make short strokes at least halfway across the mesial surface from the facial aspect.

Section 6
Skill Application

PRACTICAL FOCUS

- **Task 1:** Use the lower shank as a visual clue to determine if the correct working-end of a posterior sickle scaler is being used in the photographs shown in Figures 14-44 and 14-45. What visual clue did you use?
- **Task 2:** What is the tooth-to-face angulation of the sickle scalers shown in Figures 14-46 and 14-47?
- **Task 3:** Identify the inner and outer cutting edges in Figure 14-48. Should cutting edge A or B be used on the distal surfaces of the posterior teeth?

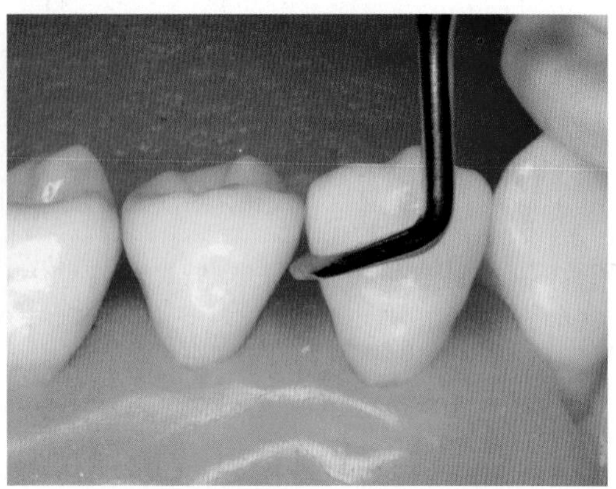

Figure 14-44. Photo 1.

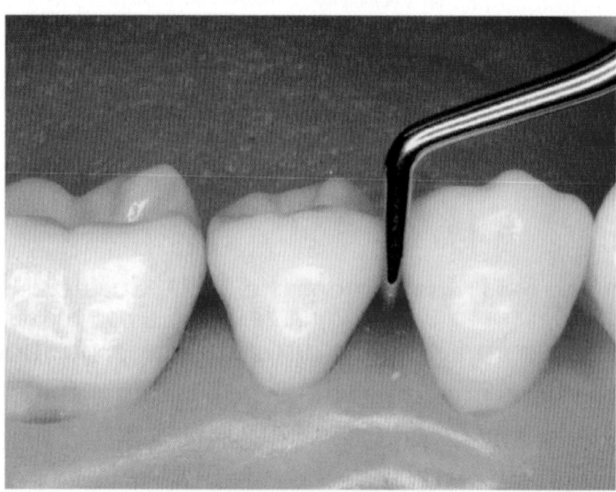

Figure 14-45. Photo 2.

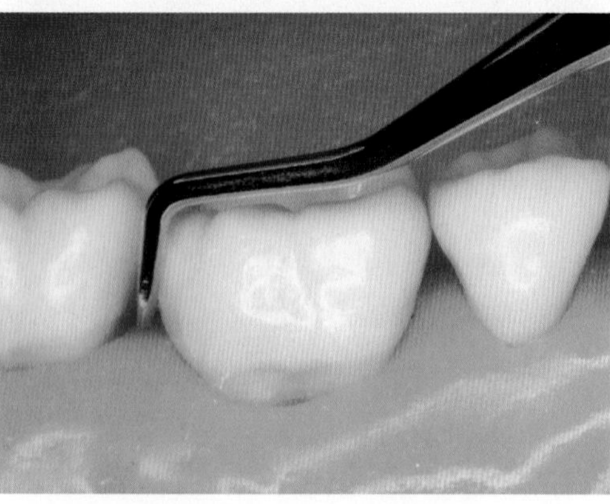

Figure 14-46. Photo 3.

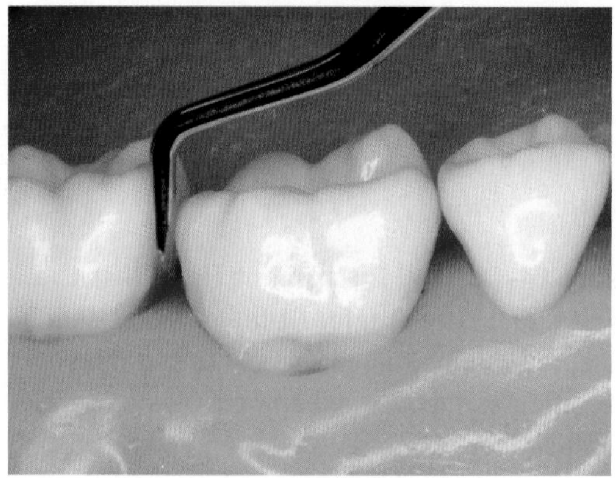

Figure 14-47. Photo 4.

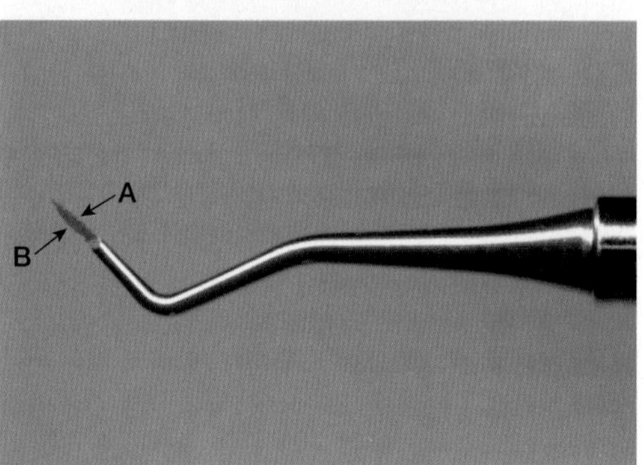

Figure 14-48. Photo 5.

REFERENCE SHEET: SICKLE SCALERS

Use of Sickle Scalers:

- Sickle scalers are used to remove medium- and large-size calculus deposits from the crowns of posterior teeth.
- The pointed tip provides good access to the proximal surfaces apical to the contact areas on posterior teeth.
- Sickle scalers are NOT recommended for use on root surfaces.

Basic Concepts:

- Tilt the lower shank slightly toward the tooth surface to establish correct face-to-tooth surface angulation.
- Maintain adaptation of the tip-third of the cutting edge to the tooth surface.
- Before initiating a calculus removal stroke, press down with your fulcrum finger and apply pressure against the instrument handle with the index finger and thumb to create lateral pressure against the tooth surface.
- Activate the calculus removal stroke using wrist motion activation.
- Relax your fingers between each calculus removal stroke.

Anterior Teeth:

- Sequence: Begin with the surfaces toward your nondominant hand. Start on the canine on the opposite side of the mouth and work toward yourself. (Right-handed clinicians start with the left canine, mesial surface; left-handed clinicians start with the right canine, mesial surface.)

Posterior Teeth:

- Sequence: Begin at the distofacial line angle of the posterior-most tooth in the sextant and work toward the distal surface. Reposition at the distofacial line angle and complete the facial (or lingual) and mesial surfaces of the tooth, working toward the front of the mouth.

Note to Course Instructor: Refer to Module 21, Calculus Removal: Concepts, Planning, and Patient Cases, for instrumentation strategies and patient cases relating to calculus removal.

STUDENT SELF-EVALUATION MODULE 14 SICKLE SCALERS

Student: ______________________ Date: ______________________

DIRECTIONS: Self-evaluate your skill level in each treatment area as: **S** (satisfactory) or **U** (unsatisfactory).

Criteria				
Positioning/Ergonomics	**Area 1**	**Area 2**	**Area 3**	**Area 4**
Adjusts clinician chair correctly				
Assumes the recommended clock position				
Positions backrest of patient chair for the specified arch and adjusts height of patient chair so that clinician's elbows remain at waist level when accessing the specified treatment area				
Asks patient to assume the head position that facilitates the clinician's view of the specified treatment area				
Directs light to illuminate the specified treatment area				
Instrument Grasp: Dominant Hand	**Area 1**	**Area 2**	**Area 3**	**Area 4**
Grasps handle with tips of finger pads of index finger and thumb				
Rests pad of middle finger lightly on instrument shank				
Positions the thumb, index, and middle fingers in the "knuckles-up" convex position; hyperextended joint position is avoided				
Holds ring finger straight so that it supports the weight of hand and instrument; ring finger position is "advanced ahead of" the other fingers in the grasp				
Maintains a relaxed grasp; fingers are NOT blanched in grasp				
Finger Rest: Dominant Hand				
Establishes secure finger rest that is appropriate for tooth to be treated				
Once finger rest is established, pauses to self-evaluate finger placement in the grasp, verbalizes to evaluator his/her self-assessment of grasp, and corrects finger placement if necessary				
Prepare for Instrumentation ("Get Ready")				
Selects correct working-end for tooth surface to be instrumented				
Places the working-end in the "Get Ready Zone" while using a correct finger rest for the treatment area				

(Note: Student Self-Evaluation continues on the next page)

STUDENT SELF-EVALUATION MODULE 14 SICKLE SCALERS (continued)

Criteria				
Adaptation, Angulation, and Instrument Stroke	**Area 1**	**Area 2**	**Area 3**	**Area 4**
Correctly orients the lower shank to the tooth surface to be instrumented				
Initiates a stroke in a coronal direction by positioning the working-end beneath a calculus deposit, "locking the tip" against tooth surface and using an angulation between 45° and 80°				
Uses rotating motion to make a short, biting stroke in a coronal direction to snap a deposit from the tooth; does NOT close face toward tooth surface during activation; uses whole hand as a unit; does NOT pull with thumb and index finger				
Maintains appropriate lateral pressure against the tooth throughout the stroke while maintaining control of the working-end				
Precisely stops each individual stroke and pauses briefly (at least 3 seconds) to relax grasp before repositioning working-end beneath calculus deposit; strokes should be short				
Maintains neutral wrist position throughout motion activation				
Maintains correct adaptation as instrument strokes progress around tooth surface; pivots and rolls instrument handle as needed				
Thoroughly instruments proximal surface under each contact area				
Uses appropriate sequence for the specified sextant				
Keeps hands steady and controlled during instrumentation so that working-end moves with precision, regardless of nervousness				
Ethics and Professionalism				
Punctuality, appearance, demeanor, attitude, composure, honesty				

Module 15

Universal Curets

Module Overview

This module presents the design characteristics of universal curets and step-by-step instructions for using universal curets to remove small- or medium-size calculus deposits from the anterior and posterior teeth. Module 13, Technique Essentials: Angulation and Calculus Removal, should be completed prior to beginning this module.

Module Outline

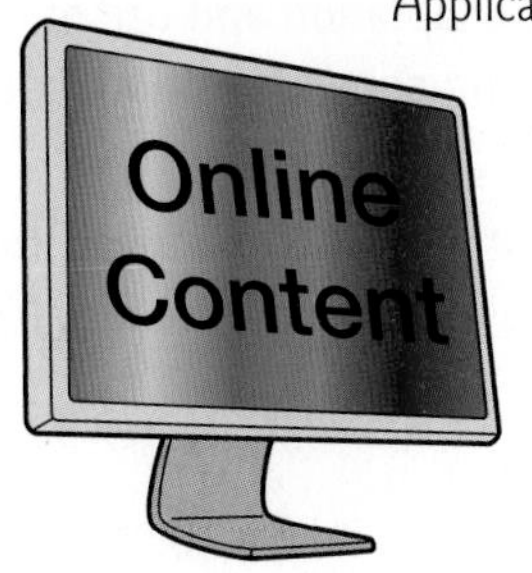

A video on the use of a universal curet can be viewed at http://thepoint.lww.com/GehrigFundamentals7e

Key Terms

Universal curet
Face at 90° to the lower shank
Outer cutting edge
Inner cutting edge

Learning Objectives

1. Given a variety of universal curets, identify the design characteristics of each instrument.
2. Discuss the advantages and limitations of the design characteristics of universal curets.
3. Name the uses of universal curets.
4. Describe how the clinician can use visual clues to select the correct working-end of a universal curet on anterior and posterior teeth.
5. Given a variety of universal curets to choose from and a task (location, depth, and size of calculus deposits), select the best instrument for the specified task.
6. Explain why the lower shank of a universal curet should be tilted slightly toward the tooth surface being instrumented to obtain correct angulation.
7. Using a universal curet, demonstrate correct adaptation and use of calculus removal strokes on the anterior teeth while maintaining correct position, correct finger rests, and precise finger placement in the grasp.
8. Using a universal curet, demonstrate correct adaptation and use of calculus removal strokes on the posterior teeth while maintaining correct position, correct finger rests, and precise finger placement in the grasp.
9. Using a universal curet, demonstrate horizontal calculus removal strokes at the distofacial line angles of posterior teeth and at the midlines on the facial and lingual surfaces of anterior teeth.

Section 1
Universal Curets

GENERAL DESIGN CHARACTERISTICS

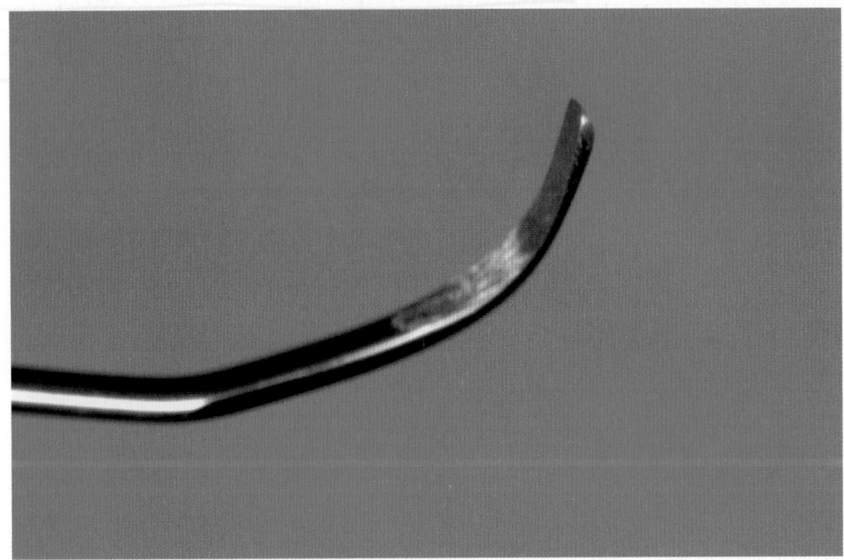

Figure 15-1. The Working-End of a Universal Curet.

1. **Functions of Universal Curets**
   a. A universal curet is a periodontal instrument used to remove small- and medium-size calculus deposits (Figs. 15-1 and 15-2).
      1. Universal curets can be used both supragingivally and subgingivally—on crown and root surfaces.
      2. A universal curet usually is a double-ended instrument with paired, mirror-image working-ends.
   b. Universal curets are one of the most frequently used and versatile of all the calculus removal instruments. This type of curet is called "universal" because it can be applied to both anterior and posterior teeth. In other words, this type of curet is used universally throughout the entire mouth.
2. **Design Characteristics.** The working-end of a universal curet has several unique design characteristics (Table 15-1):
   a. A rounded back
   b. A rounded toe
   c. A semi-circular cross section
   d. Two cutting edges per working-end
   e. The face is at a 90° angle to the lower shank, and as a result, the two cutting edges are level with one another and can be used for calculus removal
3. **Examples of Universal Curet Instruments.** Some examples of universal curet instruments are the Columbia 4R/4L, Columbia 13/14, Rule 3/4, Barnhart 1/2, Barnhart 5/6, Younger-Good 7/8, Indiana University 13/14, McCalls 13/14, Bunting 5/6, Mallery 1/2, Langer 1/2, Langer 3/4, Langer 5/6, and Langer 17/18.

WORKING-END DESIGN

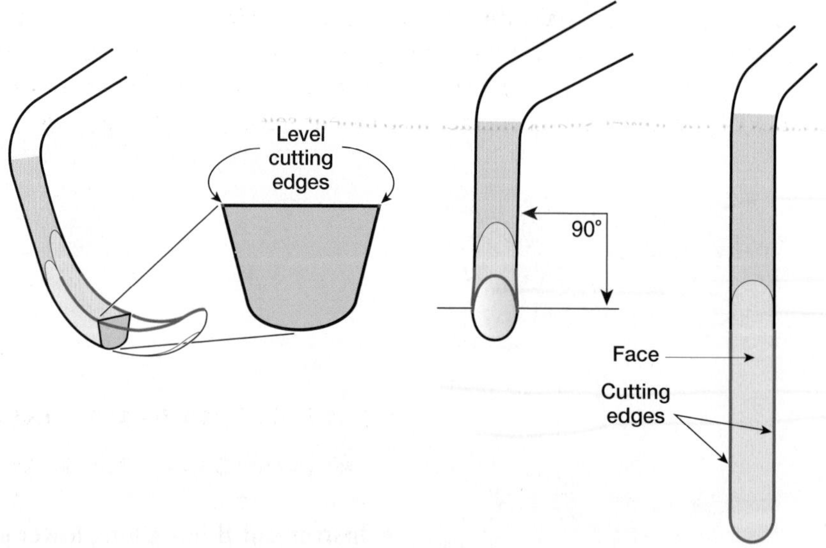

Figure 15-2. Design Characteristics of a Universal Curet.

TABLE 15-1. Reference Sheet: Universal Curet	
Cross section	Semi-circular cross section; this design allows the working-end to be used both supragingivally and subgingivally
Working-end	Rounded back and toe Two working cutting edges per working-end
Face	Face is at a 90° angle to the lower shank, and as a result, the two cutting edges on a working-end are level with one another Because the face is perpendicular to the lower shank, ***the lower shank must be tilted slightly toward the tooth surface to establish correct angulation***
Cutting edges	Two ***parallel cutting edges*** meet in a rounded toe
Application	One double-ended instrument is used on both anterior and posterior teeth
Primary functions	***Instrumentation of crown and root surfaces*** Removal of small- to medium-size calculus deposits

SELECTING A UNIVERSAL CURET FOR A PARTICULAR TASK

In selecting a universal curet for a particular calculus removal task, consider its design characteristics such as the curve of the working-end, length of the lower shank, and degree of bend in the shank. The photographs in Figures 15-3 to 15-5 compare two universal curets, demonstrating how the design characteristics of the lower shank impact instrument selection for a particular task.

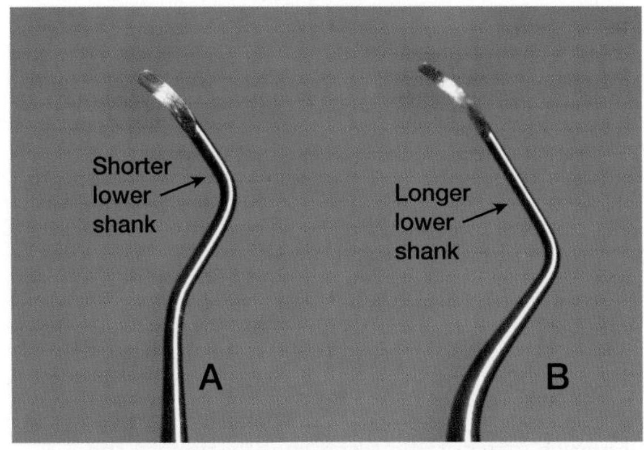

Figure 15-3. Two Universal Curet Designs.

- **Instrument** A has a short lower shank and working-end.
- **Instrument** B has a long lower shank and working-end.

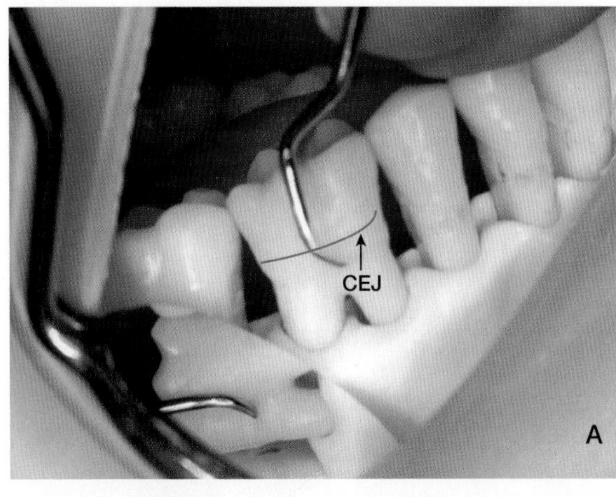

Figure 15-4. Shorter Lower Shank Length. Instrument A is an excellent choice for removal of supragingival calculus and removal of deposits in normal sulci and shallow pockets. (Key: CEJ = cementoenamel junction)

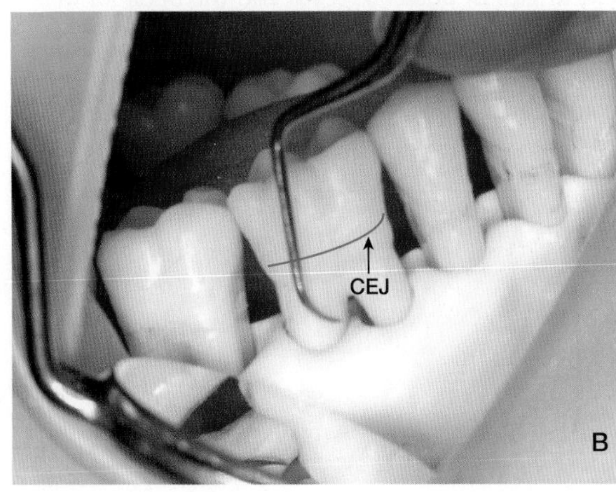

Figure 15-5. Longer Lower Shank Length. Instrument B, with its longer lower shank, is an excellent choice for removal of deposits in deep pockets.

Section 2
Calculus Removal Concepts

CHARACTERISTICS OF THE CALCULUS REMOVAL STROKE

Before beginning the step-by-step technique practice with a universal curet, review the (1) characteristics of the calculus removal stroke and (2) steps for calculus removal. These concepts are similar for use of sickle scalers and universal curets.

TABLE 15-2. The Calculus Removal Stroke with a Universal Curet

Stabilization	Apply pressure with the index finger and thumb inward against the instrument handle and press the tip of the fulcrum finger against the tooth surface
Adaptation	Toe-third of cutting edge is adapted
Angulation	70°–80°; for universal curets, the lower shank must be tilted slightly toward the tooth surface to achieve correct angulation
Lateral pressure for calculus removal	Moderate to firm pressure against the tooth surface is maintained during the short, controlled calculus removal stroke made ***away from the junctional epithelium***
Characteristics	Powerful controlled strokes, short in length
Stroke direction	Vertical strokes are most commonly used on anterior teeth and on the mesial and distal surfaces of posterior teeth Oblique strokes are most commonly used on the facial and lingual surfaces of posterior teeth Horizontal strokes are used at the line angles of posterior teeth and the midlines of the facial or lingual surfaces of anterior teeth
Stroke number	Calculus removal strokes should be limited to areas where calculus is present; use the minimum number of strokes needed to remove calculus deposits

Before beginning the step-by-step technique practice with a universal curet, review the steps for calculus removal summarized in Figure 15-6.

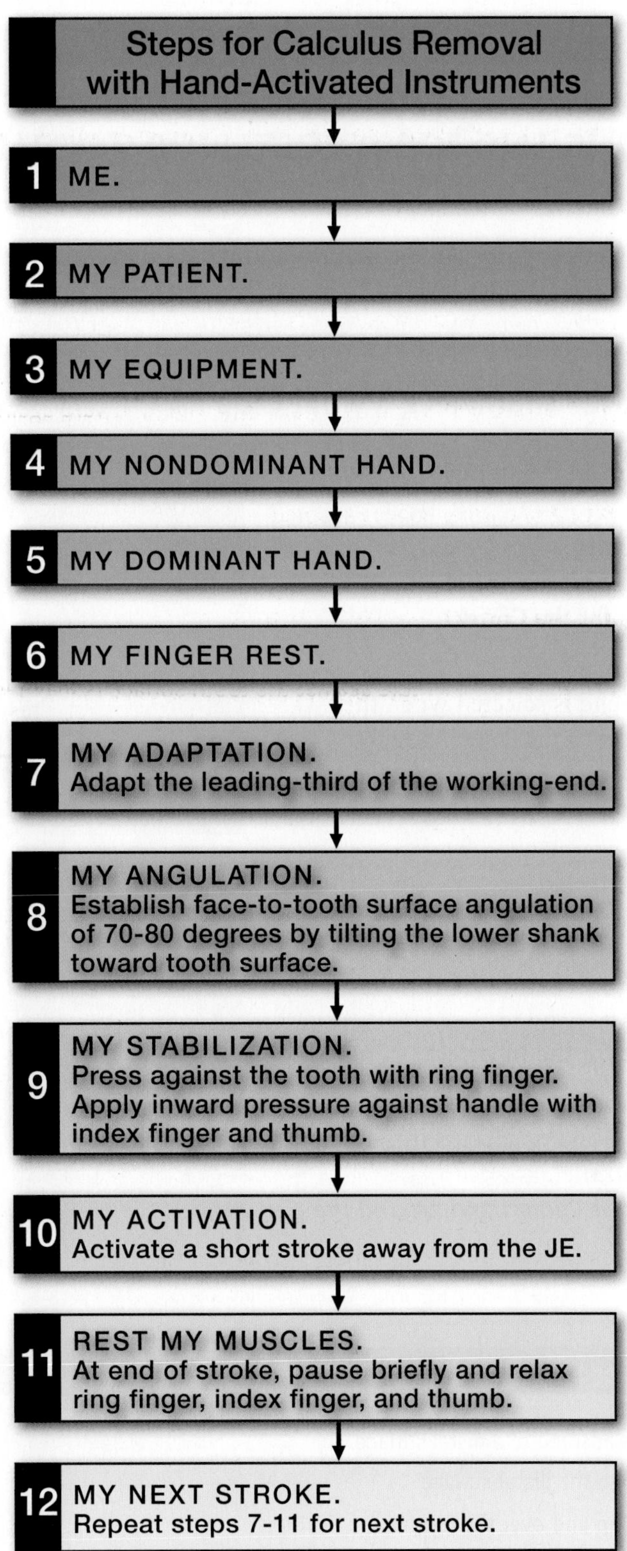

Figure 15-6. Flow Chart for Calculus Removal. (Key: JE = junctional epithelium)

Section 3
Technique Practice—Posterior Teeth

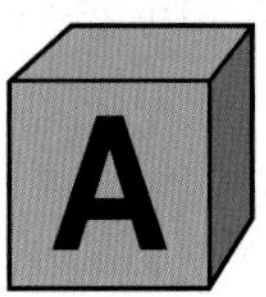

SKILL BUILDING. SELECTING THE CORRECT WORKING-END FOR A POSTERIOR TOOTH

There are two methods for recognizing the correct working-end of a universal curet. The clinician may use either the lower shank (Figs. 15-7 and 15-8) or the inner and outer cutting edges (Fig. 15-9) as a visual clue.

Method 1: The Lower Shank as a Visual Clue

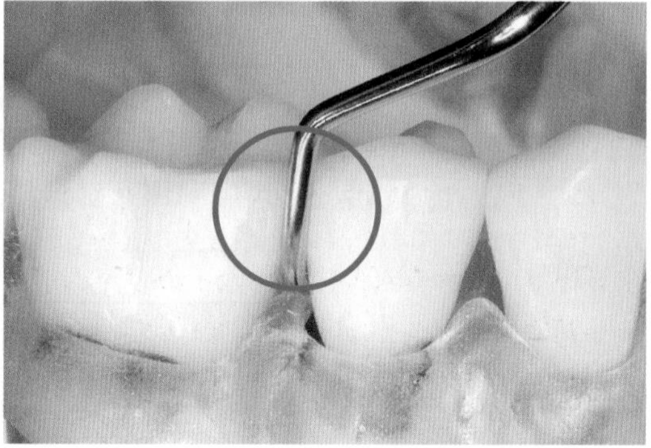

Figure 15-7. Visual Clue for the Correct Working-End.

- The correct working-end is selected when the *lower shank is parallel* to the distal surface.
- The *functional shank goes "up and over the tooth."*

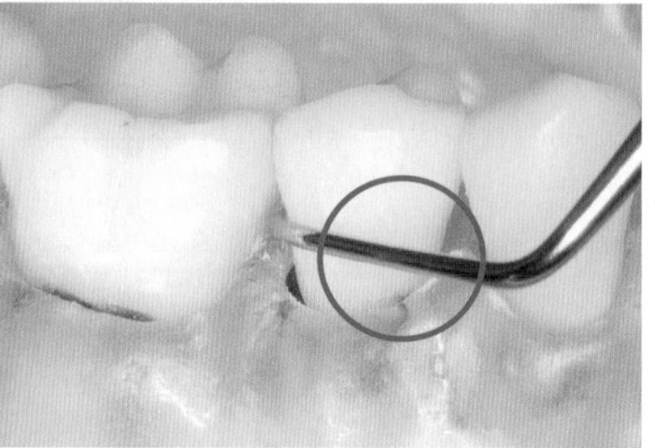

Figure 15-8. Visual Clue for the Incorrect Working-End.

- The incorrect working-end is selected if the *lower shank is not parallel.*
- The *functional shank is "down and around the tooth."*

Box 15-1. The Lower Shank as a Visual Clue

When the working-end is adapted to a distal surface:

- Lower shank is parallel to the distal surface
- Functional shank goes up and over the tooth

Think: *"Posterior = Parallel. Functional shank up and over!"*

Method 2: The Inner and Outer Cutting Edges as a Visual Clue

There is a second method for recognizing the correct working-end of a universal curet. For this method, the cutting edges provide the visual clue (Figs. 15-7 and 15-8). It is not important whether a clinician uses method 1 or method 2 to select the working-end. Each clinician should use the method that is easiest for him or her.

Method 2: ***The bends in the functional shank of a universal curet cause one of the cutting edges to be nearer to the handle than the other.*** Each working-end has two cutting edges: an inner and outer cutting edge (Fig. 15-9).

1. The outer cutting edge is the one that is *farther* from the instrument handle.
2. The inner cutting edge is the one that is *closer* to the instrument handle.

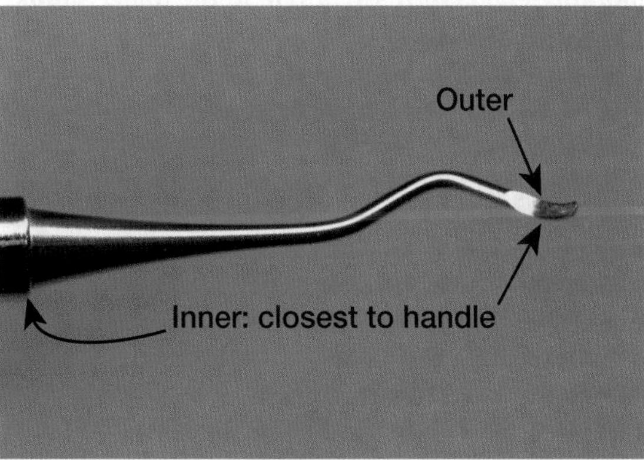

Figure 15-9. Inner and Outer Cutting Edges. To identify the cutting edges, hold the instrument ***so that you are looking down on the face of the working-end***. One of the cutting edges will be nearer to the instrument handle than the other.

Box 15-2. The Inner and Outer Cutting Edges as a Visual Clue

- The ***inner cutting edges*** are used to instrument the ***distal surfaces***.
- The ***outer cutting edges*** are used to instrument the ***facial, lingual, and mesial surfaces***.

ESTABLISHING 70° TO 80° ANGULATION

The relationship of a universal curet's face to the lower shank should be kept in mind when establishing correct angulation of the working-end to the tooth surface (Figs. 15-10 to 15-12).

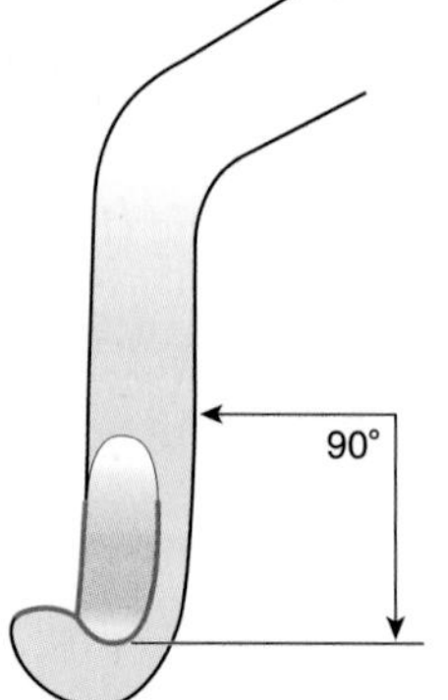

Figure 15-10. Relationship of the Face to the Lower Shank. In establishing correct angulation, it is important to remember that ***on a universal curet, the face of the working-end is at a 90° angle to the lower shank***.

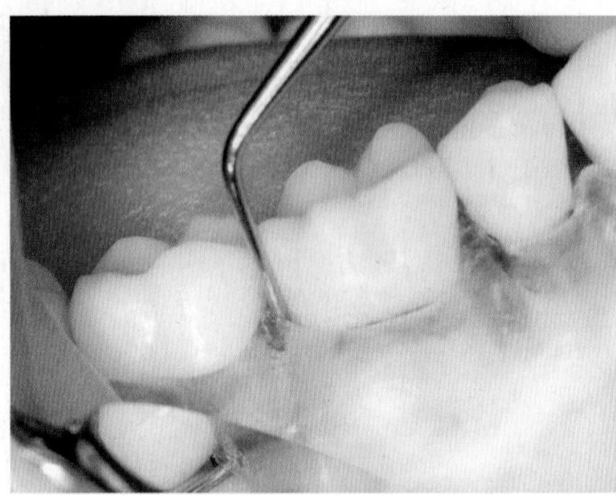

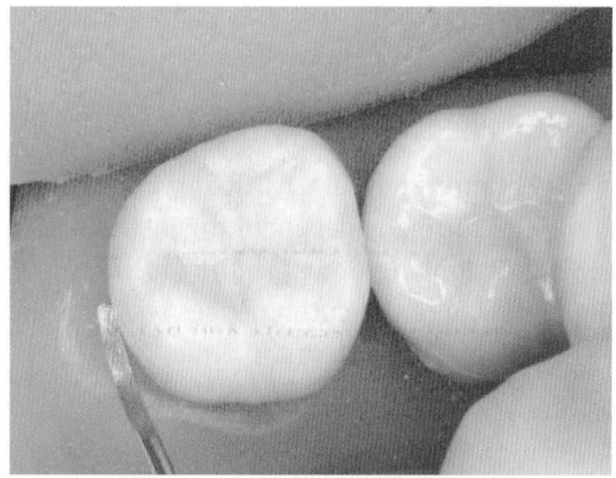

Figure 15-11. Incorrect Angulation. Because the lower shank is at a 90° angle to face, *positioning the lower shank parallel to the tooth surface results in an angulation of 90°*.

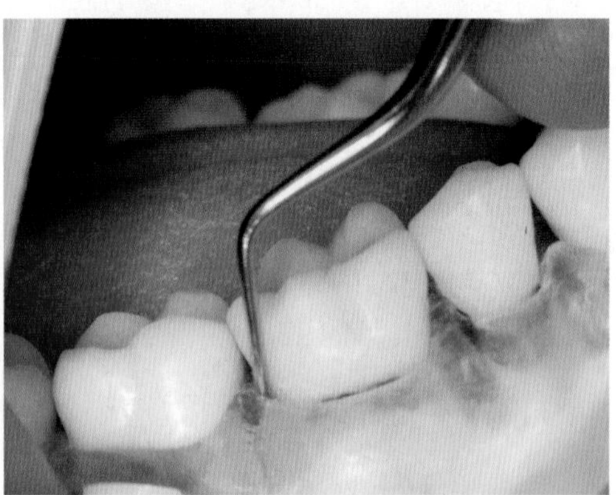

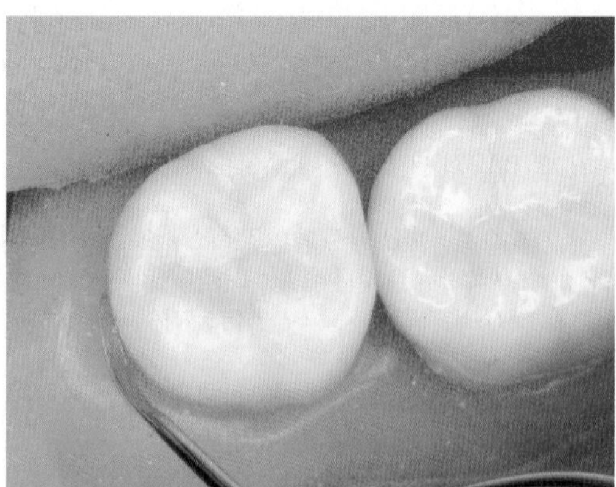

Figure 15-12. Correct Angulation. Correct angulation is *achieved by tilting the lower shank slightly toward the tooth surface* to be instrumented. In this position, the face-to-tooth surface angulation is between 70° and 80°.

APPLICATION OF THE CUTTING EDGES TO THE POSTERIOR TEETH

All four cutting edges of a universal curet are used for calculus removal on the posterior sextants. Figures 15-13 and 15-14 depict application of the cutting edges to the mandibular right posterior sextant.

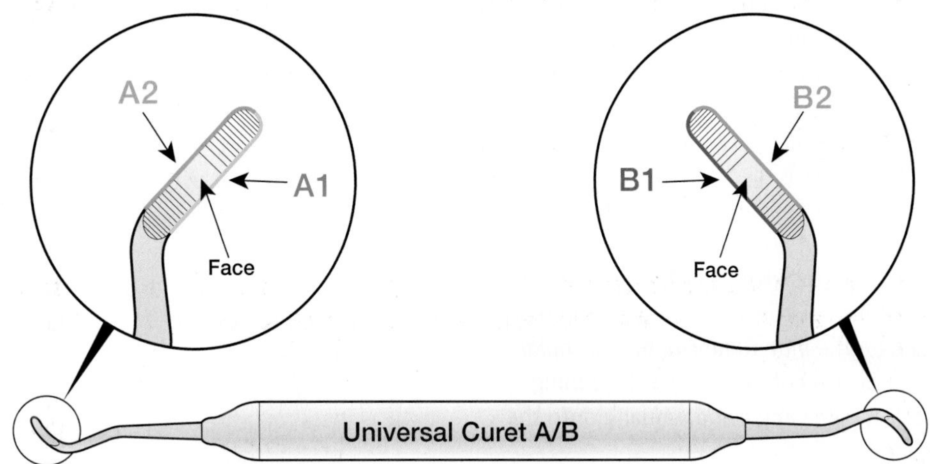

Figure 15-13. Four Cutting Edges of a Universal Curet. A universal curet has two working-ends. Working-end A has two cutting edges (A1 and A2). Working-end B has two cutting edges (B1 and B2).

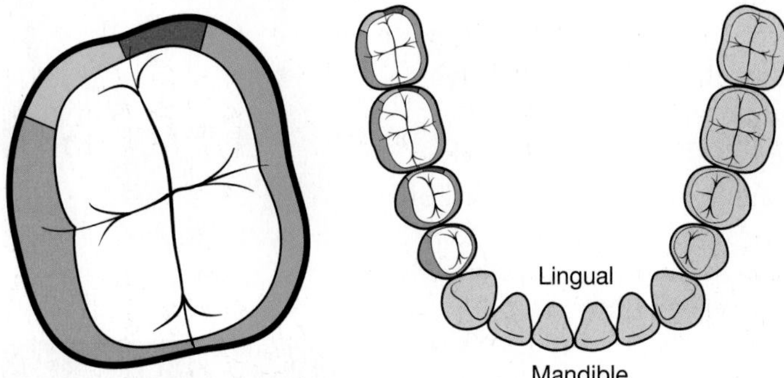

Figure 15-14. Application of Cutting Edges to Posterior Surfaces. These illustrations indicate how the cutting edges of a universal curet are applied to the tooth surfaces of the mandibular first molar and the mandibular right posterior sextant.

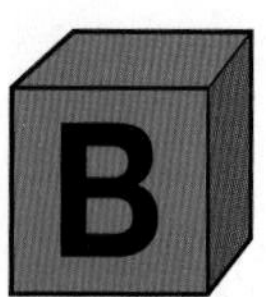

SKILL BUILDING. STEP-BY-STEP TECHNIQUE ON MANDIBULAR FIRST MOLAR

- Follow steps 1 to 19—shown in Figures 15-15 to 15-33—to practice use of a universal curet on the mandibular right posterior sextant.
- ***Use a periodontal typodont.***[1,2] ***Practice insertion with the gingiva in place, and then remove the gingiva to practice making calculus removal strokes on the cervical thirds of the roots.***
- Remember: "Me, My patient, My light, My dominant hand, My nondominant hand, My finger rest, My adaptation."

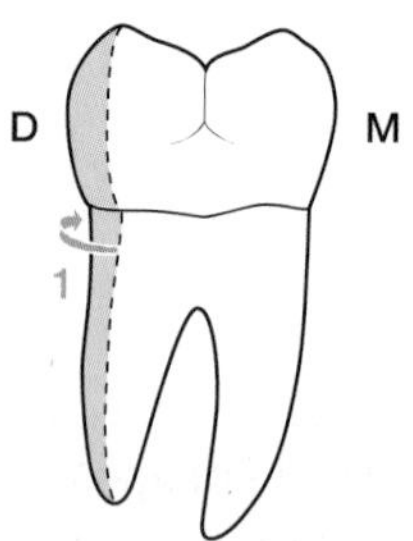

1. **Figure 15-15. Begin with Mandibular First Molar.** As an introduction to the universal curet, first practice on the *mandibular right first molar*. The distal surface is completed first, beginning at the distofacial line angle and working onto the distal surface.

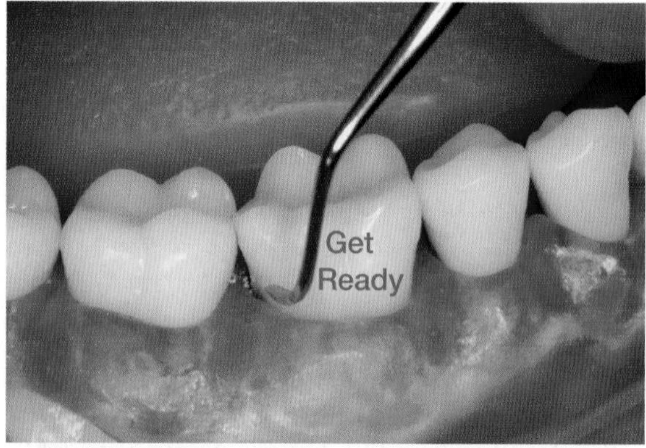

2. **Figure 15-16. Get Ready.**
   - Turn the toe of the working-end toward the distal surface.
   - Place the working-end in the **Get Ready Zone** in the middle-third of the crown. In this case, the Get Ready Zone is at the distofacial line angle in the middle-third of the crown.

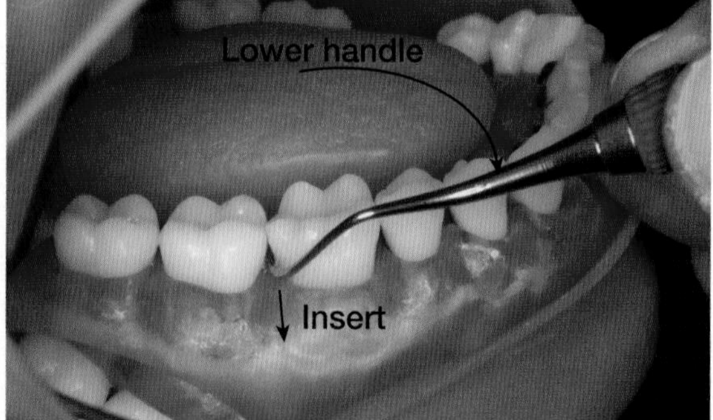

3. **Figure 15-17. Lower Handle.** Lower the instrument handle and establish a 0° angulation.

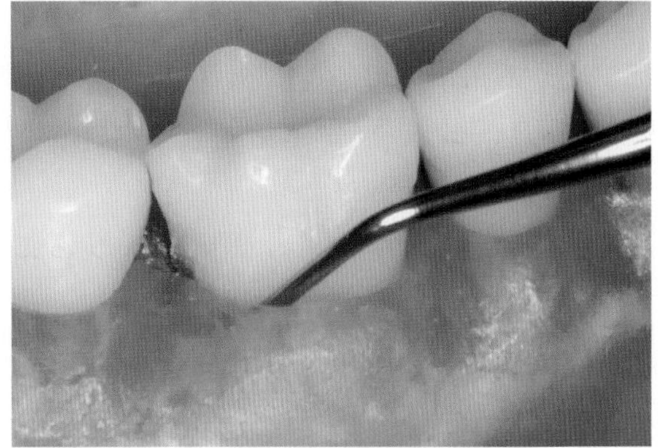

4. **Figure 15-18. Insert.** Gently slide the working-end beneath the gingival margin and onto the distal surface of the root.

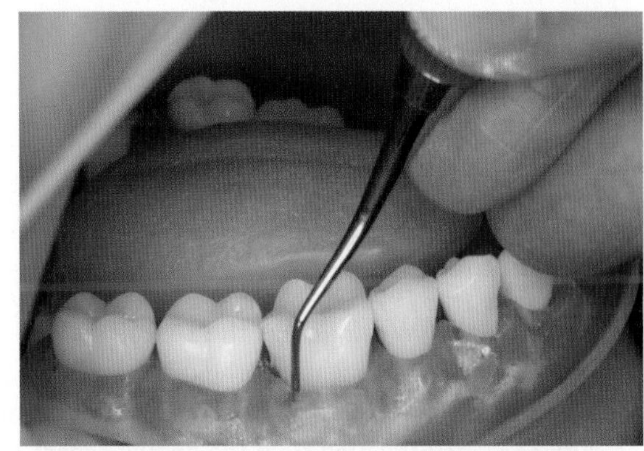

5. **Figure 15-19. Reestablish Handle Position.** Return handle to its normal upright position in preparation for initiation of calculus removal strokes.

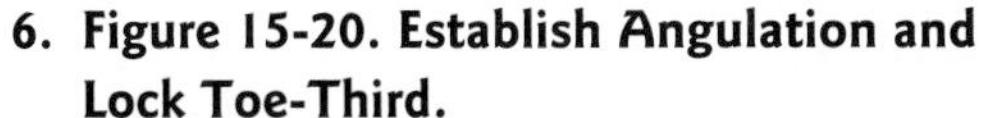

6. **Figure 15-20. Establish Angulation and Lock Toe-Third.**
    - Establish an 80° face-to-root surface angulation ***by tilting the lower shank slightly toward the distal surface.***
    - Adapt the toe-third of the working-end to the distofacial line angle. ***Imagine "locking" the toe-third against the tooth surface.***

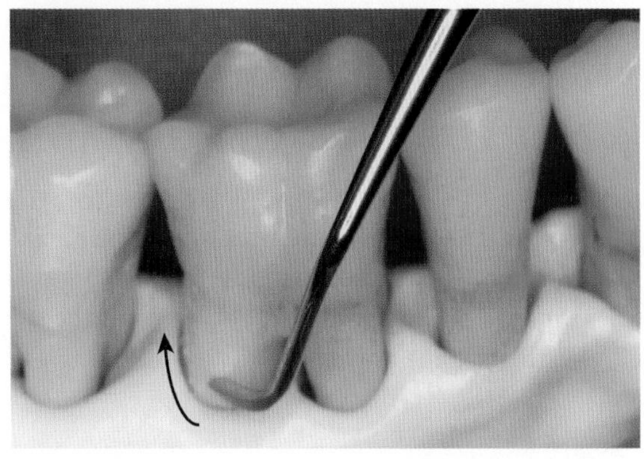

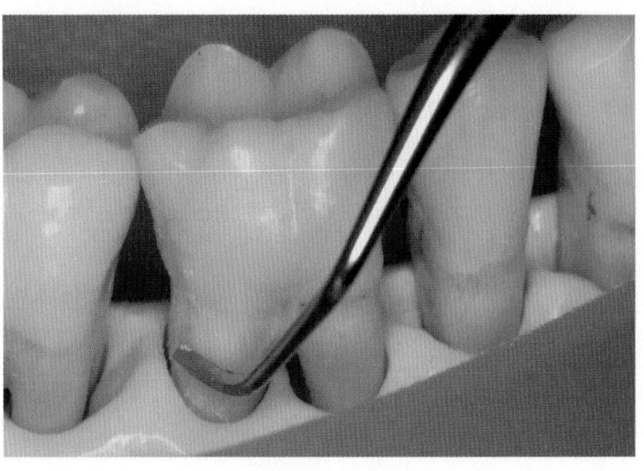

7. **Figure 15-21. Roll Handle.** Roll the instrument handle to maintain adaptation as strokes are made around the distofacial line angle.

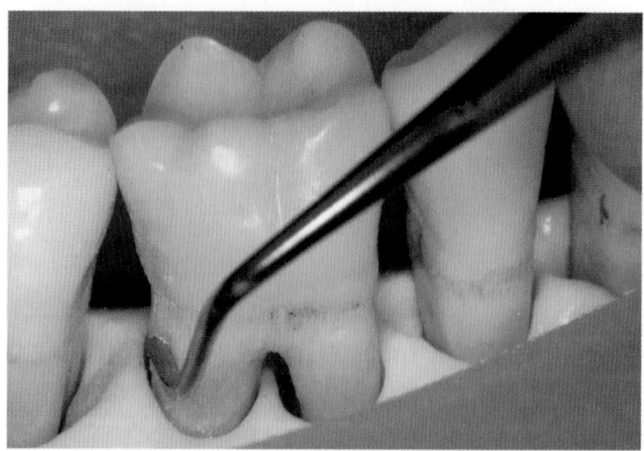

8. **Figure 15-22. Continue Strokes across Distal Surface.** Continue making short, precise strokes on the distal surface.

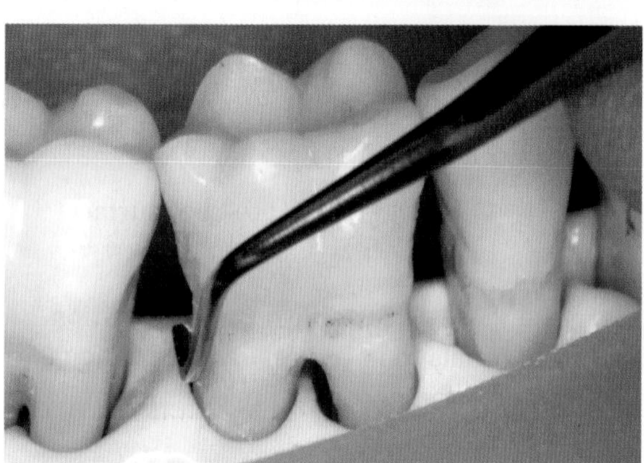

9. **Figure 15-23. Work across the Distal Surface.** Work at least halfway across the distal surface from the facial aspect. The other half of the distal surface is instrumented from the lingual aspect.

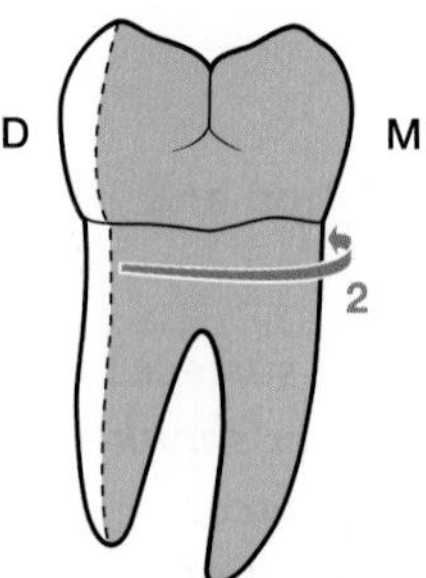

10. **Figure 15-24. Instrumentation of the Facial Surface.** Next, instrument the facial and mesial surfaces of the first molar, beginning at the distofacial line angle.

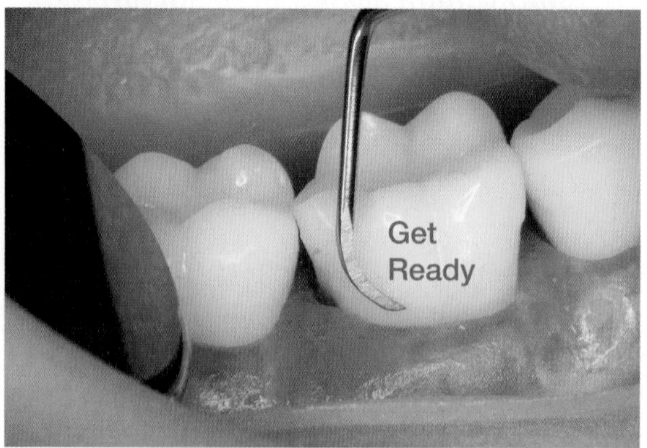

11. **Figure 15-25. Get Ready for Facial Surface.**
    - Turn the working-end so that the toe of the curet aims toward the front of the mouth.
    - Place the working-end in the Get Ready Zone on the middle-third of the facial surface near the line angle.

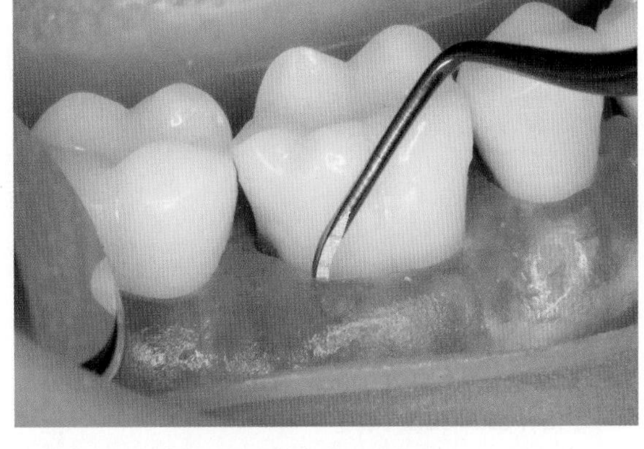

12. **Figure 15-26. Insert.**
    - Gently slide the working-end beneath the gingival margin.
    - Imagine the face sliding along the facial surface all the way to the base of the pocket.

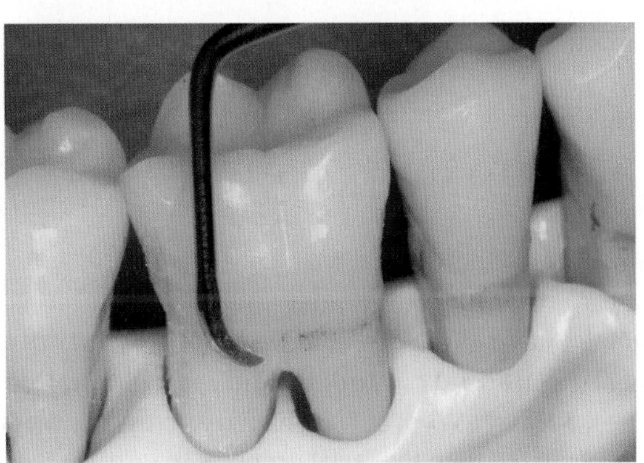

13. **Figure 15-27. Establish Angulation and Lock Toe-Third.**
    - Establish an 80° face-to-root surface angulation ***by tilting the lower shank slightly toward the facial surface.***
    - Adapt the toe-third of the working-end to the distofacial line angle. ***Imagine "locking" the toe-third against the tooth surface.***

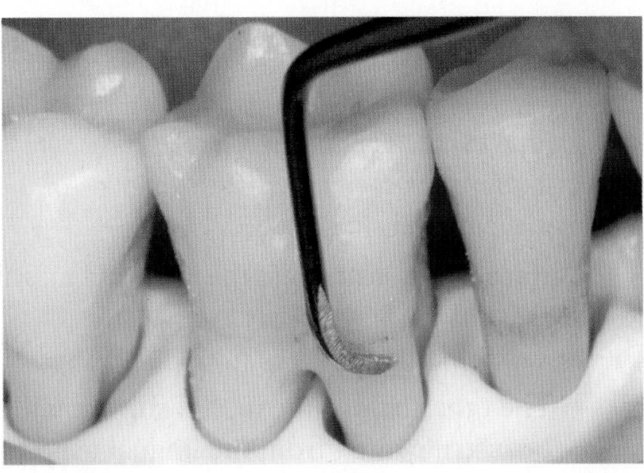

14. **Figure 15-28. Make Strokes across the Facial Surface.** Initiate a series of short, precise strokes across the facial surface.

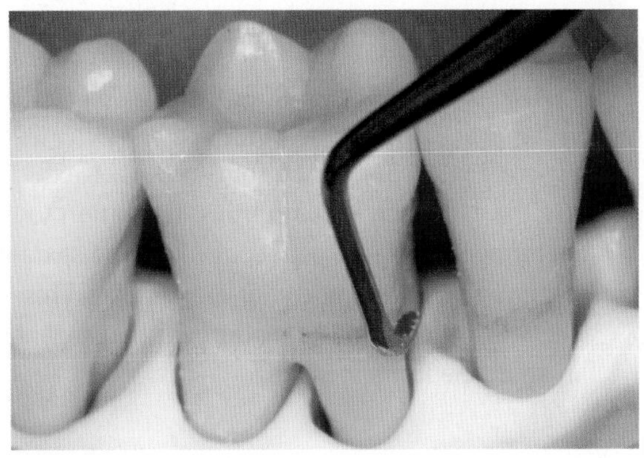

15. **Figure 15-29. Instrument the Facial Surface. Roll Handle at Line Angle.**
    - As you approach the mesiofacial line angle, roll the handle slightly to maintain adaptation.
    - Keep the toe-third "locked" against the tooth surface.

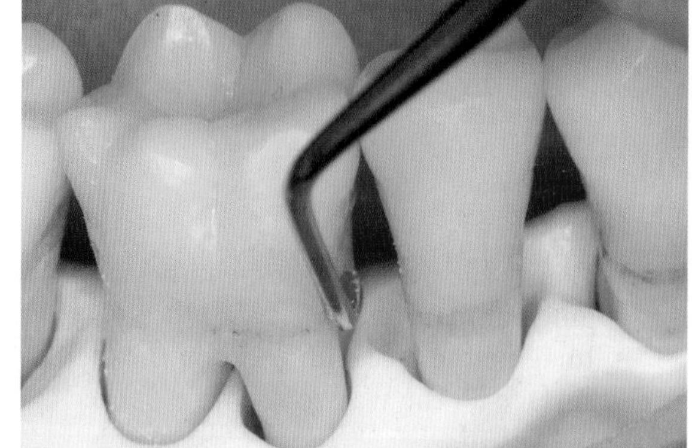

16. **Figure 15-30. Work across the Mesial Surface.** Make a series of precise strokes across the mesial surface.

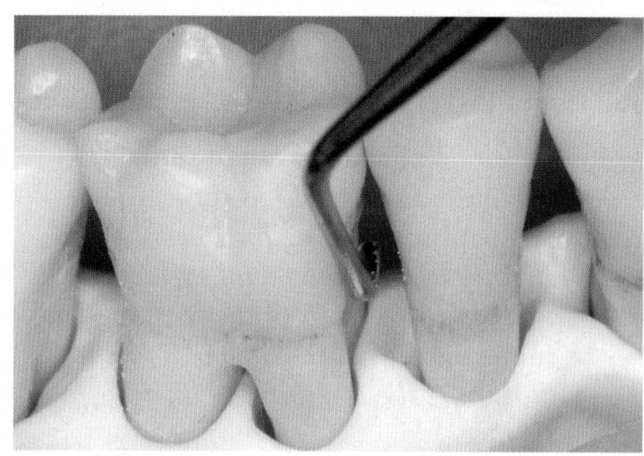

17. **Figure 15-31. Work to Midline of Mesial Surface.** Work at least halfway across the mesial surface from the facial aspect.

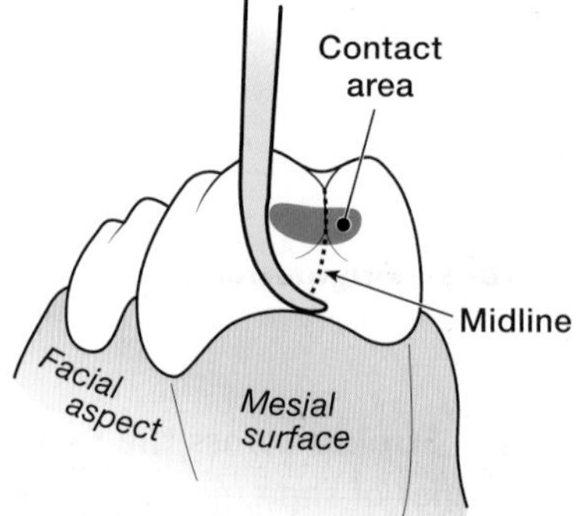

18. **Figure 15-32. Technique Check.** Make sure that your strokes extend past the midline of the mesial proximal surface.
    - Work at least halfway across the mesial surface from the facial aspect while maintaining proper angulation.
    - The other half of the mesial surface will be instrumented from the lingual aspect.

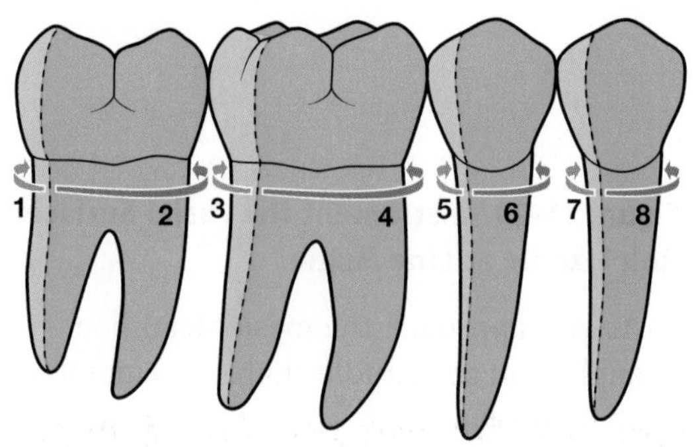

19. **Figure 15-33. Sequence for Sextant.** Next, use the sequence shown in this illustration to instrument the facial aspect of the entire sextant, beginning with the posterior-most molar. This sequence allows you to instrument the sextant in an efficient manner.

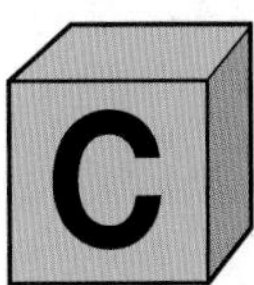

SKILL BUILDING. STEP-BY-STEP TECHNIQUE ON MAXILLARY FIRST MOLAR

- Follow steps 1 to 6—shown in Figures 15-34 to 15-39—to practice use of a universal curet on the maxillary right posterior sextant.
- Use a periodontal typodont. Practice insertion with the gingiva in place, and then remove the gingiva to practice making calculus removal strokes on the cervical thirds of the roots.[1,2]
- Remember: "Me, My patient, My light, My dominant hand, My nondominant hand, My finger rest, My adaptation."

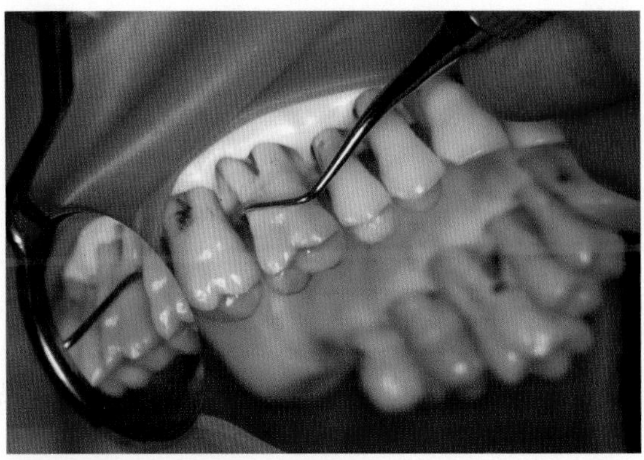

1. Figure 15-34. Get Ready and Insert.

- Turn the toe toward the distal surface. Position the working-end in the Get Ready Zone.
- Raise the instrument handle and establish a 0° angulation.
- Gently slide the working-end beneath the gingival margin.

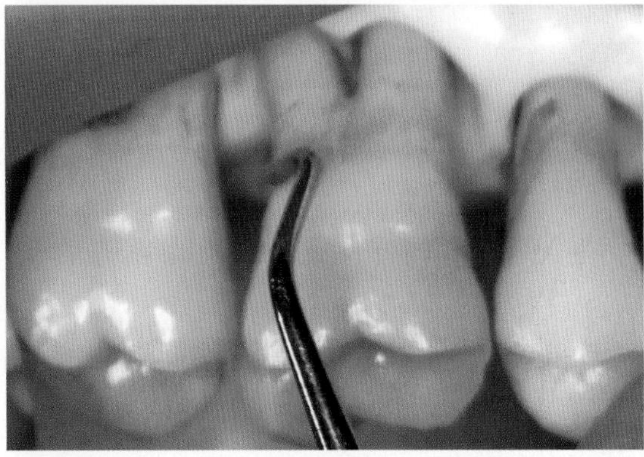

2. Figure 15-35. Establish Angulation and Lock-Toe Third.

- Establish an 80° angulation.
- Adapt the toe-third of the working-end to the distofacial line angle. Imagine "locking" the toe-third against the tooth surface.

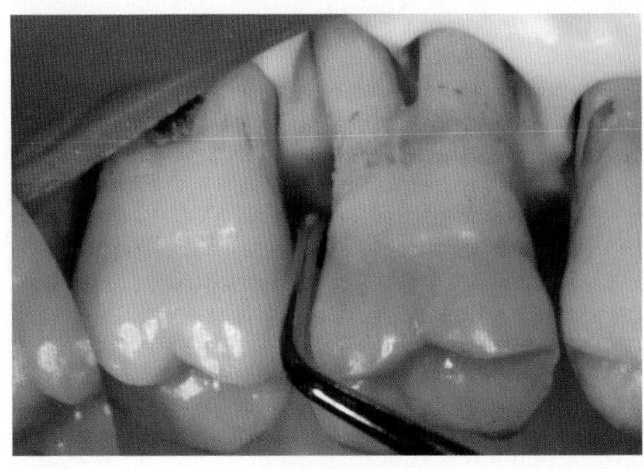

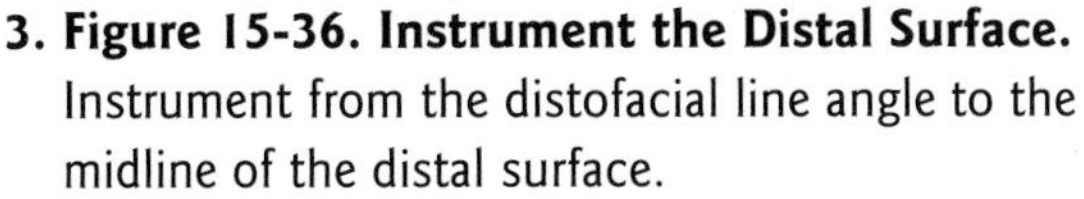

3. Figure 15-36. Instrument the Distal Surface. Instrument from the distofacial line angle to the midline of the distal surface.

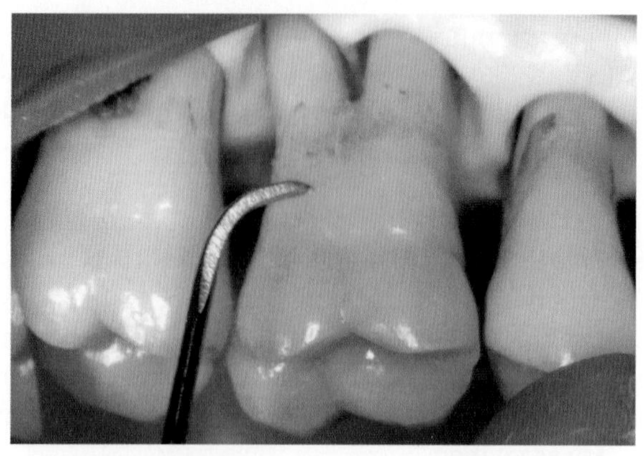

4. **Figure 15-37. Get Ready for Facial Surface.**
   - Turn the working-end so the toe aims toward the front of the mouth.
   - Place the working-end in the Get Ready Zone on the middle-third of the facial surface near the distofacial line angle.
   - Gently slide the working-end beneath the gingival margin all the way to the base of the pocket.

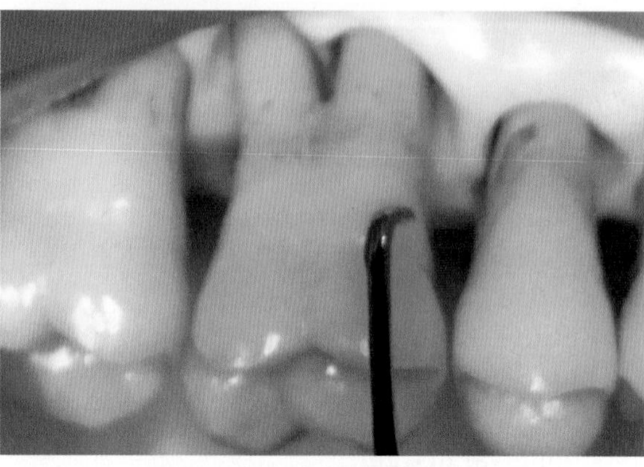

5. **Figure 15-38. Instrument the Facial Surface.**
   - Work across the facial surface.
   - As you approach the mesiofacial line angle, roll the handle slightly to maintain adaptation.

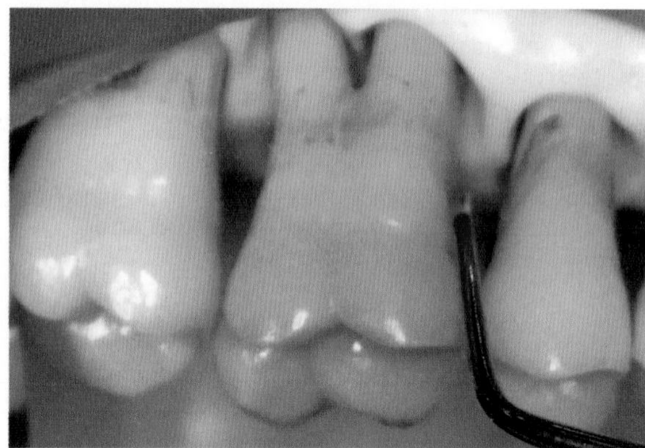

6. **Figure 15-39. Instrument the Mesial Surface.** Work from the mesiofacial line angle to the midline of the mesial surface.

Section 4
Technique Alert—Lower Shank Position

Adapting the working-end to the facial and lingual root surfaces of the mandibular posterior teeth is challenging for two reasons: (1) the clinician's hand position may block the view of the mandibular lingual surfaces, and (2) the rounded posterior crowns make it difficult to instrument the root surfaces of these teeth. Figures 15-40 to 15-44 depict incorrect and correct techniques for shank alignment to root surfaces.

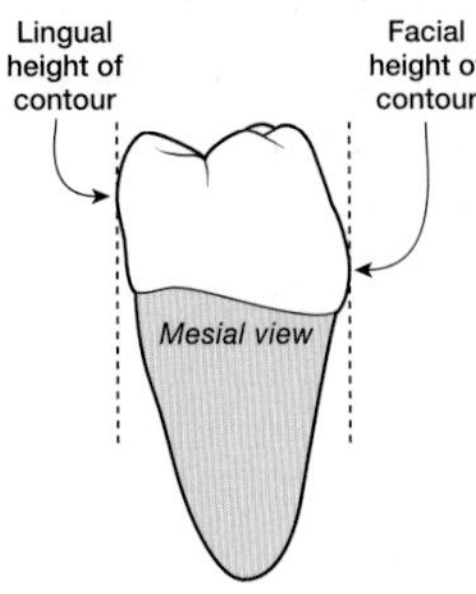

Figure 15-40. Height of Contour on Molars. ***This illustration shows a side view of a molar, looking at the mesial surface.*** Note that the crown protrudes over—overhangs—the root surface.

INCORRECT TECHNIQUE

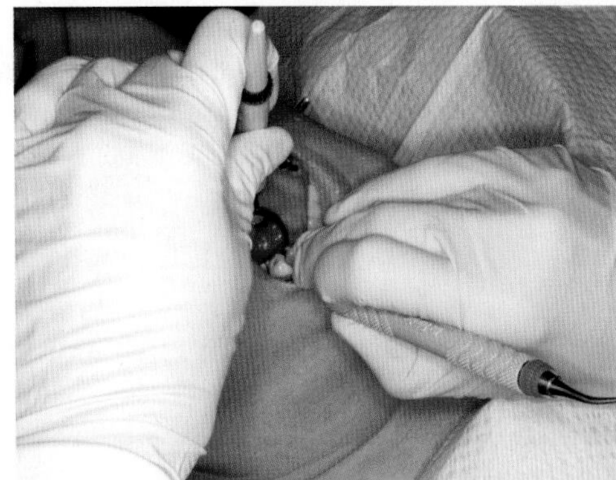

Figure 15-41. Incorrect Handle Position. Inexperienced clinicians often will tilt the instrument handle down in an attempt to obtain a better view of the mandibular lingual surfaces.

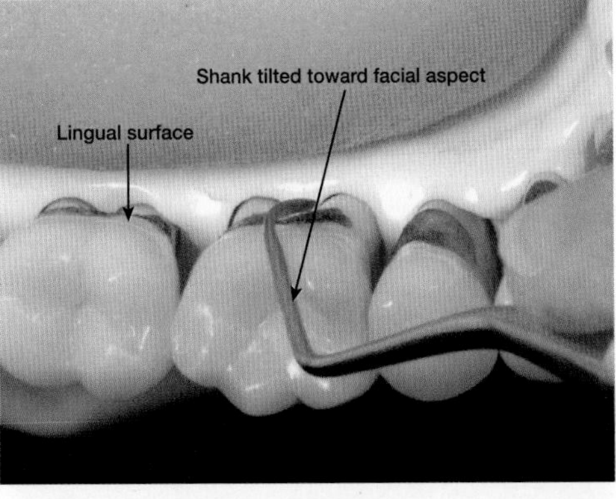

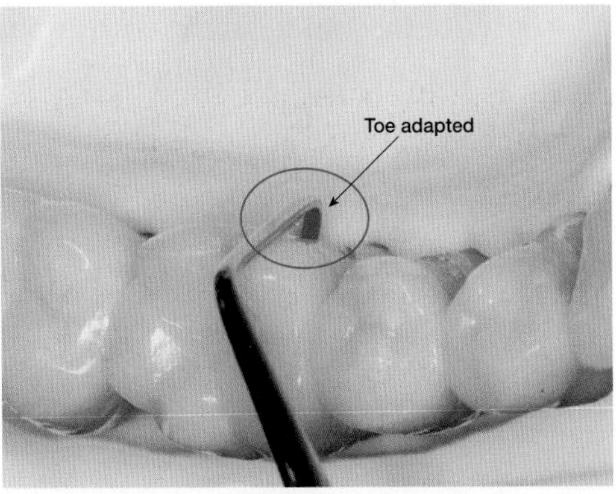

Figure 15-42. Incorrect Technique: Handle Tilted toward Clinician. Tilting the instrument handle toward the clinician causes the lower shank to hit the crown of the tooth. In this position, it is not possible to adapt the working-end to the root surface because the root is smaller in diameter than the crown. The lower shank simply rocks against the occlusal surface of the crown, causing the working-end to lift off of the root surface without engaging the calculus deposit.

CORRECT TECHNIQUE

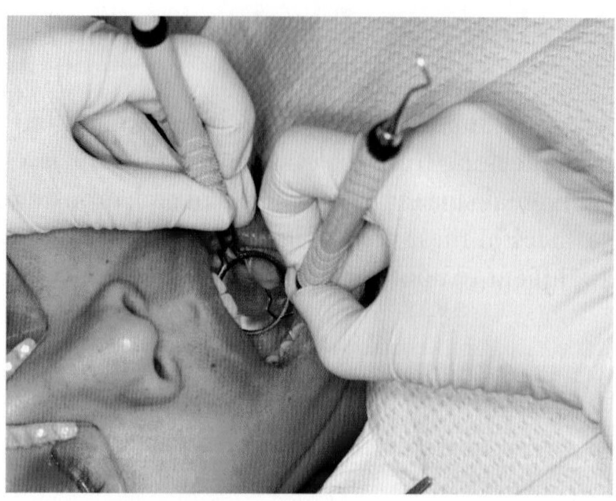

Figure 15-43. Correct Handle Position. When working on the lingual surfaces, keep the handle in the normal position and use the mirror for indirect vision.

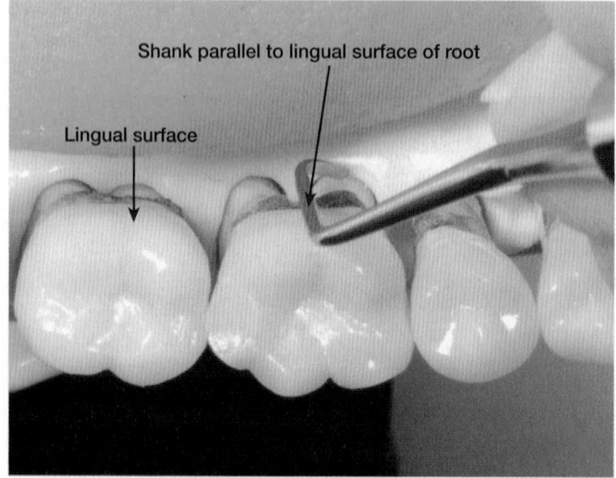

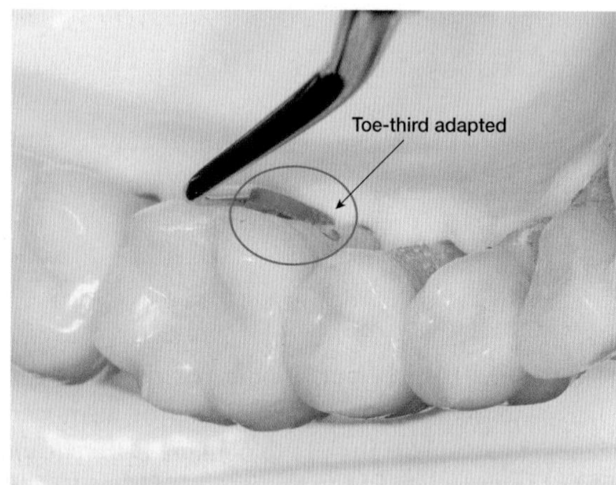

Figure 15-44. Correct Technique Produces an Unimpeded Stroke.

- With the handle in the correct position, the lower shank is not in contact with either the lingual or occlusal surfaces of the tooth crown.
- In this position, it is easy to make oblique or vertical instrumentation strokes upward along the root surface without rocking against the occlusal surface of the crown.

Section 5
Technique Practice—Anterior Teeth

Adapting a universal curet to the anterior teeth requires a technique that is different from that used with other instruments. For this reason, some clinicians prefer not to use universal curets on the anterior sextants. The complex shank design of the universal curet, however, sometimes facilitates access to the lingual root surfaces of the mandibular anterior teeth. Additionally, it is efficient to use a single instrument for both the anterior and posterior teeth.

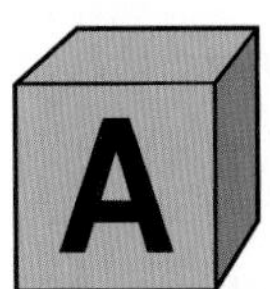

SKILL BUILDING. SELECTING THE CORRECT WORKING-END FOR AN ANTERIOR TOOTH

Method 1: Lower Shank as a Visual Clue

The first method uses the lower shank as a visual clue as shown in Figures 15-45 to 15-47.

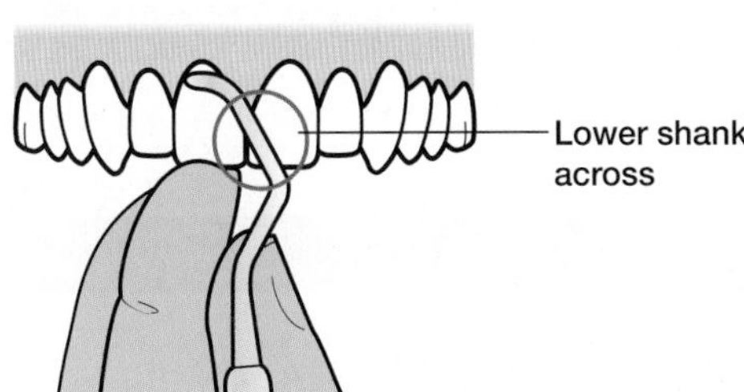

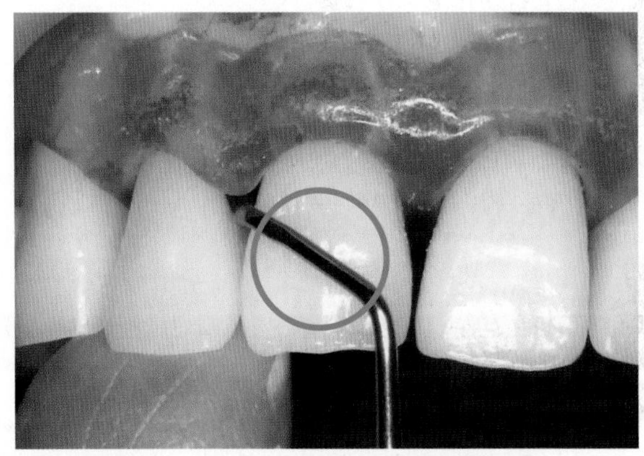

Figures 15-45 and 15-46. Lower Shank as Visual Clue: Correct Working-End.

- When using a universal curet on anterior teeth, the correct working-end is selected if the *lower shank is across the tooth surface.*
- *Think: "Universal curet = Anterior across."*

Figure 15-47. Incorrect Working-End.

- This photo shows the **incorrect** working-end of a universal curet adapted to the distal surface of the central incisor.
- In this position, the cutting edge is not correctly adapted to the tooth surface.

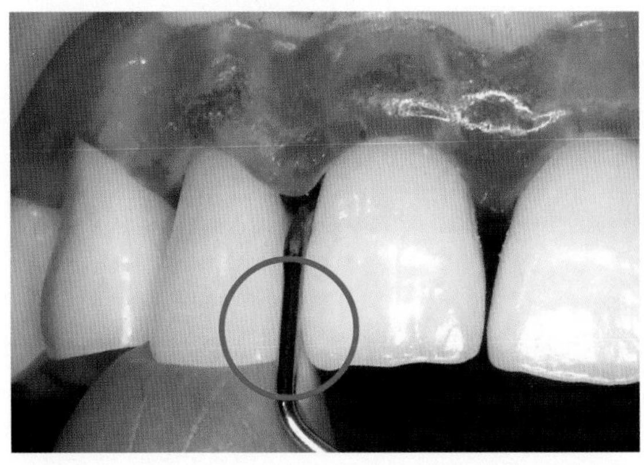

Method 2: The Inner and Outer Cutting Edges as a Visual Clue

There is a second method for selecting the correct working-end of a universal curet. For this method, the cutting edges provide the visual clue (Fig. 15-48). It is not important whether a clinician uses method 1 or method 2 to select the working-end. Each clinician should use the method that is easiest for him or her.

Method 2: *The bends in the functional shank of a universal curet cause one of the cutting edges to be nearer the handle than the other.* Each working-end has two cutting edges: an inner and an outer cutting edge.

- The **outer cutting edge** is the one that is *farther from the instrument handle.*
- ***Only the outer cutting edges—the edges farthest from the handle—are used to instrument the anterior teeth.***

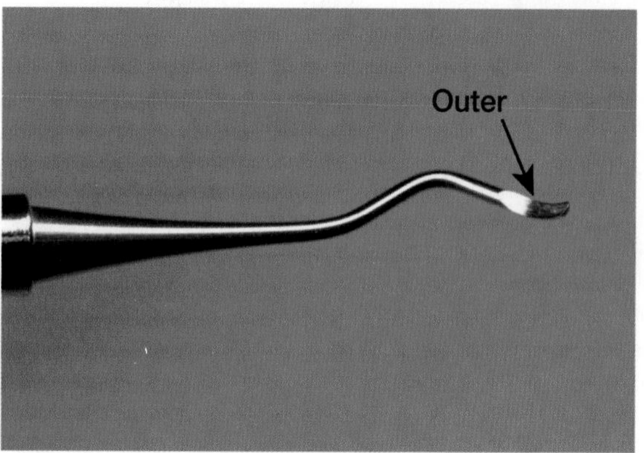

Figure 15-48. Outer Cutting Edge.

- To identify the outer cutting edge, hold the instrument so that you are looking down at the face of the working-end.
- ***Only the outer cutting edges are used to instrument the anterior teeth.***

Box 15-3. Outer Cutting Edge as Visual Clue

When using a universal curet on anterior teeth, only the ***outer cutting edges*** are used.

APPLICATION OF THE CUTTING EDGES TO THE ANTERIOR TEETH

Only one cutting edge per working-end (Fig. 15-49) is used on the anterior sextants when working with a universal curet. The visual clues for the correct working-end are (1) the lower shank goes across the tooth surface, and (2) only the outer cutting edge is used (Fig. 15-50).

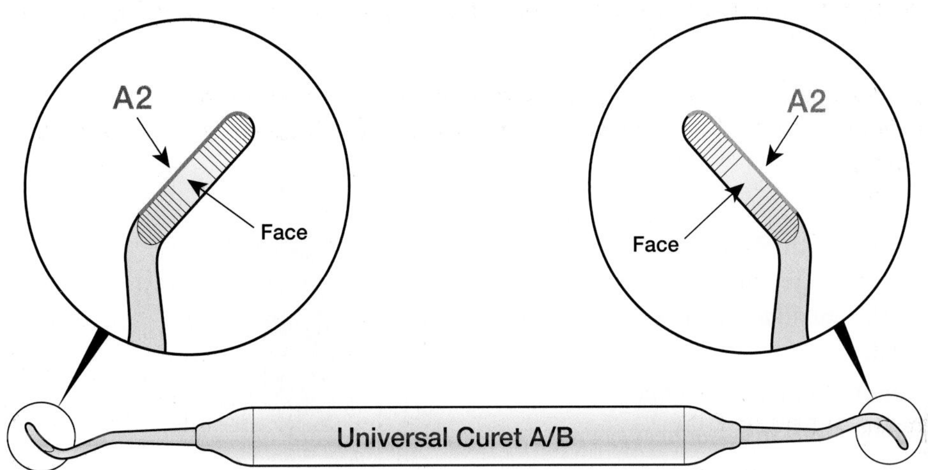

Figure 15-49. Cutting Edges. On a universal curet, ***only one cutting edge per working-end is used on anterior tooth surfaces.***

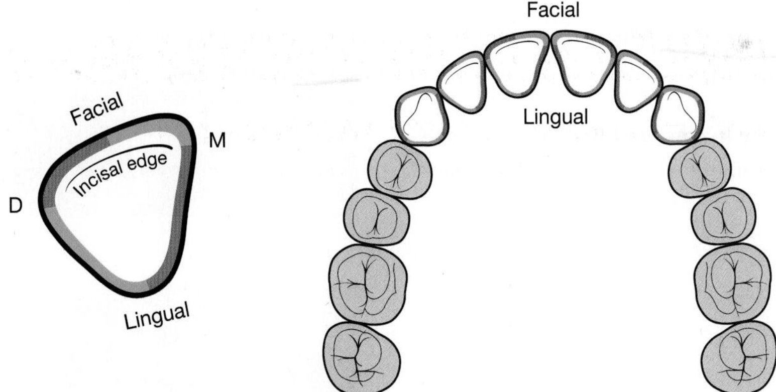

Figure 15-50. Application to Anterior Surfaces. The illustration indicates how the working-ends of a universal curet are applied to the anterior tooth surfaces. ***For each aspect, one working-end is used on the surfaces toward the clinician, and the opposite working-end is used on the surfaces away from the clinician.***

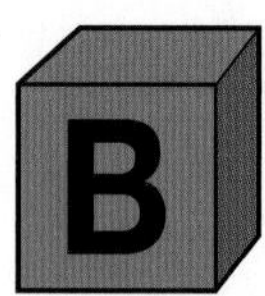

SKILL BUILDING. STEP-BY-STEP TECHNIQUE ON A MAXILLARY CENTRAL INCISOR

- Follow steps 1 to 8—shown in Figures 15-51 to 15-58—to practice use of a universal curet on the maxillary anterior teeth.
- Remember: "Me, My patient, My light, My dominant hand, My nondominant hand, My finger rest, My adaptation."

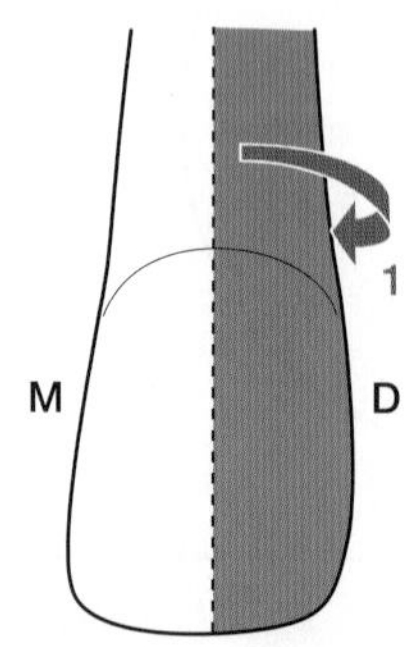

1. **Figure 15-51. Tooth.** As an introduction to using a universal curet on the anterior teeth, first practice on the ***maxillary right central incisor, facial aspect***.

   RIGHT-Handed clinicians—*surface away*.

   LEFT-Handed clinicians—*surface toward*.

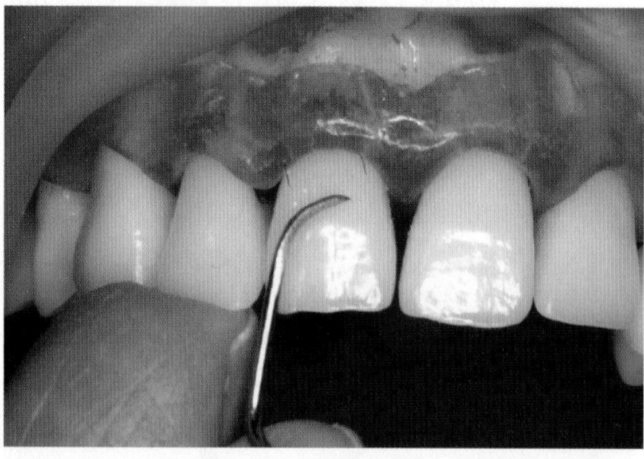

2. **Figure 15-52. Get Ready and Insert.** Select the correct working-end and place it in the Get Ready Zone.

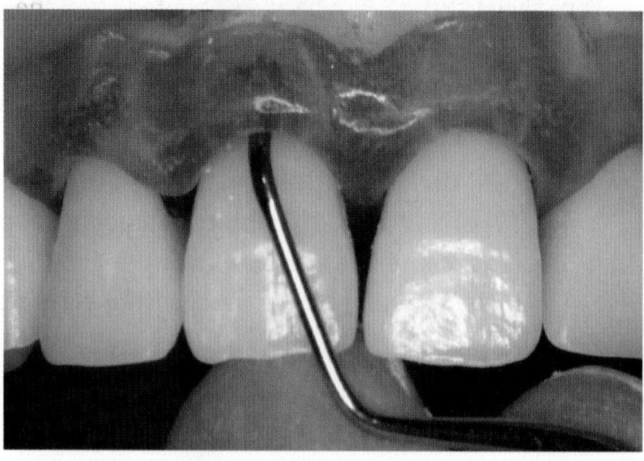

3. **Figure 15-53. Insert.** Insert the working-end to the base of the pocket.

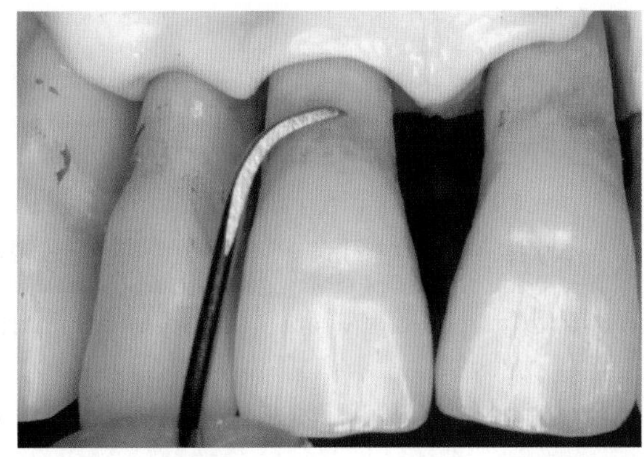

4. **Figure 15-54. Establish Correct Angulation.**
   - Adapt the toe-third to the root surface. ***Imagine "locking" the toe-third against the root surface.***
   - Instrument from the midline of the facial surface toward the mesial surface.

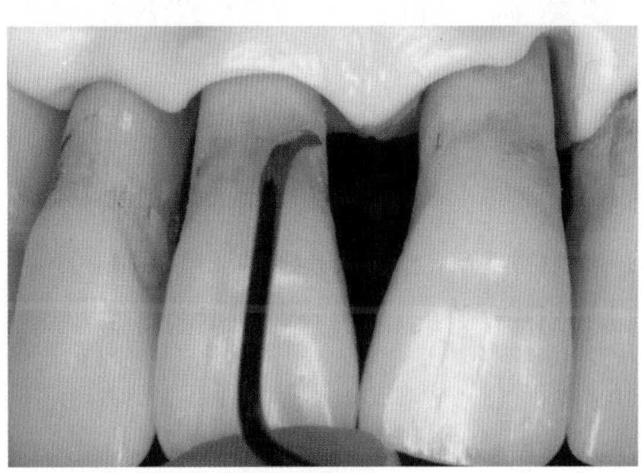

5. **Figure 15-55. Roll Handle at Line Angle.** Roll the handle slightly to maintain adaptation of the toe-third to the line angle.

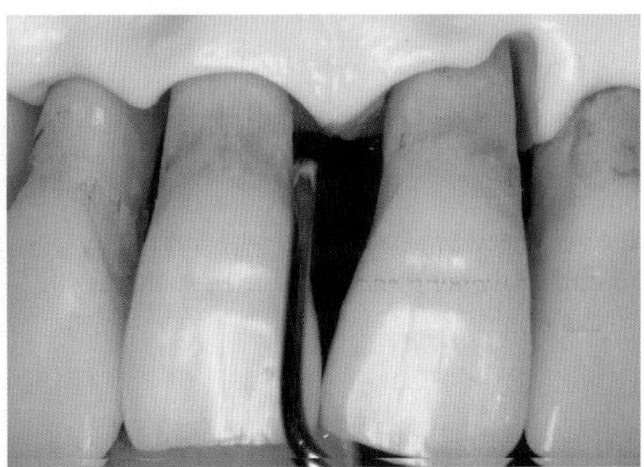

6. **Figure 15-56. Mesial Surface.** Work at least half-way across the mesial surface. The other half of the mesial surface will be instrumented from the lingual aspect of the tooth.

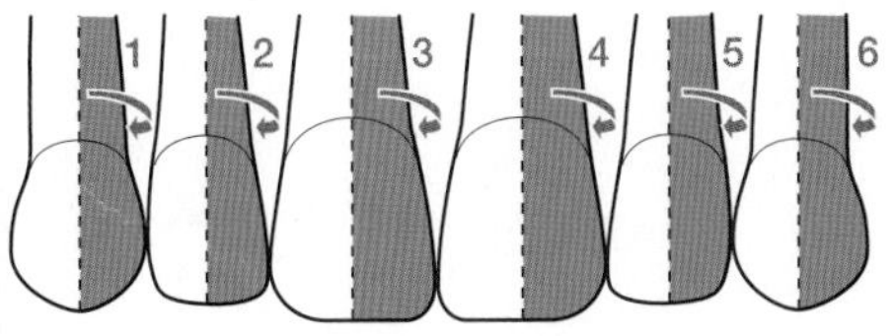

7. **Figure 15-57. Sequence.** Use the sequence shown in this illustration to instrument the colored tooth surfaces of the facial aspect. Begin with the left canine and end with the right canine.

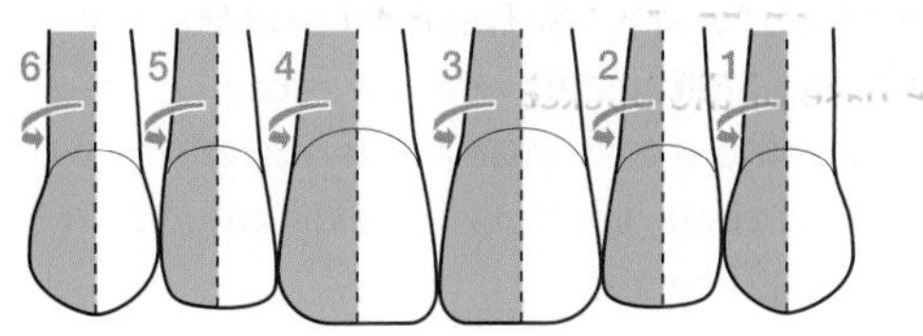

8. **Figure 15-58. Sequence.** Complete the remaining facial surfaces, beginning with the right canine and ending with the left canine.

Section 6
Technique Alert—Horizontal Strokes

- Novice clinicians often fail to remove calculus deposits that are located:
  - Near the distofacial or distolingual line angles of posterior root surfaces
  - At the midlines of the facial and lingual surfaces of anterior root surfaces
- Horizontal calculus removal strokes are extremely useful for calculus removal in these areas.

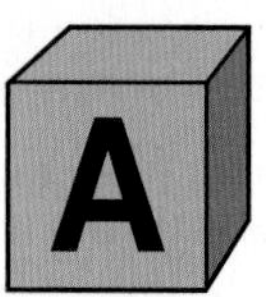

SKILL BUILDING. HORIZONTAL STROKES BELOW THE GINGIVAL MARGIN

Directions: Follow the directions below to practice making horizontal calculus removal strokes at the distofacial line angle of the mandibular first molar (Figs. 15-59 and 15-60).

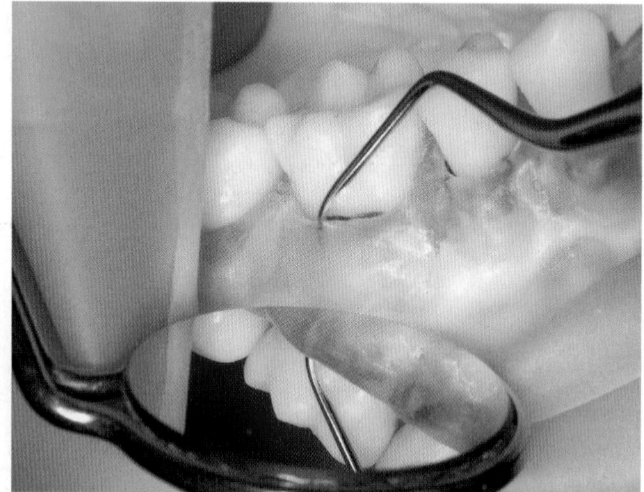

Figure 15-59. Establish Handle Position. Insert the curet slightly distal to the distofacial line angle. Lower the instrument handle until the curet working-end is oriented with the toe toward—but not touching—the base of the sulcus or pocket.

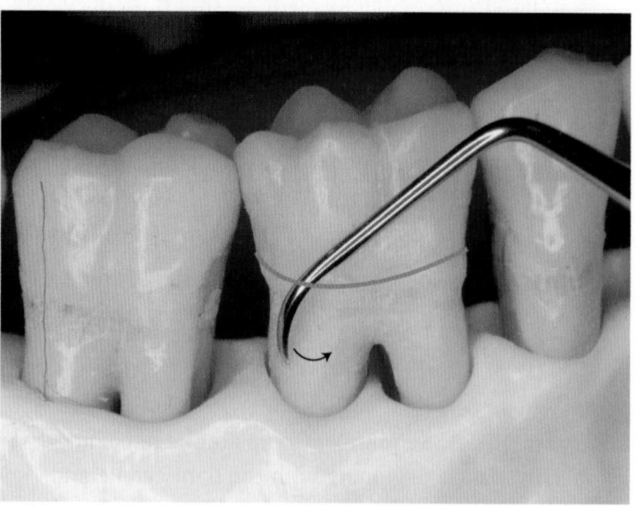

Figure 15-60. Make Several Horizontal Strokes. Begin a calculus removal stroke slightly distal to the distofacial line angle. Make several short, controlled strokes around the distofacial line angle.

Directions: Follow the directions below to practice making horizontal strokes at the midline of the facial and lingual surfaces of a central incisor (Figs. 15-61 and 15-62).

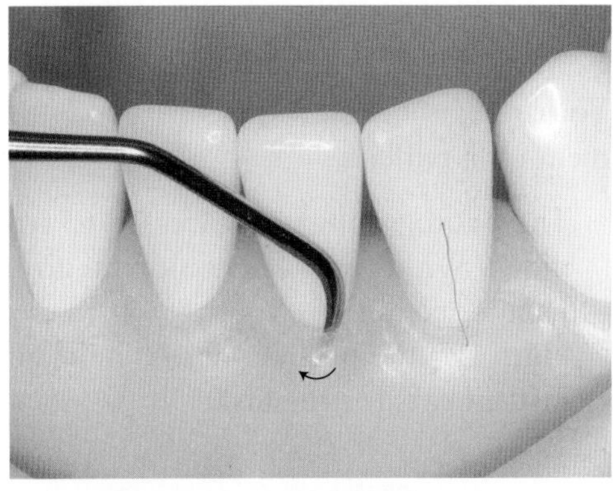

Figure 15-61. Horizontal Strokes on Facial Surface. Insert the working-end just distal to the midline.

Lower the handle until the curet toe is toward—but not touching—the base of the sulcus. Make several short, controlled horizontal strokes across the midline of the facial surface.

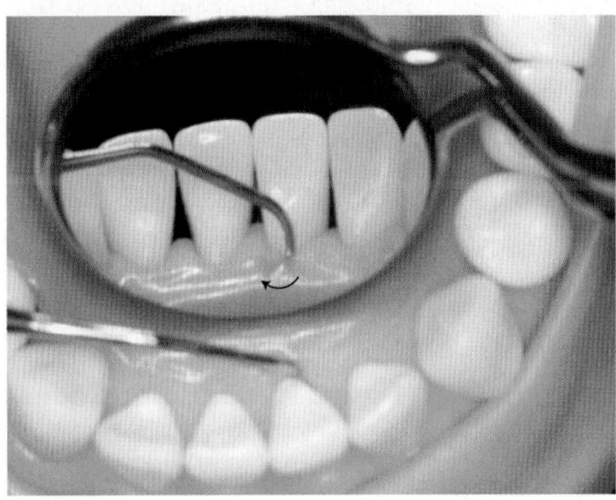

Figure 15-62. Horizontal Strokes on Lingual Surface. Lower the handle until the curet toe is toward—but not touching—the base of the sulcus. Make several short, controlled horizontal strokes across the midline of the lingual surface.

REFERENCES

1. Dufour LA, Bissell HS. Periodontal attachment loss induced by mechanical subgingival instrumentation in shallow sulci. *J Dent Hyg.* 2002;76:207–212.
2. Ruhling A, Konig J, Rolf H, Kocher T, Schwahn C, Plagmann HC. Learning root debridement with curettes and power-driven instruments. Part II: clinical results following mechanical, non-surgical therapy. *J Clin Periodontol.* 2003;30:611–615.

Section 7
Skill Application

PRACTICAL FOCUS

You have been assigned to observe a second-year student, Ling, as she performs periodontal debridement on a patient.

- The photographs in Figures 15-63 to 15-67 are characteristic of Ling's instrumentation technique. What feedback could you give to Ling about her instrumentation technique and instrument selection?
- Hint: Use the probing depths indicated in Figures 15-63 and 15-64 to evaluate Ling's choice of instruments for the task.

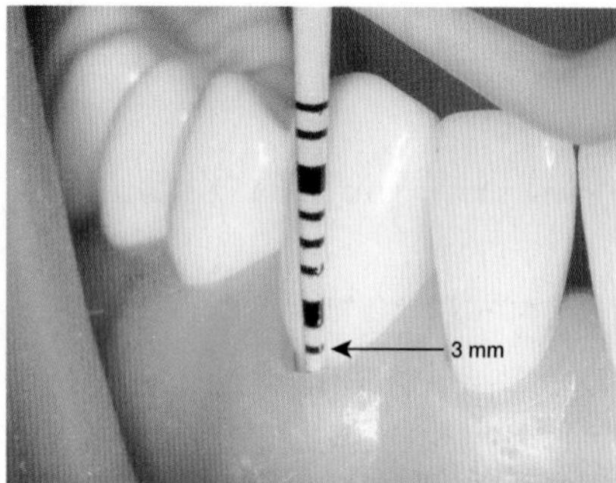

Figure 15-63. Color-Coded Probe.

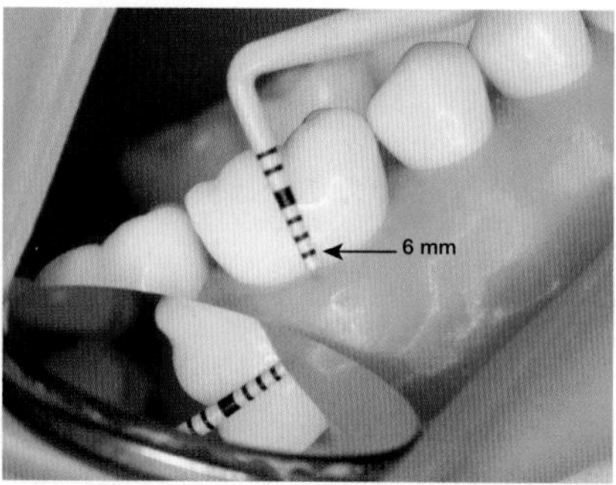

Figure 15-64. Color-Coded Probe.

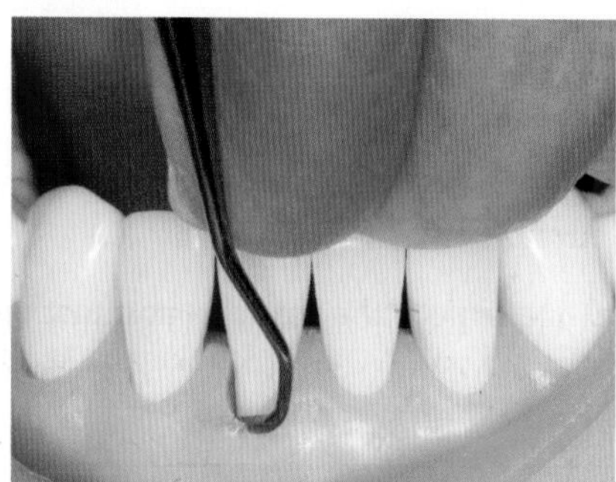

Figure 15-65. Sickle Scaler.

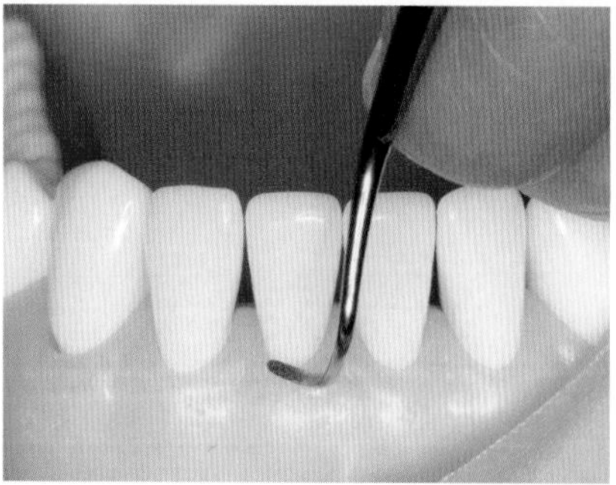

Figure 15-66. Universal Curet.

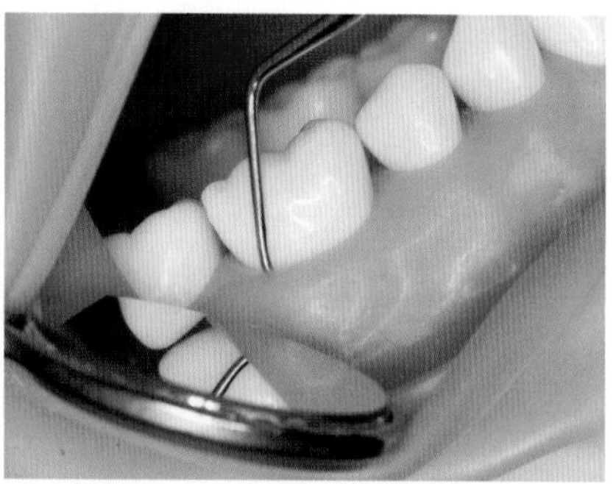

Figure 15-67. Universal Curet.

REFERENCE SHEET: UNIVERSAL CURETS

Use of Universal Curets:

A universal curet is a periodontal instrument used to remove light and medium calculus deposits from the crowns and roots of the teeth.

Basic Concepts:

1. Tilt the lower shank slightly toward the tooth surface to establish correct face-to-tooth surface angulation.
2. Insert the working-end beneath the gingival margin at a 0° to 40° angulation.
3. Maintain adaptation of the toe-third of the cutting edge to the tooth surface.
4. Activate the calculus removal stroke away from the junctional epithelium using wrist motion activation.
5. Relax your fingers between each calculus removal stroke.

Anterior Teeth:

1. Select the correct working-end:
   - Method 1: When adapted on a proximal surface, the lower shank goes across the tooth ***(Anterior = Across)***.
   - Method 2: Only the outer cutting edges are used to instrument the anterior teeth.
2. Sequence: Begin with the surfaces toward your nondominant hand. Start on the canine on the opposite side of the mouth and work toward yourself. (Right-handed clinicians start with the left canine, mesial surface; left-handed clinicians start with the right canine, mesial surface.)

Posterior Teeth:

1. Select the correct working-end:
   - Method 1: The lower shank is parallel to the tooth surface ***(Posterior = Parallel. Functional shank up and over!)***
   - Method 2: The inner cutting edges are used on the distal surfaces. The outer cutting edges are used on the facial, lingual, and mesial surfaces.
2. Sequence: Begin at the distofacial line angle of the posterior-most tooth in the sextant and work toward the distal surface. Reposition at the distofacial line angle and complete the facial (or lingual) and mesial surfaces of the tooth, working toward the front of the mouth.

STUDENT SELF-EVALUATION MODULE 15 UNIVERSAL CURETS

Student: ____________________ Date: ____________________

DIRECTIONS: Self-evaluate your skill level in each treatment area as: **S** (satisfactory) or **U** (unsatisfactory).

Criteria				
Positioning/Ergonomics	**Area 1**	**Area 2**	**Area 3**	**Area 4**
Adjusts clinician and patient chairs and equipment correctly				
Assumes the recommended clock position				
Instrument Grasp: Dominant Hand	**Area 1**	**Area 2**	**Area 3**	**Area 4**
Grasps handle with tips of finger pads of index finger and thumb				
Rests pad of middle finger lightly on instrument shank				
Positions the thumb, index, and middle fingers in the "knuckles-up" convex position; hyperextended joint position is avoided				
Finger Rest: Dominant Hand				
Establishes secure finger rest that is appropriate for tooth to be treated				
Once finger rest is established, pauses to self-evaluate finger placement in the grasp, verbalizes to evaluator his/her self-assessment of grasp, and corrects finger placement if necessary				
Prepare for Instrumentation ("Get Ready")				
Selects correct working-end for tooth surface to be instrumented				
Places the working-end in the "Get Ready Zone" while using a correct finger rest for the treatment area				
Insertion	**Area 1**	**Area 2**	**Area 3**	**Area 4**
Establishes 0° angulation (face hugs tooth surface) in preparation for insertion				
Gently inserts curet toe beneath the gingival margin to base of sulcus or pocket				
Adaptation, Angulation, and Instrument Stroke	**Area 1**	**Area 2**	**Area 3**	**Area 4**
Assesses the root surface with curet using light, sweeping assessment strokes away from the junctional epithelium				
Initiates a stroke in a coronal direction by positioning the working-end beneath a calculus deposit, "locking the toe" against tooth surface and using an angulation between 45° and 80°				
Uses rotating motion to make a short, biting stroke in a coronal direction to snap a deposit from the tooth; does NOT close face toward tooth surface during activation; uses whole hand as a unit; does NOT pull with thumb and index finger				
Maintains appropriate lateral pressure against the tooth throughout the stroke while maintaining control of the working-end				
Precisely stops each individual stroke and pauses briefly (at least 3 seconds) to relax grasp before repositioning working-end beneath calculus deposit; strokes should be short and working-end remains beneath the gingival margin (to avoid trauma to gingival margin); does NOT remove working-end from the pocket with each stroke				
Maintains neutral wrist position throughout motion activation				
Maintains correct adaptation as instrument strokes progress around tooth surface; pivots and rolls instrument handle as needed				
Thoroughly instruments proximal surface under each contact area				
Uses appropriate sequence for the specified sextant				
Keeps hands steady and controlled during instrumentation so that working-end moves with precision, regardless of nervousness				
Demonstrates horizontal strokes at the midlines of anterior teeth and the line angles of posterior teeth				
Ethics and Professionalism				
Punctuality, appearance, demeanor, attitude, composure, honesty				

Module 16

Area-Specific Curets

Module Overview

This module presents the design characteristics of area-specific curets and step-by-step instructions for using area-specific curets to remove calculus deposits from the anterior and posterior teeth. Module 13, Technique Essentials: Angulation and Calculus Removal, should be completed before beginning this module.

Module Outline

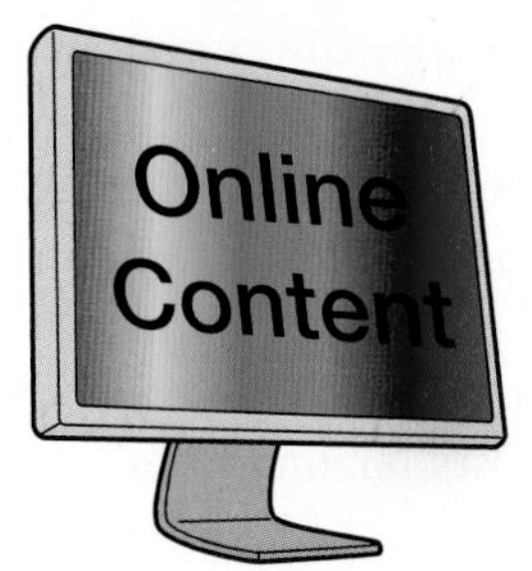

A video on the use of area-specific curets can be viewed at http://thepoint.lww.com/GehrigFundamentals7e

Section 7 **Skill Application**

Practical Focus

Reference Sheet: Area-Specific Curets

Student Self-Evaluation Module 16: Area-Specific Curets

Key Terms

Area-specific curet	Self-angulated curet
Working cutting edge	Lower cutting edge

Learning Objectives

1. Given a variety of area-specific curets, identify the design characteristics of each instrument.
2. Discuss the advantages and limitations of the design characteristics of area-specific curets.
3. Name the uses of area-specific curets.
4. Explain why a set of area-specific curets is needed to instrument the entire dentition.
5. Describe how the clinician can use visual clues to select the correct working-end of an area-specific curet on anterior and posterior teeth.
6. Using area-specific curets, demonstrate correct adaptation and use of calculus removal strokes on the anterior teeth while maintaining correct position, correct finger rests, and precise finger placement in the grasp.
7. Using area-specific curets, demonstrate correct adaptation and use of calculus removal strokes on the posterior teeth while maintaining correct position, correct finger rests, and precise finger placement in the grasp.
8. Using area-specific curets, demonstrate horizontal calculus removal strokes at the distofacial line angles of posterior teeth and at the midlines on the facial and lingual surfaces of anterior teeth.
9. Given any sickle scaler, universal curet, or area-specific curet, identify its function and where it should be used on the dentition.

Note to Course Instructor:

- Please refer to Module 19, Instruments for Advanced Root Debridement, for content on the design and use of Langer curets, Gracey designs with extended shanks and miniature working-ends, Curvettes, and debridement curets.
- Refer to Module 20, Advanced Techniques for Root Surface Debridement, for content on the anatomy of root surfaces/root concavities and instrumentation of bifurcated and trifurcated roots.
- Refer to Module 21, Calculus Removal: Concepts, Planning, and Patient Cases, for instrumentation strategies and patient cases relating to calculus removal.

Section 1
Area-Specific Curets

GENERAL DESIGN CHARACTERISTICS

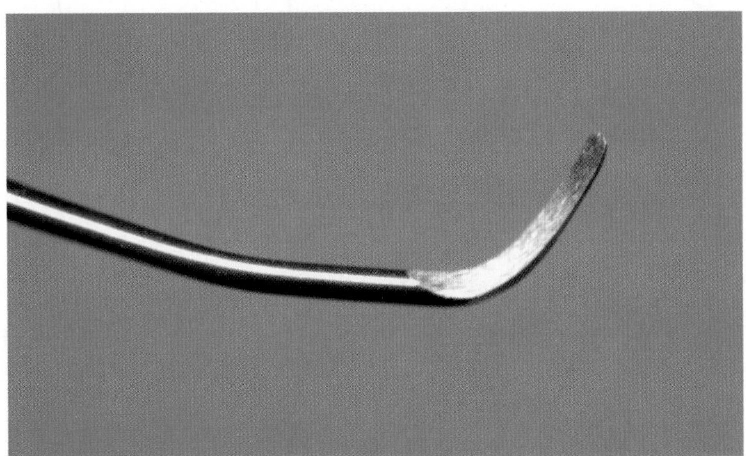

Figure 16-1. The Working-End of an Area-Specific Curet.

1. **Functions of Area-Specific Curets**
   a. An area-specific curet is a periodontal instrument used to remove light to moderate calculus deposits from the crowns and roots of the teeth (Fig. 16-1).
   b. *The name "area-specific" signifies that each instrument is designed for use only on certain teeth and certain tooth surfaces. For this reason, several area-specific curets are required to instrument the entire mouth.*

2. **Design Characteristics.** These curets represent an important breakthrough in instrument design and have unique design characteristics (Fig. 16-2 and Table 16-1).
   a. A *face that is tilted in relation to the lower shank*
      1. The face of an area-specific curet tilts at approximately a 70° angle to the lower shank.
      2. The tilted face causes one cutting edge to be lower than the other cutting edge on each working-end.
   b. *Only one cutting edge per working-end is used for periodontal instrumentation (the lower cutting edge).*
   c. A *long, complex functional shank* that is especially suited for root surface debridement within periodontal pockets
   d. Other design features of an area-specific curet are similar to those of universal curets:
      1. A *rounded back*
      2. A *rounded toe*
      3. A *semi-circular cross section.*

3. **Examples of Area-Specific Curet Instruments.** Some examples of area-specific curets are the Gracey curet series, Kramer-Nevins series, Turgeon series, After Five Gracey curet series, Gracey +3 curet series, Mini Five Gracey curet series, Gracey +3 Deep Pocket series, and Vision Curvette series.

WORKING-END DESIGN

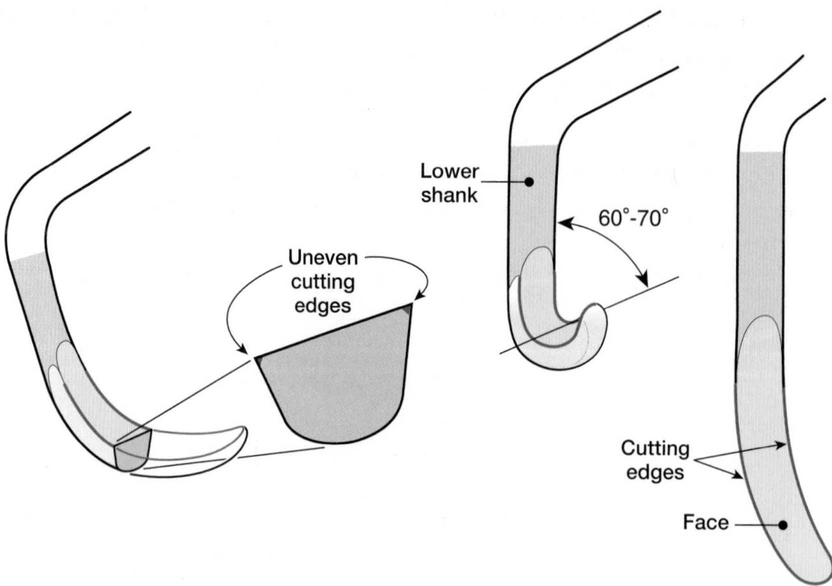

Figure 16-2. Design Characteristics of an Area-Specific Curet.

TABLE 16-1. Reference Sheet: Area-Specific Curet

Cross section	Semi-circular cross section
Working-end	Rounded back and toe One working cutting edge per working-end
Face	Face tilts at approximately a 70° angle to the lower shank; one cutting edge is lower than the other in relation to the lower shank Tilted face means that the lower cutting edge is self-angulated—***the lower cutting edge is automatically at the correct angulation when the lower shank is parallel to the tooth surface to be instrumented***
Cutting edges	***Curved cutting edges***; the curved cutting edges and rounded toe enhance adaptation to rounded root surfaces and root concavities
Application	Each instrument curet is limited to use on certain teeth and certain surfaces
Primary functions	***Instrumentation of crown and root surfaces*** Standard curets are used to remove light calculus deposits and for deplaquing; rigid Gracey curets can remove medium-size deposits

RELATIONSHIP OF FACE TO LOWER SHANK

A unique design characteristic of an area-specific curet is the relationship of the face of the working-end to the lower shank. Its design differs from that of sickle scalers and universal curets. The face of a sickle scaler or a universal curet meets the lower shank at a 90° angle (Fig 16-3). In contrast, the face of an area-specific curet is tilted in relationship to the lower shank.

- The tilted face on an area-specific curet causes one cutting edge—the working cutting edge—to be lower than the other cutting edge on each working-end.
- The nonworking cutting edge of an area-specific curet is too close to the lower shank to be used for periodontal debridement.
- ***Only the lower cutting edge of an area-specific curet is used for periodontal instrumentation*** (Fig. 16-4).

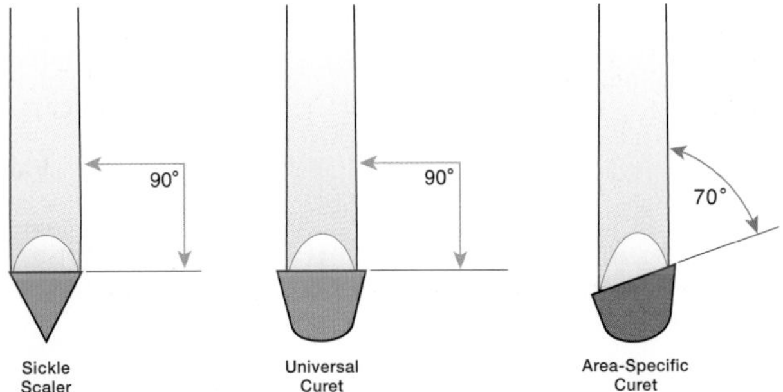

Figure 16-3. Relationship of the Face to the Lower Shank. The face of a sickle scaler or universal curet is at a 90° angle to the lower shank. The cutting edges on these instruments are level. The face of an area-specific curet is tilted in relationship to the lower shank. The tilted face causes one cutting edge—the working cutting edge—to be lower than the other cutting edge on each working-end.

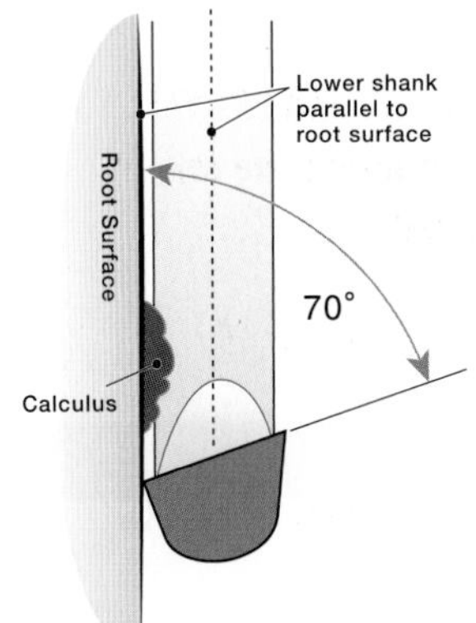

Figure 16-4. Self-Angulated Curet. ***The lower cutting edge of an area-specific curet is automatically at the correct angulation for periodontal debridement when the lower shank is parallel to the tooth surface to be instrumented.*** Instruments with this design characteristic are termed **self-angulated**.

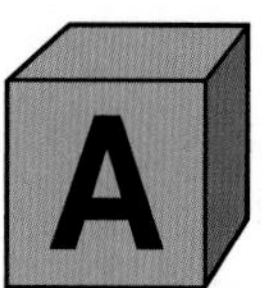

SKILL BUILDING. IDENTIFYING THE LOWER CUTTING EDGE

Because the face of an area-specific curet is tilted in relationship to the lower shank, one cutting edge is lower than the other cutting edge. The lower cutting edge tilts away from the lower shank.

- ***Only the lower cutting edge of an area-specific curet is used for periodontal instrumentation.***
- The higher cutting edge is angled away from the soft tissue wall of the periodontal pocket to facilitate subgingival instrumentation. The higher cutting edge is not used for periodontal instrumentation.
- The lower cutting edge is identified by holding the instrument with the toe facing the clinician with the lower shank perpendicular to the floor. This technique is pictured in Figure 16-5 and summarized in Box 16-1.

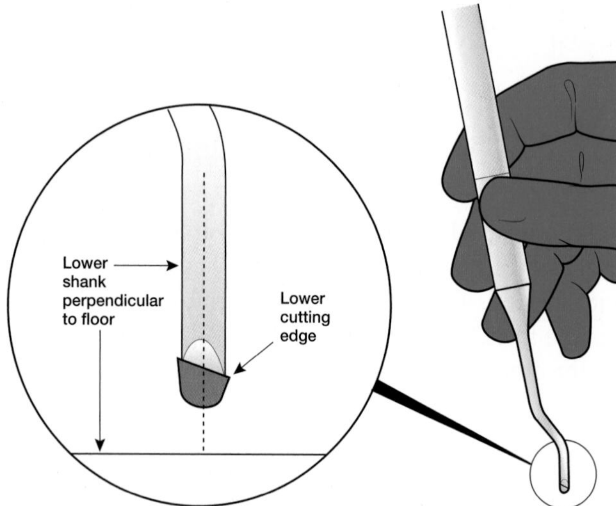

Figure 16-5. Identifying the Lower Cutting Edge. Hold the instrument as pictured here with the toe facing you and the lower shank perpendicular—at a 90° angle—to the floor.

Box 16-1. Identifying the Lower Cutting Edge

Follow these steps to identify the working cutting edge of an area-specific curet.

1. Hold the instrument so that you are ***looking directly at the toe*** of the working-end.
2. Raise or lower the instrument handle until the ***lower shank is perpendicular (⊥) to the floor***.
3. Look closely at the working-end and note that one of the cutting edges is lower—closer to the floor—than the other cutting edge.
4. The ***lower cutting edge is the working cutting edge***—the cutting edge used for instrumentation.

THE GRACEY CURET SERIES

Area-specific curets were developed through the genius of Dr. Clayton Gracey who envisioned a periodontal instrument that would reach root surfaces within deep periodontal pockets without trauma to the pocket epithelium. In the early 1940s, Dr. Gracey worked with Hugo Friedman of Hu-Friedy Manufacturing Company to develop 14 single-ended area-specific Gracey curets (Fig. 16-6). The Gracey instrument series continues to be popular today and is the basis for several other area-specific curets. The Gracey series continues to evolve and is currently available in standard, rigid, extended shank, miniature working-end, and microminiature working-end versions.

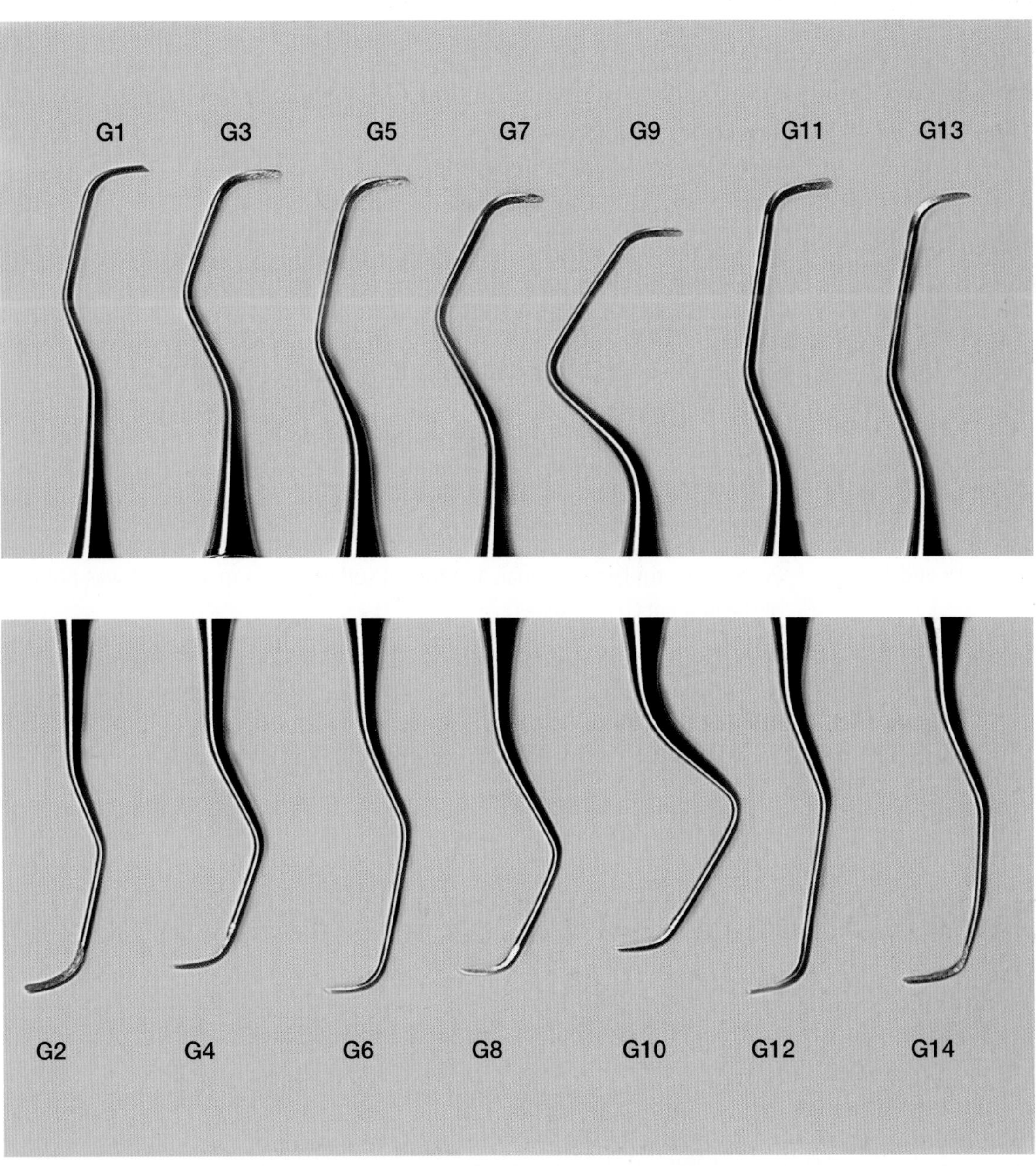

Figure 16-6. The Standard Gracey Curet Series.

APPLICATION OF GRACEY CURETS

The original Gracey series contains 14 curets, Gracey 1 to 14 (Table 16-2). In practice, rarely are all 14 curets used on a single patient's mouth. Over the years, clinicians have found that they are able to instrument the mouth using a fewer number of Gracey curets. A set of three or four Gracey curets may be adequate to instrument the entire dentition.

TABLE 16-2. The Gracey Instrument Series

Curet	Area of Application
Gracey 1 and 2 Gracey 3 and 4	Anterior teeth: all tooth surfaces[G]
Gracey 5 and 6	Anterior teeth: all tooth surfaces[G] Premolar teeth: all tooth surfaces[G] Molar teeth: facial, lingual, and mesial surfaces
Gracey 7 and 8 Gracey 9 and 10	Anterior teeth: all surfaces Premolar teeth: all surfaces Posterior teeth: facial and lingual surfaces[G]
Gracey 11 and 12	Anterior teeth: mesial and distal surfaces Posterior teeth: mesial surfaces[G] Posterior teeth: facial, lingual, and mesial surfaces
Gracey 13 and 14	Anterior teeth: mesial and distal surfaces Posterior teeth: distal surfaces[G]
Gracey 15 and 16	Posterior teeth: facial, lingual, and mesial surfaces (this instrument was not part of the original Gracey series)
Gracey 17 and 18	Posterior teeth: distal surfaces (this instrument was not part of the original Gracey series)

Table Key: The [G] symbol indicates the areas of application as originally designated by Dr. Gracey.

Over the years, many modifications have been made to the standard Gracey curet design. Table 16-3 summarizes these design modifications.

TABLE 16-3. Comparison of Gracey Designs

Instrument	Design Features
Standard	• Shank Length: standard design • Shank Diameter: standard diameter • Working-End Length: standard length • Working-End Width: standard width
Rigid	• Shank Length: standard length • Shank Diameter: increased shank diameter • Working-End Length: standard length • Working-End Width: standard width
Extended lower shank	• Shank Length: longer lower shank • Shank Diameter: standard shank diameter • Working-End Length: standard length • Working-End Width: decreased by 10% compared to standard
Rigid extended lower shank	• Shank Length: lower shank 3 mm longer than standard • Shank Diameter: increased shank diameter • Working-End Length: standard length • Working-End Width: decreased by 10% compared to standard
Extended lower shank and miniature working-end	• Shank Length: longer lower shank • Shank Diameter: standard shank diameter • Working-End Length: decreased by 50% compared to standard • Working-End Width: decreased by 10% compared to standard
Rigid extended lower shank and miniature working-end	• Shank Length: longer lower shank • Shank Diameter: increased shank diameter • Working-End Length: decreased by 50% compared to standard • Working-End Width: decreased by 10% compared to standard
Extended lower shank and microminiature working-end	• Shank Length: longer lower shank • Shank Diameter: increased functional shank diameter with tapered lower shank • Working-End Length: decreased by 50% compared to standard • Working-End Width: decreased by 20% compared to miniature working-end

Section 2
Technique Practice—Anterior Teeth

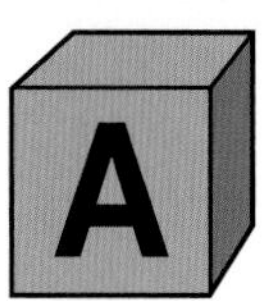

SKILL BUILDING. SELECTING THE CORRECT WORKING-END FOR AN ANTERIOR TOOTH

Only one cutting edge per working-end of an area-specific curet is used for instrumentation. The clinician observes the face of the working-end as it is adapted to the tooth surface (Figs. 16-7 and 16-8).

- When the working-end is adapted to the facial (or lingual) surface, the *face* of the correct working-end ***tilts slightly toward the tooth*** and is partially hidden from view.

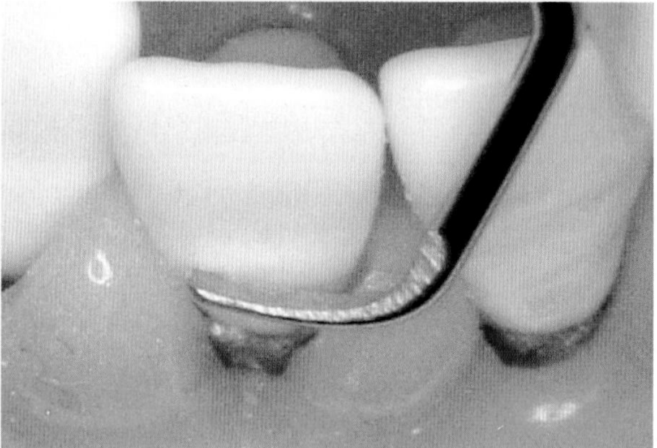

Figure 16-7. Correct Working-End.

- The correct working-end is selected if **the *instrument face* tilts toward the tooth surface** when placed against the midline of the facial (or lingual surface).
- Looking down on the working-end, the face is partially hidden.

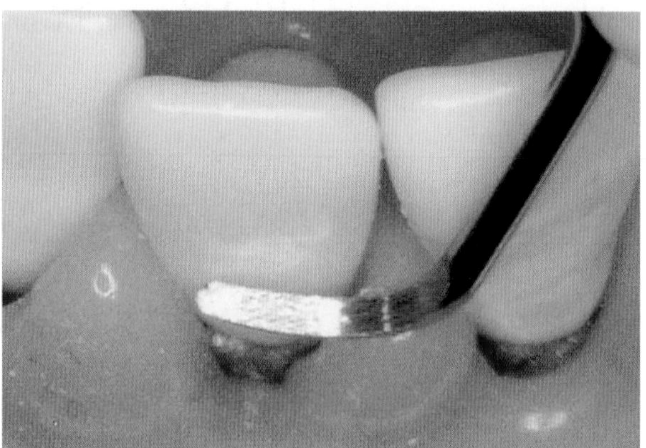

Figure 16-8. Incorrect Working-End.

- The incorrect working-end is selected if **the *instrument's face* tilts slightly away from the tooth surface** when placed against the midline of the facial (or lingual surface).
- Looking down on the working-end, the entire face is clearly visible.
- This working-end would traumatize the soft tissue if used subgingivally.

APPLICATION OF THE CUTTING EDGES TO ANTERIOR TEETH

Only one cutting edge per working-end of an area-specific curet is used for instrumentation of the anterior teeth. Figures 16-9 and 16-10 depict application of the cutting edges to the maxillary anterior teeth, facial aspect.

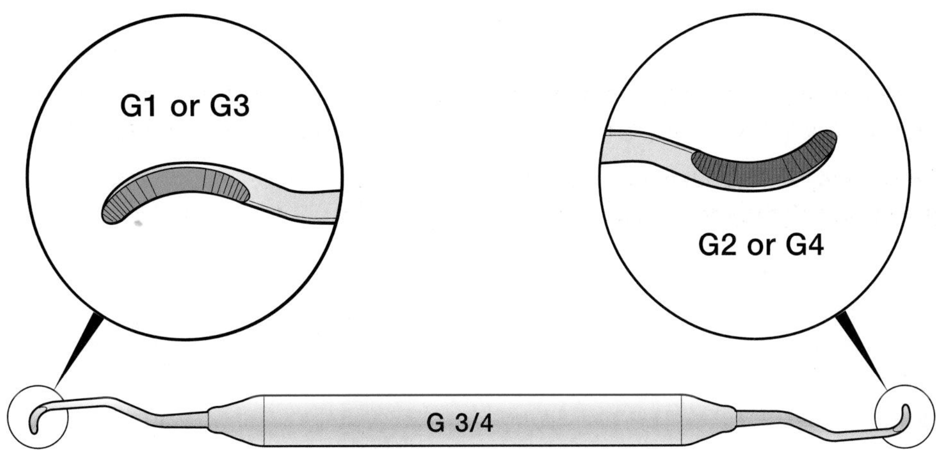

Figure 16-9. Application to Anterior Surfaces. A double-ended area-specific curet has two lower cutting edges that are used on anterior tooth surfaces.

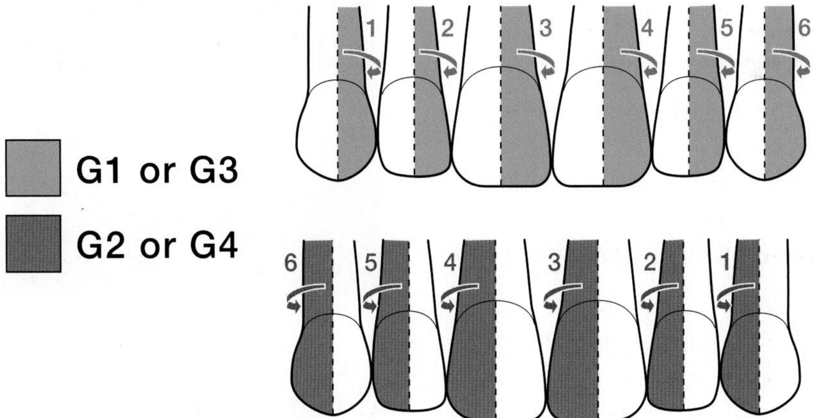

Figure 16-10. Application to Anterior Surfaces. This illustration indicates how the cutting edges of a Gracey 1/2 or Gracey 3/4 are applied to the surfaces toward and surfaces away on the facial aspect of the anterior tooth surfaces.

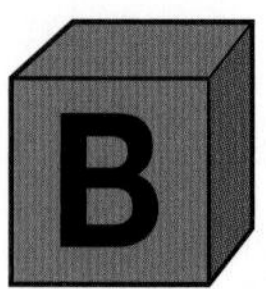

SKILL BUILDING. STEP-BY-STEP TECHNIQUE ON MAXILLARY CENTRAL INCISOR

Directions:

- Follow steps 1 to 8 to practice use of an area-specific curet on the maxillary anterior teeth (Figs. 16-11 to 16-18).
- ***Use a periodontal typodont.***[1,2] ***Practice insertion with the gingiva in place, and then remove the gingiva to practice making calculus removal strokes on the cervical thirds of the roots.***
- Remember: "Me, My patient, My light, My dominant hand, My nondominant hand, My finger rest, My adaptation."

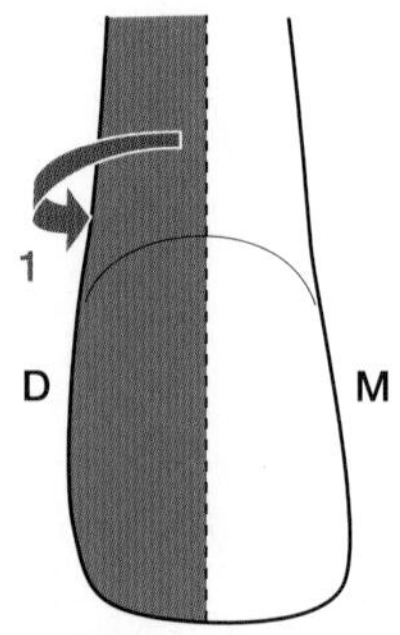

1. **Figure 16-11. Tooth.** As an introduction to using a universal curet on the anterior teeth, first practice on the ***maxillary right central incisor, facial aspect***.

   RIGHT-Handed clinicians—*surface toward.*

   LEFT-Handed clinicians—*surface away.*

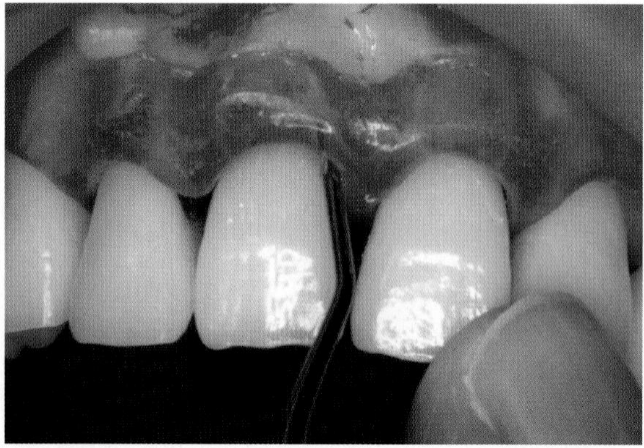

2. **Figure 16-12. Get Ready and Insert.**
   - Select the correct working-end and place it in the Get Ready Zone.
   - The toe of the working-end should aim toward the distal surface.
   - Insert the working-end to the base of the pocket.

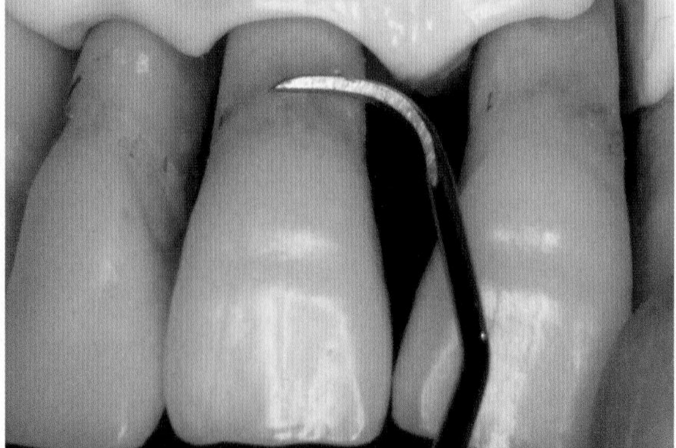

3. **Figure 16-13. Adapt the Toe-Third to the Midline.** Adapt the toe-third to the root surface. ***Imagine "locking" the toe-third against the root surface.***

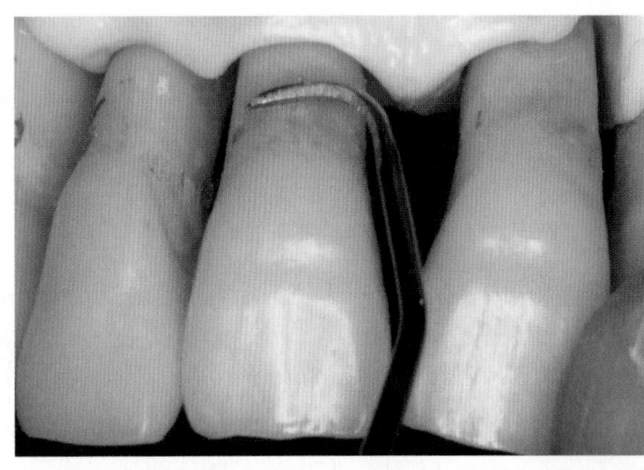

4. **Figure 16-14. Work across Facial Surface.** Make a series of short, precise strokes across the facial surface toward the distofacial line angle.

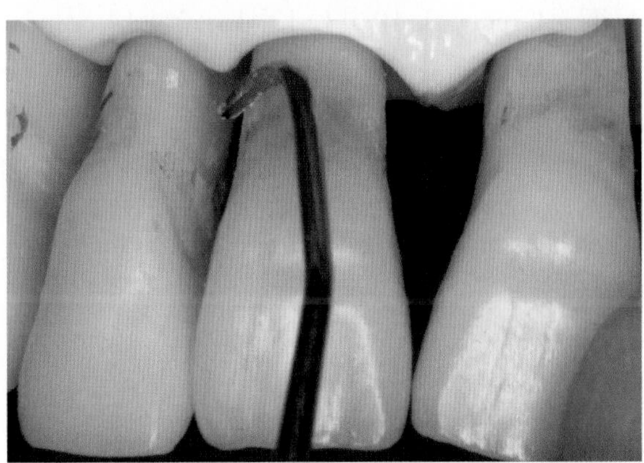

5. **Figure 16-15. Roll Handle at Line Angle.** Roll the handle slightly to maintain adaptation of the toe-third at the distofacial line angle.

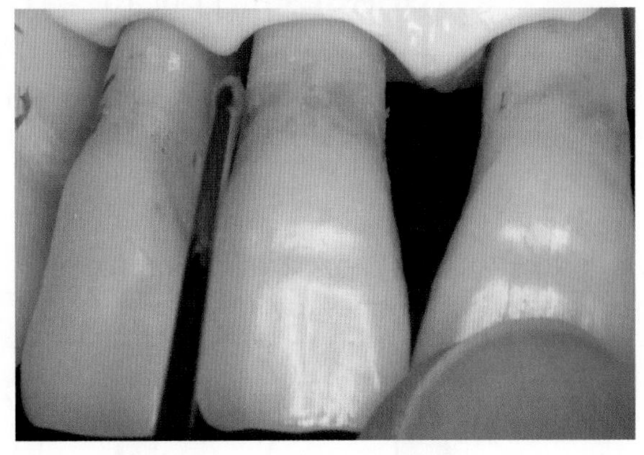

6. **Figure 16-16. Distal Surface.** Work at least halfway across the distal surface. The other half of the distal surface will be instrumented from the lingual aspect of the tooth.

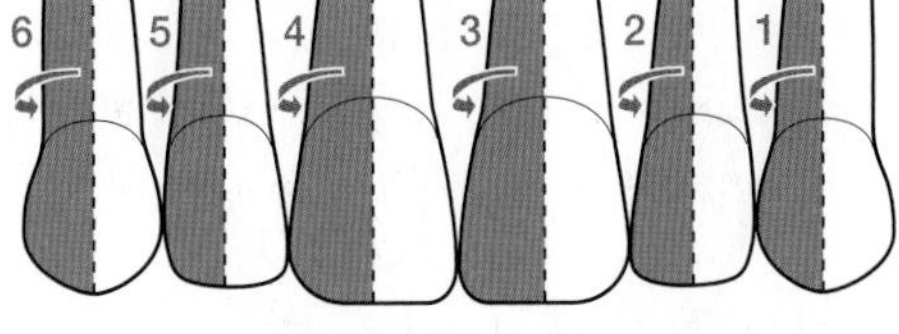

7. **Figure 16-17. Sequence.** Next, use the sequence shown in this illustration to instrument the colored tooth surfaces of the facial aspect. Begin with the left canine and end with the right canine.

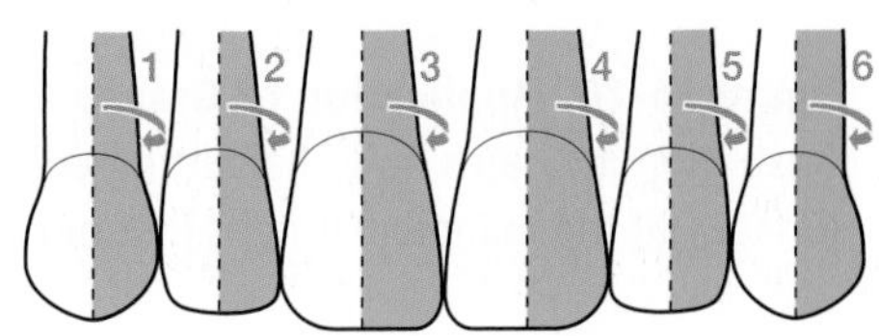

8. **Figure 16-18. Sequence.** Change your clock position and complete the remaining facial surfaces, beginning with the right canine and ending with the left canine.

Section 3
Technique Practice—Posterior Teeth

APPLICATION OF THE CUTTING EDGES TO POSTERIOR TEETH

At least two double-ended area-specific instruments are needed for instrumentation of the posterior teeth. Commonly, two to three double-ended Gracey curets are used to instrument the posterior sextants. For example, a clinician might select one of the following combinations of curet working-ends:

- The Gracey 11, 12, 13, and 14 might be selected for the posterior teeth.
- The Gracey 15, 16, 17, and 18 compose a set of curets for the posterior teeth.
- The Gracey 9, 10, 11, 12, 13, and 14 compose a set of six curets for the posterior teeth.
- The Gracey 7, 8, 15, 16, 17, and 18 compose a set of six curets for the posterior teeth.

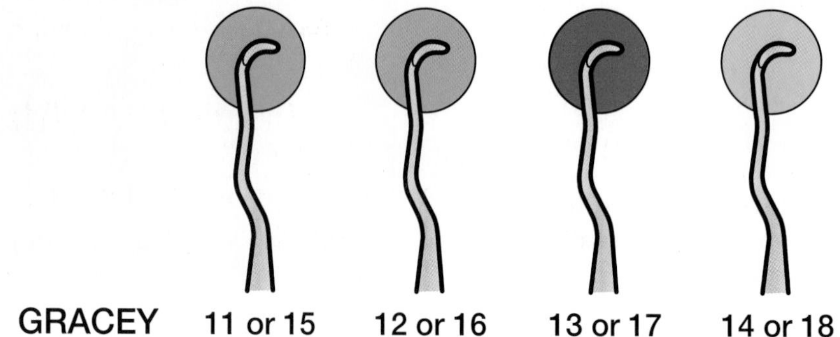

Figure 16-19. Gracey Set for Posterior Teeth. Several Gracey curets are required to instrument a posterior sextant. To instrument a posterior sextant, a clinician might select a set of Gracey curets such as the 11/12 and 13/14 or the 15/16 and 17/18.

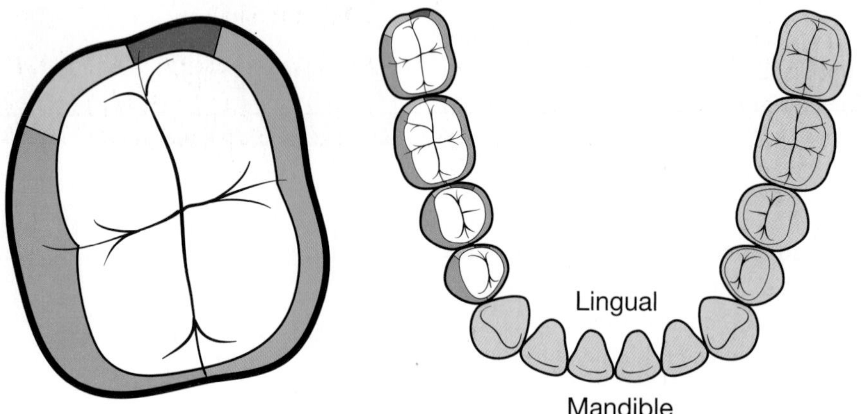

Figure 16-20. Application of Gracey Cutting Edges to Posterior Surfaces. The illustration indicates how the cutting edges of a Gracey curet are applied to the tooth surfaces of the mandibular right first molar and the mandibular right posterior sextant.

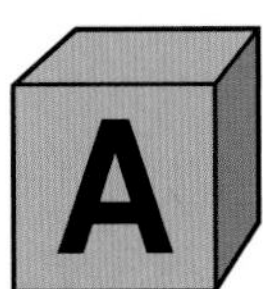

SKILL BUILDING. SELECTING THE CORRECT WORKING-END FOR A POSTERIOR TOOTH

Use the lower shank as the visual clue for selecting the correct working-end for use on a posterior tooth. ***Think: "Posterior = Parallel. Functional shank up and over!"*** Figures 16-21 and 16-22 show the visual clues for selection of an area-specific curet for use on the distal surface of a posterior tooth.

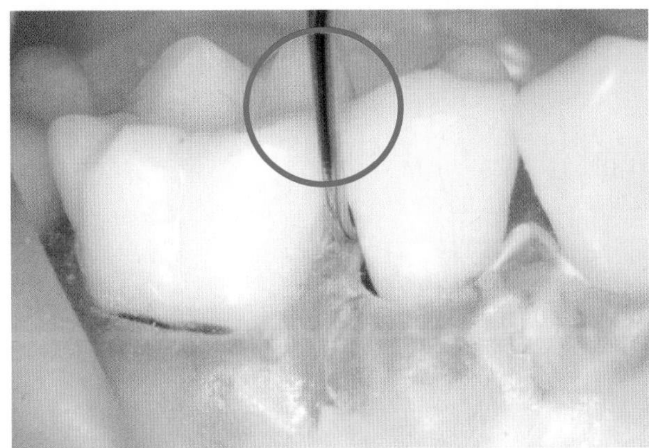

Figure 16-21. Visual Clue for the Correct Working-End. The correct working-end is selected when:

- The *lower shank is parallel* to the distal surface.
- The *functional shank goes "up and over the tooth."*

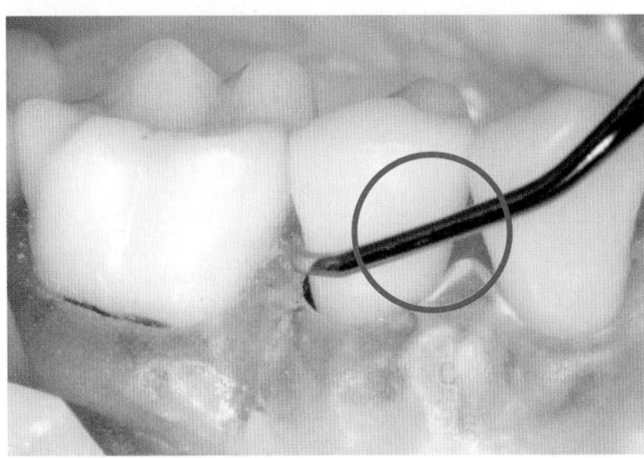

Figure 16-22. Visual Clue for the Incorrect Working-End. The incorrect working-end is selected if the:

- The *lower shank is not parallel.*
- The *functional shank is "down and around the tooth."*

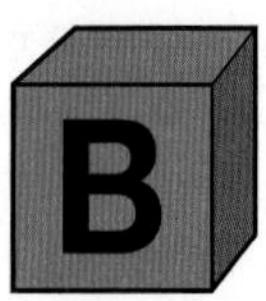

SKILL BUILDING. STEP-BY-STEP TECHNIQUE ON MANDIBULAR FIRST MOLAR

Directions:

- Follow steps 1 to 18 as shown in Figures 16-23 to 16-40 to practice use of an area-specific curet on the mandibular right posterior sextant.
- ***Use a periodontal typodont.***[1,2] ***Practice insertion with the gingiva in place, and then remove the gingiva to practice making calculus removal strokes on the cervical thirds of the roots.***
- Remember: "Me, My patient, My light, My dominant hand, My nondominant hand, My finger rest, My adaptation."

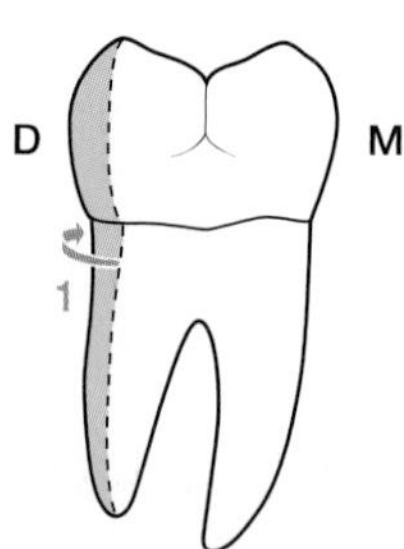

1. **Figure 16-23. Begin with the Distal Surfaces.**
   - As an introduction to the area-specific curet, first practice on the mandibular right first molar.
   - *Use a distal area-specific curet on the distal surface.*

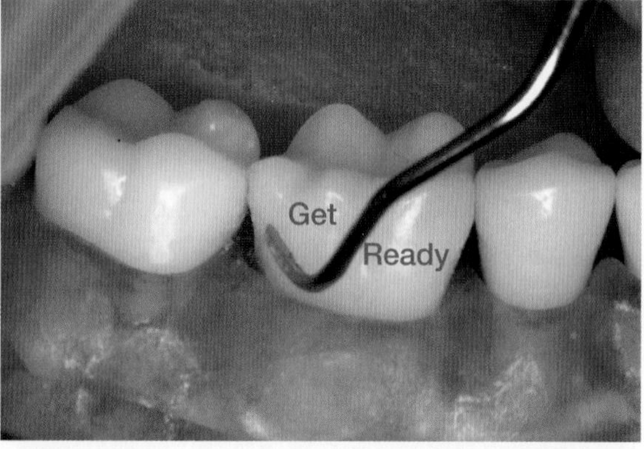

2. **Figure 16-24. Get Ready.**
   - Place the distal curet at the distofacial line angle in the Get Ready Zone.
   - The toe should aim toward the back of the mouth because this is the direction in which you are working.

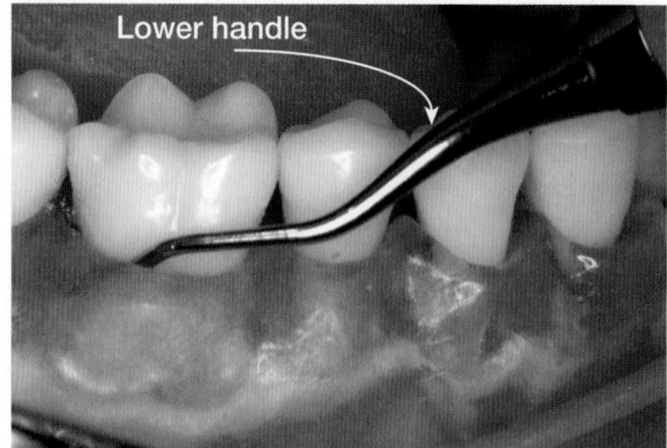

3. **Figure 16-25. Insert.** Lower handle and gently slide the working-end beneath the gingival margin.

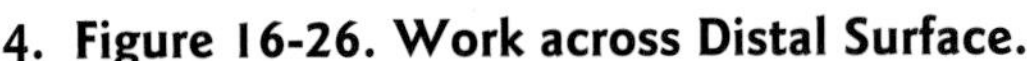

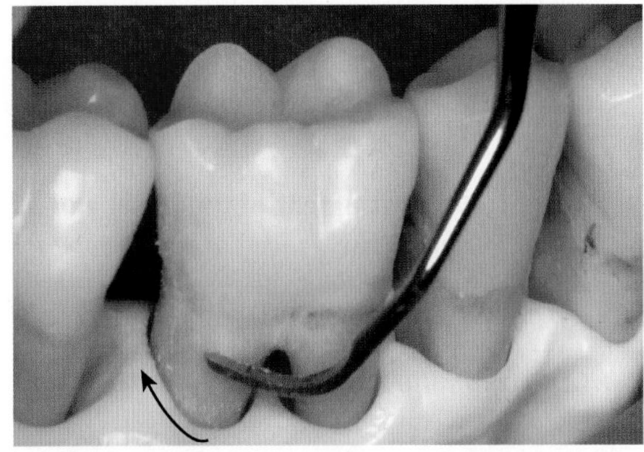

4. **Figure 16-26. Work across Distal Surface.**
    - Return the handle to an upright position.
    - "Lock" the toe-third against the distofacial line angle.
    - Instrument at least halfway across the distal surface from the facial aspect.

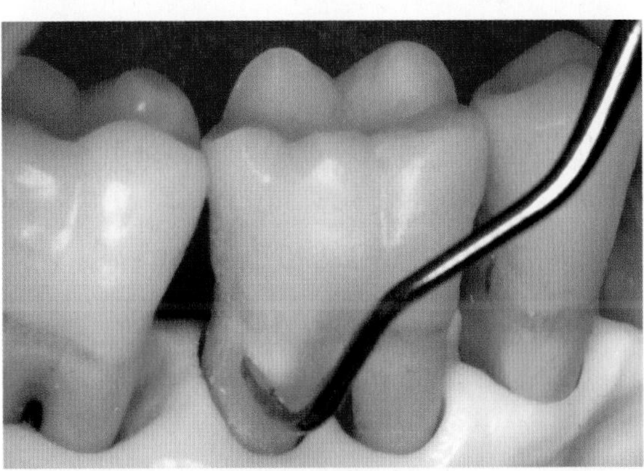

5. **Figure 16-27. Roll the Handle.** Roll the instrument handle to maintain adaptation as you work around the distofacial line angle and onto the distal surface.

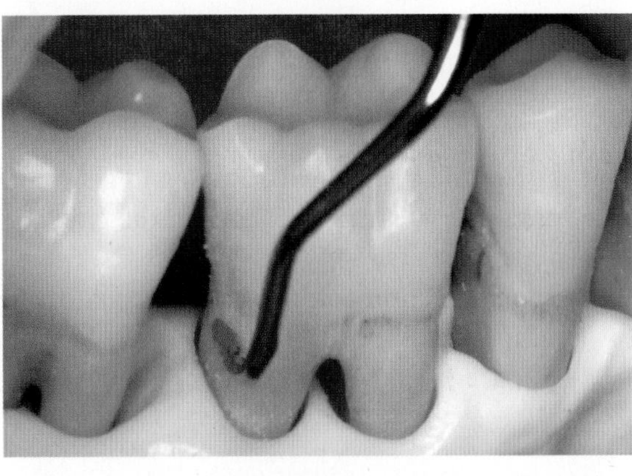

6. **Figure 16-28. Continue Strokes.** Continue making a series of short, precise strokes across the distal surface.

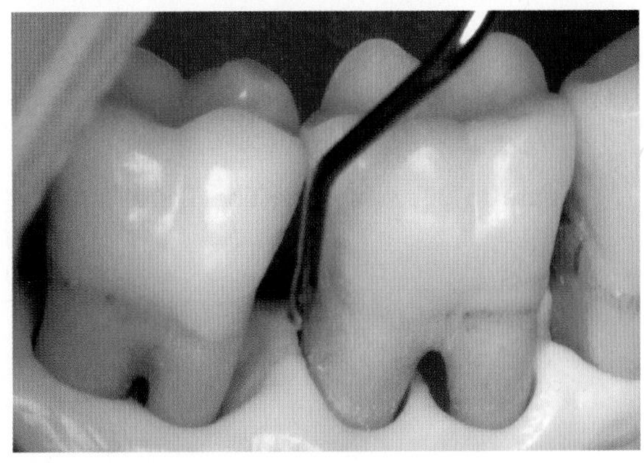

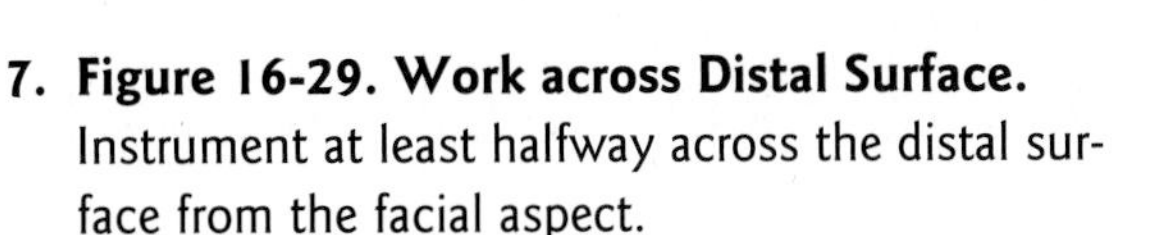

7. **Figure 16-29. Work across Distal Surface.** Instrument at least halfway across the distal surface from the facial aspect.

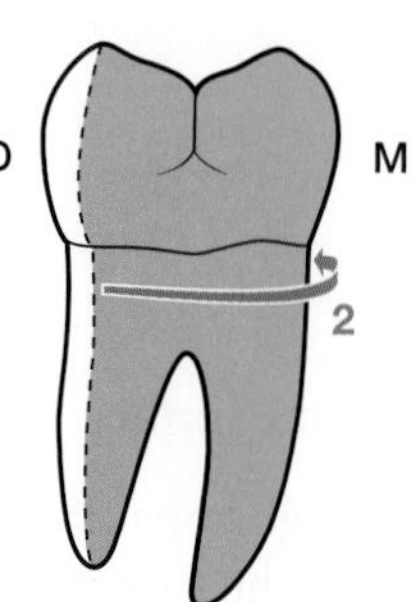

8. **Figure 16-30. Instrument of the Facial and Mesial Surfaces.** *Use a facial or mesial curet for the facial surface of the tooth, beginning at the distofacial line angle.*

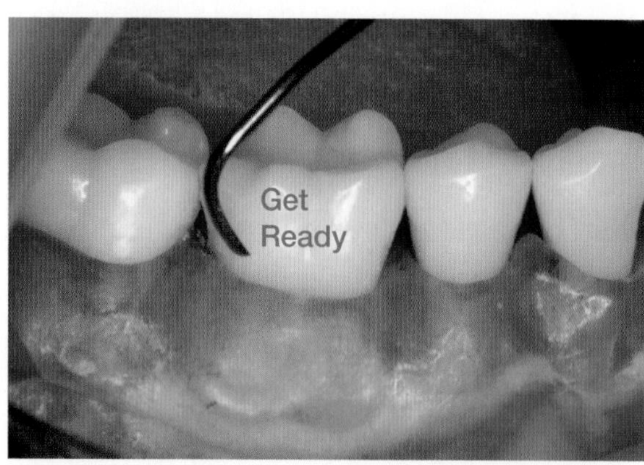

9. **Figure 16-31. Get Ready.** Place the mesial curet in the Get Ready Zone with the toe aiming toward the mesial surface in preparation for insertion.

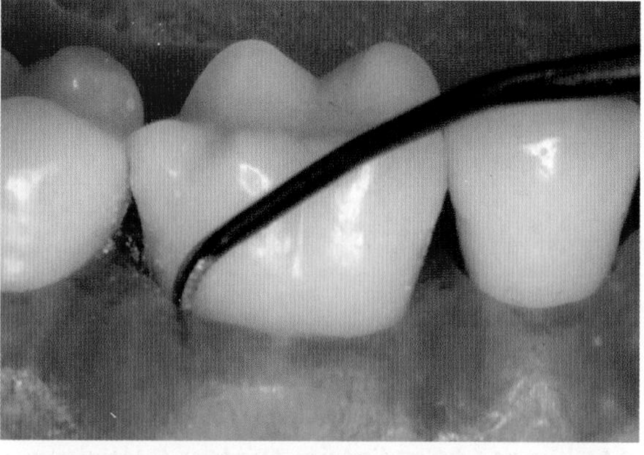

10. **Figure 16-32. Insert.**
    - Lower the instrument handle and gently slide the working-end beneath the gingival margin.
    - Insert the curet to the base of the periodontal pocket.

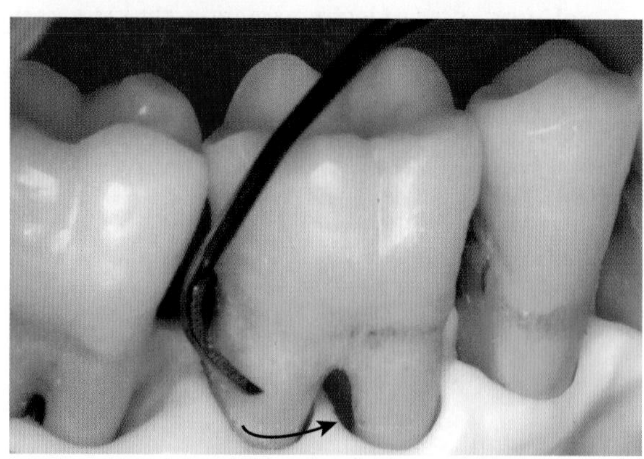

11. **Figure 16-33. Adapt the Toe-Third.**
    - Return the handle to the upright position.
    - "Lock" the toe-third to the root surface at the distofacial line angle.

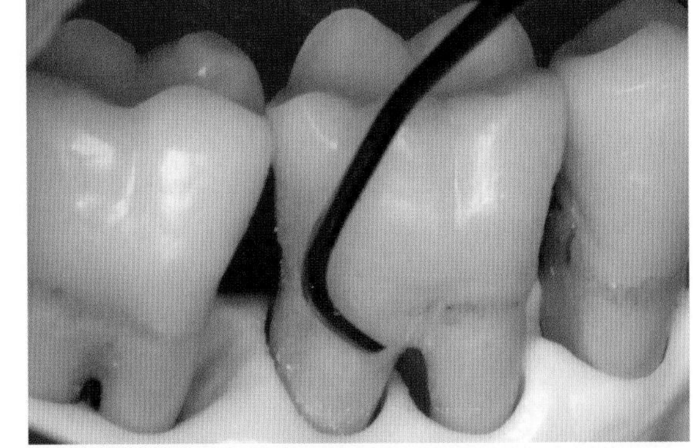

12. **Figure 16-34. Instrument the Facial Surface.** Make a series of oblique calculus removal strokes across the mesial surface.

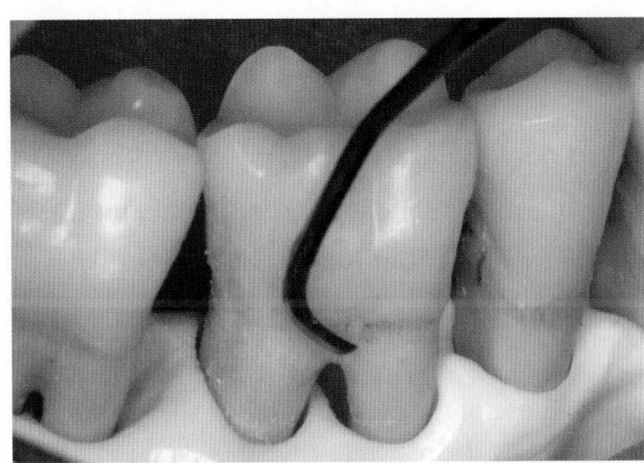

13. **Figure 16-35. Continue Strokes.** Make a series of short, precise instrumentation strokes across the facial surface.

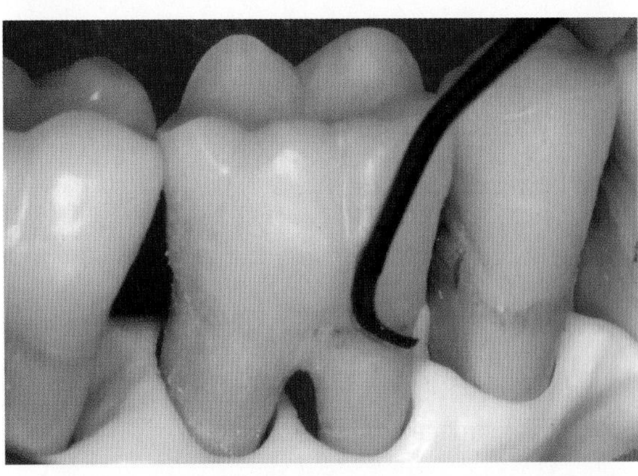

14. **Figure 16-36. Continue Strokes.** Make a series of short, precise instrumentation strokes across the facial surface.

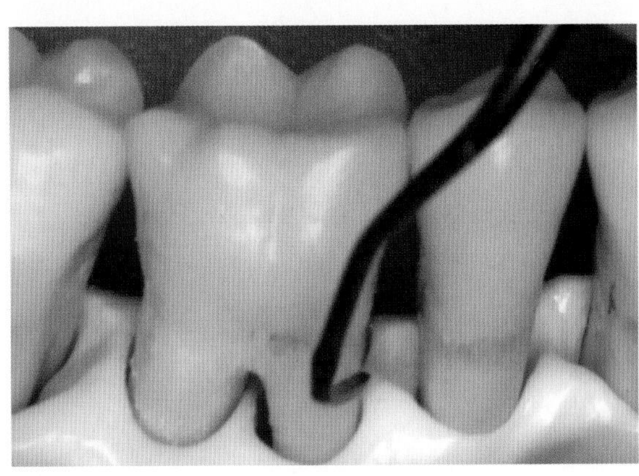

15. **Figure 16-37. Roll the Handle.** As you approach the mesiofacial line angle, roll the handle slightly to maintain adaptation.

16. **Figure 16-38. Technique Check.** Make sure that your strokes extend past the midline of the mesial proximal surface.
    - *Work at least halfway across the mesial surface from the facial aspect.*
    - The other half of the mesial surface will be instrumented from the lingual aspect.

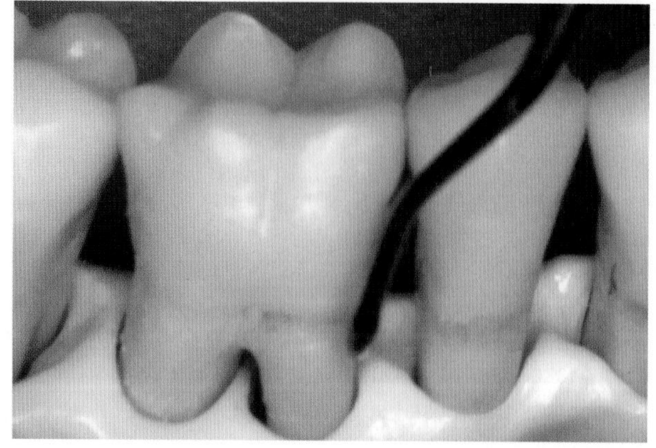

17. **Figure 16-39. Sequence for Distal Surfaces.** Use the sequence shown in this illustration for the distal surfaces in the sextant. It is easier to begin with the posterior-most molar and move forward toward the first premolar because of the pressure exerted against your hand by the patient's cheek.

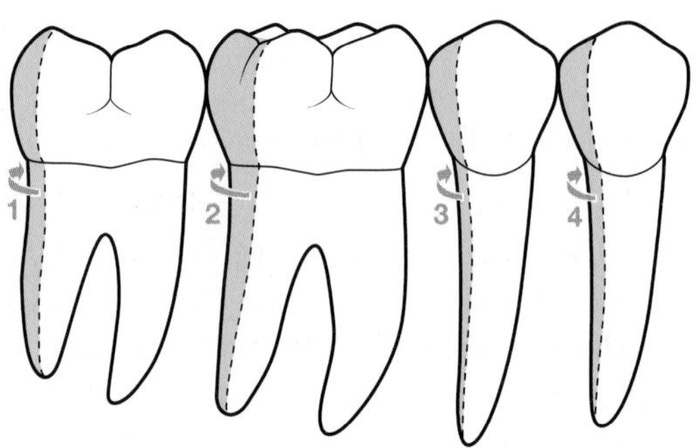

18. **Figure 16-40. Sequence for Facial and Mesial Surfaces.** Use the sequence shown in this illustration to instrument the facial and mesial surfaces in the sextant.

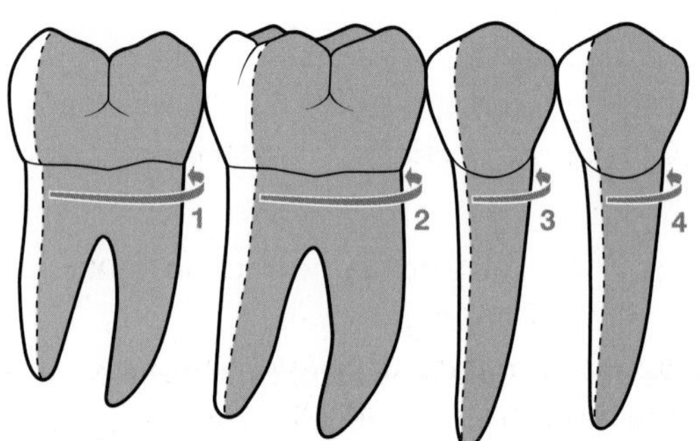

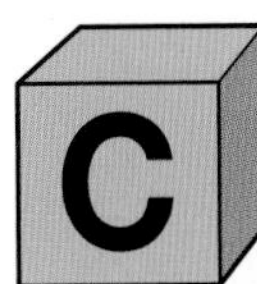

SKILL BUILDING. STEP-BY-STEP TECHNIQUE ON MAXILLARY FIRST MOLAR

Directions:

- Follow steps 1 to 10 to practice use of an area-specific curet on the maxillary left posterior sextant (Figs. 16-41 to 16-50).
- ***Use a periodontal typodont.***[1,2] ***Practice insertion with the gingiva in place, and then remove the gingiva to practice making calculus removal strokes on the cervical thirds of the roots.***
- Remember: "Me, My patient, My light, My dominant hand, My nondominant hand, My finger rest, My adaptation."

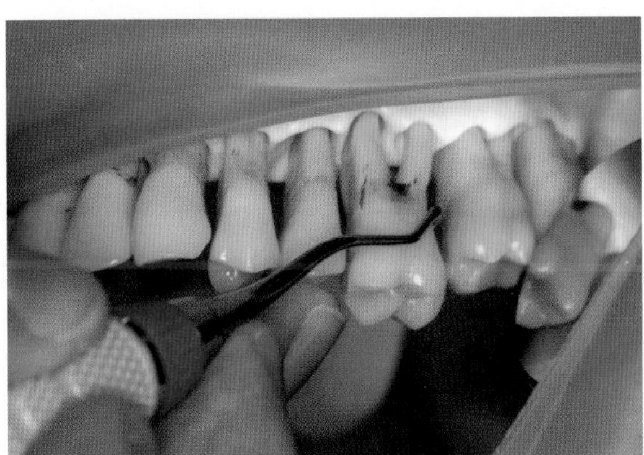

1. **Figure 16-41. Get Ready and Insert.**
    - Turn the toe toward the distal surface. Position the working-end in the Get Ready Zone.
    - Raise the instrument handle and establish a 0° angulation.
    - Gently slide the working-end beneath the gingival margin.

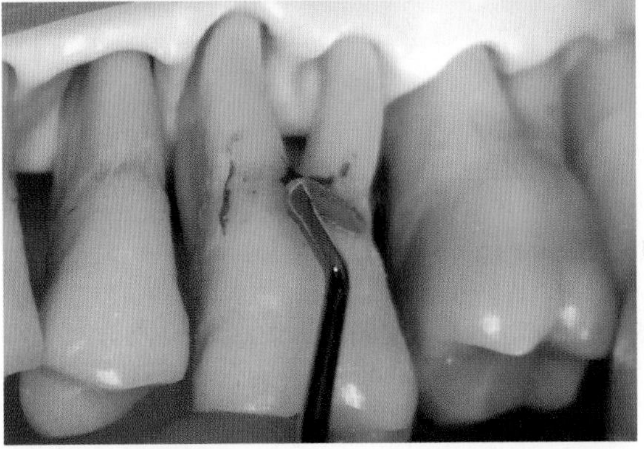

2. **Figure 16-42. Establish Angulation and Lock Toe-Third.**
    - Lower the handle to the correct position.
    - Establish an 80° angulation.
    - Adapt the toe-third of the working-end to the distofacial line angle. Imagine "locking" the toe-third against the tooth surface.

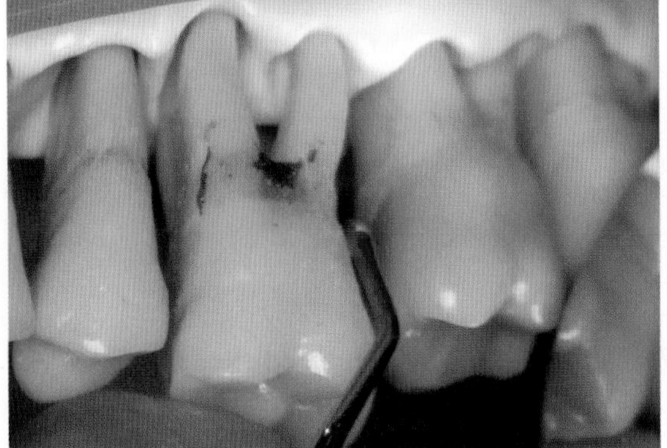

3. **Figure 16-43. Instrument the Distal Surface.** Instrument from the distofacial line angle to the midline of the distal surface.

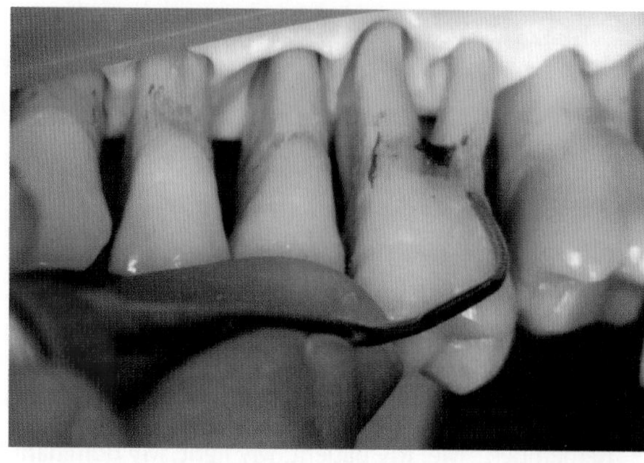

4. **Figure 16-44. Insert on Facial Surface.**
    - Use the mesial curet for the facial and mesial surfaces.
    - Place the working-end in the Get Ready Zone on the middle-third of the facial surface near the distofacial line angle.
    - Raise the handle and slide the working-end beneath the gingival margin.

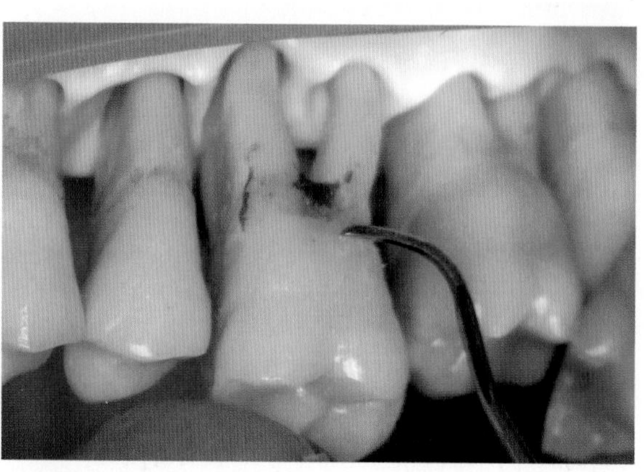

5. **Figure 16-45. Begin at Distofacial Line Angle.** Lower the handle to the correct position. Begin instrumentation of the facial surface starting at the distofacial line angle.

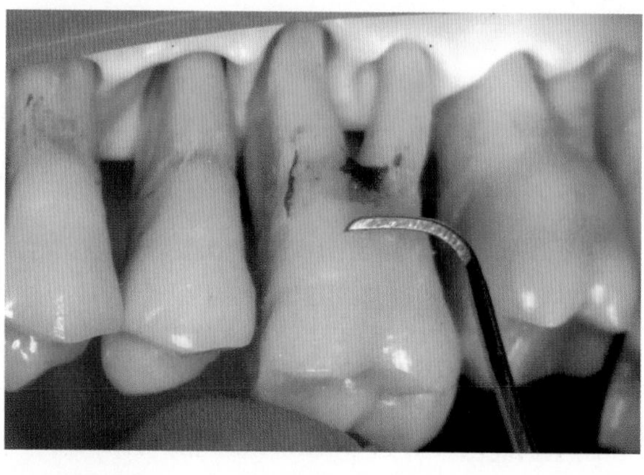

6. **Figure 16-46. Instrument the Facial Surface.** Work across the facial surface keeping the toe-third adapted.

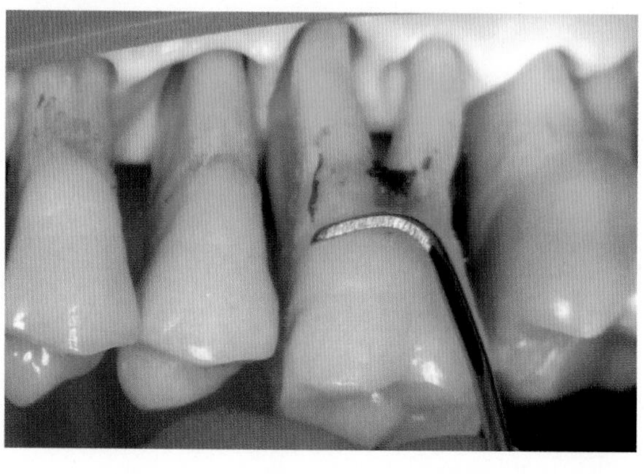

7. **Figure 16-47. Continue across the Facial Surface.** Make a series of tiny oblique calculus removal strokes across the facial surface.

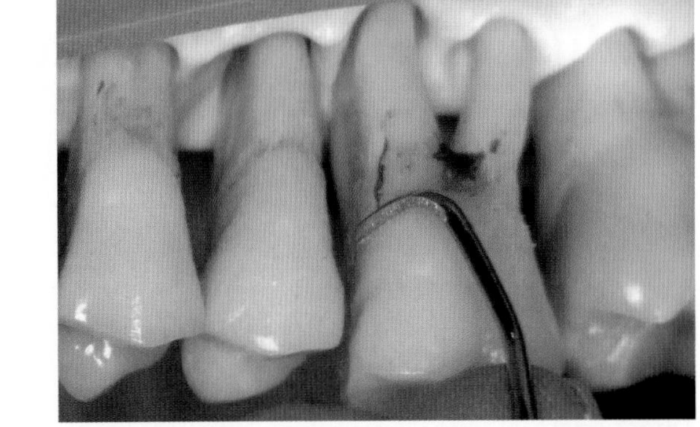

8. **Figure 16-48. Roll the Instrument Handle.** As you approach the mesiofacial line angle, roll the handle slightly to maintain adaptation.

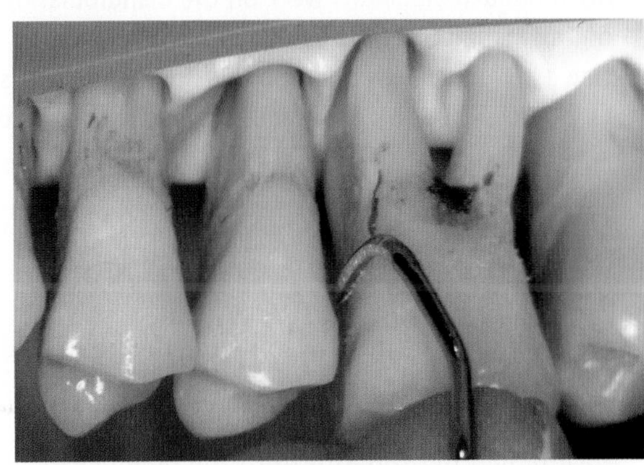

9. **Figure 16-49. Instrument the Mesial Surface.** Work across the mesial surface taking care to assure that the toe-third remains adapted.

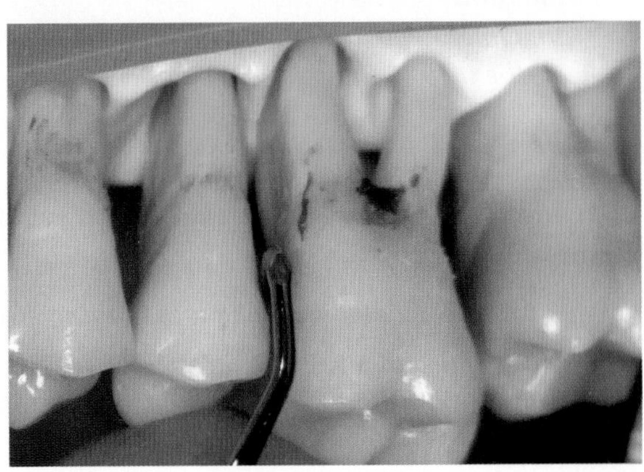

10. **Figure 16-50. Instrument to Midline of Mesial Surface.** Instrument at least halfway across the mesial surface from the facial aspect.

Section 4
Production of a Root Debridement Stroke

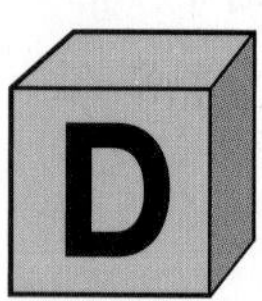

SKILL BUILDING. ROOT DEBRIDEMENT STROKES

Directions:

- *Right-handed clinicians* work on the mandibular right first molar, facial aspect. *Left-handed clinicians* work on the mandibular left first molar, facial aspect.
- Use a *periodontal typodont with flexible "gingiva"* so that you can practice as if working in a deep periodontal pocket.[2] Use an *area-specific curet* such as a *Gracey curet* for this technique practice.

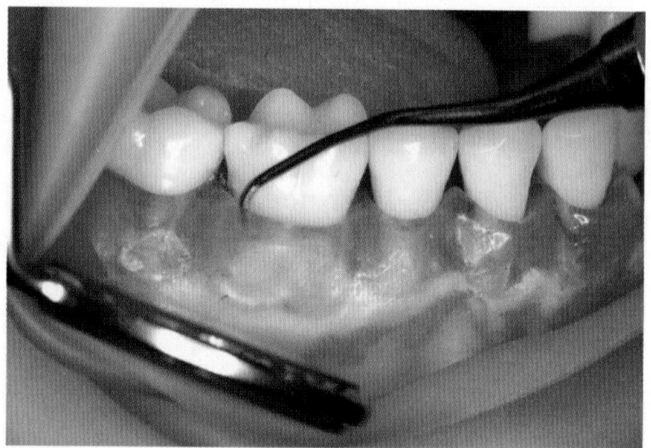

1. Figure 16-51. Insert.

- Insert at a 0° angulation with the lower shank close to the tooth surface.
- Gently slide the working-end beneath the gingival margin and onto the facial surface of the root.
- *Imagine the face sliding along the facial surface all the way to the base of the pocket.*

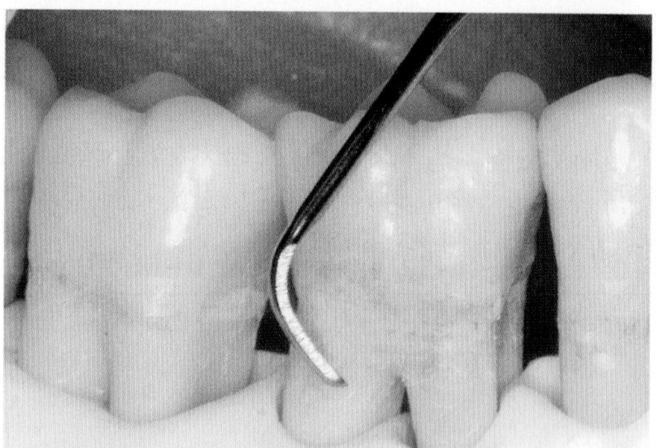

2. Figure 16-52. Prepare for Stroke: Tilt Lower Shank toward Root Surface.

- ***A root debridement stroke is a shaving stroke.***
- To accomplish a shaving stroke, the face should be approximately at a *60° angle to the tooth surface.*
- To create this angulation, simply tilt the lower shank toward the root surface.

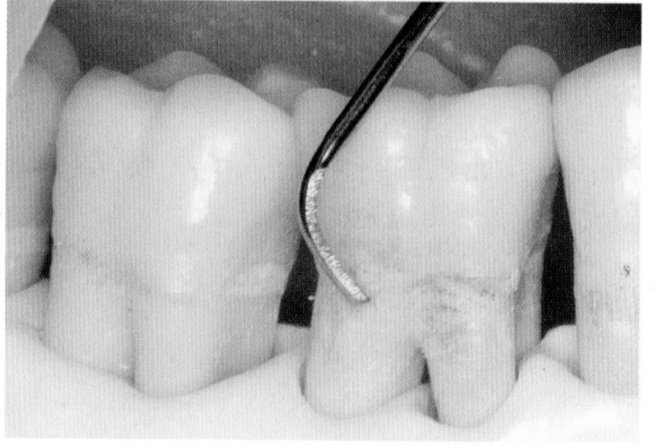

3. Figure 16-53. Make a Root Debridement Stroke.

- Initiate *a light, shaving stroke away from the base of the pocket.*
- A root debridement stroke is a *lighter* and *longer stroke* than a calculus removal stroke.

Section 5
Horizontal Strokes below the Gingival Margin

Horizontal strokes are extremely useful in removing calculus deposits that are located (1) near the distofacial or distolingual line angle of posterior teeth and (2) at the midline of the facial or lingual surfaces of anterior teeth. Figures 16-54 to 16-56 depict the use of horizontal strokes on anterior and posterior teeth.

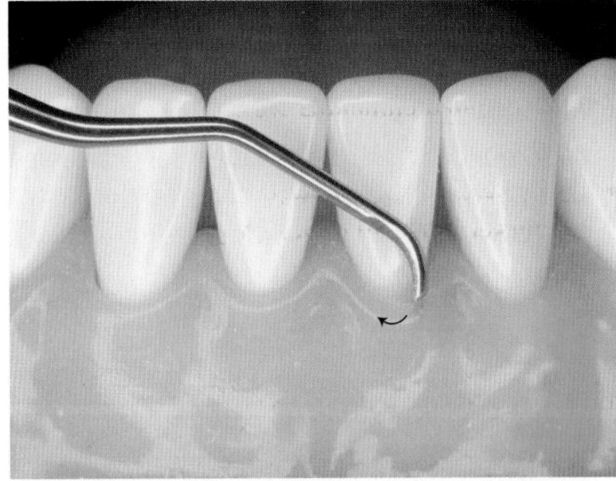

Figure 16-54. Anterior Teeth. The technique for making horizontal strokes with an area-specific curet is similar to that used with a universal curet.

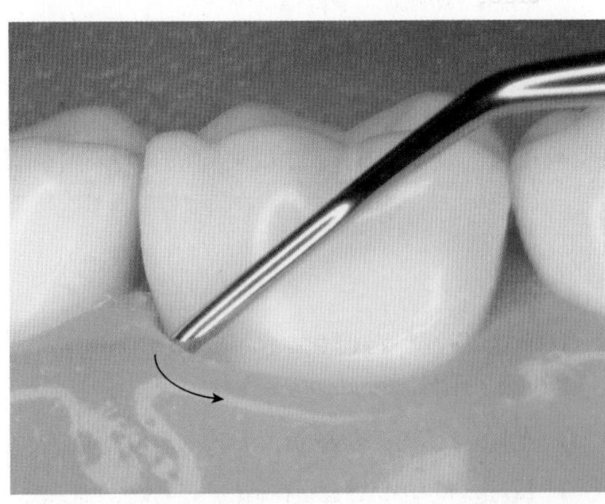

Figure 16-55. Posterior Teeth. Horizontal calculus removal strokes are very effective in removing deposits from the line angle region of posterior teeth.

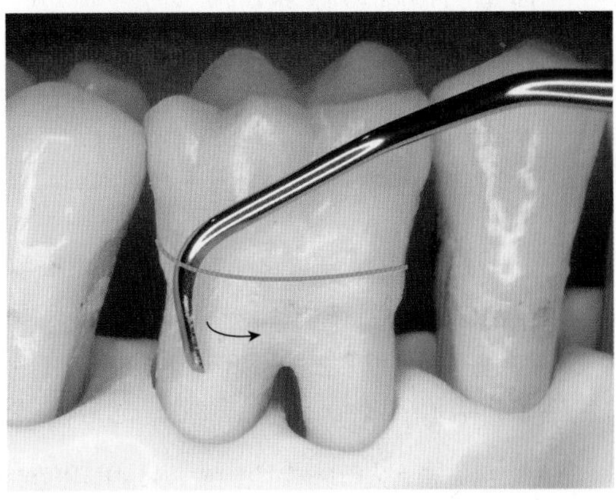

Figure 16-56. Technique Check. The gingiva has been removed from the typodont in this photograph to provide a view of the working-end of an area-specific curet during a horizontal stroke.

Section 6
Design Analysis of Scalers and Curets

TABLE 16-4. Summary Sheet: Design Analysis of Sickles and Curets

Characteristic	Instrument	Critique
Back pointed	Sickle	Advantage = strong, "bulky" working-end Disadvantage = not recommended for use on root surfaces
Back rounded	Universal & area-specific	Advantage = used subgingivally without tissue trauma Disadvantage = none
Tip (pointed)	Sickle	Advantage = provides good access to proximal surfaces on anterior crowns and enamel surfaces apical to contact areas of posterior teeth Disadvantage = sharp point can gouge cemental surfaces
Toe (rounded)	Universal & area-specific	Advantage = adapts well to convex, rounded root surfaces and root concavities Disadvantage = is wider than a pointed tip and, therefore, more difficult to adapt to proximal surfaces of anterior crowns
Curved cutting edge	Area-specific	Advantage = enhances adaptation to rounded root surfaces and root concavities Disadvantage = none
Face perpendicular to lower shank; level cutting edges	Sickle & universal	Advantage = efficient, two cutting edges per working-end, both of which can be used for calculus removal Disadvantage = level cutting edges mean that the lower shank must be titled slightly toward the tooth for correct angulation
Face tilts in relation to lower shank; uneven cutting edges	Area-specific	Advantage = working cutting edge is self-angulated Disadvantage = only one working cutting edge per working-end means frequent instrument changes

Section 7
Skill Application

PRACTICAL FOCUS

Periodontal Debridement Case: Mr. Smithfield

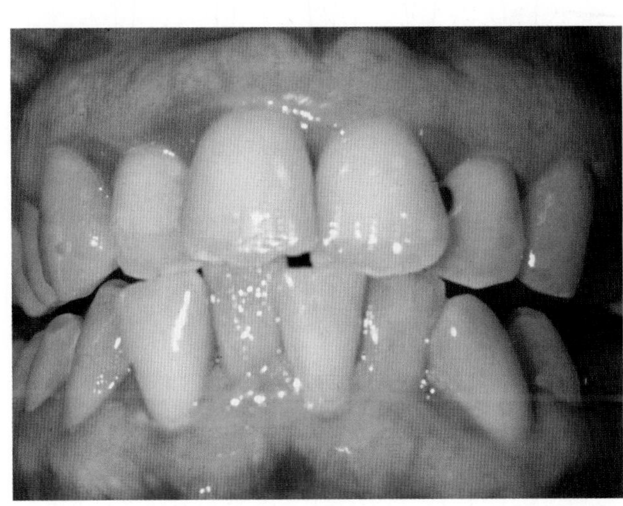

Figure 16-57. Mr. Smithfield: Intraoral Photograph.

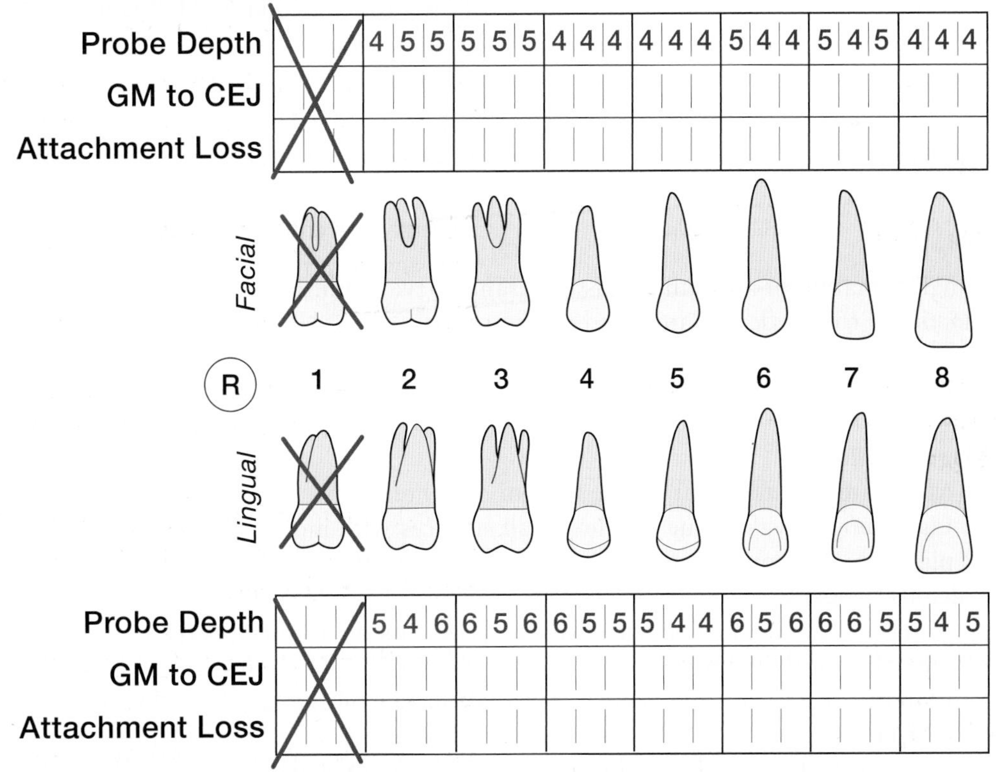

Probe Depth
GM to CEJ
Attachment Loss
4 5 5
5 5 5
4 4 4
4 4 4
5 4 4
5 4 5
4 4 4
Facial
R
1
2
3
4
5
6
7
8
Lingual
Probe Depth
GM to CEJ
Attachment Loss
5 4 6
6 5 6
6 5 5
5 4 4
6 5 6
6 6 5
5 4 5

Figure 16-58. Mr. Smithfield: Periodontal Chart for Maxillary Right Quadrant. (Key: CEJ = cementoenamel junction; GM = gingival margin)

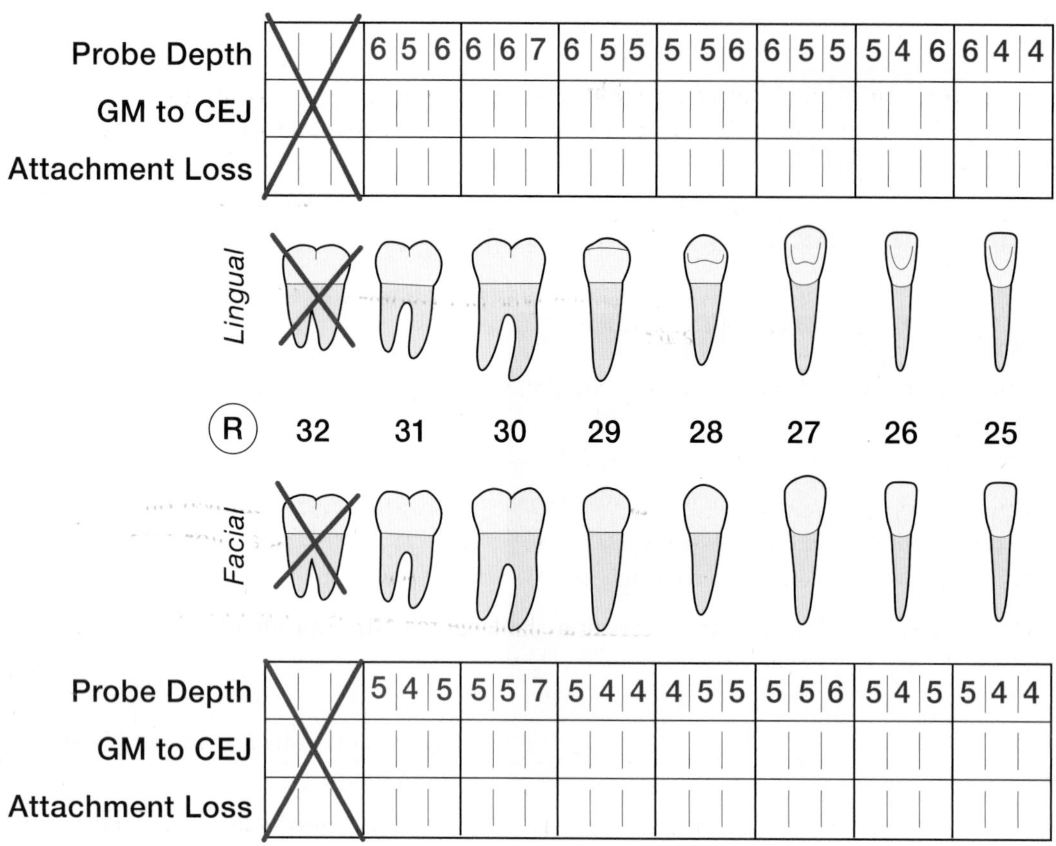

Probe Depth
GM to CEJ
Attachment Loss
6 5 6 6 6 7 6 5 5 5 5 6 6 5 5 5 4 6 6 4 4
Lingual
R
32 31 30 29 28 27 26 25
Facial
Probe Depth
GM to CEJ
Attachment Loss
5 4 5 5 5 7 5 4 4 4 5 5 5 5 6 5 4 5 5 4 4

Figure 16-59. Mr. Smithfield: Periodontal Chart for Mandibular Right Quadrant. (Key: CEJ = cementoenamel junction; GM = gingival margin)

Mr. Smithfield: Assessment Data

1. **Tissue**
   - **a.** Gingival margin of all teeth in this quadrant is level with the cementoenamel junction. Probing depths are noted on the chart.
   - **b.** Generalized bleeding upon probing.
2. **Deposits**
   - **a. Plaque Biofilm:**
     - Moderate ***supra***gingival plaque biofilm on all teeth.
     - Light ***sub***gingival plaque biofilm on all surfaces with moderate ***sub***gingival plaque biofilm on the proximal surfaces on all teeth.
   - **b. Calculus Deposits:**
     - Anterior teeth: light subgingival calculus deposits on all surfaces (facial, lingual, mesial, and distal).
     - Posterior teeth: light subgingival calculus deposits on the facial and lingual surfaces.
     - Posterior teeth: medium-size deposits on the proximal surfaces.

Mr. Smithfield: Case Questions 1–6

1. Do the assessment data indicate healthy sulci or periodontal pockets in this quadrant? Explain which data you used to determine the presence of sulci or pockets?
2. How effective is Mr. Smithfield's self-care (daily plaque control)? Explain which data helped you evaluate the effectiveness of his self-care?
3. After obtaining the probing depths, which type of explorer would you select to explore the teeth in this quadrant?
4. Which of the following instruments would you select for calculus removal on the anterior teeth in this quadrant: sickle scalers, universal curets, and/or area-specific curets? Explain your rationale for instrument selection.
5. Which of the following instruments would you select for calculus removal on the posterior teeth in this quadrant: sickle scalers, universal curets, and/or area-specific curets? Explain your rationale for instrument selection.
6. What anatomical characteristics present a challenge for Mr. Smithfield in his daily self-care and to the hygienist for instrumentation?

REFERENCES

1. Dufour LA, Bissell HS. Periodontal attachment loss induced by mechanical subgingival instrumentation in shallow sulci. *J Dent Hyg*. 2002;76:207–212.
2. Ruhling A, Konig J, Rolf H, Kocher T, Schwahn C, Plagmann HC. Learning root debridement with curettes and power-driven instruments. Part II: clinical results following mechanical, non-surgical therapy. *J Clin Periodontol*. 2003;30:611–615.

REFERENCE SHEET: AREA-SPECIFIC CURETS

Use of Area-Specific Curets:

An area-specific curet is a periodontal instrument used to remove light to moderate calculus deposits from the crowns and roots of the teeth and to deplaque (remove plaque biofilm from) the root surfaces.

Basic Concepts:

- Insert the working-end beneath the gingival margin at a 0° to 40° angulation.
- Maintain adaptation of the toe-third of the cutting edge to the tooth surface.
- Before initiating a calculus removal stroke, press down with your fulcrum finger and apply pressure against the instrument handle with the index finger and thumb to create lateral pressure against the tooth surface.
- Activate the calculus removal stroke using wrist motion activation. Use digital activation in areas where movement is restricted, such as furcation areas and narrow, deep pockets.
- Relax your fingers between each calculus removal stroke.

Anterior Teeth:

- Select the correct working-end:
  - Use only the lower cutting edges for periodontal instrumentation.
  - The lower shank is parallel to the tooth surface being instrumented.
- Sequence: Begin with the surfaces toward your nondominant hand. Start on the canine on the opposite side of the mouth and work toward yourself. (Right-handed clinicians start with the left canine, mesial surface; left-handed clinicians start with the right canine, mesial surface.)

Posterior Teeth:

- Select the correct working-end:
  - Use only the lower cutting edges for periodontal instrumentation.
  - The lower shank is parallel to the tooth surface.
- Use a distal curet (G13, G14, G17, G18) for distal surfaces. Use a mesial curet (G11, G12, G15, G16) for mesial surfaces. For facial and lingual surfaces, a mesial curet or the G7, G8, G9, and G10 curets may be used.
- Sequence: Complete all distal surfaces first; next, instrument the facial and mesial surfaces (or the lingual and mesial surfaces).

STUDENT SELF-EVALUATION MODULE 16 AREA-SPECIFIC CURETS

Student: ____________________ Area 1 = ____________________

Date: ____________________ Area 2 = ____________________

Area 3 = ____________________

Area 4 = ____________________

DIRECTIONS: Self-evaluate your skill level in each treatment area as: **S** (satisfactory) or **U** (unsatisfactory).

Criteria				
Positioning/Ergonomics	**Area 1**	**Area 2**	**Area 3**	**Area 4**
Adjusts clinician chair correctly				
Reclines patient chair and assures that patient's head is even with top of headrest				
Positions instrument tray within easy reach for front, side, or rear delivery as appropriate for operatory configuration				
Positions unit light at arm's length or dons dental headlight and adjusts it for use				
Assumes the recommended clock position				
Positions backrest of patient chair for the specified arch and adjusts height of patient chair so that clinician's elbows remain at waist level when accessing the specified treatment area				
Asks patient to assume the head position that facilitates the clinician's view of the specified treatment area				
Maintains neutral position				
Directs light to illuminate the specified treatment area				
Instrument Grasp: Dominant Hand	**Area 1**	**Area 2**	**Area 3**	**Area 4**
Grasps handle with tips of finger pads of index finger and thumb so that these fingers are opposite each other on the handle, but do NOT touch or overlap				
Rests pad of middle finger lightly on instrument shank; middle finger makes contact with ring finger				
Positions the thumb, index, and middle fingers in the "knuckles-up" convex position; hyperextended joint position is avoided				
Holds ring finger straight so that it supports the weight of hand and instrument; ring finger position is "advanced ahead of" the other fingers in the grasp				
Keeps index, middle, ring, and little fingers in contact; "like fingers inside a mitten"				
Maintains a relaxed grasp; fingers are NOT blanched in grasp				
Finger Rest: Dominant Hand	**Area 1**	**Area 2**	**Area 3**	**Area 4**
Establishes secure finger rest that is appropriate for tooth to be treated				
Once finger rest is established, pauses to self-evaluate finger placement in the grasp, verbalizes to evaluator his/her self-assessment of grasp, and corrects finger placement if necessary				
Prepare for Instrumentation ("Get Ready")	**Area 1**	**Area 2**	**Area 3**	**Area 4**
Selects correct working-end for tooth surface to be instrumented				
Places the working-end in the "Get Ready Zone" while using a correct finger rest for the treatment area				

(Note student self-evaluation continues on the next page)

STUDENT SELF-EVALUATION MODULE 16 AREA-SPECIFIC CURETS *(continued)*

Insertion	Area 1	Area 2	Area 3	Area 4
Establishes 0° angulation (face hugs tooth surface) in preparation for insertion				
Gently inserts curet toe beneath the gingival margin to base of sulcus or pocket				
Adaptation, Angulation, Calculus Removal Stroke	**Area 1**	**Area 2**	**Area 3**	**Area 4**
Assesses the root surface using light, sweeping assessment strokes away from the junctional epithelium				
Correctly orients the lower shank to the tooth surface to be instrumented				
Initiates a stroke away from the junctional epithelium by positioning the working-end beneath a calculus deposit, "locking the toe" against tooth surface and using an angulation between 45° and 80°				
Uses rotating motion to make a short, biting stroke in a coronal direction to snap a deposit from the tooth; does NOT close face toward tooth surface during activation; uses whole hand as a unit; does NOT pull with thumb and index finger				
Maintains appropriate lateral pressure against the tooth throughout the stroke while maintaining control of the working-end				
Precisely stops each individual stroke and pauses briefly (at least 3 seconds) to relax grasp before repositioning working-end beneath calculus deposit; strokes should be short and working-end remains beneath the gingival margin (to avoid trauma to gingival margin); does NOT remove working-end from the pocket with each stroke				
Maintains neutral wrist position throughout motion activation				
Maintains correct adaptation as instrument strokes progress around tooth surface; pivots and rolls instrument handle as needed				
Thoroughly instruments proximal surface under each contact area				
Uses appropriate sequence for the specified sextant				
Demonstrates horizontal strokes at the midlines of anterior teeth and the line angles of posterior teeth				
Keeps hands steady and controlled during instrumentation so that working-end moves with precision, regardless of nervousness				
Root Debridement Stroke	**Area 1**	**Area 2**	**Area 3**	**Area 4**
Establishes a 60° angle to the tooth surface				
Demonstrates a series of lighter, longer, shaving strokes away from the base of the periodontal pocket				
Ethics and Professionalism				
Punctuality, appearance, demeanor, attitude, composure, honesty				

Module 17

Periodontal Files

Module Overview

This module presents the design characteristics and techniques for use of periodontal files. The periodontal file is restricted in its use, serving only as a supplement to other periodontal instruments.

Module Outline

Key Terms

Periodontal file
Two-point contact

Learning Objectives

1. Discuss the advantages and limitations of the design characteristics of periodontal files.
2. Name the uses of periodontal files.
3. Given any periodontal file, identify where it should be used on the dentition.
4. Demonstrate what is meant by a "two-point contact" when using a periodontal file.
5. Using periodontal files, demonstrate correct adaptation and use of calculus removal strokes on the anterior teeth while maintaining correct position, correct finger rests, and precise finger placement in the grasp.
6. Using periodontal files, demonstrate correct adaptation and use of calculus removal strokes on the posterior teeth while maintaining correct position, correct finger rests, and precise finger placement in the grasp.

Section 1
Periodontal Files

GENERAL DESIGN CHARACTERISTICS

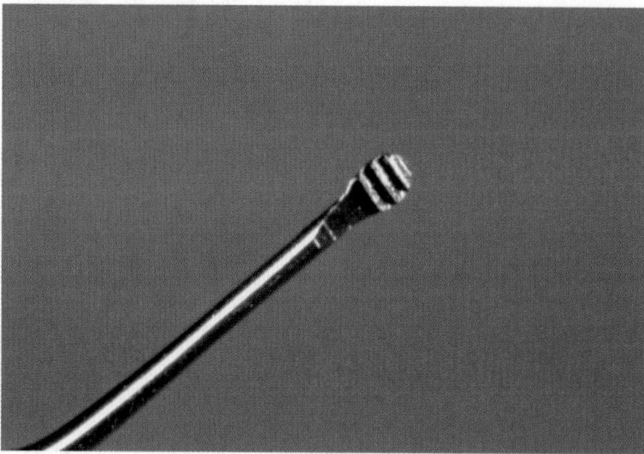

Figure 17-1. The Working-End of a Periodontal File.

1. **Functions of Periodontal Files**
   - **a.** A periodontal file is a periodontal instrument that is used to prepare calculus deposits before removal with another instrument (Fig. 17-1). A periodontal file is used to crush or roughen a heavy calculus deposit so that it can be removed with a sickle scaler or curet.
   - **b.** Periodontal files are restricted in use, serving only as a supplement to sickle scalers or curets.
   - **c.** Files are limited to use on enamel surfaces or the outer surface of a calculus deposit. The flat base and straight cutting edges do not adapt well to curved root surfaces.
   - **d.** They are used to crush large, tenacious subgingival calculus deposits that are not accessible to the sickle scalers that are usually used to remove heavy calculus deposits. Once the deposit has been crushed, it is then removed by a curet.
   - **e.** Files are used to roughen the surface of burnished calculus deposits to facilitate removal of these deposits with a curet.
   - **f.** Periodontal files can be used to smooth overhanging amalgam restorations.
   - **g.** Because of their design limitations, periodontal files have been replaced to a great extent by ultrasonic instruments. Ultrasonic instruments are very effective at removing large calculus deposits.
2. **Design Characteristics.** The working-end of a periodontal file has several unique design characteristics (Fig. 17-2 and Table 17-1).
   - **a.** A *series of cutting edges lined up on a base*
   - **b.** *Cuttings edges at a 90° to 105° angle to the base*
   - **c.** A *rectangular, round, or oblong base*
   - **d.** A *rounded back* to permit subgingival use
   - **e.** A *rigid shank* that transmits limited tactile information to the clinician's fingers
   - **f.** *Area-specific use.* Each file is designed for use only on certain tooth surfaces; therefore, a set of files is needed to instrument the entire mouth.
3. **Examples of Periodontal File Instruments.** Some examples of periodontal files include the Hirschfeld 3/7, 5/11, and 9/10 files and the Orban 10/11 and 12/13 files.

WORKING-END DESIGN

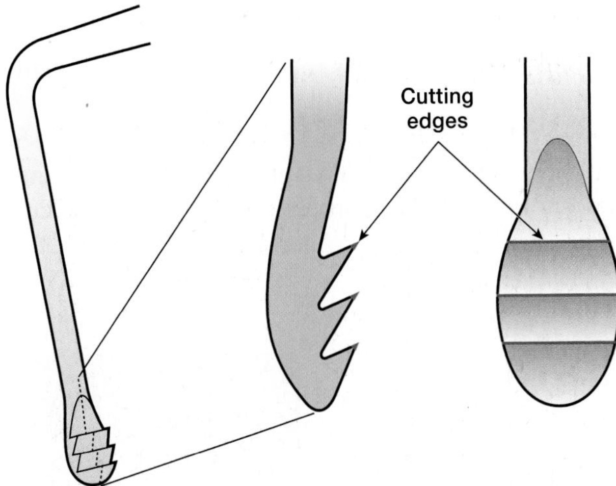

Figure 17-2. Design Characteristics. The working-end of a file has multiple, straight cutting edges.

TABLE 17-1. Reference Sheet: Periodontal File

Working-end	Thin in width and round, rectangular, or oblong in shape
Face	Has a series of cutting edges lined up on a base
Cutting Edges	Multiple edges, at a 90° to 105° angulation to the base
Application	Each working-end is designed for single-surface use; a set of files is required to instrument the entire mouth
Primary Functions	• Crush large calculus deposit • Roughen burnished calculus deposit • Smooth overhanging amalgam restoration • Limited to use on enamel surfaces or the outer surface of a calculus deposit; the flat base does not adapt well to curved root surfaces

ADAPTATION: TWO-POINT CONTACT

1. Two-point contact with a periodontal file involves adaptation of the working-end to a calculus deposit while resting the lower shank against the tooth (Fig. 17-3). This two-point contact provides the additional stability and leverage needed when making an instrumentation stroke with a file.
2. The *entire face* of the working-end should be flat against the calculus deposit (parallel to the root surface). The face should not be applied at an angle to the tooth surface; in this position, the sharp corners on one side of the cutting edges can gouge the cementum, while the sharp corners on the opposite end can traumatize the soft tissue.

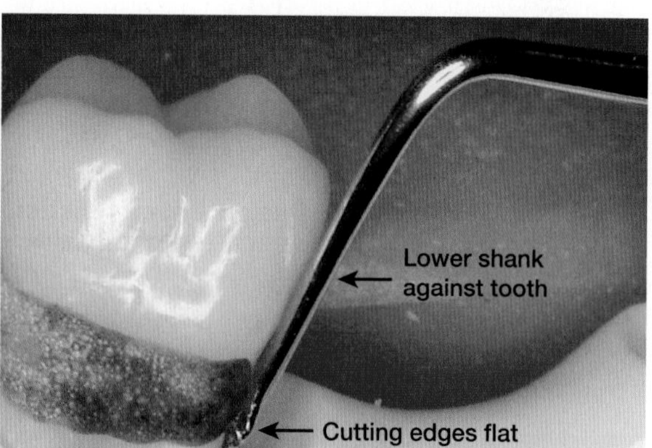

Figure 17-3. Two-Point Contact.

- Point One: The face of the working-end should be flat against the calculus deposit so that the corners of the straight cutting edges do not gouge the root surface or the soft tissue.
- Point Two: The lower shank should rest against the tooth surface.

FILE SELECTION

Each periodontal file is designed for use only on certain tooth surfaces; therefore, a set of files is needed to instrument the entire mouth. One of the most versatile series of files is the Hirschfeld series (Table 17-2). A set of Hirschfeld periodontal files includes the Hirschfeld 9/10, 3/7, and 5/11 files. Another common file series is the Orban series. There are two Orban files, the Orban 10/11 and 12/13.

TABLE 17-2. Application of Periodontal Files

Instrument	Area of Application
Hirschfeld 9/10	Facial and lingual surfaces of the anterior teeth
Hirschfeld 3/7	Facial and lingual surfaces of the posterior teeth
Hirschfeld 5/11	Mesial and distal surfaces of the posterior teeth
Orban 10/11	Facial and lingual surfaces of the posterior teeth
Orban 12/13	Mesial and distal surfaces of the posterior teeth

Section 2
Technique Practice—Posterior Teeth

APPLICATION OF THE CUTTING EDGES

A minimum of two double-ended periodontal files is required to instrument the tooth surfaces of the posterior teeth (Figs. 17-4 and 17-5).

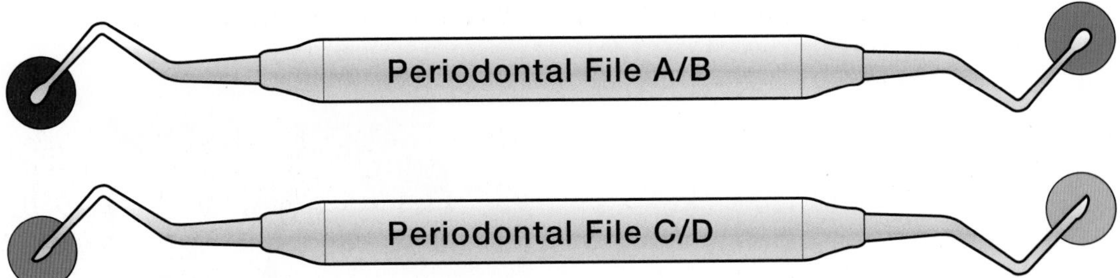

Figure 17-4. Application of Hirschfeld Files to Posterior Surfaces. Two files are used on the posterior teeth: the H 3/7 for facial and lingual surfaces and the H 5/11 for the proximal surfaces.

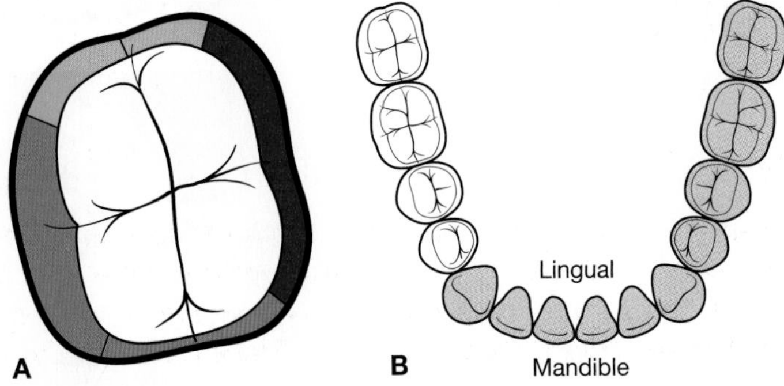

Figure 17-5. Application to Posterior Surfaces. This illustration indicates how the Hirschfeld files are applied to the posterior tooth surfaces.

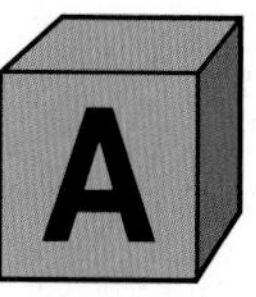

SKILL BUILDING. STEP-BY-STEP TECHNIQUE ON FACIAL AND LINGUAL SURFACES

Directions:

- Follow steps 1 to 5 to practice use of a periodontal file on the facial and lingual tooth surfaces (Figs. 17-6 to 17-10).

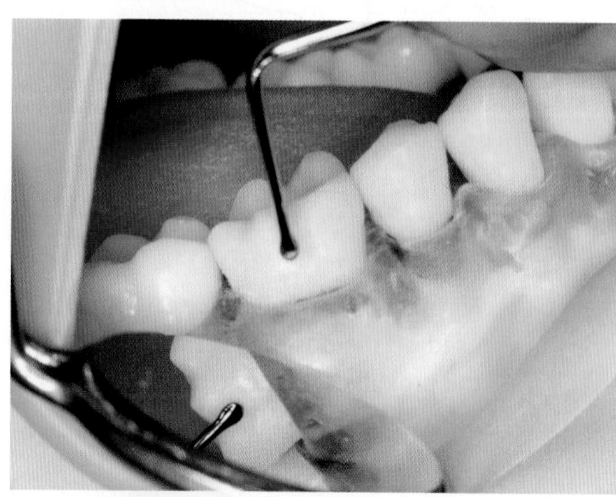

1. **Figure 17-6. Get Ready.** Select the correct file for use on the facial aspect of the mandibular right first molar. In preparation for insertion, place the working-end against the facial surface.

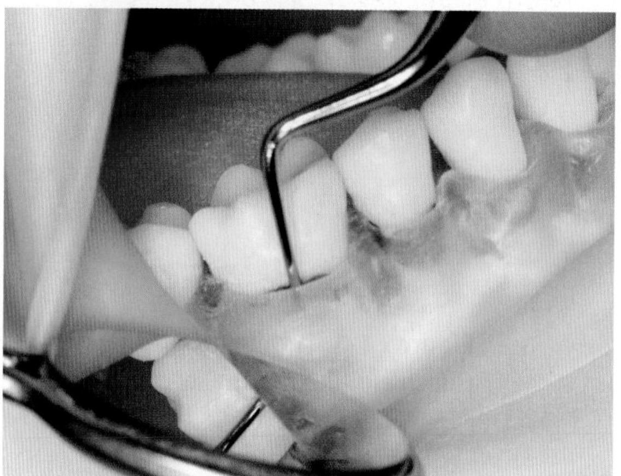

2. **Figure 17-7. Insert.** Gently insert the working-end beneath the gingival margin.

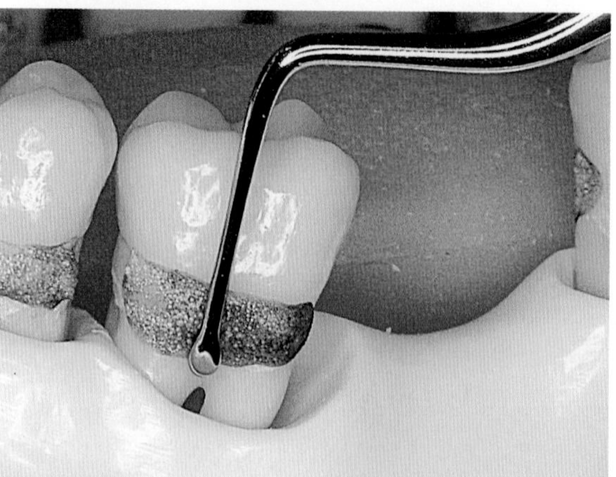

3. **Figure 17-8. Adapt to the Calculus Deposit.** Move the file along the root surface until it is adapted to the calculus deposit.

- *Remember to establish a two-point contact with the working-end and the lower shank.*
- Activate pull strokes in a vertical direction.

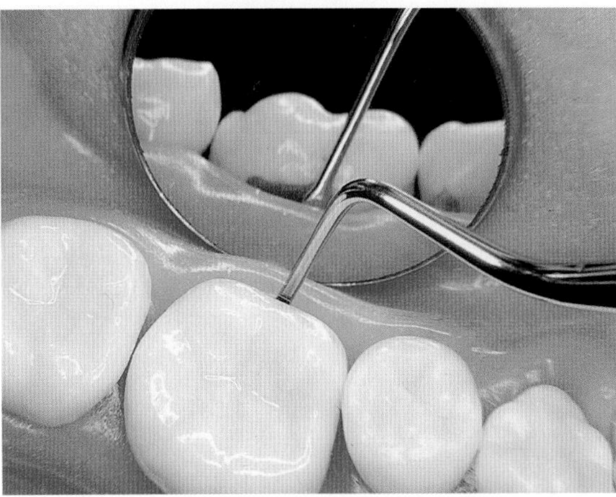

4. **Figure 17-9. Lingual Surface.** Select the correct file for use on the lingual surface. Gently slip the working-end beneath the gingival margin. Establish two-point contact. Use indirect vision to check the placement of the periodontal file.

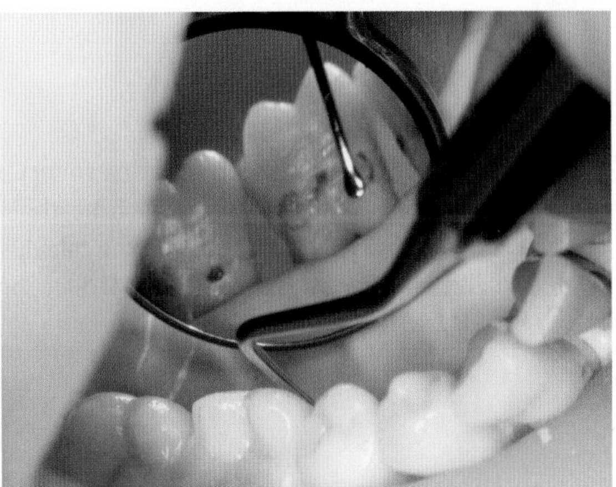

5. **Figure 17-10. Adapt to the Calculus Deposit.** Move the file along the root surface until it is adapted to the calculus deposit. Activate pull strokes in a vertical direction.

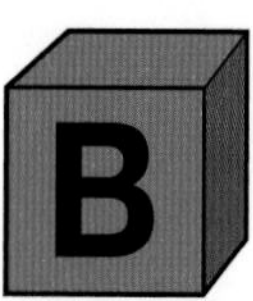

SKILL BUILDING. STEP-BY-STEP TECHNIQUE ON MESIAL AND DISTAL SURFACES

- Follow steps 1 and 2 to practice use of a periodontal file on the mesial and distal tooth surfaces (Figs. 17-11 and 17-12).

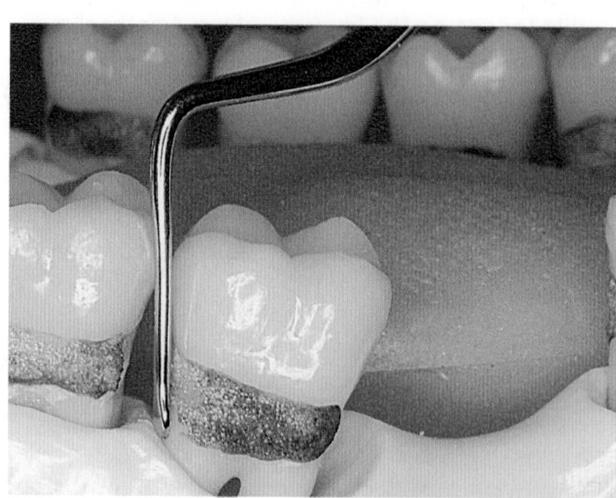

1. **Figure 17-11. Distal Surface.** Select the correct file for the distal surface. Insert the file beneath the gingival margin and position it on the calculus deposit. Activate pull strokes in a vertical direction.

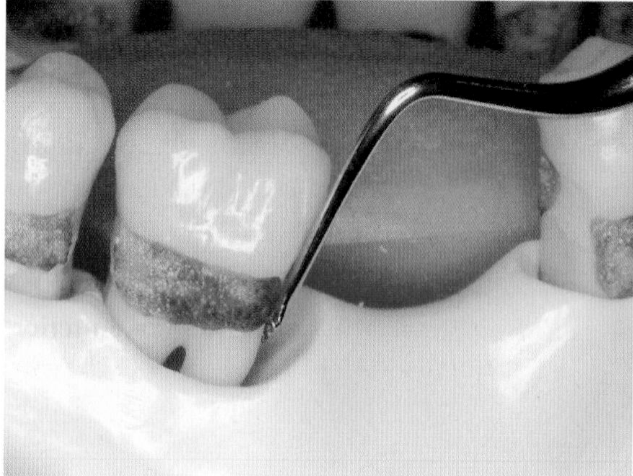

2. **Figure 17-12. Mesial Surface.** Using the correct file for the mesial surface, position the working-end on the calculus deposit. Remember to maintain two-point contact. Activate pull strokes in a vertical direction.

Section 3
Technique Practice—Anterior Teeth

APPLICATION OF THE CUTTING EDGES

A minimum of one double-ended periodontal file is required to instrument the facial and lingual surfaces of anterior teeth (Figs. 17-13 and 17-14).

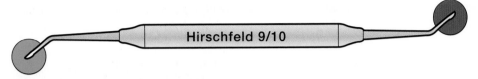

Figure 17-13. Application of a Hirschfeld File to Anterior Teeth. The Hirschfeld 9/10 periodontal file is used to instrument the anterior teeth.

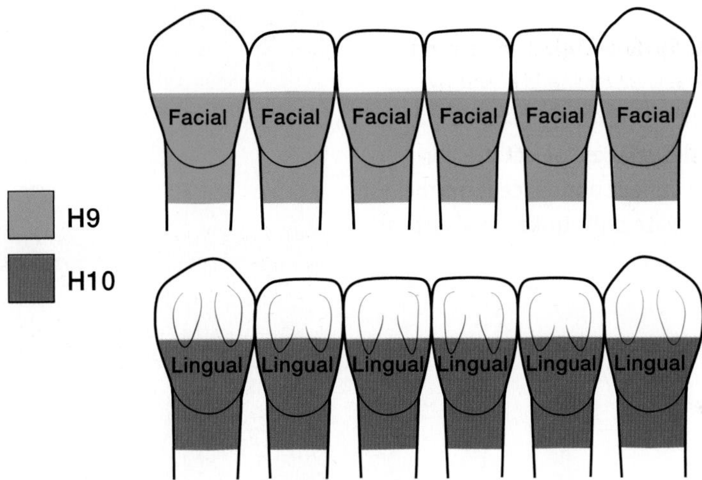

Figure 17-14. Application to Anterior Surfaces. This illustration indicates how the Hirschfeld 9/10 file is applied to the anterior tooth surfaces.

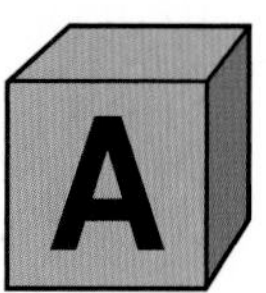

SKILL BUILDING. STEP-BY-STEP TECHNIQUE ON CENTRAL INCISOR

Directions:

- Follow steps 1 and 2 to practice use of a periodontal file on the facial and lingual tooth surfaces of anterior teeth (Figs. 17-15 and 17-16).
- Remember: ***"Me, My patient, My light, My dominant hand, My nondominant hand, My finger rest, My adaptation."***

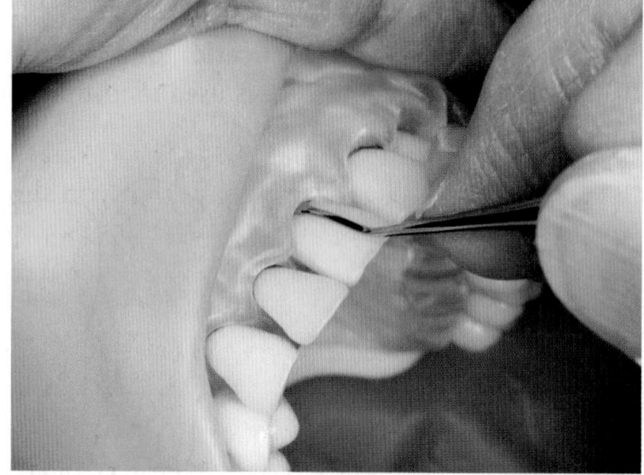

1. **Figure 17-15. Facial Surfaces.** Select the correct file for the facial surface and place it on the calculus deposit. Activate pull strokes in a vertical direction.

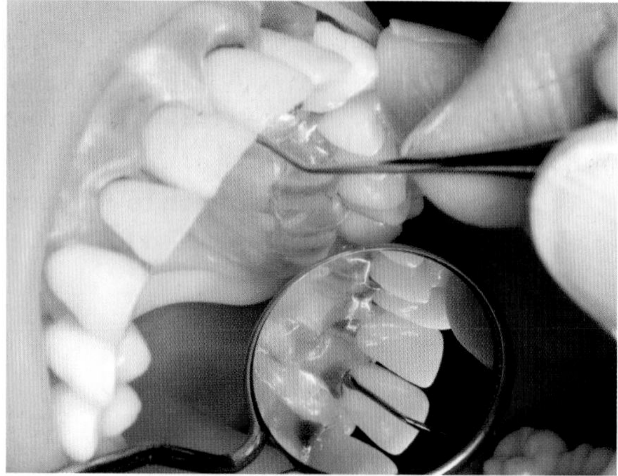

2. **Figure 17-16. Lingual Surfaces.** Insert the correct file beneath the gingival margin. Adapt to the calculus deposit and activate a series of pull strokes in a vertical direction.

Section 4
Skill Application

PRACTICAL FOCUS

Case 1: You have been assigned to observe a second-year student, Lawanda, as she performs periodontal instrumentation on a patient. You observe Lawanda using a periodontal file on the facial aspect of the maxillary right first molar. She is working within a periodontal pocket. Lawanda makes several vertical strokes with the file and then uses an area-specific curet to remove a calculus deposit. What reason would Lawanda have to use both a file and an area-specific curet on the facial aspect of this molar?

Case 2: You have been assigned to work as a team with a second-year student, Henry, to provide care for Mr. Wilson. Mr. Wilson has ledges of subgingival calculus throughout his dentition. The calculus deposits are located in 5- to 6-mm pockets. Today, the mandibular left posterior quadrant will be instrumented. Henry tries to remove the calculus ledges using area-specific curets but is unsuccessful because the deposits are so tenacious. So, Henry uses periodontal files to instrument the teeth. At this point, Henry says that you should be able to take over and finish instrumentation on this quadrant. What do you expect to find when you explore the teeth? After exploring the teeth, what do you plan to do next?

Case 3: You have been assigned to observe a second-year student, Wynne, as she performs periodontal debridement on a patient. Wynne spends considerable time instrumenting the maxillary right second molar with an area-specific curet. This tooth has a pocket, and Wynne says that there is a ledge of calculus that she just cannot budge. You suggest that she try a periodontal file. As you and Wynne walk to the clinic dispensary to obtain a set of periodontal files, Wynne confesses that she has never used a file on a patient. Wynne uses the file in the area and is successful in breaking up the calculus ledge. When she checks the facial surface with an explorer, Wynne is surprised to find several long gouges in the root surface. You also notice that the soft tissue began to bleed heavily after Wynne used the file. What technique error might have produced the gouges in the cementum and traumatized the tissue wall of the pocket?

STUDENT SELF-EVALUATION MODULE 17 PERIODONTAL FILES

Student: ______________________ Date: ______________________

DIRECTIONS: Self-evaluate your skill level in each treatment area as: **S** (satisfactory) or **U** (unsatisfactory).

Criteria				
Positioning/Ergonomics	**Area 1**	**Area 2**	**Area 3**	**Area 4**
Adjusts clinician and patient chairs and equipment correctly				
Assumes the recommended clock position				
Instrument Grasp: Dominant Hand	**Area 1**	**Area 2**	**Area 3**	**Area 4**
Grasps handle with tips of finger pads of index finger and thumb				
Rests pad of middle finger lightly on instrument shank				
Positions the thumb, index, and middle fingers in the "knuckles-up" convex position; hyperextended joint position is avoided				
Finger Rest: Dominant Hand				
Establishes secure finger rest that is appropriate for tooth to be treated				
Once finger rest is established, pauses to self-evaluate finger placement in the grasp, verbalizes to evaluator his/her self-assessment of grasp, and corrects finger placement if necessary				
Prepare for Instrumentation ("Get Ready")				
Selects correct working-end for tooth surface to be instrumented				
Places the working-end in the "Get Ready Zone" while using a correct finger rest for the treatment area				
Adaptation, Angulation, and Instrument Stroke	**Area 1**	**Area 2**	**Area 3**	**Area 4**
Establishes two-point contact				
Uses vertical strokes				
Applies appropriate stroke pressure in a coronal direction				
Maintains appropriate lateral pressure against the tooth throughout the stroke while maintaining control of the working-end				
Keeps hands steady and controlled during instrumentation so that working-end moves with precision, regardless of nervousness				
Ethics and Professionalism				
Punctuality, appearance, demeanor, attitude, composure, honesty				

Module 18

Advanced Probing Techniques

Module Overview

The comprehensive periodontal assessment is one of the most important functions performed by dental hygienists. This module begins with a review of the periodontal attachment system in health and attachment loss in disease. Other module sections describe techniques for advanced assessments with periodontal probes including (1) bleeding on gentle probing, (2) level of the free gingival margin, (3) oral deviations, (4) tooth mobility, (5) furcation involvement, (6) clinical attachment levels, and (7) width of the attached gingiva.

Module Outline

Section 5	Skill Application	457
	Practical Focus: Calculation of Clinical Loss of Attachment Practical Focus: Fictitious Patient Case, Mr. Temple Practical Focus: Fictitious Patient Case, Mrs. Blanchard Student Self-Evaluation Module 18: Angulation and Calculus Removal	

Key Terms

Comprehensive periodontal assessment
Periodontal attachment system
Junctional epithelium
Fibers of the gingiva
Periodontal ligament fibers
Alveolar bone
Loss of attachment (LOA)
Recession of the gingival margin
Mobility
Horizontal tooth mobility
Vertical tooth mobility
Mobility rating scales
Bifurcation
Trifurcation
Furcation area
Root trunk
Furcation involvement
Furcation arrows
Furcation probe
Clinical attachment level (CAL)
Clinical attachment loss (CAL)
Attached gingiva
Width of the attached gingiva

Learning Objectives

1. Discuss the uses of calibrated and furcation probes in performing a periodontal assessment.
2. Describe the rationale for assessing tooth mobility.
3. Demonstrate the technique for assessing tooth mobility and use a mobility rating scale to classify the extent of mobility.
4. Describe the rationale and technique for determining the level of the gingival margin.
5. Describe the consequences of loss of attachment to the tooth.
6. Given the probing depth measurements and gingival margin levels for a tooth, compute the clinical attachment loss.
7. Describe the rationale for furcation detection.
8. Demonstrate correct technique for use of a furcation probe on a periodontal typodont and classify furcation involvement according to severity.
9. Use advanced probing techniques to accurately assess a student partner's periodontium.
10. For simulated patient cases, use periodontal measurements to differentiate a healthy periodontium from periodontitis and record these findings on a periodontal chart.

Note to Course Instructor: The Skill Application section includes two fictitious patient cases for analysis and practice in calculation of clinical attachment levels. Additional fictitious patient cases and practice opportunities in calculating clinical attachment levels are found in Modules 19 and 21.

Section I
Assessment and the Periodontal Attachment System

COMPREHENSIVE PERIODONTAL ASSESSMENT

A comprehensive periodontal assessment is an intensive clinical periodontal evaluation used to gather information about the periodontium. The comprehensive periodontal assessment normally includes clinical features such as probing depth measurements, bleeding on probing, presence of exudate, level of the free gingival margin and the mucogingival junction, tooth mobility, furcation involvement, presence of calculus and bacterial plaque, gingival inflammation, radiographic evidence of alveolar bone loss, and presence of local contributing factors.[1,2] ***Much of the information collected during the comprehensive periodontal assessment involves the use of periodontal probes.*** Table 18-1 summarizes the role of periodontal probes in the comprehensive periodontal assessment.

TABLE 18-1. Uses of Periodontal Probes in the Comprehensive Periodontal Assessment

Assessment	Technique
Intraoral lesions	• Measurement of the size of pathologic lesions
Bleeding on probing	• Bleeding on gentle probing indicates gingival inflammation
Recession of the gingival margin	• Measurement from the free gingival margin to the cementoenamel junction (CEJ) • A clinical indicator of loss of attachment
Amount of attached gingiva	• Determination of the width of the **attached gingiva** (the part of the gingiva that is tightly connected to the cementum on the cervical-third of the root and to the periosteum of the alveolar bone)
Probing depth	• Measurement from free marginal gingiva to the base of the sulcus or periodontal pocket; deepest reading is recorded for each of six surfaces (distofacial, facial, mesiofacial, distolingual, lingual, mesiolingual)
Clinical attachment level	• Measurement from the CEJ to the base of the sulcus or periodontal pocket • Measuring from a fixed point—the CEJ—more accurately reflects the true extent of the bone support, especially when recession of the free gingival margin is present
Distance between teeth	• Measurement of distances between teeth or migration of teeth with severe periodontal disease
Furcation involvement	• Detection of bone loss between the roots of multirooted teeth • A specialized curved furcation probe—the Nabers probe—is used to detect furcation involvement

ATTACHMENT IN HEALTH

The periodontal attachment system is a group of structures that work together *to attach* the teeth to the maxilla and mandible (Fig. 18-1). To remain in the oral cavity, each tooth must be attached by:

1. Junctional epithelium—the epithelium that attaches the gingiva to the tooth.
2. Fibers of the gingiva—a network of fibers that brace the free gingiva against the tooth and unite the free gingiva with the tooth root and alveolar bone.
3. Periodontal ligament fibers—the fibers that surround the root of the tooth. These fibers attach to the bone of the socket on one side and to the cementum of the root on the other side.
4. Alveolar bone—the bone that surrounds the roots of the teeth. It forms the bony sockets that support and protect the roots of the teeth.

LOSS OF ATTACHMENT IN DISEASE

Loss of attachment (LOA) is damage to the structures that support the tooth. Loss of attachment occurs in periodontitis and is characterized by (1) relocation of the junctional epithelium to the tooth root, (2) destruction of the fibers of the gingiva, (3) destruction of the periodontal ligament fibers, and (4) loss of alveolar bone support from around the tooth. The changes that occur in the alveolar bone in periodontal disease are significant because loss of bone height eventually can result in tooth loss. Table 18-2 summarizes the status of the attachment structures in health versus in disease. Figures 18-2 to 18-5 depict the changes in the level of the alveolar bone and gingival margin in health and disease.

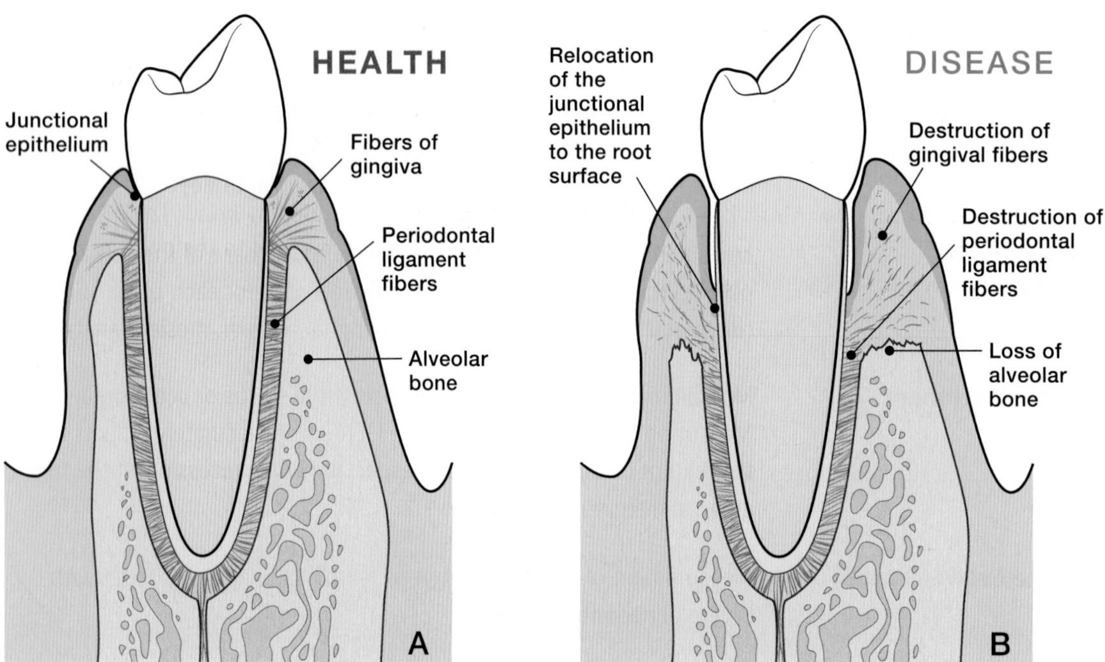

Figure 18-1. Cross Section of the Periodontal Attachment System. A. The periodontal attachment system in health. **B.** Destruction of the periodontal attachment system in disease.

TABLE 18-2. Attachment Structures in Health and Disease

Attachment in Health	Attachment in Disease
• Junctional epithelium attaches to enamel at base of sulcus	• Junctional epithelium attaches to cementum at base of periodontal pocket
• Fibers brace the tissue against the crown	• Fiber destruction, tissue lacks firmness
• Many fibers attach root to bone of socket	• Fewer fibers remain to hold tooth in socket
• Most of the root is surrounded by bone; the tooth is firmly held in its socket	• Part of the root is surrounded by bone; the tooth may be movable in its socket

ALVEOLAR BONE SUPPORT IN HEALTH AND DISEASE

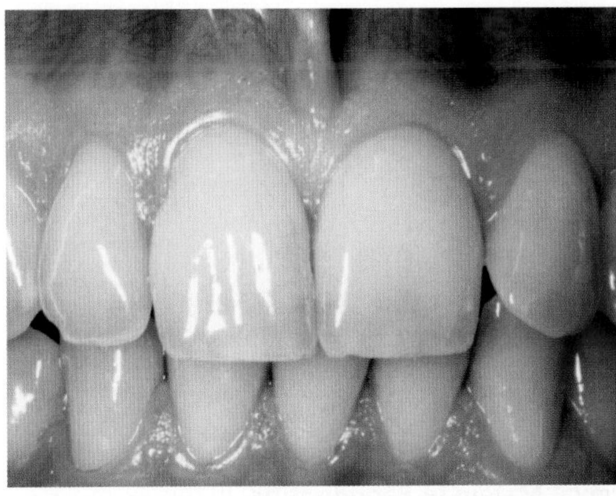

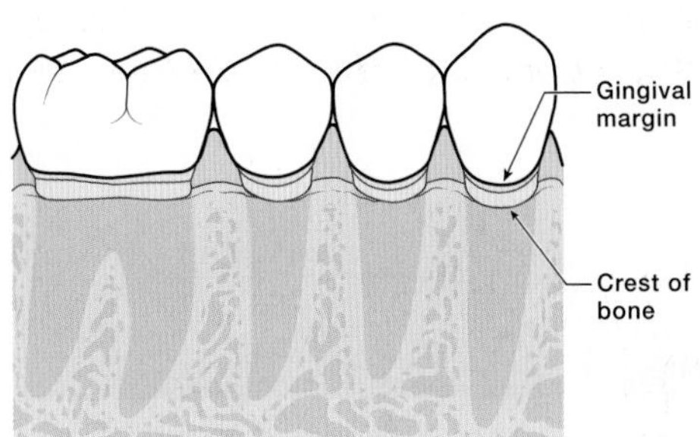

Figure 18-2. Bone Support in Health. In health, most of the root is surrounded by bone. The crest of the alveolar bone is located very close to the crowns, only 1 to 2 mm apical to (below) the cementoenamel junctions (CEJs) of the teeth.

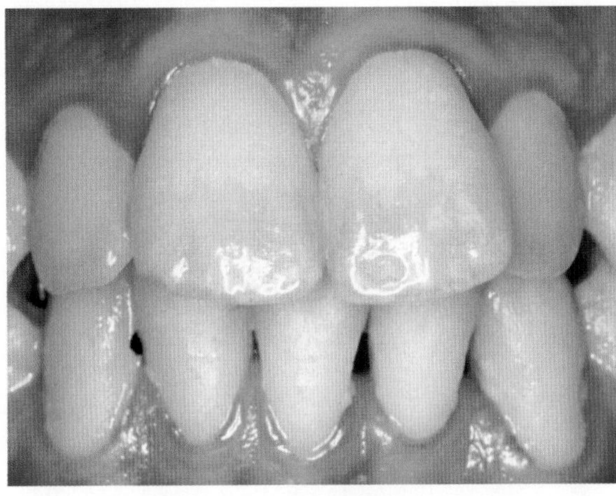

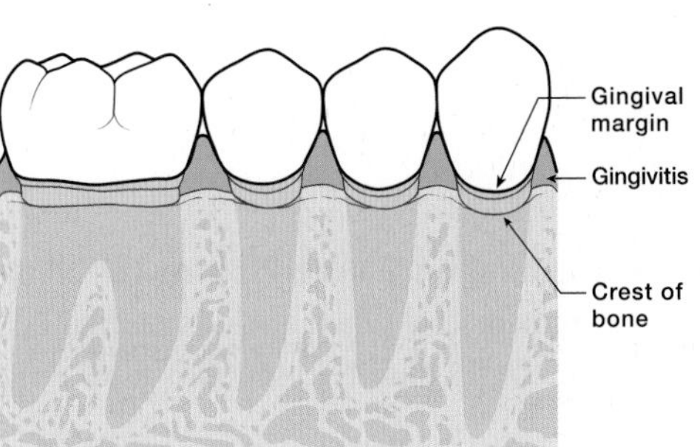

Figure 18-3. Bone Support in Gingivitis. In gingival disease, there is no loss of alveolar bone, and the crest of the alveolar bone remains only 1 to 2 mm apical to (below) the CEJs of the teeth.

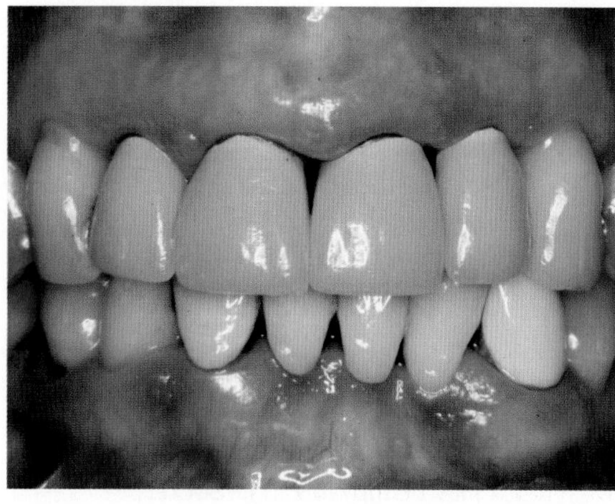

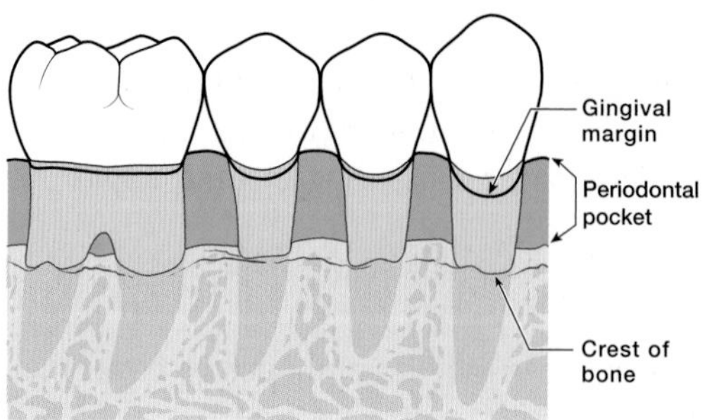

Figure 18-4. Bone Loss and Pocket Formation in Periodontitis. In periodontitis, bone is destroyed and the teeth are not well supported in the arch. In this example of bone loss, the gingival margin has remained near the CEJ, creating deep periodontal pockets.

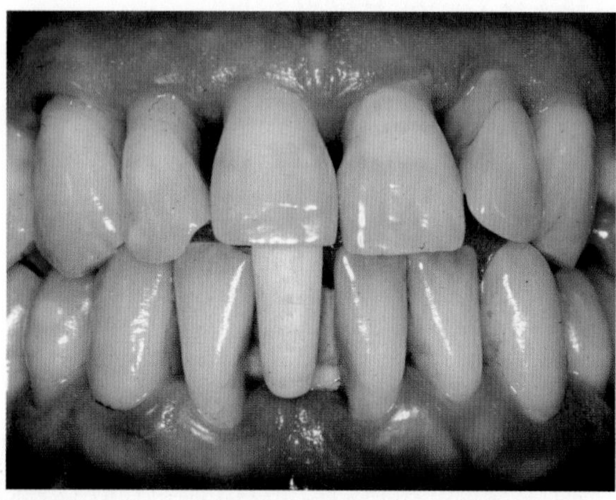

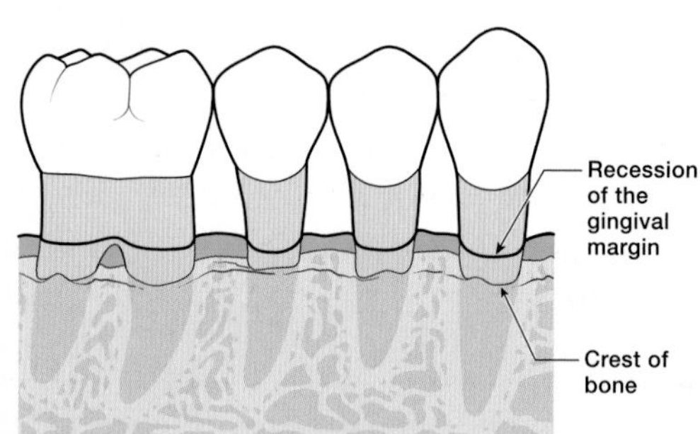

Figure 18-5. Loss of Bone and Recession of the Gingival Margin in Periodontitis. In this example of periodontitis, the gingival margin has receded, and the tooth roots are visible in the mouth. Note that the probing depth is less in this example; however, the alveolar bone is at the same level. Only the level of the gingival margin differs between Figures 18-4 and 18-5.

BLEEDING ON GENTLE PROBING

Bleeding on gentle probing is a clinical sign of gingival inflammation (Fig. 18-6).

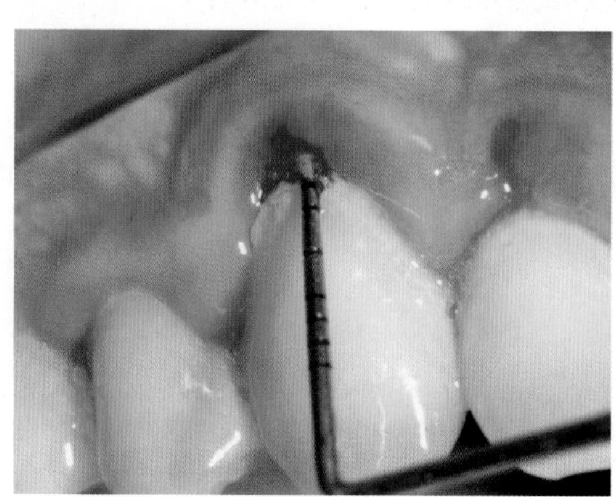

Figure 18-6. Bleeding on Gentle Probing. Bleeding may be visible immediately when a site is probed or might not be evident for about 10 seconds after a site is probed.

Most periodontal charts have a row of boxes that are used to document sites that bleed; bleeding may be indicated with a red dot.

Section 2
Assessments with Calibrated Probes

LEVEL OF THE FREE GINGIVAL MARGIN

The level of the free gingival margin can change over time in response to trauma, medications, or disease. Three possible relationships exist between the gingival margin and the CEJ of the tooth (Figs. 18-7 to 18-9).

1. **Gingival Margin Is Slightly Coronal to the CEJ.** The natural position of the gingival margin is slightly coronal to the CEJ.
2. **Gingival Margin Significantly Covers the CEJ.**
   a. In this instance, the gingiva covers a significant portion of the tooth crown, with the gingival margin being significantly coronal to the CEJ.
   b. The position of the gingival margin may be coronal to the CEJ due to (1) swelling (edema), (2) an overgrowth of the gingival tissues caused by certain medications that a patient takes to treat a medical condition, and/or (3) an increase in the fibrous connective tissue of the gingiva due to a long-standing inflammation of the tissue.
3. **Gingival Margin Is Significantly Apical to the CEJ.**
   a. When the gingival margin is significantly apical to the CEJ, a portion of the root surface is exposed in the mouth. This relationship is known as recession of the gingival margin.
   b. Recession of the gingival margin is the movement of the gingival margin from its normal position—usually with underlying loss of bone—resulting in the exposure of a portion of the root surface. In recession, the gingival margin is apical to the CEJ, and the papillae may be rounded or blunted.

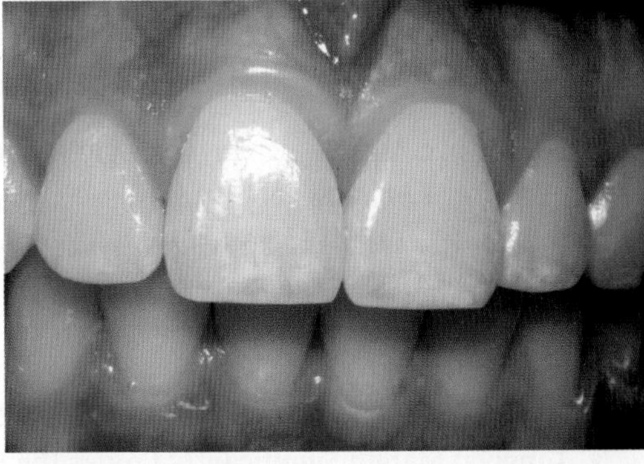

Figure 18-7. Gingival Margin Slightly Coronal to the CEJ. The gingival margin is at its normal position, slightly coronal to the CEJ in this photograph.

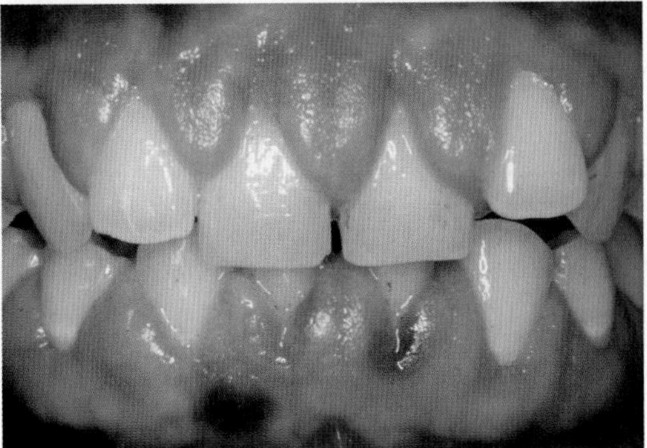

Figure 18-8. Gingival Margin Significantly Covers the CEJ. The gingival margin is significantly coronal to the CEJ in this photograph.

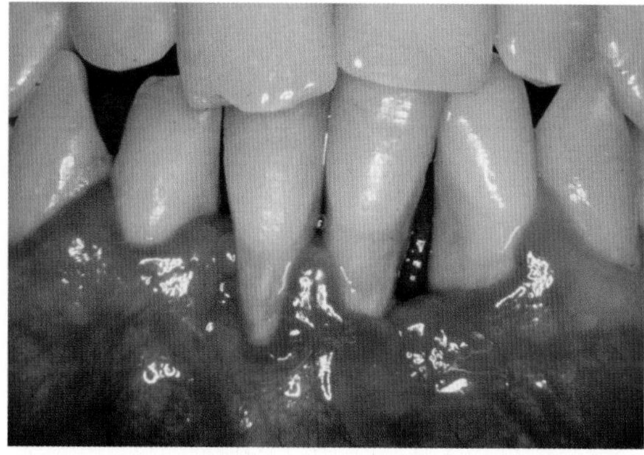

A

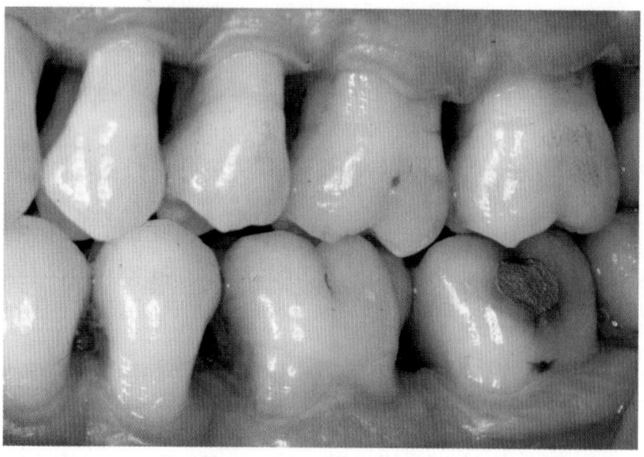

B

Figure 18-9. Gingival Margin Significantly Apical to CEJ. This relationship, known as recession of the gingival margin, leads to exposure of the root surface. **A.** Recession of the gingival margin on the facial aspect of three anterior teeth. **B.** Recession of the gingival margin on the facial aspect of the posterior teeth.

DOCUMENTING FREE GINGIVAL MARGIN LEVEL ON A CHART

Most periodontal charts include rows of boxes that are used to record the level of the free gingival margin on the facial and lingual aspects. In addition, the level may be indicated on the facial and lingual aspects of the teeth by a line (Fig. 18-10).

Box 18-1. Recording the Gingival Margin Level

Customarily, the following notations indicate the gingival margin level on a periodontal chart:

1. **Gingival Margin at Normal Level (Slightly Coronal to the CEJ).** A zero (**0**) is entered on the chart to indicate that the gingiva is slightly coronal to the CEJ (normal level of gingival margin).
2. **Gingival Margin Is Apical to the CEJ (Recession of the Gingival Margin)**
   - In this case, the clinician records the millimeters that the gingival margin would need to move coronally along the root for the margin to be at the normal position.
   - *Think: "How much gingival tissue would **be added** (+) to return the gingival margin to its normal position slightly coronal to the CEJ?"*
   - Record the number of millimeters that "need to be added" to bring the margin to its normal position as a positive (+) number.
   - Example: 4 mm of gingival recession is recorded as +4 to indicate that the margin would need to move coronally 4 mm to be at the normal position.
3. **Gingival Margin Significantly Covers the CEJ (Margin Is Coronal to Normal Position)**
   - In this case, the gingiva would need to be reduced in height in order to be at its normal position slightly coronal to the CEJ.
   - *Think: "How much gingival tissue would **be taken away** (−) to return the margin to its normal position?"*
   - Record the number of millimeters that "need to be taken away" to lower the margin to its normal position as a negative (−) number.
   - Example: a gingival margin that is 3 mm coronal to the CEJ is recorded on the periodontal chart as −3.

Sample Periodontal Chart

On the sample periodontal chart shown below (Fig. 18-10), the gingival margin level is charted in the row of boxes labeled *"GM to CEJ"—gingival margin to cementoenamel junction*. In addition, the level of the gingival margin may be drawn across the teeth on a periodontal chart.

In this example chart, the level of the gingival margin is significantly coronal to the CEJ on teeth 22, 23, and 24. The gingival margin level is normal for teeth 20 and 21. Recession of the gingival margin is present on teeth 18 and 19.

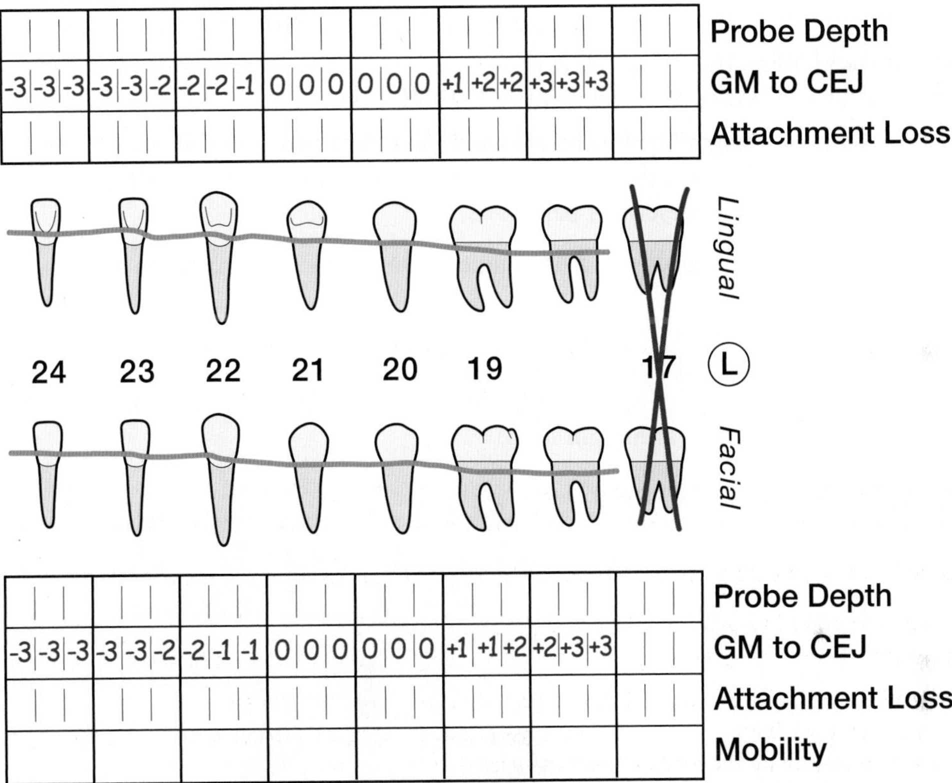

Figure 18-10. Sample Periodontal Chart. Shown above is an example of how the level of the free gingival margin might be indicated on a periodontal chart for the mandibular left quadrant. (Key: GM to CEJ = measurement from the gingival margin to the cementoenamel junction.)

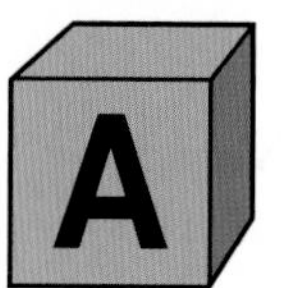

SKILL BUILDING. DETERMINING THE LEVEL OF THE GINGIVAL MARGIN

When tissue swelling or recession of the gingival margin is present, a periodontal probe is used to measure the distance the gingival margin is apical or coronal to the CEJ.

1. **For Areas Exhibiting Recession of the Gingival Margin.**
   a. If recession of the gingival margin is present, the distance between the CEJ and the gingival margin is measured using a calibrated periodontal probe as pictured in Figure 18-11.
   b. This distance is recorded as the gingival margin level.
2. **When the Gingival Margin Significantly Covers the CEJ.** If the gingival margin significantly covers the CEJ, the distance between the margin and the CEJ is estimated using the steps described below.
   a. Position the tip of the probe at a 45° angle to the tooth in preparation for insertion.
   b. Slowly move the probe beneath the gingival margin until the junction between the enamel and cementum is detected.
   c. Measure the distance between the gingival margin and the CEJ. This distance is recorded as the gingival margin level.

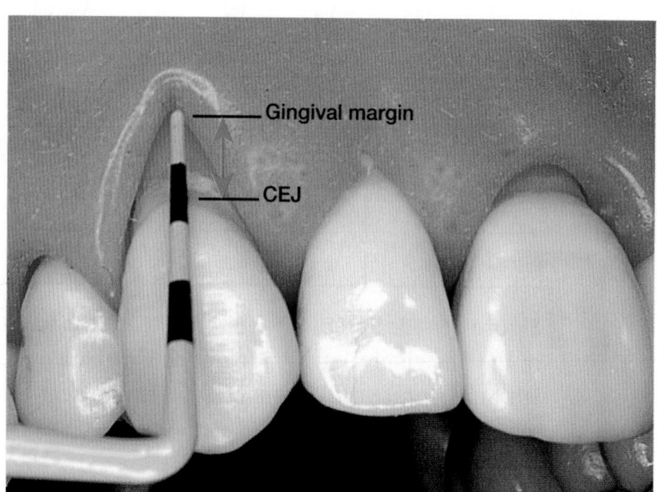

Figure 18-11. Measuring Recession of the Gingival Margin. The extent of recession of the gingival margin is measured in millimeters from the gingival margin to the CEJ.

ORAL DEVIATIONS

A calibrated probe is used to determine the size of an intraoral lesion or deviation. Figures 18-12 to 18-14 depict the use of a periodontal probe to determine the size of pathologic intraoral lesions.

- When an oral lesion is observed in a patient's mouth, this finding should be recorded in the patient's chart. Information recorded should include (1) the date, (2) size, (3) location, (4) color, (5) character of the lesion, and (6) any information provided by the patient (e.g., duration, sensation, or oral habits).
- For example: *"January 12, 2012: a soft, red, papillary lesion located on the buccal mucosa opposite the maxillary left first premolar; measuring 5 mm in an anterior–posterior direction and 6 mm in a superior–inferior direction."*
- It is best to use anatomic references, rather than "length" or "width," to document your measurements on the chart (e.g., as the anterior–posterior measurement and the superior–inferior measurement).

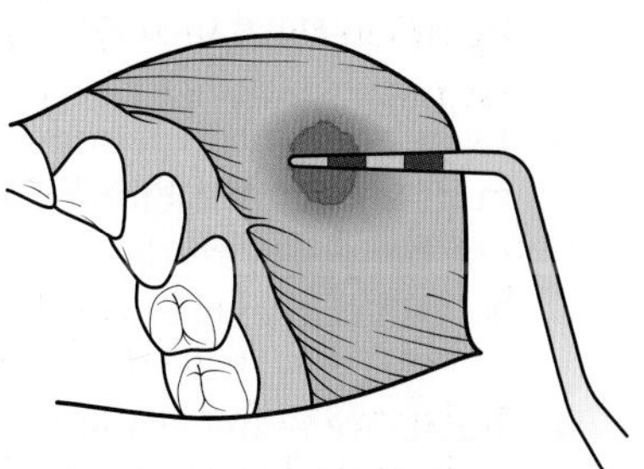

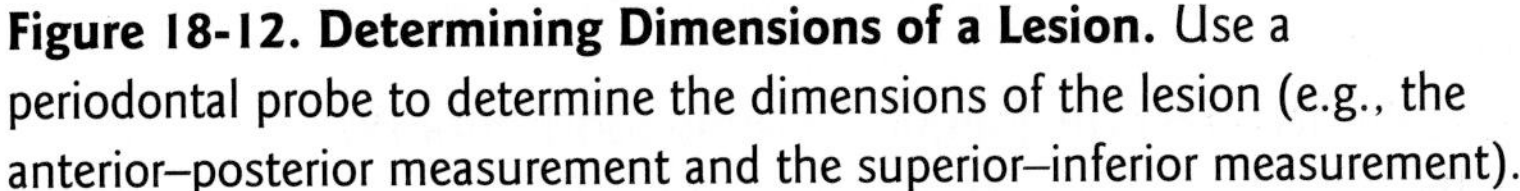

Figure 18-12. Determining Dimensions of a Lesion. Use a periodontal probe to determine the dimensions of the lesion (e.g., the anterior–posterior measurement and the superior–inferior measurement).

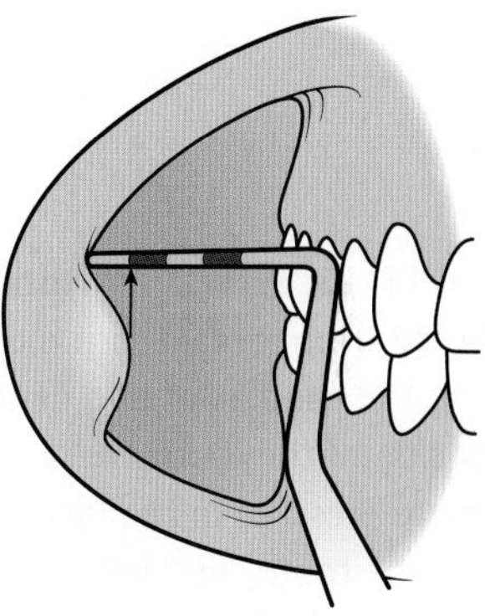

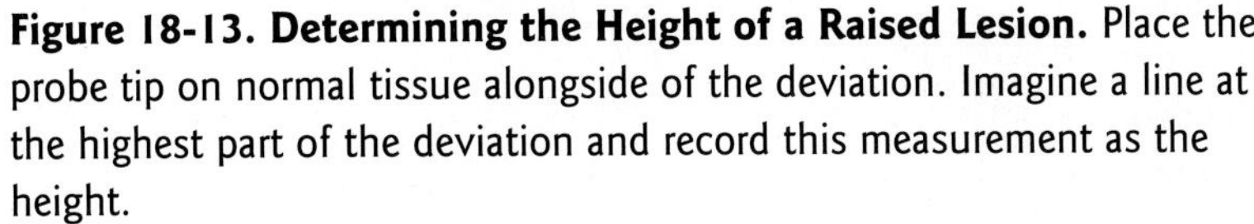

Figure 18-13. Determining the Height of a Raised Lesion. Place the probe tip on normal tissue alongside of the deviation. Imagine a line at the highest part of the deviation and record this measurement as the height.

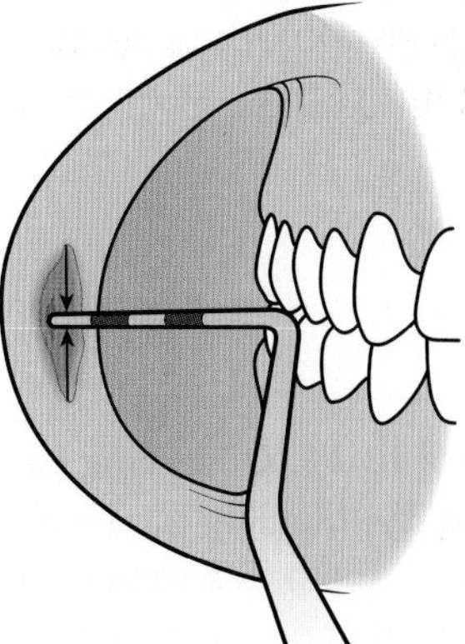

Figure 18-14. Determining the Depth of a Sunken Lesion. Carefully place the probe tip in the deepest part. Imagine a line running from edge to edge of the deviation. The depth is the distance from this imaginary line to the base of the deviation.

TOOTH MOBILITY

Mobility is the loosening of a tooth in its socket. Mobility may result from loss of bone support around the tooth. Most periodontal charts include boxes for documenting tooth mobility.

1. Horizontal tooth mobility is the ability to move the tooth in a facial to lingual direction in its socket.
   - **a.** Horizontal tooth mobility is assessed by putting the handles of two dental instruments on either side of the tooth and applying alternating moderate pressure in the facial–lingual direction against the tooth, first with one and then the other instrument handle (Figs. 18-15 and 18-16).
   - **b.** Mobility can be observed by using an adjacent tooth as a stationary point of reference during attempts to move the tooth being examined.
2. Vertical tooth mobility—the ability to depress the tooth in its socket—is assessed using the end of an instrument handle to exert pressure against the occlusal or incisal surface of the tooth (Fig. 18-17).
3. Even though the periodontal ligament allows some slight movement of the tooth in its socket, the amount of this natural tooth movement is so slight that it cannot be seen with the naked eye. Thus, when visually assessing mobility, the clinician should expect to find no visible movement in a periodontally healthy tooth.
4. There are many mobility rating scales for recording clinical visible tooth mobility on a periodontal chart. One useful rating scale is indicated in Table 18-3.

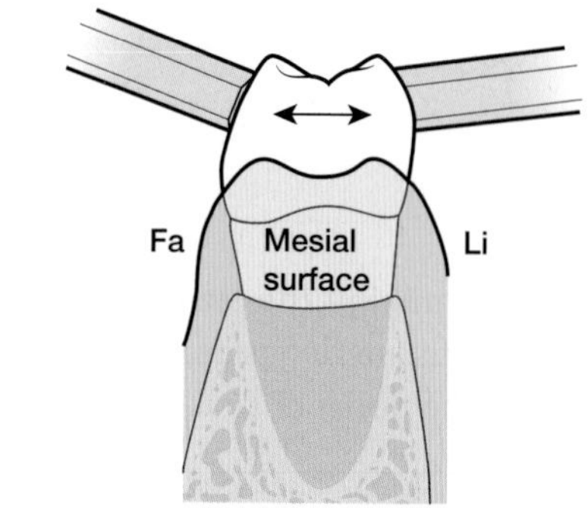

Figure 18-15. Assessing Horizontal Tooth Mobility. Horizontal tooth mobility is assessed by putting the handles of two dental instruments on either side of the tooth and applying alternating moderate pressure in the facial–lingual direction against the tooth, first with one and then the other instrument handle.

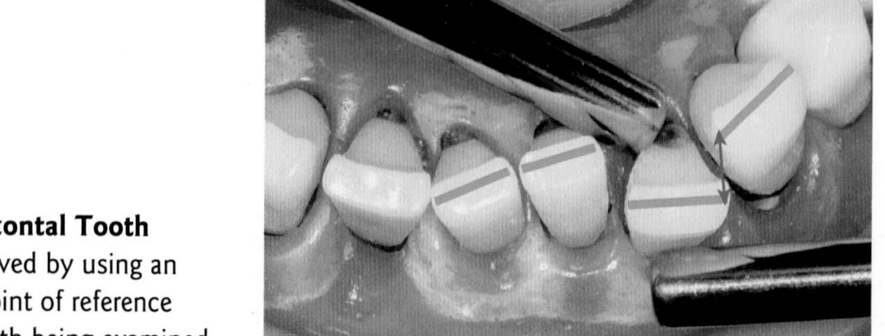

Figure 18-16. Observing Horizontal Tooth Mobility. Mobility can be observed by using an adjacent tooth as a stationary point of reference during attempts to move the tooth being examined.

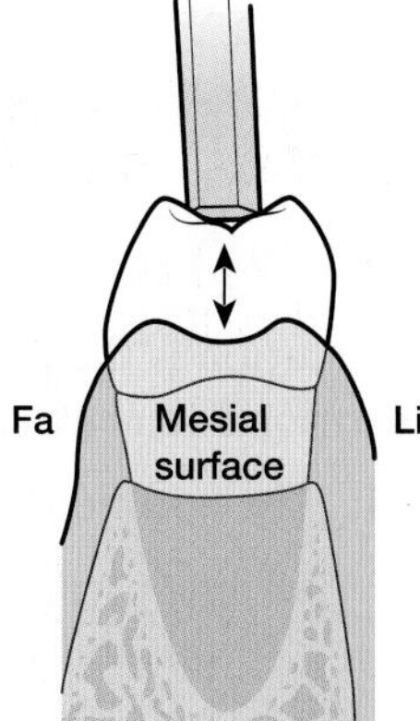

Figure 18-17. Assessing Vertical Tooth Mobility. Use the end of an instrument handle to exert pressure against the occlusal surface or incisal edge of the tooth.

TABLE 18-3. Scale for Rating Visible Tooth Mobility

Classification	Description
Class 1	Slight mobility; up to 1 mm of horizontal displacement in a facial–lingual direction
Class 2	Moderate mobility; greater than 1 mm but less than 2 mm of horizontal displacement in a facial–lingual direction
Class 3	Severe mobility, greater than 2 mm of displacement in a facial–lingual direction or vertical displacement (tooth depressible in the socket)

Section 3
Assessments with Furcation Probes

FURCATION INVOLVEMENT

A furcation is the place on a multirooted tooth where the root trunk divides into separate roots. The furcation is termed a bifurcation on a two-rooted tooth and a trifurcation on a three-rooted tooth.

1. The furcation area is the space—apical to the root trunk—between two or more roots.
   a. Teeth typically have one, two, or three roots. Anterior teeth usually have one root. Mandibular molars have two roots. Typically, maxillary molars have three roots.
   b. The area of a multirooted tooth that extends from the CEJ to the entrance of the furcation is termed the root trunk (Fig. 18-18).
   c. The entrance to a furcation may be as little as 3 to 4 mm apical to (below) the CEJ.
2. In health, the furcation area cannot be probed because it is filled with alveolar bone and periodontal ligament fibers.
3. Furcation involvement is a loss of alveolar bone and periodontal ligament fibers in the space between the roots of a multirooted tooth. Bone loss in the furcation area may be hidden beneath the gingival tissue, or when recession of the gingival margin is present, the furcation area may be clinically visible in the mouth (Fig. 18-19).
   a. Furcation involvement occurs on a multirooted tooth when periodontal infection invades the area between and around the roots, resulting in a loss of attachment and loss of alveolar bone between the roots of the tooth.
      1. Mandibular molars are usually bifurcated (mesial and distal roots), with potential furcation involvement on both the facial and lingual aspects of the tooth.
      2. Maxillary molar teeth are usually trifurcated (mesiobuccal, distobuccal, and palatal roots) with potential furcation involvement on the facial, mesial, and distal aspects of the tooth.
      3. Maxillary first premolars can have bifurcated roots (buccal and palatal roots) with the potential for furcation involvement on the mesial and distal aspects of the tooth. Approximately 60% of maxillary first molars have a buccal and lingual root.[3]
   b. Furcation involvement frequently signals a need for periodontal surgery after completion of nonsurgical therapy, so detection and documentation of furcation involvement are critical components of the comprehensive periodontal assessment.
4. The ability to mentally visualize root furcation morphology is important for effective assessment and instrumentation of periodontal patients. The location of root furcations (Box 18-2) has been the subject of several studies.[3–7]

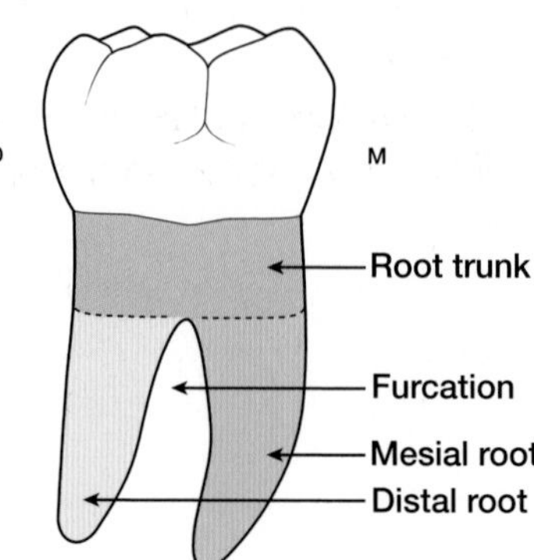

Figure 18-18. Anatomy of a Mandibular First Molar. The root trunk extends from the CEJ to the entrance of the bifurcation. Mandibular molars have distal and mesial roots.

REVIEW OF ROOT FURCATION MORPHOLOGY

Box 18-2. Root Furcation Morphology

Mandibular Molars

Mandibular molars have two roots with furcations on the facial and lingual surfaces between the mesial and distal roots.

Maxillary First Premolars

Maxillary first premolars that are bifurcated have a buccal and palatal root. When bifurcated, the roots of a maxillary first premolar separate many millimeters apical to the cementoenamel junction.

Maxillary Molars (Buccal View)

Maxillary molar teeth usually are trifurcated with ***mesiobuccal (MB), distobuccal (DB), and palatal*** (lingual) ***roots.***

Maxillary Molars (Proximal View)

On the mesial surface of a maxillary molar, the furcation is located more toward the lingual surface.

On the distal surface of a maxillary molar, the furcation is located near the center of the tooth.

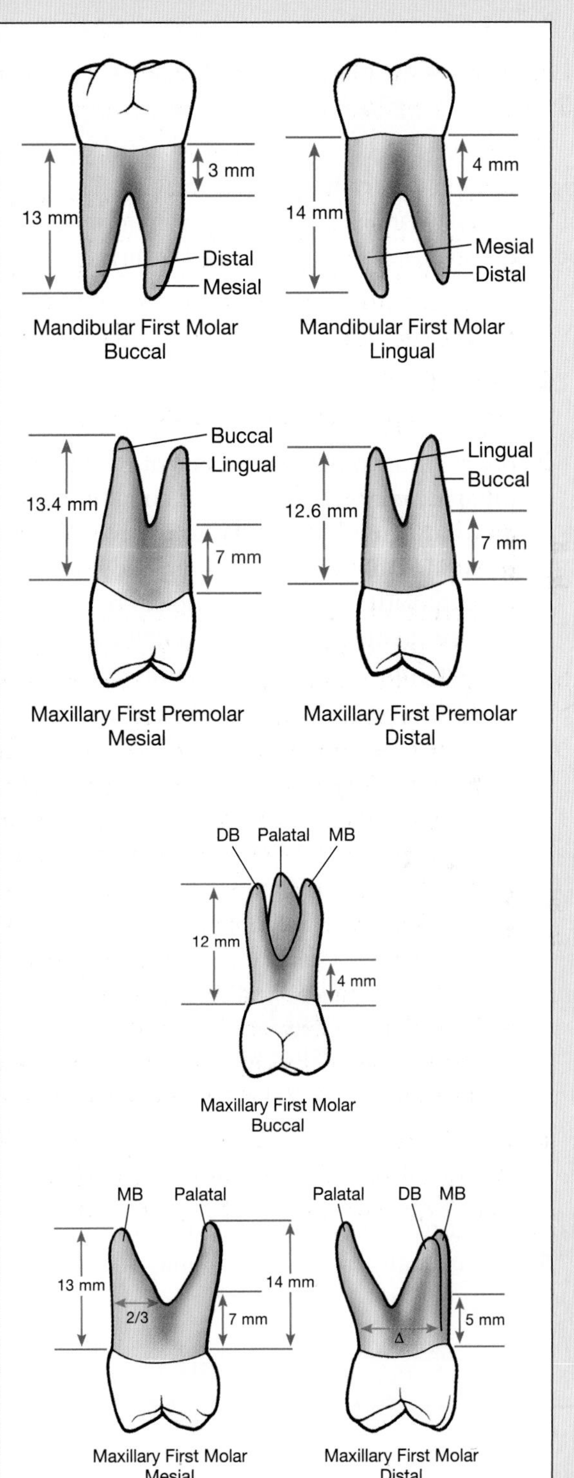

Mandibular First Molar Buccal

Mandibular First Molar Lingual

Maxillary First Premolar Mesial

Maxillary First Premolar Distal

Maxillary First Molar Buccal

Maxillary First Molar Mesial

Maxillary First Molar Distal

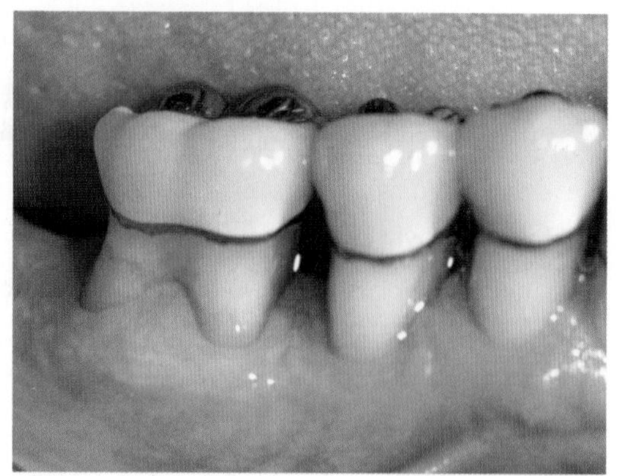

Figure 18-19. Clinically Visible Furcation. The furcation of this mandibular first molar is visible in the mouth due to bone loss and recession of the gingival margin.

RADIOGRAPHIC EVIDENCE OF FURCATION INVOLVEMENT

1. A classic study by Ross and Thompson showed that furcation involvement occurs three times more frequently among maxillary molars than among mandibular molars.[8]
   a. Many molars with furcation involvement functioned well from 5 to 24 years.[8]
   b. In the Ross and Thompson study, furcation involvement was detected more frequently in maxillary molars by radiographic examination than by clinical examination. However, furcation involvement was detected more frequently in mandibular molars by clinical examination than by radiographic examination.
2. In health, the furcation area cannot be probed because it is filled with alveolar bone and periodontal ligament fibers (Fig. 18-20).
3. When radiographs of maxillary molars are observed, ***a small, triangular radiographic shadow pointing toward the furcation*** is sometimes noted over either the mesial or distal roots in the ***proximal*** furcation area. These small triangular radiographic shadows are called furcation arrows. Figures 18-21 to 18-25 show examples of furcation arrows on radiographs.
   a. Because the furcation arrow seldom appears over uninvolved furcations, the appearance of a furcation arrow indicates that there is proximal bony furcation involvement.[9]
   b. However, absence of the furcation arrow image does not necessarily mean an absence of a bony furcation involvement because the arrow was not seen in a large number of furcations with involvement.[9]
4. On a radiograph, a triangular radiolucency in the furcation of a molar indicates furcation involvement. Figures 18-21 to 18-25 show examples of radiographic evidence of furcation involvement.
5. Occasionally, a radiograph may show evidence of a molar with fused roots (Fig. 18-26).

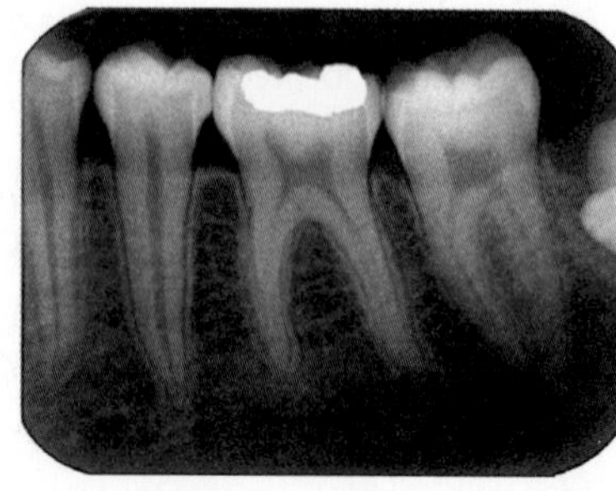

Figure 18-20. Periodontium in Health. In health, the alveolar bone and periodontal ligament fill the furcation area between the roots.

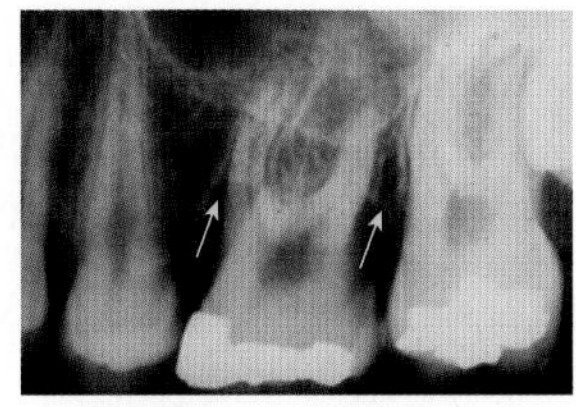

Figure 18-21. Furcation Involvement: Radiolucent Arrows on Proximal Surfaces. The yellow arrows on this radiograph indicate the furcation arrows on the proximal surfaces of a maxillary first molar.

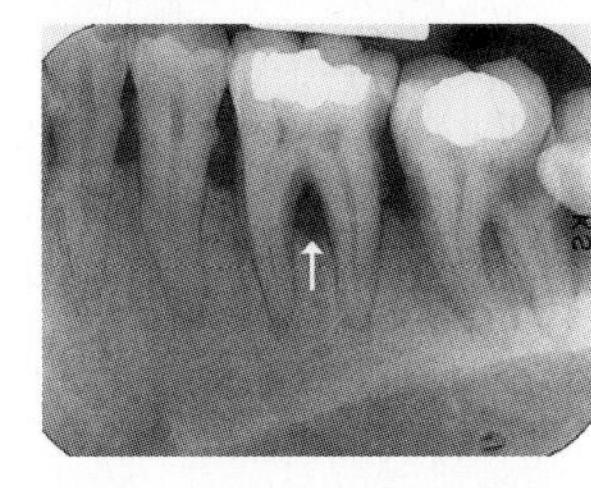

Figure 18-22. Furcation Involvement: Triangular Radiolucency. A triangular radiolucency in the bifurcation of a mandibular first molar indicates furcation involvement.

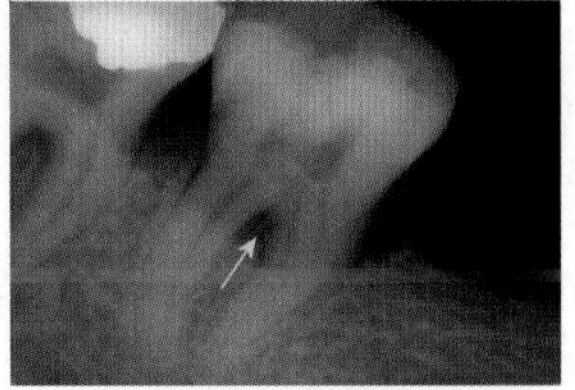

Figure 18-23. Furcation Involvement: Triangular Radiolucency. A triangular radiolucency in the bifurcation of a mandibular molar indicates furcation involvement.

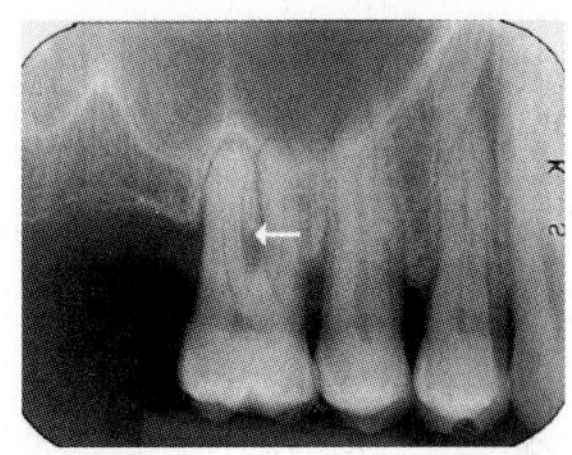

Figure 18-24. Furcation Involvement: Triangular Radiolucency. This radiograph shows furcation involvement on a maxillary first molar. (Courtesy of Dr. Robert P. Langlais.)

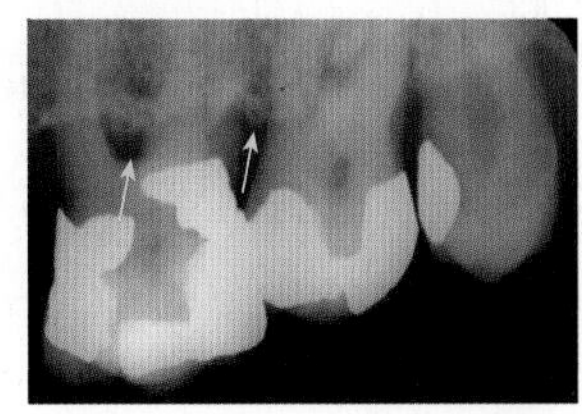

Figure 18-25. Furcation Involvement. The maxillary second molar on this radiograph shows a radiolucent arrow on the distal proximal surface and a triangular radiolucency in the furcation.

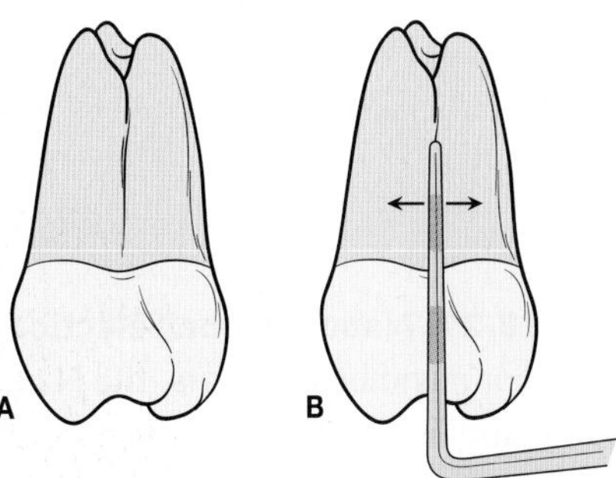

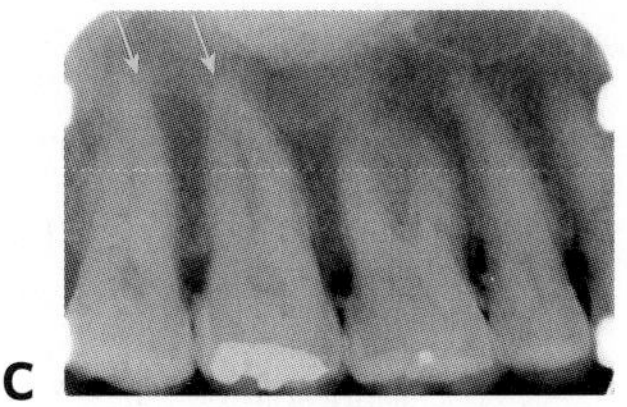

Figure 18-26. Fused Maxillary Roots. A. The concavity formed by fused roots on the distal proximal surface of a maxillary molar. **B.** Probe tip in the concavity. **C.** Radiograph showing fused roots on maxillary molars.

DESIGN CHARACTERISTICS OF FURCATION PROBES

A furcation probe is a type of periodontal probe used to evaluate the bone support in the furcation areas of bifurcated and trifurcated teeth.

1. Furcation probes have curved, blunt-tipped working-ends that allow easy access to the furcation areas.
2. The Nabers N1 and N2 furcation probes are the traditional instruments used for measuring the horizontal depth of bone loss in a furcation area (Figs. 18-27 to 18-29).

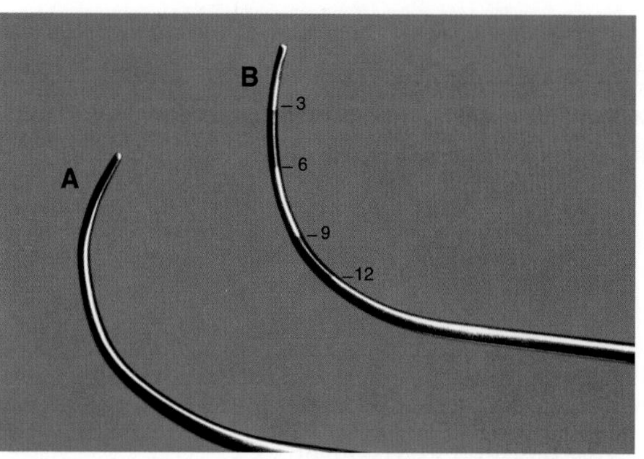

Figure 18-27. Nabors N2 Furcation Probes. Probe **B** has black bands from 3 to 6 mm and 9 to 12 mm. Furcation probes with millimeter markings often are used in research studies.

Other furcation probes, like probe **A**, do not have millimeter markings.

WORKING-END SELECTION: NABERS PROBES

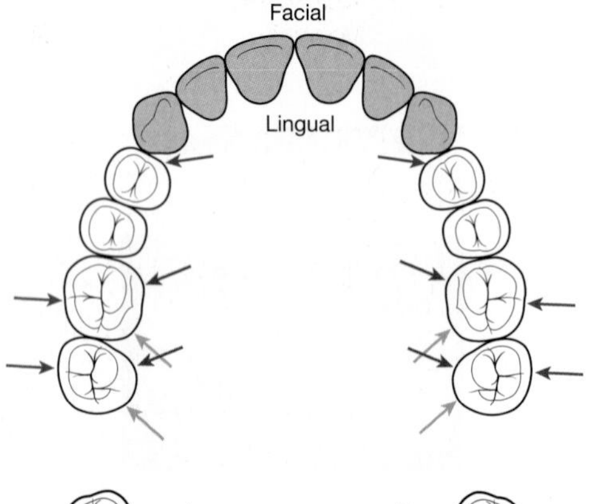

Figure 18-28. Nabers Probe Selection for the Maxillary Teeth.

For maxillary first premolars and molars:

- The N2 is used for assessment of facial and lingual furcation areas.
- The N1 is used for assessment of mesial and distal furcation areas.

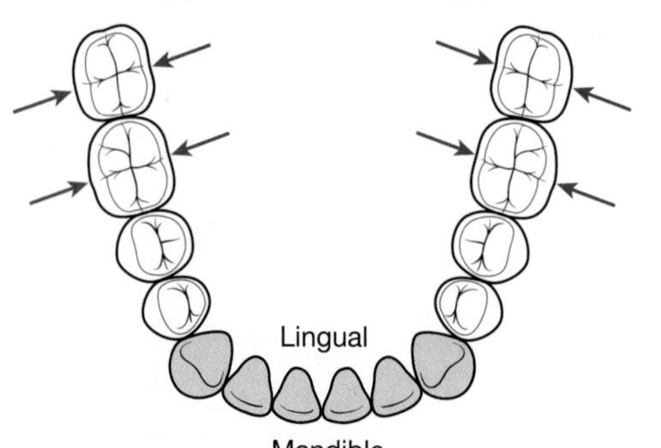

Figure 18-29. Nabers Probe Selection for the Mandibular Teeth. For mandibular molars, the N2 is used for assessment of facial and lingual furcation areas.

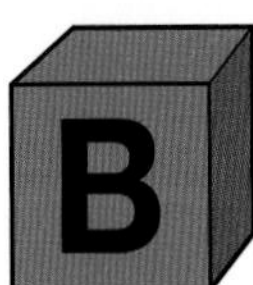

SKILL BUILDING. TECHNIQUE PRACTICE WITH FURCATION PROBES

Directions:

1. Practice with a periodontal typodont or mount an acrylic mandibular molar, maxillary first premolar, and maxillary first molar in modeling clay or plaster. Mount the teeth so that the furcation areas are exposed.
2. Position the probe at the gingival line at a location near where the furcation is suspected.
3. Direct the probe beneath the gingival margin. At the base of the pocket, rotate the probe tip toward the tooth to turn the tip into the entrance of the furcation.
4. Refer to the diagrams and photographs shown in Figures 18-30 to 18-34 for guidance in accessing the furcation areas of mandibular and maxillary molars and the maxillary first premolars.

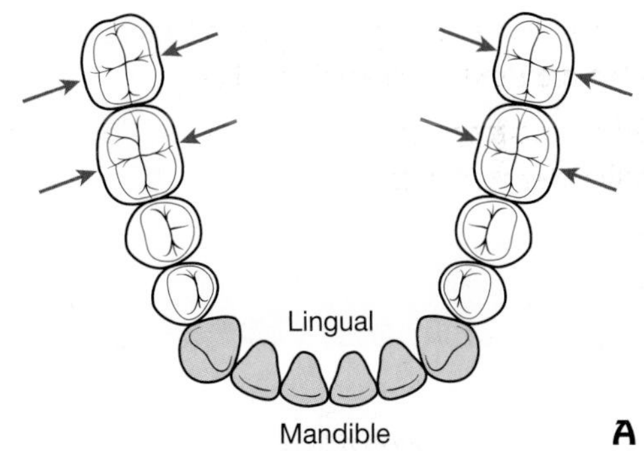

Figure 18-30, A–C. Access to the Furcation on the Buccal and Lingual Aspects of a Mandibular Molar. The furcation area of a mandibular molar is located between the mesial and distal roots. The furcation area can be entered from both the buccal and lingual aspects of the molar tooth.

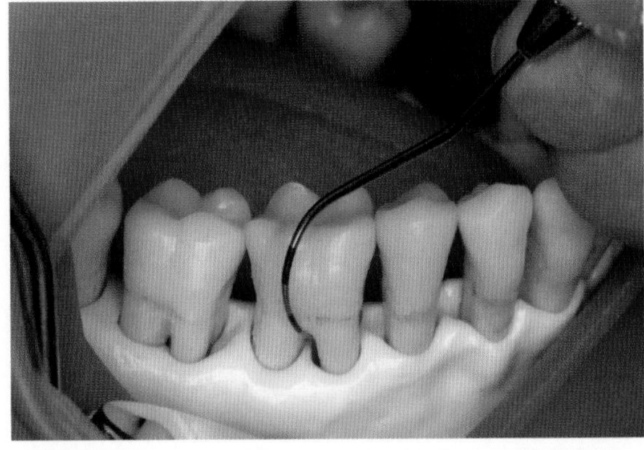

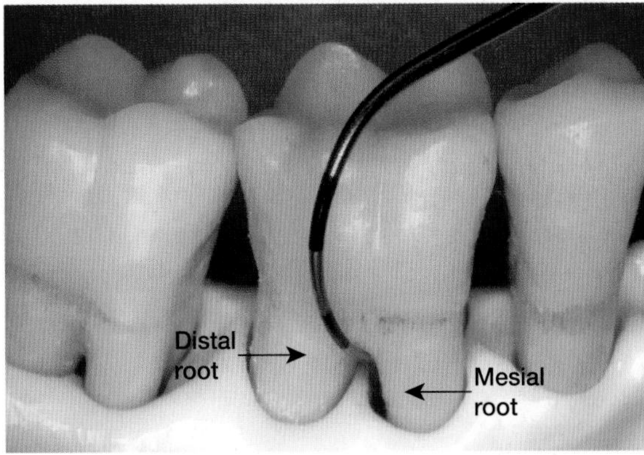

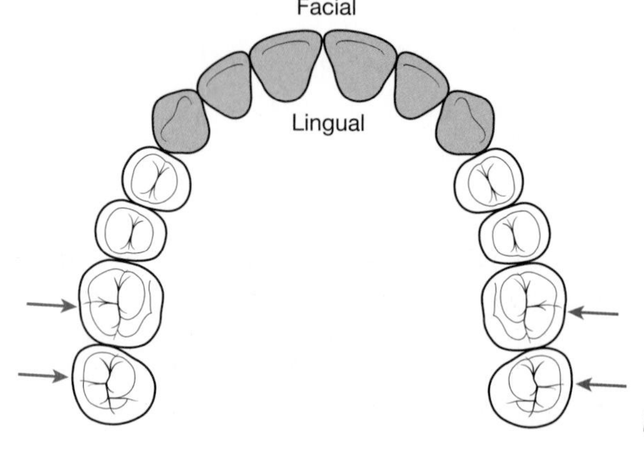

Figure 18-31, A–C. Access to the Furcation on the Buccal Aspect of a Maxillary Molar. Maxillary molars have three roots: a distobuccal, mesiobuccal, and palatal (lingual) root. Enter the furcation between the distobuccal and mesiobuccal roots from the facial aspect.

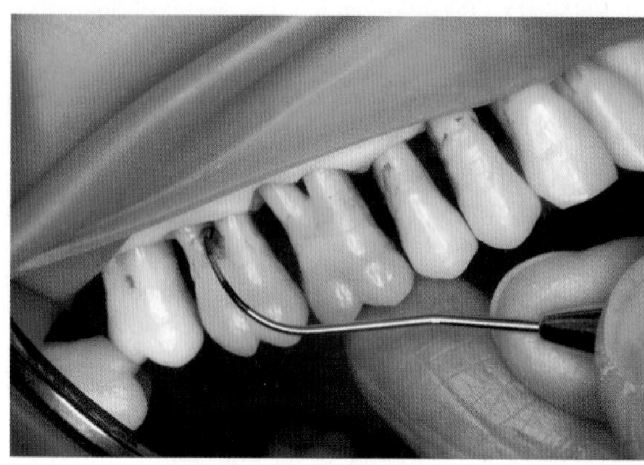

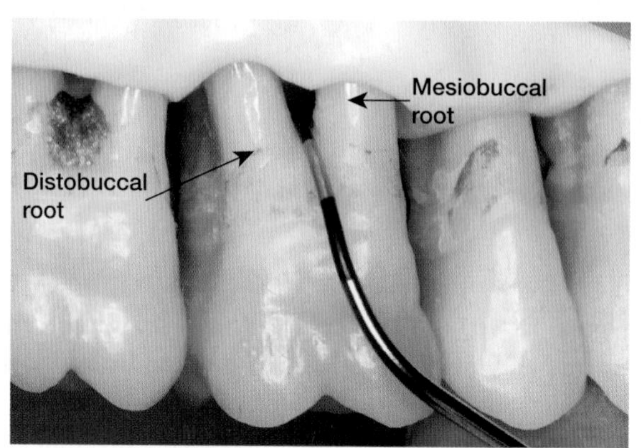

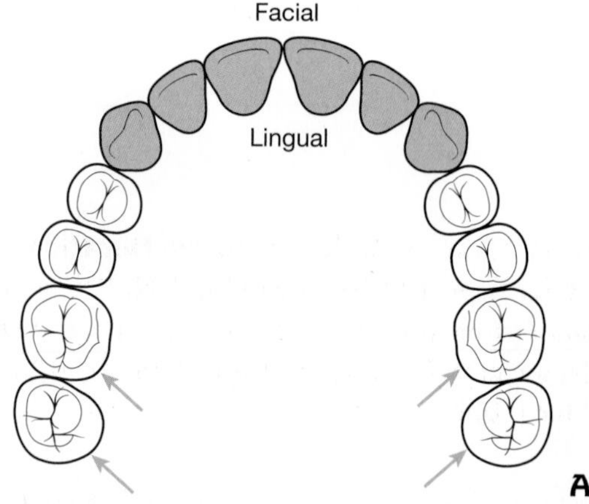

Figure 18-32, A–C. Access to the Furcation on the Distal Aspect of a Maxillary Molar. The distal proximal furcation of a maxillary molar is accessed from the lingual aspect. The N1 furcation probe wraps around the palatal root to enter the furcation between the distobuccal and palatal roots.

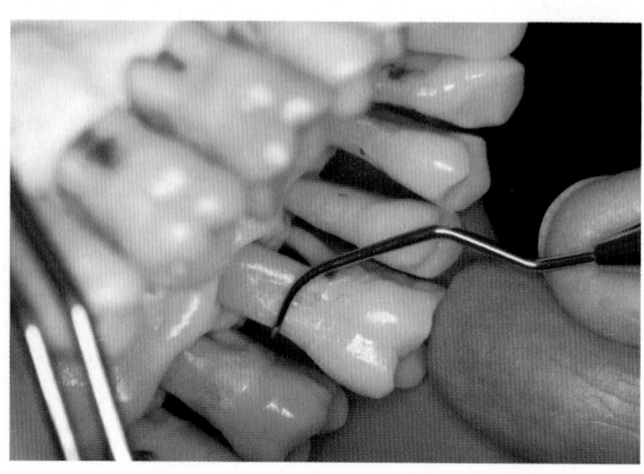

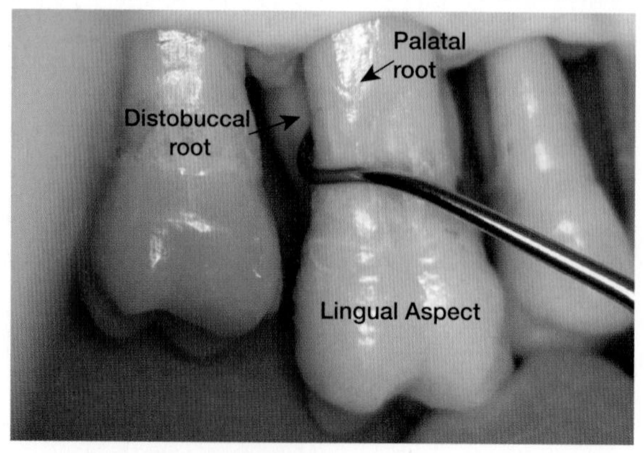

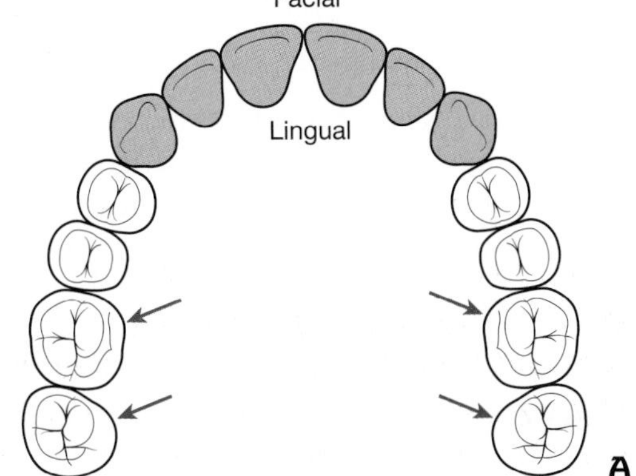

Figure 18-33, A–C. Access to the Furcation on the Mesial Aspect of a Maxillary Molar. The mesial proximal furcation of a maxillary molar is accessed from the lingual aspect. The N1 furcation probe is inserted between the mesiobuccal and palatal roots.

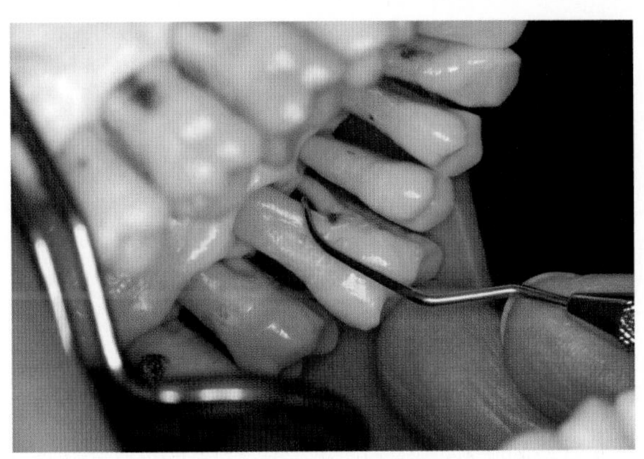

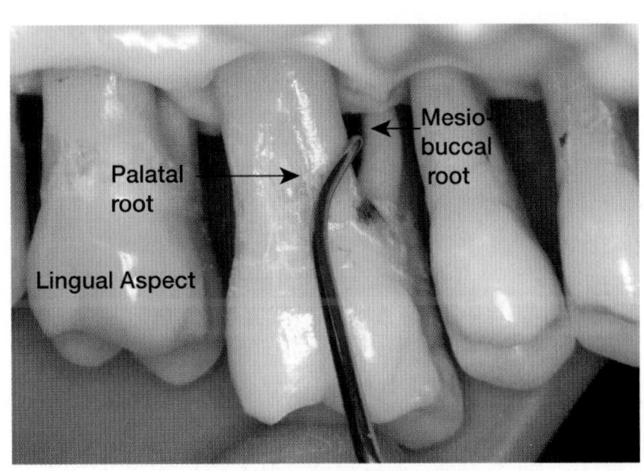

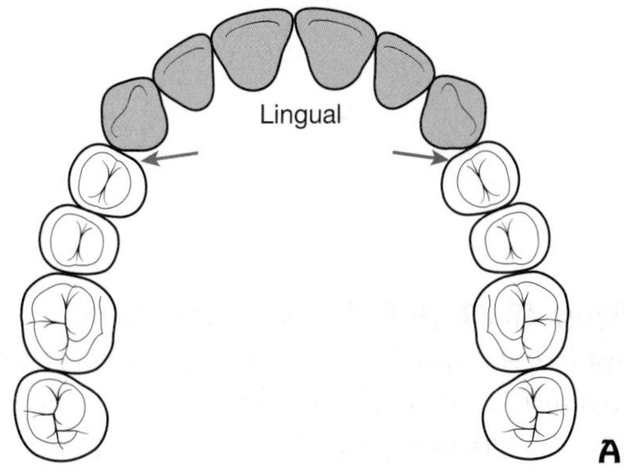

Figure 18-34, A–C. Access to the Furcation on the Mesial Aspect of the Maxillary First Premolar. A maxillary first premolar may have a buccal and a palatal root. The proximal furcation is entered from the lingual aspect of the tooth.

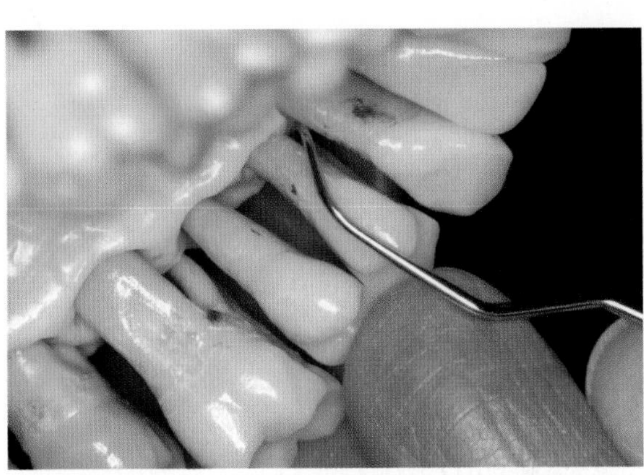

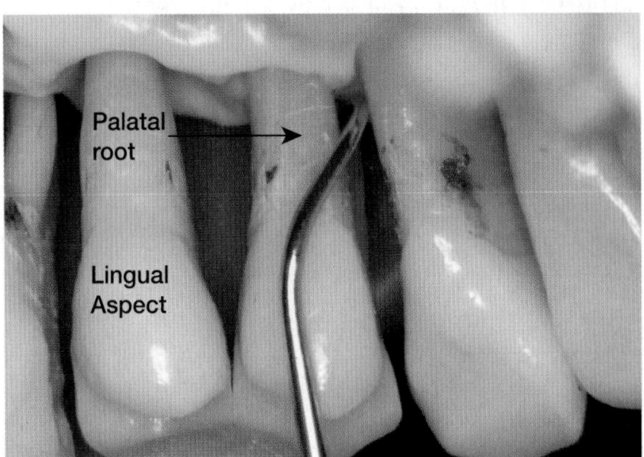

FOUR CLASSIFICATIONS OF FURCATION INVOLVEMENT

Furcation involvement should be recorded on a periodontal chart using a scale that quantifies the ***severity (or extent) of the furcation invasion.*** Furcation involvement rating scales are based on the horizontal measurement of attachment loss in the furcation.[10,11] Table 18-4 shows a common furcation rating scale based on four grades and charting symbols that may be used to indicate the grade on a periodontal chart.[12]

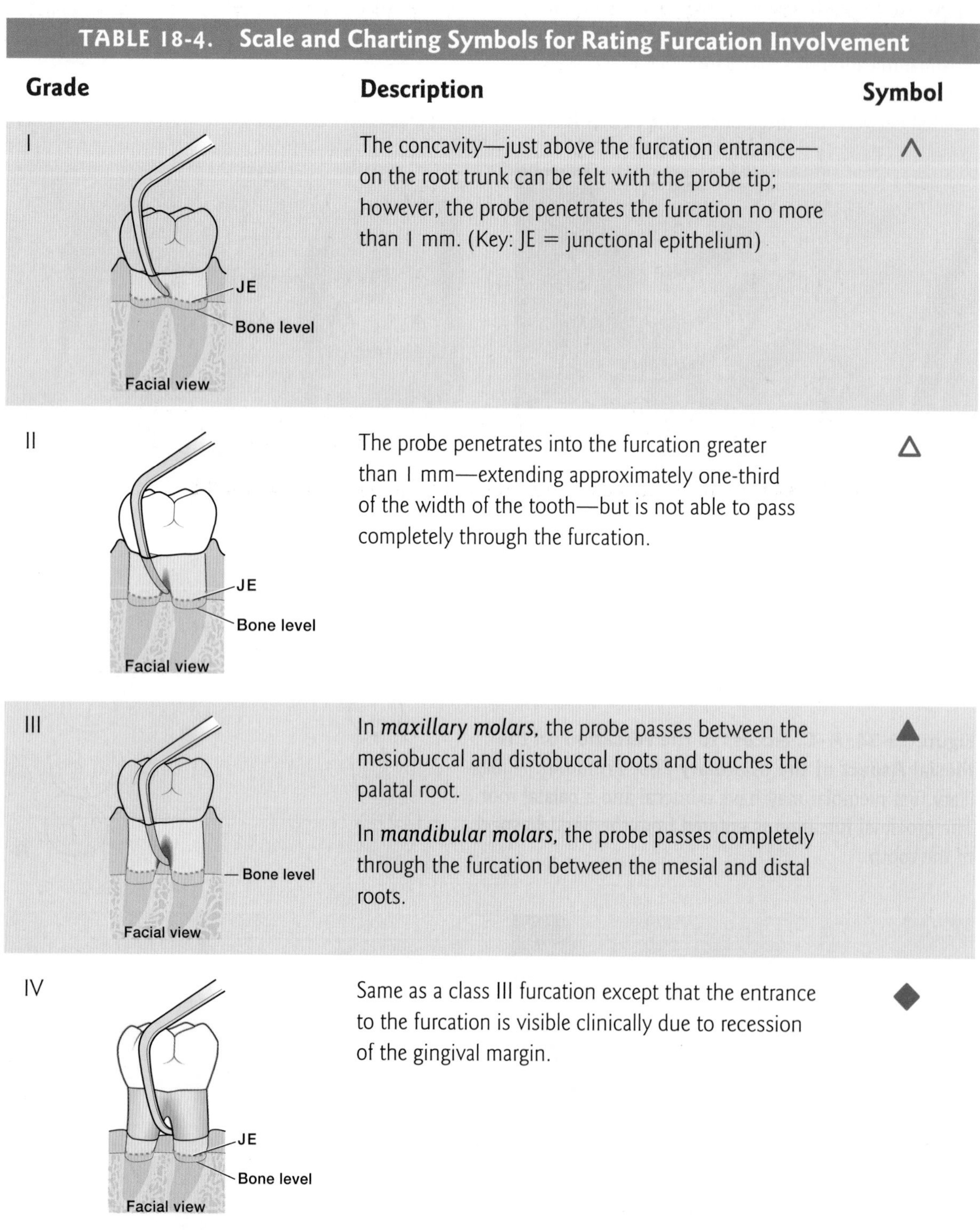

TABLE 18-4. Scale and Charting Symbols for Rating Furcation Involvement

Grade	Description	Symbol
I	The concavity—just above the furcation entrance—on the root trunk can be felt with the probe tip; however, the probe penetrates the furcation no more than 1 mm. (Key: JE = junctional epithelium)	^
II	The probe penetrates into the furcation greater than 1 mm—extending approximately one-third of the width of the tooth—but is not able to pass completely through the furcation.	△
III	In *maxillary molars,* the probe passes between the mesiobuccal and distobuccal roots and touches the palatal root. In *mandibular molars,* the probe passes completely through the furcation between the mesial and distal roots.	▲
IV	Same as a class III furcation except that the entrance to the furcation is visible clinically due to recession of the gingival margin.	◆

DOCUMENTATION OF FURCATION INVOLVEMENT

On the sample periodontal chart shown in Figure 18-35, all four classes of furcation involvement are represented.

- Tooth 2 has a class IV furcation involvement on the facial aspect.
- Tooth 3 has a class I furcation involvement on the facial aspect between the mesiobuccal and distobuccal roots.
- On the lingual aspect, tooth 2 has a class III furcation involvement between the distobuccal and palatal roots and a class II furcation involvement between the mesiobuccal and palatal roots.

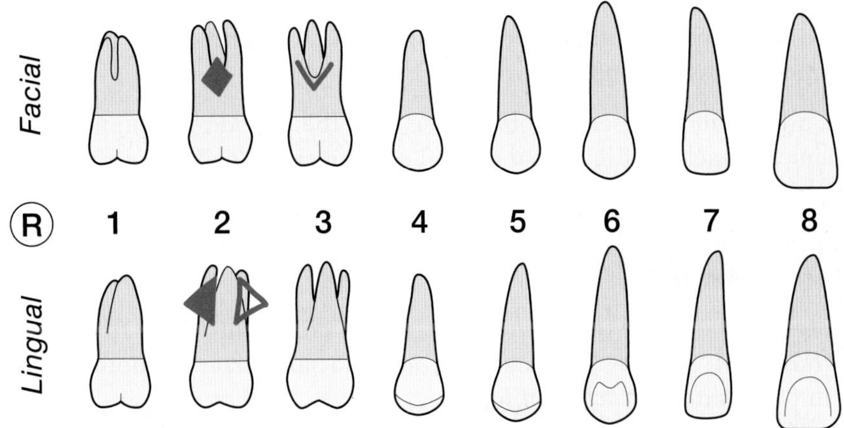

Figure 18-35. Periodontal Chart Indicating Furcation Involvement.

Section 4
Assessments That Require Calculations

Information collected during the comprehensive periodontal assessment is used to make certain calculations that provide valuable information about the health of the periodontal tissues. The most common calculations are the clinical attachment level and width of the attached gingiva.

CLINICAL ATTACHMENT LEVEL

The clinical attachment level (CAL) refers to the estimated position of the structures that support the tooth as measured with a periodontal probe. The clinical attachment level provides an estimate of a tooth's stability and the loss of bone support (Box 18-3).

1. Two terms are commonly used in conjunction with the periodontal support system—clinical attachment level and clinical attachment loss. Both of these terms may be abbreviated as CAL and can be used synonymously.
2. Clinical attachment loss (CAL) is the extent of periodontal support that has been destroyed around a tooth.
3. As an example of the use of these two terms, a clinician might report that the "*clinical attachment levels* were calculated for the facial surface of tooth 32 and there is 6 mm of *clinical attachment loss.*"

Box 18-3. Rationale for Computing CAL

- ***Probing depths*** are not reliable indicators of the extent of bone support because these measurements are made from the gingival margin. The position of gingival margin changes with tissue swelling, overgrowth, and tissue recession.
- ***Clinical attachment levels*** are calculated from measurements made from a fixed point that does not change—the CEJ. Because the bone level in health is approximately 2 mm apical to the CEJ, clinical attachment levels provide a reliable indication of the extent of bone support for a tooth.

CALCULATING CLINICAL ATTACHMENT LEVEL

A competent clinician must understand the procedure for determining the clinical attachment level (CAL) for the three possible relationships of the gingival margin to the CEJ. Figures 18-36 to 18-38 depict the three relationships.

1. The gingival margin may be (a) apical to the CEJ, (b) cover the CEJ, or (c) at its normal level, coronal to the CEJ.
2. Two measurements are used to calculate the clinical attachment level:
   (a) the probing depth and
   (b) the level of the gingival margin (distance from CEJ to gingival margin).
3. Note that both of these measurements are routinely taken and documented on a periodontal chart.

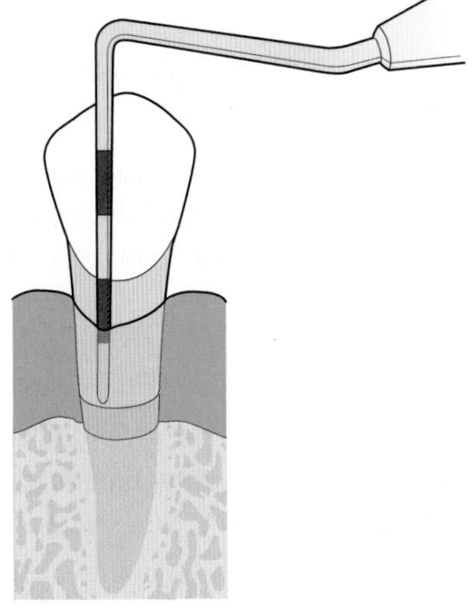

Figure 18-36. Calculating CAL in the Presence of Recession of the Gingival Margin. When recession of the gingival margin is present, the CAL is calculated by ADDING the probing depth to the gingival margin level.

For example:

Probing depth measurement:	4 mm
Gingival margin level:	+2 mm*
Clinical attachment loss:	6 mm

* = 2 mm of tissue needs ***to be added*** for the gingival margin to be at its normal level.

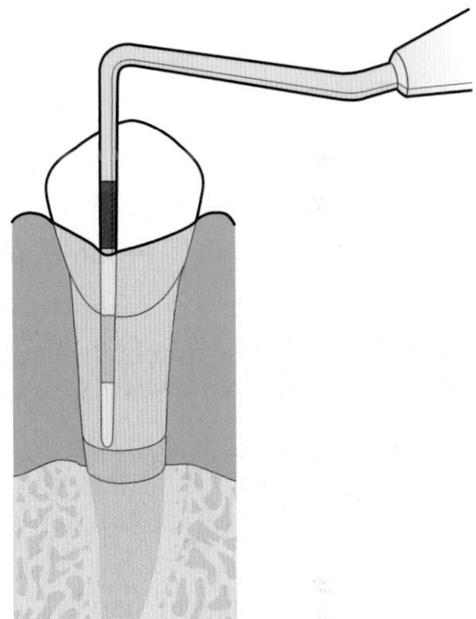

Figure 18-37. Calculating CAL when the Gingival Margin Covers the CEJ. When the gingival margin is coronal to the CEJ, the CAL is calculated by SUBTRACTING the gingival margin level from the probing depth.

For example:

Probing depth measurement:	9 mm
Gingival margin level:	−3 mm*
Clinical attachment loss:	6 mm

* = 3 mm of tissue needs ***to be taken away*** for the gingival margin to be at its normal level.

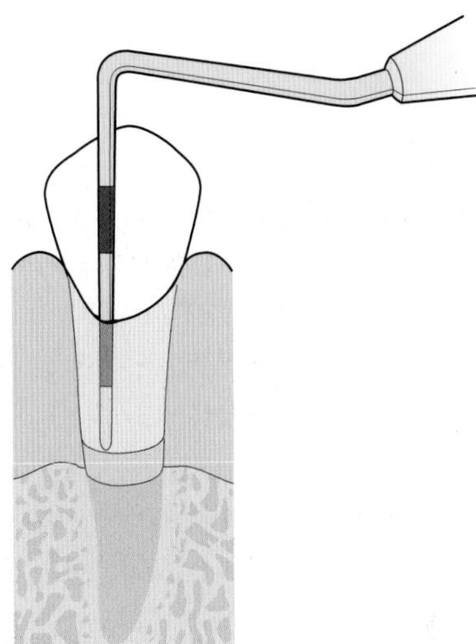

Figure 18-38. Calculating CAL when the Gingival Margin Is at the Normal Level. When the gingival margin is slightly coronal to the CEJ, no calculations are needed since the probing depth and the clinical attachment level are equal.

For example:

Probing depth measurement:	6 mm
Gingival margin level:	0 mm*
Clinical attachment loss:	6 mm

* = gingival margin is at the normal level; therefore, no gingival tissue needs to added or taken away (0).

DOCUMENTING CLINICAL ATTACHMENT LEVELS

On the sample periodontal chart shown in Figure 18-39, all three possible relationships of the gingival margin to the CEJ are demonstrated.

- On tooth 28—the gingival margin is at the level of the CEJ.
- On teeth 25 to 27—the gingival margin covers the CEJ.
- On teeth 29 and 31—the gingival margin is apical to (below) the CEJ

Lingual	32	31	30	29	28	27	26	25
Probe Depth		4 3 3		3 2 3	3 3 4	4 5 5	5 5 6	6 6 6
GM to CEJ		+5 +4 +3		+2 +2 +1	0 0 0	-1 -2 -2	-2 -2 -3	-3 -4 -4
Attachment Loss		9 7 6		5 4 4	3 3 4	3 3 3	3 3 3	3 2 2

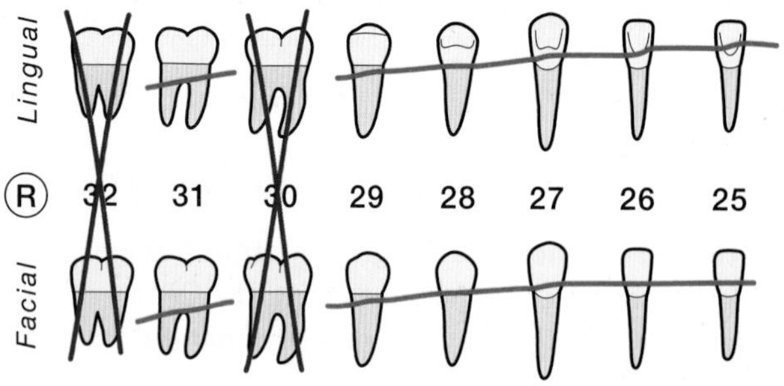

Ⓡ

Facial	32	31	30	29	28	27	26	25
Probe Depth		3 3 2		2 1 2	2 2 3	3 4 4	4 4 5	5 5 5
GM to CEJ		+4 +4 +3		+2 +2 +1	0 0 0	-1 -2 -2	-2 -2 -2	-2 -2 -2
Attachment Loss		7 7 5		4 3 3	2 2 3	2 2 2	2 2 3	3 3 3
Mobility								

Figure 18-39. Sample Periodontal Chart. The chart shown above depicts how the following information might be indicated on a periodontal charting of the mandibular right sextant: (1) probing depth measurements, (2) measurement of the level of the free gingival margin (GM) to the cementoenamel junction (CEJ), and (3) calculated clinical attachment levels. The clinical attachment levels are calculated based on the measurements for the probing depths and level of the free gingival margin.

WIDTH OF THE ATTACHED GINGIVA

The attached gingiva is the part of the gingiva that is tightly connected to the cementum on the cervical-third of the root and to the periosteum (connective tissue cover) of the alveolar bone. The function of the attached gingiva is to keep the free gingiva from being pulled away from the tooth. The width of the attached gingiva is an important clinical feature for the dentist to keep in mind when planning restorative procedures. If there is no attached gingiva on a tooth surface, the dentist is limited in the types of restorations that can be placed on the tooth. Adequate attached gingiva is an important factor in preventing mucogingival defects and recession of the gingival margin in the presence of bone loss.

1. The attached gingiva extends from the base of the sulcus to the mucogingival junction. The alveolar mucosa can be detected visually by its deep red color and shiny appearance.
2. The width of the attached gingiva on the facial aspect varies in different areas of the mouth.
    a. It is widest in the anterior teeth (3.5 to 4.5 mm in the maxilla and 3.3 to 3.9 mm in the mandible).
    b. It is narrowest in premolar regions (1.8 mm on mandible and 1.9 mm on maxilla).
    c. The width of the attached gingiva is not measured on the palate because clinically it is not possible to determine where the attached gingiva ends and the palatal mucosa begins.
3. The formula for calculating the width of attached gingiva is shown in Box 18-4.

Box 18-4. Width of the Attached Gingiva

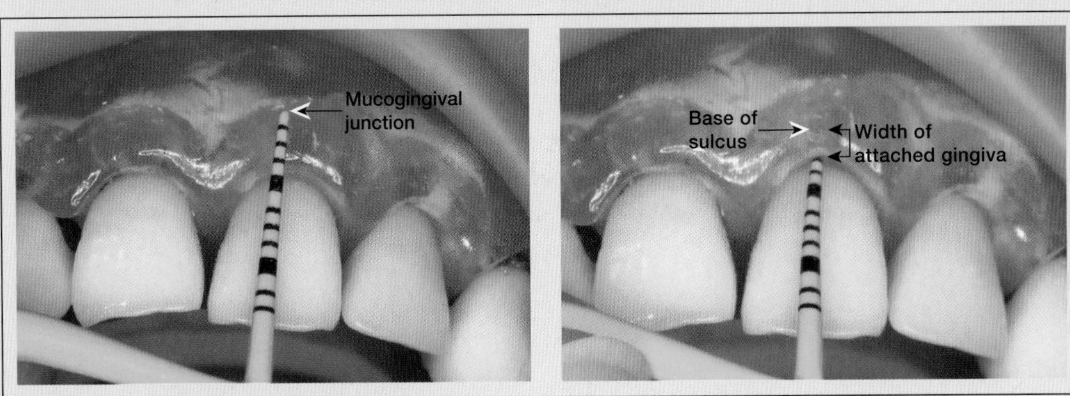

Figure 18-40A. Total Width of Gingiva.

Figure 18-40B. Probing Depth.

Formula: Calculate the width of the attached gingiva by subtracting the probing depth from the total width of the gingiva.

Step 1: Measure the total width of the gingiva from the gingival margin to the mucogingival junction. ***In the example shown in Figure 18-44A, this measurement is 4 mm.***

Step 2: Measure the probing depth (from the gingival margin to the base of the pocket). ***In the example shown in Figure 18-44B, this measurement is 2 mm.***

Step 3: Calculate the width of the attached gingiva by subtracting the probing depth from the total width of the gingiva. ***In the example, the width of the attached gingiva is 4 mm minus 2 mm, equaling 2 mm of attached gingiva.***

REFERENCES

1. Armitage GC. Diagnosis of periodontal diseases. *J Periodontol.* 2003;74:1237–1247.
2. American Dental Hygienists' Association. *Standards for Clinical Dental Hygiene Practice.* Chicago, IL: American Dental Hygienists' Association; 2008.
3. Scheid R, Weiss G. *Woelfel's Dental Anatomy: Its Relevance to Dentistry.* 8th ed. Philadelphia, PA: Lippincott Williams & Wilkins; 2011.
4. Dunlap RM, Gher ME. Root surface measurements of the mandibular first molar. *J Periodontol.* 1985;56:234–238.
5. Gher MW Jr, Dunlap RW. Linear variation of the root surface area of the maxillary first molar. *J Periodontol.* 1985;56:39–43.
6. Plagmann HC, Holtorf S, Kocher T. A study on the imaging of complex furcation forms in upper and lower molars. *J Clin Periodontol.* 2000;27:926–931.
7. Santana RB, Uzel MI, Gusman H, Gunaydin Y, Jones JA, Leone CW. Morphometric analysis of the furcation anatomy of mandibular molars. *J Periodontol.* 2004;75:824–829.
8. Ross IF, Thompson RH Jr. Furcation involvement in maxillary and mandibular molars. *J Periodontol.* 1980;51:450–454.
9. Hardekopf JD, Dunlap RM, Ahl DR, Pelleu GB Jr. The "furcation arrow." A reliable radiographic image? *J Periodontol.* 1987;58:258–261.
10. Glickman I. *Clinical Periodontology: The Periodontium in Health and Disease—Recognition, Diagnosis and Treatment of Periodontal Disease in the Practice of General Dentistry.* Philadelphia, PA: Saunders; 1953.
11. Hamp SE, Nyman S, Lindhe J. Periodontal treatment of multirooted teeth. Results after 5 years. *J Clin Periodontol.* 1975;2:126–135.
12. Newman MG, Takei HH, Klokkevold PR, Carranza FA. *Carranza's Clinical Periodontology.* 11th ed. St. Louis, MO: Saunders Elsevier; 2012.

Section 5
Skill Application

PRACTICAL FOCUS: CALCULATION OF CLINICAL LOSS OF ATTACHMENT

Using the probe shown in Figure 18-41, calculate the CAL for the teeth depicted in Figure 18-42A–C.

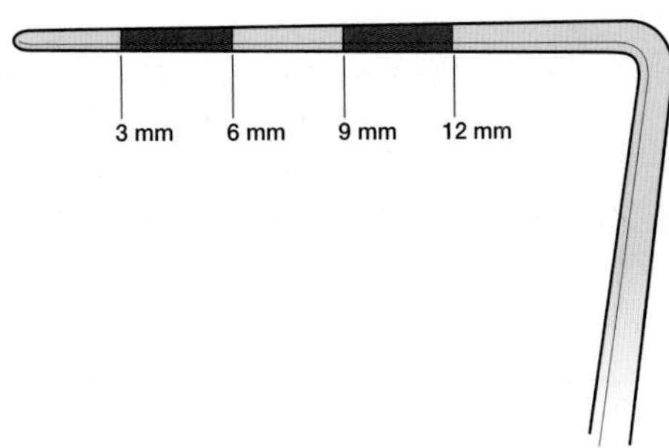

Figure 18-41. Probe Calibrations.

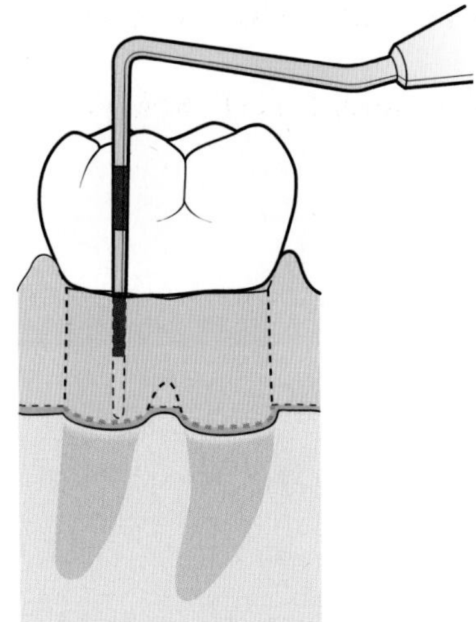

Figure 18-42A. Tooth A.

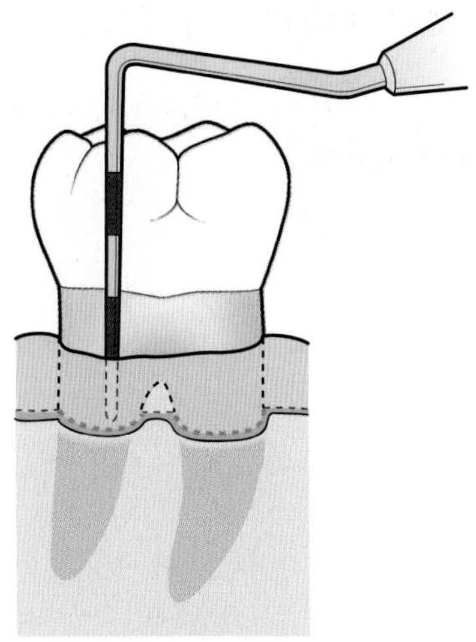

Figure 18-42B. Tooth B.

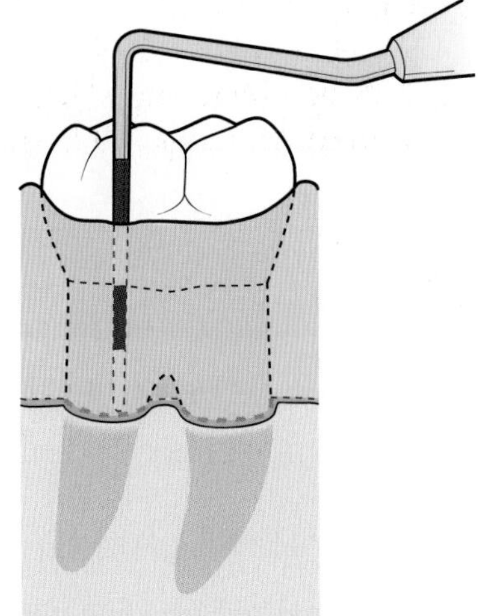

Figure 18-42C. Tooth C.

Tooth A		**Tooth B**		**Tooth C**	
Probing Depth	=	Probing Depth	=	Probing Depth	=
GM to CEJ	=	GM to CEJ	=	GM to CEJ	=
Attachment Loss	=	Attachment Loss	=	Attachment Loss	=

PRACTICAL FOCUS: FICTITIOUS PATIENT CASE, MR. TEMPLE

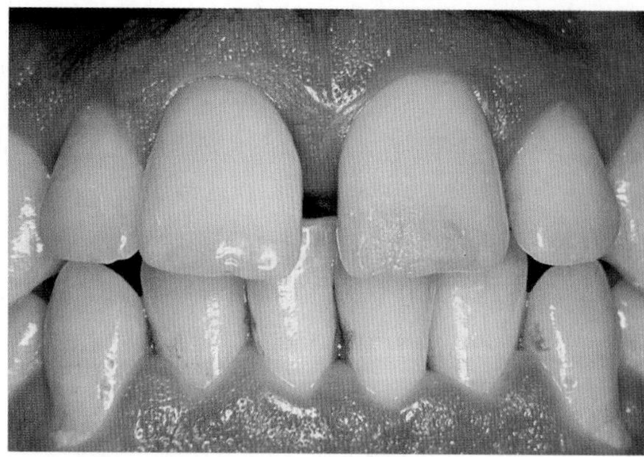

Figure 18-43A

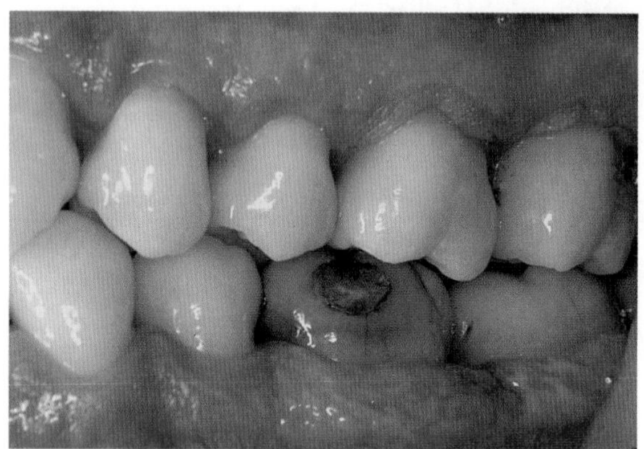

Figure 18-43B

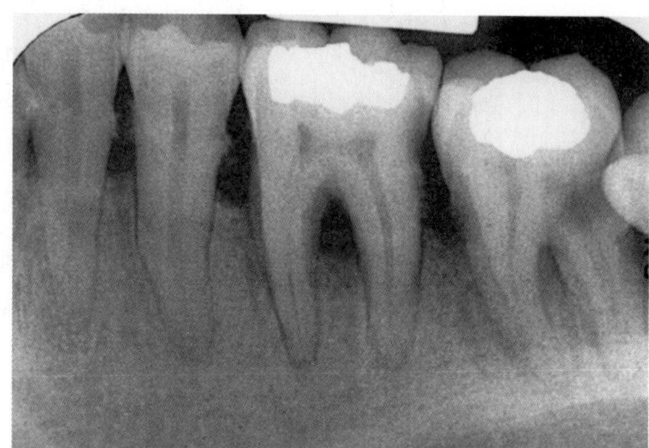

Figure 18-43C

Mr. Temple: Assessment Data

1. Generalized bleeding upon probing.
2. Deposits
   a. Moderate supragingival plaque on all teeth. Light subgingival plaque on all surfaces with moderate subgingival plaque on the proximal surfaces of all teeth.
   b. Supragingival calculus deposits—light calculus on lingual surfaces of mandibular anteriors.
   c. Subgingival calculus deposits—small-sized deposits on all teeth; medium-sized deposits on all proximal surfaces.

Mr. Temple: Periodontal Chart

4 3 5	5 4 6	6 6 6	6 5 6	6 6 6	8 9 8	8 7 7		Probe Depth
0 0 0	0 0 0	0 0 0	0 0 0	0 0 0	0 0 0	0 0 0		GM to CEJ
								Attachment Loss

Lingual

24 23 22 21 20 19 18 17 (L)

Facial

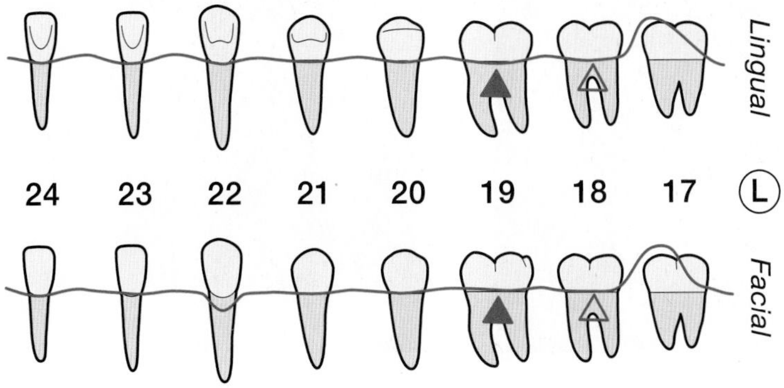

4 3 4	4 4 5	4 2 4	5 4 5	5 5 6	7 8 7	7 6 7		Probe Depth
0 0 0	0 0 0	+1 +3 +1	0 0 0	0 0 0	0 0 0	0 0 0		GM to CEJ
								Attachment Loss
					2	1		Mobility

Figure 18-43D. Mr. Temple's Periodontal Chart. Mr. Temple's periodontal chart for the mandibular left quadrant. (Key: GM = gingival margin; CEJ = cementoeanmel junction)

Mr. Temple: Case Questions

1. *Use the information recorded on Mr. Temple's periodontal chart to calculate the clinical attachment loss on the facial and lingual aspects for teeth 18 to 24 and enter this information on Mr. Temple's periodontal chart in Figure 18-43D.*
2. Describe the characteristics of the class I mobility on tooth 18. Describe the characteristics of the class II mobility on tooth 19.
3. Describe the characteristics of the furcation involvement on teeth 18 and 19 (i.e., what does this level of furcation involvement look like in the mouth?).
4. Do the assessment data indicate healthy sulci or periodontal pockets in this quadrant? Explain which data you used to determine the presence of sulci or pockets?
5. If the gingival margin level information had NOT been documented on this chart, would the probing depth measurements alone be an accurate indicator of the level of bone support present? Why?
6. Based on the assessment information, which type of explorer would you select to explore the teeth in this quadrant? Which instruments would you select for calculus removal in this quadrant: sickle scalers, universal curets, and/or area-specific curets? Explain your rationale for instrument selection.

PRACTICAL FOCUS: FICTITIOUS PATIENT CASE, MRS. BLANCHARD

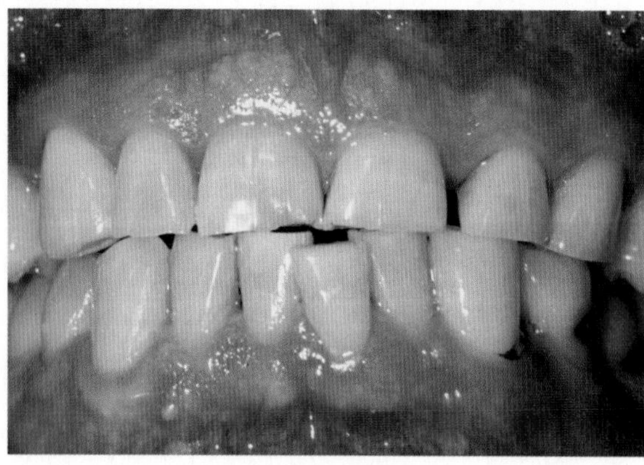

Figure 18-44A

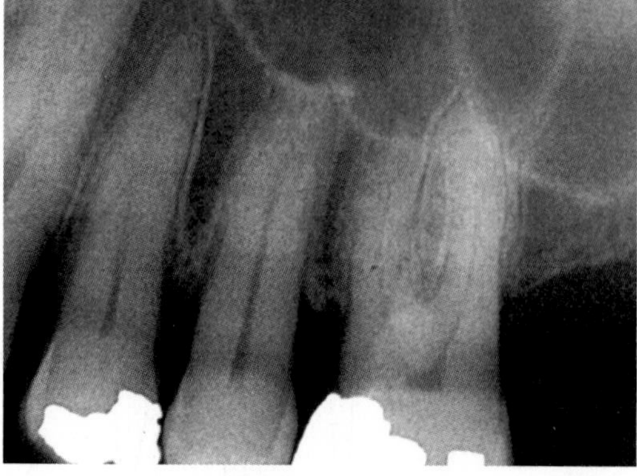

Figure 18-44B

Mrs. Blanchard: Assessment Data

1. Generalized bleeding upon probing.
2. Deposits
   a. Light supragingival plaque on all teeth. Light subgingival plaque on all surfaces.
   b. Supragingival calculus deposits—light calculus on lingual surfaces of mandibular anteriors and facial surfaces of maxillary molar.
   c. Subgingival calculus deposits—small-sized deposits on all teeth

Note to Course Instructor: Additional fictitious patient cases and opportunities for practice in calculating clinical attachment levels are found in Modules 19 and 21.

Mrs. Blanchard: Periodontal Chart

9	10	11	12	13	14	15	16	
								Mobility
3 2 3	2 1 3	3 2 4	5 5 3	4 3 5	4 5 6			Probe Depth
+4 +5 +4	+5 +6 +5	+4 +5 +4	+3 +4 +3	+2 +2 +1	+1 +1 +1			GM to CEJ
								Attachment Loss

Facial

9 10 11 12 13 14 15 16 (L)

Lingual

9	10	11	12	13	14	15	16	
4 3 4	3 3 4	4 3 5	6 5 4	5 4 5	5 6 7			Probe Depth
+4 +5 +4	+5 +6 +5	+4 +5 +4	+3 +4 +3	+2 +2 +1	+1 +1 +1			GM to CEJ
								Attachment Loss

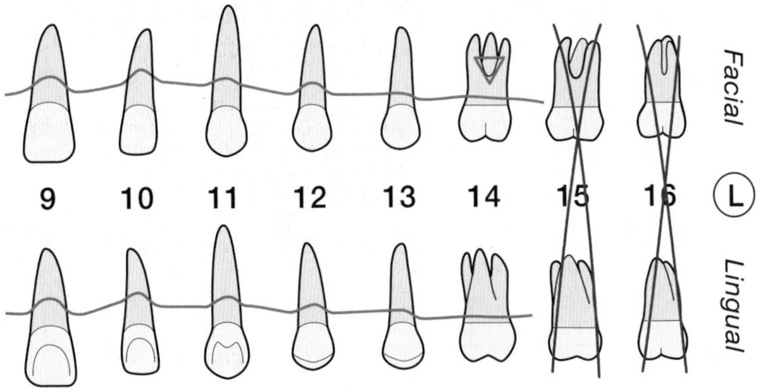

Figure 18-44C. Mrs. Blanchard's Periodontal Chart. Mrs. Blanchard's periodontal chart for the mandibular left quadrant. (Key: GM = gingival margin; CEJ = cementoenamel junction)

Mrs. Blanchard: Case Questions

1. *Use the information recorded on Mrs. Blanchard's chart to calculate the clinical attachment loss on the facial and lingual aspects for teeth 9 to 14 and enter this information on Mrs. Blanchard's periodontal chart in Figure 18-48C.*
2. When assessing tooth 14 for mobility, up to 1 mm of horizontal movement in a facial–lingual direction was evident. Determine the classification of mobility for tooth 14 and enter it on the chart.
3. What class furcation involvement is present on the facial aspect of tooth 14? No furcation involvement is present between the mesiobuccal root and the palatal root. In addition, there is no furcation involvement between the distobuccal root and the palatal root. How would you explain this finding?
4. Do the assessment data indicate healthy sulci or periodontal pockets in this quadrant? Explain which data you used to determine the presence of sulci or pockets?
5. If the gingival margin level information had NOT been documented on this chart, would the probing depth measurements alone be an accurate indicator of the level of bone support present? Why?
6. Based on the assessment information, which type of explorer would you select to explore the teeth in this quadrant? Which instruments would you select for calculus removal in this quadrant: sickle scalers, universal curets, and/or area-specific curets? Explain your rationale for instrument selection.

STUDENT SELF-EVALUATION MODULE 18 ANGULATION AND CALCULUS REMOVAL

Student: ______________________ Date: ______________________

Evaluator: ______________________

PART 1—PROBING DEPTH MEASUREMENTS ON STUDENT PARTNER

Evaluator assigns a tooth number in each quadrant to be probed on student partner (six readings per tooth).
S = student probing depth reading is within 1 mm of the evaluator's finding for the tooth.
U = student probing depth reading is not within 1 mm of the evaluator's finding for the tooth

QUADRANT	ASPECT	TOOTH #	STUDENT READINGS			EVALUATOR READINGS		
1	Facial	#						
	Lingual							
2	Facial	#						
	Lingual							
3	Facial	#						
	Lingual							
4	Facial	#						
	Lingual							

OPTIONAL GRADE PERCENTAGE CALCULATION—PART 1
Total number of readings within 1 mm of evaluator's measurement ______. (Possible 24 pts.)

PART 2A—FURCATIONS ASSESSMENT ON PERIODONTAL TYPODONT

On a periodontal typodont, uses furcation probe to assess a mandibular first molar (2 possible points) and a maxillary first molar (3 possible points). S = correct technique. U = incorrect technique.

PART 2B—CALCULATING ATTACHMENT LOSS

Calculate the clinical attachment loss for teeth A, B, and C below. S = correct calculation. U = incorrect calculation.

Tooth A		Tooth B		Tooth C	
Probing Depth	=2 mm	Probing Depth	=3 mm	Probing Depth	=6 mm
GM to CEJ	=+5 mm	GM to CEJ	=+4 mm	GM to CEJ	=−3 mm
Attachment Loss	=	Attachment Loss	=	Attachment Loss	=

OPTIONAL GRADE PERCENTAGE CALCULATION—PART 2
Total number of S evaluations for technique with furcation probe ______. (Possible 5 pts.)
Total number of correct CAL calculations ______. (Possible 3 pts.)

Module 19

Instruments for Advanced Root Debridement

Module Overview

Periodontitis causes alveolar bone loss that exposes the teeth roots to dental plaque biofilm. The effectiveness of instrumentation decreases with increasing probing depths, especially when probing depths exceed 5 mm.[1] ***Treatment of periodontally involved patients requires specialized instruments with longer shank lengths and miniature working-ends for instrumentation of root concavities and furcation areas.*** This module presents a variety of periodontal instruments that have been developed to increase treatment effectiveness on root surfaces within deep periodontal pockets.

Module Outline

Key Terms

Root concavity
Extended shanks
Miniature working-ends
Micro-miniature working-ends
Diamond-coated instruments
Dental endoscope

Learning Objectives

1. Describe characteristics of root morphology that make root instrumentation challenging.
2. Identify instruments that are appropriate for instrumentation of root surfaces within deep periodontal pockets.
3. Compare and contrast standard curets, extended shank curets, miniature curets, and micro-miniature curets.
4. Given any instrument, identify where and how it may be used on the dentition.
5. Demonstrate the use of an explorer on extracted or acrylic teeth, including exploration of root concavities and the furcations of multirooted teeth.

Section 1
Root Surface Anatomy

ROOT CONCAVITIES AND FURCATIONS

Instrumentation of a periodontally involved patient requires advanced instrumentation skills because of the concavities found on the roots of most teeth and the furcation areas exposed on some posterior teeth. In health, most of the tooth root is surrounded by alveolar bone. In disease, bone support is lost, exposing the root to dental plaque biofilm and requiring instrumentation of these surfaces.

Effective debridement of the root surfaces requires the clinician to have a complete knowledge of root morphology. ***The majority of instrumentation on roots is performed on surfaces that are hidden beneath the gingival margin. A clear mental picture of root anatomy and a keen tactile sense are necessary for subgingival instrumentation to be successful.***

1. A root concavity is a linear developmental depression in the root surface. Two examples of root concavities are pictured in Figure 19-1A,B. Figure 19-2 demonstrates the cross section of a root showing the concavity. Root concavities commonly occur on the: AQ2
   a. Proximal surfaces of anterior and posterior teeth
   b. Facial and lingual surfaces of molar teeth
2. In health, root concavities are covered with alveolar bone and help to secure the tooth in the bone.
3. In periodontitis, bone loss exposes the root concavities.
   a. If the gingival margin has receded, these concavities can be seen in the mouth.
   b. If the gingival margin is near the cementoenamel junction, the root concavities remain hidden beneath the tissue in a periodontal pocket.
4. It is difficult for a patient to successfully remove plaque from root surface concavities. Likewise, instrumentation of these areas by a clinician requires skill and an attention to root anatomy. Figures 19-3 and 19-4 show the importance of correct adaptation technique for exploration and instrumentation of root concavities.

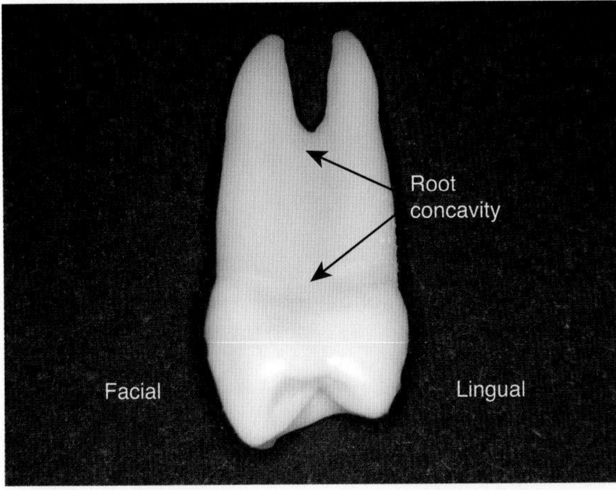

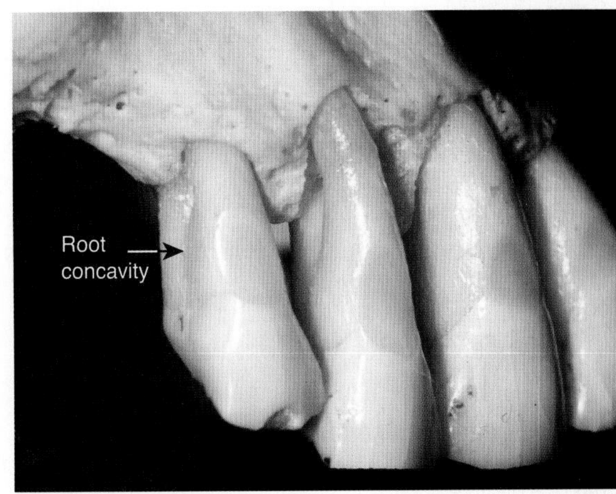

Figure 19-1. Concavity on the Mesial Surface of a Maxillary Premolar Tooth. A. Maxillary right first premolar showing the linear mesial concavity commonly found on this tooth. **B.** This photograph shows the mesial root concavity on a maxillary first premolar.

REVIEW OF ROOT MORPHOLOGY

TABLE 19-1. Root Concavities and Furcations

Teeth	Characteristics
Mandibular Anteriors Single-rooted teeth that frequently have shallow, linear concavities on the mesial and distal surfaces	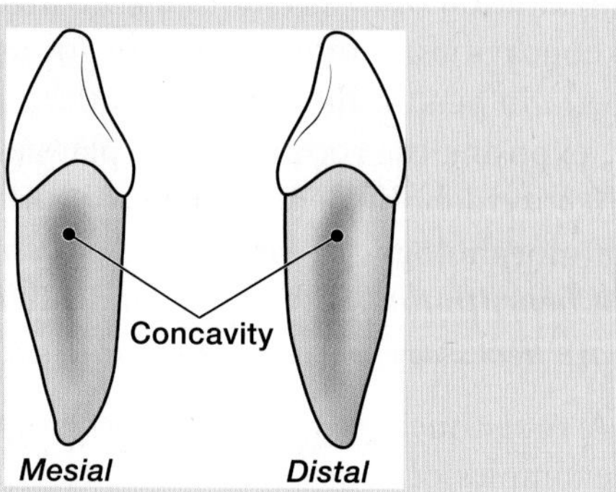
Maxillary Anteriors Single-rooted teeth that may have proximal root concavities; canines generally have proximal root concavities Lateral incisors may have a palatal groove on the cingulum that extends onto the cervical-third of the lingual surface.	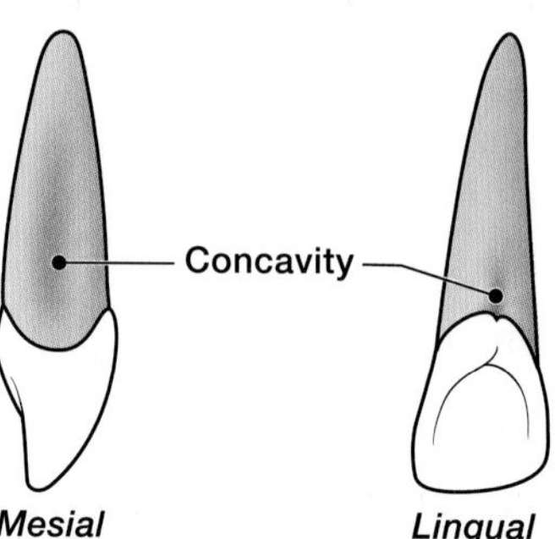
Premolars The mandibular premolars and the maxillary second premolars are single-rooted teeth that may have deep linear concavities on the mesial and distal surfaces.	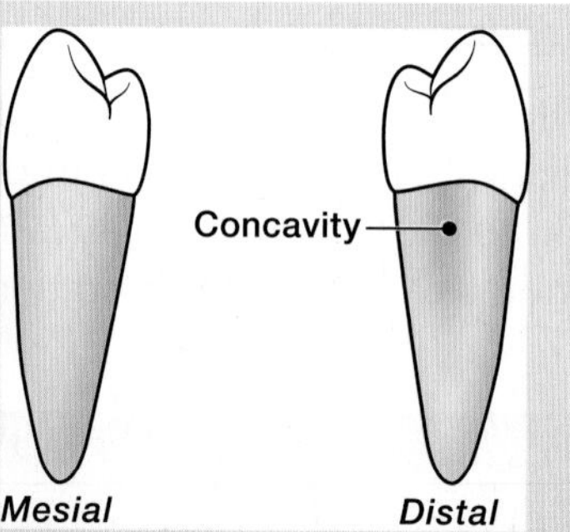
Maxillary First Premolar The root of this tooth may be bifurcated and has a deep linear mesial concavity. The distal concavity is less pronounced. When bifurcated, the roots of a maxillary first premolar separate many millimeters apical to the cementoenamel junction.	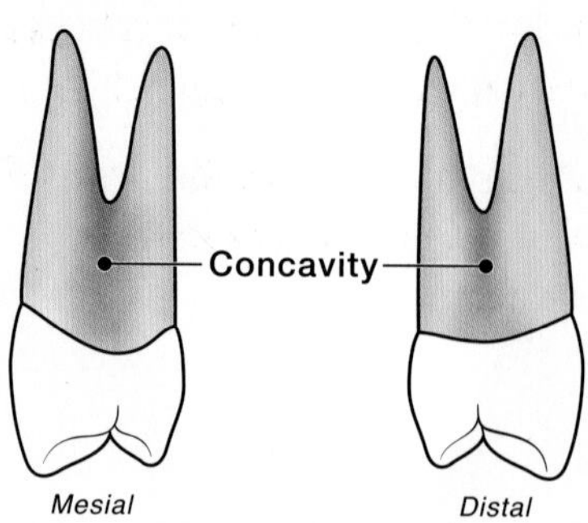

continues

TABLE 19-1. Root Concavities and Furcations (*continued*)

Teeth	Characteristics
Mandibular First Molar: Facial and Lingual Aspects Bifurcated, mesial, and distal roots The root trunk has a deep depression that extends from cervical line to the bifurcation. This depression deepens near the furcation.	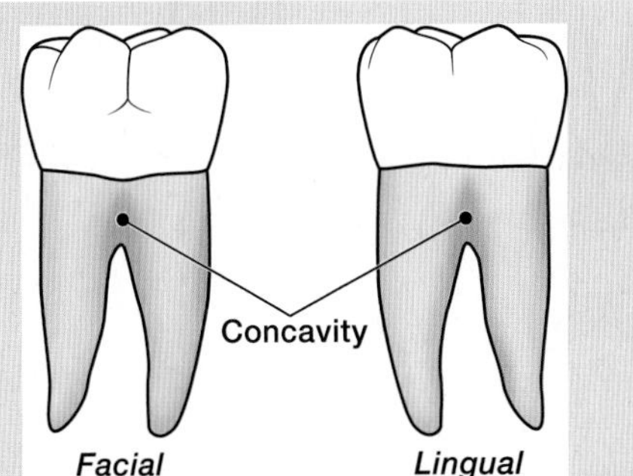
Mandibular First Molar: Proximal Aspects The mesial root has a wide, shallow concavity.	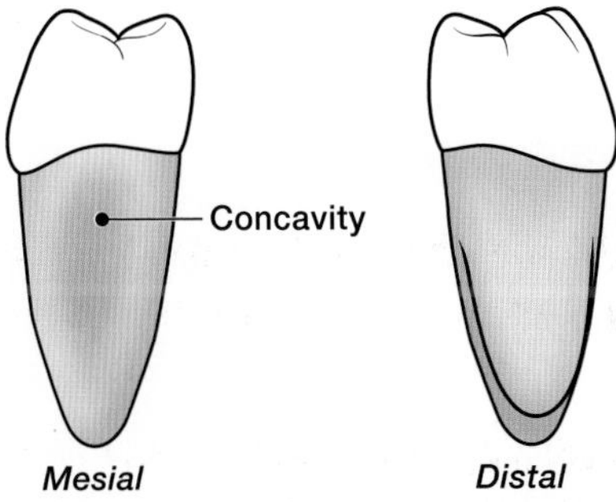
Maxillary First Molar: Facial and Lingual Aspects Trifurcated mesiobuccal, distobuccal, and palatal (lingual) roots The root trunk has a deep depression that extends from cervical line to the bifurcation. A longitudinal groove extends the length of the palatal root.	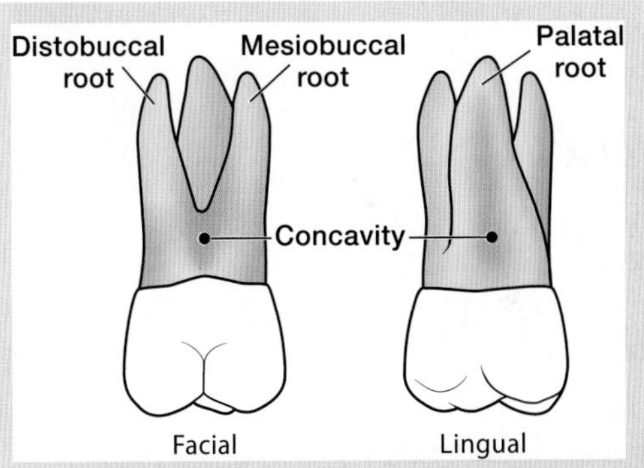
Maxillary First Molar: Proximal Aspects Mesial and distal surfaces have concavities extending from the furcation toward the cervical line. The mesial furcation is located more toward the lingual surface. The distal furcation is located near the center of the tooth.	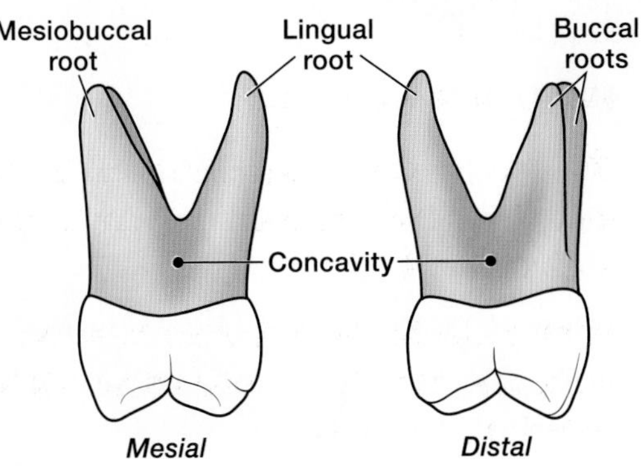

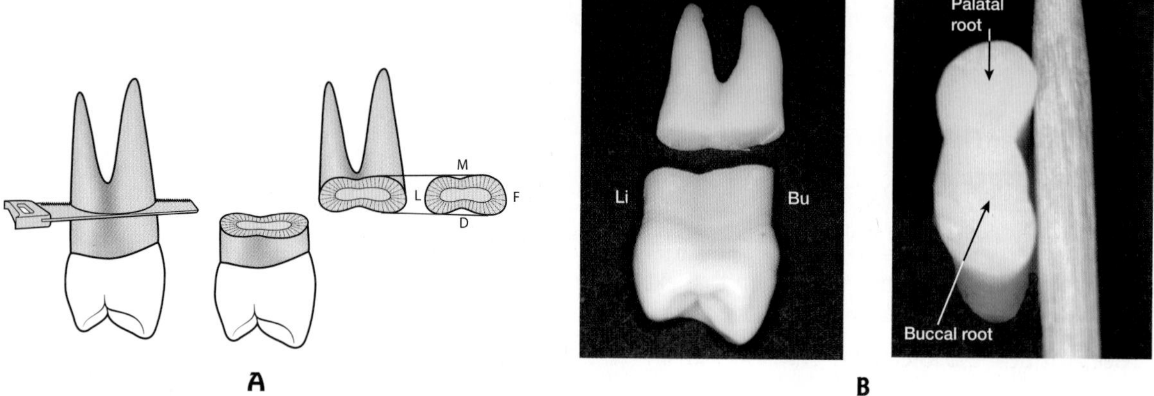

Figure 19-2. Root Concavity in Cross Section. A. A tooth is cut to expose the cross section of the root. **B.** The root of the maxillary first premolar in cross section. A toothpick spans the depression of the mesial root concavity.

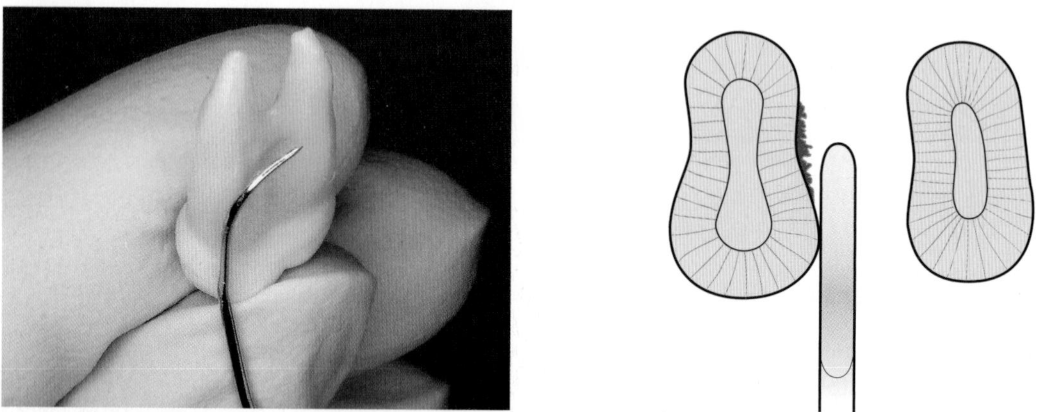

Figure 19-3. Incorrect Technique Causes the Working-End to Span the Concavity. A problem can occur during instrumentation when the clinician does not consider root morphology. The length of the working-end will span the depression, leaving the concavity untouched.

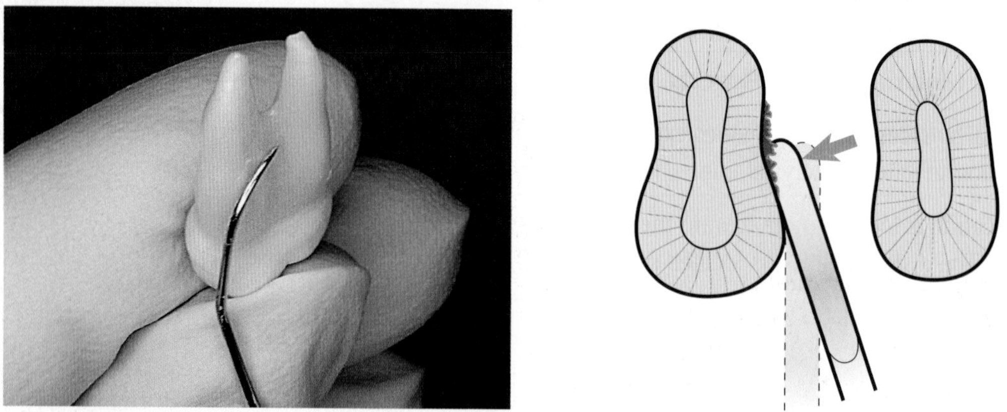

Figure 19-4. Correct Technique for Adaptation to the Concavity. Correct instrumentation technique involves rolling the handle to direct the leading-third of the explorer tip into the root concavity. Note that the middle- and heel-thirds of the working-end are rotated toward the adjacent tooth.

Section 2
Technique Practice

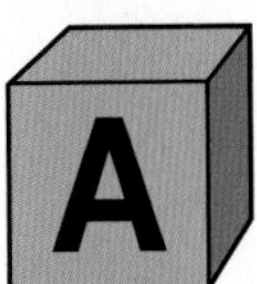

SKILL BUILDING. EXPLORATION OF ROOT CONCAVITIES AND FURCATIONS

Directions: For this technique practice, you will need the following items:

- An appropriate explorer for root exploration such as an 11/12-type explorer with an extended shank.
- The following acrylic or extracted teeth: maxillary first premolar, maxillary first molar, and mandibular first molar.

Note to Course Instructor: A source of acrylic teeth with anatomically correct roots is Kilgore International, Inc.: 800-892-9999 or online at http://www.kilgoreinternational.com.

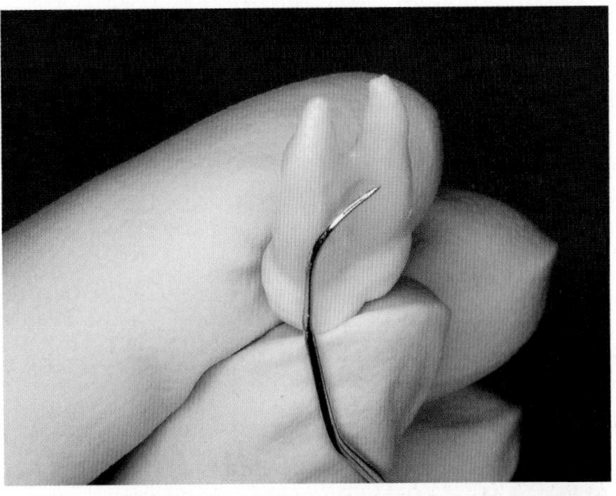

Figure 19-5. Adaptation to Proximal Concavity—Incorrect. First, span the concavity and explore the root surface. To experience working in a periodontal pocket, close your eyes as you explore. Notice how the explorer seems to slip across the surface of the root.

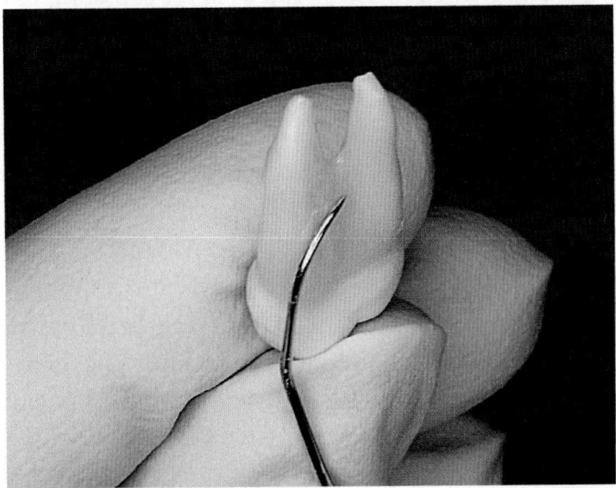

Figure 19-6. Adaptation to Proximal Concavity—Correct. Roll the handle slightly to direct the tip-third of the explorer into the concavity. Close your eyes and feel the difference as the tip explores the concavity, rather than just spanning the depression. This is the sensation that you should feel when working within a deep periodontal pocket.

MAXILLARY FIRST PREMOLAR—PROXIMAL CONCAVITY

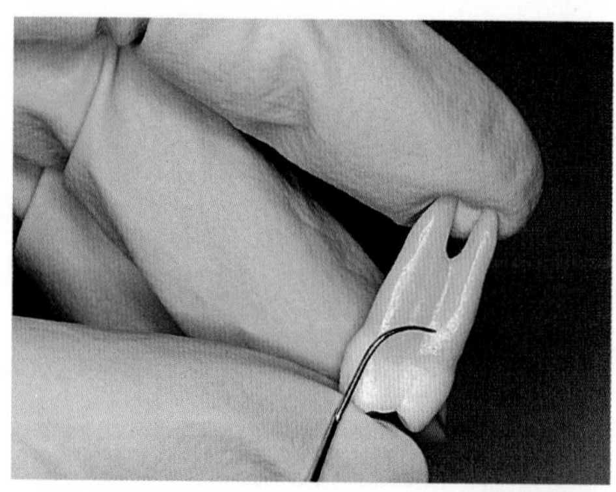

1. **Figure 19-7. Explore the Mesial Surface from Facial Aspect.** It is important to explore the mesial surface from both the facial and lingual aspects. First, practice exploring the mesial surface from the facial aspect as pictured here.

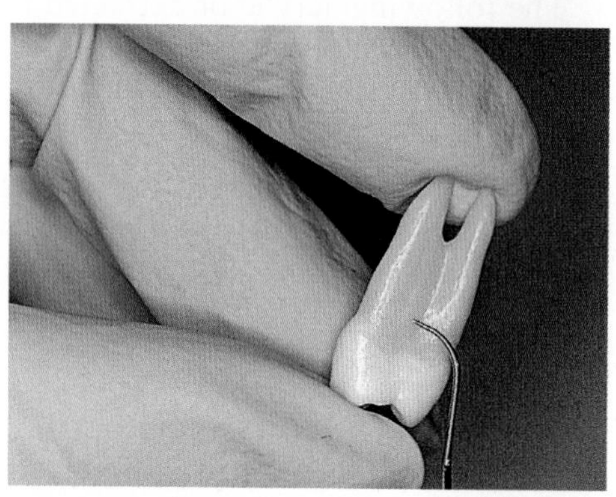

2. **Figure 19-8. Explore the Mesial Surface from Lingual Aspect.** Next, practice exploring the mesial surface from the lingual aspect as pictured here.

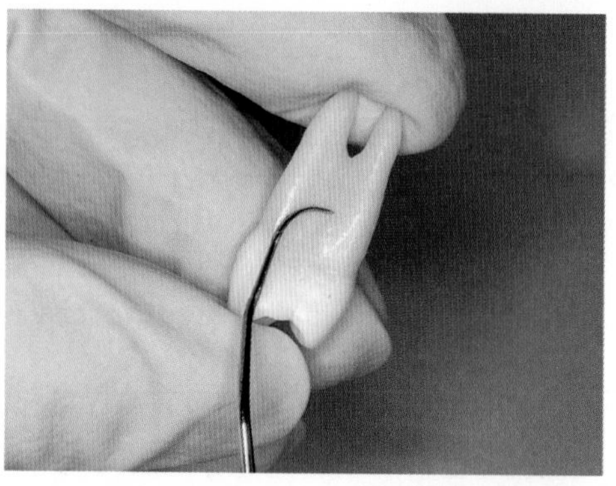

3. **Figure 19-9. Basic Working-End Position.** As you explore the concavity, note how difficult it is to completely adapt the explorer tip to the concavity using the basic instrumentation technique used for exploring tooth crowns.

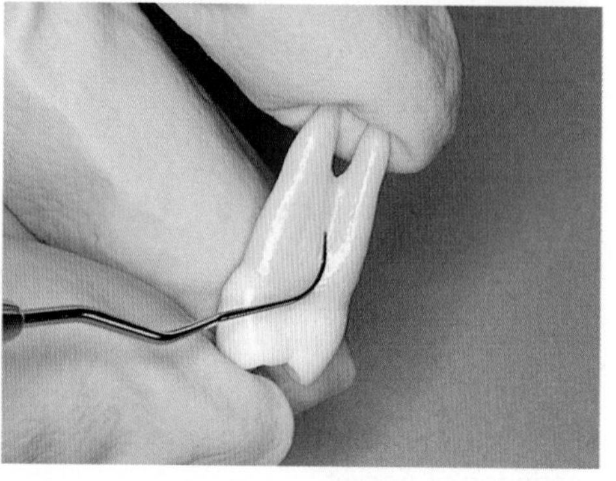

4. **Figure 19-10. Advanced Working-End Position.** Proximal root concavities can be more effectively explored by positioning the working-end in a tip-up position. Use horizontal strokes to explore the concavity.

MANDIBULAR FIRST MOLAR—CONCAVITIES AND FURCATION

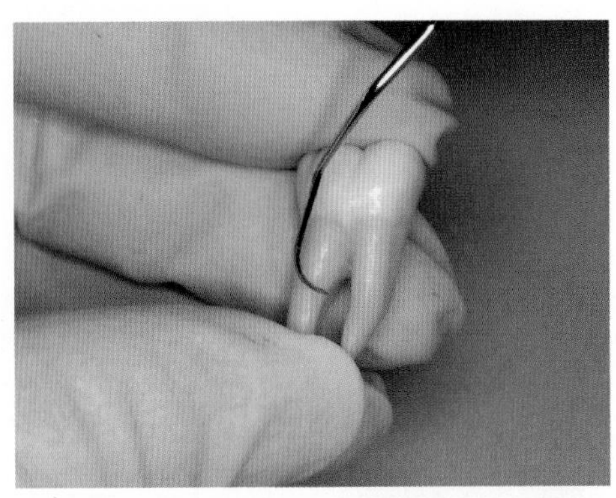

1. **Figure 19-11. Furcation—Mesial Portion of Distal Root.** Use the leading-third of the tip to explore the mesial portion of the distal root.

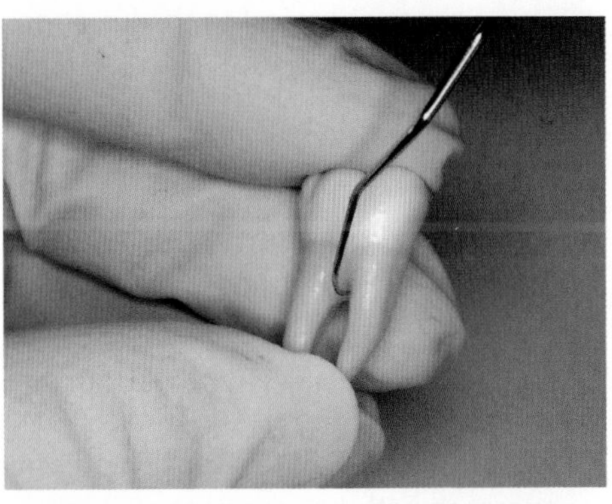

2. **Figure 19-12. Roof of the Furcation.** Use the explorer tip to explore the roof of the furcation.

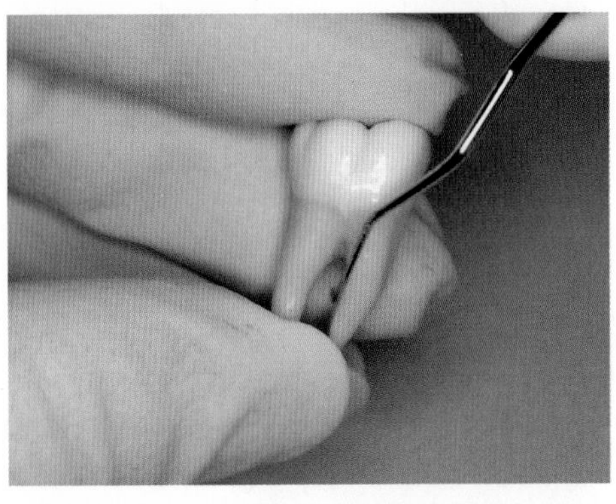

3. **Figure 19-13. Furcation—Distal Portion of Mesial Root.** Explore the distal portion of the mesial root.

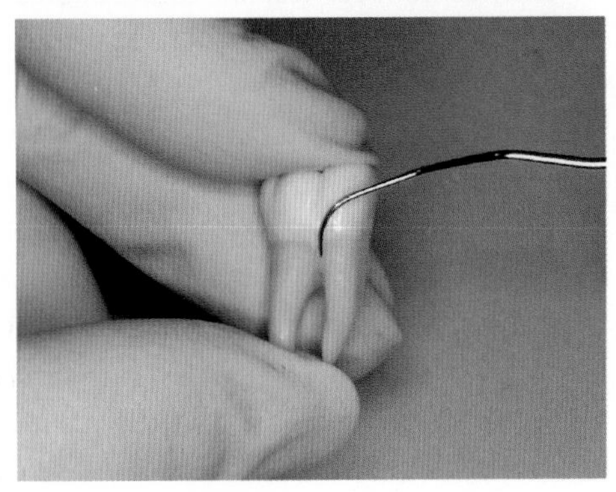

4. **Figure 19-14. Facial Depression.** Most mandibular molars have a deep depression on the root trunk that extends from cervical line to the bifurcation. A tip-down position of the explorer is most effective for exploring this depression. As you explore, note that the depression deepens near the furcation.

MAXILLARY FIRST MOLAR—CONCAVITIES AND FURCATIONS

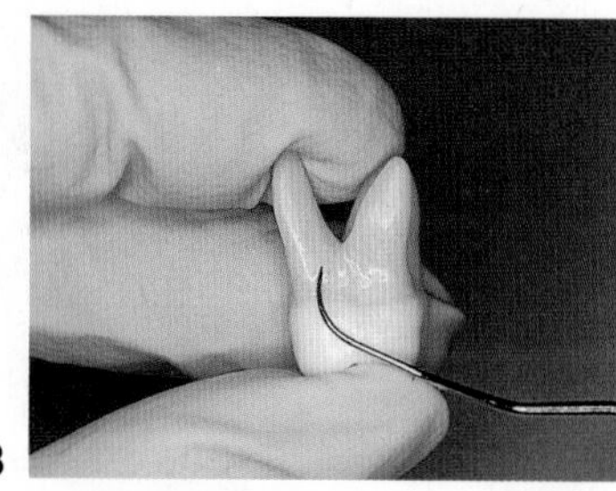
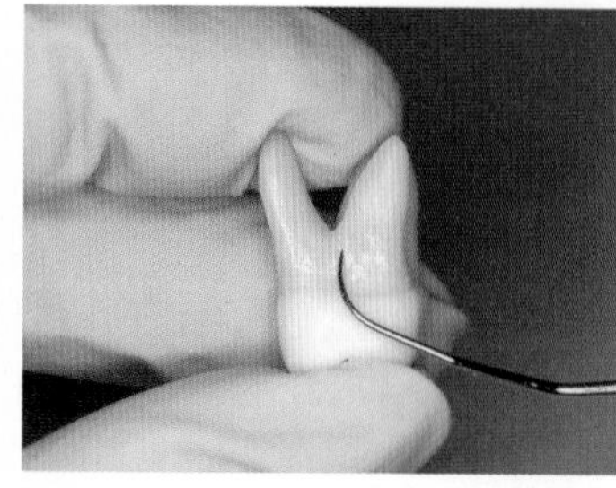
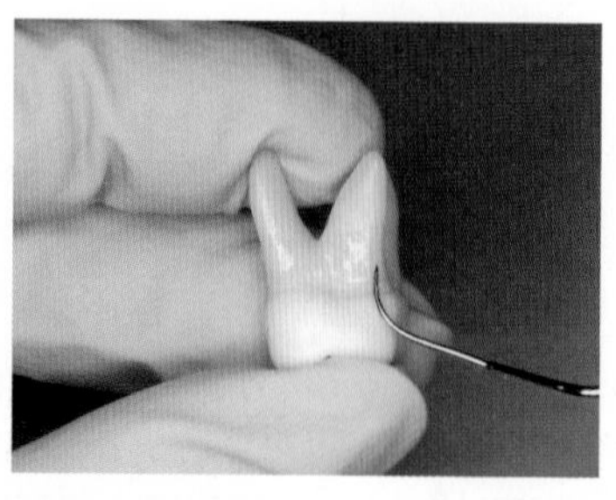

A, B C

1. **Figures 19-15, A–C. Concavity—Advanced Technique.** Practice using the explorer in a tip-up position to explore the distal surface of the maxillary first molar using a horizontal stroke. This is the most effective approach for adapting to the concavity apical to the furcation.

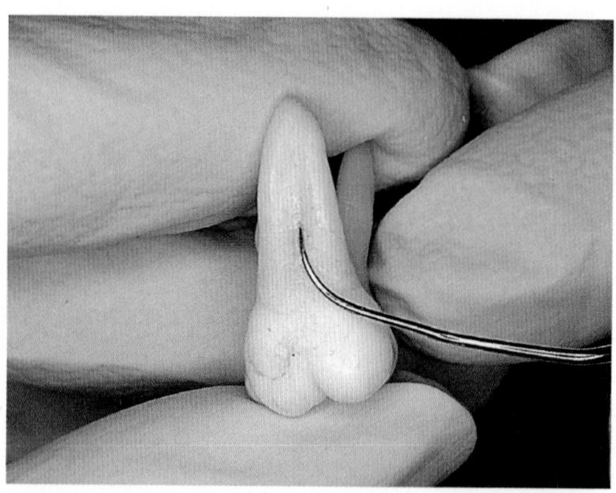

2. **Figure 19-16. Palatal Root Depression.** A tip-up approach with horizontal strokes is most effective when exploring the narrow linear depression on the palatal (lingual) root of a maxillary molar.

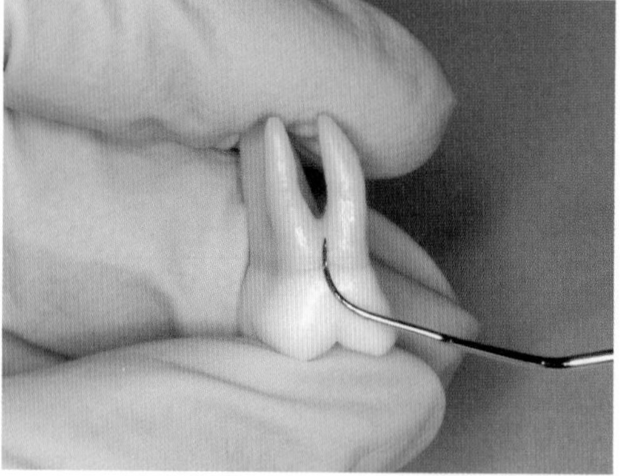

3. **Figure 19-17. Facial Depression.** Most maxillary molars have a deep depression on the root trunk that extends from cervical line to the bifurcation. Use a tip-up position and horizontal strokes to explore this area of the molar.

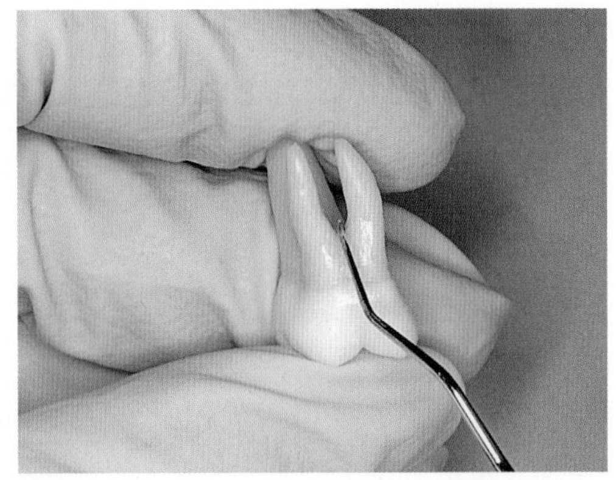

4. **Figure 19-18. Floor of the Furcation.** Use the explorer tip to explore the floor of the furcation.

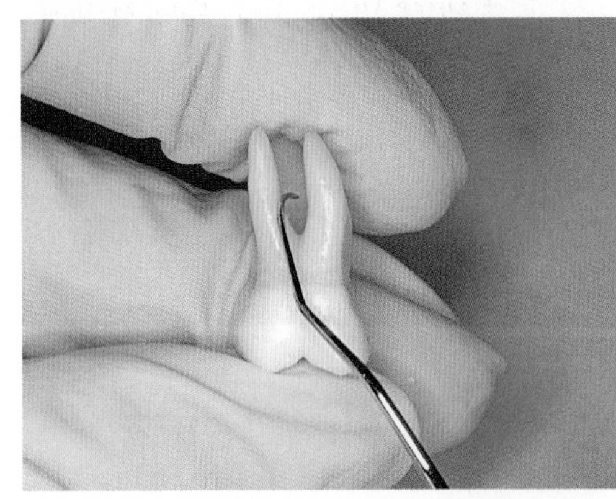

5. **Figure 19-19. Furcation—Mesial Portion of Distal Root.** Use the leading-third of the tip to explore the mesial portion of the distal root.

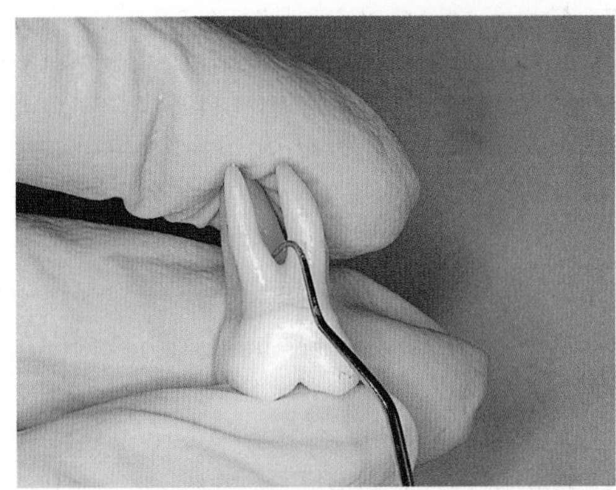

6. **Figure 19-20. Furcation—Distal Portion of Mesial Root.** Explore the distal portion of the mesial root.

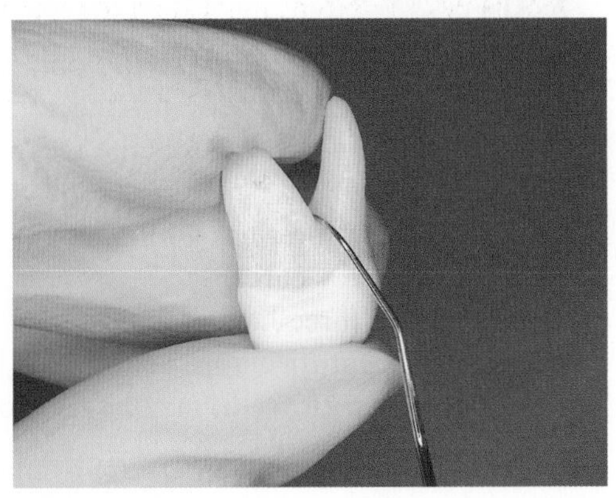

7. **Figure 19-21. Furcation—Mesial Surface.** The mesial furcation between the mesiobuccal and palatal roots is located more toward the lingual surface. Therefore, the mesial furcation is explored more easily from the lingual aspect. The distal furcation is located near the center of the tooth and may be explored from either the facial or lingual approach.

Section 3
Universal Curets for Root Debridement

LANGER MINIATURE CURETS

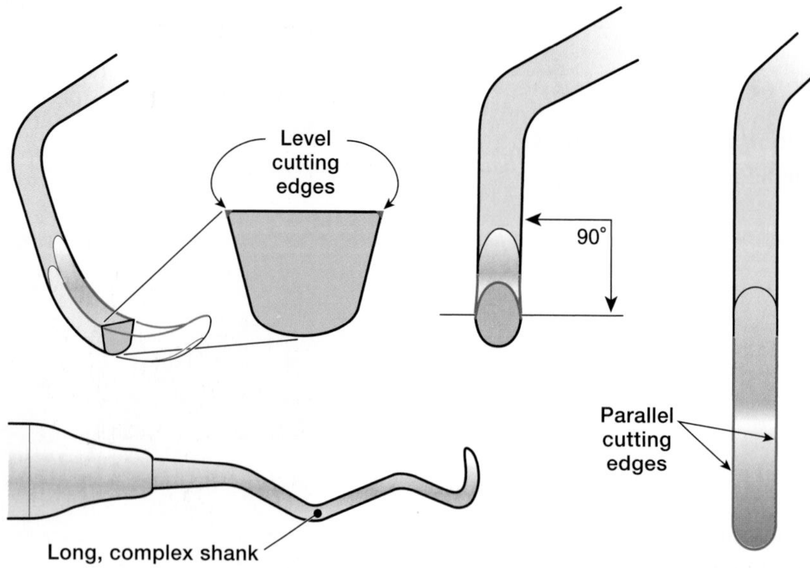

Figure 19-22. Miniature Langer Curet.

Langer curets with extended shanks and miniature working-ends are universal curets that have been modified to increase their effectiveness on root surfaces (Fig. 19-22). ***The Langer curet may be thought of as a hybrid design that combines features of a universal curet with features typical of an area-specific curet.*** This combination of design features allows an instrument to be used on all surfaces of a tooth and provides improved access to root surfaces through the shank design.[2]

1. **Design Characteristics of a Miniature Langer Curet.**
   a. **Longer Lower Shank.** The extended lower shank is designed for instrumenting pockets greater than 4 mm in depth.
   b. **Smaller Working-End.** A miniature working-end designed for access into deep narrow pockets.
2. **Use.**
   a. Each curet is limited to use only on certain teeth and certain tooth surfaces. For this reason, several Langer curets are required to instrument the entire mouth. Table 19-2 lists the recommended area of use for each curet in the Langer series.
   b. A Langer curet has a long, complex, functional shank design similar to that of a Gracey curet.
   c. A set of three Langer curets—the Langer 5/6, 1/2, and 3/4—is needed to instrument the entire dentition. The Langer 17/18, which facilitates access to the posterior teeth, may be used on molar teeth.
3. **Availability.** Langer curets are available in standard, rigid, extended shank, and miniature curet designs.

TABLE 19-2. Langer Curet Application

Curet	Area of Use
Langer 5/6	Anterior teeth
Langer 1/2	Mandibular posterior teeth
Langer 3/4	Maxillary posterior teeth
Langer 17/18	Posterior teeth

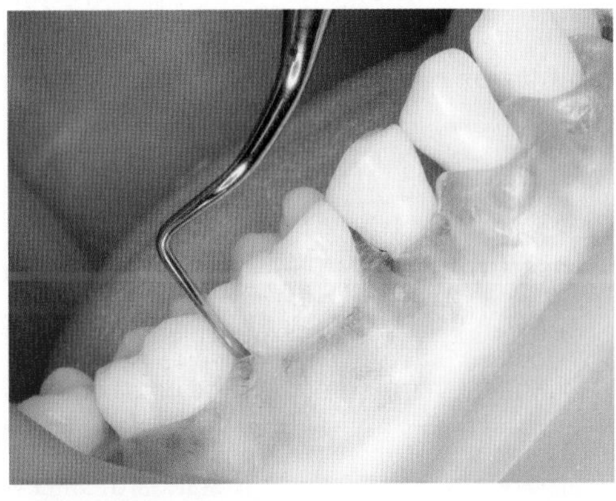

Figure 19-23. Langer 17/18. The modified shank design of the Langer 17/18 makes it easier to position the lower shank parallel to the distal surfaces of molar teeth.

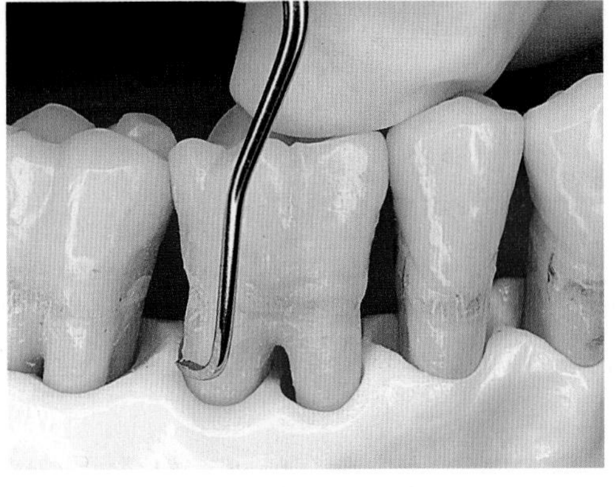

Figure 19-24. Adaptation to Line Angles. ***Within its recommended area of use, each Langer curet is used like any other universal curet.*** The extended shank and miniature working-end of the Langer 1/2 miniature curet facilitate adaptation to the distofacial line angle.

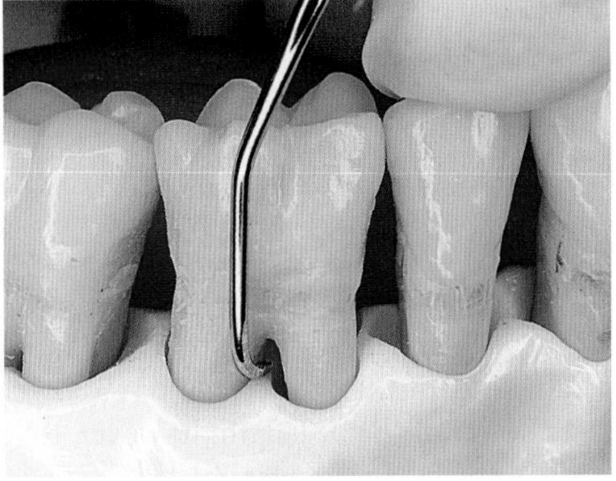

Figure 19-25. Adaptation to Furcation Area. The miniature working-end of this miniature Langer curet facilitates adaptation to the furcation area.

Section 4
Modified Gracey Curets for Advanced Root Debridement

INTRODUCTION TO MODIFIED GRACEY CURET DESIGNS

Standard area-specific curets are designed for instrumenting root surfaces in periodontal pockets that are 4 mm or less in depth. To increase treatment effectiveness on root surfaces in periodontal pockets greater than 4 mm in depth, modified Gracey curet designs were developed. Table 19-3 summarizes the design modifications of curets designed for use in deep periodontal pockets.

- Modified curet designs with extended shanks are designed to debride root surfaces within deep pockets over 4 mm in depth (Fig. 19-26).
- Modified curets with miniature working-ends and micro-miniature working-ends are designed for use in narrow deep pockets over 4 mm in depth to debride root branches, midlines of anterior roots, root concavities, and furcation areas.

TABLE 19-3. Comparison of Standard and Modified Gracey Curet Designs

Instrument	Shank Design	Working-End Length	Working-End Width
Extended shank curet	Lower shank is 3 mm longer than that of a standard Gracey curet	Same length as a standard Gracey curet	10% thinner than a standard Gracey curet
Miniature working-end curet	Lower shank is 3 mm longer than that of a standard Gracey curet	Half the length of a standard Gracey curet	10% thinner than a standard Gracey curet
Micro-miniature working-end curet	Lower shank is 3 mm longer than that of a standard Gracey curet	Half the length of a standard Gracey curet	20% thinner than a standard Gracey curet

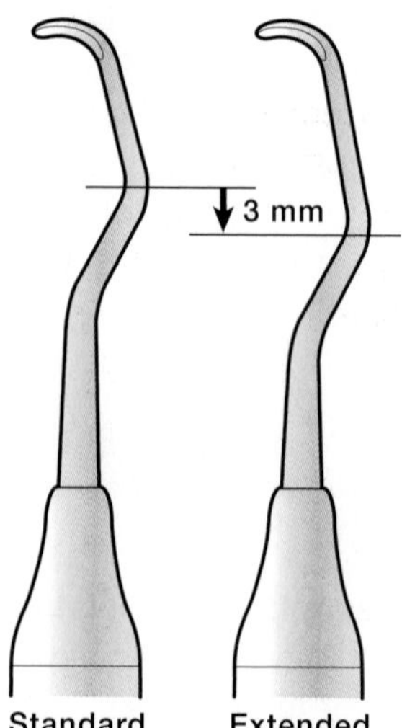

Figure 19-26. Comparison of Standard and Extended Shank Gracey Curets.

- The instrument on the left has a standard shank.
- The instrument on the right has a lower shank that is 3 mm longer. The overall shank length, however, for the instrument on the right is the same as that of a standard Gracey curet.

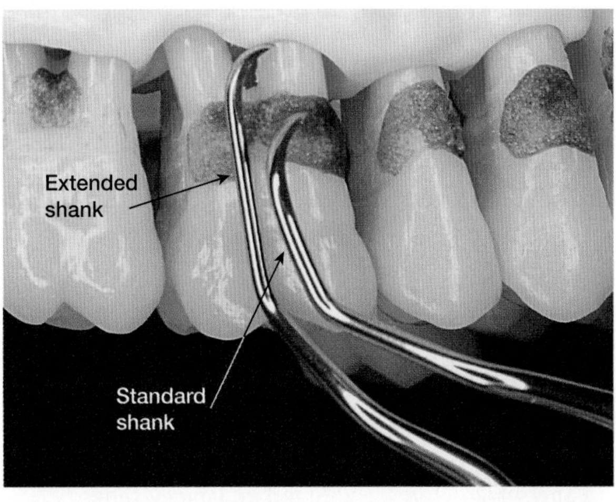

Figure 19-27. Comparison of Extended and Standard Lower Shanks.

- The curet on the left has an extended lower shank. Instruments with extended shanks are used to instrument root surfaces in periodontal pockets over 4 mm in depth.
- The curet on the right has a standard lower shank. It is recommended for use in normal sulci and periodontal pockets that are less than 4 mm in depth.

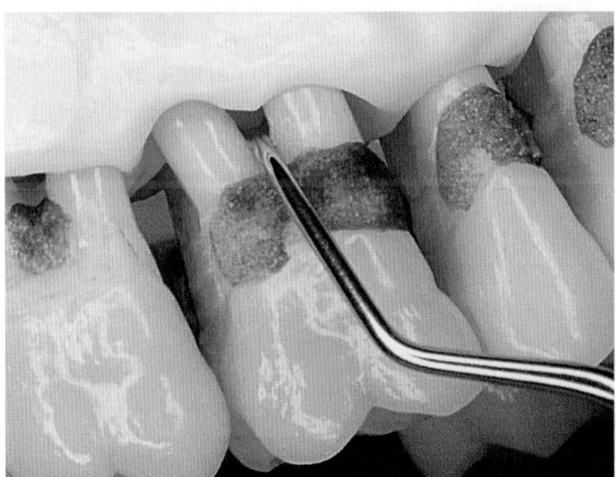

Figure 19-28. Extended Shank Length. The extended lower shank of this modified curet facilitates access to the furcation area of this molar.

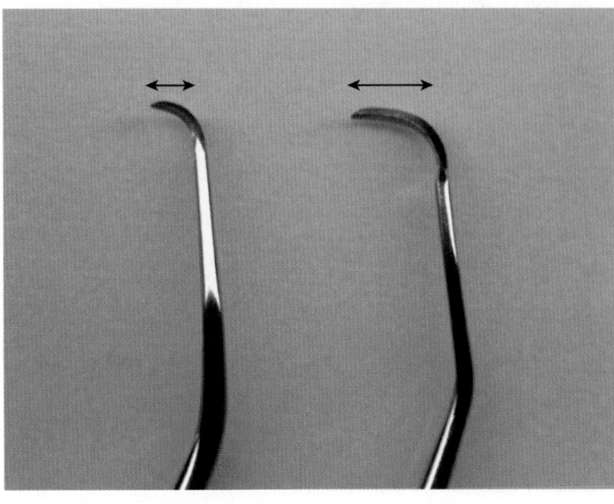

Figure 19-29. Micro-Miniature and Standard Working-Ends. The instrument on the left, a micro-miniature curet, has a working-end that is approximately half the length of that of the standard Gracey curet on the right side of the photo.

AVAILABILITY AND APPLICATION OF GRACEY DESIGNS

Area-specific curets with extended shanks and miniature working-ends are modifications of the standard Gracey series. The modified Gracey curets can be applied to the same tooth surfaces as the original Gracey series. Table 19-4 lists the availability of the various curet series in standard and modified designs and their area of application.

TABLE 19-4. Gracey Curet Availability and Application

Curet	Curet Availability	Tooth Application
Curets 1/2 Curets 3/4	• Standard Gracey series • Extended shank Gracey series • Miniature Gracey series • Micro-miniature series: Gracey 1/2 curet only	• Anterior teeth: all tooth surfaces
Curets 5/6	• Standard Gracey series • Extended shank Gracey series • Miniature Gracey series	• Anterior teeth: all tooth surfaces • Premolar teeth: all tooth surfaces • Molar teeth: facial, lingual, and mesial surfaces
Curets 7/8 Curets 9/10	• Standard Gracey series • Extended shank Gracey series • Miniature Gracey series • Micro-miniature series: Gracey 7/8 curet only	• Anterior teeth: all surfaces • Premolar teeth: all surfaces • Posterior teeth: facial and lingual surfaces
Curets 11/12	• Standard Gracey series • Extended shank Gracey series • Miniature Gracey series • Micro-miniature series	• Anterior teeth: mesial and distal surfaces • Posterior teeth: mesial surfaces • Posterior teeth: facial, lingual, and mesial surfaces
Curets 13/14	• Standard Gracey series • Extended shank Gracey series • Miniature Gracey series • Micro-miniature series	• Anterior teeth: mesial and distal surfaces • Posterior teeth: distal surfaces
Curets 15/16	• Standard Gracey series • Extended shank Gracey series	• Posterior teeth: facial, lingual, and mesial surfaces
Curets 17/18	• Standard Gracey series	• Posterior teeth: distal surfaces

MODIFIED GRACEY CURETS WITH EXTENDED SHANKS

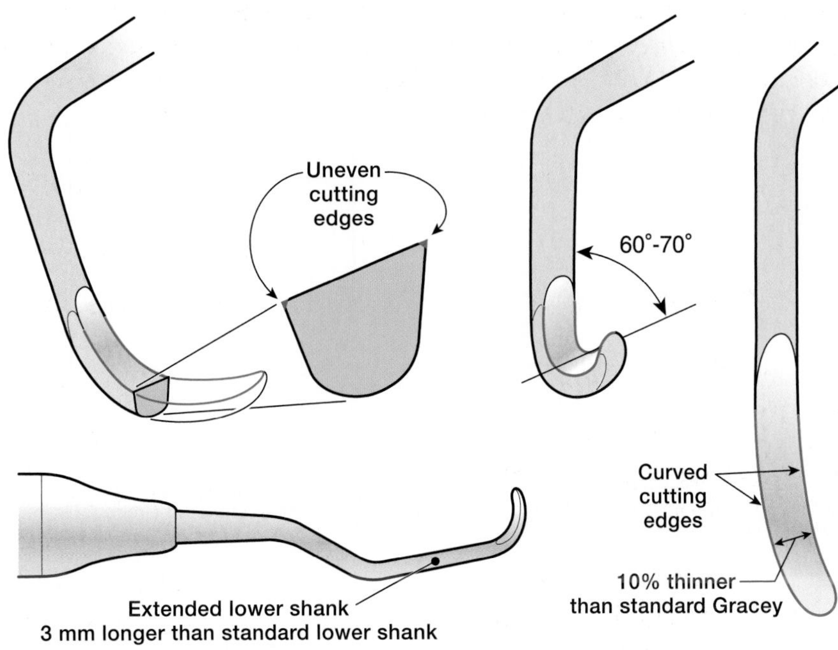

Figure 19-30. Modified Gracey Curet with Extended Shank Length.

1. **Design Modifications.** The design characteristics of the extended shank curets differ from those of standard Gracey curets in two important respects (Fig. 19-30):
   a. **Longer Lower Shank.**
      1. The extended lower shank is 3 mm longer than the lower shank of a standard Gracey curet.
      2. The longer lower shank permits access to root surfaces within periodontal pockets greater than 4 mm in depth.

   b. **Thinner Working-End.**
      1. The working-end is 10% thinner than that of a standard Gracey curet.
      2. The thinner working-end facilitates insertion beneath the gingival margin and reduces tissue distention away from the root surface.
2. **Use.** Modified Gracey curets with extended shanks are designed to debride root surfaces within deep pockets over 4 mm in depth.
3. **Examples.** Examples of extended shank Gracey curets include the Hu-Friedy Manufacturing Company's After Five curets, American Eagle Instruments' Gracey +3 Deep Pocket curets, and G. Hartzell's Extended Gracey Curettes.

MODIFIED GRACEY CURETS WITH MINIATURE WORKING-ENDS

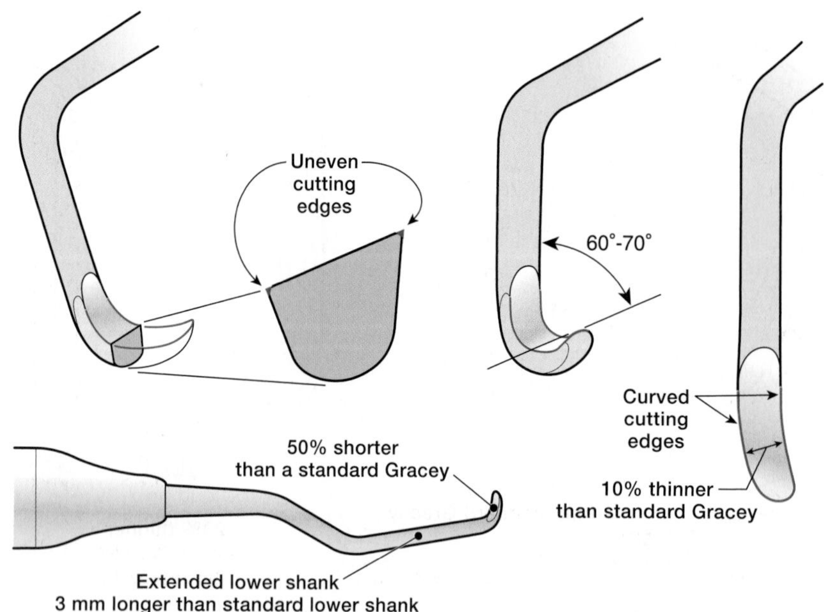

Figure 19-31. Miniature Gracey Curet.

1. **Design Modifications.** The design characteristics of the miniature curets differ from those of standard Gracey curets in three important respects (Fig. 19-31):
   a. **Extended Shank Length.**
      1. The extended lower shank is 3 mm longer than the lower shank of a standard Gracey curet.
      2. The longer lower shank permits access to root surfaces within periodontal pockets greater than 4 mm in depth.
   b. **Thinner Working-End.**
      1. The working-end is 10% thinner than that of a standard Gracey curet.
      2. The thinner working-end facilitates insertion beneath the gingival margin and reduces tissue distention away from the root surface.
   c. **Shorter Working-End.** The miniature working-end is half the length of a standard Gracey curet. The working-end does not curve up.[3] Compare this design to that of the Vision Curvette discussed later in this chapter.
2. **Uses.**
   a. Miniature Gracey curets are designed for use in narrow deep pockets over 4 mm in depth to debride root branches, midlines of anterior roots, root concavities, and furcation areas.
   b. ***The miniature curets are not intended to replace either the standard or extended shank Gracey curets for routine instrumentation of all tooth surfaces.*** Rather, miniature curets are used instead of standard curets for instrumentation of areas that are extremely difficult to reach with standard working-ends such as furcations, line angles, and deep narrow pockets.
   c. The miniature curets adapt well to narrow facial and lingual surfaces of anterior teeth, furcations, and root surfaces in narrow and deep periodontal pockets.
3. **Examples.** Examples of miniature curets include the Hu-Friedy Mini Five, American Eagle Instruments' Gracey +3 Access curets, and G. Hartzell Slim Gracey Curettes.

MODIFIED GRACEY CURETS WITH MICRO-MINIATURE WORKING-ENDS

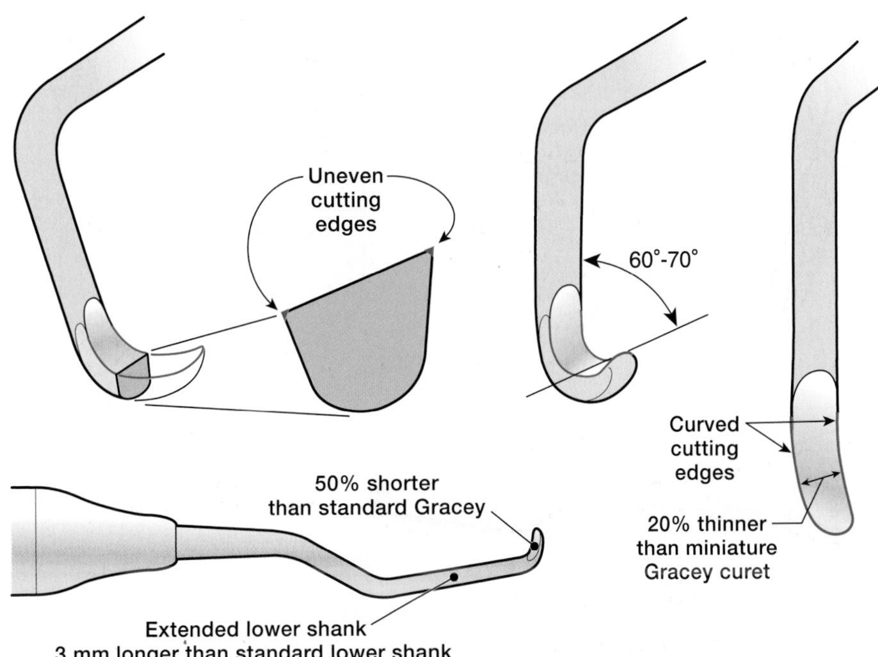

Figure 19-32. Micro-Miniature Gracey Curet.

1. **Design Modifications.** The design characteristics of the micro-miniature curets differ from those of standard Gracey curets in three important respects (Fig. 19-32):
   a. **Longer Shank Length.**
      1. The extended lower shank is 3 mm longer than the lower shank of a standard Gracey curet.
      2. The shank has slightly increased rigidity compared to miniature curets.

   b. **Thinner Working-End.**
      1. The working-end is 20% thinner than that of a miniature Gracey curet.
      2. The thinner working-end facilitates insertion beneath the gingival margin and reduces tissue distention away from the root surface.

   c. **Shorter Working-End.** The miniature working-end is half the length of a standard Gracey curet.

   d. **Availability.** The micro-miniature set includes four instruments: 1/2, 7/8, 11/12, and 13/14.

2. **Uses.**
   a. They facilitate insertion and adaptation into very tight, deep, or narrow pockets and facilitate access to narrow furcations; developmental depressions; line angles; and deep pockets on facial, lingual, or palatal surfaces, especially when the tissue is tight and/or thin.

   b. ***Micro-miniature curets are not used routinely instead of the standard Gracey curets, but rather, in special areas of difficult access.*** These curets are ideal for fine deposit removal following instrumentation with other curets.

   c. Vertical or oblique strokes work well with these instruments. Horizontal strokes might not extend far enough subgingivally and may gouge the root surface.

3. **Examples.** An example is the Hu-Friedy Micro Mini Fives.

VISION CURVETTE MINIATURE CURETS

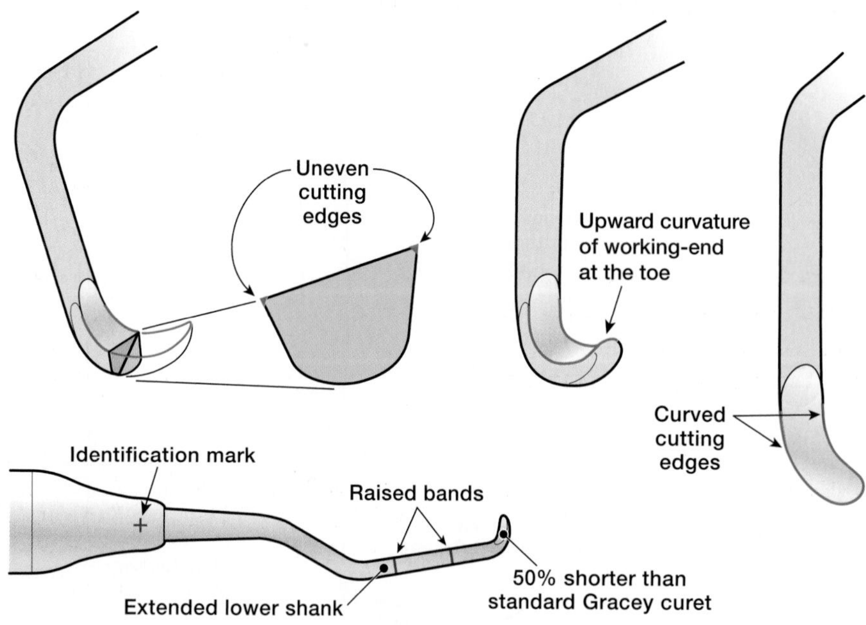

Figure 19-33. The Vision Curvette Curet.

1. **Design Modifications.** The design characteristics of Vision Curvette area-specific curets (Hu-Friedy Manufacturing) differ from those of standard Gracey curets in several important respects (Fig. 19-33):
   a. **Extended Shank Design.**
      1. Extended lower shank on the Vision Curvette 11/12 and 13/14 curets allows access to root surfaces within periodontal pockets greater than 4 mm in depth.
      2. The lower shank has two ***raised bands*** at 5 and 10 mm. These raised bands provide a means to visually estimate the pocket depth during instrumentation.
   b. **Shorter Working-End.** The Vision Curvette working-end is shortened to half the length of a standard Gracey curet.
      1. The shorter working-end allows the entire length of the working-end to be adapted to the root surface.
      2. The miniature working-end provides improved access to root concavities, furcation areas of posterior teeth, and midlines of anterior teeth.
   c. **Working-End Curvature.** The working-end has a slight upward curvature at the toe. This curvature facilitates adaptation to curved root surfaces, particularly at line angles.
   d. **Working Cutting Edge Identification Mark.** An identification mark ("+") on the handle near the junction of the shank indicates the lower cutting edge.
2. **Uses.**
   a. The Vision Curvette series facilitates access to areas that are extremely difficult to reach with standard curets such as narrow deep pockets over 4 mm in depth, root branches, midlines of anterior roots, root concavities, and furcation areas and are very effective for the palatal surfaces of maxillary anterior teeth.
   b. *Vision Curvette curets are not used routinely instead of the standard Gracey curets, but rather, in special areas of difficult access.*

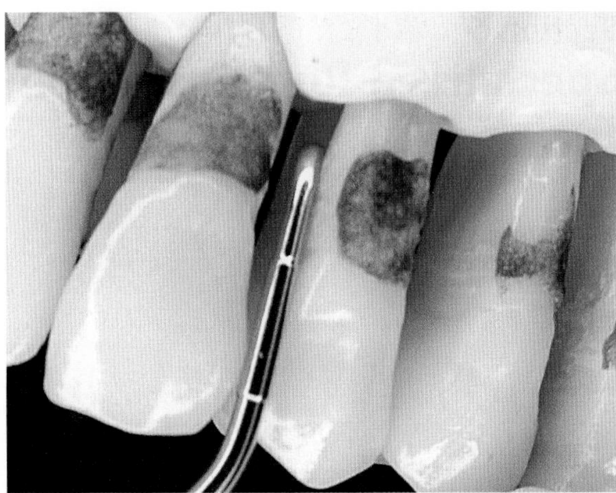

Figure 19-34. Vision Curvette Curet. The lower shank on a Vision Curvette curet has raised bands at 5 and 10 mm that provide a means to visually estimate the pocket depth during instrumentation.

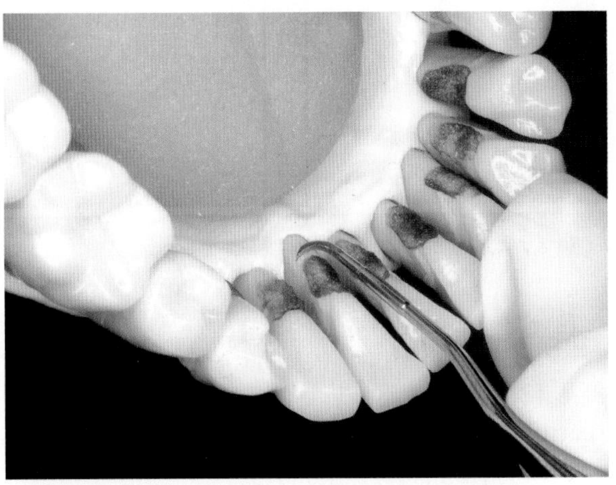

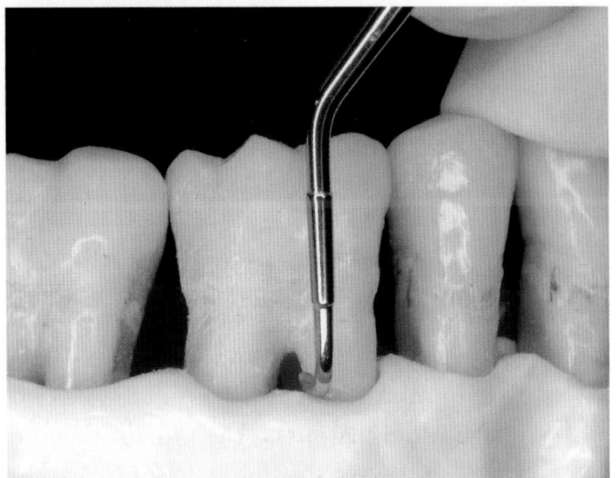

Figure 19-35. Vision Curvette Working-End. The shorter working-end of a Vision Curvette curet facilitates adaptation to narrow anterior root surfaces and the furcation areas of molar teeth.

TABLE 19-5. Vision Curvette Curet Application

Curet	Area of Use
Vision Curvette Sub-Zero	Anterior teeth
Vision Curvette 1/2	Anterior and premolar teeth
Vision Curvette 11/12	Mesial, facial, and lingual surfaces of molars
Vision Curvette 13/14	Distal surfaces of molar teeth

Section 5
Specialized Root Instruments

QUÉTIN FURCATION CURETS

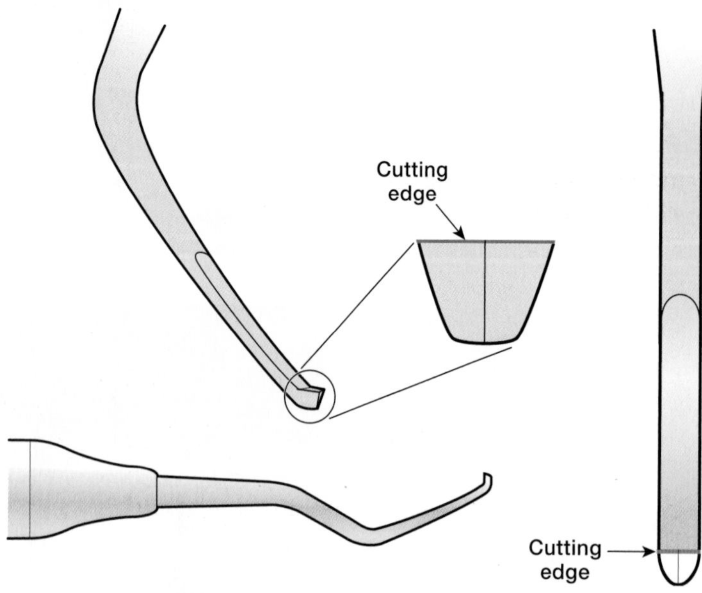

Figure 19-36. Quétin Furcation Curet.

1. **Design Modifications.** The Quétin (kee-tan) furcation curets have very unique design characteristics (Fig. 19-36).
   a. **Working-End Design.**
      1. Each miniature working-end is a miniature hoe with a single, semi-circular cutting edge.
      2. The corners of the cutting edges and back of the working-end are rounded to minimize the potential for gouging the tooth surface.
   b. **Working-End Size.** Each working-end is available in either the 0.9- or 1.3-mm size.
2. **Uses.** Quétin furcation curets are specialized instruments used to debride furcation areas and developmental depressions on the inner aspects of the roots.
3. **Availability.** Quétin curets are available in facial-lingual and mesial-distal instruments.
   a. The shallow semi-circular cutting edge fits into the roof or floor of furcation areas. The curvature of the tip also fits into developmental depressions on the inner aspects of the roots.
   b. These instruments remove calculus from recessed areas of the furcation where other curets, even Graceys with miniature working-ends, can be too large to gain access.

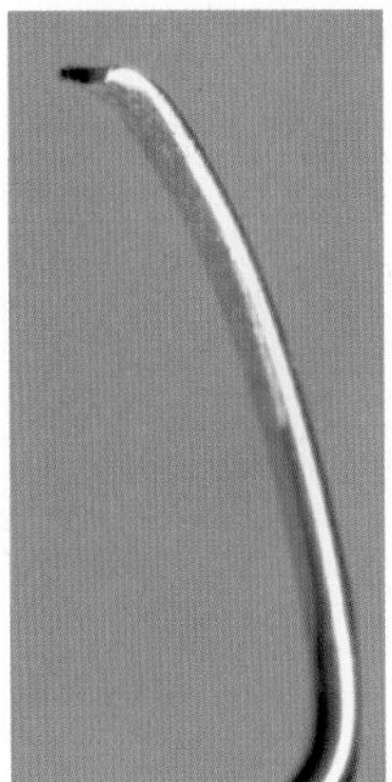

Figure 19-37. Quétin Furcation Curet. A close-up view of the working-end of a Quétin curet.

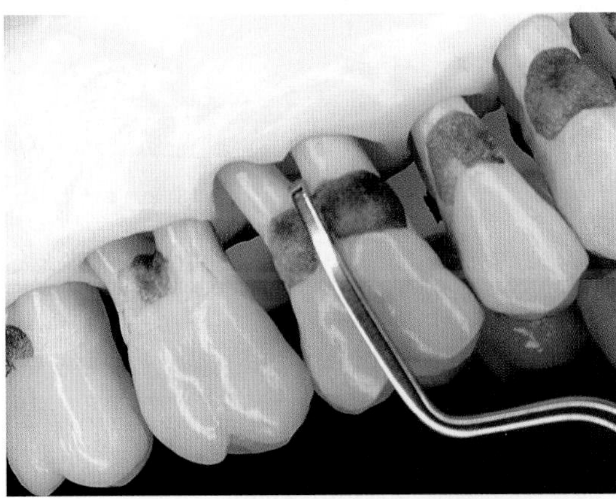

Figure 19-38. Quétin Curet in Furcation. The Quétin 1 curet used on the furcation roof of a maxillary first molar.

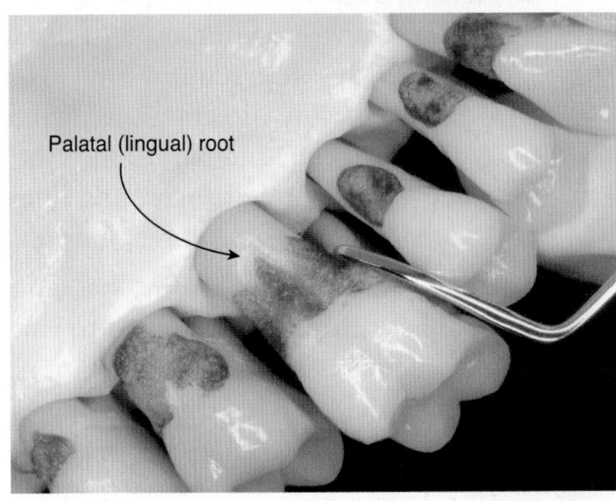

Figure 19-39. Quétin Curet in the Mesial Furcation. The Quétin 2 curet used in the mesial furcation of a maxillary first molar. The mesial furcation is accessed from the lingual aspect of the molar.

TABLE 19-6. Quétin Curet Application

Curet	Area of Use
Quétin 1	Facial and lingual surfaces of posterior teeth
Quétin 2	Mesial and distal surfaces of posterior teeth
Quétin 3	Facial and lingual surfaces of anterior teeth

O'HEHIR DEBRIDEMENT CURETS/DEMARCO CURETS

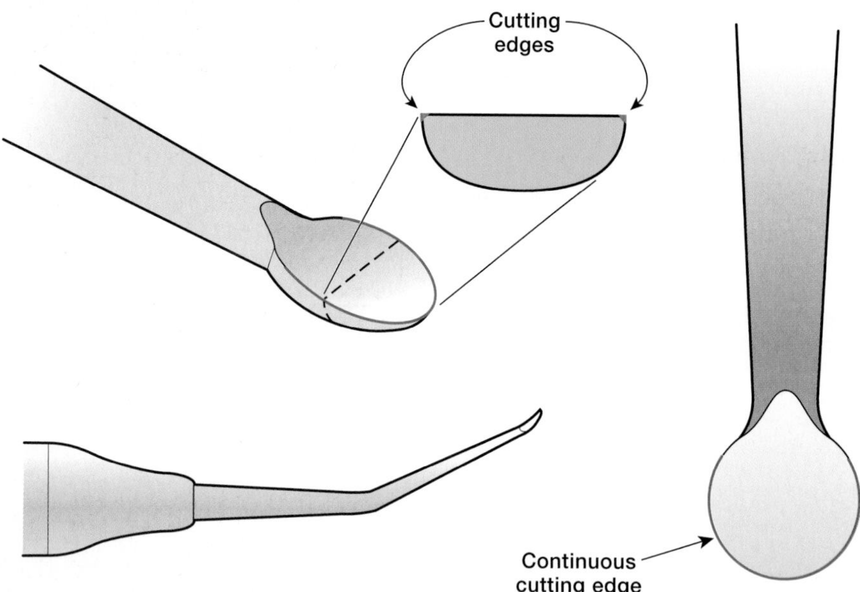

Figure 19-40. The O'Hehir Curet.

1. **Design Modifications.** The O'Hehir Debridement curets and DeMarco curets are examples of a new type of area-specific curet.
   a. **Shape of Working-End.** The working-end of an O'Hehir or DeMarco curet is a tiny circular disk.
   b. **Cutting Edge.**
      1. The entire circumference of the working-end is one continuous cutting edge. This design allows the instrument to be used with a push or pull stroke in any direction: vertical, horizontal, or oblique.
      2. The working-end curves into the tooth for easy adaptation in furcations, developmental grooves, and line angles.
   c. **Shank Design.** These curets have extended lower shanks for easy access into deep periodontal pockets.
2. **Uses.** These curets are designed to smooth root surfaces and remove small residual deposits after instrumentation with curets. They are ideal for furcations, developmental grooves, and line angles.
3. **Examples.** Examples include O'Hehir Debridement curets and DeMarco curets.

TABLE 19-7. O'Hehir Debridement Curet Application

Curet	Area of Use
O'Hehir 1/2	Facial and lingual surfaces of posterior teeth
O'Hehir 3/4	Mesial and distal surfaces of posterior teeth
O'Hehir 5/6	Anterior teeth
O'Hehir 7/8	Anterior teeth with deep pockets

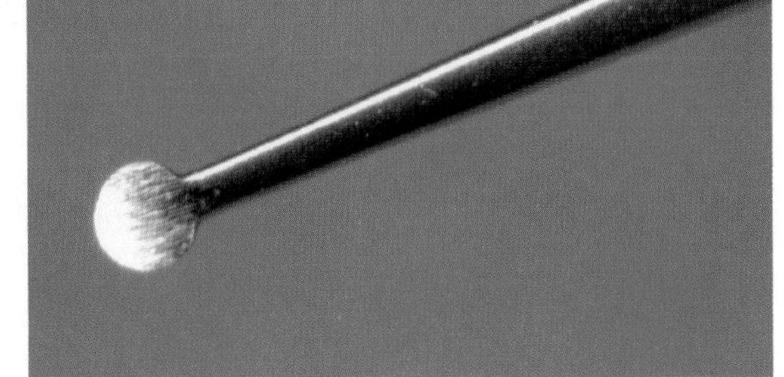

Figure 19-41. O'Hehir Debridement Curet. Close-up view of the disk-shaped working-end of an O'Hehir Debridement curet.

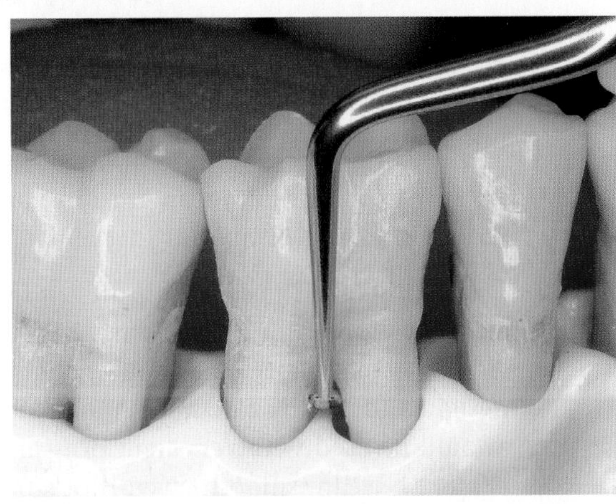

Figure 19-42. Adaptation to a Furcation Area. The tiny disk-shaped working-end of the debridement curet curves toward the tooth surface to adapt to the furcation.

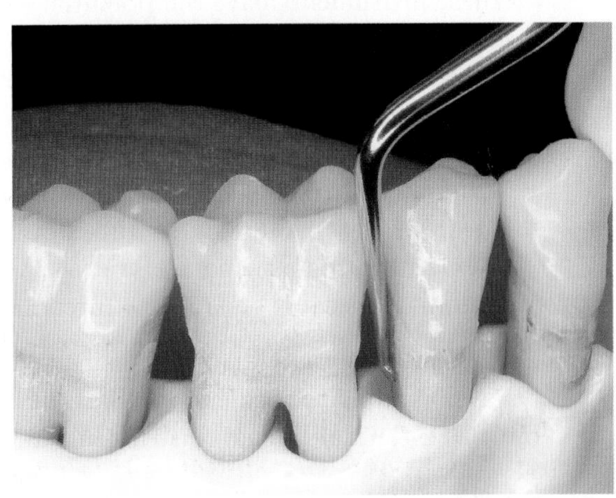

Figure 19-43. Adaptation to a Distal Concavity. The disk-shaped working-end of a debridement curet adapts well to the distal root concavity on the mandibular second premolar.

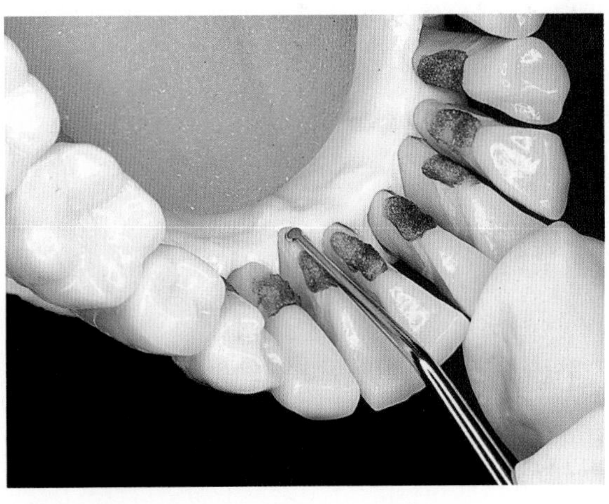

Figure 19-44. Access to the Lingual Surfaces of the Mandibular Anteriors. The O'Hehir 7/8 curet is excellent for adaptation to the lingual surfaces of the mandibular anterior teeth. This instrument features a 15 mm long shank that provides access to the base of even the deepest periodontal pocket.

DIAMOND-COATED INSTRUMENTS

1. **Design Modifications.** The design characteristics of diamond-coated instruments are truly unique:
   a. **No Cutting Edges.** Diamond-coated instruments have no cutting edges; instead, the working-end is coated with a very fine diamond grit. The diamond-coated instruments from Hu-Friedy Manufacturing Company have diamond coating placed 360° around the tip. On the Brasseler USA, G. Hartzell & Son instruments, the diamond coating is placed 180° around the tip; the back of the 180° instrument is smooth for placement against the tissue.
   b. **Pronounced Working-End Curvature.** The working-end design is similar to that of a Nabers furcation probe for easy insertion between the roots of bifurcated and trifurcated teeth.
2. **Uses.** Diamond instruments are used like an emery board to remove small, embedded remnants of calculus that remain on the root surface after instrumentation.
   a. Diamond-coated instruments are finishing instruments for use after deposit removal with other instruments in narrow, inaccessible areas, like furcations.
   b. Used for final debridement and polishing of root surfaces and furcations; not designed for heavy calculus removal.
   c. Should be used with very light pressure and multidirectional strokes to achieve a clean, smooth, even root surface. Caution is indicated because these instruments have the potential to cause overinstrumentation of the root surfaces.
   d. Light strokes in various directions remove the last bits of embedded/burnished calculus from roots in developmental depressions, deep pockets, and furcations. Activation of the instrument is with both a push and pull stroke with very light pressure in a multidirectional fashion.
   e. Ideal for class III furcations and root surfaces on both sides of the furcation area and for debridement of a class IV furcation between the mesiobuccal and distobuccal roots and the furcation roof.
3. **Examples.** Hu-Friedy diamond instruments are the Nabors and the MD (mesial-distal) DiamondTec Scalers; the Brasseler Diamond Files F (fine) series includes the F1/F2 (buccal-lingual) instruments and F3/F4 (mesial-distal) instruments.

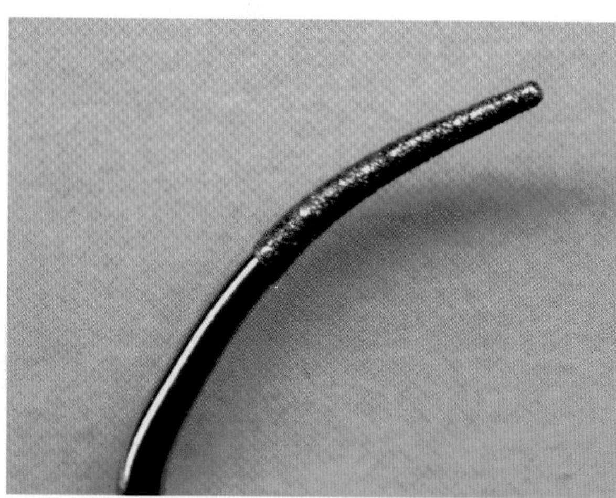

Figure 19-45. Diamond-Coated Instrument. A close-up view of a working-end on an MD DiamondTec scaler. Note the textured coating on the working-end.

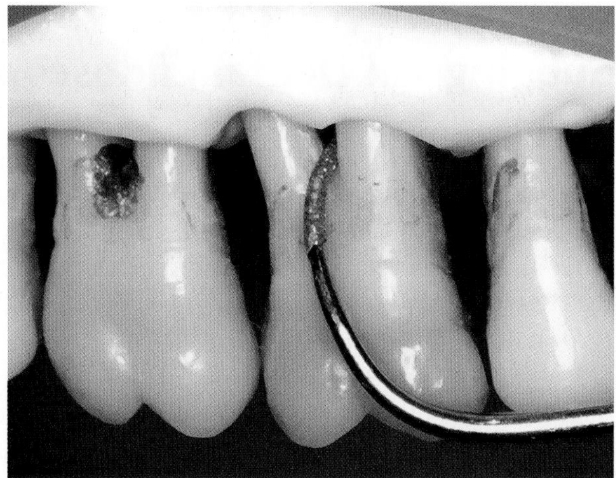

Figure 19-46. Diamond-Coated Instrument in Facial Furcation. The thin, curved working-end of this diamond-coated instrument inserts easily between the distobuccal and mesiobuccal roots of this maxillary first molar.

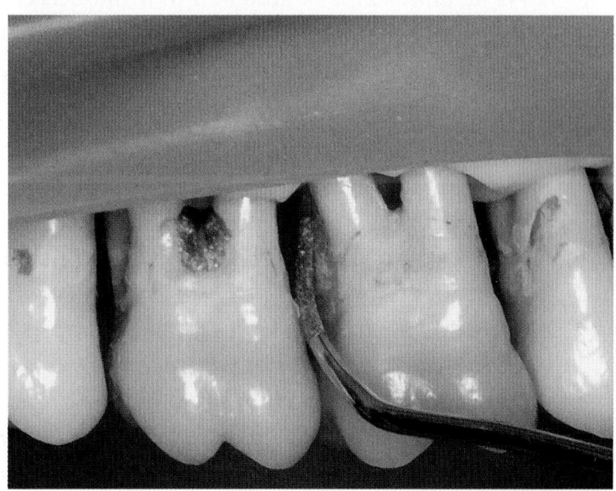

Figure 19-47. Diamond-Coated Instrument. A mesial-distal diamond-coated instrument adapted to the distal root concavity of a maxillary first molar.

Section 6
Subgingival Dental Endoscope

A dental endoscope is a long, flexible tubular device that has a fiber optic light and video camera attached. The endoscope is used to view and examine inside a periodontal pocket. Once inserted in a periodontal pocket, images of the root are transmitted from the endoscope and projected on a flat-screen monitor. First introduced by DentalView, Inc., ownership of the dental endoscope has recently been acquired by Perioscopy Incorporated, Oakland, California.

1. **Description of Dental Endoscope.** The dental endoscope is about 1 m in length and 0.99 mm in diameter (Fig. 19-48). To maintain sterility, a disposable sterile sheath is placed around the endoscope for each patient use.
   - **a.** The dental endoscope allows for subgingival visualization of the root surface at magnifications of 20× to 40×.[4,5]
   - **b.** The endoscope is attached to a flat-screen monitor (Fig. 19-49) that provides a highly magnified picture of subgingival conditions. With the dental endoscope, clinicians actually can see subgingival deposits instead of only detecting deposits with an explorer (Fig. 19-51).
2. **Technique.**
   - **a.** A limitation of the dental endoscope is that the technique takes time and effort to master.[5,6] In his article, "Enhanced Periodontal Debridement with the Use of Micro Ultrasonic, Periodontal Endoscopy,"[5] Dr. John Y. Kwan, President and CEO of Perioscopy Incorporated, describes mastery of the dental endoscope as "*a difficult task to master. It requires a desire to learn, focused attention, lots of practice, and much patience.*"
   - **b.** Dr. Kwan recommends a two-handed technique for use of the dental endoscope.[5] ***For the two-handed technique, the clinician holds the endoscope in the non-dominant hand and an instrument in the dominant hand.*** With this technique, the root surface is viewed and instrumented at the same time (Fig. 19-50).
3. **Recommended Use.** ***The dental endoscope is not recommended for routine subgingival instrumentation because this process would be too time consuming.*** Candidates for endoscopy include patients being treated for sites that did not respond to traditional periodontal instrumentation, patients in whom periodontal surgical therapy is contraindicated, and patients receiving maintenance for chronically inflamed or increasing pockets.[5]

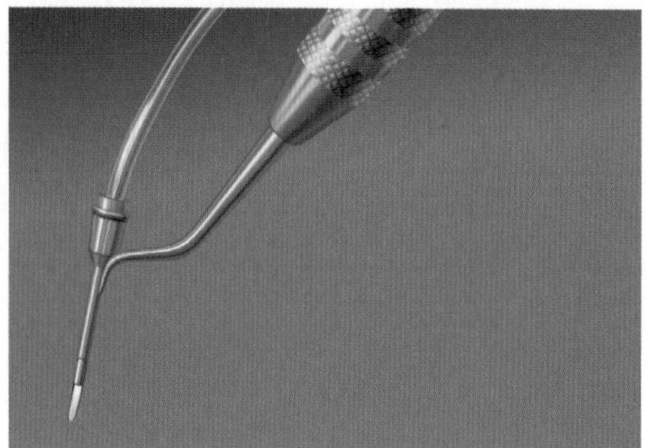

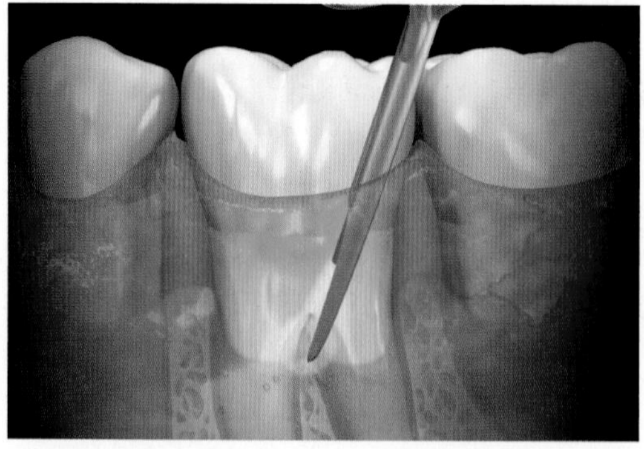

Figure 19-48. Modified Endoscopic Instruments. A modified periodontal instrument is used to guide the endoscope subgingivally. The modified periodontal instruments are about the size of a periodontal probe and are easily inserted into a periodontal pocket.

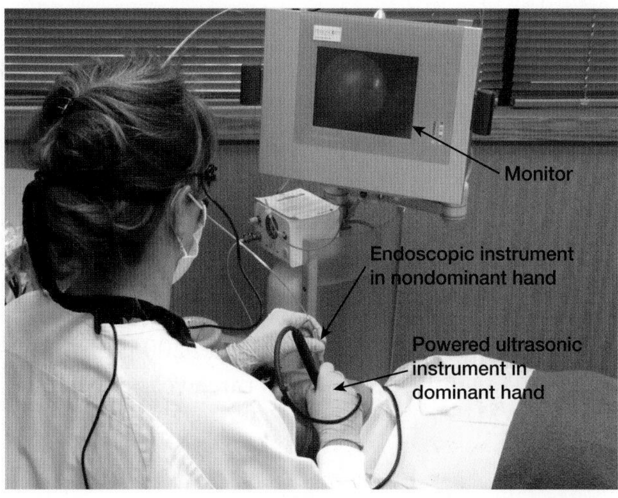

Figure 19-49. Dental Endoscopic System.

- The clinician holds the endoscopic instrument in her nondominant hand.
- In this photo, the clinician uses a powered calculus removal instrument (ultrasonic tip) in her dominant hand.
- Note that the clinician indirectly views the root surface in the monitor, rather than looking in the oral cavity. (Courtesy of John Y. Kwan.)

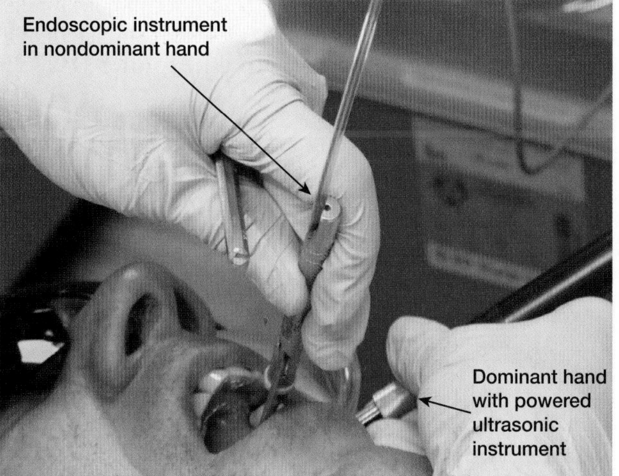

Figure 19-50. Two-Handed Technique. Efficient use of a dental endoscope requires a two-handed technique.

- The clinician uses the dental endoscope with the nondominant hand.
- The periodontal instrument is held in the dominant hand. (Courtesy of John Y. Kwan.)

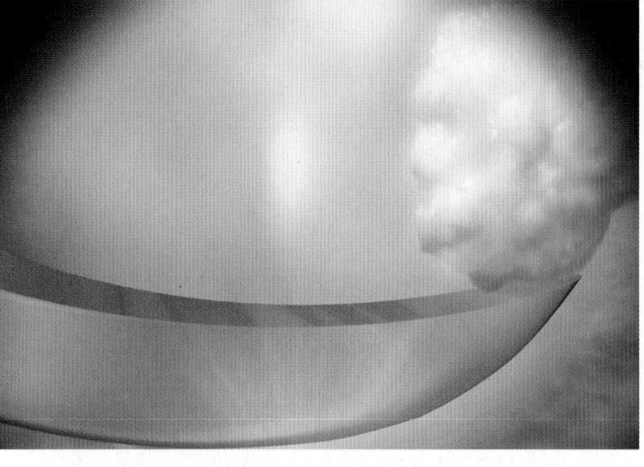

Figure 19-51. Tooth Surface as Seen on Monitor Screen. The endoscope is attached to a flat-screen monitor that provides a highly magnified picture of subgingival conditions. Real-time images of the actual subgingival conditions are displayed on the monitor.

REFERENCES

1. Cobb CM. Clinical significance of non-surgical periodontal therapy: an evidence-based perspective of scaling and root planing. *J Clinical Periodontol.* 2002;29(suppl 2):6–16.
2. Scaramucci M. The versatility of the universal curet. A review of a hand instrumentation staple. *Dimen Dent Hyg.* 2010;8:32, 36, 38.
3. Long B. Hand instrumentation: what are our options? Part 2. *Access.* 2010:35–36.
4. Stambaugh RV, Myers G, Ebling W, Beckman B, Stambaugh K. Endoscopic visualization of the submarginal gingiva dental sulcus and tooth root surfaces. *J Periodontol.* 2002;73:374–382.
5. Kwan JY. Enhanced periodontal debridement with the use of micro ultrasonic, periodontal endoscopy. *J Calif Dental Assoc.* 2005;33:241–248.
6. Stambaugh R. A clinician's three year experience with perioscopy. *Compend Contin Educ Dent.* 2002;23:1061–1070.

Note to Course Instructor: Advanced techniques for instrumentation of root surfaces are covered in Module 20, Advanced Techniques for Root Surface Debridement.

Section 7
Skill Application

PRACTICAL FOCUS: FICTITIOUS PATIENT CASE, MRS. JEFFERSON

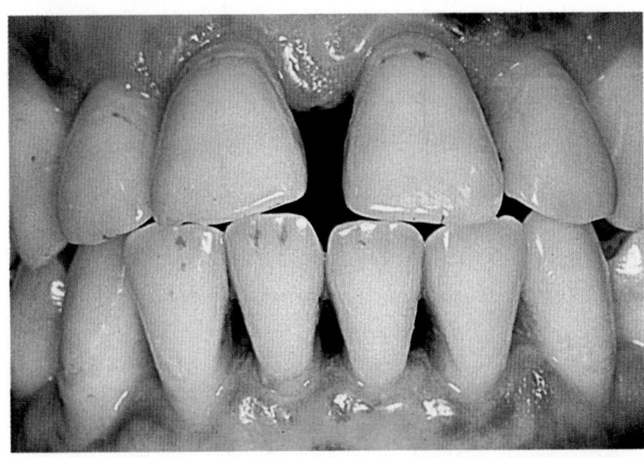

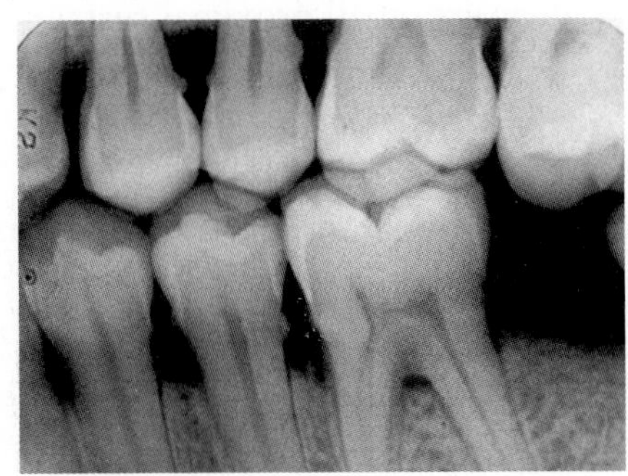

Figure 19-52. Intraoral Photo and Radiograph for Mrs. Jefferson.

Lingual

	24	23	22	21	20	19	18	17
Probe Depth	3 3 3	3 2 3	3 2 3	5 6 6	6 6 6	7 6 6		
GM to CEJ	+1 +1 +1	+2 +2 +2	+2 +4 +2	+1 0 0	0 0 0	0 0 0		
Attachment Loss								

24 23 22 21 20 19 18 17 (L)

Facial

	24	23	22	21	20	19	18	17
Probe Depth	3 2 3	2 2 2	2 1 3	4 5 5	5 5 5	6 5 5		
GM to CEJ	+1 +1 +1	+2 +2 +2	+2 +4 +2	+1 0 0	0 0 0	0 0 0		
Attachment Loss								
Mobility								

Figure 19-53. Periodontal Chart for Mrs. Jefferson.
(Key: GM = gingival margin; CEJ = cementoenamel junction.)

Mrs. Jefferson: Assessment Data

1. Generalized bleeding upon probing.
2. **Deposits.**
   a. Moderate supragingival plaque on all teeth.
   b. Supragingival calculus deposits—light calculus on lingual surfaces of the mandibular anteriors and molar teeth.
   c. Subgingival calculus deposits—small-sized deposits on all teeth; medium-sized deposits on all proximal surfaces.

Mrs. Jefferson: Case Questions

1. *Use the information recorded on Mrs. Jefferson's periodontal chart to calculate the clinical attachment loss on the facial and lingual aspects for teeth 19 to 24 and enter this information on her periodontal chart in Figure 19-53.*
2. Is there mobility or furcation involvement present on Mrs. Jefferson's periodontal chart? If so, which teeth are involved, and what is the extent of the mobility and/or furcation involvement?
3. Do the assessment data indicate normal bone levels or bone loss in this quadrant? Do the assessment data indicate healthy sulci or periodontal pockets in this quadrant? Explain which data you used to make these determinations.
4. The gingival margin is located at the cementoenamel junction for teeth 19 and 20. There is no gingival recession present on these teeth. Does the location of the gingival margin make the instrumentation of these teeth more difficult or less difficult?
5. Do you expect to encounter any root concavities or furcation involvement while instrumenting the teeth in this quadrant? If so, indicate which teeth will probably have root concavities and/or furcation areas to be instrumented.
6. Based on the assessment information, select explorer(s), probe(s), and calculus removal instruments that would be appropriate for instrumentation of this quadrant. List the instruments you would select and explain your rationale for instrument selection.

Module 20

Advanced Techniques for Root Surface Debridement

Module Overview

Treating root surfaces located within deep periodontal pockets is challenging, especially on maxillary posterior teeth. Advanced fulcruming techniques can facilitate access and adaptation to these root surfaces. Instrumentation of root surfaces within deep periodontal pockets is further complicated by root surface anatomy including root concavities, fissures, and furcation areas. This module presents advanced fulcruming techniques and strategies for debridement of root surfaces.

Module Outline

Key Terms

Cross arch fulcrum
Opposite arch fulcrum
Finger-on-finger fulcrum
"Palm facing out" technique
"Chin-cup" technique
Instrumentation stroke with a finger assist

Learning Objectives

1. Select instruments that are appropriate for root instrumentation in the presence of attachment loss.
2. Discuss anatomical features that complicate the instrumentation of root surfaces in the presence of attachment loss.
3. Demonstrate each of the following advanced intraoral fulcrums on a periodontal typodont in an appropriate sextant of the dentition for the fulcrum: finger-on-finger intraoral, cross arch, and opposite arch, and instrumentation strokes with a finger assist technique.
4. Demonstrate each of the following extraoral fulcrums on a periodontal typodont in an appropriate sextant of the dentition for the fulcrum: extraoral "palm facing out" technique, extraoral "chin-cup" technique, and instrumentation strokes with a finger assist technique.

5. Select the correct working-end of an area-specific curet for use with horizontal strokes in mesial and distal root concavities (toe-down or toe-up positions).
6. Demonstrate horizontal strokes in a proximal root concavity on an acrylic tooth or periodontal typodont and explain the rationale for using horizontal strokes in concavities.
7. Demonstrate horizontal strokes in the facial concavity located between the cementoenamel junction and furcation area of multirooted teeth and explain the rationale for using horizontal strokes in this area.
8. Demonstrate horizontal strokes at the distofacial and distolingual line angles on acrylic teeth or periodontal typodont and explain the rationale for using horizontal strokes at line angles.
9. Demonstrate instrumentation of the furcation area on a mandibular first molar on an acrylic tooth or periodontal typodont.
10. Demonstrate instrumentation of the furcations on a maxillary first molar from the facial aspect. Instrument only those furcations that are best accessed from the facial aspect.
11. Demonstrate instrumentation of the furcations on a maxillary first molar from the lingual aspect. Instrument only those furcations that are best accessed from the lingual aspect.

Section 1
Introduction to Root Instrumentation

ANATOMICAL FEATURES THAT COMPLICATE ROOT INSTRUMENTATION

Root surface morphology can greatly complicate instrumentation, especially when the roots are hidden from view within deep periodontal pockets. These anatomical features include root concavities and depressions and, occasionally, root fissures (Fig. 20-1).

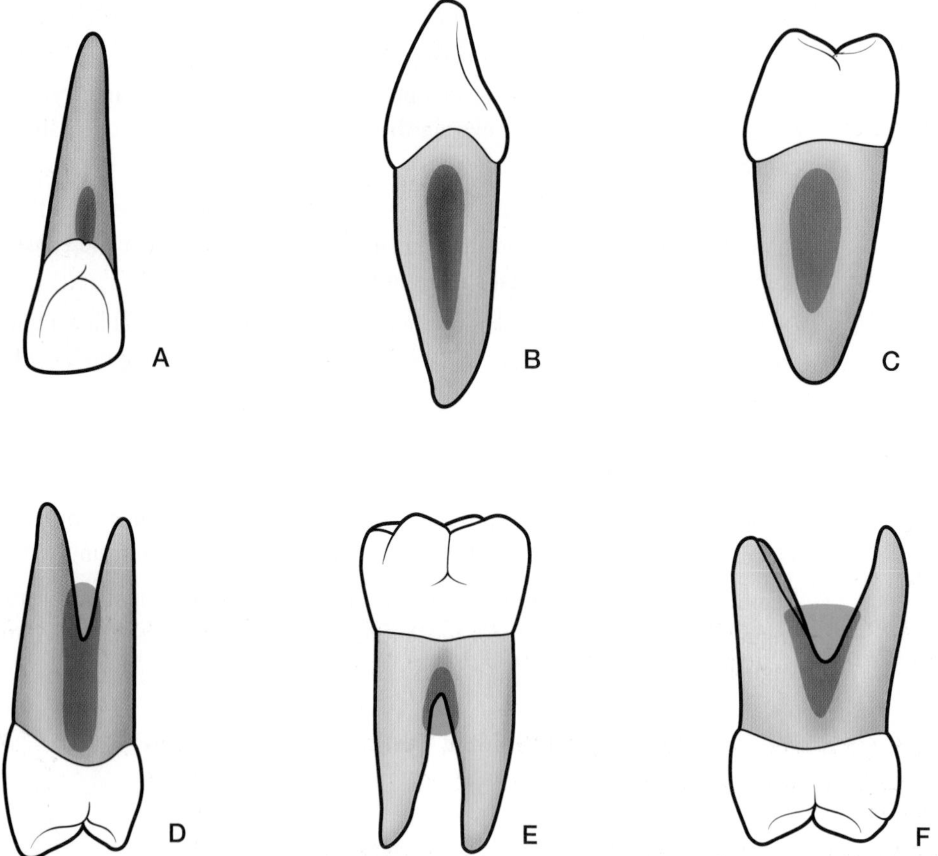

Figure 20-1. Root Concavities, Depressions, and Grooves. Examples of root surface morphology (shaded areas) that can hinder instrumentation of root surfaces.

- **A.** ***Palatal groove*** on mandibular lateral incisor that extends onto the cervical-third of the root surface.
- **B.** ***Deep linear root concavities*** on the proximal surfaces of mandibular canine.
- **C.** ***Wide shallow root concavity*** on the mesial surface of mandibular molar.
- **D.** ***Deep linear proximal root concavities* and *furcation*** on maxillary first premolar.
- **E.** ***Deep depression on root trunk* and *furcation*** on mandibular molar.
- **F.** ***Proximal concavities*** extending from the furcation to cementoenamel junction (CEJ) on maxillary molar.

ROOT FURCATIONS

Instrumentation is complicated on molar teeth when furcation areas are exposed due to bone loss. Furcation exposure can be encountered in pockets as shallow as 4 mm in depth. Gher and Vernino[1] demonstrated that furcations could be located at as little as 3 mm from the CEJ (Table 20-1).

TABLE 20-1. Location of Furcations

Tooth	Roots	Furcation	Distance from CEJ
Maxillary first premolar	2	Mid-mesial	7 mm
		Mid-distal	7 mm
Mandibular molar	2	Mid-facial	3 mm
		Mid-lingual	4 mm
Maxillary molar	3	Mid-facial	4 mm
		Mesial toward lingual	3 mm
		Mid-distal	5 mm

INSTRUMENTATION SEQUENCE ON MULTIROOTED TEETH

Successful debridement of a multirooted tooth is dependent on a systematic approach to instrumentation. A recommended approach is summarized in Figure 20-2.

Figure 20-2. Sequence for Instrumenting Multirooted Teeth. Follow the steps below when using an area-specific curet to instrument a root.

1. Debride the root trunk using the distal curet and then mesial curet.
2. Treat each root as a separate tooth. Use the distal curet on the distal portion of each root.
3. Use the mesial curet on the mesial portions of each root.
4. Treat the roof of the furcation and the concavity coronal to the furcation entrance with the mesial curet.
   - Use the toe of the curet against the roof of the furcation on a mandibular tooth.
   - Position the curet in a toe-down position, and use horizontal strokes in the concavity.

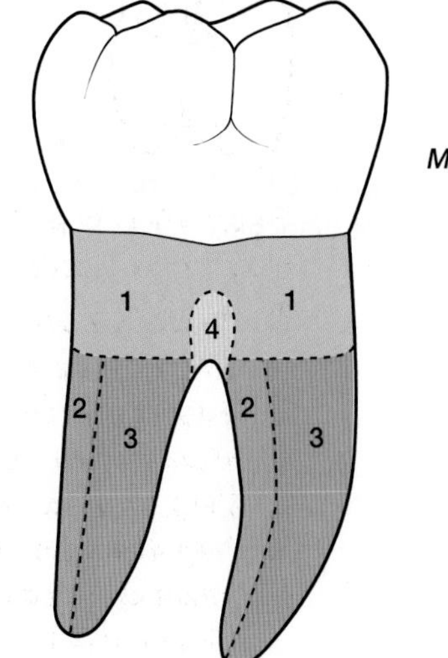

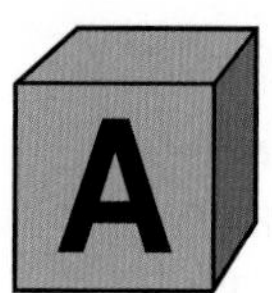

SKILL BUILDING. BASIC INSTRUMENTATION OF MULTIROOTED TEETH

Periodontal debridement is complicated when furcation areas, root concavities, and multiple roots have been exposed due to the loss of alveolar bone. With multirooted teeth, the best approach is to instrument each root as a separate tooth. For example, imagine that the two roots of a mandibular molar tooth are the single roots of two premolar teeth. A combination of vertical, horizontal, and oblique strokes is used for root instrumentation.

STEP-BY-STEP TECHNIQUE ON MULTIROOTED TEETH

Directions. Miniature area-specific curets with extended shanks and a periodontal typodont or acrylic tooth model are recommended for this technique practice. Follow steps 1 to 7 in Figures 20-3 to 20-9 to practice instrumentation on root surfaces.

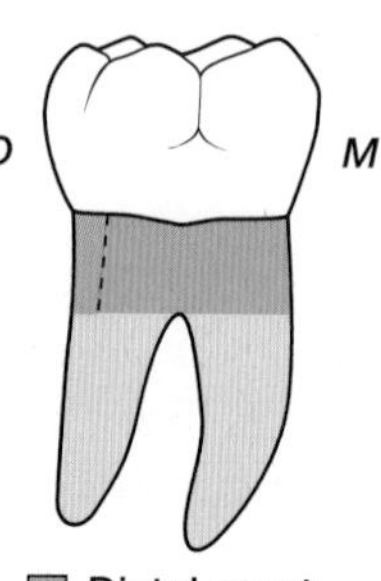

1. **Figure 20-3. Begin with the Root Trunk.** Debride the root trunk using the distal curet on the distal surface and the mesial curet on the facial and mesial surfaces.

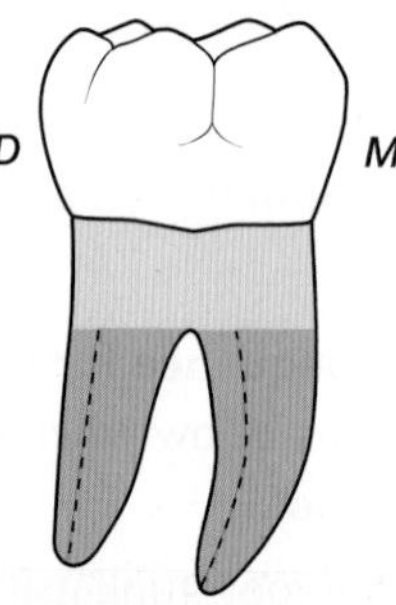

2. **Figure 20-4. Instrument the Root Branches.** Treat each root branch as if it were the root of a single-rooted tooth.

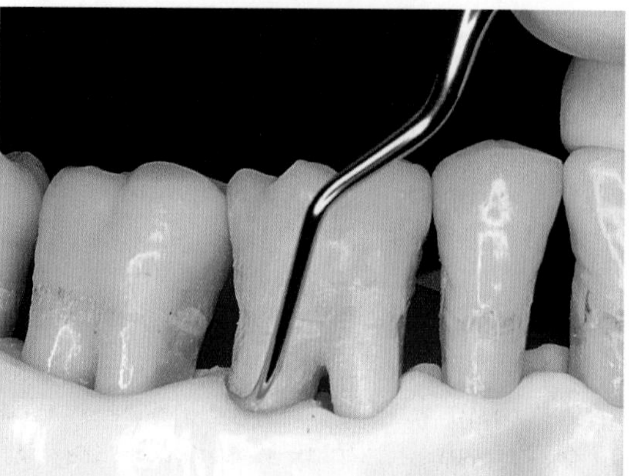

3. **Figure 20-5. Distal Portion of Distal Root.** Use the ***distal*** curet to instrument the distal portion of the distal root, beginning at the line angle.

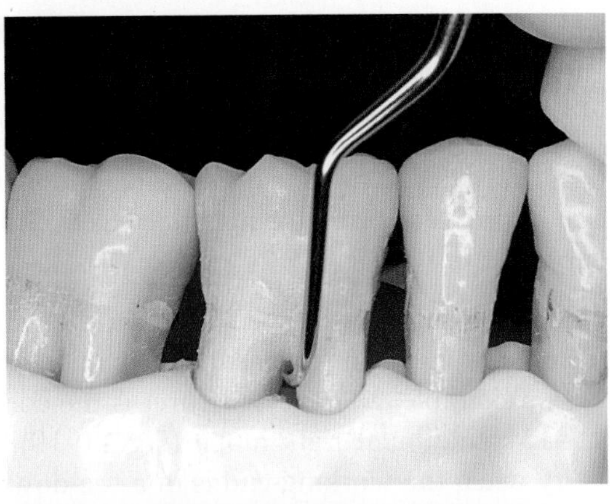

4. **Figure 20-6. Distal Portion of Mesial Root.** Using the ***distal*** curet, instrument the distal portion of the mesial root.

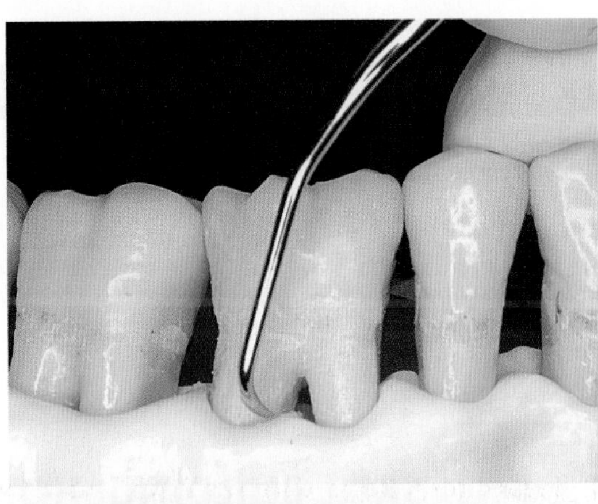

5. **Figure 20-7. Mesial Portion of Distal Root.** Beginning at the line angle, use the ***mesial*** curet to debride the mesial portion of the distal root.

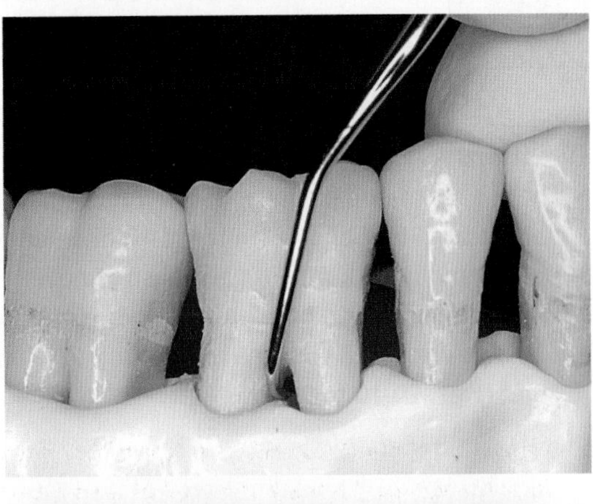

6. **Figure 20-8. Furcation**. Instrument the mesial side of the furcation using the ***mesial*** curet.

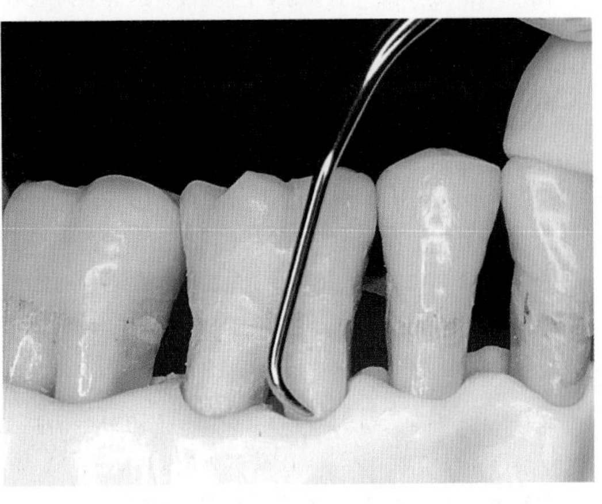

7. **Figure 20-9. Mesial Portion of Mesial Root.** Use the ***mesial*** curet to debride the mesial portion of the mesial root and the mesial surface of the root.

USE OF HORIZONTAL STROKES IN ROOT CONCAVITIES

Horizontal strokes are helpful when instrumenting proximal root concavities on the mesial and distal surfaces of roots. The working-end is used in a toe-down position for mandibular teeth and a top-up position for maxillary teeth. In this position, the working-end fits nicely in the root depression.

- When using an area-specific curet, the working-end selection for a horizontal stroke requires some thought on the part of the clinician (Box 20-1).
- For example, a Gracey 11 curet is the correct working-end for vertical strokes on the mesial root of a mandibular right molar (Fig. 20-10). The Gracey 12 curet adapts to the mesial root concavity when the working-end is in a toe-down position for a horizontal stroke (Fig. 20-11)

Box 20-1. Horizontal Strokes on Proximal Surfaces

Switch working-ends to make horizontal strokes on either the distal or mesial surface of a tooth.

- For distal surfaces, if the G13 is used for vertical strokes, use the G14 for horizontal strokes.
- For mesial surfaces, if the G11 is used for vertical strokes, use the G12 for horizontal strokes.

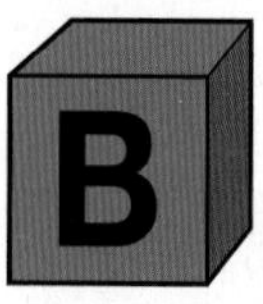

SKILL BUILDING. HORIZONTAL STROKES IN ROOT CONCAVITIES

Directions:

- For this technique practice, you will need (1) a periodontal typodont or an acrylic mandibular molar, (2) Gracey 11/12 and 13/14 standard or extended shank curets, (3) a container of brightly colored nail polish, and (4) a bottle of nail polish remover.
- On each working-end, paint the ***lower cutting edge and its lateral surface*** with nail polish.
- Follow steps 1 to 3 to practice selecting the correct working-end for horizontal strokes with an area-specific curet (Figs. 20-10 to 20-12).

1. **Figure 20-10. Vertical Strokes on Mesial Root Surface.**
   - *Adapt the Gracey 11 curet to the mesial surface of a mandibular right molar in position for a VERTICAL stroke.*
   - Note that the lower cutting edge with the nail polish is adapted against the mesial surface.
   - *The Gracey 11 is the correct working-end for making vertical strokes across the mesial surface.*

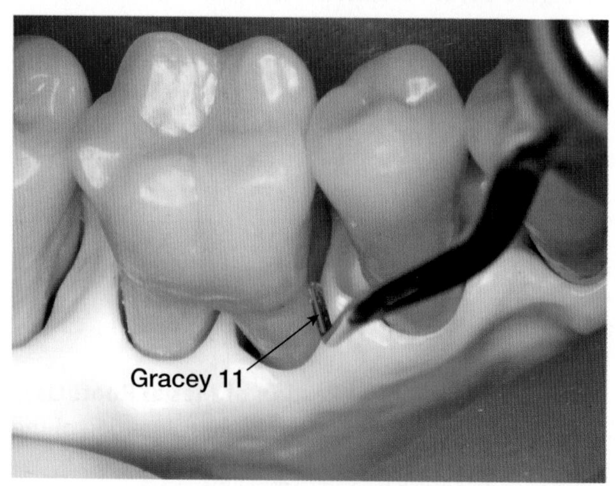

2. **Figure 20-11. Horizontal Strokes on the Mesial Proximal Surface.**
    - ***Next, position the Gracey 12 in a toe-down position for a HORIZONTAL stroke and adapt it to the mesial surface.***
    - *The correct working-end is the Gracey 12 when making horizontal strokes on the mesial proximal surface of the mandibular right molar from the facial aspect.*

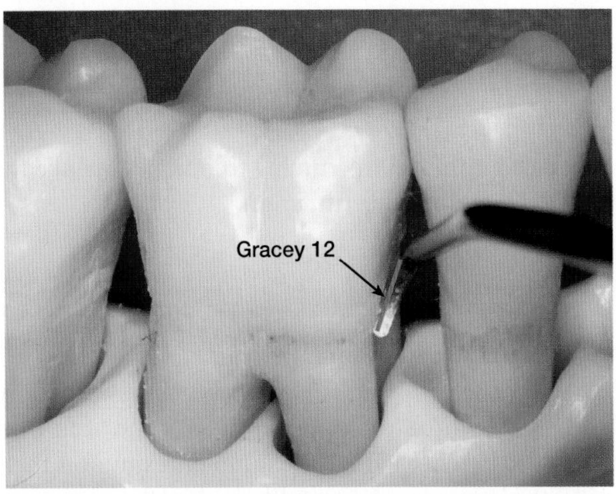

3. **Figure 20-12. Horizontal Strokes on the Distal Proximal Surface.**
    - Select the correct working-end of a Gracey 13/14 curet for use on the distal surface when making vertical strokes.
    - ***For VERTICAL strokes, the correct curet is the Gracey 14.***
    - *For HORIZONTAL strokes, the correct working-end is the Gracey 13 on the distal proximal surface of the mandibular right molar from the facial aspect.*

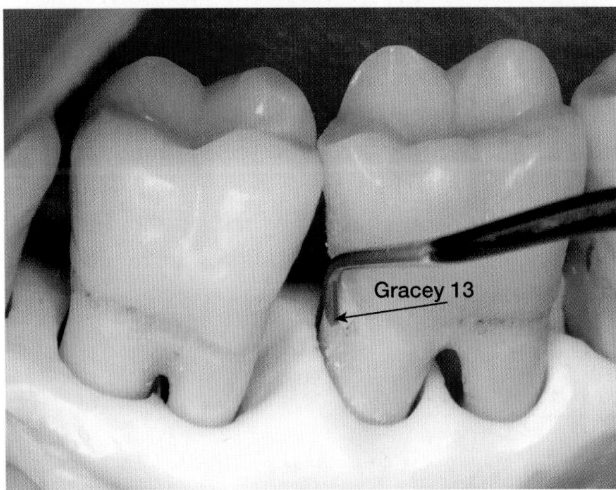

Section 2
Advanced Intraoral Techniques for Root Debridement

Advanced intraoral fulcruming techniques include the (1) cross arch fulcrum, (2) opposite arch fulcrum, and (3) finger-on-finger fulcrum.

CROSS ARCH AND OPPOSITE ARCH FULCRUMS

1. **Cross Arch Intraoral Fulcrum**
   a. The cross arch fulcrum is accomplished by resting the ring finger on a tooth on the opposite side of the arch from the teeth being instrumented (Fig. 20-13)—for example, resting on the left side of the mandible to instrument a mandibular right molar.
   b. ***Cross arch fulcrums are most useful when using horizontal strokes in proximal root concavities with the curet in either a toe-up or toe-down position.***
2. **Opposite Arch Intraoral Fulcrum**
   a. The opposite arch fulcrum is an advanced fulcrum used to improve access to deep pockets and to facilitate parallelism to proximal root surfaces (Fig. 20-14).
   b. It is accomplished by resting the ring finger on the opposite arch from the treatment area (e.g., resting on the mandibular arch to instrument maxillary teeth).

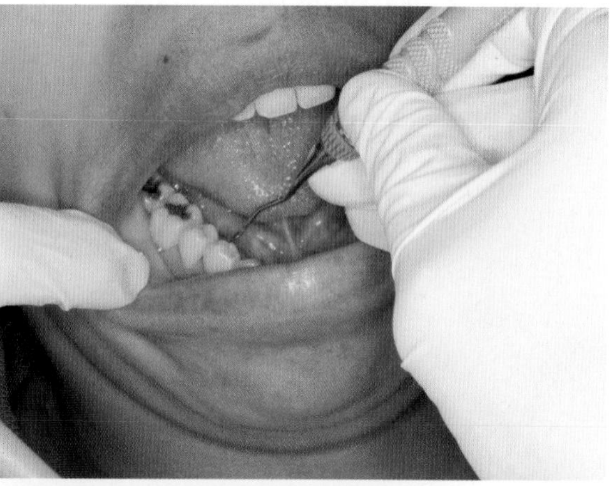

Figure 20-13. Cross Arch Fulcrum. The photograph shows a cross arch fulcrum demonstrated by a right-handed clinician. The clinician fulcrums on the mandibular left premolars while instrumenting the lingual aspect of the mandibular right posteriors.

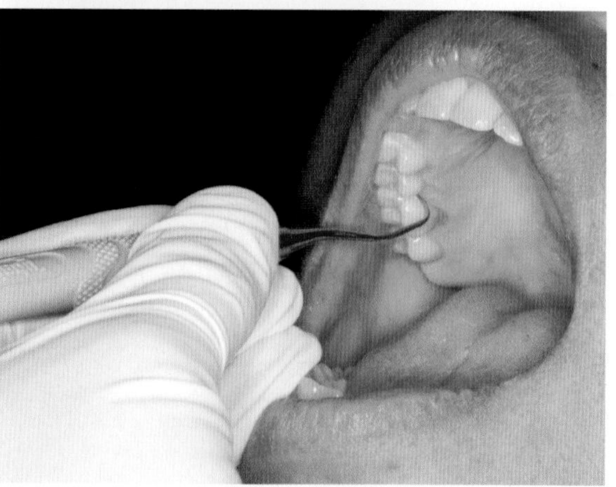

Figure 20-14. Opposite Arch Fulcrum. In this example, an opposite arch fulcrum is being used on the mandibular anterior teeth.

FINGER-ON-FINGER FULCRUM

The finger-on-finger fulcrum is accomplished by resting the ring finger of the dominant hand on a finger of the ***nondominant*** hand.

- This technique allows the clinician to fulcrum in line with the long axis of the tooth to improve parallelism of the lower shank to the tooth surface.
- The nondominant index finger provides a stable rest for the clinician's dominant hand and provides improved access to deep periodontal pockets.
- Figures 20-15 to 20-17 depict a finger-on-finger fulcrum for the maxillary right posterior teeth, maxillary left posterior teeth, and mandibular left posterior teeth.

Example 1: Maxillary Right Posteriors, Facial Aspect

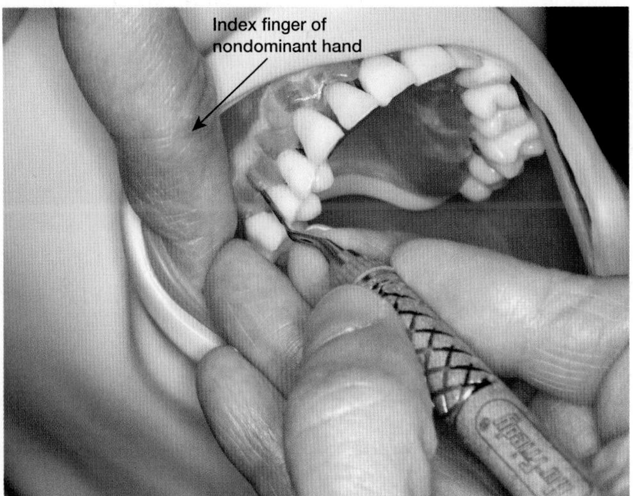

Figure 20-15A. Finger-on-Finger Fulcrum for the Maxillary Right Posteriors, Facial Aspect.

- In this example, the ***right-handed clinician*** establishes a finger rest on the index finger of the nondominant hand.
- The index finger of the nondominant hand is positioned in the mucobuccal fold, resting against the attached gingiva, alveolar mucosa, and underlying alveolar bone.

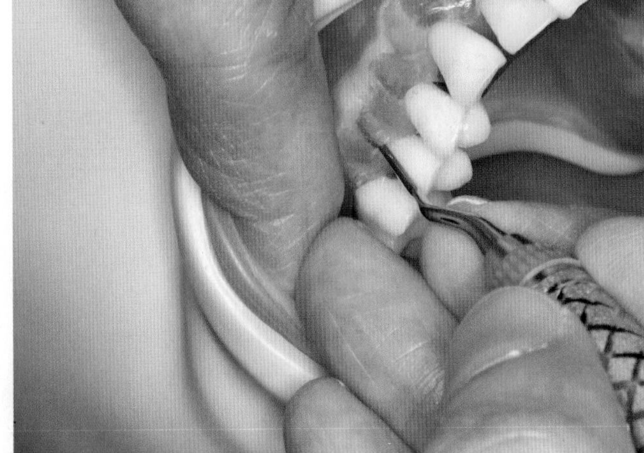

Figure 20-15B. Close-up View: Finger-on-Finger Fulcrum for the Maxillary Right Posteriors, Facial Aspect. This photograph provides a closer view of the finger-on-finger fulcrum shown above in Figure 20-15A.

Example 2: Maxillary Left Posteriors, Facial Aspect

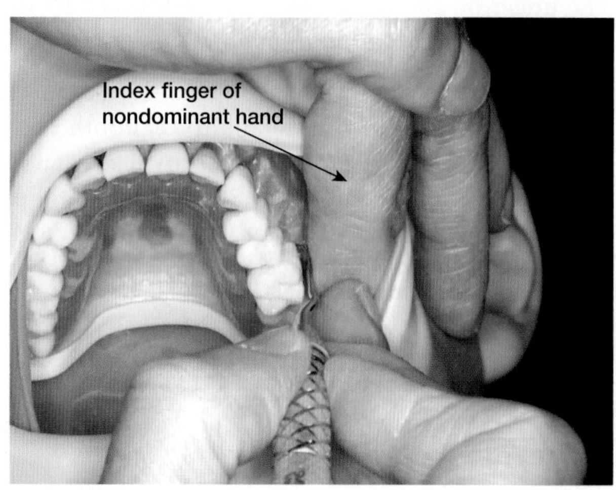

Figure 20-16A. Finger-on-Finger Fulcrum for the Maxillary Left Posteriors, Facial Aspect.

- In this example, the ***right-handed clinician*** establishes a finger rest on the index finger of the nondominant hand.
- The index finger of the nondominant hand is positioned in the mucobuccal fold, resting against the attached gingiva, alveolar mucosa, and underlying alveolar bone.

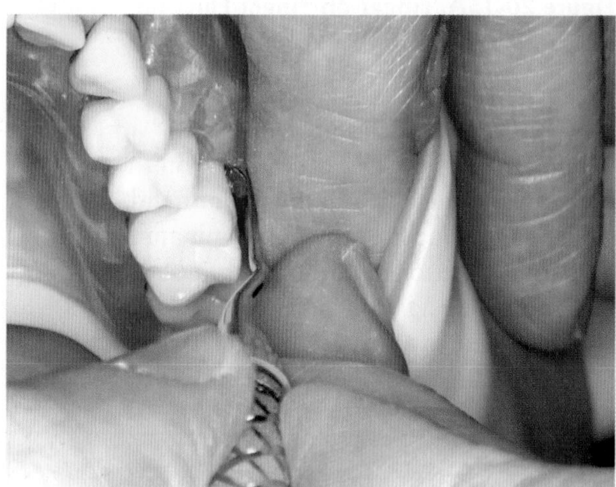

Figure 20-16B. Close-up View: Finger-on-Finger Fulcrum for the Maxillary Right Posteriors, Facial Aspect. This photograph provides a closer view of the finger-on-finger fulcrum shown above in Figure 20-16A.

Example 3: Mandibular Left Posteriors, Facial Aspect

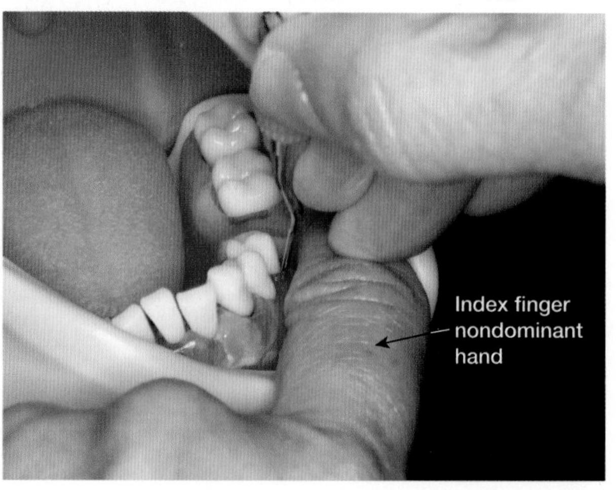

Figure 20-17. Finger-on-Finger Fulcrum for the Mandibular Left Posteriors, Facial Aspect.

- In this example, the ***right-handed clinician*** establishes a finger rest on the index finger of the nondominant hand.
- The index finger of the nondominant hand is positioned in the mucobuccal fold, resting against the attached gingiva, alveolar mucosa, and underlying alveolar bone.

Section 3
Extraoral Fulcruming Techniques

There are times when it is difficult to obtain parallelism with the lower shank or to adapt the cutting edge when using a standard intraoral fulcrum. In instances when a standard intraoral fulcrum does not seem to work well, an advanced extraoral fulcruming technique can improve access to the tooth surface.

1. **When to Use an Advanced Extraoral Fulcrum.** Advanced extraoral fulcrums are required when working in a deep periodontal pocket, especially when instrumenting the maxillary posterior teeth. Advanced extraoral fulcrums facilitate:
   a. **Proper Adaptation.** Advanced extraoral fulcrums facilitate positioning of the lower shank of a Gracey extended shank curet so that the extended shank is parallel to the root surface to be instrumented.
   b. **Complete Coverage with Instrumentation Strokes.** Advanced extraoral fulcrums facilitate insertion of the curet working-end all the way to the base of a deep periodontal pocket. Insertion to the base of a deep pocket allows the clinician to cover every millimeter of the root surface with instrumentation strokes.
2. **Considerations and Cautions for Use of Advanced Extraoral Fulcrums**
   a. **Clinician Skill Level.** Advanced extraoral fulcruming techniques require greater clinician skill and psychomotor control.
      1. Before attempting advanced fulcruming techniques, the clinician should have mastered the fundamentals of neutral position and standard fulcruming technique.
         a. Bad habits with fundamental techniques and intraoral fulcrums cannot be corrected by the use of advanced fulcrums.
         b. *A clinician with poor skill attainment of fundamental techniques will compound his or her problems by attempting to use advanced fulcrums. Unorthodox methods of instrumentation may serve as a quick fix for achieving an end product, but usually at the expense of the clinician's musculoskeletal system.*
      2. Before attempting advanced fulcruming techniques, the student should self-evaluate his or her skill level with a standard intraoral fulcrum and request a critique from an instructor.
   b. **Selective Use of Advanced Extraoral Fulcrums**
      1. *Advanced fulcruming techniques are NOT intended to replace the intraoral fulcrum.* Intraoral fulcrums provide the best stability for instrumentation. An advanced extraoral fulcrum should be used if an intraoral fulcrum is not effective or possible.
      2. *Advanced fulcrums should be used selectively in areas of limited access and/or in order to maintain neutral body position.*

MAXILLARY POSTERIOR TEETH WITH DEEP POCKETS

An intraoral fulcrum usually is effective in most treatment areas of the mouth. One exception is maxillary posterior teeth with deep periodontal pockets. Within a deep periodontal pocket, an intraoral fulcrum makes it difficult to position the lower shank of an extended Gracey curet parallel to the root surface. An effective intraoral fulcrum requires the clinician's fingers to be positioned so that the index, middle, and ring fingers are in contact and the use of wrist motion activation. This technique is effective for normal sulci and shallow periodontal pockets on the maxillary molar teeth. Unfortunately, the intraoral fulcrum makes it difficult to effectively instrument deep periodontal pockets on the maxillary teeth. The solution to the problem of instrumentation of maxillary posterior teeth with deep periodontal pockets is to use an advanced extraoral fulcrum. Table 20-2 summarizes the advantages and disadvantages of extraoral fulcruming techniques.

TABLE 20-2. Advantages and Disadvantages of Extraoral Fulcruming Techniques

Advantages	Disadvantages
• Easier access to maxillary second and third molars	• Require a greater degree of muscle coordination and instrumentation skill to achieve calculus removal
• Easier access to deep pockets on molar teeth	• Greater risk for instrument stick
• Improved parallelism of the lower shank to molar teeth	• Reduce tactile information to the fingers
• Facilitate neutral wrist position for molar teeth	• Not well tolerated by patients with temporomandibular joint problems

BASIC EXTRAORAL FULCRUMING TECHNIQUES: RIGHT-HANDED CLINICIANS

Basic extraoral fulcruming techniques involve resting the fingers or palm of the hand against the patient's chin or cheeks and underlying bone of the mandible.

The "Palm Facing Out" Extraoral Technique for Maxillary Right Posterior Sextants

When working on the maxillary right posterior sextants, the clinician rests the fingers against the patient's chin. The "palm-facing out" technique involves resting the front surfaces of the middle, ring, and little fingers against the skin and underlying bone of the mandibular arch (Fig. 20-18). The fingers should remain straight—not curved like a fist—and together in the grasp. As much of the length of the fingers as possible should be kept in contact with the mandible.

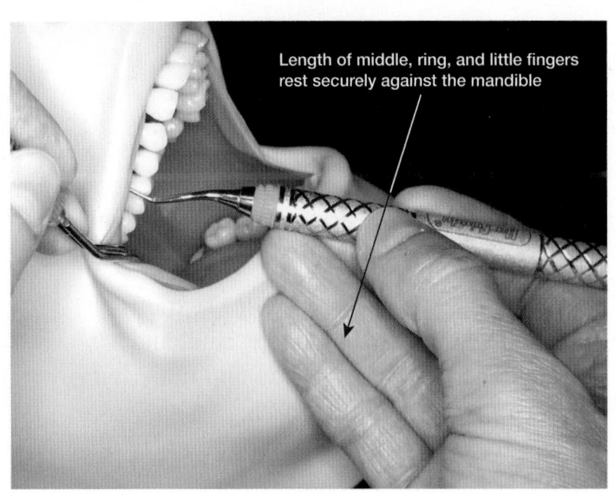
Length of middle, ring, and little fingers rest securely against the mandible

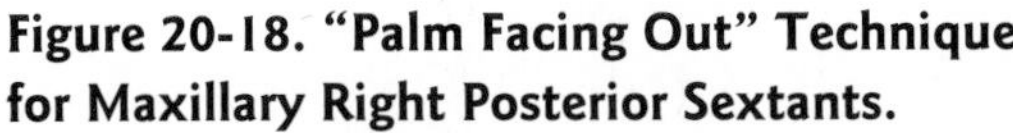

Figure 20-18. "Palm Facing Out" Technique for Maxillary Right Posterior Sextants.

- For the maxillary right posterior sextants, the clinician rests the middle, ring, and little fingers against the skin and underlying bone of the mandibular arch.
- Note that the palm is facing out, away from the patient's face.

The "Chin-Cup" Extraoral Technique for Maxillary Left Posterior Sextants

When working on the maxillary left posterior sextants, the patient's chin and mandible are cupped with the palm of the clinician's hand in the "chin-cup" technique (Fig. 20-19).

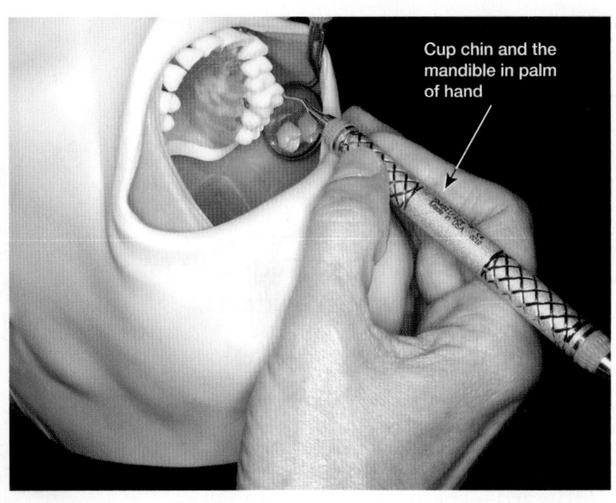
Cup chin and the mandible in palm of hand

Figure 20-19. "Chin-Cup" Technique for Maxillary Left Posterior Sextants.

- For the maxillary left posterior sextants, the clinician cups the patient's chin and mandible with the palm of his or her hand.
- Note that the palm of the hand is against—toward—the patient's mandible.

BASIC EXTRAORAL FULCRUMING TECHNIQUES: LEFT-HANDED CLINICIANS

Basic extraoral fulcruming techniques involve resting the fingers or palm of the hand against the patient's chin or cheeks and underlying bone of the mandible.

The "Palm Facing Out" Extraoral Technique for Maxillary Left Posterior Sextants

When working on the maxillary left posterior sextants, the clinician cups the mandible in the palm of his or her hand. The "palm facing out" technique involves resting the front surfaces of the middle, ring, and little fingers against the skin and underlying bone of the mandibular arch (Fig. 20-20). The fingers should remain straight—not curved like a fist—and together in the grasp. As much of the length of the fingers as possible should be kept in contact with the mandible.

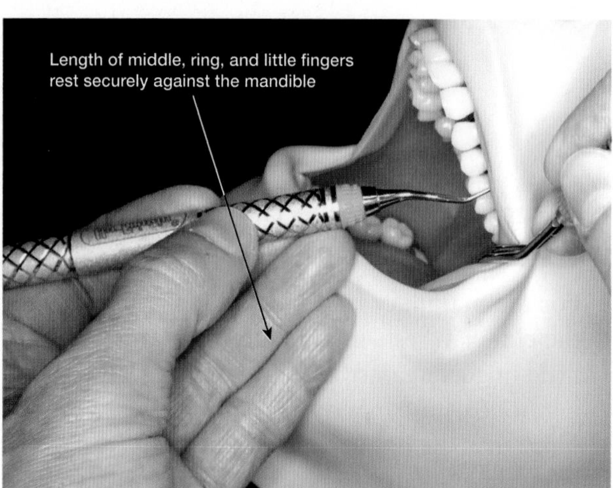
Length of middle, ring, and little fingers rest securely against the mandible

Figure 20-20. "Palm Facing Out" Technique for Maxillary Left Posterior Sextants.

- For the maxillary left posterior sextants, the clinician rests the middle, ring, and little fingers against the skin and underlying bone of the mandibular arch.
- Note that the palm is facing out, away from the patient's face.

The "Chin-Cup" Extraoral Technique for Maxillary Right Posterior Sextants

When working on the maxillary right posterior sextants, the patient's chin and mandible are cupped with the palm of the clinician's hand (Fig. 20-21).

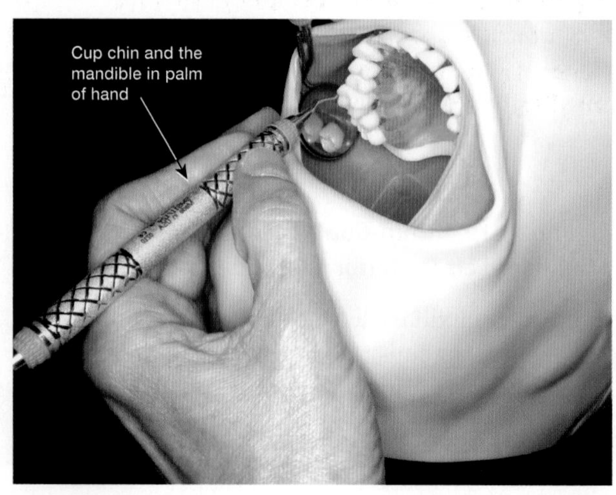
Cup chin and the mandible in palm of hand

Figure 20-21. "Chin-Cup" Technique for Maxillary Right Posterior Sextants.

- For the maxillary right posterior sextants, the clinician cups the patient's chin and mandible with the palm of his or her hand.
- Note that the palm of the hand is against—toward—the patient's mandible.

CRITERIA FOR AN EFFECTIVE EXTRAORAL FULCRUM

Effective fulcruming technique for an extraoral fulcrum differs from that of an intraoral fulcrum in two important ways. These technique differences involve the instrument grasp and the technique used to stabilize the hand. Table 20-3 summarizes the techniques used for each type of finger rest. Figure 20-22 shows the modified grasp used with an extraoral fulcrum.

TABLE 20-3. Technique Comparison for Intraoral and Extraoral Fulcrums

	Intraoral Fulcrum	Extraoral Fulcrum
Grasp	• Handle held in a modified pen grasp near the junction of the handle and the shank, close to the working-end	• Handle grasped lower on the handle, farther away from the working-end (Fig. 20-22)
Stabilization	• Pad of ring finger rests securely on a stable tooth • Ringer finger acts as a "support beam" for the hand • Middle, ring, and little fingers are in contact acting as a unit	• Lengths of middle, ring, and little fingers rest securely against the skin and underlying bone of the mandible • All three fingers press against the mandible; one-finger contact is not effective • Middle, ring, and little fingers are in contact acting as a unit

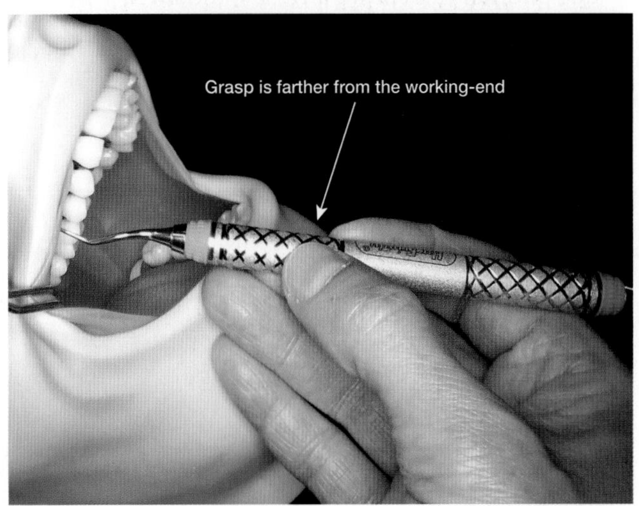

Figure 20-22. Grasp for Extraoral Fulcrum. The clinician should grasp the instrument handle farther away from the working-end for an effective extraoral fulcruming technique.

MODIFICATIONS TO BASIC EXTRAORAL FULCRUMS: INSTRUMENTATION STROKE WITH A FINGER ASSIST

An instrumentation stroke with a finger assist is accomplished by using the index finger of the nondominant hand ***against the shank of a periodontal instrument to assist in the instrumentation stroke*** (Figs. 20-23 to 20-25).

- For this advanced technique, the index finger of the nondominant hand is placed against the instrument shank to (1) concentrate lateral pressure against the tooth surface and (2) help control the working-end throughout the instrumentation stroke.
- The *instrumentation stroke with a finger assist* can be combined with a basic intraoral fulcrum and extraoral fulcrum.
- The *instrumentation stroke with finger assist* is an extremely effective technique for removing calculus deposits from root surfaces located within deep periodontal pockets.
- ***For this technique, the clinician applies pressure against the shank of the instrument. The index finger of the nondominant hand moves with the instrument shank throughout a short, controlled instrumentation stroke.*** As long as the nondominant finger remains securely against the shank, the risk of an instrument stick is limited.

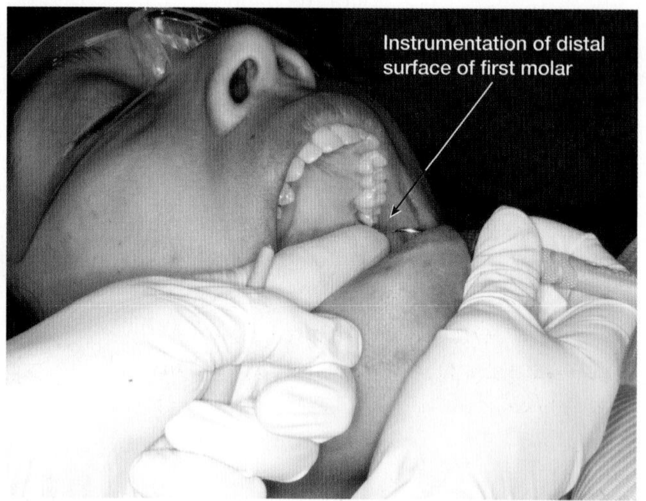
Instrumentation of distal
surface of first molar

Figure 20-23A. Finger Assist on the Distal Surface.

- The photograph shows a right-handed clinician applying a finger assist behind the instrument shank.
- In this case, the clinician is instrumenting the *distal surface* of the maxillary first molar.
- The clinician is using an extraoral arch fulcrum on the mandibular arch.

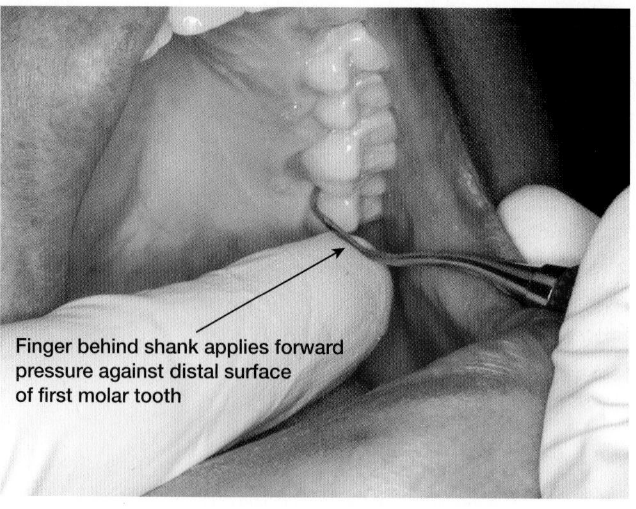
Finger behind shank applies forward
pressure against distal surface
of first molar tooth

Figure 20-23B. Closer View of Finger Assist on the Distal Surface.

- This photograph is a closer view of the finger assist in Figure 20-23A.
- The clinician is using the index finger of the left hand to apply pressure behind the shank, ***thus concentrating lateral pressure with the cutting edge forward against the distal surface of the first molar.***

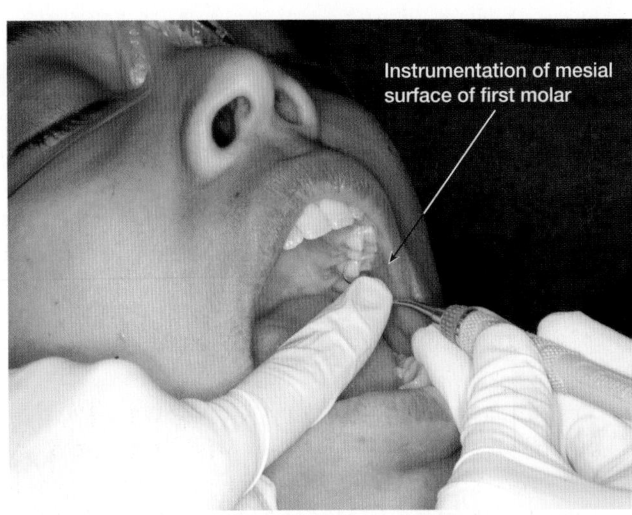
Instrumentation of mesial
surface of first molar

Figure 20-24A. Finger Assist on the Mesial Surface.

- The photograph shows a right-handed clinician applying a finger assist against the instrument shank.
- In this case, the clinician is instrumenting the ***mesial surface*** of the maxillary first molar.
- The clinician is using an extraoral arch fulcrum on the mandibular arch.

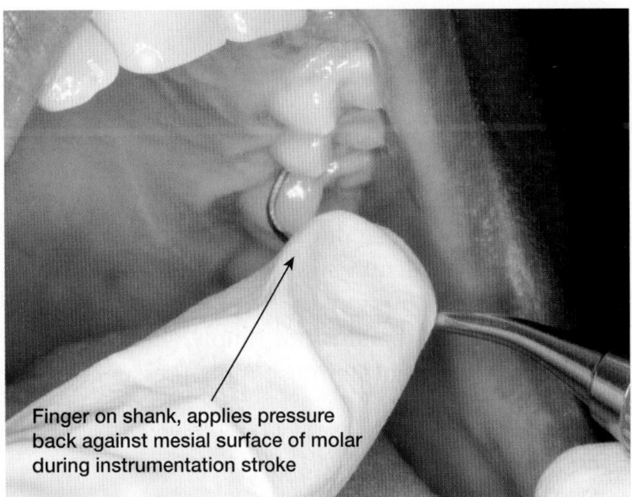
Finger on shank, applies pressure
back against mesial surface of molar
during instrumentation stroke

Figure 20-24B. Closer View of Finger Assist on the Mesial Surface.

- This photograph is a closer view of the finger assist in Figure 20-24A.
- The clinician is using the index finger of the left hand to apply pressure against the shank, ***thus concentrating lateral pressure with the cutting edge backward against the mesial surface of the first molar.***

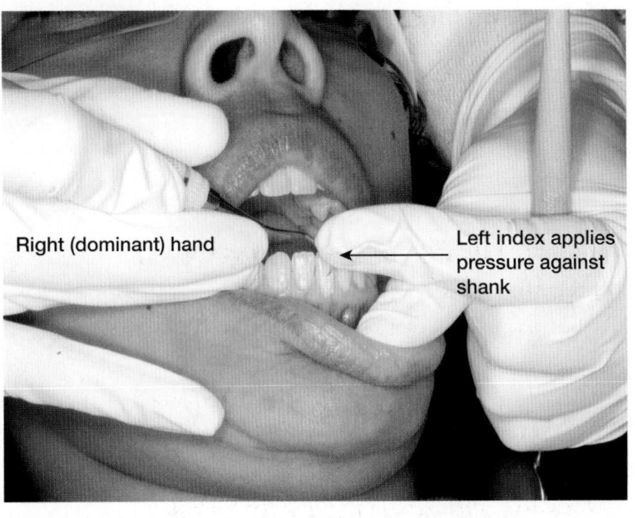
Right (dominant) hand
Left index applies
pressure against
shank

Figure 20-25. Finger Assist on Mandibular Arch.

- The right-handed clinician—seated behind the patient—positions the left index finger on the shank to stabilize a short horizontal stroke.
- The finger assist helps the clinician to control a short horizontal stroke by concentrating pressure precisely on the cutting edge.

Section 4
Technique Practice: Extraoral Finger Rests for Right-Handed Clinician

Directions: Miniature area-specific curets with extended shanks, such as the Hu-Friedy Mini Five, are recommended for this technique practice. This technique practice is best accomplished on a dental manikin and periodontal typodont.

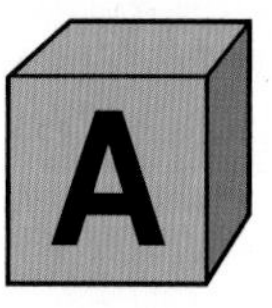

SKILL BUILDING. "PALM FACING OUT" EXTRAORAL FULCRUM: MAXILLARY RIGHT POSTERIOR SEXTANTS

Basic Extraoral Finger Rest for Maxillary Right Posterior Sextants

- Rest the front surfaces of the middle, ring, and little fingers against the skin and underlying bone of the mandible (Fig. 20-26).
- Keep the fingers straight and together in the grasp; as much of the length of the fingers as possible should be kept in contact with the mandible.
- Apply pressure against the bone of the mandible to stabilize your hand and the instrument during instrumentation.
  - Note that the hand is not simply "hovering" over the skin of the mandible.
  - Rather, the clinician must apply pressure against the underlying bone to stabilize the grasp.

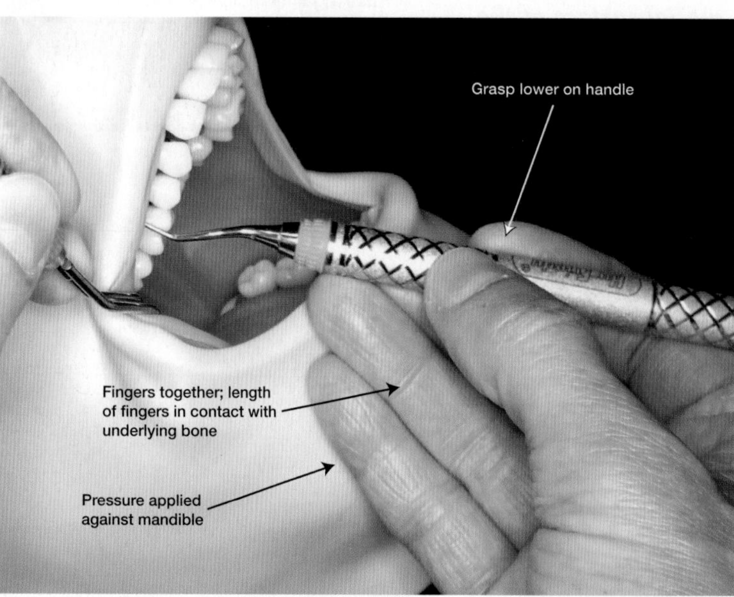

Figure 20-26. Basic Extraoral Finger Rest for Maxillary Right Posterior Sextants.

Maxillary Right Posteriors, Facial Aspect—Distal Surfaces

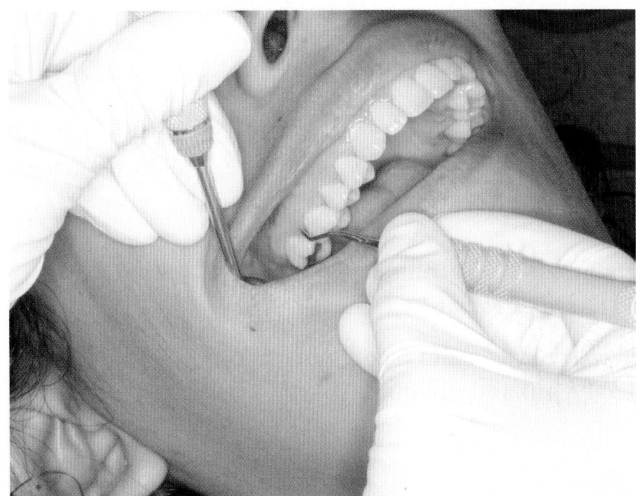

Figure 20-27. Technique Summary for Distal Surfaces of Facial Aspect.

- Extraoral "palm facing out" fulcrum
- Vertical and oblique strokes

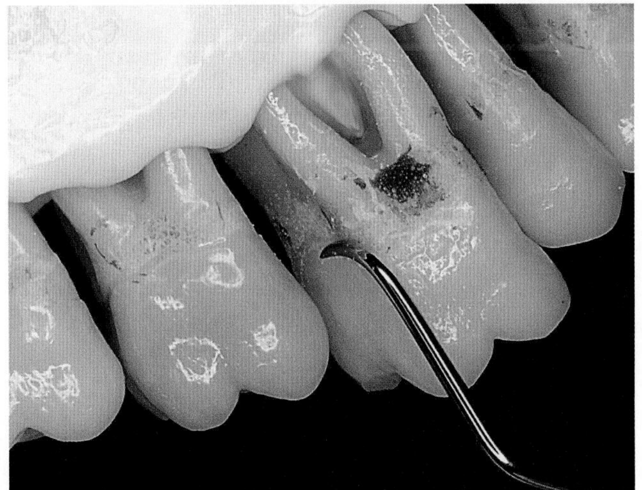

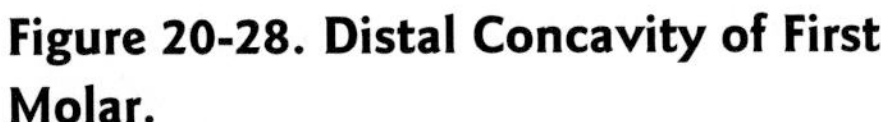

Figure 20-28. Distal Concavity of First Molar.

- Use the *distal curet.*
- Rotate the handle slightly to adapt the toe-third of the cutting edge to the distal concavity.

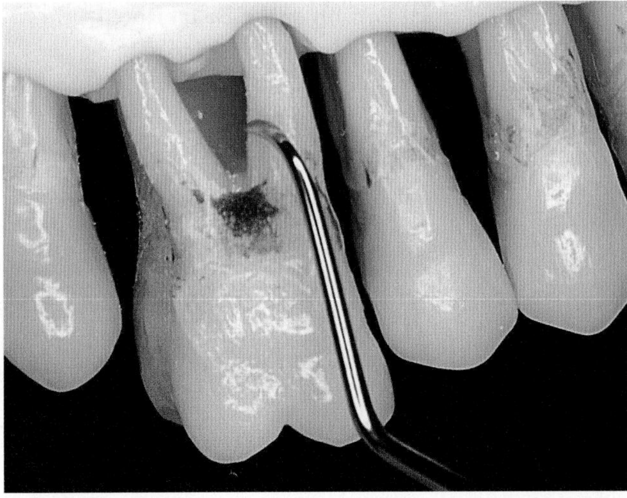

Figure 20-29. Distal Portion of the Mesial Root.

Use the ***distal curet*** on the distal portion of the mesial root.

Maxillary Right Posteriors, Facial Aspect—Mesial Surfaces

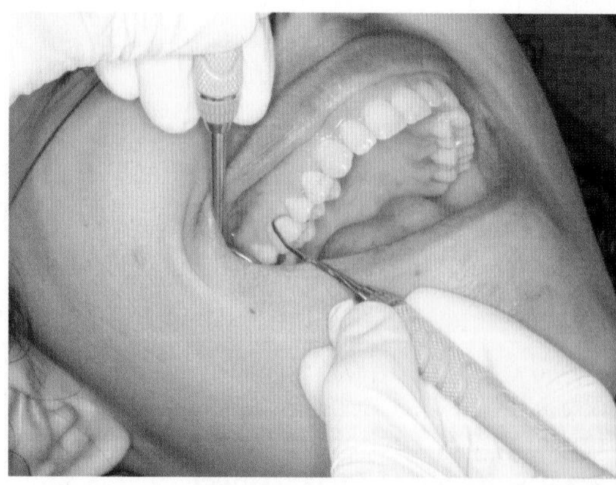

Figure 20-30. Technique Summary for Mesial Surfaces of Facial Aspect.

- Extraoral "palm facing out" fulcrum
- Vertical and oblique strokes

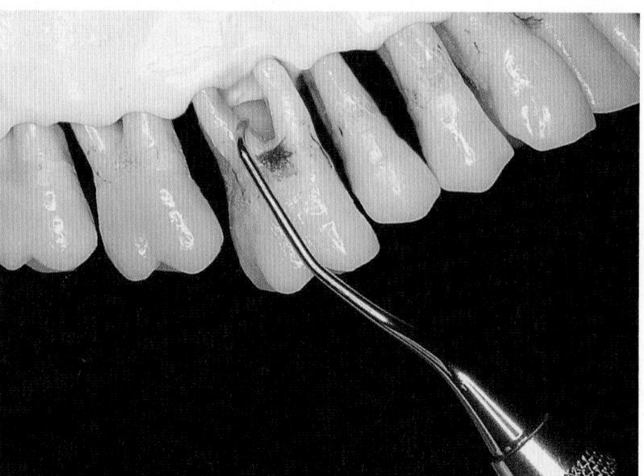

Figure 20-31. Mesial Portion of the Distal Root. Use the ***mesial curet*** on the mesial portion of the distal root.

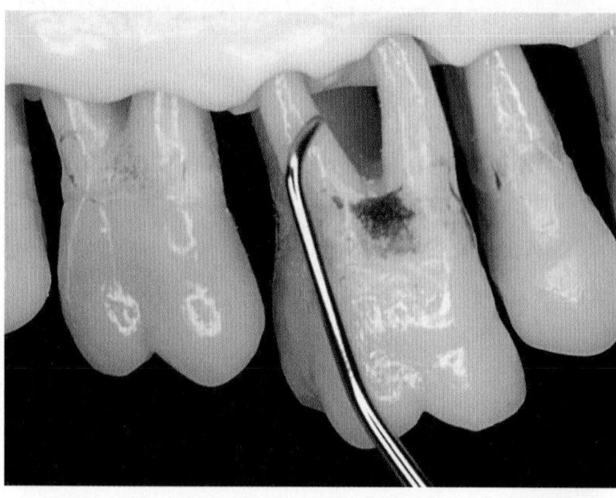

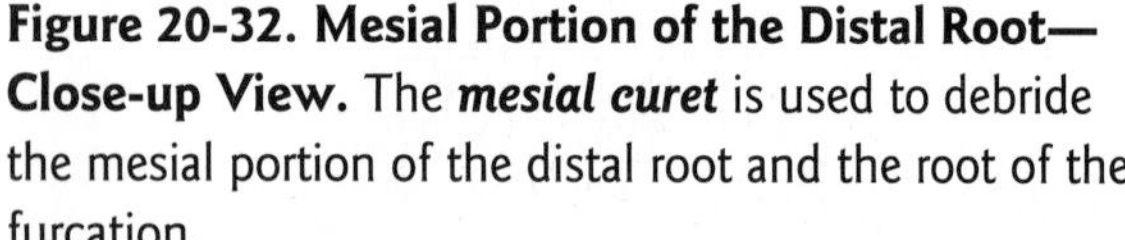

Figure 20-32. Mesial Portion of the Distal Root—Close-up View. The ***mesial curet*** is used to debride the mesial portion of the distal root and the root of the furcation.

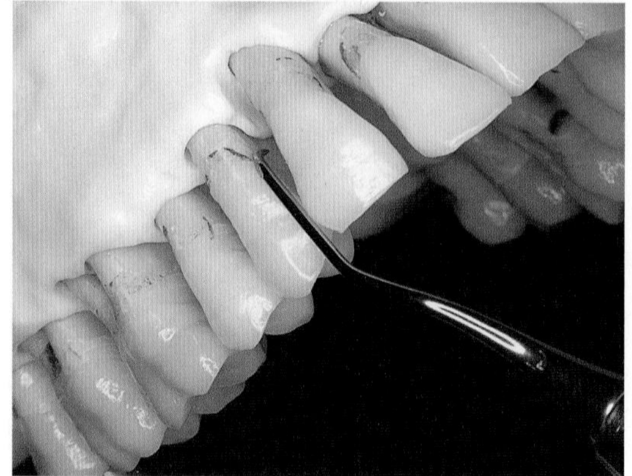

Figure 20-33. Mesial Surface of the First Premolar.

- The maxillary first premolar has the deepest concavity in the entire dentition.
- Use the mesial curet to debride the mesial concavity.
- *Rotate the toe-third of the cutting edge toward the root surface to adapt to the concavity.*

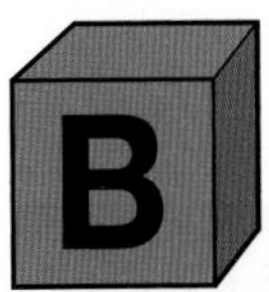

SKILL BUILDING. "CHIN-CUP" EXTRAORAL FULCRUM: MAXILLARY LEFT POSTERIOR SEXTANTS

When working on the maxillary left posterior sextants, the patient's chin and mandible are cupped with the palm of the clinician's hand (Fig. 20-34).

Basic Extraoral Finger Rest for Maxillary Left Posterior Sextants

- Cup the patient's chin and mandible in the palm of the hand.
- Rest the palmer surfaces of the middle, ring, and little fingers against the skin and underlying bone of the mandible.
- Keep the fingers straight and together in the grasp; as much of the length of the fingers as possible should be kept in contact with the mandible.
- Apply pressure against the bone of the mandible to stabilize your hand and the instrument during instrumentation.
  - Note that the hand is not simply "hovering" over the skin of the mandible.
  - Rather, the clinician must apply pressure against the underlying bone to stabilize the grasp.

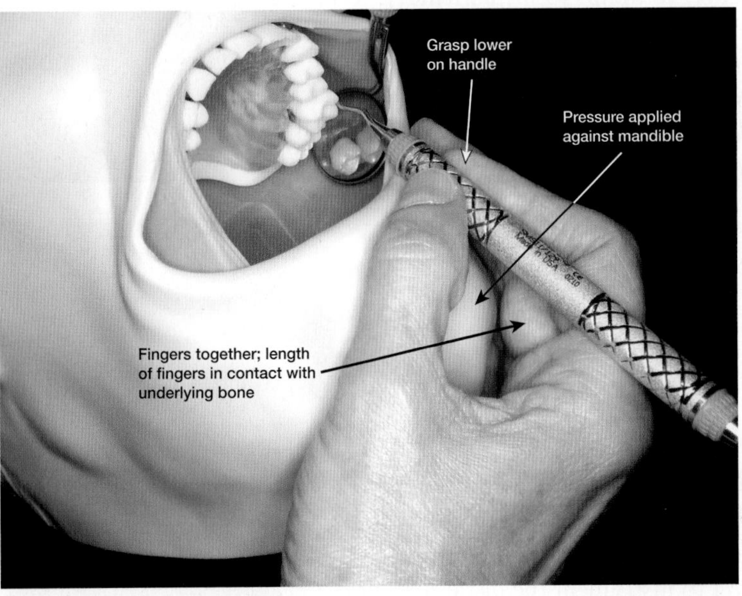

Figure 20-34. Basic Extraoral Finger Rest for Maxillary Left Posterior Sextants.

Maxillary Left Posteriors, Lingual Aspect—Distal Surfaces

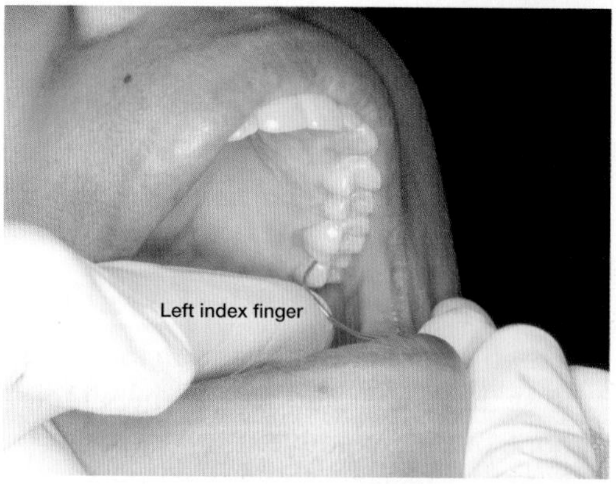

Figure 20-35. Technique Summary for Distal Surfaces.

- Extraoral "chin-cup" fulcrum with a finger assist
- Vertical strokes

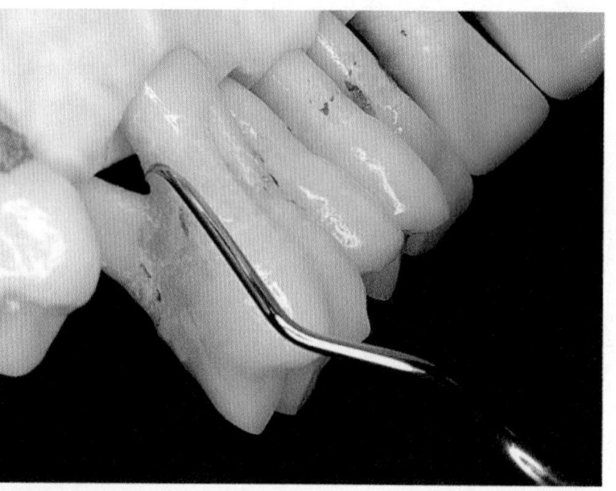

Figure 20-36. Distal Concavity.

- Use a ***distal curet*** to debride the distal concavity with vertical strokes. ***It is important to rotate the toe-third of the curet to adapt to the concavity.***
- Use the index finger of your nondominant hand to apply pressure behind the shank, thus ***concentrating pressure with the cutting edge forward against the distal surface*** of the first molar. (See Figure 20-35.)

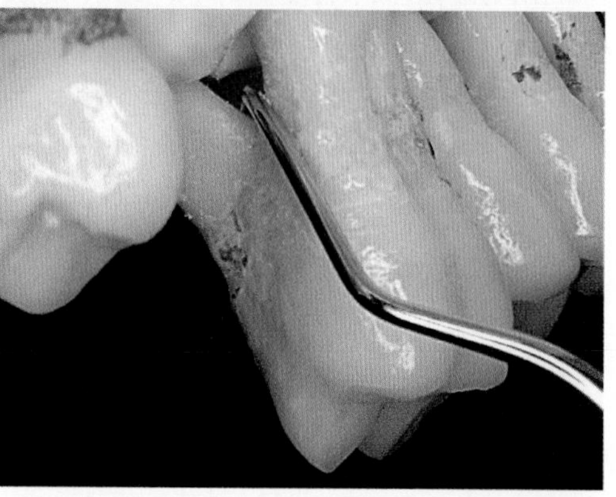

Figure 20-37. Distal Furcation.

- The distal furcation entrance is located near the midline of the tooth and, therefore, can be instrumented from both the facial and lingual aspects.
- Use the ***distal curet*** to instrument the distal furcation.

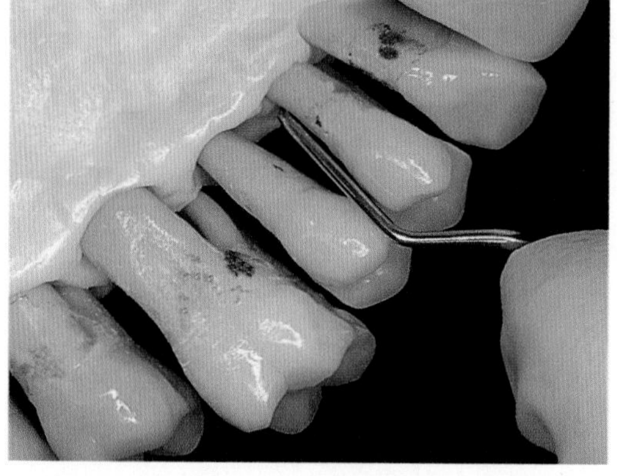

Figure 20-38. Distal Surface of Premolar.

- Use the ***distal curet*** on the distal surface of the premolar.
- Use the index finger of your nondominant hand to apply pressure behind the shank, thus ***concentrating pressure with the cutting edge forward against the distal surface*** of the premolar.

Maxillary Left Posteriors, Lingual Aspect—Mesial Surfaces

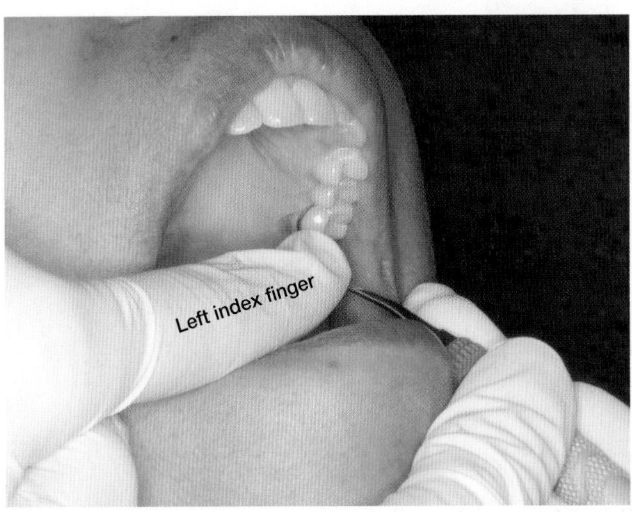

Figure 20-39. Technique Summary for Mesial Surfaces.

- Extraoral "chin-cup" fulcrum with a finger assist
- Index finger of nondominant hand provides lateral pressure back against mesial surface
- Vertical strokes

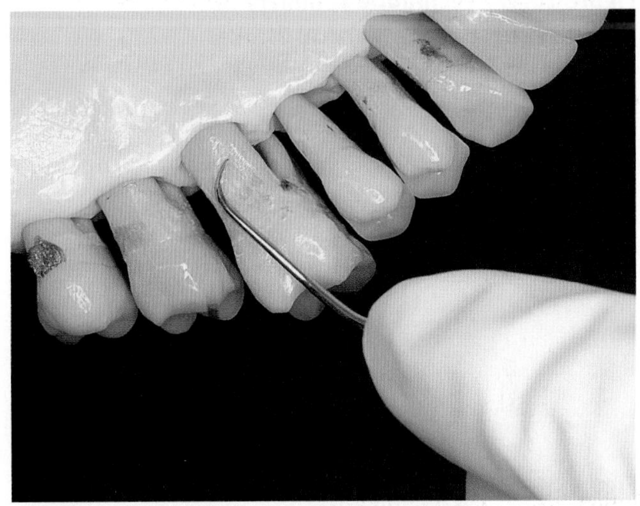

Figure 20-40. Lingual Surface of Palatal Root.

- The palatal root commonly has a deep depression.
- Use the *mesial curet.*
- Use the index finger of your nondominant hand to apply pressure against the shank, thus ***concentrating pressure with the cutting edge against the lingual surface*** of the first molar. (See Figure 20-39.)

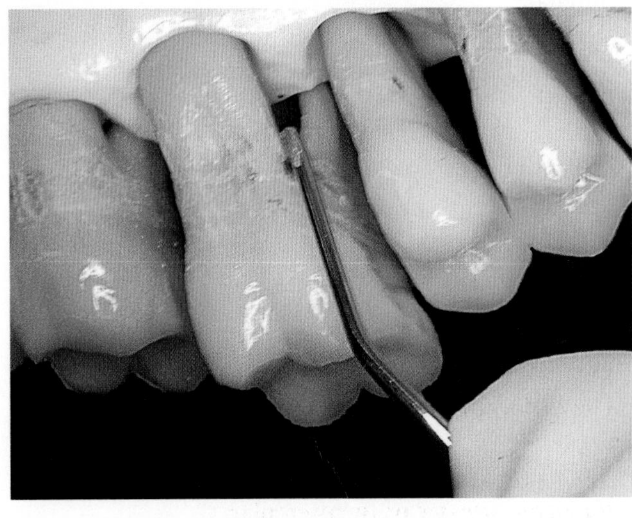

Figure 20-41. Mesial Furcation.

- The entrance to the mesial furcation is located toward the lingual aspect, rather than being located at the midline of the mesial surface.
- Due to its location, the entrance is best accessed from the lingual aspect using a mesial curet.

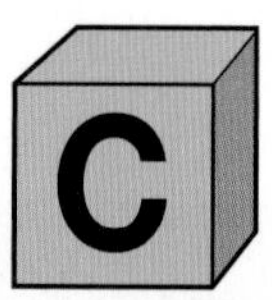

SKILL BUILDING. MAXILLARY ANTERIORS

Maxillary Anteriors, Lingual Aspect

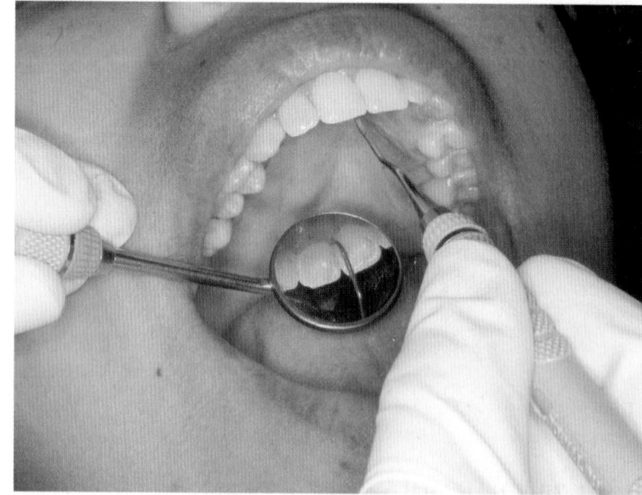

Figure 20-42. Technique Summary for Lingual Aspect Using Vertical Strokes.

- Extraoral fulcrum
- Vertical strokes

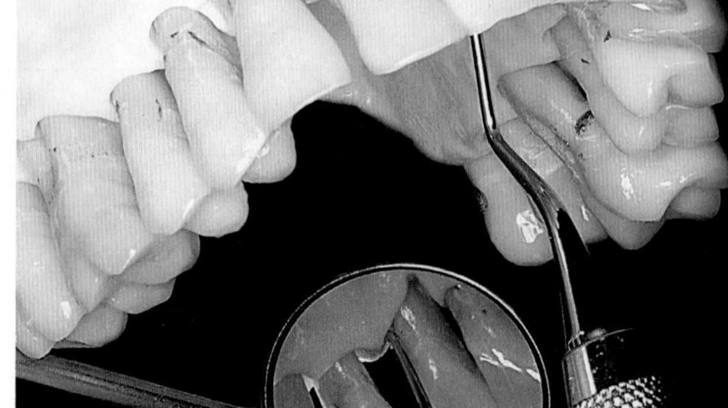

Figure 20-43. Lingual and Mesial Surfaces.

- Note that the root tapers toward the lingual.
- Use the index finger of your nondominant hand to apply pressure against the shank.

Section 5
Technique Practice: Horizontal Strokes for Right-Handed Clinician

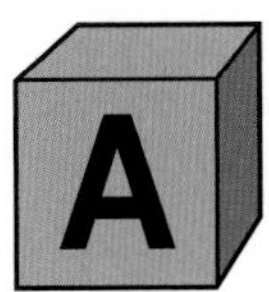

SKILL BUILDING. HORIZONTAL STROKES: MAXILLARY RIGHT

Curet Toe-Up—Distal Concavities

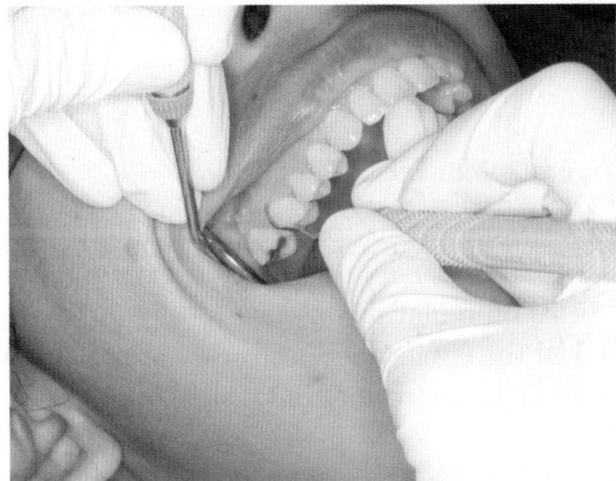

Figure 20-44. Technique Summary for Distal Concavities.

- Intraoral fulcrum
- Working-end in the toe-up position with Gracey miniature 7 or 13 curets
- Very short, controlled horizontal strokes

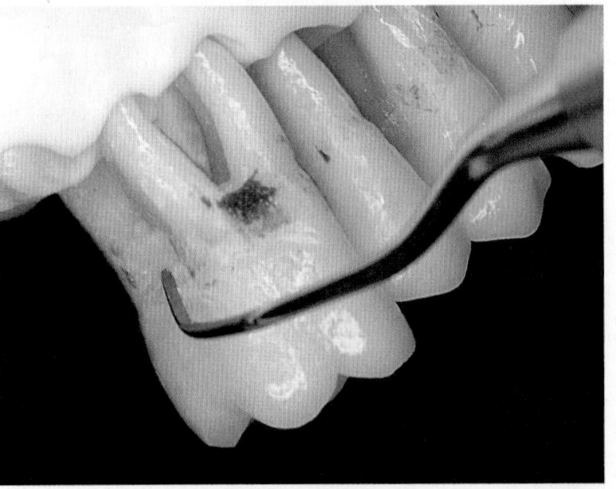

Figure 20-45. Distal Concavity of First Molar.

- The Gracey miniature 7/8 works well in this area.
- Use the opposite working-end from the one that you used to make vertical strokes on the distal.
- Use the curet in a toe-up position, adapt the lower cutting edge, and make a series of horizontal strokes. This technique facilitates calculus removal from the concavity.

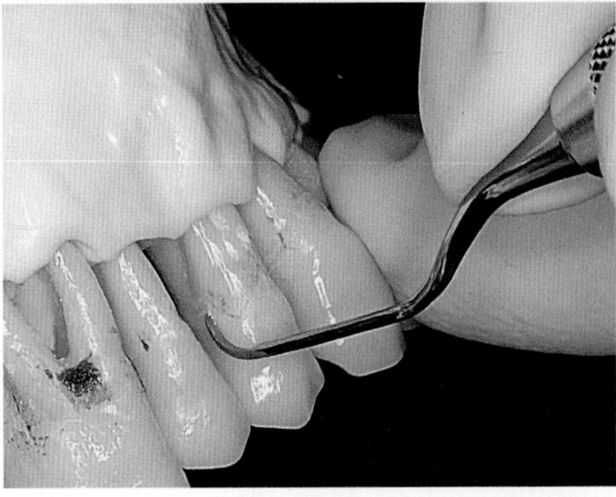

Figure 20-46. Distal Concavity of First Premolar. Use the curet in a toe-up position to make a series of short controlled horizontal strokes in the distal concavity.

Curet Toe-Up—Mesial Concavities

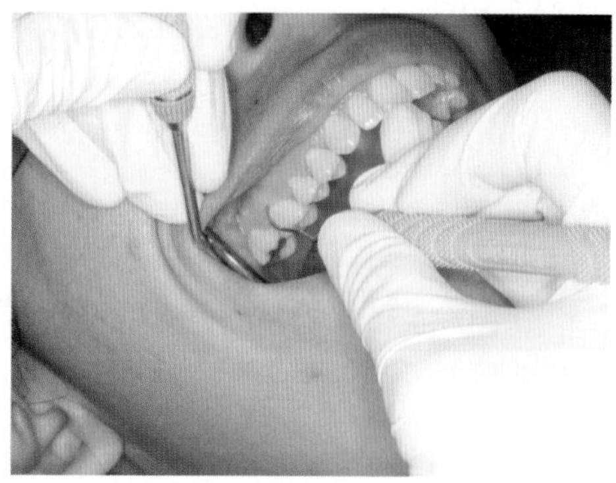

Figure 20-47. Technique Summary for Facial and Mesial Concavities.

- Intraoral fulcrum
- Working-end in the toe-up position
- Short horizontal strokes

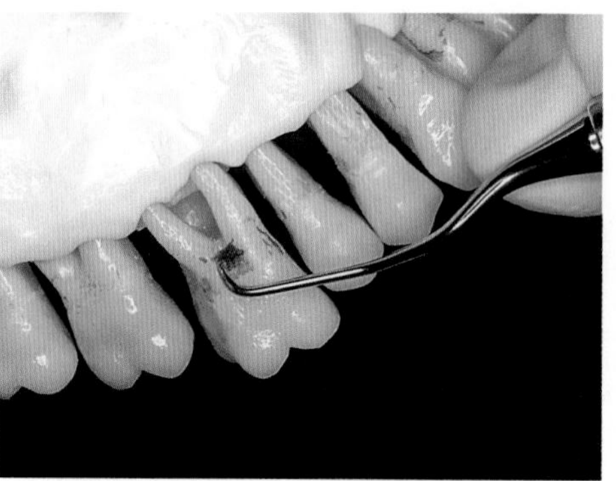

Figure 20-48. Facial Concavity.

- A common area for missed calculus deposits is the broad concavity that extends from the furcation to the CEJ on molar teeth.
- Use the Gracey miniature 12 curet in a toe-up position to make short horizontal strokes in the depression.

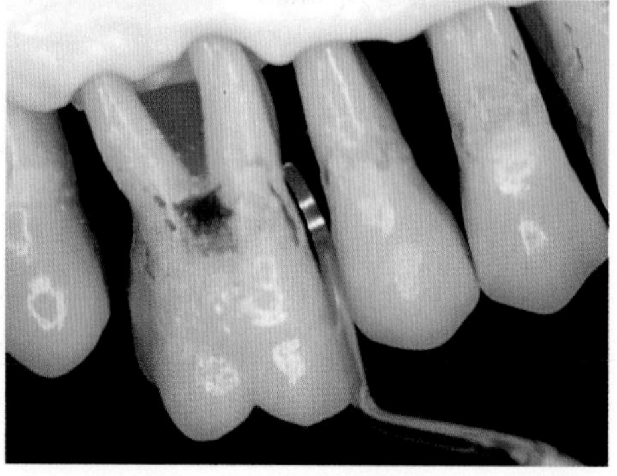

Figure 20-49. Mesial Concavity of Molar.

- Use the Gracey miniature 11 curet in a toe-up position to make horizontal strokes in the concavity.
- This is the opposite working-end from the one you would use to make vertical strokes on the mesial surface.

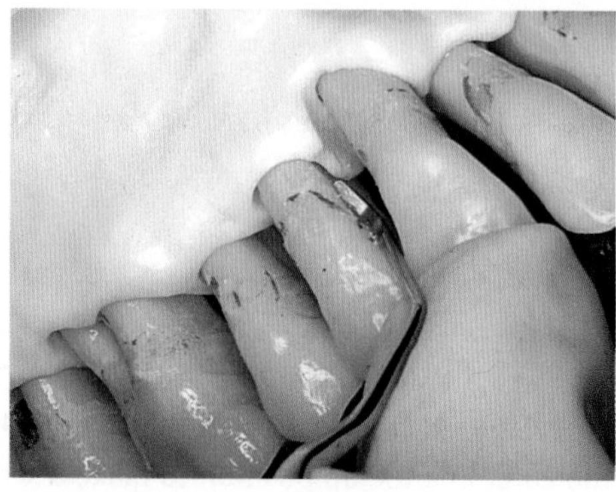

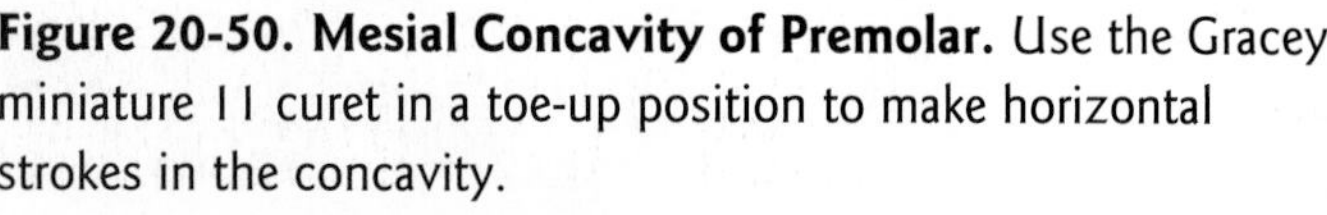

Figure 20-50. Mesial Concavity of Premolar. Use the Gracey miniature 11 curet in a toe-up position to make horizontal strokes in the concavity.

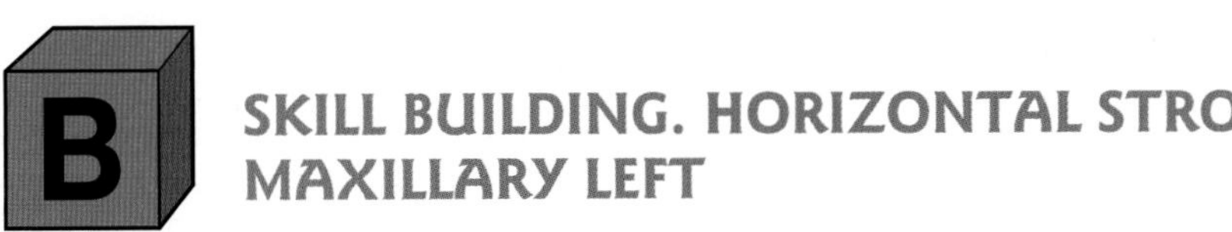

B SKILL BUILDING. HORIZONTAL STROKES: MAXILLARY LEFT

Curet Toe-Up—Mesial Concavities

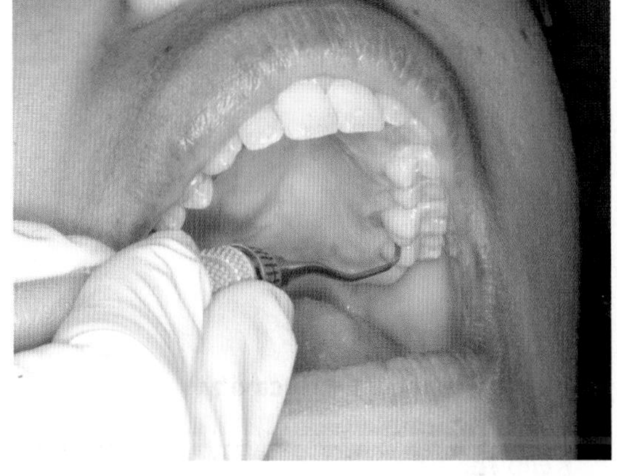

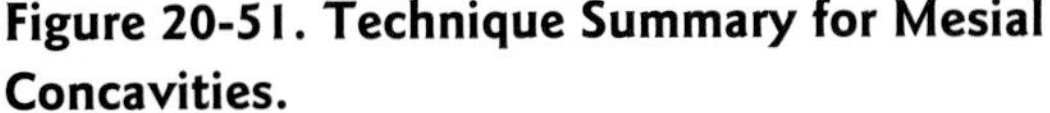

Figure 20-51. Technique Summary for Mesial Concavities.

- Cross arch fulcrum
- Working-end in the toe-up position
- Short horizontal strokes

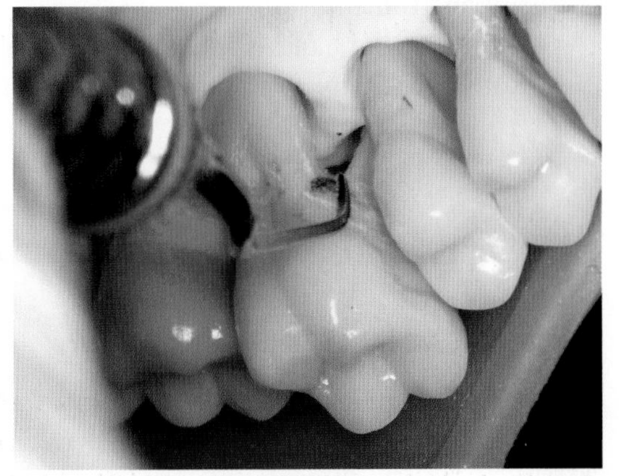

Figure 20-52. Mesial Concavity of Molar.

- The linear concavities often are difficult to debride using vertical strokes.
- Use the miniature curet in a toe-up position (toward the palate) with horizontal strokes to debride the concavity. This is the opposite working-end from the one you would use to make vertical strokes on the mesial surface.

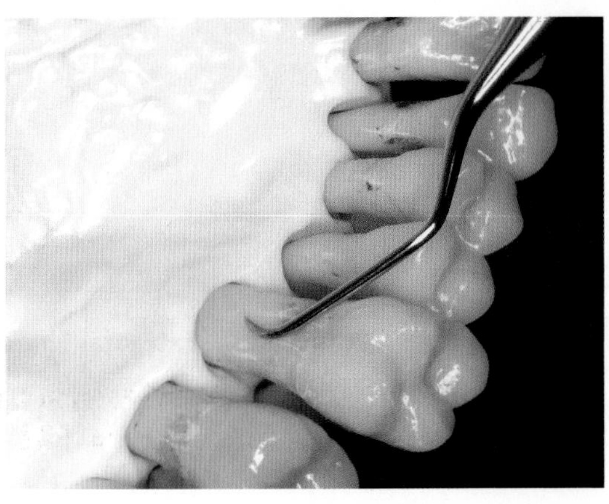

Figure 20-53. Palatal Root Depression.

- The palatal root has a narrow root depression that is difficult to instrument using vertical strokes.
- Use a miniature curet in a toe-up position with a series of short horizontal strokes. Begin making strokes at the base of the pocket, then move coronally slightly, and repeat the process.

Section 6
Technique Practice: Extraoral Finger Rests for Left-Handed Clinician

Directions: Miniature area-specific curets with extended shanks, such as the Hu-Friedy Mini Five or Micro Mini, are recommended for this technique practice. This technique practice is best accomplished on a dental manikin and periodontal typodont.

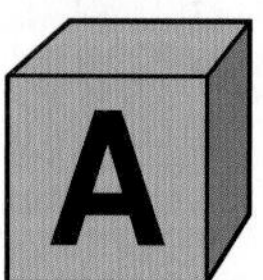

SKILL BUILDING. "PALM FACING OUT" EXTRAORAL FULCRUM: MAXILLARY LEFT POSTERIOR SEXTANTS

Basic Extraoral Finger Rest for Maxillary Left Posterior Sextants

- Rest the front surfaces of the middle, ring, and little fingers against the skin and underlying bone of the mandible (Fig. 20-54).
- Keep the fingers straight and together in the grasp; as much of the length of the fingers as possible should be kept in contact with the mandible.
- Apply pressure against the bone of the mandible to stabilize your hand and the instrument during instrumentation.
  - Note that the hand is not simply "hovering" over the skin of the mandible.
  - Rather, the clinician must apply pressure against the underlying bone to stabilize the grasp.

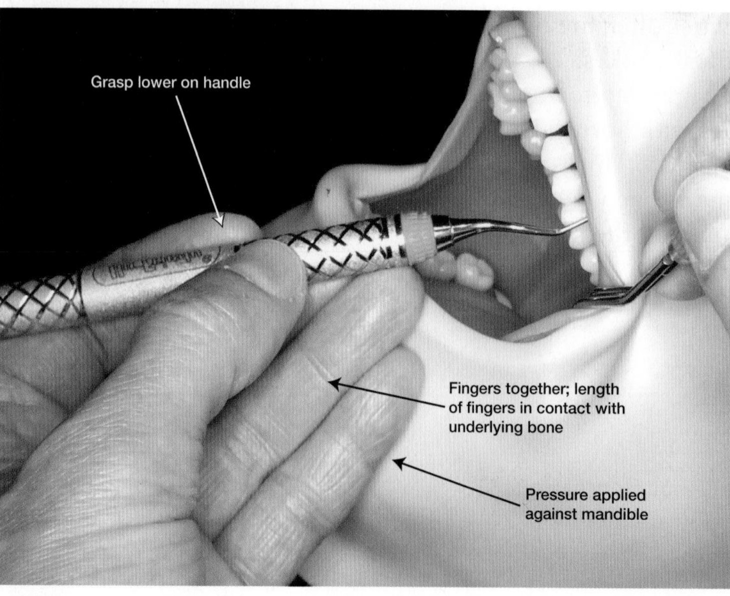

Figure 20-54. Basic Extraoral Finger Rest for Maxillary Left Posterior Sextants.

LEFT-Handed Clinician

Maxillary Left Posteriors, Facial Aspect—Distal Surfaces

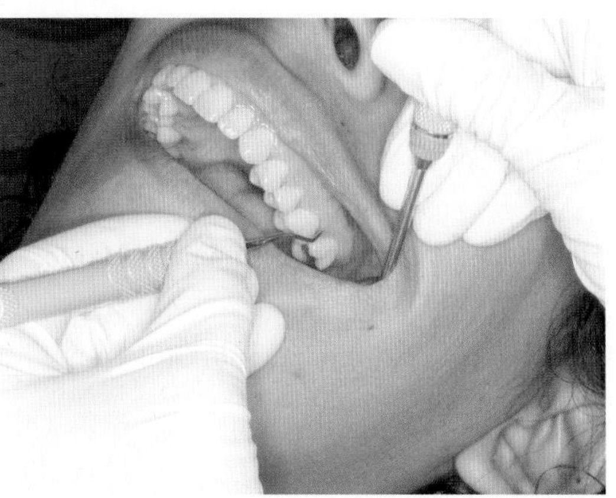

Figure 20-55. Technique Summary for Distal Surfaces of Facial Aspect.

- Extraoral "palm facing out" fulcrum
- Vertical and oblique strokes

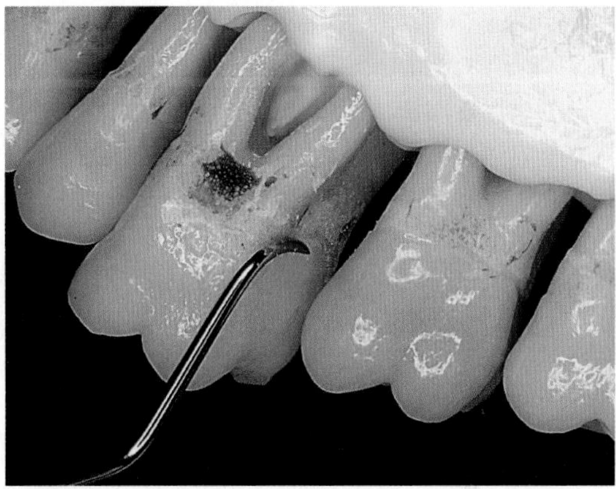

Figure 20-56. Distal Concavity of First Molar.

- Use the ***distal curet.***
- Rotate the handle slightly to adapt the toe-third of the cutting edge to the distal concavity.

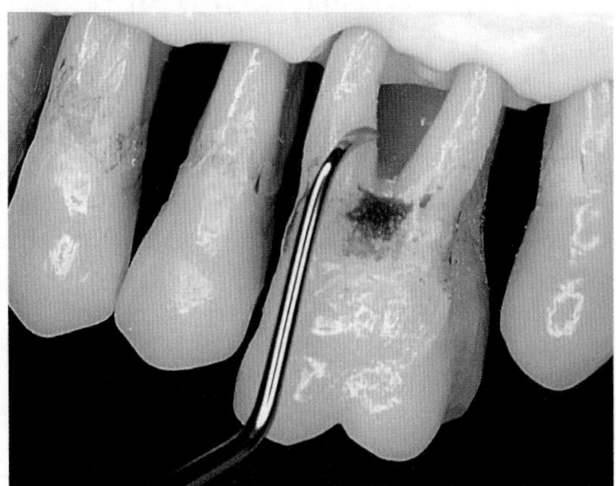

Figure 20-57. Distal Portion of the Mesial Root.

Use the ***distal curet*** on the distal portion of the mesial root.

Maxillary Left Posteriors, Facial Aspect—Mesial Surfaces

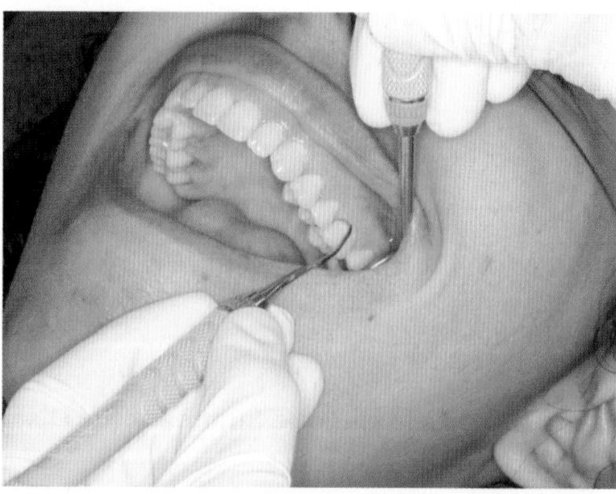

Figure 20-58. Technique Summary for Mesial Surfaces of Facial Aspect.

- Extraoral "palm facing out" fulcrum
- Vertical and oblique strokes

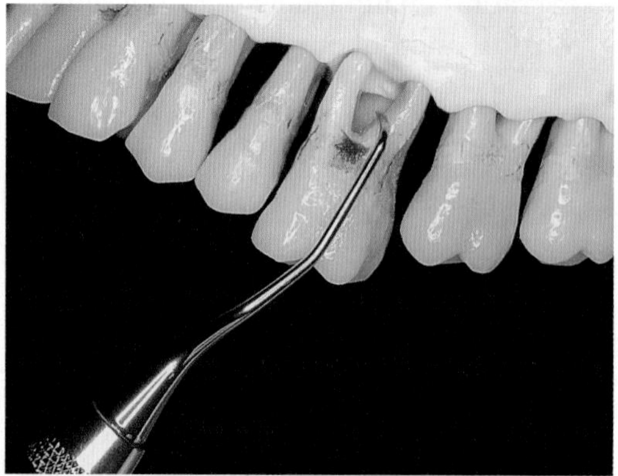

Figure 20-59. Mesial Portion of the Distal Root. Use the ***mesial curet*** on the mesial portion of the distal root.

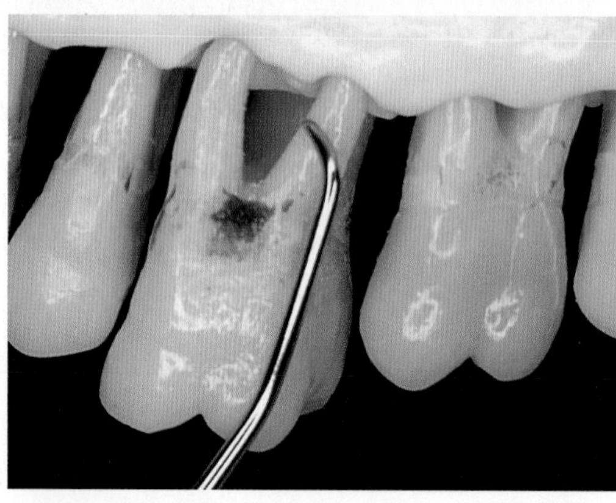

Figure 20-60. Mesial Portion of the Distal Root—Close-up View. The ***mesial curet*** is used to debride the mesial portion of the distal root and the root of the furcation.

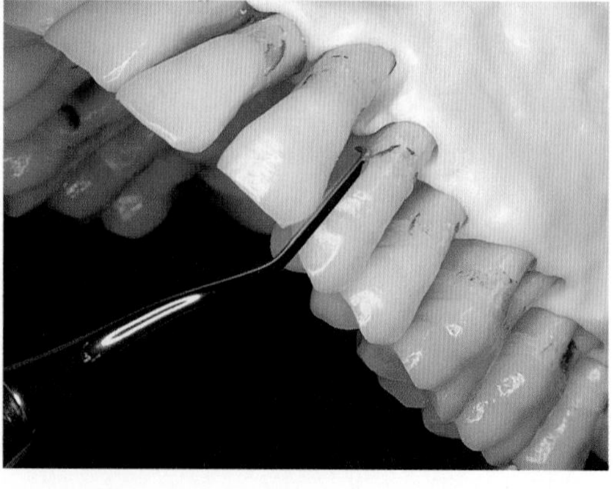

Figure 20-61. Mesial Surface of the First Premolar.

- The maxillary first premolar has the deepest concavity in the entire dentition.
- Use the mesial curet to debride the mesial concavity.
- *Rotate the toe-third of the cutting edge toward the root surface to adapt to the concavity.*

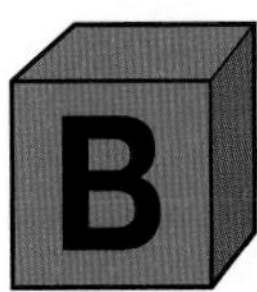

SKILL BUILDING. "CHIN-CUP" EXTRAORAL FULCRUM: MAXILLARY RIGHT POSTERIOR SEXTANTS

When working on the maxillary right posterior sextants, the patient's chin and mandible are cupped with the palm of the clinician's hand (Fig. 20-62).

Basic Extraoral Finger Rest for Maxillary Right Posterior Sextants

- Cup the patient's chin and mandible in the palm of the hand.
- Rest the palmer surfaces of the middle, ring, and little fingers against the skin and underlying bone of the mandible.
- Keep the fingers straight and together in the grasp; as much of the length of the fingers as possible should be kept in contact with the mandible.
- Apply pressure against the bone of the mandible to stabilize your hand and the instrument during instrumentation.
  - Note that the hand is not simply "hovering" over the skin of the mandible.
  - Rather, the clinician must apply pressure against the underlying bone to stabilize the grasp.

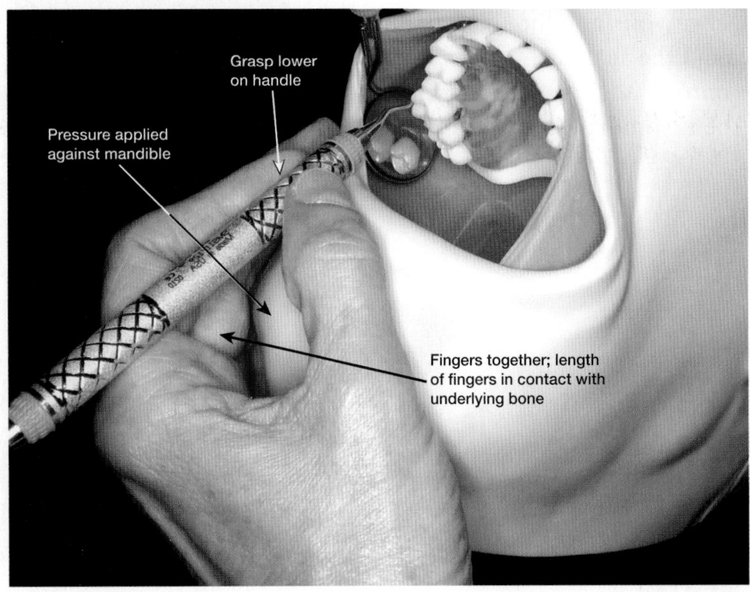

Figure 20-62. Basic Extraoral Finger Rest for Maxillary Right Posterior Sextants.

Maxillary Right Posteriors, Lingual Aspect—Distal Surfaces

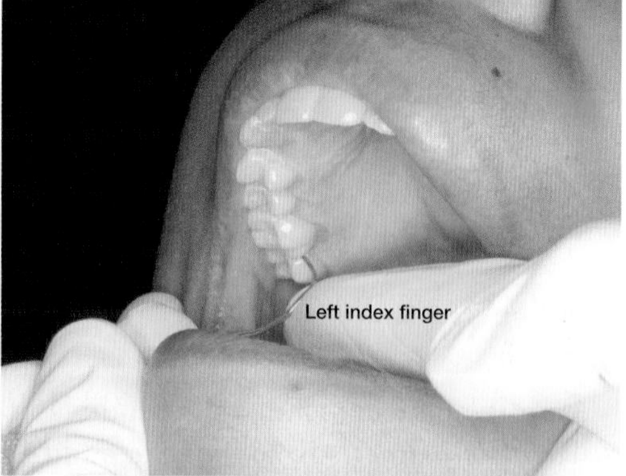

Figure 20-63. Technique Summary for Distal Surfaces.

- Extraoral "chin-cup" fulcrum with a finger assist
- Vertical strokes

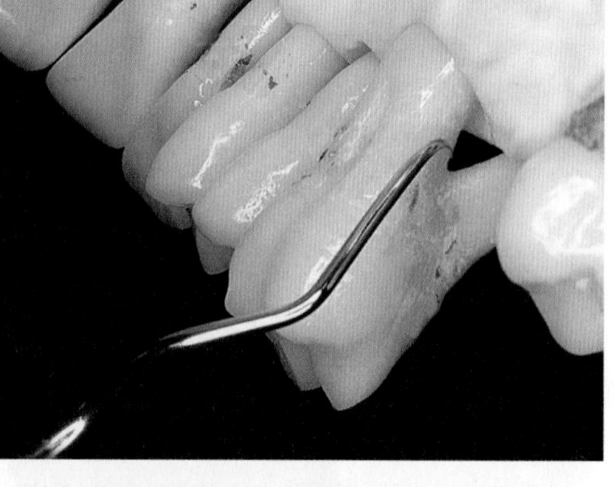

Figure 20-64. Distal Concavity.

- Use a ***distal curet*** to debride the distal concavity with vertical strokes. ***It is important to rotate the toe-third of the curet to adapt to the concavity.***
- Use the index finger of your nondominant hand to apply pressure behind the shank, thus ***concentrating pressure with the cutting edge forward against the distal surface*** of the first molar. (See Figure 20-63.)

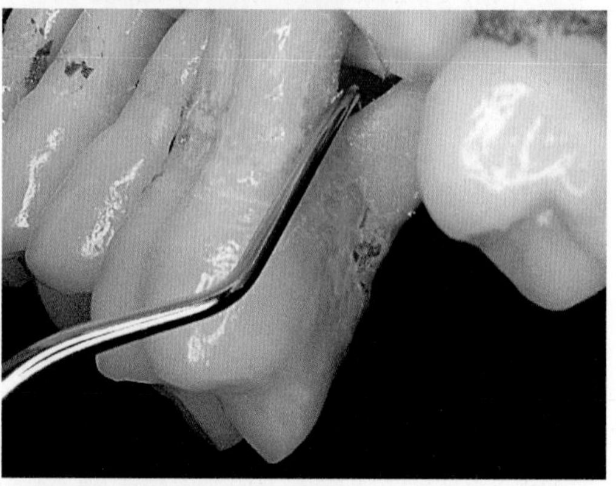

Figure 20-65. Distal Furcation.

- The distal furcation entrance is located near the midline of the tooth and, therefore, can be instrumented from both the facial and lingual aspects.
- Use the ***distal curet*** to instrument the distal furcation.

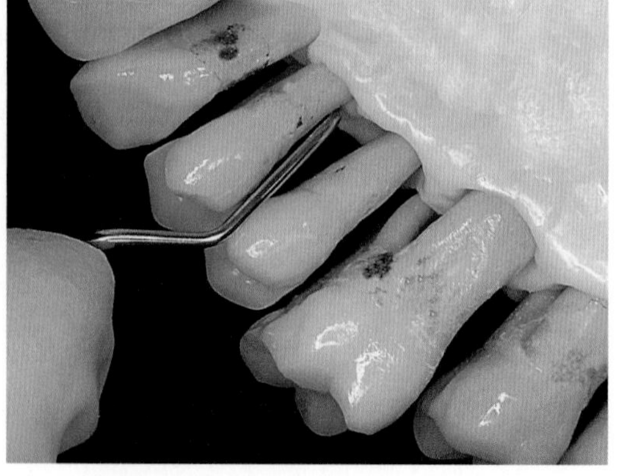

Figure 20-66. Distal Surface of Premolar.

- Use the ***distal curet*** on the distal surface of the premolar.
- Use the index finger of your nondominant hand to apply pressure behind the shank, thus ***concentrating pressure with the cutting edge forward against the distal surface*** of the premolar.

Maxillary Right Posteriors, Lingual Aspect—Mesial Surfaces

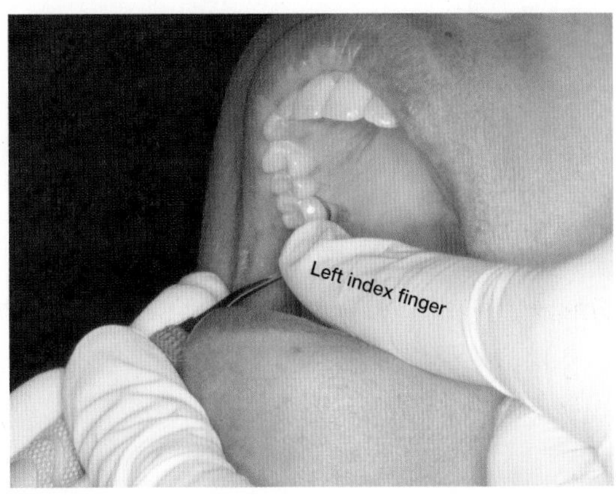

Figure 20-67. Technique Summary for Mesial Surfaces.

- Extraoral "chin-cup" fulcrum with a finger assist
- Index finger of nondominant hand provides lateral pressure back against mesial surface.
- Vertical strokes

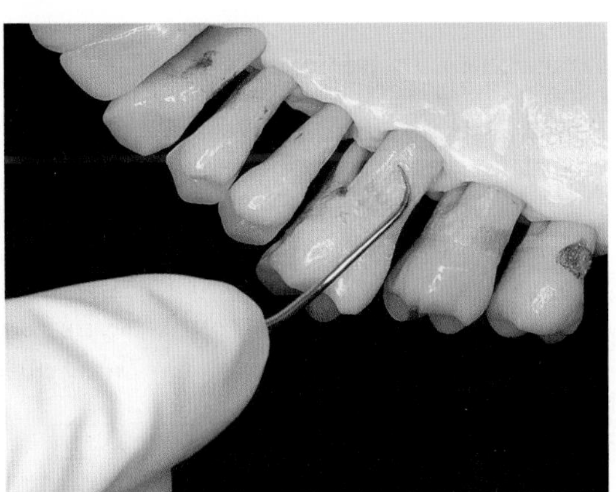

Figure 20-68. Lingual Surface of Palatal Root.

- The palatal root commonly has a deep depression.
- Use the ***mesial curet.***
- Use the index finger of your nondominant hand to apply pressure against the shank, thus ***concentrating pressure with the cutting edge against the lingual surface*** of the first molar. (See Figure 20-67.)

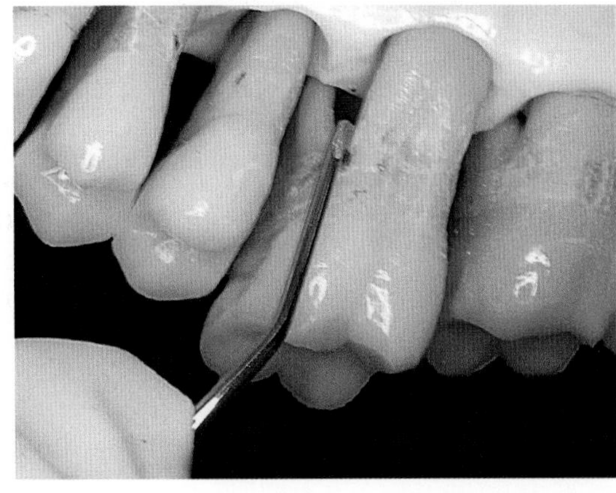

Figure 20-69. Mesial Furcation.

- The entrance to the mesial furcation is located toward the lingual aspect, rather than being located at the midline of the mesial surface.
- Due to its location, the entrance is best accessed from the lingual aspect using a mesial curet.

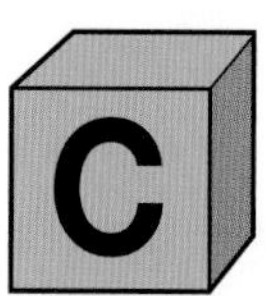

SKILL BUILDING. MAXILLARY ANTERIORS

Maxillary Anteriors, Lingual Aspect

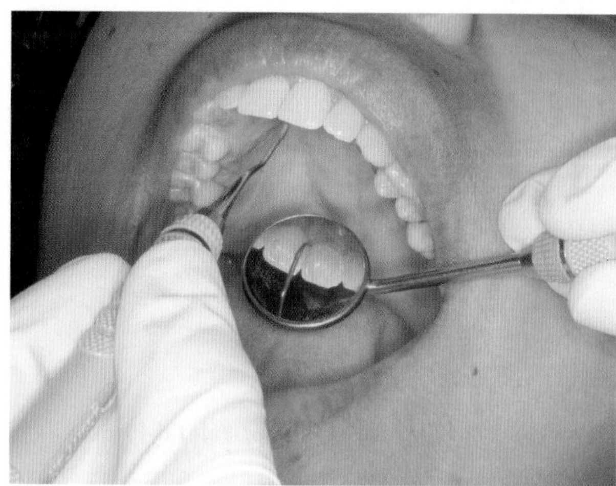

Figure 20-70. Technique Summary for Lingual Aspect Using Vertical Strokes.

- Extraoral fulcrum
- Vertical strokes

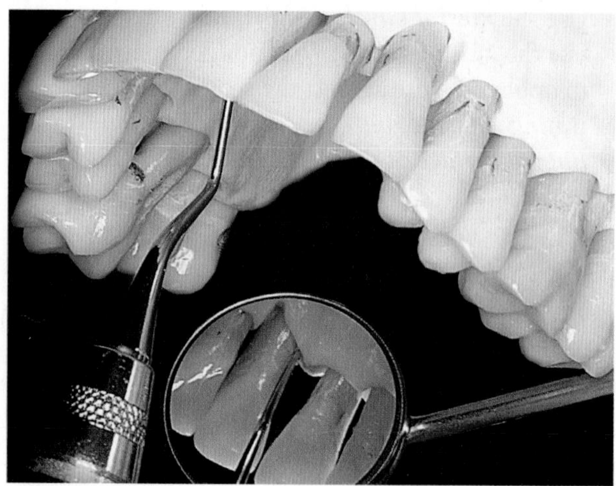

Figure 20-71. Lingual and Mesial Surfaces.

- Note that the root tapers toward the lingual.
- Use the index finger of your nondominant hand to apply pressure against the shank.

Section 7
Technique Practice: Horizontal Strokes for Left-Handed Clinician

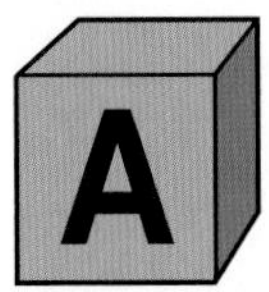

SKILL BUILDING. HORIZONTAL STROKES: MAXILLARY LEFT

Curet Toe-Up—Distal Concavities

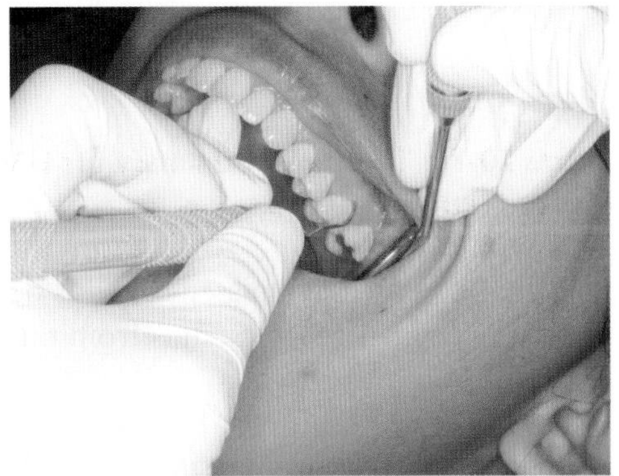

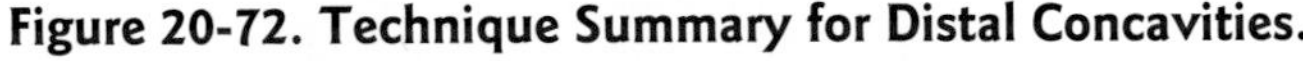

Figure 20-72. Technique Summary for Distal Concavities.

- Intraoral fulcrum
- Working-end in the toe-up position with Gracey miniature 7 or 13 curets
- Very short, controlled horizontal strokes

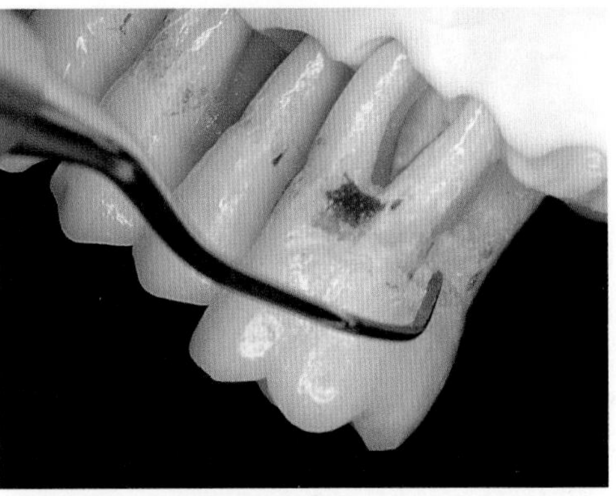

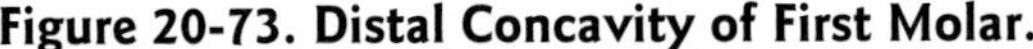

Figure 20-73. Distal Concavity of First Molar.

- The Gracey miniature 7/8 works well in this area.
- Use the opposite working-end from the one that you used to make vertical strokes on the distal.
- Use the curet in a toe-up position, adapt the lower cutting edge, and make a series of horizontal strokes. This technique facilitates calculus removal from the concavity.

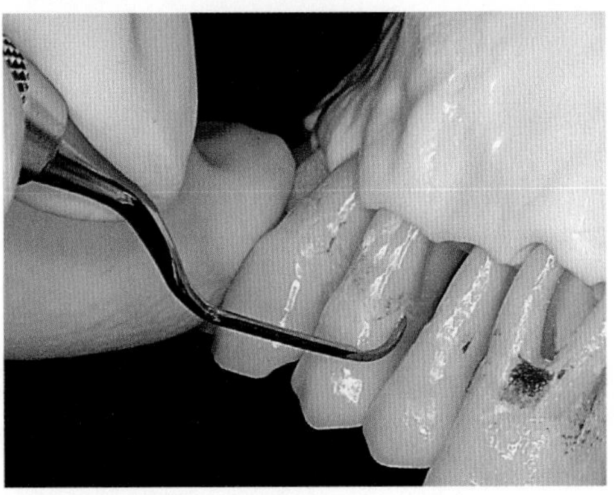

Figure 20-74. Distal Concavity of First Premolar. Use the curet in a toe-up position to make a series of short, controlled horizontal strokes in the distal concavity.

Curet Toe-Up—Mesial Concavities

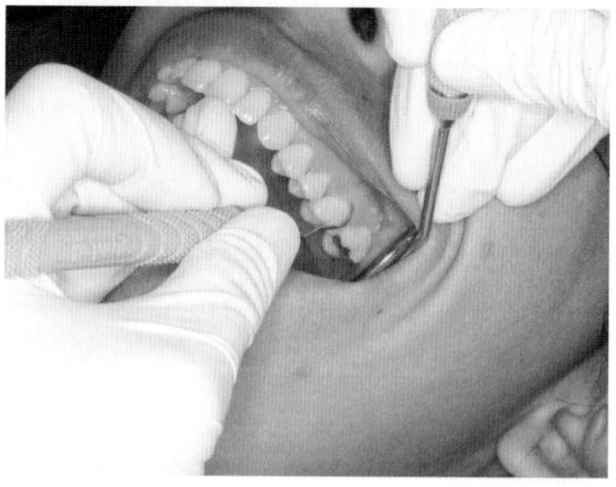

Figure 20-75. Technique Summary for Facial and Mesial Concavities.

- Intraoral fulcrum
- Working-end in the toe-up position
- Short horizontal strokes

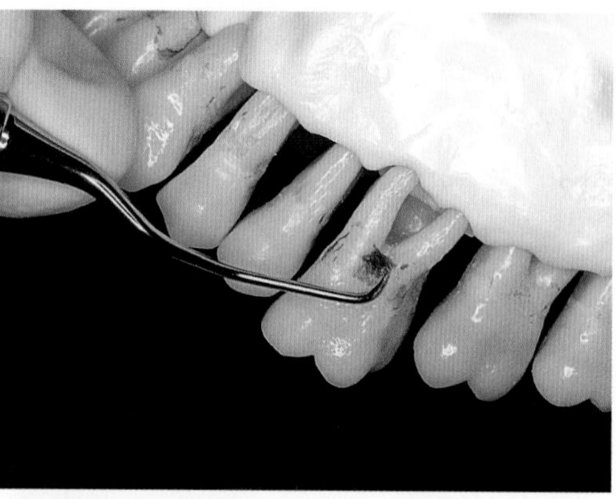

Figure 20-76. Facial Concavity.

- A common area for missed calculus deposits is the broad concavity that extends from the furcation to the CEJ on molar teeth.
- Use the Gracey miniature 12 curet in a toe-up position to make short, horizontal strokes in the depression.

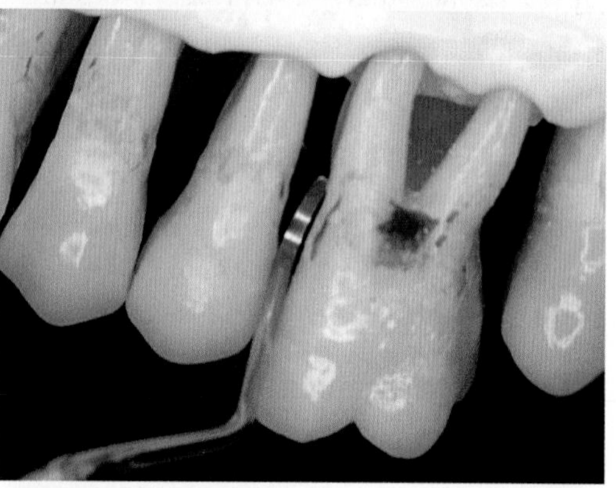

Figure 20-77. Mesial Concavity of Molar.

- Use the Gracey miniature 11 curet in a toe-up position to make horizontal strokes in the concavity.
- This is the opposite working-end from the one you would use to make vertical strokes on the mesial surface.

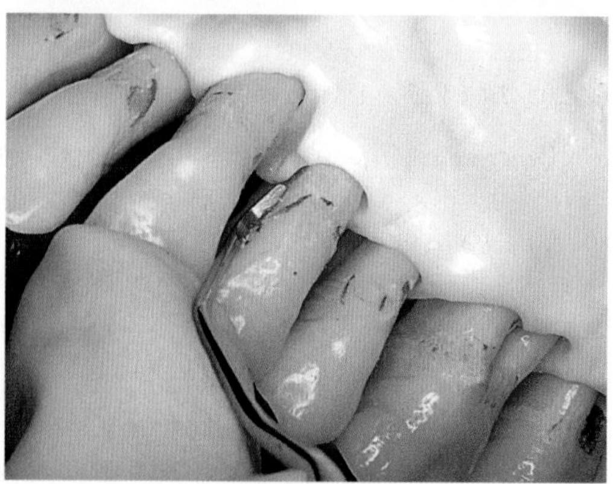

Figure 20-78. Mesial Concavity of Premolar. Use the Gracey miniature 11 curet in a toe-up position to make horizontal strokes in the concavity.

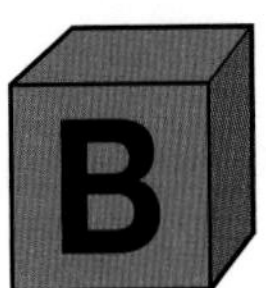

SKILL BUILDING. HORIZONTAL STROKES: MAXILLARY RIGHT

Curet Toe-Up—Mesial Concavities

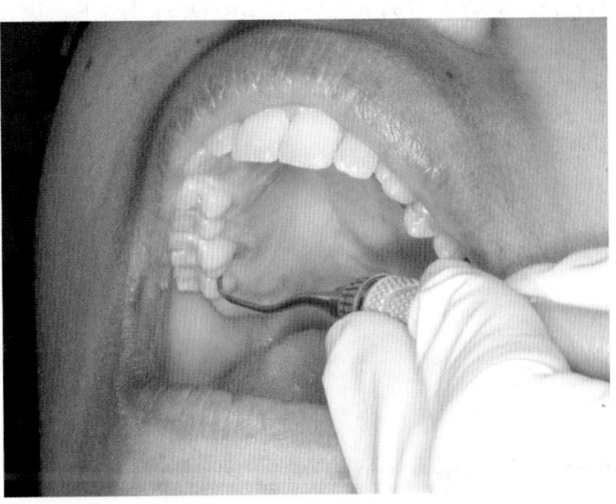

Figure 20-79. Technique Summary for Mesial Concavities.

- Cross arch fulcrum
- Working-end in the toe-up position
- Short horizontal strokes

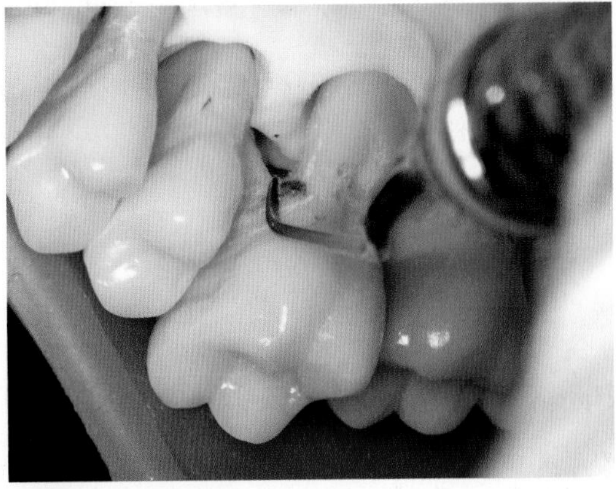

Figure 20-80. Mesial Concavity of Molar.

- The linear concavities often are difficult to debride using vertical strokes.
- Use the miniature curet in a toe-up position (toward the palate) with horizontal strokes to debride the concavity. This is the opposite working-end from the one you would use to make vertical strokes on the mesial surface.

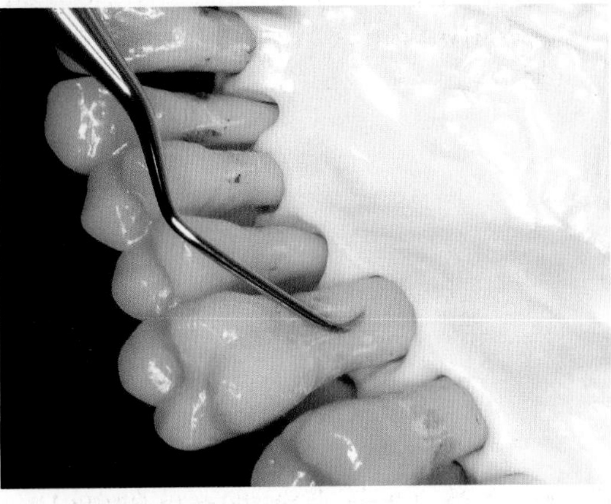

Figure 20-81. Palatal Root Depression.

- The palatal root has a narrow root depression that is difficult to instrument using vertical strokes.
- Use a miniature curet in a toe-up position with a series of short horizontal strokes. Begin making strokes at the base of the pocket, then move coronally slightly, and repeat the process.

REFERENCE

1. Gher ME, Vernino AR. Root morphology—clinical significance in pathogenesis and treatment of periodontal disease. *J Am Dent Assoc.* 1980;101:627–633.

RECOMMENDED READING

Bower RC. Furcation morphology relative to periodontal treatment. Furcation root surface anatomy. *J Periodontol.* 1979;50:366–374.

Cosaboom-FitzSimons ME, Tolle SL, Darby ML, Walker ML. Effects of 5 different finger rest positions on arm muscle activity during scaling by dental hygiene students. *J Dent Hyg.* 2008;82:34.

Section 8
Skill Application

STUDENT SELF-EVALUATION MODULE 20 ADVANCED TECHNIQUES FOR ROOT SURFACE DEBRIDEMENT

Student: ______________________ Date: ______________________

DIRECTIONS FOR STUDENT: Evaluate your skill level as: **S** (satisfactory) or **U** (unsatisfactory).

Criteria	Eval.
Right-Handed Clinicians—Maxillary Right Posteriors, Facial Aspect: **Left-Handed Clinicians—Maxillary Left Posteriors, Facial Aspect:**	
Selects an appropriate curet and demonstrates a "palm facing out" fulcrum for this sextant	
Selects an appropriate curet and demonstrates instrumentation of the broad facial concavity adjacent to the furcation area on the facial aspect	
Selects an appropriate curet and demonstrates the toe-up technique for the instrumentation of the mesial concavity on the first premolar	
Right-Handed Clinicians—Maxillary Left Posteriors, Lingual Aspect: **Left-Handed Clinicians—Maxillary Right Posteriors, Lingual Aspect:**	
Selects an appropriate curet and demonstrates a "chin-cup" fulcrum with a finger assist for the distal surface of the first molar	
Selects an appropriate curet and demonstrates instrumentation of the mesial surface of the first molar	
Selects an appropriate curet and demonstrates instrumentation of the distal furcation on the first molar tooth	
Selects an appropriate curet and demonstrates instrumentation of the mesial furcation on the first molar tooth; states whether the mesial furcation should be accessed from the facial or lingual aspect and explains the rationale	
Right-Handed Clinicians—Maxillary Left Posteriors, Lingual Aspect: **Left-Handed Clinicians—Maxillary Right Posteriors, Lingual Aspect:**	
Selects an appropriate curet and demonstrates a cross arch fulcrum for this sextant	
Selects an appropriate curet and demonstrates the toe-up technique for the instrumentation of the distal root concavity on the first molar	
Selects an appropriate curet and demonstrates the toe-up technique for the instrumentation of the palatal root depression	
Mandibular Anteriors, Lingual Aspect	
Selects an appropriate curet, and using an extraoral fulcrum, instruments the lingual aspect	

Module 21

Calculus Removal: Concepts, Planning, and Patient Cases

Module Overview

Periodontal instrumentation for the removal of plaque biofilm and dental calculus is an important component of nonsurgical periodontal therapy. This module begins with a discussion of the (1) objective and rationale for periodontal instrumentation, (2) terminology used to describe periodontal instrumentation, (3) healing after instrumentation, and (4) dental hypersensitivity. The second part of the module presents information on appointment planning and instrument sequencing for calculus removal. Section 4 contains six fictitious patient cases for practice in appointment planning for multiple calculus removal appointments.

Module Outline

Key Terms

Periodontal maintenance
Long junctional epithelium
Dentinal hypersensitivity
Dentinal tubules
Odontoblastic process
Scaling
Root planing
Periodontal debridement
Deplaquing
Informed consent
Capacity for consent
Written consent
Verbal consent
Implied consent
Informed refusal
Gross scaling
Circuit scaling

Learning Objectives

1. List two objectives of periodontal instrumentation.
2. Discuss how terminology related to calculus removal has evolved and give several examples.
3. Discuss the rational for periodontal instrumentation in the treatment of patients.
4. Define the term *periodontal debridement* as defined in the dental hygiene literature.
5. Discuss the ways in which a clinician's choice of words can facilitate or hinder communication with patients regarding dental hygiene care.
6. Define and discuss the terms *informed consent, capacity for consent, written consent,* and *informed refusal* as these terms apply to periodontal instrumentation.
7. Describe the type of healing to be expected following successful instrumentation of root surfaces.
8. Explain the origin of the condition called dental hypersensitivity.

Section 1
Concepts of Periodontal Instrumentation

OBJECTIVE AND RATIONALE FOR PERIODONTAL INSTRUMENTATION

1. Objective of Periodontal Instrumentation

a. The objective of periodontal instrumentation is the mechanical removal of microorganisms and their products for the prevention and treatment of periodontal diseases.
   1. ***Because of the structure of biofilms, physical removal of bacterial plaque biofilm is the most effective mechanism of control.***
   2. Most subgingival plaque biofilm located within periodontal pockets cannot be reached by brushes, floss, or mouth rinses.
      a) For this reason, frequent periodontal debridement of subgingival root surfaces to remove or disrupt bacterial plaque mechanically is an essential component of the treatment of periodontitis.
      b) In fact, periodontal instrumentation is likely to remain the most important component of nonsurgical periodontal therapy for the foreseeable future.

b. The removal of calculus deposits from tooth surfaces is a critical step in any plan for nonsurgical periodontal therapy.
   1. Calculus deposits harbor living bacterial biofilms; thus, if the calculus remains, so do the pathogenic bacteria, making it impossible to reestablish periodontal health.[1–3]
   2. ***In order to reestablish periodontal health, root surfaces must be free of plaque biofilm and all calculus deposits.*** Periodontal instrumentation must cover every square millimeter of the root surface.
   3. Calculus removal is always a fundamental part of periodontal therapy.

2. Rationale for Periodontal Instrumentation. The scientific basis for performing periodontal instrumentation includes all points listed below.

a. To arrest the progress of periodontal disease by removing plaque biofilms and plaque biofilm–retentive calculus deposits.
b. To induce positive changes in the subgingival bacterial flora (count and content).
c. To create an environment that assists in maintaining tissue health and/or permits the gingival tissue to heal, thus eliminating inflammation in the periodontium.
d. To increase the effectiveness of patient self-care by eliminating areas of plaque biofilm retention that are difficult or impossible for the patient to clean.
e. To prevent recurrence of disease during periodontal maintenance. Periodontal maintenance refers to continuing patient care provided by the dental team to help the periodontitis patient maintain periodontal health following complete nonsurgical or surgical periodontal therapy.

3. Healing after Periodontal Instrumentation

a. After thorough periodontal instrumentation, some healing of the periodontal tissues normally occurs. Tissue healing does not occur overnight, and in most cases, it is not possible to assess the true tissue response for at least 1 month after the completion of instrumentation.

b. Clinically, periodontal instrumentation can result in reduced probing depths. Tissue response to periodontal instrumentation is depicted in Figure 21-1. ***It is important to realize that following periodontal instrumentation, normally there is no formation of new alveolar bone, new cementum, or new periodontal ligament.***

1. Reduced probing depth due to formation of a long junctional epithelium.

a) As inflammation in the periodontium resolves, the junctional epithelium can readapt to the root surface as shown in Figure 21-2.

b) This readaptation of the epithelial cells to the root surface is referred to as a long junctional epithelium.

2. Reduced probing depth due to resolution of tissue swelling and shrinkage of the tissue.

3. There can be very little change in the level of the soft tissues, resulting in a residual periodontal pocket.

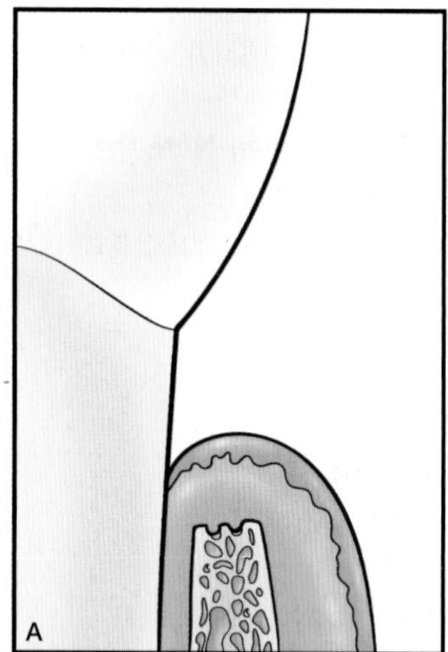

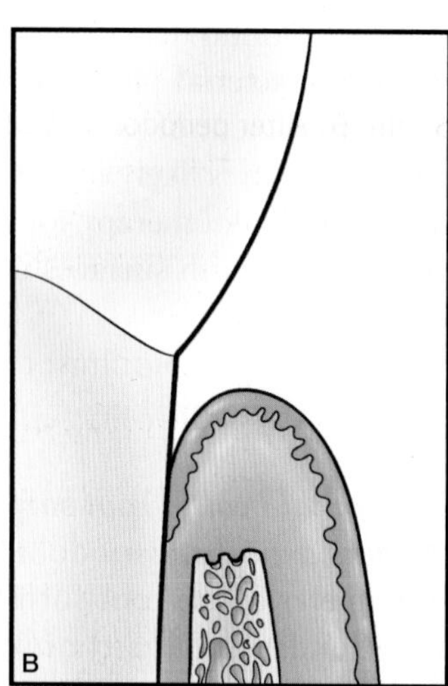

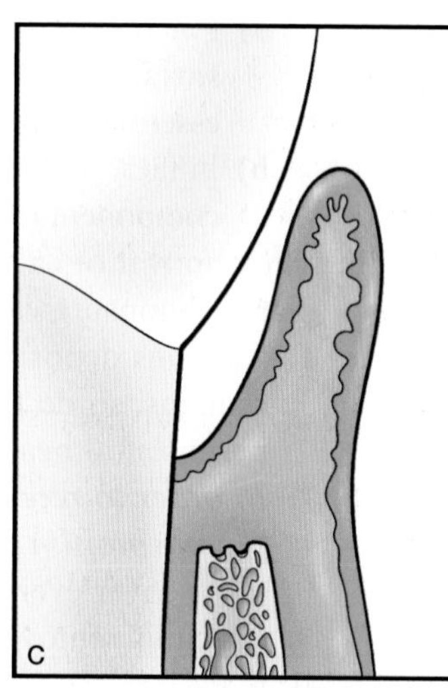

Figure 21-1. Soft Tissue Responses to Thorough Periodontal Debridement. This figure shows some of the possible tissue changes that can occur following thorough periodontal debridement. **A.** There can be complete resolution of the inflammation resulting in shrinkage of the tissue and a shallow probing depth. **B.** There can be readaptation of the tissues to the root surface forming a long junctional epithelium. **C.** There can be very little change in the level of the soft tissues resulting in a residual periodontal pocket. (Used with permission from Nield-Gehrig JS. *Foundations of Periodontics for the Dental Hygienist*. 3rd ed. Philadelphia, PA: Lippincott Williams & Wilkins; 2011.)

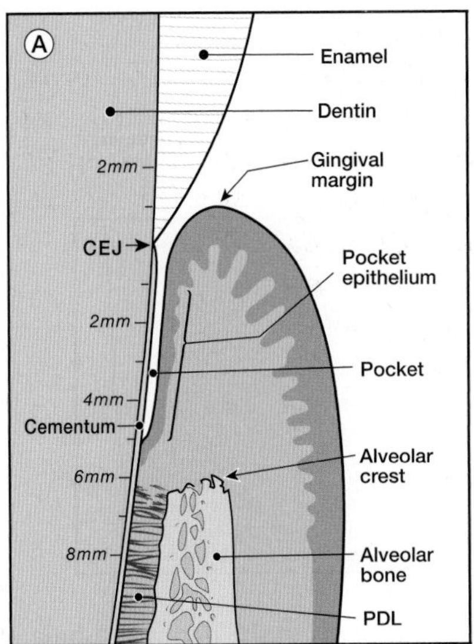

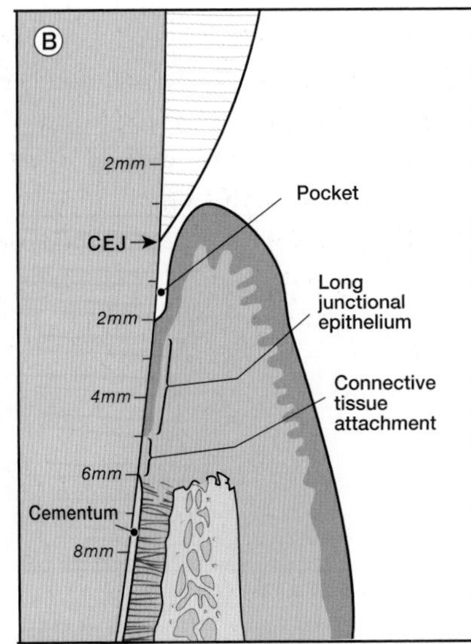

Figure 21-2. Healing by Formation of a Long Junctional Epithelium. A. Before therapy, the periodontal pocket depicted has a probing depth of 6 mm. **B.** After periodontal instrumentation, the tissue healing is through the formation of a long junctional epithelium. This results in a probing depth of 2 mm. Note that there is no formation of new bone, cementum, or periodontal ligament during the healing process that occurs after periodontal debridement. (Used with permission from Nield-Gehrig JS. *Foundations of Periodontics for the Dental Hygienist*. 3rd ed. Philadelphia, PA: Lippincott Williams & Wilkins; 2011.)

4. **Dentinal Hypersensitivity after Periodontal Instrumentation**
   a. **Description.** Dentinal hypersensitivity is a short, sharp painful reaction that occurs when some areas of exposed dentin are subjected to mechanical (touch of toothbrush bristles), thermal (ice cream), or chemical (acidic grapefruit) stimuli. For example, an individual may experience pain when brushing a certain tooth or when eating sweet, sour, or acidic foods. In some patients with this condition, breathing in cold air while walking outside on a cold day can produce a similar painful reaction.
   b. **Precipitating Factors for the Sensitivity**
      1. Hypersensitivity is associated with exposed dentin; however, not all exposed dentin is hypersensitive.
      2. The pain of hypersensitivity is sporadic. A patient may experience sensitivity for a period of time, but may experience other periods when sensitivity is not a problem.
      3. Instrumentation of root surfaces can result in dentinal hypersensitivity. The possibility of creating dentinal hypersensitivity underscores that conservation of cementum should be a goal of nonsurgical instrumentation.
   c. **Fundamental Origin of Hypersensitivity**
      1. Evidence suggests that the origin of dentinal hypersensitivity is explained by the hydrodynamic theory of dentin sensitivity.[4] Important elements of this theory are outlined below.
         a) The dentinal tubules penetrate the dentin like long, miniature tunnels extending throughout the thickness of the dentin.
         b) The part of a dentinal tubule closest to the pulp contains an odontoblastic process, which is a thin tail of cytoplasm from a cell in the tooth pulp called an odontoblast (Fig. 21-3).

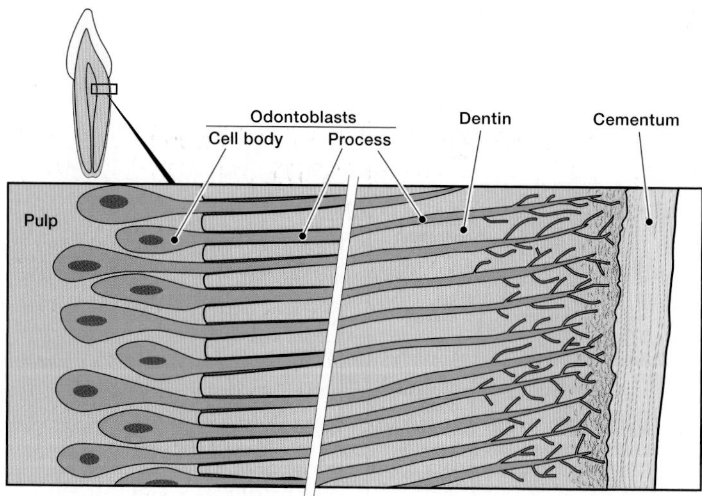

Figure 21-3. Odontoblastic Process. The odontoblastic cell process in the dentinal tubule often fills the part of the dentinal tubule closest to the pulp but can extend farther from the pulp toward the junction of the dentin with the enamel or cementum.

- **c)** Disturbances to the surface of exposed dentin where the tubules remain open can result in movement of the fluids within the tubules themselves. As already discussed, examples of disturbances to the surface of the tooth can be mechanical, thermal, or chemical stimuli. Cold temperature is one of the most common triggers for dentinal hypersensitivity.
- **d)** Fluid movement within open dentinal tubules can stimulate certain nerve endings that are associated with the odontoblastic processes, resulting in a short, sharp pain in the tooth.

2. Periodontal instrumentation and hypersensitivity can be closely related.
- **a)** For teeth with existing dentinal hypersensitivity, instrumentation of root surfaces can result in eliciting the sharp pain. During instrumentation, local anesthesia can be used to control any discomfort that might arise during thorough instrumentation.
- **b)** Most dentinal hypersensitivity resulting from periodontal instrumentation is mild and resolves within a few weeks if the exposed root surfaces are kept plaque biofilm free.
- **c)** In its more severe forms, however, dentinal hypersensitivity can result in a patient's inability to perform complete self-care.

d. Patient Education. The dental hygienist can provide the patient with the following facts regarding dentinal hypersensitivity:

1. Sensitivity to cold can increase following periodontal instrumentation.
2. If sensitivity resulting from periodontal instrumentation occurs, it usually gradually disappear over a few weeks.
3. Thorough daily removal of plaque biofilm is one of the most important factors in the prevention and control of sensitivity. Without meticulous plaque control, treatments for dentinal hypersensitivity are usually not successful.
4. If dentinal hypersensitivity becomes a problem, recommendations for special toothpastes can be made that can enhance its resolution, but immediate results should not be expected.

TERMINOLOGY USED TO DESCRIBE PERIODONTAL INSTRUMENTATION

1. **Periodontal Instrumentation Terminology.** There has been some evolution in the terminology associated with dental calculus removal and dental plaque biofilm removal over the past years. The careful reader will be wise to note that there are different sets of terminology that appear in the dental hygiene journals and textbooks compared to the terminology in dental journals and textbooks. The differences in this terminology revolve around the terms described below.

   a. **Traditional Instrumentation Terminology.** Traditionally, the terms scaling and root planing were used to describe periodontal instrumentation.

      1. Scaling is defined as the instrumentation of the crown and root surfaces of the teeth to remove plaque, calculus, and stains.
      2. Root planing is defined as a treatment procedure designed to remove cementum or surface dentin that is rough, impregnated with calculus, or contaminated with toxins or microorganisms.
         a) As traditionally defined, root planing involves the routine, intentional removal of cementum and the instrumenting of all root surfaces to a glassy smooth texture.
         b) Until relatively recently, it was thought that bacterial products were firmly held in cemental surfaces exposed by attachment loss occurring as a result of periodontitis. It was believed that vigorous root planing with intentional removal of most cementum was always needed to ensure the removal of all calculus as well as all bacterial products from the root surfaces.
         c) It is now understood that vigorous root planing is not universally needed to reestablish periodontal health in all sites of periodontitis. Rather than vigorous root planing and removal of most or all of the cementum, it is now known that the bacterial products can be removed from the root surfaces with a minimal amount of actual cementum removal.[5–8]

   b. **Emerging Terminology**

      1. Periodontal debridement is a newer term that has been used in the dental hygiene literature since 1993 to replace the terms scaling and root planing.
         a) Periodontal debridement is defined as the removal or disruption of bacterial plaque biofilm, its by-products, and plaque biofilm–retentive calculus deposits from coronal tooth surfaces and tooth root surfaces to reestablish periodontal health and restore a balance between the bacterial flora and the host's immune responses.
         b) ***Periodontal debridement includes instrumentation of every square millimeter of root surface for removal of plaque biofilm and calculus, but does not include the deliberate, aggressive removal of cementum.***
         c) Conservation of cementum is one goal of periodontal debridement. It is currently believed that conservation of cementum enhances periodontal healing in the form of either repair or regeneration. In periodontal health, an important function of cementum is to attach the periodontal ligament fibers to the root surface. During the healing process after disease, cementum is thought to contribute to repair of the periodontium.
      2. Deplaquing is the disruption or removal of subgingival microbial plaque biofilm and its by-products from cemental surfaces and the pocket space.

WORD CHOICE WHEN COMMUNICATING WITH PATIENTS

There are several aspects relating to word choice—or terminology—to consider when talking with patients about dental hygiene care and periodontal instrumentation.

1. **Word Choice Pertaining to Dental Hygiene Care.** Dental hygienists hope that patients will value the care that they provide. The value a patient perceives may be influenced by the way that the hygienist refers to those services.
   - **a.** Using words such as "dental cleaning" or "prophy" minimizes the perceived value of hygiene care. Hygienists do not simply "shine the teeth" as the phrase "clean the teeth" implies.
   - **b.** Word choices such as "dental hygiene services" or "dental hygiene therapies" better convey the complex, therapeutic nature of dental hygiene care.
   - **c.** Instead of saying, "Can we set up your next cleaning appointment?" consider a statement such as, "Let's set up your next dental hygiene appointment to care for the health of your mouth and prevent disease."
2. **Word Choice Pertaining to Periodontal Instrumentation.** A second consideration is the mental images that the hygienist's words create in the patient's mind.
   - **a.** Words such as "scale" and "root plane" do not clarify the treatment procedure for the patient, but they may conjure up very negative mental pictures. For example, hearing that his teeth are going to be "root planed" might cause a patient to picture layers of his teeth being shaved away the way a wood plane shaves off layers of wood. The phrase "scale and root plane your teeth" might cause the patient to envision the planned treatment as something very aggressive and uncomfortable.
   - **b.** Even the phrase "instrument the teeth" does nothing to explain the procedure to the patient. On the positive side, "instrument" does not produce the negative mental images that the forceful sounding terms "scale and root planing" elicit.
   - **c.** The ideal solution to word use when explaining periodontal instrumentation is simply to EXPLAIN in everyday words how the patient will benefit from the procedure.

INFORMED CONSENT FOR PERIODONTAL INSTRUMENTATION

The core value of "Individual Autonomy and Respect for Human Beings" within the Code of Ethics for the American Dental Hygienists' Association (ADHA) discusses informed consent.[9] According to this core value, "People. . .have the right to full disclosure of all relevant information so they can make informed choices about their care."[9]

1. **Consent as it Relates to Periodontal Instrumentation**
   - **a.** It is the responsibility of the dental hygienist to provide complete and comprehensive information about the recommended plan for periodontal instrumentation so that the patient can make a well-informed decision about either accepting or rejecting the proposed treatment.
   - **b.** **Informed consent** involves informing the patient not only about the expected successful outcomes of periodontal instrumentation, but also about the possible risks, unanticipated outcomes, and alternative treatments as well.

Box 21-1. Ethical Considerations for Informed Consent for the Patient

- Reasoning/importance of proposed periodontal instrumentation
- Expected outcomes of the proposed periodontal instrumentation
- Risks involved in the proposed periodontal instrumentation
- Possible unexpected results of periodontal instrumentation
- Alternative approaches to periodontal instrumentation
- Possible consequences of refusal of treatment
- Costs of proposed treatment and alternatives
- Patient's capacity to consent (age, mental capacity, language comprehension)
- Written consent by patient

The patient should be made aware of the costs for each of the options involved, which may influence the patient's ultimate decision. Box 21-1 summarizes some of the ethical considerations for informed consent.

2. **Capacity for Consent.** A patient must also have the capacity to consent.
   a. Capacity for consent—the ability of a patient to fully understand the proposed treatment, possible risks, unanticipated outcomes, and alternative treatments—takes into account the patient's age, mental capacity, and language comprehension.
   b. The patient would expect that the dental hygienist would carry out the proposed periodontal instrumentation according to the proper standard of care, or that of the "reasonably prudent hygienist," and perform the services in a manner that "any hygienist would do in the same or similar situation."
   c. A dialogue between the patient and the hygienist is the best way to initiate the informed consent process.

3. **Documenting Consent**
   a. Once the patient is satisfied and agrees to the proposed plan for periodontal instrumentation, it is best if it is written in the patient's chart and signed by the patient and hygienist. This is an example of written consent. Written consent is legally binding and will hold up in a court of law.
   b. Both verbal consent (verbally agreeing to a proposed treatment without any formal written documentation) and implied consent (sitting in a dental chair and opening one's mouth for the hygienist), although acceptable for certain procedures, are not as legally sound as written consent.
   c. Figure 21-4 shows an example of an informed consent/informed refusal form.

4. **Informed Refusal.** Despite being informed of the proposed treatments, risks, and alternatives, the patient may decide to refuse the treatment plan. This is called informed refusal.
   a. Autonomy, as defined by the ADHA Code of Ethics, guarantees "self-determination" of the patient and is linked to informed consent.[9]
   b. Only after the patient has received informed consent can a decision be made to either accept or reject the proposed treatment.

c. Although refusal may not be the optimal choice of the treating hygienist, the patient has a right to make any decisions about his or her treatments that only affect him or her personally and do not pose a threat to others. Radiographs, fluoride treatments, and sealants are a few services for which patients have exercised informed refusal.
d. As a result, each dental office should include an informed consent/refusal form as part of the patient treatment record to ensure proper documentation.
e. Figure 21-4 shows an example of an informed consent/informed refusal form.

Informed Consent/Informed Refusal Form

1. I ______________________________, (name) agree to the proposed dental treatment by ______________________________, (name) RDH.

2. I fully understand the importance of the proposed treatment. ___Yes ___No

3. I understand that ____________________ is the expected outcome of the proposed treatment.

4. I understand that the possible risks and/or unanticipated outcomes of the proposed treatment are ____.

5. The possible treatment alternatives to the proposed treatment are ____________________.

6. I have been informed of the costs of the proposed and alternative treatments. ___Yes ___No

7. I understand the possible consequence(s) of refusal of the proposed treatment is/are ____.

8. I have the capacity to consent to the proposed treatment. ___Yes ___No

9. I refuse the proposed treatment. ___Yes ___No

10. Please list the treatment you are refusing. ______________________________

______________________ ______________ ______________________

Patient Signature Date RDH Signature

Figure 21-4. Sample Informed Consent/Informed Refusal Form.

Section 2
Planning for Calculus Removal

Frequently, it is not possible to remove calculus deposits from all the teeth in a single appointment. In this instance, calculus removal is completed using multiple appointments.

1. *The multiple appointment approach to calculus removal is based on the concept of complete calculus removal on the teeth treated at each appointment.*
2. *At each appointment, the clinician should treat only as many teeth, sextants, or quadrants as he or she can render calculus free during that appointment.* For example, the clinician may complete a single sextant (facial and lingual aspects) on a patient with periodontitis or complete two quadrants (half the mouth) on a patient with gingivitis.

GROSS CALCULUS REMOVAL—A HISTORICAL PERSPECTIVE

1. **A Historical Perspective on Calculus Removal**
   a. In the past, one common method of planning multiple calculus removal appointments involved instrumentation of all the teeth in the mouth with the goal of only partially removing some calculus deposits at the first appointment.
      1. The gross scaling approach involved devoting the first calculus removal appointment to removal of only the large-sized calculus deposits from the entire mouth. In this approach, medium and smaller calculus deposits were intentionally left on the teeth.
      2. The second appointment would involve instrumentation of the entire mouth to remove medium-sized deposits.
      3. Thus in this approach, all the teeth were instrumented at each appointment, "whittling away" the calculus deposits bit by bit at appointment after appointment.

   b. This intentional incomplete removal of calculus is commonly known as gross scaling because treatment began with removal of large, "gross" calculus deposits. This approach is sometimes called circuit scaling (because the clinician works around and around the mouth at appointment after appointment).
   c. This approach to calculus removal was common in the past but is no longer recommended. Gross scaling is discussed here because clinicians may encounter patients who have undergone gross scaling procedures and some clinicians still use this method of appointment planning for calculus removal.
2. **The Dangers of Incomplete Calculus Removal.** *The gross scaling approach is not recommended because of the undesirable consequences that can result from incomplete calculus removal.*
   a. **Proliferation of Microorganisms.** Gross scaling leaves behind partially removed deposits that are rough, irregular, and covered with bacterial plaque biofilm. As the marginal tissue shrinks, it closes off the entrance to the pocket, providing a protected environment within the pocket in which the microorganisms continue to multiply.

b. **Abscess Formation.** Incomplete calculus removal has been implicated in the formation of an abscess of the periodontium. An abscess of the periodontium is a localized collection of pus in the periodontal tissues.
   1. Abscesses may occur on teeth with a deep probing depth where gross scaling removes only the calculus deposits located above and slightly beneath the gingival margin.
   2. It is theorized that this incomplete calculus removal allows the gingival margin to tighten around the tooth, like a drawstring pouch, preventing drainage of bacterial waste products from the pocket.
   3. Medically compromised individuals—such as uncontrolled diabetics—and those with deep periodontal pockets are especially prone to abscess formation.

c. **Difficult Instrumentation.** Insertion beneath the gingival margin is often more difficult at those appointments following the initial gross scaling appointment because the gingival margin is more closely adapted to the tooth surface.

d. **Decreased Patient Motivation for Treatment.** Many patients are motivated to seek treatment for esthetic (appearance) reasons. Removal of the visible *supra*gingival deposits combined with the improved appearance of the gingival tissues may influence the patient to forego further treatment. It is hard for patients to recognize that "what they can't see can hurt them."

e. **Patient Frustration.** When the patient undergoes multiple appointments at which the entire mouth is instrumented, he begins to feel that nothing is being accomplished by the treatment. All he knows is that the clinician goes around and around his mouth at each appointment, seemly without end. ("I thought you cleaned all of my teeth at the LAST appointment!")

COMPLETE CALCULUS REMOVAL—THE GOLD STANDARD FOR CARE

When multiple appointments are needed for calculus removal, the clinician must decide how to divide up the work. ***At each appointment, the clinician should treat only as many teeth, sextants, or quadrants as he or she can render calculus free during that appointment.***

1. **Complete Several Teeth**
   a. With extremely difficult cases, the student clinician may only complete a few teeth (both facial and lingual aspects).
   b. In most instances, however, the clinician will be able to complete the facial and lingual aspects of a sextant or quadrant.

2. **Complete One Sextant or Quadrant**
   a. Usually, it is possible to complete one sextant or quadrant at an appointment.
   b. For example, the clinician might begin by treating the facial and lingual aspects of a posterior sextant. Treatment can end here for the appointment, or if time permits, the adjacent anterior teeth are completed to the midline of the arch (resulting in completion of the quadrant).

3. **Complete Two Quadrants on the Same Side of the Mouth**
   a. When two quadrants are completed at one appointment, treatment of *a maxillary and mandibular quadrant on the same side of the mouth* is recommended (versus treating the entire maxillary arch or the entire mandibular arch).

b. Completing a maxillary and mandibular quadrant on one side of the mouth is preferred for several reasons.

1. This approach gives the patient an untreated side on which to chew comfortably.

2. Completing quadrants on one side of the mouth usually divides the work more evenly because the maxillary arch is more difficult for most clinicians.

3. When local anesthesia is indicated for two quadrants, it is recommended that a maxillary and mandibular quadrant on the same side of the mouth be selected.

Section 3
Appointment Planning for Calculus Removal

INSTRUMENT SELECTION FOR CALCULUS REMOVAL

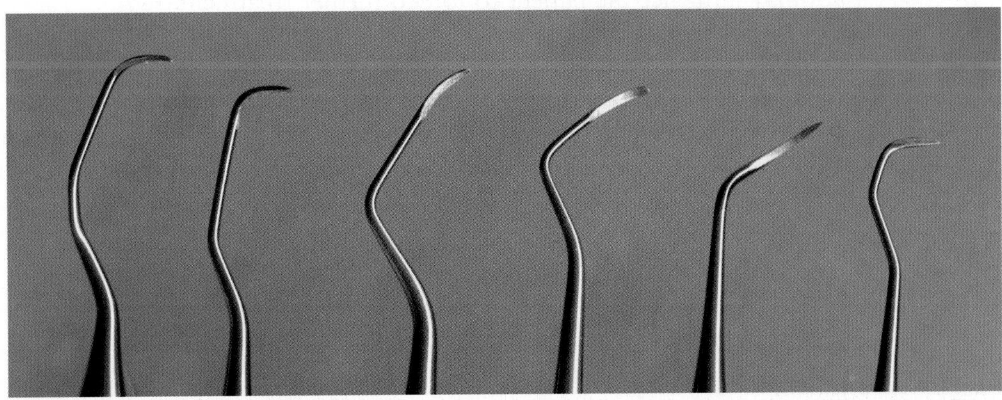

Figure 21-5. Calculus Removal Instruments. An important component of periodontal debridement is selecting the correct instrument for the task.

For calculus removal, periodontal instruments (Fig. 21-5) are selected based on the size and location of the calculus deposits (Table 21-1).

1. Large-sized calculus deposits most commonly are located above the gingival margin and can be removed using sickle scalers.
2. Small- or medium-sized calculus deposits usually are located below the gingival margin and can be removed using either universal or area-specific curets.
   - Small- or medium-sized deposits on root surfaces located within sulci or shallow periodontal pockets can be removed with a universal curet.
   - Small- or medium-sized deposits located on root surfaces within deep periodontal pockets can be removed with area-specific curets.
   - Tenacious and large-sized deposits can be removed with rigid curets, ultrasonic instruments, or sonic instruments.

TABLE 21-1. General Guide for Selection of Calculus Removal Instruments

Size of Deposit	Location of Deposit	Instrument
Large deposits	Above the gingival margin	Sickle scalers
Medium deposits	Above and below the gingival margin	Universal curets
Small deposits	Above the gingival margin	Universal curets
Small deposits	On cervical-third of root	Universal curets
Small deposits	On middle or apical-third of root	Area-specific curets

PLAN FOR CALCULUS REMOVAL

Although it is critical for the clinician to develop a calculus removal plan that will meet the needs of each individual patient, beginning clinicians often find it helpful to review an example of a typical plan for calculus removal (Table 21-2). In Section 4, patient profiles and examples of typical calculus removal plans are provided. Each calculus removal plan shown simply provides an example of one approach to calculus removal; other acceptable plans for calculus removal could be developed.

FICTITIOUS PATIENT EXAMPLE

Patient Assessment Data Example

- 28 teeth (third molars have not erupted)
- Gingival margin is at the cementoenamel junction (CEJ) on all teeth; probing depths vary between 4 and 5 mm
- **Supragingival deposits**—heavy deposits above the gingival margin on the lingual surface of the mandibular anterior teeth and the facial aspect of the maxillary molars
- **Subgingival deposits**—medium-sized deposits on the cervical-third of the roots of all teeth; small-sized deposits generalized on all teeth

TABLE 21-2. Typical Calculus Removal Plan for Example

Treatment Area	Instrument(s)—Listed in the Order of Use
Appt. 1: Mandibular anterior sextant	1. Anterior sickle for supragingival deposits 2. Universal curet for medium-sized deposits 3. Area-specific curets for small-sized deposits
Appt. 2: Mandibular right posterior sextant	1. Universal curet for medium-sized deposits 2. Area-specific curets for small-sized deposits
Appt. 3: Maxillary right posterior sextant	1. Posterior sickle for supragingival deposits on molar teeth 2. Universal curet for medium-sized deposits 3. Area-specific curets for small-sized deposits
Appt. 4: Maxillary anterior sextant	1. Universal curet for medium-sized deposits 2. Area-specific curets for small-sized deposits
Appt. 5: Maxillary left posterior sextant	1. Posterior sickle for supragingival deposits on molar teeth 2. Universal curet for medium-sized deposits 3. Area-specific curets for small-sized deposits
Appt. 6: Mandibular left posterior sextant	1. Universal curet for medium-sized deposits 2. Area-specific curets for small-sized deposits

Fictitious Patient Cases are found in Section 4 of this module.

REFERENCES

1. Checchi L, Montevecchi M, Checchi V, Zappulla F. The relationship between bleeding on probing and subgingival deposits. An endoscopical evaluation. *Open Dent J.* 2009;3:154–160.
2. Fujikawa K, O'Leary TJ, Kafrawy AH. The effect of retained subgingival calculus on healing after flap surgery. *J Periodontol.* 1988;59:170–175.
3. Wilson TG, Harrel SK, Nunn ME, Francis B, Webb K. The relationship between the presence of tooth-borne subgingival deposits and inflammation found with a dental endoscope. *J Periodontol.* 2008;79:2029–2035.
4. Burwell A, Jennings D, Muscle D, Greenspan DC. NovaMin and dentin hypersensitivity–in vitro evidence of efficacy. *J Clin Dent.* 2010;21:66–71.
5. Hughes FJ, Smales FC. Immunohistochemical investigation of the presence and distribution of cementum-associated lipopolysaccharides in periodontal disease. *J Periodontal Res.* 1986;21:660–667.
6. Moore J, Wilson M, Kieser JB. The distribution of bacterial lipopolysaccharide (endotoxin) in relation to periodontally involved root surfaces. *J Clin Periodontol.* 1986;13:748–751.
7. Nakib NM, Bissada NF, Simmelink JW, Goldstine SN. Endotoxin penetration into root cementum of periodontally healthy and diseased human teeth. *J Periodontol.* 1982;53:368–378.
8. O'Leary TJ. The impact of research on scaling and root planing. *J Periodontol.* 1986;57:69–75.
9. American Dental Hygienists' Association. *Bylaws and Code of Ethics.* Chicago, IL: American Dental Hygienists' Association; 2009.

RECOMMENDED READING

Darby ML, Walsh MM. *Dental Hygiene: Theory and Practice.* 3rd ed. St. Louis, MO: Saunders/Elsevier; 2010.

Dougall A, Fiske J. Access to special care dentistry, part 3. Consent and capacity. *Br Dent J.* 2008;205:71–81.

Fitch P. Cultural competence and dental hygiene care delivery: integrating cultural care into the dental hygiene process of care. *J Dent Hyg.* 2004;78:11–21.

Kimbrough-Walls V, Jautar C. *Ethics, Jurisprudence and Practice Management in Dental Hygiene.* 3rd ed. Upper Saddle River, NJ: Pearson; 2012.

Ozar DT, Sokol DJ. *Dental Ethics at Chairside: Professional Principles and Practical Applications.* 2nd ed. Washington, DC: Georgetown University Press; 2002.

Rule JT, Veatch RM. *Ethical Questions in Dentistry.* 2nd ed. Chicago, IL: Quintessence Publishing; 2004.

Section 4
Practical Focus—Fictitious Patient Cases

Instruments for Fictitious Patient Cases

For the fictitious patient cases in this section, you may select calculus removal instruments from your school's instrument kit or any of the instruments found in Modules 11 to 19 of this book.

Case Questions

Directions: Photocopy the **Calculus Removal Plan** form in Table 21-3 (or create a similar form yourself on tablet paper).

For each fictitious patient case:

1. *Use the information recorded on the periodontal chart to calculate the clinical attachment loss on the facial and lingual aspects and enter this information on the patient's periodontal chart.*
2. Determine how many appointments you will need for calculus removal.
3. List the treatment area(s) to be completed at each appointment. For example, at a single appointment, can you complete (1) the entire mouth, (2) the maxillary and mandibular right quadrants (half the mouth), (3) the mandibular right quadrant (half the mandibular arch), (4) the mandibular right sextant, or (5) the mandibular anterior sextant?
4. Select appropriate instruments for use at each appointment. Indicate the sequence the instruments will be used in and the use of each instrument.
5. On the back of the form, explain your rationale for instrument selection and sequence.

TABLE 21-3. Calculus Removal Plan

Treatment Area	Instrument(s)—Listed in the Order of Use
Appt. 1:	
Appt. 2 (if needed):	
Appt. 3 (if needed):	
Appt. 4 (if needed):	
Appt. 5 (if needed):	
Appt. 6 (if needed):	

FICTITIOUS PATIENT CASE 1

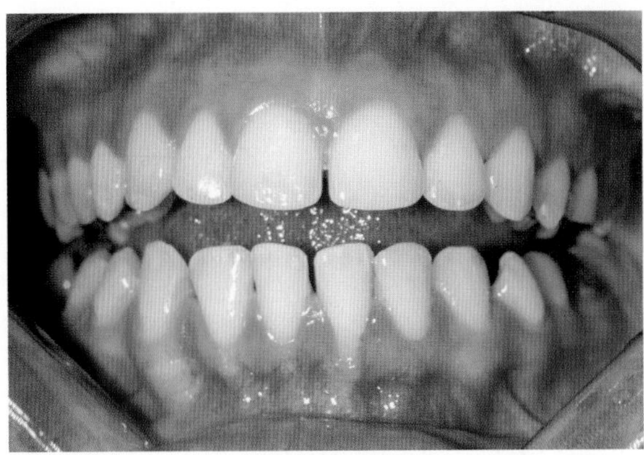

Figure 21-6A

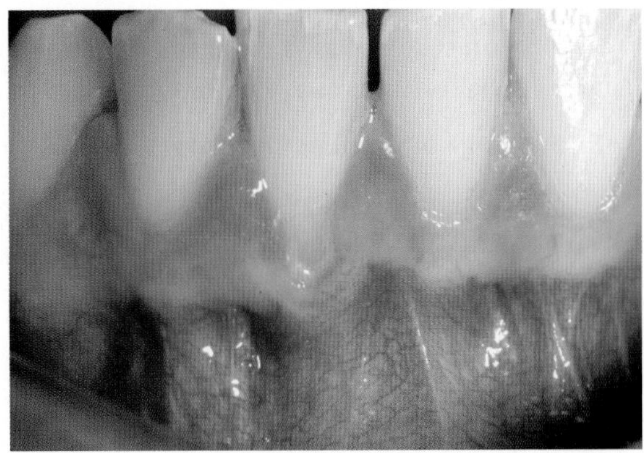

Figure 21-6B

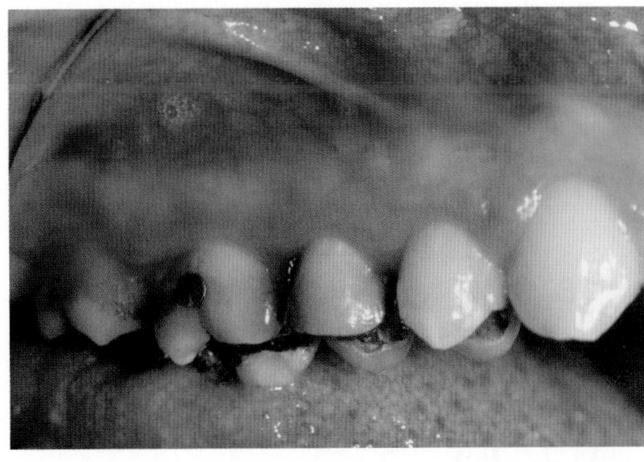

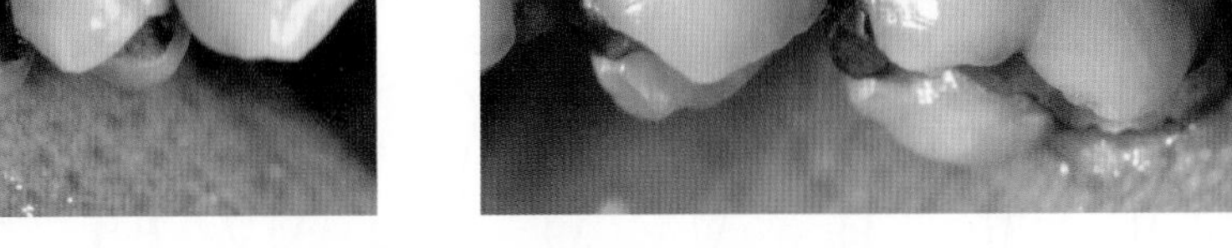

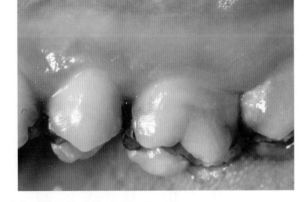

Figure 21-6, C and D. Facial Aspects of the Maxillary Posterior Sextants.

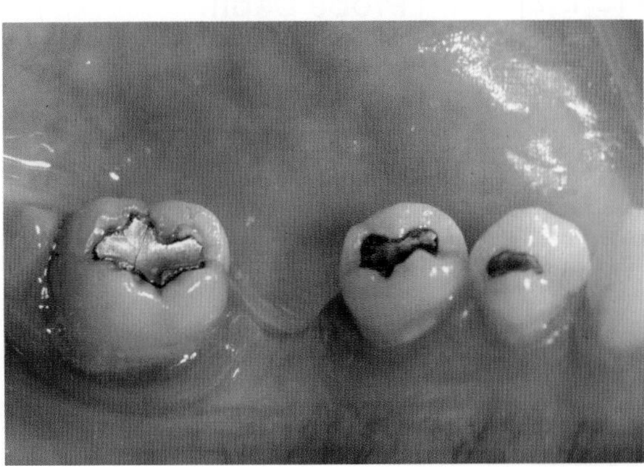

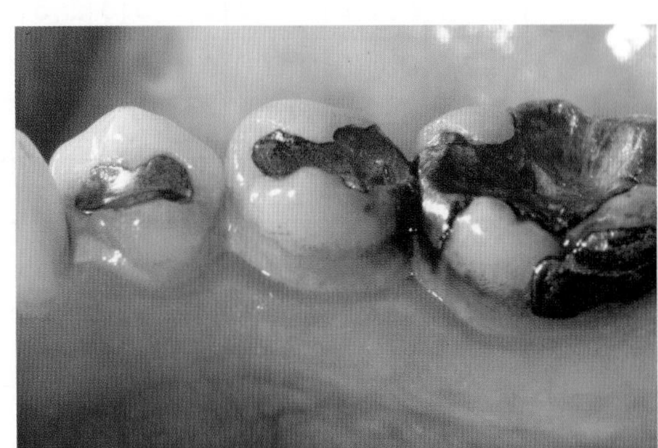

Figure 21-6, E and F. Lingual Aspects of the Mandibular Posterior Sextants.

Patient Case 1: Assessment Data

1. Supragingival Calculus Deposits

- Moderate deposits generalized on the lingual aspect of the mandibular arch
- Moderate deposits on lingual aspect of the maxillary first and second molars

2. Subgingival Calculus Deposits

- Medium-sized deposits on the lingual aspects of maxillary and mandibular arches
- Light deposits on facial aspect of maxillary and mandibular arches

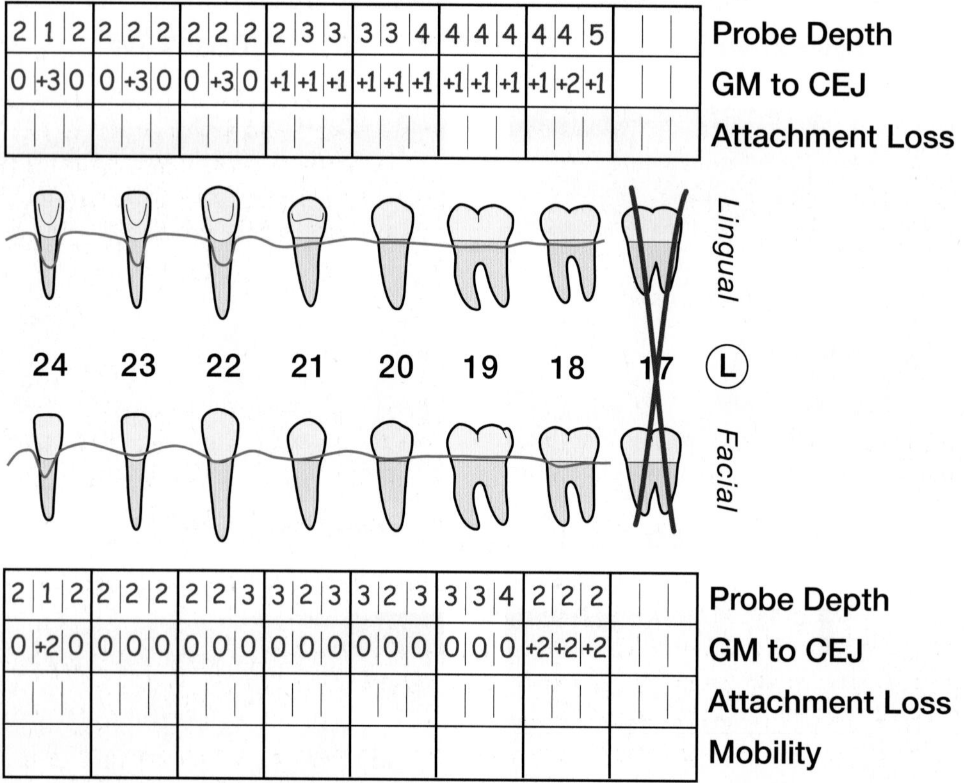

Lingual	24	23	22	21	20	19	18	17
Probe Depth	2 1 2	2 2 2	2 2 2	2 3 3	3 3 4	4 4 4	4 4 5	
GM to CEJ	0 +3 0	0 +3 0	0 +3 0	+1 +1 +1	+1 +1 +1	+1 +1 +1	+1 +2 +1	
Attachment Loss								

Facial	24	23	22	21	20	19	18	17
Probe Depth	2 1 2	2 2 2	2 2 3	3 2 3	3 2 3	3 3 4	2 2 2	
GM to CEJ	0 +2 0	0 0 0	0 0 0	0 0 0	0 0 0	0 0 0	+2 +2 +2	
Attachment Loss								
Mobility								

Figure 21-6G. Partial Periodontal Chart for Patient 1. (Key: GM = gingival margin; CEJ = cementoenamel junction.)

FICTITIOUS PATIENT CASE 2

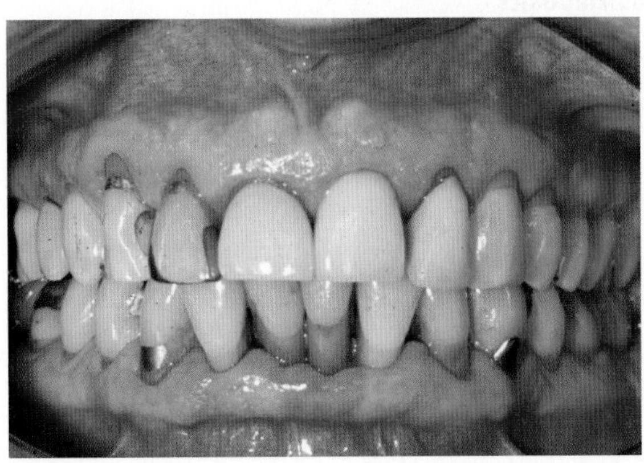

Figure 21-7A

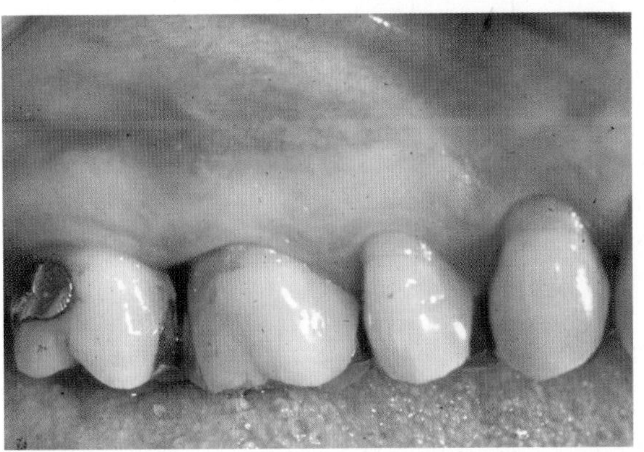

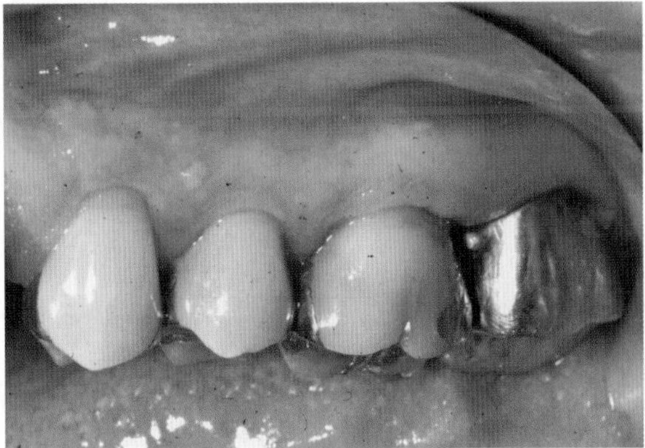

Figure 21-7, B and C. Facial Aspects of Maxillary Posterior Sextants.

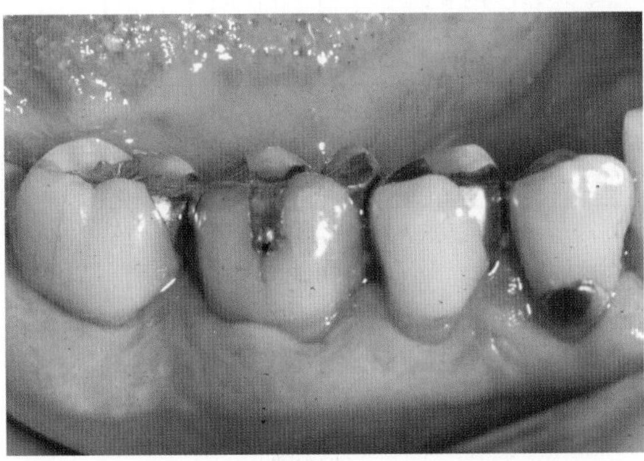

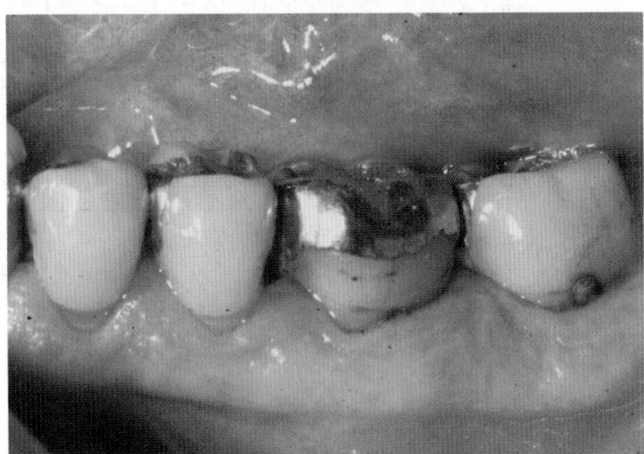

Figure 21-7, D and E. Facial Aspects of Mandibular Posterior Sextants.

Patient Case 2: Assessment Data

1. Supragingival Calculus Deposits

- No supragingival calculus present; patient self-care is excellent

2. Subgingival Calculus Deposits

- Light deposits throughout entire mouth

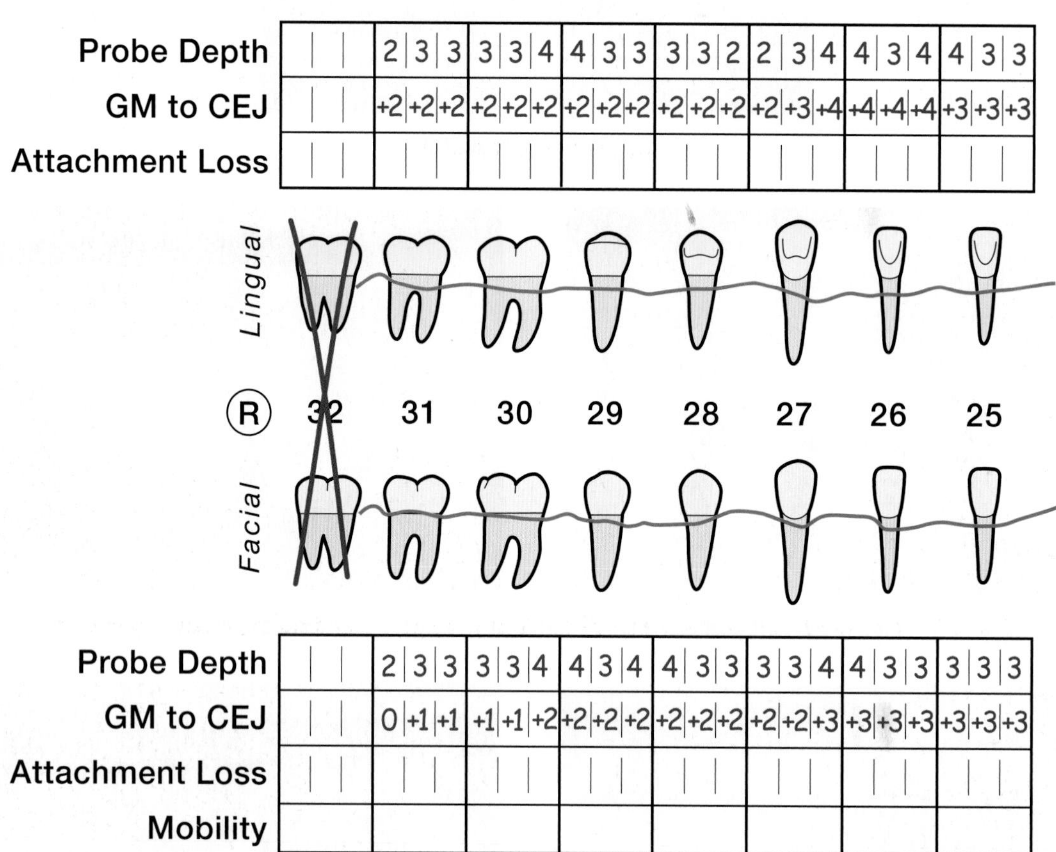

Lingual

	32	31	30	29	28	27	26	25
Probe Depth		2 3 3	3 3 4	4 3 3	3 3 2	2 3 4	4 3 4	4 3 3
GM to CEJ		+2 +2 +2	+2 +2 +2	+2 +2 +2	+2 +2 +2	+2 +3 +4	+4 +4 +4	+3 +3 +3
Attachment Loss								

Facial

	32	31	30	29	28	27	26	25
Probe Depth		2 3 3	3 3 4	4 3 4	4 3 3	3 3 4	4 3 3	3 3 3
GM to CEJ		0 +1 +1	+1 +1 +2	+2 +2 +2	+2 +2 +2	+2 +2 +3	+3 +3 +3	+3 +3 +3
Attachment Loss								
Mobility								

Figure 21-7F. Partial Periodontal Chart for Patient 2. (Key: GM = gingival margin; CEJ = cementoenamel junction.)

FICTITIOUS PATIENT CASE 3

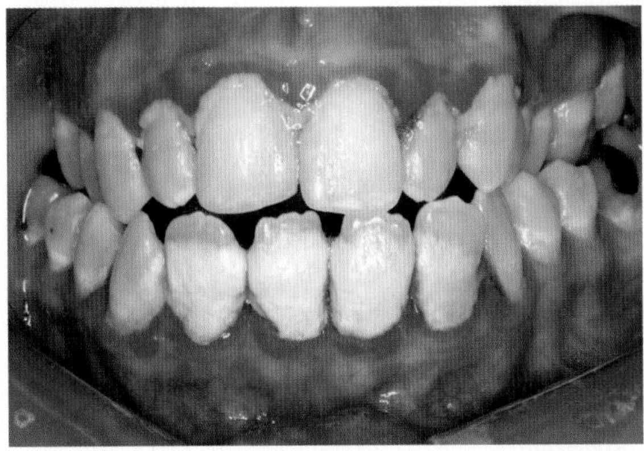

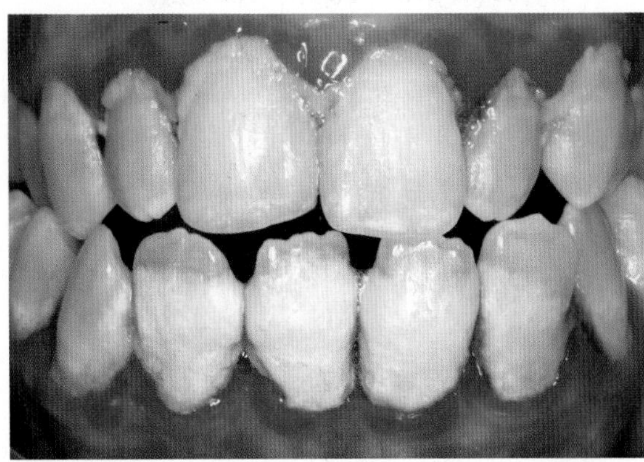

Figure 21-8, A and B

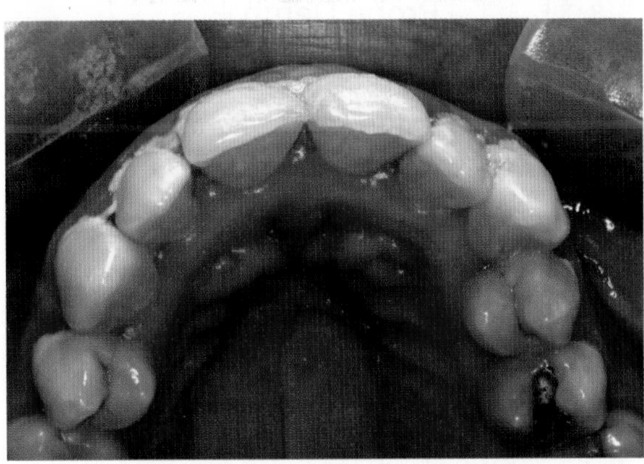

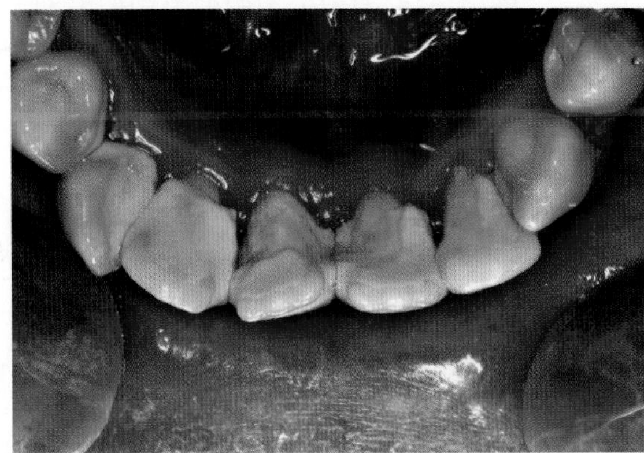

Figure 21-8, C and D. Lingual Aspects of the Maxillary and Mandibular Anterior Sextants.

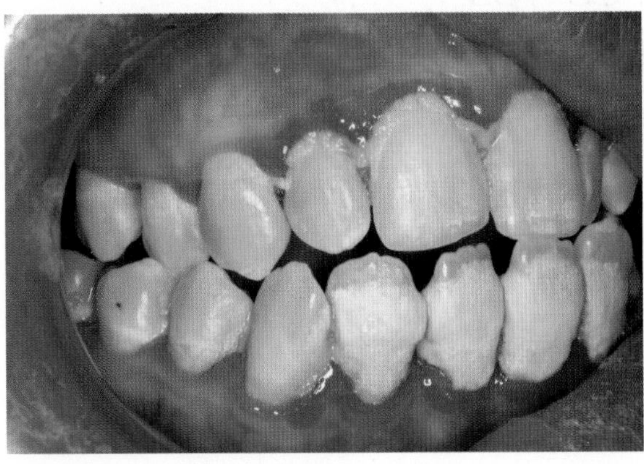

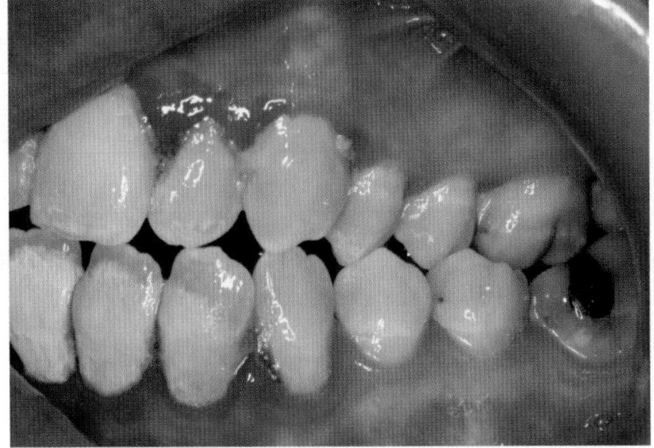

Figure 21-8, E and F. Right and Left Sides of Mouth. (Courtesy of Dr. Richard Foster, Guilford Technical Community College, Jamestown, NC.)

Patient Case 3: Assessment Data

1. Supragingival Calculus Deposits

- Heavy deposits on the mandibular anterior sextant
- Moderate deposits on the maxillary anterior sextant
- Light deposits on the maxillary and mandibular posterior sextants

2. Subgingival Calculus Deposits

- Medium-sized deposits throughout the mouth

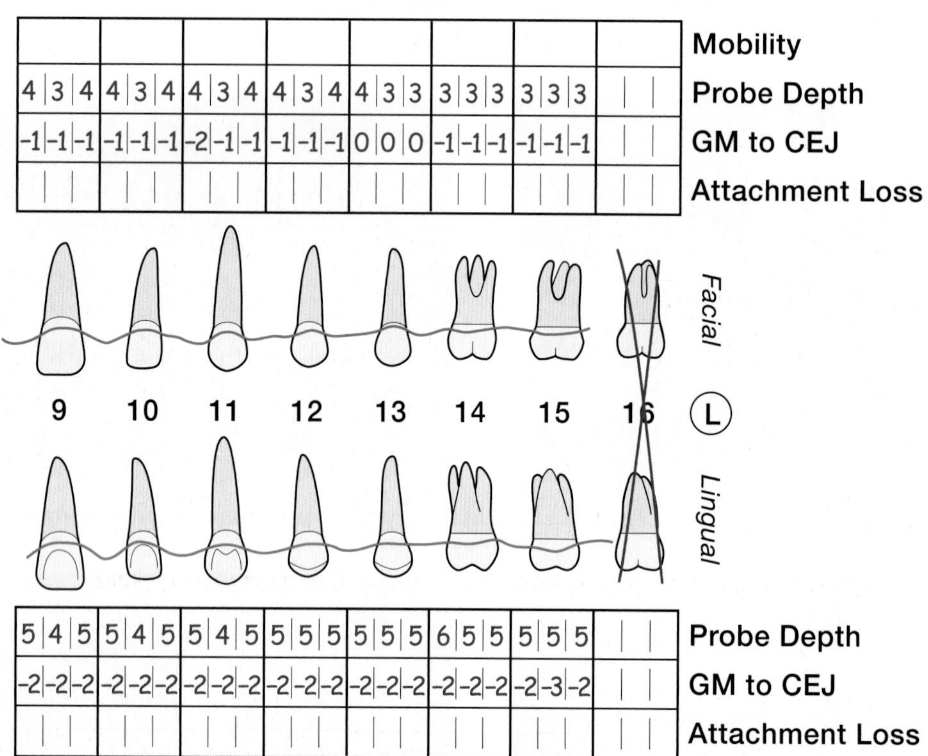

	9	10	11	12	13	14	15	16
Mobility								
Probe Depth	4 3 4	4 3 4	4 3 4	4 3 4	4 3 3	3 3 3	3 3 3	
GM to CEJ	-1 -1 -1	-1 -1 -1	-2 -1 -1	-1 -1 -1	0 0 0	-1 -1 -1	-1 -1 -1	
Attachment Loss								

	9	10	11	12	13	14	15	16
Probe Depth	5 4 5	5 4 5	5 4 5	5 5 5	5 5 5	6 5 5	5 5 5	
GM to CEJ	-2 -2 -2	-2 -2 -2	-2 -2 -2	-2 -2 -2	-2 -2 -2	-2 -2 -2	-2 -3 -2	
Attachment Loss								

Figure 21-8G. Partial Periodontal Chart for Patient 3. (Key: GM = gingival margin; CEJ = cementoenamel junction.)

FICTITIOUS PATIENT CASE 4

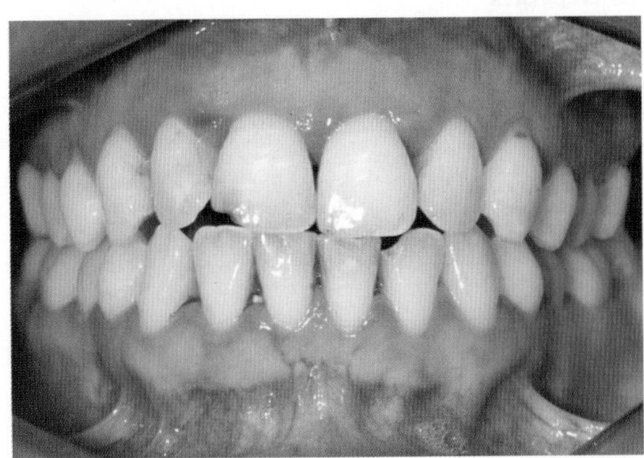

Figure 21-9A

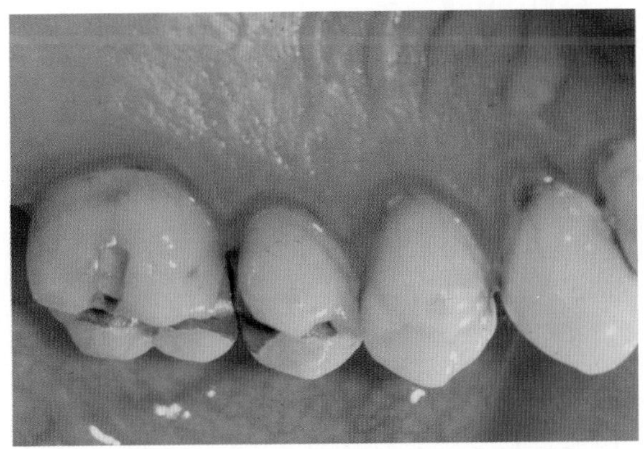

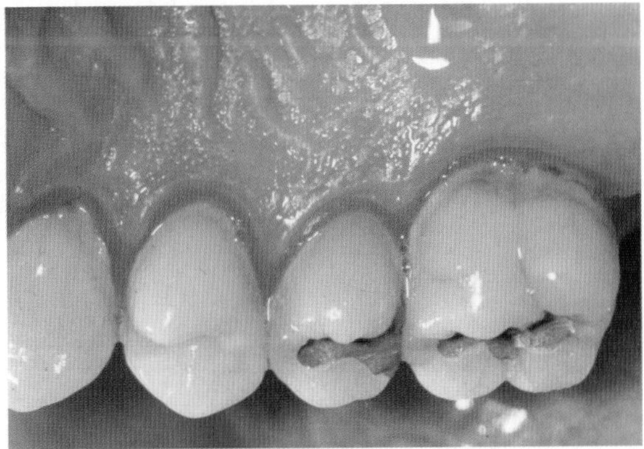

Figure 21-9, B and C. Lingual Aspects of the Maxillary Posterior Sextants.

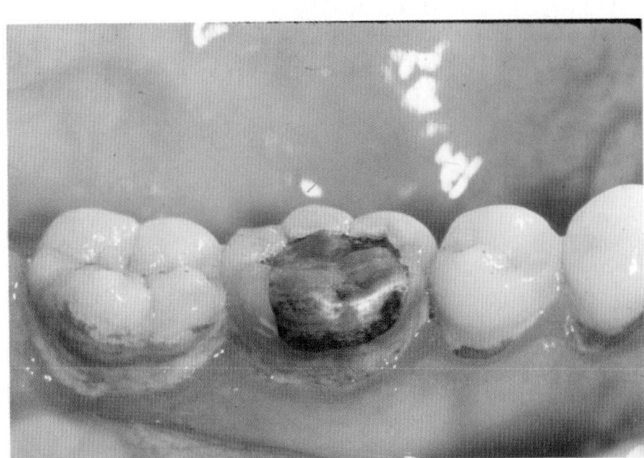

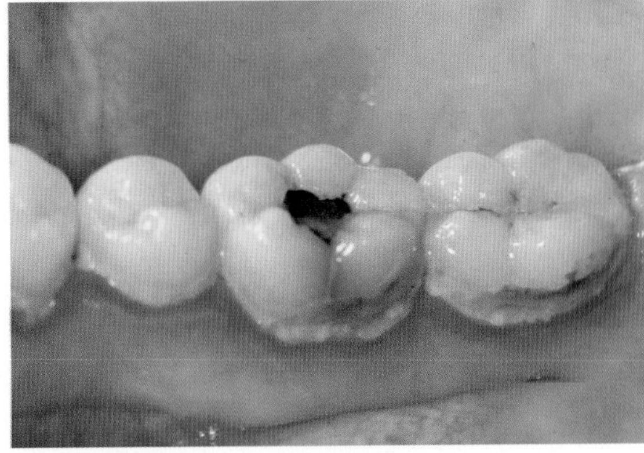

Figure 21-9, D and E. Lingual Aspects of the Mandibular Posterior Sextants.

Patient Case 4: Assessment Data

1. **Supragingival Calculus Deposits**
   - Light to moderate deposits on lingual aspect throughout the entire mouth
2. **Subgingival Calculus Deposits**
   - Medium-sized deposits throughout the entire mouth

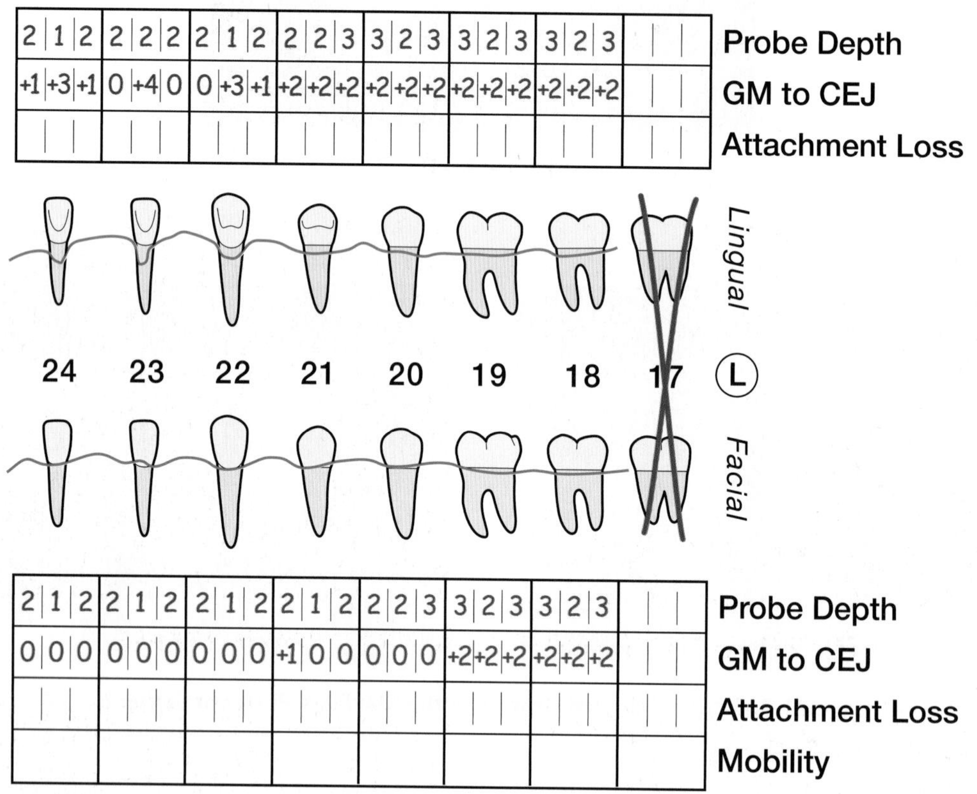

2 1 2 | 2 2 2 | 2 1 2 | 2 2 3 | 3 2 3 | 3 2 3 | 3 2 3 | Probe Depth
+1 +3 +1 | 0 +4 0 | 0 +3 +1 | +2 +2 +2 | +2 +2 +2 | +2 +2 +2 | +2 +2 +2 | GM to CEJ
Attachment Loss
Lingual
24 23 22 21 20 19 18 17
L
Facial
2 1 2 | 2 1 2 | 2 1 2 | 2 1 2 | 2 2 3 | 3 2 3 | 3 2 3 | Probe Depth
0 0 0 | 0 0 0 | 0 0 0 | +1 0 0 | 0 0 0 | +2 +2 +2 | +2 +2 +2 | GM to CEJ
Attachment Loss
Mobility

Figure 21-9F. Partial Periodontal Chart for Patient 4. (Key: GM = gingival margin; CEJ = cementoenamel junction.)

FICTITIOUS PATIENT CASE 5

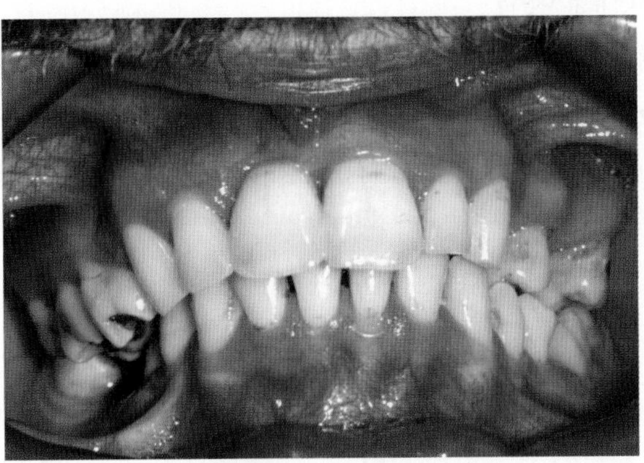

Figure 21-10A

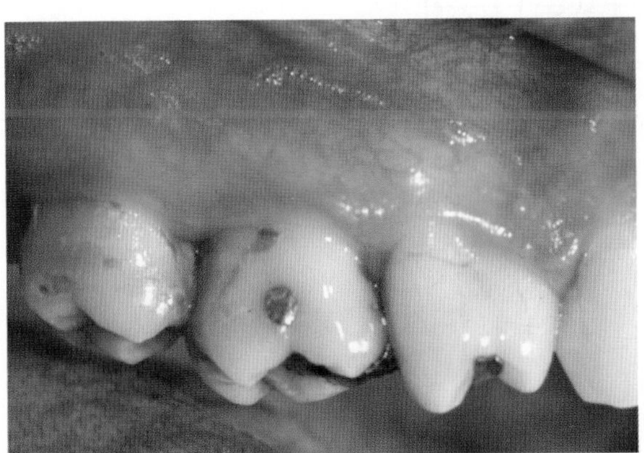

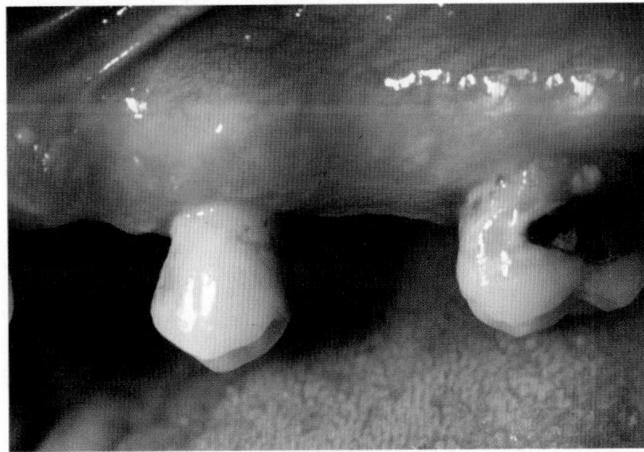

Figure 21-10, B and C. Facial Aspect of Maxillary Posterior Sextants.

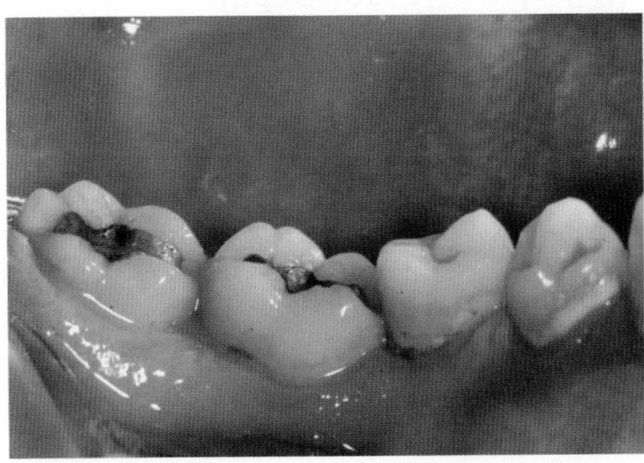

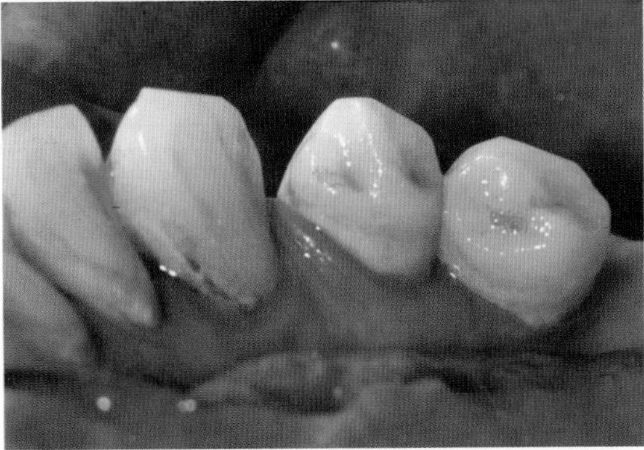

Figure 21-10, D and E. Mandibular Right Posterior Sextant and Mandibular Left Incisors, Canine, and Premolar Teeth.

Patient Case 5: Assessment Data

1. Supragingival Calculus Deposits

- Moderate deposits generalized on the lingual aspect throughout the mouth

2. Subgingival Calculus Deposits

- Medium-sized deposits on the lingual aspects of maxillary and mandibular arches
- Light deposits on facial aspect of maxillary and mandibular arches

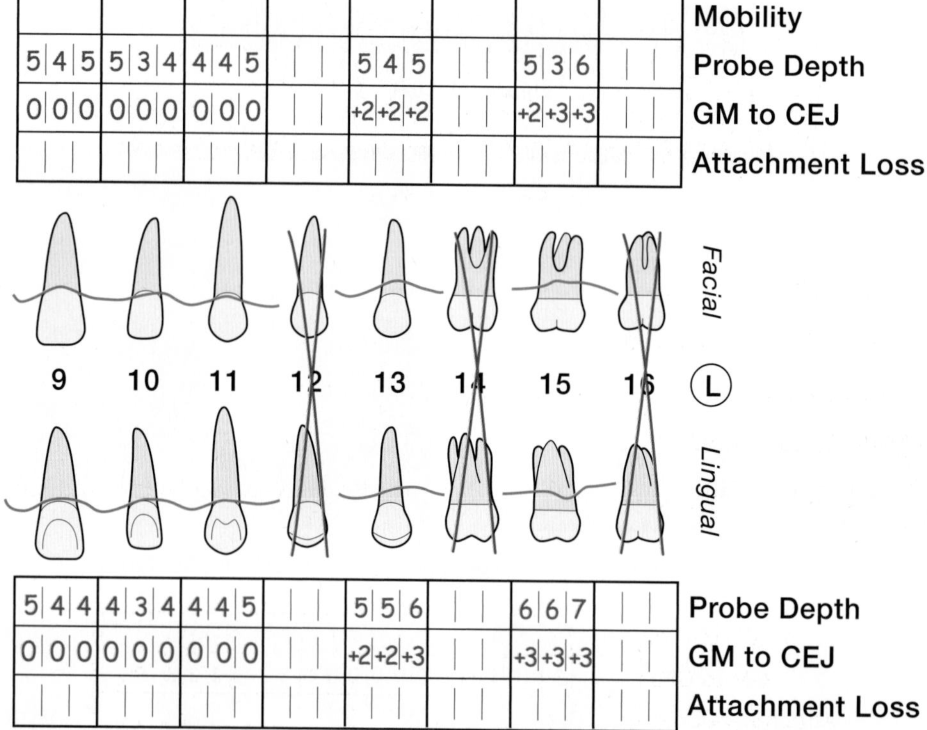

Mobility
5 4 5 | 5 3 4 | 4 4 5 | | 5 4 5 | | 5 3 6 | Probe Depth
0 0 0 | 0 0 0 | 0 0 0 | | +2 +2 +2 | | +2 +3 +3 | GM to CEJ
Attachment Loss
Facial
9 10 11 12 13 14 15 16
L
Lingual
5 4 4 | 4 3 4 | 4 4 5 | | 5 5 6 | | 6 6 7 | Probe Depth
0 0 0 | 0 0 0 | 0 0 0 | | +2 +2 +3 | | +3 +3 +3 | GM to CEJ
Attachment Loss

Figure 21-10F. Partial Periodontal Chart for Patient 5. (Key: GM = gingival margin; CEJ = cementoenamel junction.)

FICTITIOUS PATIENT CASE 6

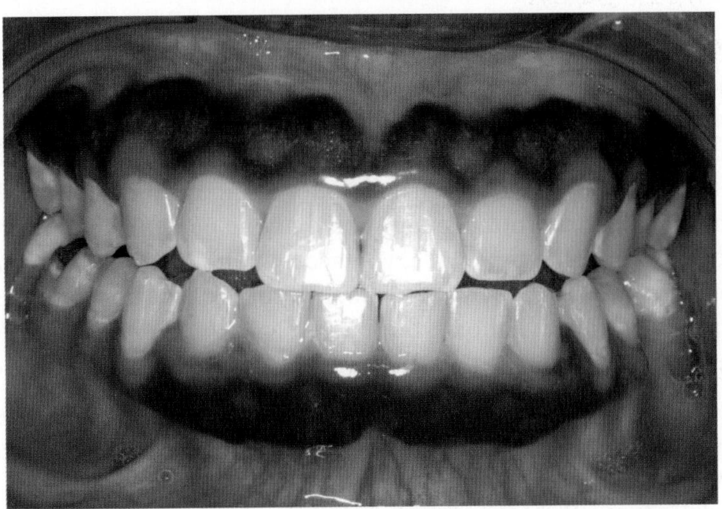

Figure 21-11A

Patient Case 6: Assessment Data

1. **Supragingival Calculus Deposits**
   - Light deposits on lingual aspect of mandibular anteriors
2. **Subgingival Calculus Deposits**
   - Light deposits on the proximal tooth surfaces of the posterior sextants throughout the mouth

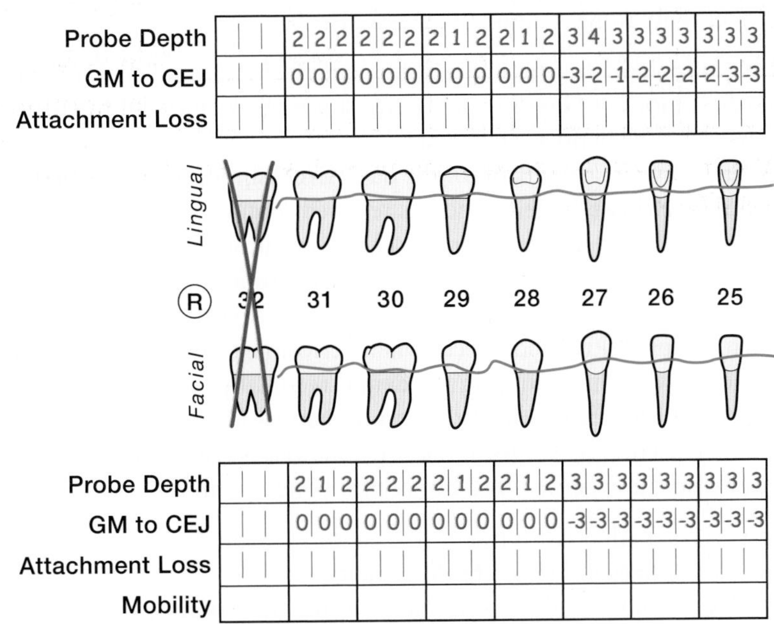

Probe Depth | | 2 2 2 | 2 2 2 | 2 1 2 | 2 1 2 | 3 4 3 | 3 3 3 | 3 3 3
GM to CEJ | | 0 0 0 | 0 0 0 | 0 0 0 | 0 0 0 | -3 -2 -1 | -2 -2 -2 | -2 -3 -3
Attachment Loss
Lingual
R
32
31
30
29
28
27
26
25
Facial
Probe Depth | | 2 1 2 | 2 2 2 | 2 1 2 | 2 1 2 | 3 3 3 | 3 3 3 | 3 3 3
GM to CEJ | | 0 0 0 | 0 0 0 | 0 0 0 | 0 0 0 | -3 -3 -3 | -3 -3 -3 | -3 -3 -3
Attachment Loss
Mobility

Figure 21-11B. Partial Periodontal Chart for Patient 6. (Key: GM = gingival margin; CEJ = cementoenamel junction.)

Section 5
Practical Focus—Professional Development Scenarios

Situation 1. You are a recent graduate of a dental hygiene program and have just started working in a new dental office. You learn that the other dental hygienist in the practice, Samantha, believes that aggressive root planing should be completed on all periodontally involved teeth. Samantha states she has been practicing for 20 years and removal of cementum is what she learned in school. You feel a little intimidated because you just graduated 5 months ago; nevertheless, you mention to her that you were taught that vigorous root planing should not be performed as a routine procedure on all teeth with periodontal pockets. For a while, you accept that you and Samantha have a difference of opinion about cementum removal, but you and Samantha see the same patients, and it is not unusual for a patient to question you about your instrumentation. For example, Mr. Riveras asked, "Why don't you use a lot of pressure against my teeth and scrape, scrape, scrape over each tooth like Samantha always does? Are you getting my teeth clean?"

- These patients' questions make you feel that you should discuss periodontal debridement with Samantha.
- How would you approach this issue with Samantha?

Situation 2. Mr. Rothenburger is a regular patient in the dental office. You saw him for periodontal debridement yesterday, and today he returned to the office complaining of a sensation "like a tiny electric shock" every time he brushes his maxillary right first molar. He also experiences "a sharp tingle" when he consumes cold water.

- What do you think is causing the sensations that Mr. Rothenburger is experiencing?
- How would you explain the problem to Mr. Rothenburger?
- What self-care instructions should you give Mr. Rothenburger in regard to dentinal sensitivity?

Situation 3. Mrs. Starnes has bone loss and periodontal pockets throughout her mouth. She has agreed to a treatment plan consisting of patient education and periodontal debridement. Mrs. Starnes asks you if the bone support around her teeth will improve after you have finished "cleaning her teeth."

- How would you reply to Mrs. Starnes' question?

Situation 4. You have accepted a full-time dental hygiene position in a general dental practice and are completing your first month of employment. You thoroughly enjoy all the office personnel and respect the clinical work of the dentist, Dr. Stuart.

You review the chart of your last patient for the day, Allie Ashton, who is 35 years old. She has been a patient of the practice for the last 10 years and has received routine dental and regular 6-month recall periodontal debridement. Allie is a lawyer. There is nothing eventful about her chart/dental history.

After you seat Allie and review her medical history, she mentions in passing that you are not to treat any of her first molars, because they are extremely sensitive. She says that every hygienist in the office has abided by her wishes to simply "skip" those teeth when performing their dental hygiene services.

You see no mention or documentation in the dental record by the previous hygienists. Furthermore, upon probing Allie's mouth, you note that on numerous locations on the first molar teeth, the probe readings have increased to 6 mm from the previous year's readings of 5 mm. The bitewings that were taken today also show generalized horizontal bone loss in those areas.

- How should you treat Allie Ashton?
- What are her alternatives in her dental hygiene therapies?
- Does her profession play a role in your decision-making process?
- How can you document that Allie is aware of her treatment options?
- What discussions would you have with her about the previous dental care she received in the office?

Module 22

Concepts for Instrument Sharpening

Module Overview

This module discusses the importance and advantages of using sharp periodontal instruments. Topics include methods for evaluating sharpness and reestablishing sharp cutting edges without altering the original design characteristics of the working-end.

Module Outline

Key Terms

Sharp cutting edge
Dull cutting edge
Visual evaluation of sharpness
Tactile evaluation of sharpness
Sharpening test stick
Straight cutting edges
Curved cutting edges
Limited use-life
Sharpening stone
Lubricant

Learning Objectives

1. List the benefits of using instruments with sharp cutting edges for periodontal instrumentation.
2. Define and differentiate the terms *sharp cutting edge* and *dull cutting edge.*
3. Given a variety of periodontal instruments, distinguish between those with sharp cutting edges and those with dull cutting edges.
4. Demonstrate two methods for determining if a cutting edge is sharp.
5. Describe important design characteristics to be maintained when sickle scalers and universal and area-specific curets are sharpened.
6. Differentiate the following sharpening stones according to grain, recommended use, and preferred lubricant: composition synthetic stone, India stone, Arkansas stone, and ceramic stone.
7. Demonstrate the correct care of a sharpening stone.
8. Describe common sharpening errors.
9. Value the practice of sharpening at the first sign of dullness.

Section 1
Introduction to Sharpening Concepts

ADVANTAGES OF SHARP INSTRUMENTS

Effective periodontal instrumentation with hand-activated instruments is possible only with properly maintained sharp cutting edges. New periodontal instruments have precise, sharp cutting edges and working-ends that have been carefully designed to facilitate calculus removal. ***It is impossible to overemphasize the importance of mastering the techniques for instrument sharpening.*** In 1908, one of the founders of modern dentistry, G. V. Black, stated that "*Nothing in the technical procedures of dental practice is more important than the care of the cutting edges of instruments. . . The student who can not, or will not learn this should abandon the study of dentistry.*"[1] Instrument sharpening is a skill needed on a daily basis. Effective periodontal debridement cannot be achieved with dull periodontal instruments.

Calculus removal involves the use of firm lateral pressure against the tooth surface. ***As an instrument is used, minute particles of metal are worn away from the working-end.*** Studies indicate that the cutting edges of curets should probably be sharpened after 15 to 40 calculus removal strokes.[2,3] ***Loss of metal from the working-end changes the cutting edge from a fine line to a rounded surface, resulting in a dull, ineffective cutting edge.*** A sharp cutting edge allows:

1. **Easier Calculus Removal**
   a. A sharp cutting edge "bites into" the calculus deposit, removing it in an efficient manner.
   b. A dull cutting edge will slide over the calculus deposit and may burnish it.
2. **Improved Stroke Control**
   a. A sharp cutting edge grabs a calculus deposit, making it easier to detect and remove.
   b. A dull cutting edge tends to slide over the tooth surface.
      1. A dull cutting edge is likely to burnish a calculus deposit, removing only the outer layer of calculus rather than the entire deposit.
      2. A dull cutting edge must be pressed with greater force against a deposit to achieve calculus removal.
      3. Excessive force used with a dull cutting edge increases the likelihood of losing control of the stroke. The clinician is more likely to slip or sustain an instrument stick when using a dull instrument.
3. **Reduced Number of Strokes/Working Efficiency**
   a. It takes fewer strokes to remove a calculus deposit with a sharp cutting edge.
   b. Sharp instruments reduce the overall treatment time.
   c. Sharp instruments decrease the likelihood of burnished calculus deposits.
4. **Increased Patient Comfort and Satisfaction**
   a. More lateral pressure must be exerted against the tooth when using a dull instrument. A sharp instrument allows the clinician to use less force, making the instrumentation process more comfortable for the patient.
   b. A sharp cutting edge permits the clinician to make fewer, better controlled instrument strokes. Therefore, sharp instruments decrease the time required for calculus removal. Patients appreciate shorter appointments.
5. **Reduced Clinician Fatigue**
   a. A dull cutting edge requires greater stroke pressure and more instrumentation strokes for calculus removal.
   b. The excessive lateral pressure and extra number of strokes needed with a dull instrument place unnecessary strain on the clinician's musculoskeletal system.

THE SHARP CUTTING EDGE

Correct sharpening technique requires knowledge of the design characteristics of sickle scalers and curets. It is important to understand the cross-sectional design of sickle scalers and curets and to recognize that the relationship of the face to the lateral surface is the same for all these instruments. On all sickle scalers and curets, a sharp cutting edge (Figs. 22-1 and 22-2) is a fine line formed by the pointed junction of the instrument face and lateral surface. Figures 22-2 to 22-5 depict the cross section of the working-end.

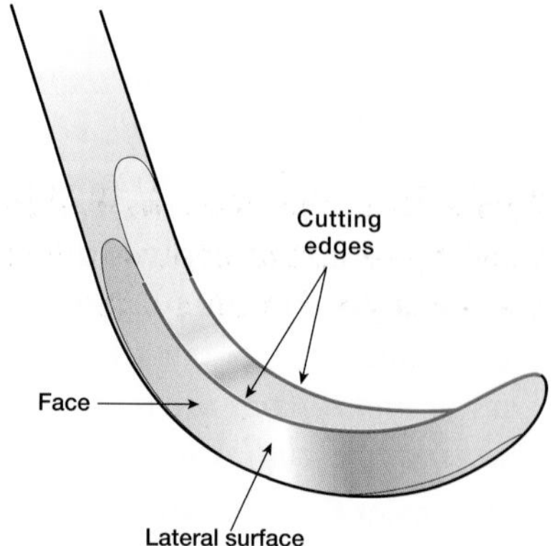

Figure 22-1. The Sharp Cutting Edge. A sharp cutting edge is a line. It has length but no width.

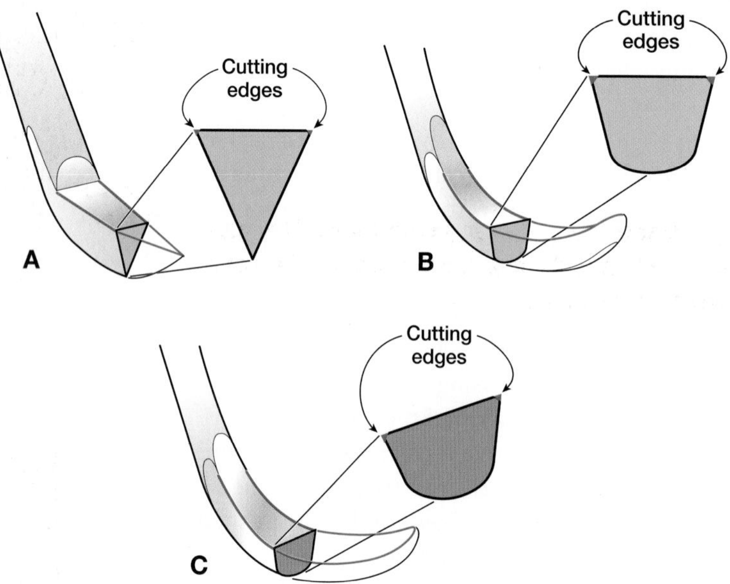

Figure 22-2. Cutting Edges on Sickle Scalers and Curets. For all sickle scalers and curets, the cutting edge is formed by the junction of the instrument face and lateral surface. **A. Sickle Scaler in Cross Section.** This illustration depicts a sickle scaler in cross section. **B. Universal Curet in Cross Section.** This illustration shows a universal curet in cross section. **C. Area-Specific Curet in Cross Section.** The cross section of an area-specific curet is shown in this illustration.

THE WORKING-END IN CROSS SECTION

When sharpening, it is vital to maintain the relationship between the instrument face and lateral surfaces (Figs. 22-3 to 22-5). ***For sickle scalers, universal curets, and area-specific curets, the internal angle formed between the face and a lateral surface is an angle between 70° and 80°.***

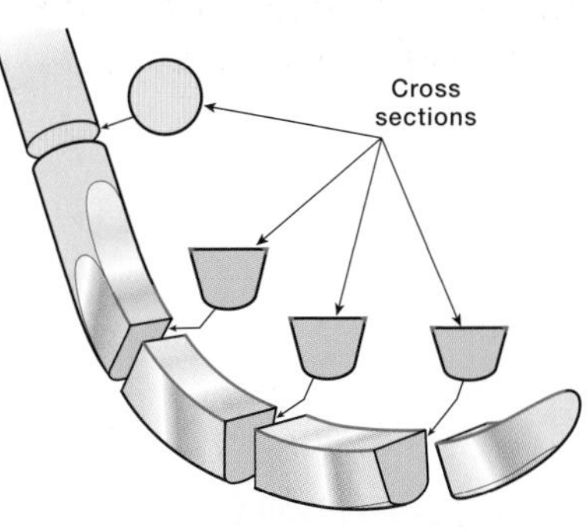

Figure 22-3. The Working-End in Cross Section. The key to understanding the cutting edge of an instrument is the ability to visualize the working-end in cross section.

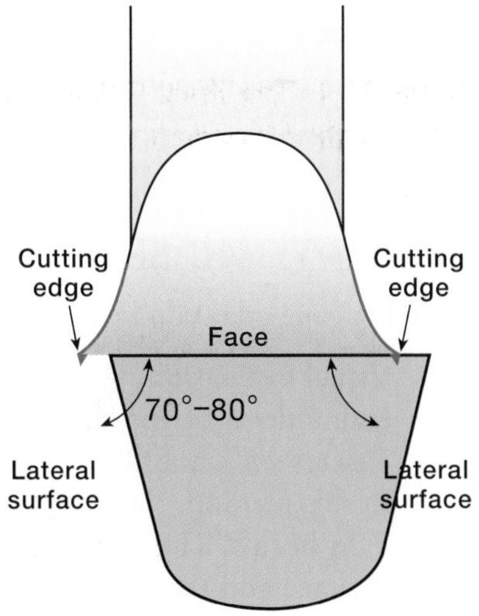

Figure 22-4. A Sharp Cutting Edge on a Universal Curet. The internal angle formed by the junction of the face and the lateral surface of a universal curet is between 70° and 80°.

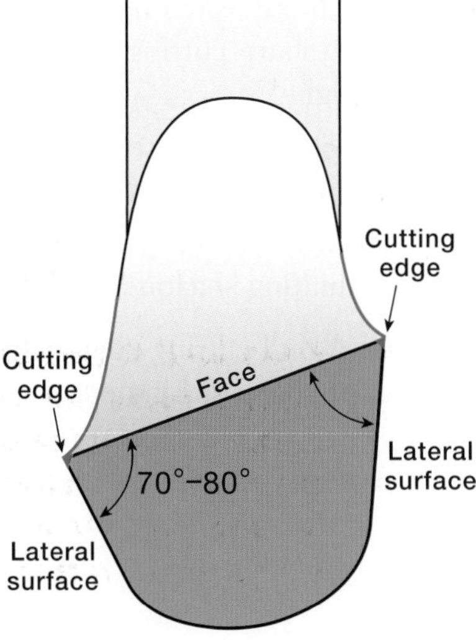

Figure 22-5. A Sharp Cutting Edge on an Area-Specific Curet. The relationship of the face to the lower shank is unique for area-specific curets. Just as for a universal curet, however, the internal angle formed by the junction of the face and the lateral surface of an area-specific curet is between 70° and 80°.

THE DULL CUTTING EDGE

As the working-end is used against the tooth surface, over time, the metal of the cutting edge is worn away. A dull cutting edge results when metal is worn away from the cutting edge until the junction between the face and lateral surface becomes a rounded surface instead of a fine line (Fig. 22-6).

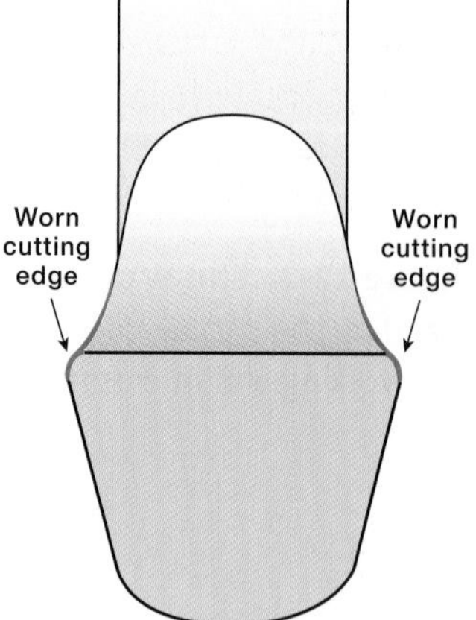

Figure 22-6. A Dull Cutting Edge. With use against the tooth surface, metal is worn away from the cutting edge until it becomes a ***rounded surface*** instead of a fine line.

A dull cutting edge is a rounded junction between the instrument face and the lateral surface.

EVALUATING SHARPNESS

A dull cutting edge can be detected by visual or tactile evaluation.

1. **Visual Evaluation.** A cutting edge is evaluated visually by holding the working-end under a bright light source, such as the dental light or a high-intensity lamp. Figures 22-7 and 22-8 depict cutting edges examined under a strong light source. In this method, the instrument face is held approximately perpendicular to the light beams. The working-end is slowly rotated while looking at the junction of the face and the lateral surface.
    - **a.** A dull cutting edge will reflect light because it is rounded and thick. The reflected light appears as a bright line running along the edge of the face.
    - **b.** A sharp cutting edge is a line—with no thickness—and does not reflect the light.
2. **Tactile Evaluation with a Test Stick.** Another method of evaluating sharpness is with tactile means by testing the cutting edge against a plastic or acrylic rod known as a sharpening test stick. Test sticks are designed specifically for use in evaluating sharpness (Fig. 22-9).
    - **a.** A dull cutting edge will slide over the surface of the stick.
    - **b.** A sharp cutting edge will bite into—grab—the surface of the test stick.

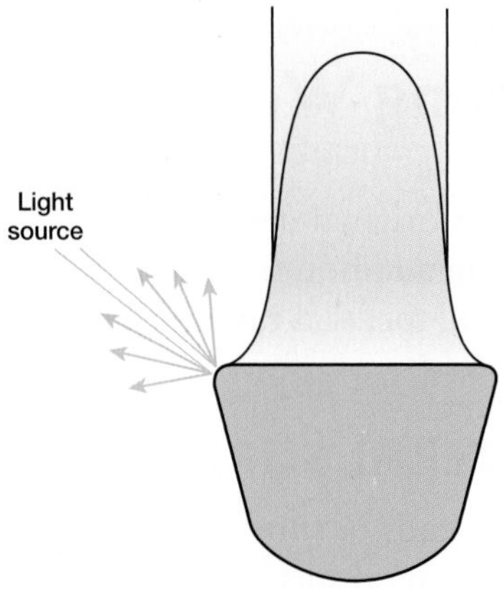

Light source

Figure 22-7. Visual Detection of a Dull Cutting Edge. The rounded surface of a dull cutting edge has thickness and thus will reflect light back to the viewer.

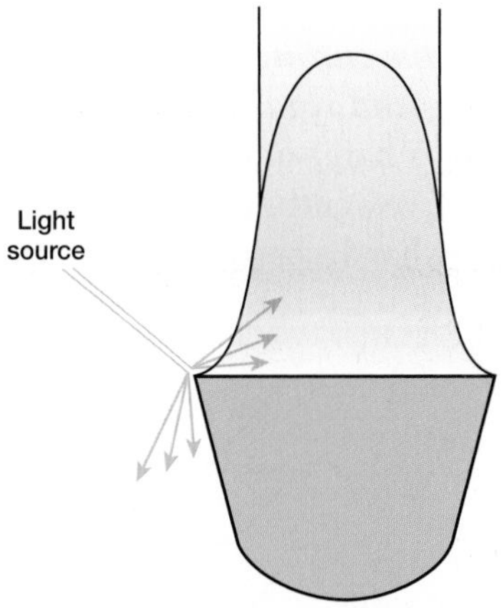

Light source

Figure 22-8. Visual Detection of a Sharp Cutting Edge. A sharp cutting edge has no thickness and therefore does not reflect light.

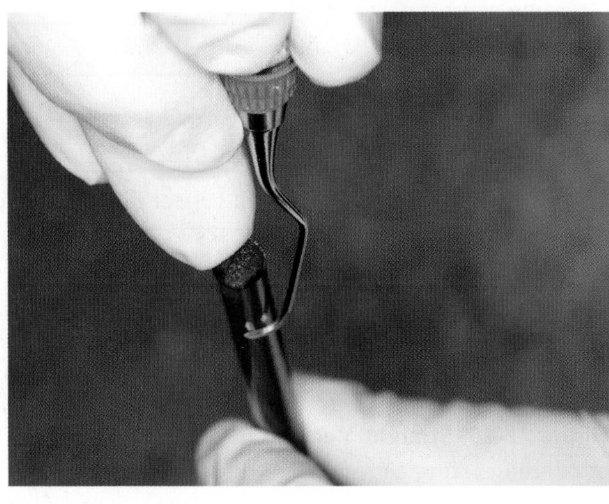

Figure 22-9. Tactile Detection with a Sharpening Test Stick. Sharpness can be evaluated using a test stick. A test stick is a cylindrical rod made of plastic or acrylic. Sharpening test sticks are autoclavable.

Section 2
Preserving Working-End Design

Preserving the original design characteristics of the working-end is an essential goal of instrument sharpening. In addition to the 70° to 80° internal angle of the working-end, the design of the lateral surfaces, back, toe, and tip must be maintained.

THE LATERAL SURFACES AND TIP OR TOE

The working-ends of some periodontal instruments have curved lateral surfaces, whereas others have straight lateral surfaces. Shown in Figure 22-10 are a variety of instrument working-ends, some with straight cutting edges and others with curved cutting edges.

- ***Sharpening the cutting edges in sections is a strategy that preserves the design characteristics of any working-end regardless of whether it has straight or curved cutting edges.***
- If you make a habit of consistently sharpening the cutting edge in sections, you will never destroy a curved cutting edge by flattening the lateral surface (Figs. 22-11 and 22-12).
- On the other hand, sharpening a straight cutting edge in sections still results in a straight cutting edge.

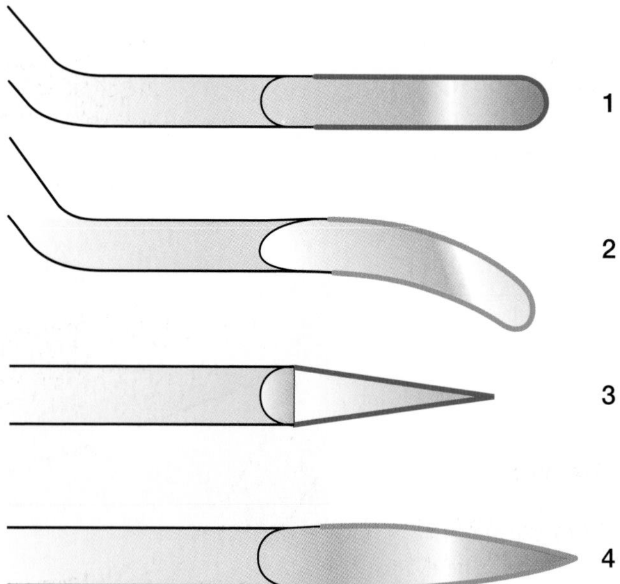

Figure 22-10. Straight Versus Curved Cutting Edges. The working-end may have **straight cutting edges** or **curved cutting edges**.

This design feature refers to the lateral surfaces being either straight or curved in design—not to whether the instrument has a rounded toe or pointed tip. To determine if the cutting edges are straight or curved, look down at the working-end from a bird's-eye view.

1. Instrument 1 is a universal curet with straight, parallel cutting edges.
2. Instrument 2 is an area-specific curet with curved working and nonworking cutting edges.
3. Instrument 3 is a sickle scaler with straight cutting edges.
4. Instrument 4 is a sickle scaler with curved cutting edges. This type of sickle scaler often is referred to as a flame-shaped sickle scaler.

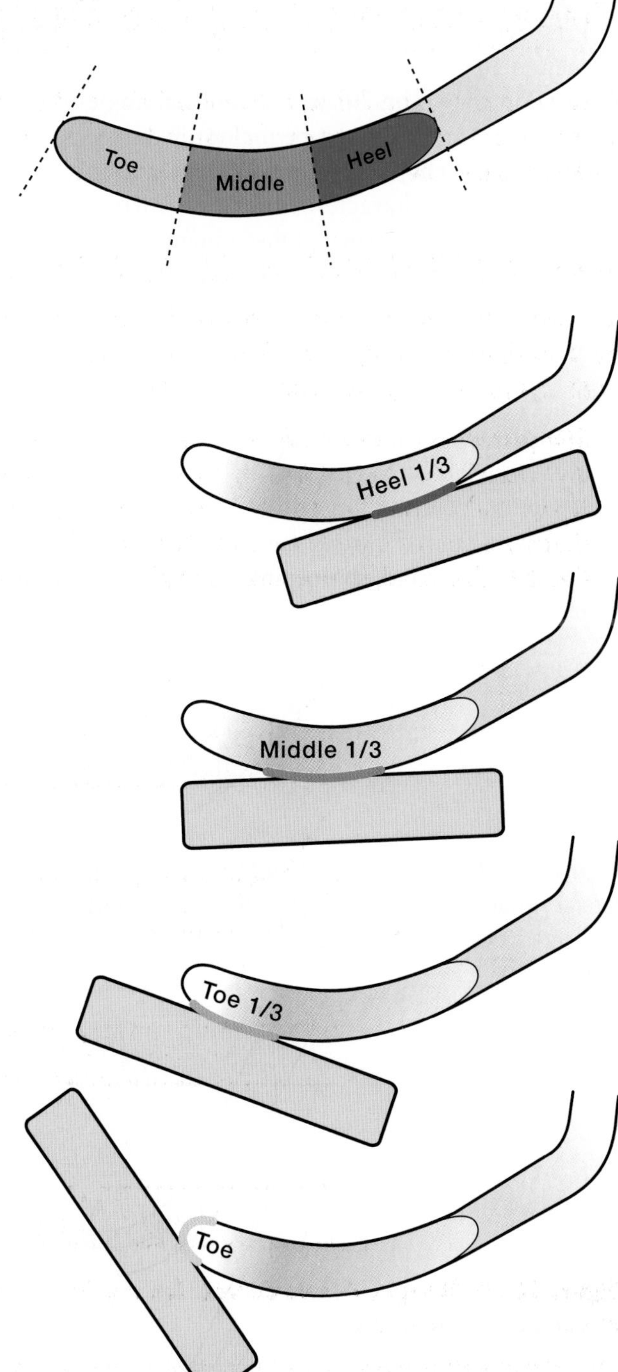

Figure 22-11. Cutting Edge Sections. Divide the cutting edge into three imaginary sections for sharpening: the heel-third, middle-third, and tip- or toe-third.

Figure 22-12. Sharpen in Sections.

- The sharpening stone is applied to only a third of the cutting edge at a time to maintain a curved cutting edge.
- Sharpen the (1) heel-third, (2) middle-third, and (3) toe- or tip-third of the cutting edge. If the instrument is a curet, (4) sharpen the toe.

COMMON SHARPENING ERRORS

- Preserving the original design characteristics of the working-end is an essential goal of instrument sharpening.
- In addition to the 70° to 80° internal angle of the working-end, the design of the lateral surfaces, back, toe, and tip must be maintained.
- A clinician who is not knowledgeable about working-end design can radically alter an instrument's design characteristics with incorrect sharpening technique.
- An incorrectly sharpened instrument will be ineffective for calculus removal and may fracture easily. Figures 22-13 to 22-16 depict how the original design characteristics of the working-end can be altered through incorrect sharpening technique.

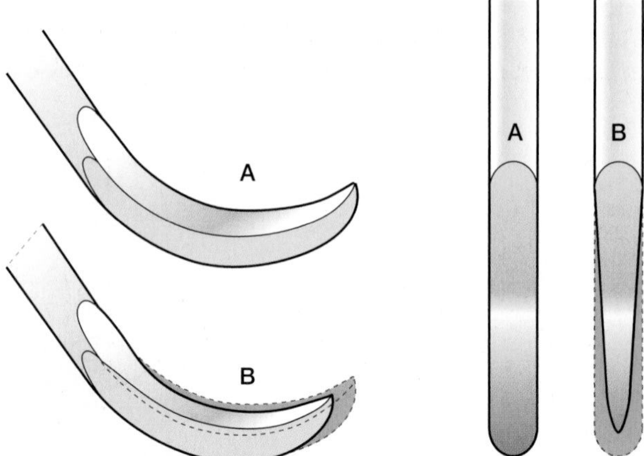

Figure 22-13. Alteration of Working-End Design. A. A new universal curet. Note that curet A has straight lateral surfaces and a rounded toe. **B.** In sharpening the curet shown in A, the clinician has altered its design characteristics. It is thinner and shorter than the original, and the curet toe has been sharpened to a point.

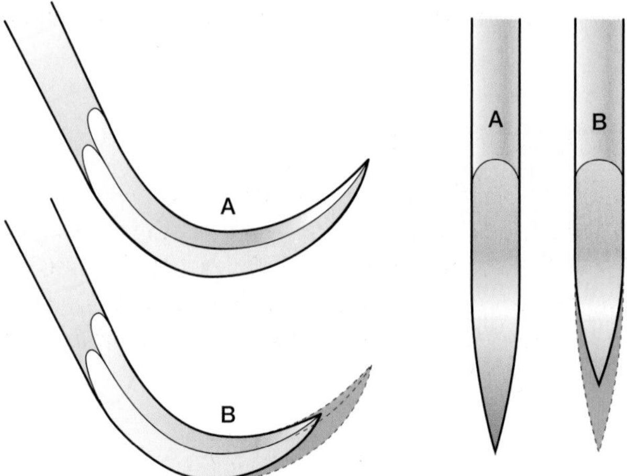

Figure 22-14. Unnecessary Metal Removal. A. A new sickle scaler. **B.** The working-end of this scaler has been excessively shortened in length by sharpening.

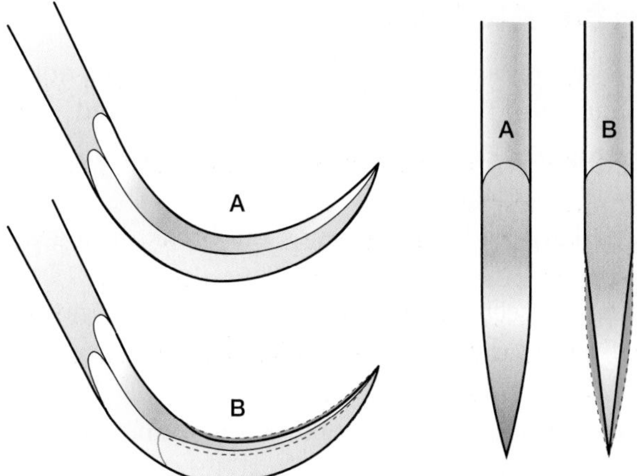

Figure 22-15. Altered Shape. A. A new sickle scaler. **B.** In this example, incorrect sharpening technique resulted in straight cutting edges, whereas the cutting edges on the original sickle were curved (flame-shaped).

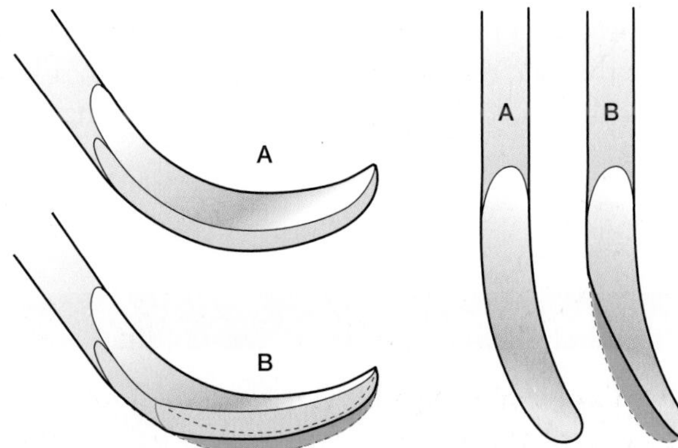

Figured 22-16. Flattened Cutting Edge. A. A new area-specific curet with curved cutting edges. **B.** In this example, incorrect sharpening technique created a straight lateral surface and a pointed tip. The original design characteristics of the instrument were curved lateral surfaces and a rounded toe.

INSTRUMENT REPLACEMENT

It is important to recognize that sickle scalers and curets have a limited use-life and must eventually be discarded. Frequent sharpening that preserves the working-end design combined with care during handling and sterilization will prolong an instrument's use-life. Eventually, every instrument will need to be replaced. When a working-end becomes thin from use and sharpening, the instrument should be discarded. One research study reports that a 20% reduction in size results in a significant reduction in working-end strength.[4]

INSTRUMENT TIP BREAKAGE

A broken instrument tip is a serious situation that all hygienists hope not to encounter. When the working-end breaks, the remnant of the working-end must be located.

1. **Maintenance for Prevention of Breakage.** The instrument's working-ends should be carefully inspected under magnification after each use.
   a. Thin or improperly sharpened working-ends can break during calculus removal.
   b. Frequent sharpening, correct sharpening technique, and discarding of instruments with thin or poorly sharpened working-ends minimize the possibility of a broken tip.
2. **Management of a Broken Working-End.** Breaking a working-end during instrumentation creates a serious problem.
   a. If not removed, the metal fragment can cause tissue inflammation and abscess formation. If the tip is aspirated (inhaled) into the lungs, a serious infection is likely to develop. If swallowed, the tip probably will pass harmlessly through the gastrointestinal system.
   b. If the tip cannot be located in the mouth, the patient should be referred for a chest X-ray to ensure that the tip has not been aspirated into a lung.
   c. Refer to Box 22-1 for the procedure for finding and retrieving a broken working-end.

Box 22-1. Retrieving a Broken Working-End

1. Stop instrumentation immediately, remain calm, and inform the patient of the problem.
2. Maintain retraction and patient head position.
   a. Do NOT use compressed air to attempt to locate the metal fragment. Compressed air could move the metal fragment around the mouth or drive it into the soft tissues.
   b. Do NOT use suction to attempt to remove the metal fragment. Suction could remove the tip but also eliminates the ability to confirm that the metal fragment has been removed.
3. Examine the location where the fracture occurred, mucobuccal fold, and the floor of the mouth. If the metal fragment is located on the surface of the tissue, blot the area with a gauze square. The metal fragment will catch in the gauze material for easy removal.
4. If the fragment cannot be located on the outer surfaces of the tissues, examine the sulci or pockets in the area.
   a. Insert a curet into the sulcus or pocket at the distofacial or distolingual line angle and move slowly forward until the fragment is located.
   b. Once located, use the curet like a scoop to remove the tip from beneath the gingival margin and catch it with a gauze square.
5. If the fragment cannot be located, take a periapical radiograph of the area. If located, use a curet as described above to remove the tip. If this fails, refer the patient to a periodontist for surgical removal of the metal fragment.
6. If the fragment still cannot be located in the mouth, the patient should be referred for a chest X-ray to ensure that the tip has not been aspirated into a lung. After referral, it is important to follow up with the patient to confirm that a chest X-ray was obtained.

Section 3
Planning for Instrument Maintenance

WHEN TO SHARPEN

Sickle scalers, curets, and periodontal files should be sharpened after each use or as needed during periodontal instrumentation. Instruments should be sharpened lightly after each use. Neglected cutting edges require extensive sharpening, increasing the likelihood of damaging the working-end.

1. **Sharpening after Instrument Use**
   a. Each sickle scaler or curet used during the appointment should be sharpened.
   b. Instruments that were not used do not need to be sharpened; modern stainless steel instruments are not dulled by autoclaving or other sterilization methods.
   c. Ideally, instruments used for treatment should be sterilized before sharpening to decrease the risk of disease transmission. Sterilized instruments are sharpened and sterilized a second time prior to use.
2. **Sharpening during Treatment**
   a. Depending on the extent of calculus deposits present, instruments may have to be sharpened during treatment.
   b. Sharpening contaminated instruments presents an increased risk of disease transmission through an instrument stick. Ideally, it is best to have a variety of individually wrapped, sterilized sharp instruments to replace instruments dulled during treatment.
   c. If contaminated instruments must be sharpened, take steps to diminish risk for disease transmission.
      1. Sharpening stones should be a part of each instrument cassette so that sterile sharpening stones are always available. If instrument cassette tray setups are not used, sharpening stones should be kept in sealed sterilized packages until needed.
      2. Use safe sharpening techniques: gloves, good lighting, and stabilize hand on flat, stable working surface.
      3. The work area should be disinfected and covered with a barrier such as plastic wrap or an impervious-backed paper. The barrier should cover both the top and edge of the countertop.
      4. Any sharpening aid or device used at chairside must be dissembled and sterilized after each use.
      5. A natural stone is not recommended for sharpening during treatment because these stones require lubrication with oil. Oil lubricants cannot undergo sterilization. Ceramic stones are best for chairside sharpening because water can be used as a lubricant with these stones.

TABLE 22-1. Frequency of Sharpening

Immediate Sharpening	Infrequent Sharpening
• Maintained cutting edges need only a few light sharpening strokes and minor recontouring. • Calculus removal is easier for both clinician and patient. • Instruments have a long use-life.	• Dull neglected cutting edges require many firm sharpening strokes and extensive recontouring. • Calculus removal is difficult and tiring for both the clinician and patient. • Instruments have a short use-life.

Section 4
Sharpening Armamentarium

WORK AREA AND EQUIPMENT

A sharpening work area must be a part of every treatment room so that periodontal instruments can be sharpened at the first sign of dullness. The right work area is important in ensuring an efficient and safe sharpening procedure.

1. A stable, flat work surface is essential for good sharpening technique. A countertop in the treatment room makes a good surface. A bracket table or other unstable surface is not appropriate for the sharpening procedure.
2. A good light source, such as the dental unit light or a high-intensity lamp, should illuminate the sharpening work area.
3. All equipment required for sharpening should be assembled and ready for use in the treatment room (Fig. 22-17).

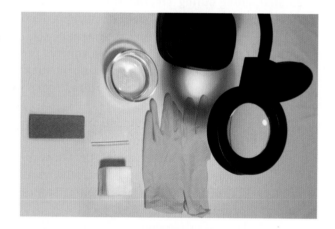

Figure 22-17. Sharpening Equipment.

- Sharpening stone(s)
- Plastic sharpening test stick
- Magnifying light, lens, or loops
- Gauze
- Lubricant
- Gloves
- Safety glasses

SHARPENING STONES

A sharpening stone is used to remove metal from the lateral surfaces of the working-end to restore a sharp, fine cutting edge (Fig. 22-18). Sharpening stones are made of abrasive particles that are harder than the metal of the instruments to be sharpened. Sharpening stones may be made from natural stone or synthetic, man-made materials.[3,5,6] The grain—or abrasiveness—is an important characteristic of sharpening stones. Fine-grain stones—400 grit or higher—produce significantly sharper cutting edges that will stay sharper longer.[7] Table 22-2 summarizes information on various types and uses of sharpening stones.

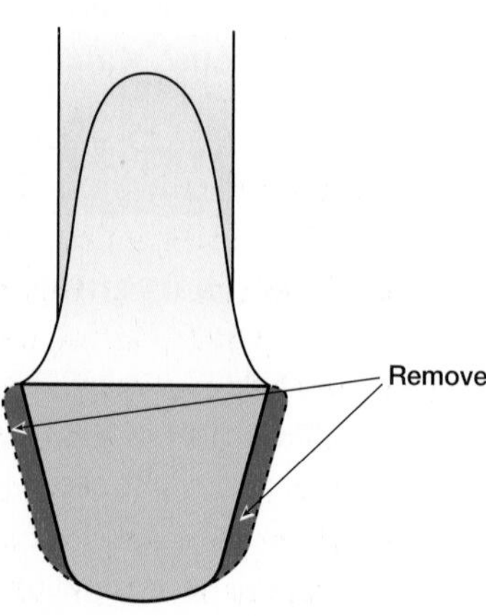

Figure 22-18. Remove Metal from the Lateral Surfaces to Restore a Sharp Cutting Edge. The recommended sharpening method for reestablishing the fine cutting edge is to remove metal from the lateral surfaces of the working-end. This illustration shows a universal curet; the portion of the working-end shaded in dark green would be removed from the lateral surfaces during sharpening.

TABLE 22-2. Sharpening Stones and Tools

Type	Grit	Use	Lubricant	Sterilization*
Ceramic synthetic stone	Fine	• Routine sharpening of metal and some plastic implant instruments	Water	All methods
Arkansas natural stone	Fine	• Routine sharpening of metal instruments	Mineral oil	All methods†
Neivert Whittler	—	• Routine sharpening of metal instruments	Water	All methods
India synthetic stone	Medium	• Sharpening of metal instruments that are dull	Water or oil	All methods
Composition synthetic stone	Coarse	• Sharpening of metal instruments that are extremely dull or that need reshaping	Water	All methods
Power devices and honing machines	Varies	• Routine sharpening and sharpening of instruments that are extremely dull	As directed by maker	As directed by maker
Test stick	Smooth	• Evaluate sharpness	None	All methods

*Includes autoclave, dry heat, or chemical sterilization.
†Natural stones become brittle over time with heat exposure.

LUBRICATION AND CARE OF STONES

1. **Lubrication of Sharpening Stone**
   - **a.** A lubricant is a substance, such as water or oil, applied to the surface of a sharpening stone to reduce friction between the stone and the instrument.
   - **b.** Lubrication helps to prevent the metal shavings from sticking to the surface of the stone. These metal shavings can become embedded in the surface of the sharpening stone and reduce its effectiveness.
   - **c.** Lubrication reduces frictional heat between the metal instrument and the stone. Stones that are used without lubrication will need to be replaced more frequently than stones used with lubricant.
   - **d.** A synthetic stone that can be lubricated with water is recommended for use when sharpening instruments during patient treatment.
   - **e.** A natural stone that must be lubricated with oil is not recommended for use when sharpening during patient treatment because the oil cannot be effectively sterilized.
2. **Care of Sharpening Stone**
   - **a.** The sharpening stone should be cleaned in an ultrasonic cleaner or scrubbed with a brush and hot water to remove metal particles from the surface of the stone.
   - **b.** After cleaning, the stone should be dried on a paper towel and placed in an autoclave bag or on an instrument cassette to be sterilized.

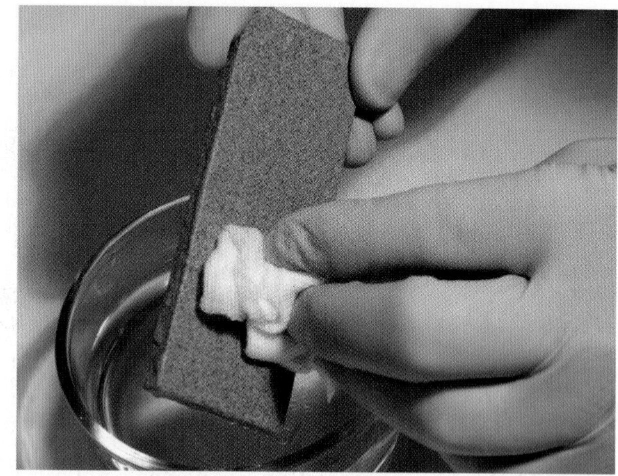

Figure 22-19. Lubrication of Sharpening Stone. The sharpening stone is lubricated with water or oil to help prevent metal shavings from becoming embedded in the surface of the stone.

SHARPENING METHODS

There are many different sharpening techniques. Two of the most common approaches to restoring a sharp cutting edge include sharpening using (1) the moving stone technique and (2) the moving instrument technique. Sharpening techniques are presented in the next module, Module 23.

REFERENCES

1. Black G. *A Work on Operative Dentistry. The Technical Procedures in Filling Teeth*. Chicago, IL: Medico-Dental Publishing Company; 1908.
2. Balevi B. Engineering specifics of the periodontal curet's cutting edge. *J Periodontol.* 1996;67:374–378.
3. Tal H, Panno JM, Vaidyanathan TK. Scanning electron microscope evaluation of wear of dental curettes during standardized root planing. *J Periodontol.* 1985;56:532–536.
4. Murray GH, Lubow RM, Mayhew RB, Summitt JB, Usseglio RJ. The effects of two sharpening methods on the strength of a periodontal scaling instrument. *J Periodontol.* 1984;55:410–413.
5. Andrade Acevedo RA, Cardozo AK, Sampaio JE. Scanning electron microscopic and profilometric study of different sharpening stones. *Braz Dent J.* 2006;17:237–242.
6. Huang CC, Tseng CC. Effect of different sharpening stones on periodontal curettes evaluated by scanning electron microscopy. *J Formos Med Assoc.* 1991;90:782–787.
7. Rossi R, Smukler H. A scanning electron microscope study comparing the effectiveness of different types of sharpening stones and curets. *J Periodontol.* 1995;66:956–961.

Section 5
Skill Application

PRACTICAL FOCUS

Nola has asked you to evaluate her instrumentation technique because she says that all her patients complain that she is "so rough." Nola hopes that you can tell her what she is doing wrong. Nola is about to begin periodontal debridement on a patient with medium-size supragingival and subgingival calculus deposits. The working-ends of her instruments are pictured below.

- Evaluate each working-end shown in Figures 22-20 to 22-25, and if problems are found, identify them.
- How efficient and effective do you think calculus removal will be using these instruments?
- What recommendations would you give Nola?

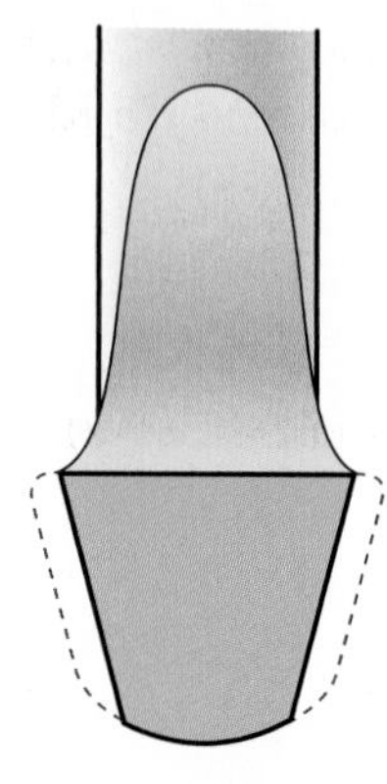

Figure 22-20. Universal Curet.

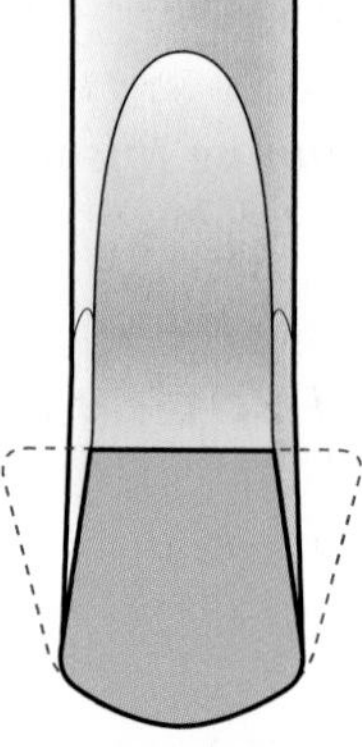

Figure 22-21. Universal Curet.

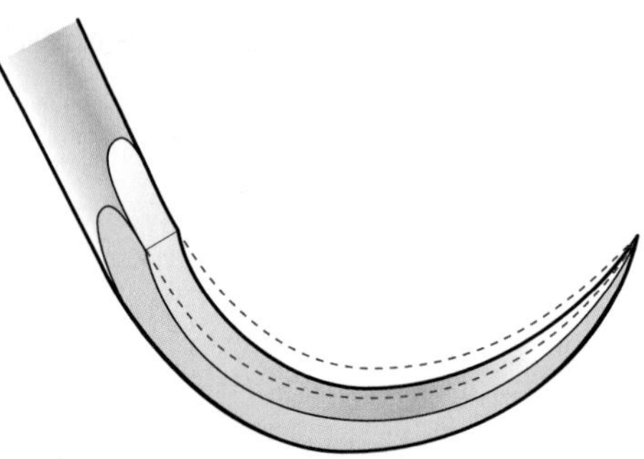

Figure 22-22. Sickle Scaler.

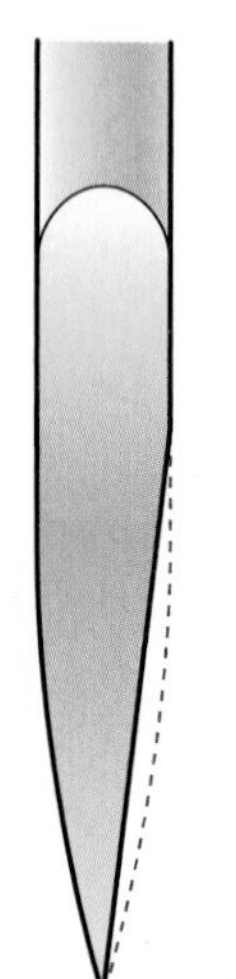

Figure 22-23. Sickle Scaler.

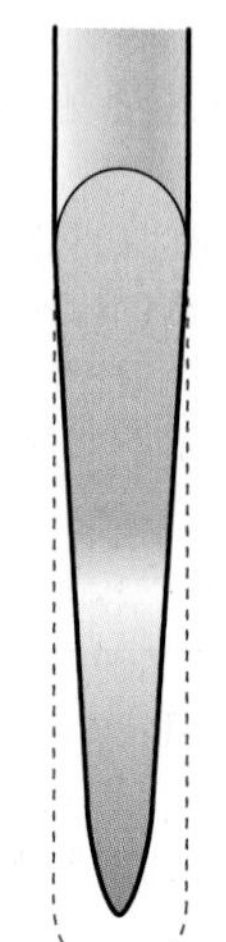

Figure 22-24. Universal Curet.

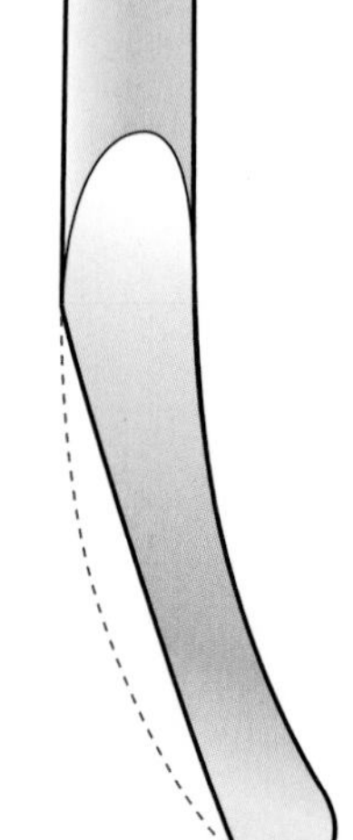

Figure 22-25. Area-Specific Curet.

Module 23

Instrument Sharpening Techniques

Module Overview

This module discusses three commonly used methods for sharpening periodontal instruments: the moving stone technique, the moving instrument technique, and a powered sharpening device. Skill practice sections provide experience in positioning the instrument and sharpening stone. Step-by-step instructions are provided in the moving stone and moving instrument techniques. ***Module 22 should be completed before beginning this module.***

Module Outline

Key Terms

Moving instrument technique
Moving stone technique
Powered sharpening device
Metal burs
Wire edge
Recontouring
Tanged file

Learning Objectives

1. Compare and contrast the moving stone and moving instrument techniques for instrument sharpening.
2. Describe and demonstrate the proper relationship of the instrument's working-end to the sharpening stone.
3. Demonstrate the correct grasp for both the instrument and the sharpening stone when using the moving stone technique.
4. Demonstrate the correct finger rest and grasp when using the moving instrument technique.
5. Describe and demonstrate the sharpening procedure for sickle scalers, universal curets, and area-specific curets using the moving stone technique.
6. Describe and demonstrate the sharpening procedure for sickle scalers, universal curets, and area-specific curets using the moving instrument technique.
7. Sharpen a dull sickle scaler, universal curet, and area-specific curet to produce a sharp, fine cutting edge while preserving all of the original design characteristics of the working-ends.
8. If applicable, sharpen a dull periodontal file with a tanged file to restore sharp cutting edges while preserving all the original design characteristics of the working-end.
9. Demonstrate the procedure for using a plastic sharpening stick to determine whether the entire length of a cutting edge is sharp.
10. Value sharp instruments and the practice of sharpening at the first sign of dullness or after each use of an instrument.

Section 1
Removing Metal to Restore a Sharp Cutting Edge

GOAL OF INSTRUMENT SHARPENING

The goal of instrument sharpening is to restore a fine, sharp cutting edge to a dull working-end. To be successful, a sharpening technique should remove a minimum amount of metal from the instrument and maintain the original design characteristics of the working-end.

A review of the literature reveals a variety of techniques for sharpening periodontal instruments.[1–10] Various authors have described the criteria of an ideal sharpening method:

- Is easy to learn[11,12]
- Relies on inexpensive equipment[11,12]
- Employs a technique that provides good visibility of the working-end and good control during the sharpening process[13]
- Removes a minimum amount of metal from the instrument's working-end
- Maintains the original design characteristics of the working-end

This module presents three commonly used sharpening techniques:

1. The moving instrument technique, which involves moving the working-end of the periodontal instrument across a stationary sharpening stone.
2. The moving stone technique, which involves holding the instrument stationary and moving a sharpening stone over a lateral surface of the working-end.
3. A powered sharpening device for sharpening periodontal instruments.

RECONTOURING THE WORKING-END

Regardless of the sharpening method used, the process of restoring a sharp cutting edge involves removing metal from the lateral surfaces of the working-end.

- Metal is removed from a lateral surface until the junction with the face is restored to a fine line with no width.
- Figure 23-1 indicates the metal (shaded in dark green) that would be removed from a universal curet to restore sharp cutting edges.

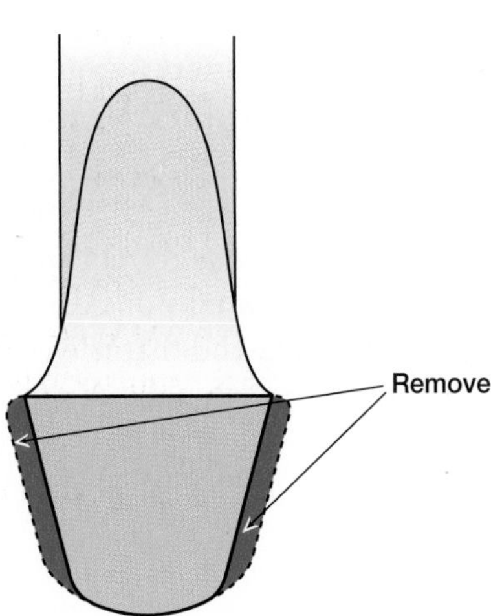

Figure 23-1. Metal Is Removed from the Lateral Surfaces to Restore a Sharp Cutting Edge. Sharp cutting edges are restored on a universal curet by removing the portion of the lateral surfaces shaded in dark green from the working-end. Removing this metal restores sharp cutting edges to the working-end.

RELATIONSHIP BETWEEN THE SHARPENING STONE AND INSTRUMENT FACE

It is vital to retain the original design characteristics of the working-end when removing metal from the lateral surfaces during sharpening. ***A sharp cutting edge is restored by removing metal from the lateral surface while maintaining the 70° to 80° internal junction between the face and the lateral surface.*** Figures 23-2 and 23-3 illustrate the consequences of correct and incorrect angulation between the instrument face and the sharpening stone.

Figure 23-2. Correct Recontouring of Working-End.

- The dark green shading in this illustration indicates the portions of the working-end to be removed during sharpening.
- By placing the sharpening stone at a 70° to 80° angle to the face, the ideal design characteristics of the working-end will be maintained after sharpening.

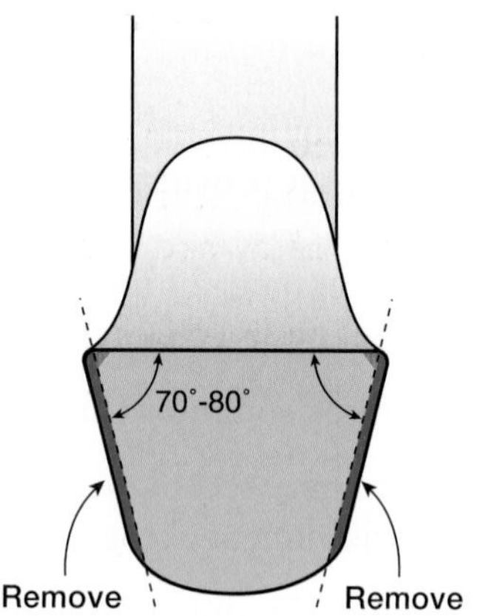

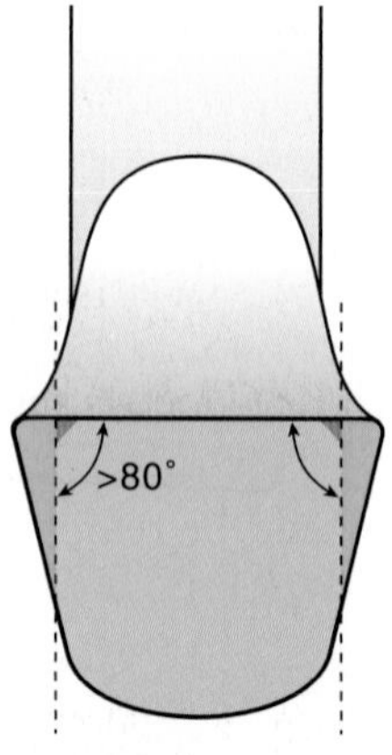

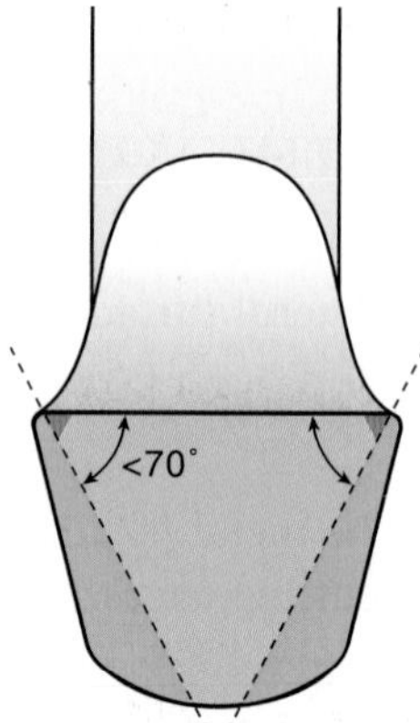

Figure 23-3. Incorrect Recontouring of Working-End. The red shading in these illustrations indicates the portions of the working-end removed during incorrect sharpening technique.

- If the stone contacts the lateral surface at an angle greater than 80°, the end result is a bulky working-end that is difficult to adapt to the tooth surface (left image). Heavy lateral pressure would be needed to remove any calculus deposits with this working-end.
- If the sharpening stone contacts the lateral surface at an angulation less than 70°, the end result is a working-end that is weakened due to excessive removal of metal (right image). Such a working-end would dull quickly and could break during calculus removal.

SHARPENING THE CUTTING EDGE IN SECTIONS

Regardless of the sharpening method used, the cutting edges should be sharpened in sections to preserve the original design characteristics of the cutting edge. Figures 23-4 and 23-5 depict the concept of sharpening the cutting edge in sections.

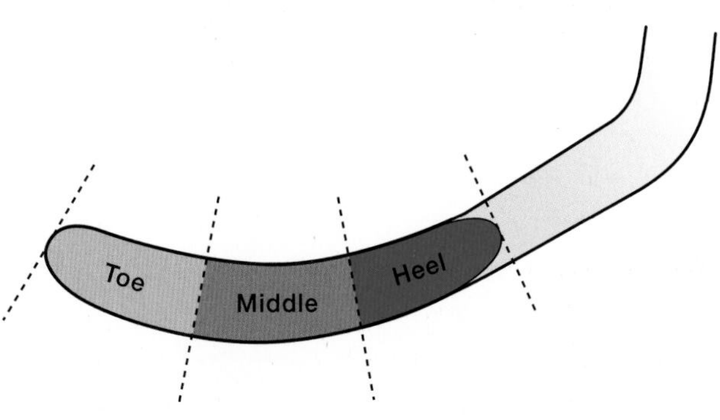

Figure 23-4. Cutting Edge Sections. Divide the cutting edge into three imaginary sections for sharpening: the heel-third, middle-third, and tip- or toe-third.

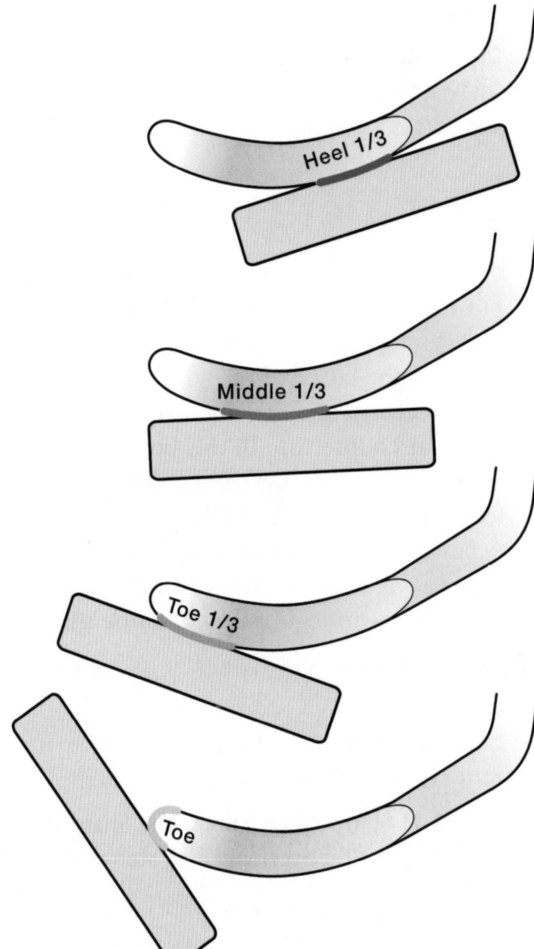

Figure 23-5. Sharpen in Sections.

- The sharpening stone is applied to only a third of the cutting edge at a time to maintain a curved cutting edge.
- Sharpen the (1) heel-third, (2) middle-third, and (3) toe- or tip-third of the cutting edge. If the instrument is a curet, (4) sharpen the toe.

Section 2
The Moving Instrument Technique

OVERVIEW OF THE MOVING INSTRUMENT TECHNIQUE

As the name suggests, the moving instrument technique involves removing metal from the lateral surface by moving the working-end across the surface of a stabilized sharpening stone (Fig. 23-6).

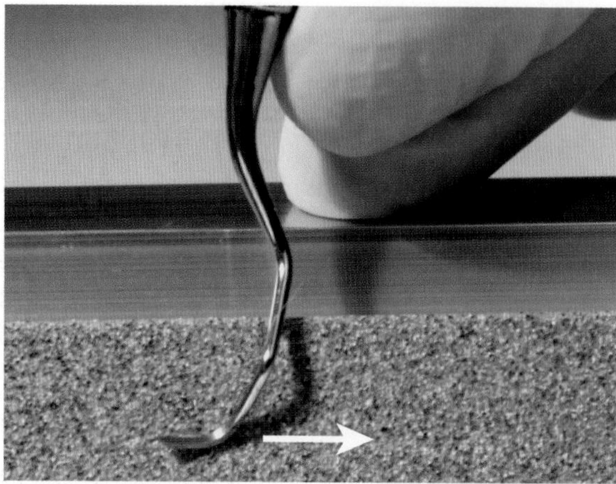

Figure 23-6. Moving Instrument Technique. For the moving instrument technique, the working-end is moved across a stationary sharpening stone.

INNOVATIONS IN THE MOVING INSTRUMENT TECHNIQUE

- For many years, the moving *stone* technique has been the most common method of instrument sharpening taught in dental hygiene programs. The fact that it is easy to see the angle formed between the face and the stone probably accounts for the popularity of the moving *stone* method.
- Until recently, the moving *instrument* method used the technique of placing the sharpening stone on a flat countertop. In this position, it is not possible to view the angle between the stone and the instrument face. The inability to see the face-to-stone angulation made the moving instrument technique difficult to teach to novice clinicians.
- A new sharpening tool, called the Sharpening Horse, is changing the way that clinicians regard the moving instrument technique (Fig. 23-7). ***The Sharpening Horse allows the clinician to see the face-to-stone angulation while using the moving instrument technique.***[14]

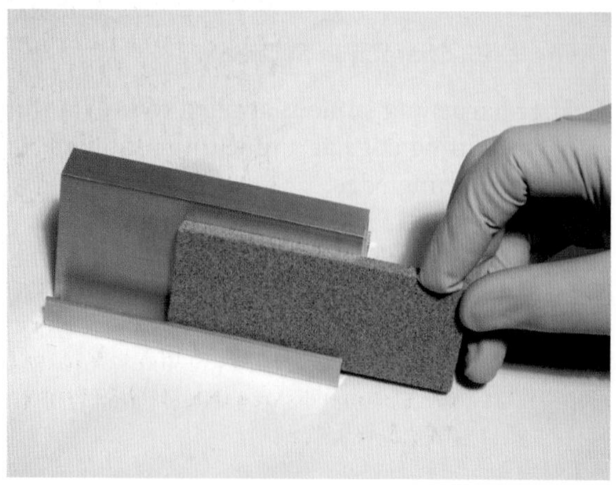

Figure 23-7. Sharpening Horse. The Sharpening Horse tool for holding a sharpening stone in a fixed position.

- The Sharpening Horse allows the clinician to view the face-to-stone angulation.
- This tool facilitates use of the moving instrument technique.
- Information on the Sharpening Horse tool is available at http://www.dhmethed.com.

EFFECTIVENESS OF THE MOVING INSTRUMENT TECHNIQUE

A recent study examined the results of many different sharpening methods. ***Researchers found that the technique that produces the most precise cutting edge without wire edges and irregularities is the moving instrument technique.***[1] For the study, experienced clinicians sharpened instruments using nine different sharpening techniques including moving stone, moving instrument, Neivert Whittler, and powered sharpening techniques. Figures 23-8 and 23-9 compare the results obtained with the moving instrument and the moving stone techniques.

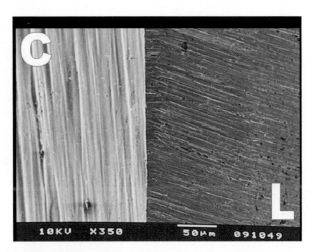

Figure 23-8. Moving Instrument Technique. A scanning electron microscopy image shows that the moving *instrument* technique produced a precise, defined cutting edge with an exact junction between the coronal (*C*) surface—instrument face—and the lateral (*L*) surface. (Used with permission from Acevedo R, Sampaio J, Shibli J. Scanning electron microscope assessment of several resharpening techniques on the cutting edges of Gracey curettes. *J Contemp Dent Pract.* 2007;8:70–77.)

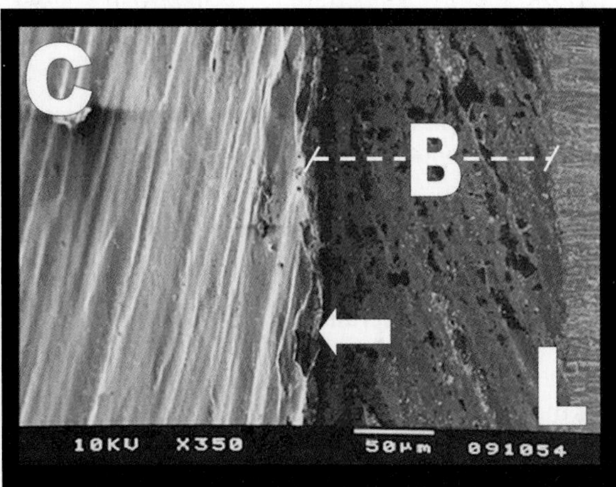

Figure 23-9. Moving Stone Technique. A scanning electron microscopy image shows that the moving *stone* technique produced a bevel and wire edges between the coronal (*C*) surface—instrument face—and the lateral (*L*) surface. (Used with permission from Acevedo R, Sampaio J, Shibli J. Scanning electron microscope assessment of several resharpening techniques on the cutting edges of Gracey curettes. *J Contemp Dent Pract.* 2007;8:70–77.)

ESSENTIAL SKILL COMPONENTS OF THE MOVING INSTRUMENT TECHNIQUE

Essential skill components of the moving instrument technique are (1) using a modified pen grasp, (2) using the ring finger as a support beam for the hand, and (3) sliding the ring finger along the top of the Sharpening Horse tool during sharpening (Figs. 23-10 to 23-12).

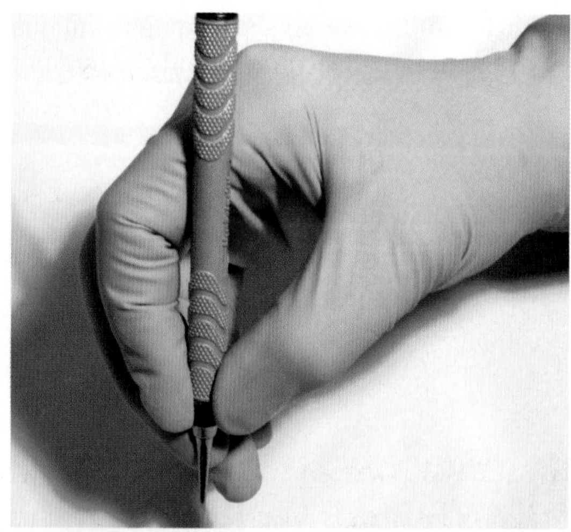

Figure 23-10. Skill Component 1: Instrument Grasp. A modified pen grasp is used to hold the instrument for the moving instrument sharpening technique.

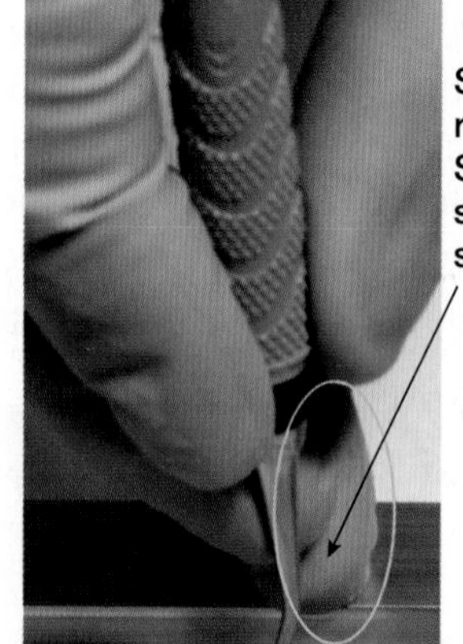
Straight fulcrum finger rests on top of the Sharpening Horse to support the hand during sharpening

Figure 23-11. Skill Component 2: Ring Finger as Support Beam.

- The ring finger is a critical element for use of the Sharpening Horse.
- *The ring finger acts as a support beam and rests on top of the Sharpening Horse tool throughout the sharpening process.*

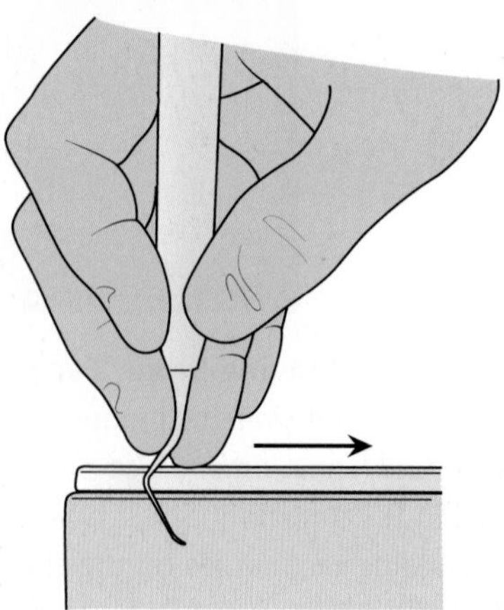

Figure 23-12. Skill Component 3: Slide on Fulcrum as You Work.

- The ring finger slides along the beam of the Sharpening Horse during the sharpening procedure.
- *Right-handed clinicians* move from left to right along the beam, sharpening the heel-third, then the middle-third, and finally the toe-/tip-third of the cutting edge.
- *Left-handed clinicians* move from right to left along the beam, sharpening from heel to toe-/tip-third.

SETTING UP THE SHARPENING HORSE

Figure 23-13 shows the components of the Sharpening Horse system. Figures 23-14 shows a simple way to adjust the height of the sharpening stone in the horse.

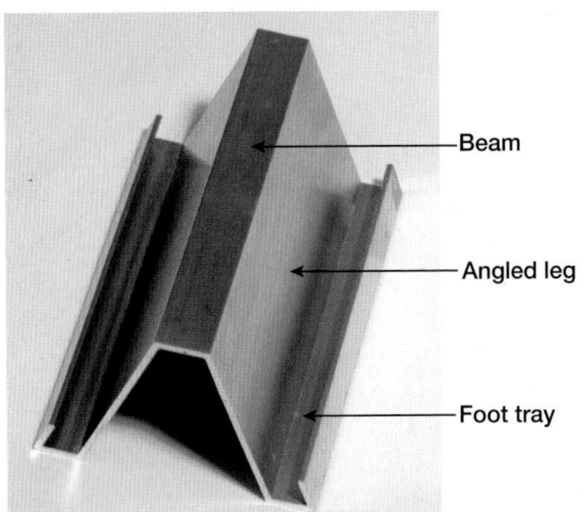

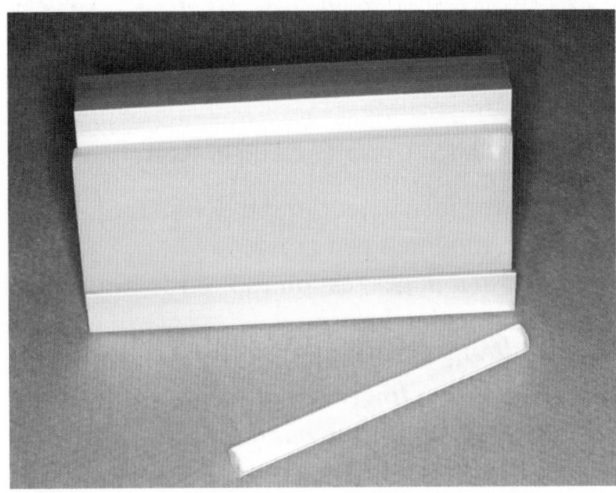

Figure 23-13. Components of the Sharpening Horse System.

- The sharpening horse system consists of a metal device that holds a sharpening stone at a fixed angle, a ceramic sharpening stone, and an acrylic test stick.
- The ceramic stone should be lubricated with water prior to sharpening.

Figure 23-14. Modifying Stone Height. For most clinicians, the sharpening stone is at an ideal height as it rests in the foot tray.

- Clinicians with petite hands or short fingers may find it helpful to raise the height of the stone in the holder.
- Sliding a test stick into the foot tray and resting the stone on top of the test stick easily raises the height of the stone in the holder.

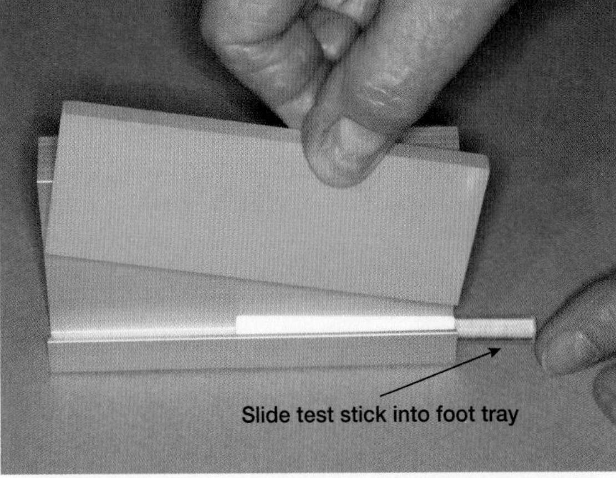

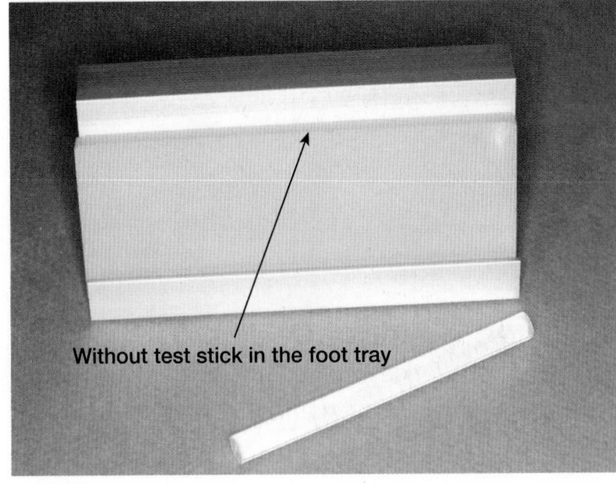

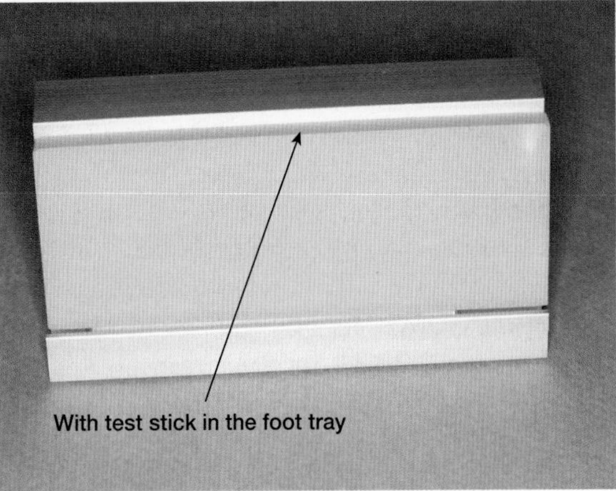

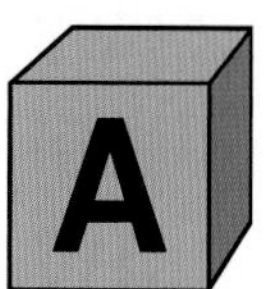

SKILL BUILDING. MOVING INSTRUMENT TECHNIQUE: STEP-BY-STEP FOR CURETS

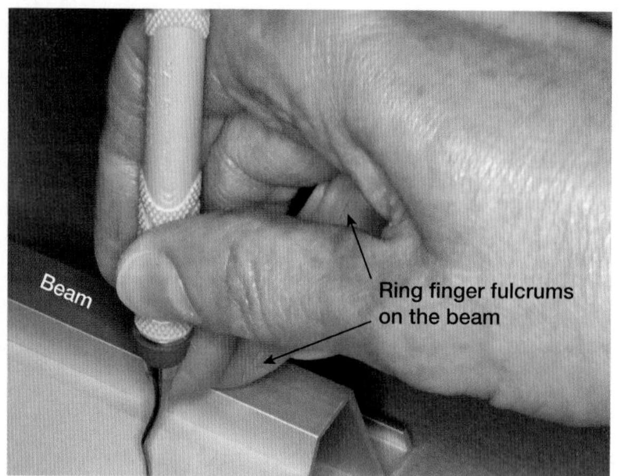

1. Figure 23-15. Grasp and Finger Rest.

- Grasp the instrument in the dominant hand using a modified pen grasp.
- Establish a finger rest on top of the beam of the Sharpening Horse.
- Stabilize the horse with the nondominant hand.
- ***Hold the ring finger straight and use it as a support beam for the hand throughout the entire sharpening procedure.***

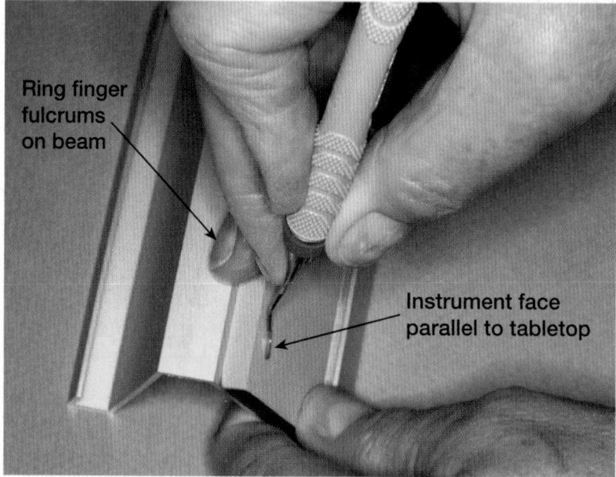

2. Figure 23-16. Face-to-Stone Angulation.

- ***Position the instrument face parallel to the tabletop.***
- With the face in this position, the Sharpening Horse device holds the stone at the correct angulation for sharpening.
- Note that the position of the face is the same—parallel to the tabletop—when sharpening both sickle scalers and curets.

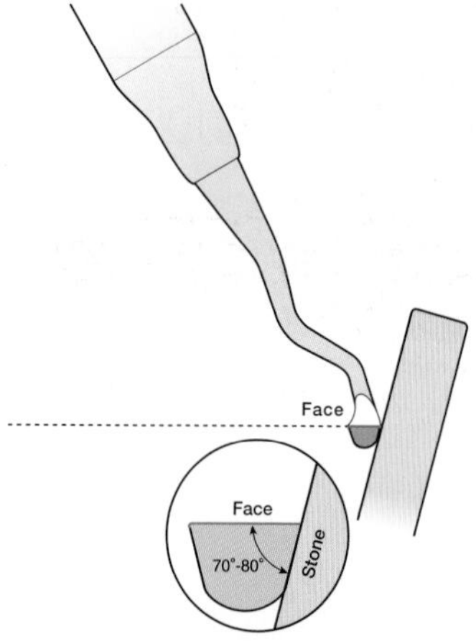

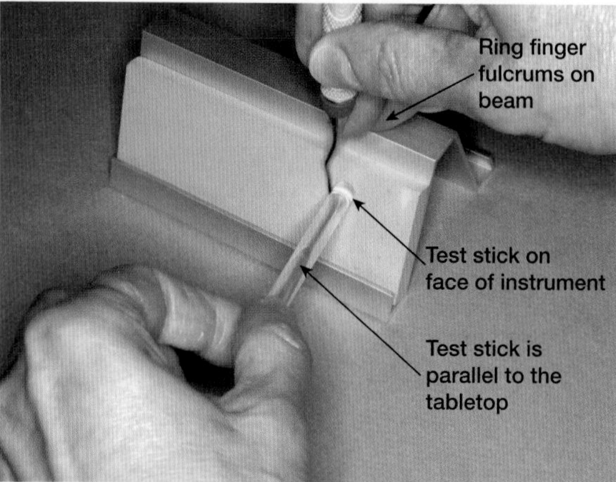

Figure 23-17. Technique Check. For all sickle scalers and curets, the working-end is properly positioned if ***the face is parallel to the tabletop***. One technique for checking for parallelism is to place a sharpening stick on the face and verify that the stick is parallel to the tabletop.

3. Figure 23-18. Begin with Heel-Third.

- Holding the ring finger straight, position the heel-third of the cutting edge against the sharpening stone.
- ***Slide both the finger rest and instrument a short distance along the stone to sharpen the heel-third of the cutting edge.***

4. Figure 23-19. Sharpen Cutting Edge in Sections.

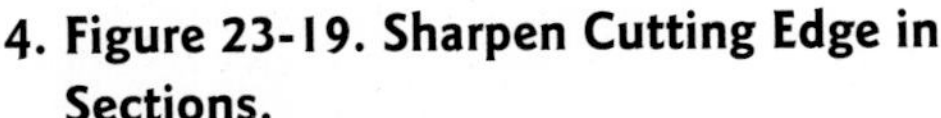

- Start at one end of the stone. Adapt the *heel-third* of the cutting edge to the stone.
- ***Slide the finger rest and instrument a short distance along the beam to sharpen the heel-third of the cutting edge.***

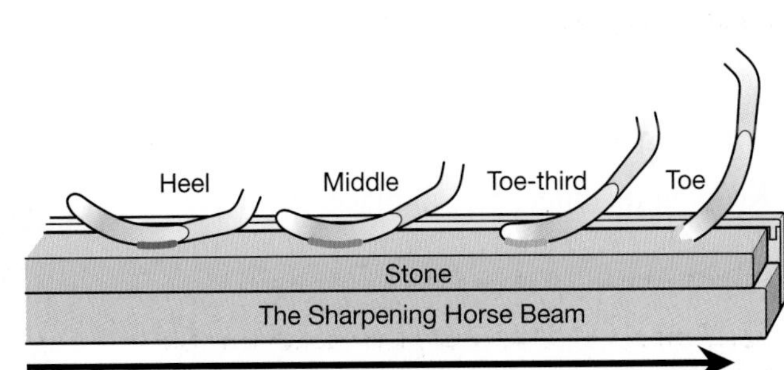

5. Figure 23-20. Slide the Fulcrum along the Beam.

- Throughout the sharpening process, slide the fulcrum finger along the beam of the Sharpening Horse.
- As the cutting edge moves along the stone, pivot the working-end to sharpen the middle-third and toe-third of the cutting edge.

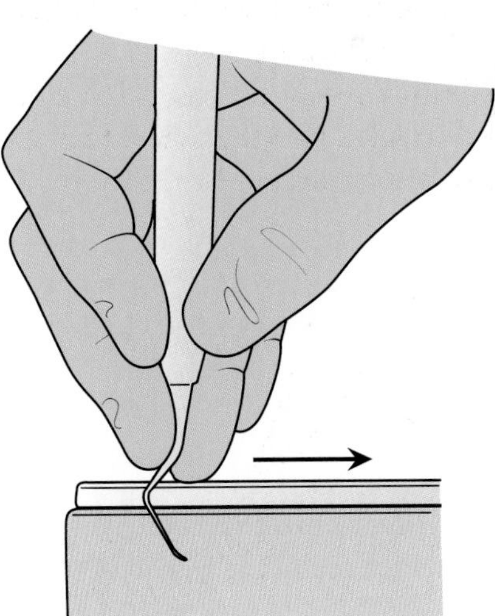

The steps for sharpening a curet continue on the next page.

6. Figure 23-21. Pivot the Working-End.

- Keeping the finger rest in place, pivot the working-end slightly so that the ***middle-third*** of the cutting edge is against the stone.
- Slide both the finger rest and instrument a short distance along the stone to sharpen the middle-third of the cutting edge.

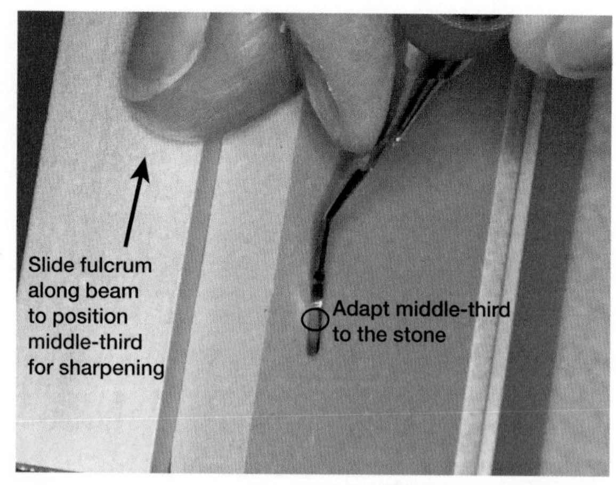

7. Figure 23-22. Pivot the Working-End.

- Keeping the finger rest in place, pivot the working-end slightly so that the ***toe-third*** of the cutting edge is against the stone.
- Slide both the finger rest and instrument a short distance along the stone to sharpen the toe-third of the cutting edge.

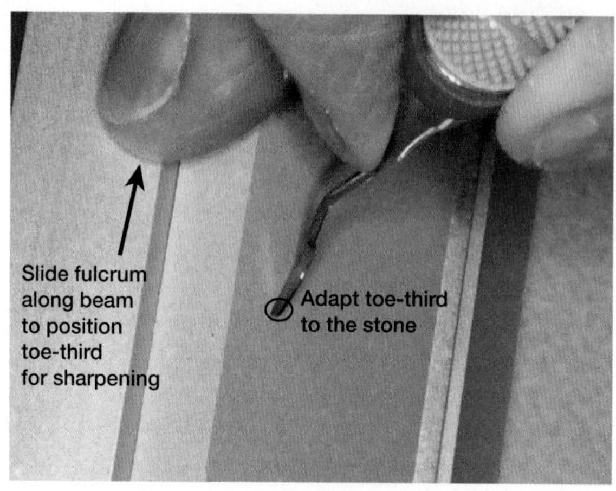

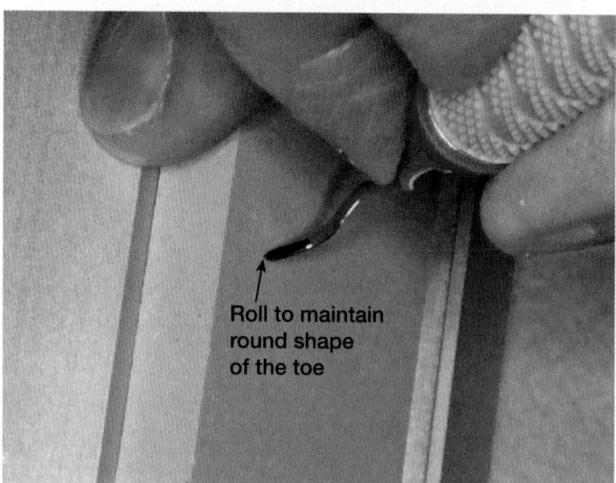

8. Figure 23-23. Pivot onto the Toe. Pivot to sharpen and round the ***toe*** of the working-end.

9. Complete the Sharpening Process:

- Complete the sharpening process by recontouring the back of the working-end on the top edge of the sharpening stone.
- Turn the Sharpening Horse around to sharpen the opposite cutting edge of a universal curet or sickle scaler.
- *After sharpening, turn to Section 4 of this module to evaluate sharpness.*

B SKILL BUILDING. MOVING INSTRUMENT TECHNIQUE: STEP-BY-STEP FOR SICKLE SCALERS

The sharpening technique for a sickle scaler is essentially the same as that used with a curet (Figs. 23-24 and 23-25). The cutting edges of a sickle scaler meet in a point; therefore, on a sickle scaler, there is no rounded toe to recontour.

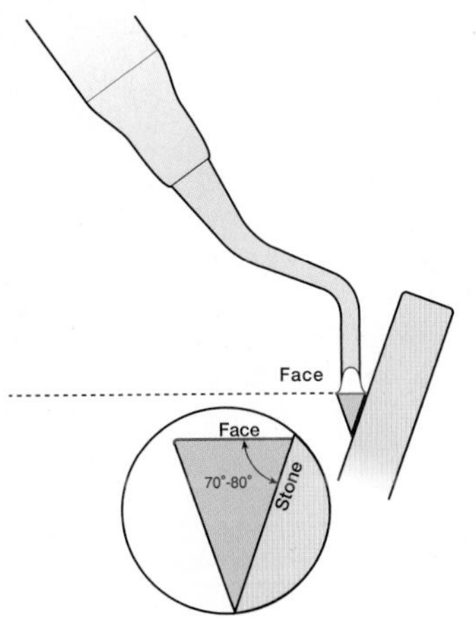

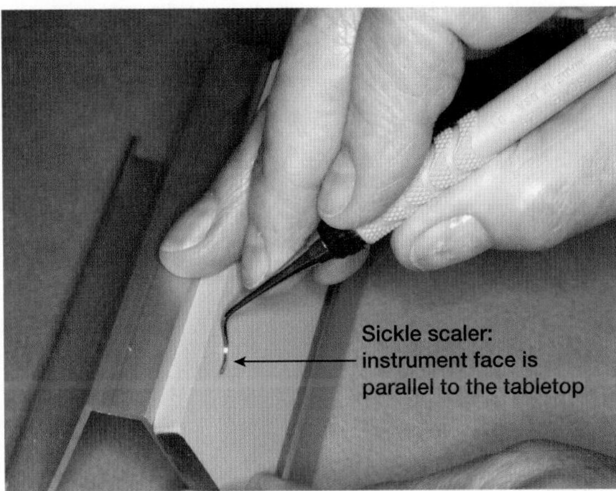

Figure 23-24. Sharpening Technique for a Sickle Scaler.

- **Adapt Sickle to Stone.** Establish the correct face-to-stone angulation by positioning the face parallel to the tabletop.
- **Establish Fulcrum.** The complex shank bend of some posterior sickles—such as the Nevi sickle pictured here—means that the clinician lowers the hand to obtain parallelism of the face to the tabletop.
- **Sharpen.** Slide the finger rest along the top of the Sharpening Horse while moving the working-end across the stone.

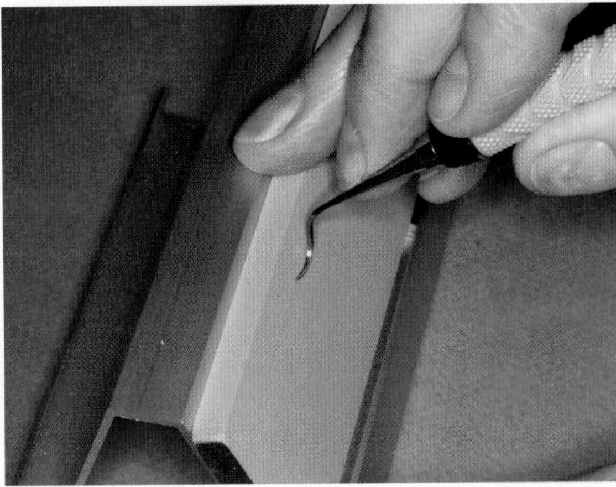

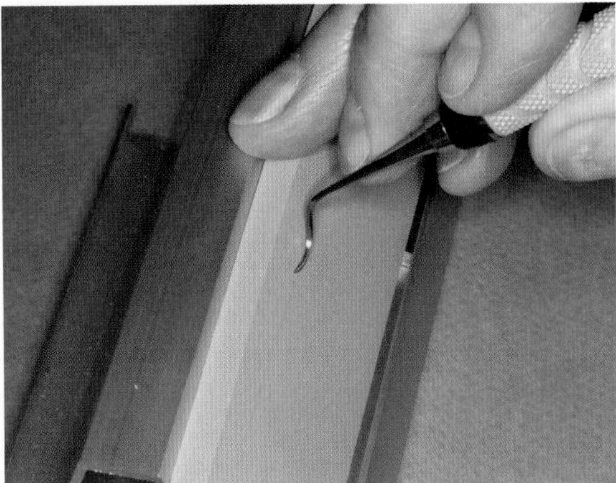

Figures 23-25. A and B. Sharpen Cutting Edge of a Sickle in Thirds. Using a similar technique to that used for a curet, sharpen the heel-third, middle-third, and tip-third of a sickle scaler.

Section 3
The Moving Stone Technique

OVERVIEW OF THE MOVING STONE TECHNIQUE

As the name suggests, the moving stone technique involves removing metal from the working-end by moving a sharpening stone over a lateral surface of a stabilized instrument (Figs. 23-26 and 23-27).

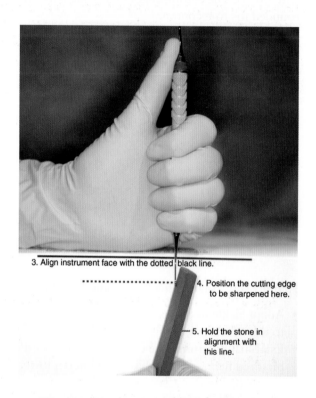

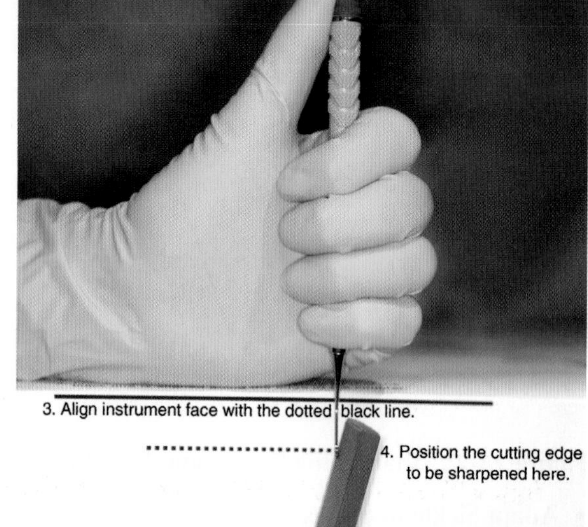

5. Hold the stone in alignment with this line.

Figure 23-26. Moving Stone Technique.

- The moving stone technique involves grasping the instrument and stabilizing it against a countertop.
- The sharpening stone is held in the clinician's other hand and is moved over the lateral surface of the working-end.

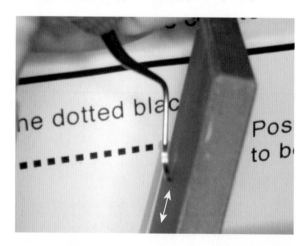

Figure 23-27. Movement of Stone. The sharpening stone is positioned against the lateral surface and moved up and down to remove metal from the working-end.

ESSENTIAL SKILL COMPONENTS OF THE MOVING STONE TECHNIQUE

Skill Component 1: Positioning the Instrument against a Stable Surface

An important component of correct sharpening technique is the position of the instrument face. *The instrument face is positioned parallel to the countertop for sharpening. Position the working-end of a sickle scaler, universal curet, or area-specific curet so that the face is parallel (=) to the countertop.* Figures 23-28 and 23-29 show the face of a sickle scaler, universal curet, and area-specific curet positioned parallel to the countertop.

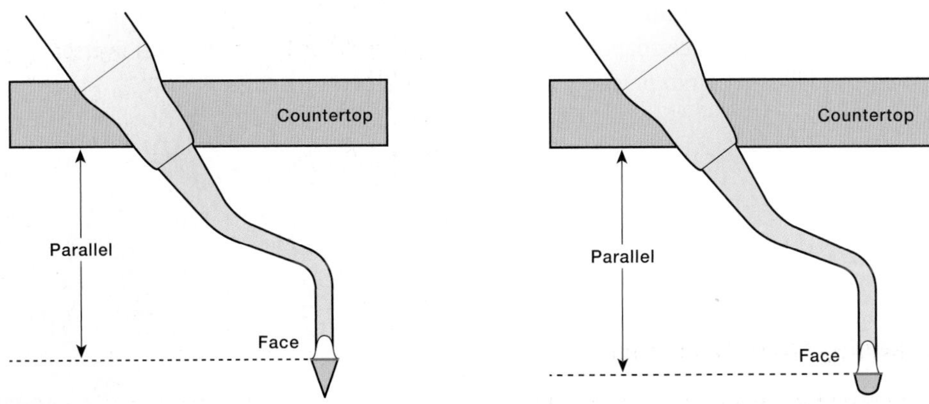

Figure 23-28. Face of a Sickle Scaler or Universal Curet.

- For sharpening a sickle scaler or a universal curet, position the instrument face parallel (=) to the countertop.
- When positioned with the face parallel to the countertop, the lower shanks of these instruments are perpendicular (⊥) to the countertop.
- *Two cutting edges are sharpened on each working-end of a sickle scaler or a universal curet.*

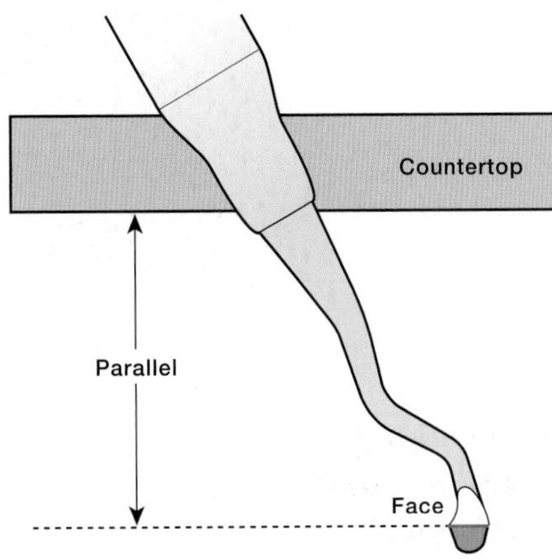

Figure 23-29. Face of an Area-Specific Curet.

- For sharpening an area-specific curet, position the instrument face parallel (=) to the countertop.
- When positioned with the face parallel to the countertop, the lower shank of an area-specific curet is NOT perpendicular to the countertop.
- *One cutting edge, the working cutting edge, is sharpened on each area-specific curet.*

Skill Component 2: Establishing Angulation of the Stone to the Instrument Face

To maintain the original design characteristics of the working-end, ***the angulation between the instrument face and the sharpening stone should be between 70° and 80°.***

- Beginning clinicians often experience difficulty in visualizing the 70° to 80° angle used in instrument sharpening.
- Follow the directions in Figures 23-30 and 23-31 to gain experience in establishing the correct angulation between the sharpening stone and the instrument face.

Directions:

- For this Skill Practice, you will need a rectangular sharpening stone and the illustrations in Figures 23-32 and 23-33 located on the next page of this module.
- Use the first illustration to practice adapting the stone to the right cutting edge of a universal curet.
- Next, use the second illustration to practice adapting to the left cutting edge.

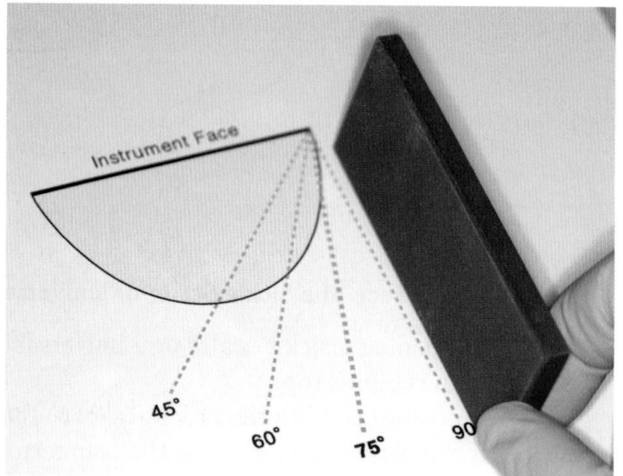

Figure 23-30. Step 1: Establish a 90° Angle.

- Place your sharpening stone on the dotted line labeled as a 90° angle. Your sharpening stone is now positioned at a 90° angle to the instrument face.
- This position gives you a visual starting point from which to establish the correct angulation.

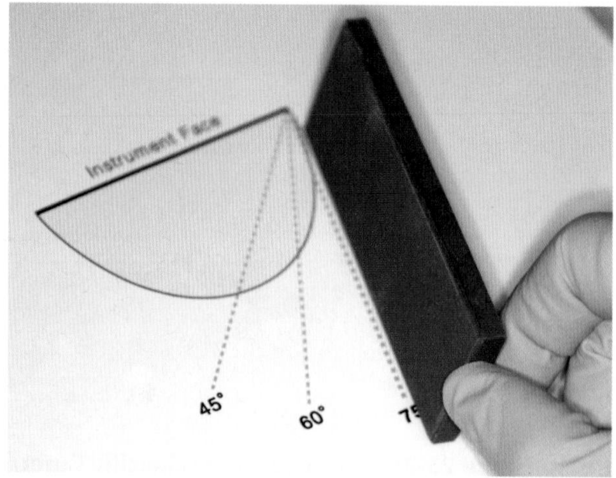

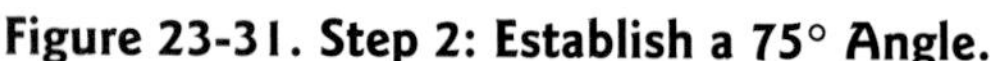

Figure 23-31. Step 2: Establish a 75° Angle.

- Swing the lower end of the sharpening stone toward the instrument back.
- Align your stone with the dotted line labeled as a 75° angle. Your sharpening stone is now at the proper angle to the face.

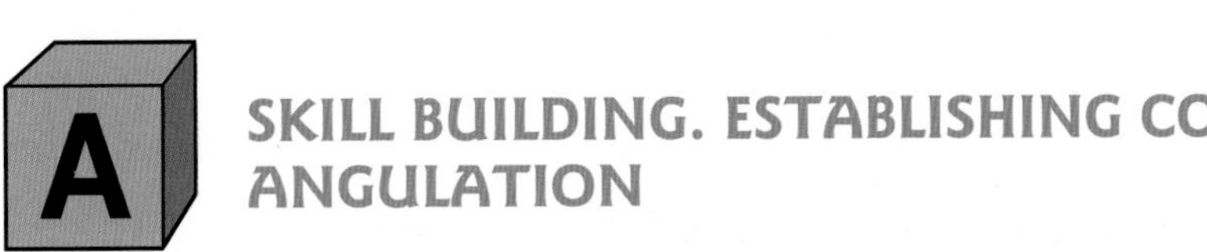

SKILL BUILDING. ESTABLISHING CORRECT ANGULATION

Use Figures 23-32 and 23-33 below to practice establishing correct angulation of a sharpening stone to the instrument face.

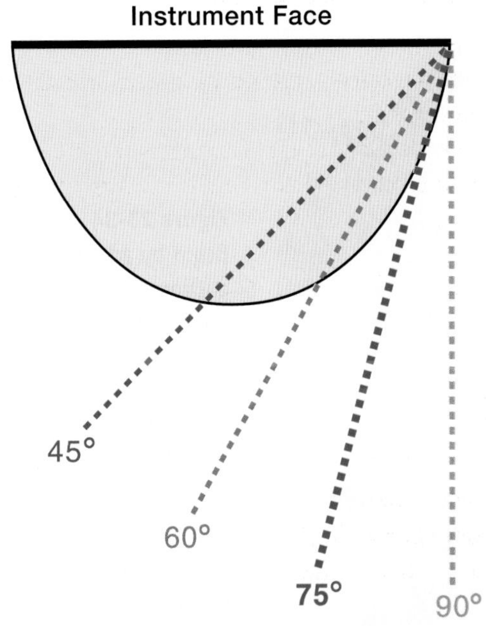

Figure 23-32. Angle for Right Cutting Edge.

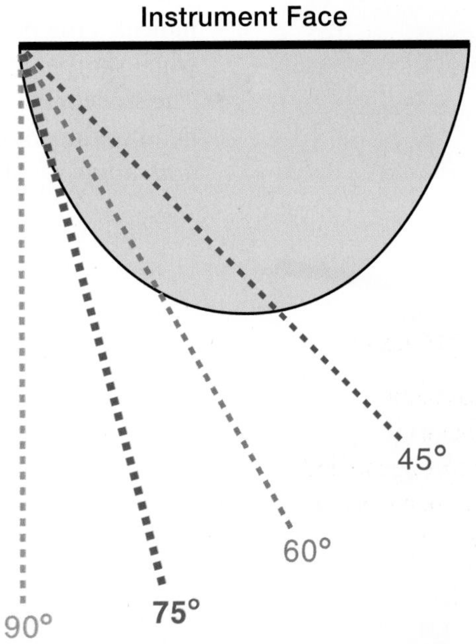

Figure 23-33. Angle for Left Cutting Edge.

Skill Component 3: Sharpen the Cutting Edge in Sections

A technique of rotating the sharpening stone is used to sharpen the cutting edge in sections (Figs. 23-34 to 23-36). First, the stone is adapted to the heel-third of the cutting edge. Next, the middle-third is sharpened. After sharpening the middle-third, the stone is rotated again to adapt to the toe- or tip-third of the cutting edge. For this technique, the stone is rotated away from the palm of the hand *while maintaining correct angulation of the stone to the instrument face.*

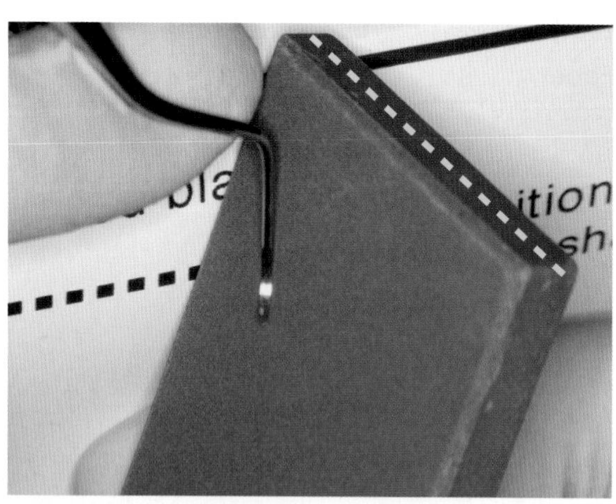

Figure 23-34. Step 1: Sharpen the Heel-Third. Begin by adapting the stone to the heel-third of the cutting edge. Note that the middle- and toe-thirds of the cutting edge are not in contact with the sharpening stone. Use a sharpening guide to establish a 75° angle with the sharpening stone.

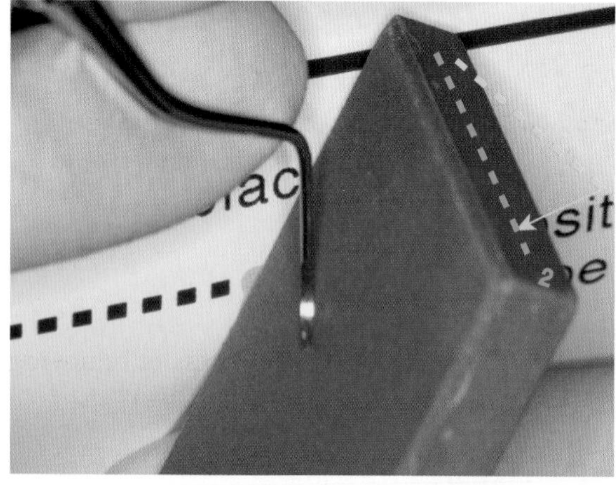

Figure 23-35. Step 2: Sharpen the Middle-Third. While maintaining correct angulation, rotate the stone away from the palm of your hand slightly. The stone is now positioned to sharpen the middle-third of the cutting edge.

- The *yellow dotted line* on the photograph indicates the position of the sharpening stone when sharpening the *heel-third.*
- The stone is rotated away from the palm of the hand to the position indicated by the *orange dotted line* for sharpening the *middle-third.*

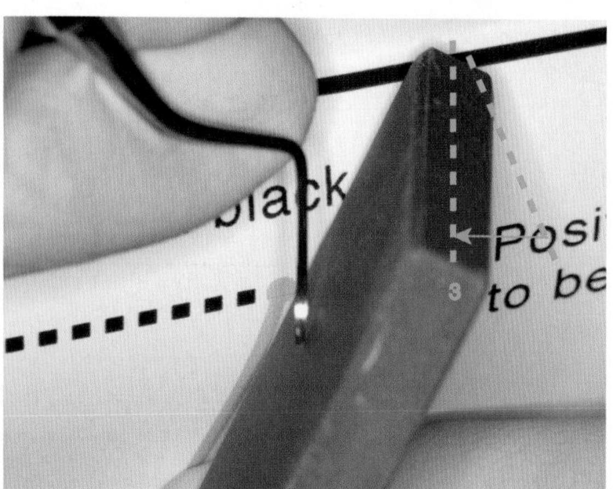

Figure 23-36. Step 3: Sharpen the Toe-Third. Rotate the stone away from the palm of your hand again. Sharpen the toe-third of the cutting edge.

- The *green dotted line* on the photograph indicates the position of the sharpening stone when sharpening the *toe-third.*

Skill Component 4: Removing Metal Burs from the Cutting Edge

Sharpening can produce minute metal burs that project from the cutting edge (Fig. 23-37A).

1. A cutting edge with metal burs is sometimes termed a wire edge because the metal burs are like tiny wire projections. The use of a wire edge on the root surfaces can result in gouging of the cementum.
2. The metal burs are impossible to see with the naked eye but can be seen using magnification.
3. Burs can be avoided by finishing with a down stroke toward the cutting edge (Fig. 23-37B).
4. Burs can easily be seen under magnification and removed using a light stroke with a cylindrical sharpening stone.

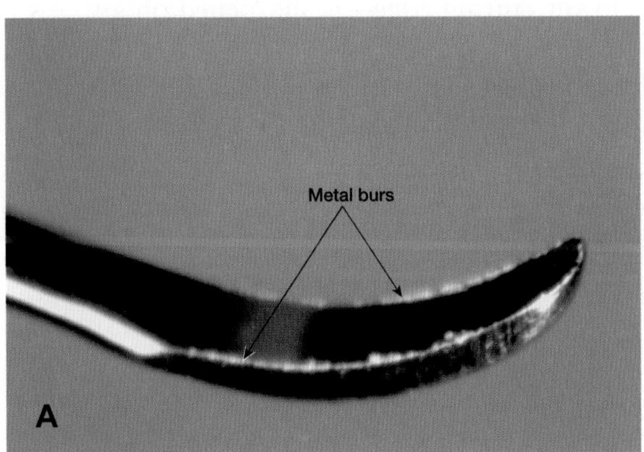

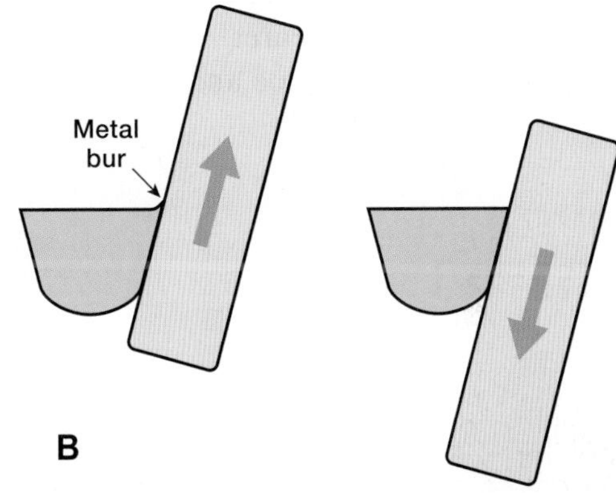

Figure 23-37. Metal Burs. A. Sharpening can produce minute metal burs that project from the cutting edge. **B.** Burs can be prevented by finishing with a down stroke of the sharpening stone toward the cutting edge.

Skill Component 5: Recontouring the Toe and Back of the Working-End

The rounded toes and backs of curets must be recontoured. Recontouring is the process of removing metal from the toe and back to restore the curved surfaces of a curet (Figs. 23-38 and 23-39).

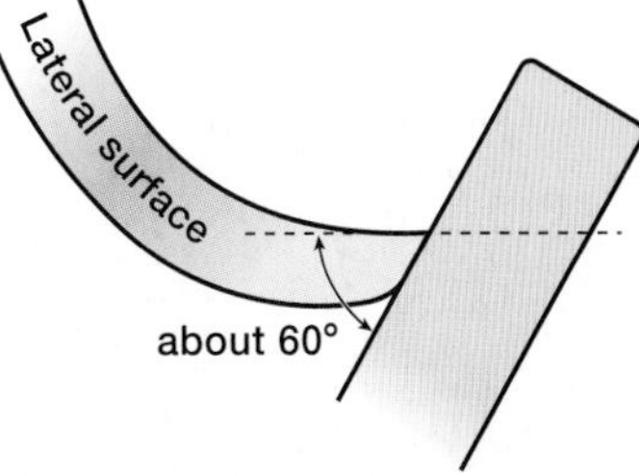

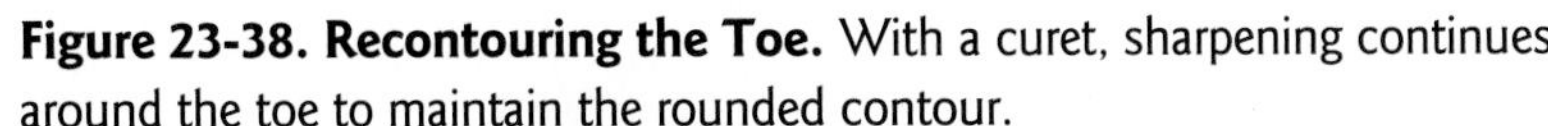

Figure 23-38. Recontouring the Toe. With a curet, sharpening continues around the toe to maintain the rounded contour.

Figure 23-39. Recontouring the Back. The back of a curet must be recontoured slightly to maintain a smooth rounded back.

BASIC PRINCIPLES WITH CURETS AND SICKLE SCALERS

1. **Consistent Basic Principles.** *The basic steps in the moving stone technique are the same for all area-specific curets, universal curets, and sickle scalers. The relationship of the face of the working-end to the countertop is the same for all area-specific curets, universal curets, and sickle scalers.*
   - The working-end is positioned so that the face is parallel to the countertop.
   - Once the face is parallel to the countertop, the stone is positioned at a 70° to 80° angle to the face (Fig. 23-40).

2. **Minor Differences.** Only a few differences apply to the techniques used with these three instruments.
   - Two sharpening edges per working-end are sharpened for universal curets and sickle scalers.
   - Only one cutting edge per working-end—the lower cutting edge—is sharpened on an area-specific curet
   - The rounded toe and back should be recontoured on area-specific and universal curets.

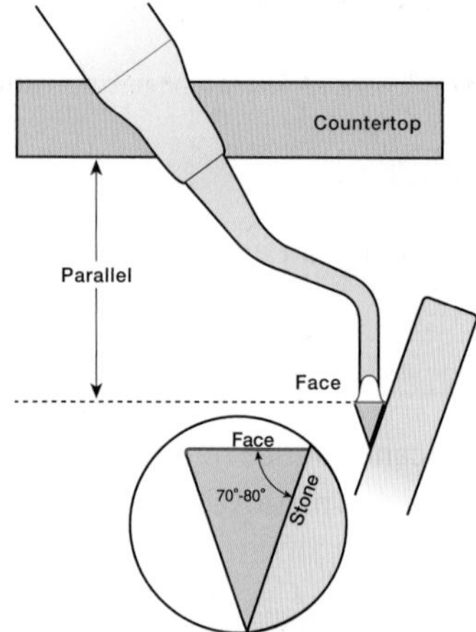

A. Sickle Scaler.

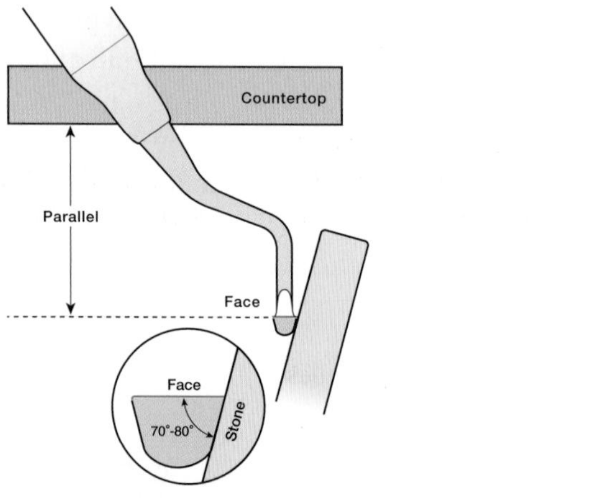

B. Universal Curet.

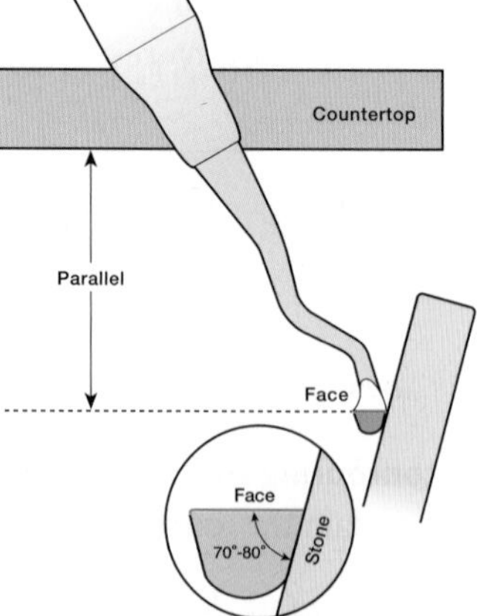

C. Area-Specific Curet.

Figure 23-40. Basic Principles for Moving Stone Technique. Preparation for the moving stone technique includes (1) positioning the face parallel to the countertop and (2) establishing a 70° to 80° angle between the face and the stone. These principles apply to all sickle scalers, universal curets, and area-specific curets.

SHARPENING GUIDE R

Directions for Use of Sharpening Guides: Photocopy **Sharpening Guide R** (Fig. 23-41) and **Sharpening Guide L** (Fig. 23-42) and place them back-to-back in a single plastic page protector or have them laminated. Another way to use a photocopied sharpening guide is to tape it to the countertop and cover it with a piece of plastic wrap.

Use Sharpening Guide R for:

- The right cutting edge of a universal curet or sickle scaler
- For ODD-numbered Gracey curets, such as a G11 and G13

Sharpening Guide - R

1. Fold this page in half along the solid black line.
2. Place the folded edge on a countertop so that the black line is aligned along the edge of the counter.

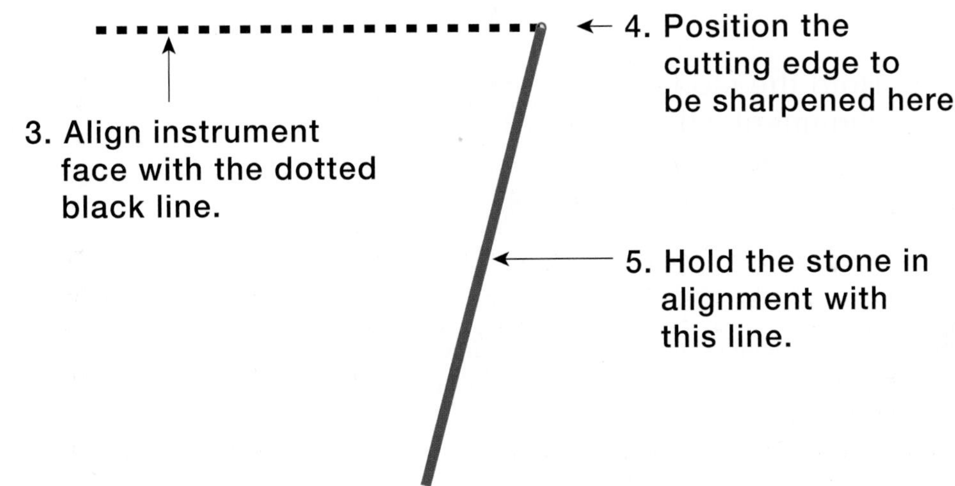
4. Position the cutting edge to be sharpened here.
3. Align instrument face with the dotted black line.
5. Hold the stone in alignment with this line.

Figure 23-41. Sharpening Guide R. Use this sharpening guide for the right cutting edge of a universal curet or sickle scaler and for odd-numbered Gracey curets, such as a Gracey 11 or 13.

SHARPENING GUIDE L

Use Sharpening Guide L for:

- The left cutting edge of a universal curet or sickle scaler
- For EVEN-numbered Gracey curets, such as a G12 and G14

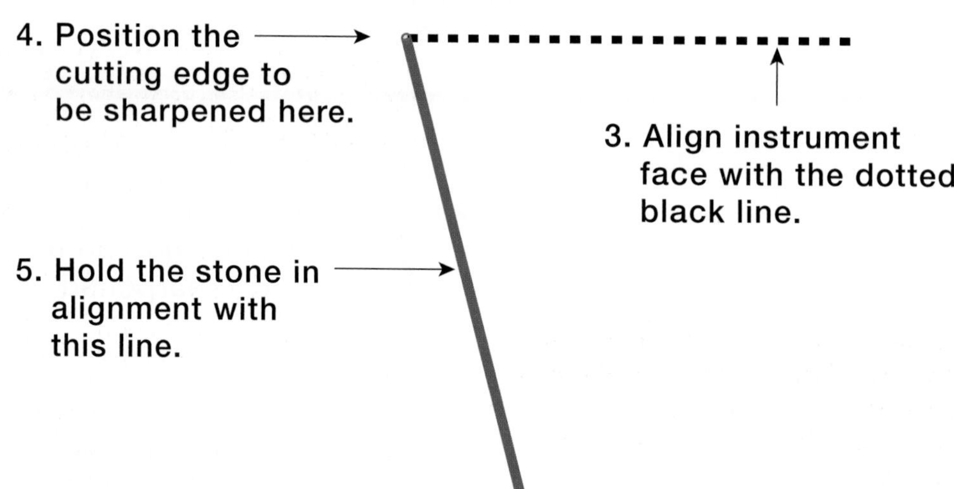
Sharpening Guide - L
1. Fold this page in half along the solid black line.
2. Place the folded edge on a countertop so that the black line is aligned along the edge of the counter.
4. Position the cutting edge to be sharpened here.
3. Align instrument face with the dotted black line.
5. Hold the stone in alignment with this line.

Figure 23-42. Sharpening Guide L. Use this sharpening guide for the left cutting edge of a universal curet or sickle scaler and for even-numbered Gracey curets, such as a Gracey 12 or 14.

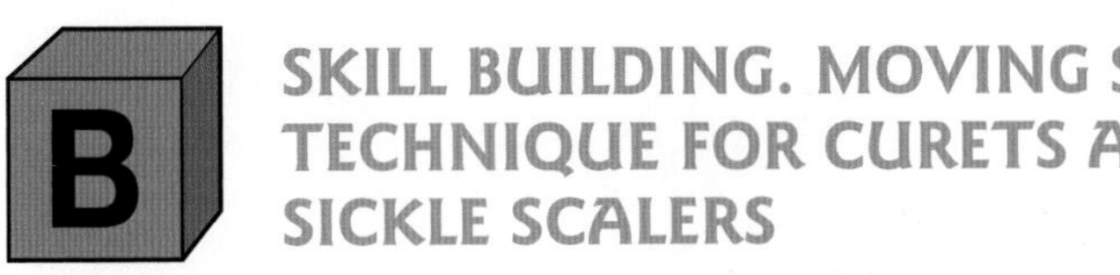

SKILL BUILDING. MOVING STONE TECHNIQUE FOR CURETS AND SICKLE SCALERS

Directions:

- Cover the top and front surfaces of the counter with a barrier such as plastic wrap. Secure the barrier to the countertop with autoclave or masking tape.
- Place ***Sharpening Guide R*** on the counter so that the heavy black line falls along the edge of the counter. Secure the guide to the countertop with autoclave or masking tape. ***Begin by sharpening the right cutting edge of a universal curet.*** Follow the steps 1 to 10 shown in Figures 23-43 to 23-52 to practice the moving stone sharpening technique.
- Lubricate the stone. If the stone is synthetic, lubricate it on both sides with a few drops of water. Synthetic stones are recommended for sharpening during treatment. If the stone is natural, lubricate it on both sides with a few drops of oil.

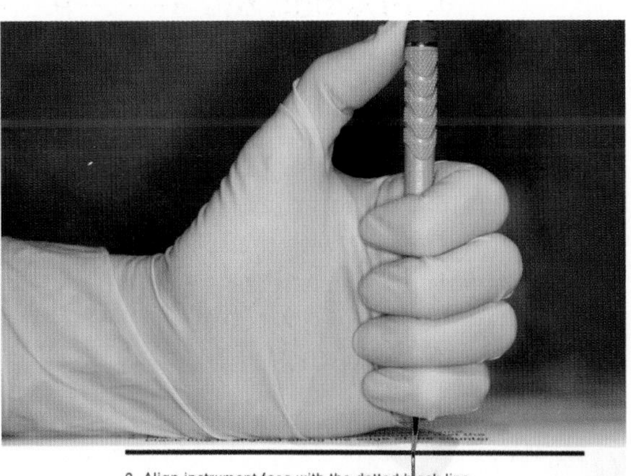
3. Align instrument face with the dotted black line.

1. **Figure 23-43. Grasp the Instrument.** ***Grasp the instrument handle in the palm of your nondominant hand.*** Rest your hand and arm on the countertop. Stabilize the instrument handle with your thumb.

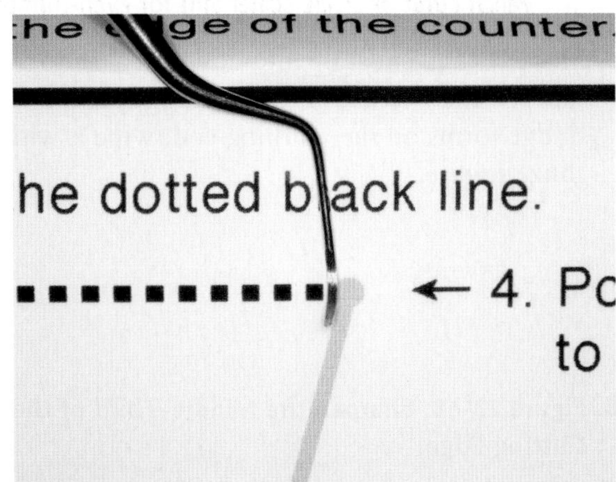
he dotted black line.

2. **Figure 23-44. Position the Instrument Face.**
   - Align the instrument face with the dotted line on the sharpening guide. This will position the working-end so that the face is parallel (=) to the countertop.
   - Keeping the face aligned with the dotted line, slide your nondominant hand over until the cutting edge to be sharpened is positioned *at the far right-hand side* of the dotted line.

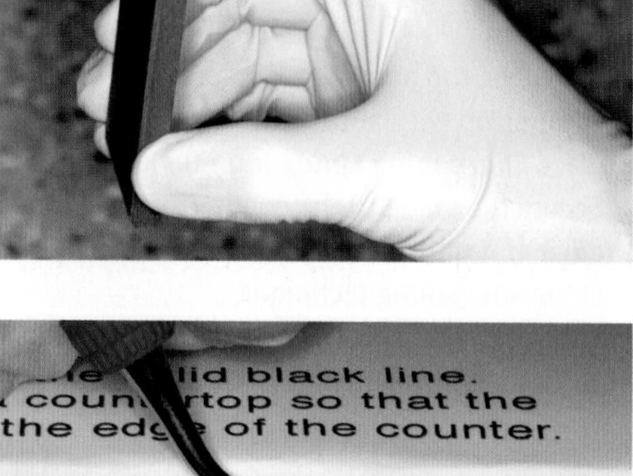

3. Figure 23-45. Grasp the Sharpening Stone.

- *Grasp the sharpening stone with your dominant hand.*
- Hold the stone on the edges so that your fingers do not get in the way when sharpening.

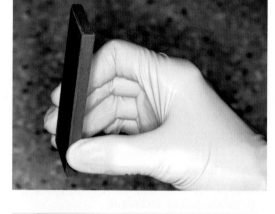

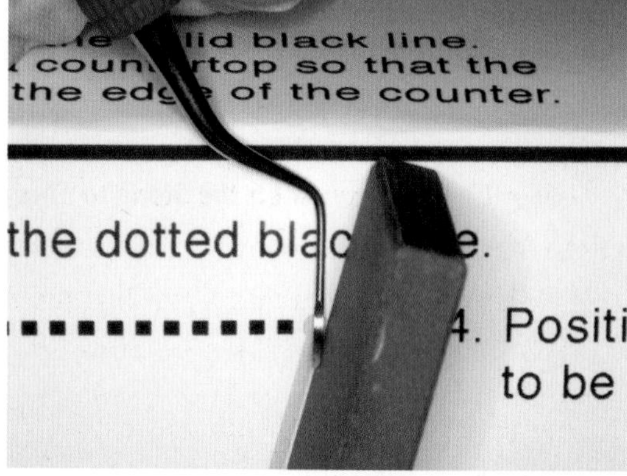

4. Figure 23-46. Position the Sharpening Stone. Align the sharpening stone with the solid line. This is the correct angulation for sharpening.

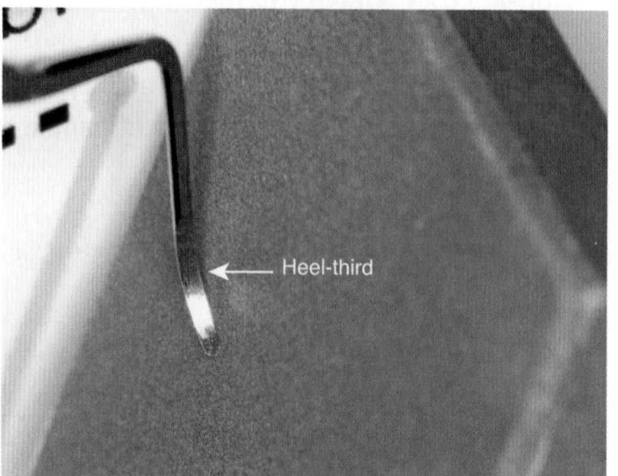

5. Figure 23-47. Adapt the Stone to the Heel-Third of the Cutting Edge.

- The photograph shows a bird's-eye view looking down at the instrument face.
- Make several short up and down strokes to sharpen this section of the cutting edge. If a metal sludge forms on the working-end, wipe it with a gauze square.

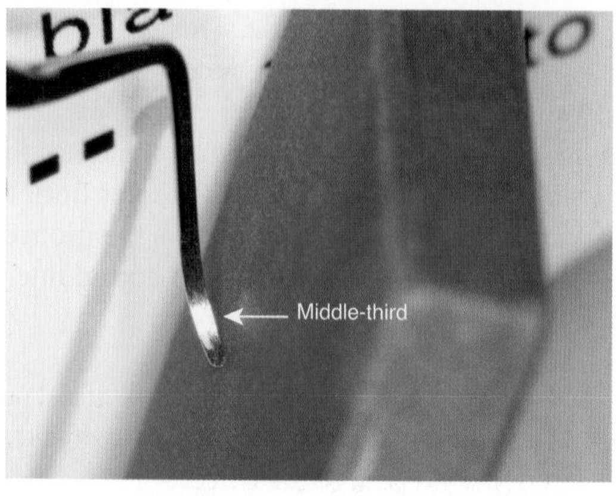

6. Figure 23-48. Sharpen the Middle-Third of the Cutting Edge.

- When the heel section is sharp, rotate the stone so that it is in contact with the middle-third of the cutting edge.
- Make several short up and down strokes to sharpen this section of the cutting edge.

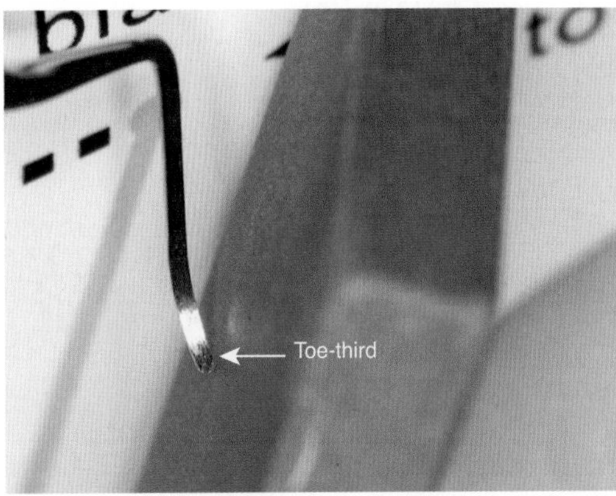

7. **Figure 23-49. Sharpen the Toe-Third of the Cutting Edge.**
   - Rotate the stone so that it is in contact with the toe-third of the cutting edge.
   - Make several short up and down strokes to sharpen this section of the cutting edge.

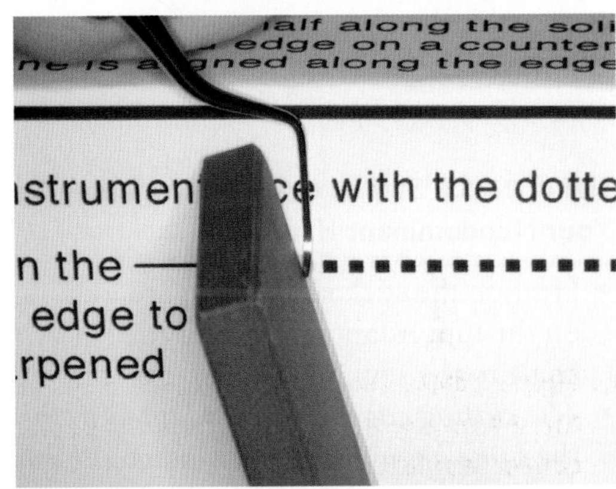

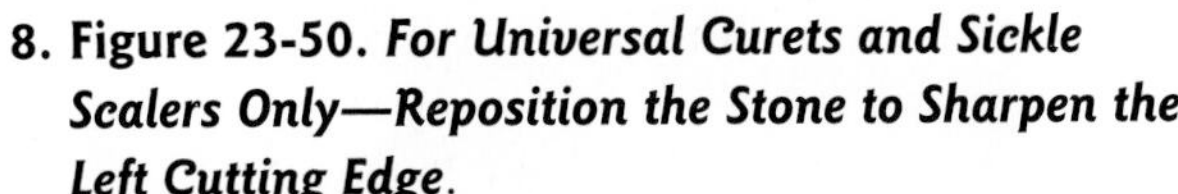

8. **Figure 23-50. *For Universal Curets and Sickle Scalers Only—Reposition the Stone to Sharpen the Left Cutting Edge*.**
   - Use **Sharpening Guide L** to position the stone for sharpening the left cutting edge on a universal curet or sickle scaler.
   - Sharpen the left cutting edge using the same technique as for the right cutting edge.

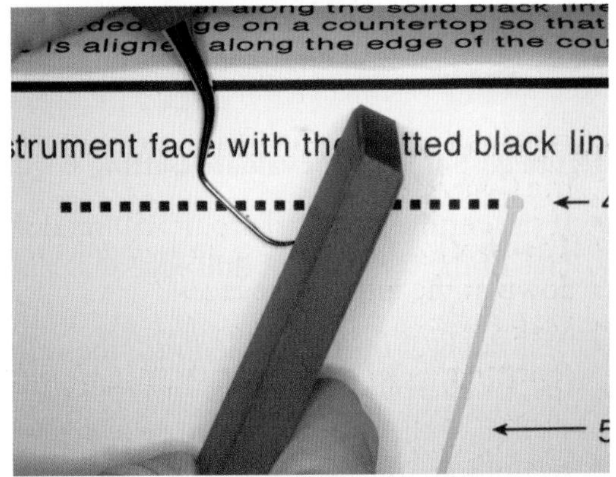

9. **Figure 23-51. *For Curets Only—Sharpen the Curet Toe.***
   - To recontour the curet toe, make a series of sharpening strokes around the toe. Be careful to keep the face parallel (=) to the countertop.
   - Move the stone in up and down strokes as you work your way around the toe.

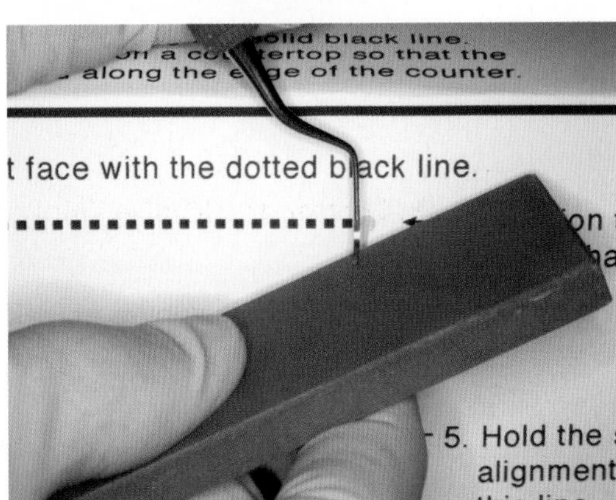

10. **Figure 23-52. *For Curets Only—Recontour the Back.*** To recontour the back, use semi-circular strokes around the back of the curet.

Section 4
Evaluating Sharpness

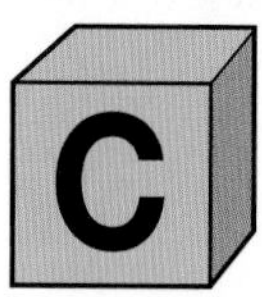

SKILL BUILDING. EVALUATING SHARPNESS OF CUTTING EDGE

After sharpening, follow steps 1 to 3 shown in Figures 23-53 to 23-55 to evaluate the sharpening process.

Figure 23-53. Step 1: Grasp a Sharpening Test Stick in Your Nondominant Hand.

- Position the stick so that you are looking down on the top. Adapt the cutting edge at a 70° to 80° angle to the stick.
- *The cutting edge must be adapted to the stick at the same angulation that you would use against a tooth surface.*

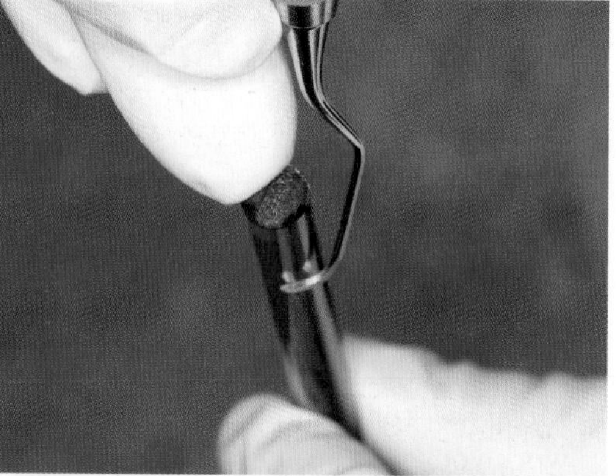

Figure 23-54. Step 2: Evaluate Cutting Edge.

- If the cutting edge is sharp, it will scratch the surface of the test stick. A dull edge will slide over the surface of the test stick.
- Test the heel-third, middle-third, toe-third, and toe for sharpness. Note that it is possible for one section of the cutting edge to be sharp while other sections are dull.

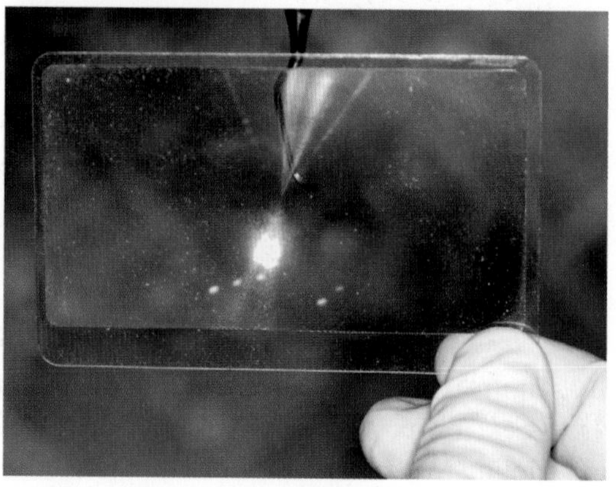

Figure 23-55. Step 3: Examine under Magnification.

- Use a magnifying lens or loops to examine the working-end.
- Evaluate the working-end to ensure that its original design has been preserved.

Section 5
Sharpening a Periodontal File

The working-end of a periodontal file is difficult to sharpen due to the multiple cutting edges. For this reason, many clinicians send files to professional instrument sharpening services to be sharpened. To sharpen a file, the clinician will need to use a metal file known as a tanged file.

- Use your nondominant hand to stabilize the file on a countertop. Grasp the tanged file with your dominant hand.
- Lay the tanged file in a horizontal position against the first cutting edge. Move the file back and forth across the cutting edge (Fig. 23-56).
- Repeat the same procedure for each of the cutting edges. Use a sharpening test stick to evaluate the sharpness of the cutting edges.

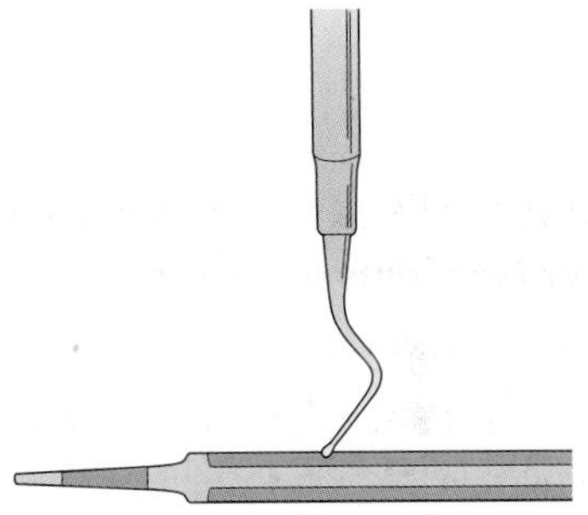

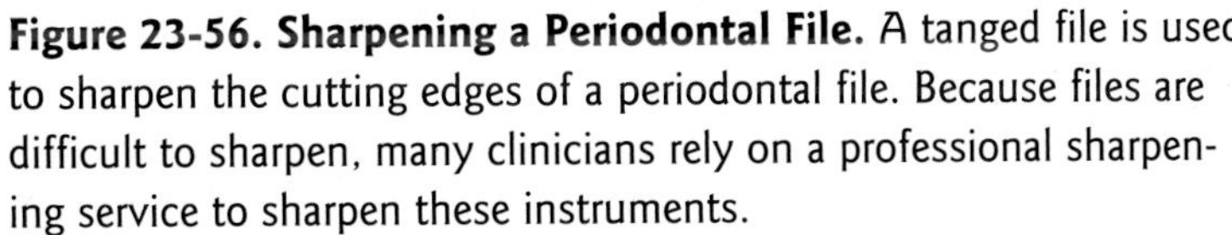

Figure 23-56. Sharpening a Periodontal File. A tanged file is used to sharpen the cutting edges of a periodontal file. Because files are difficult to sharpen, many clinicians rely on a professional sharpening service to sharpen these instruments.

REFERENCES

1. Acevedo R, Sampaio J, Shibli J. Scanning electron microscope assessment of several resharpening techniques on the cutting edges of Gracey curettes. *J Contemp Dent Pract.* 2007;8:70–77.
2. Andrade Acevedo RA, Cardozo AK, Sampaio JE. Scanning electron microscopic and profilometric study of different sharpening stones. *Braz Dent J.* 2006;17:237–242.
3. Daniel SJ, Harfst SA. *Mosby's Dental Hygiene: Concepts, Cases, and Competencies.* St. Louis, MO: Mosby; 2004.
4. Darby ML. *Mosby's Comprehensive Review of Dental Hygiene.* 6th ed. St. Louis, MO: Mosby; 2010.
5. Darby ML, Walsh MM. *Dental Hygiene: Theory and Practice.* 3rd ed. St. Louis, MO: Saunders/Elsevier; 2010.
6. Huang CC, Tseng CC. Effect of different sharpening stones on periodontal curettes evaluated by scanning electron microscopy. *J Formos Med Assoc.* 1991;90:782–787.
7. Moses O, Tal H, Artzi Z, Sperling A, Zohar R, Nemcovsky CE. Scanning electron microscope evaluation of two methods of resharpening periodontal curets: a comparative study. *J Periodontol.* 2003;74:1032–1037.
8. Rossi R, Smukler H. A scanning electron microscope study comparing the effectiveness of different types of sharpening stones and curets. *J Periodontol.* 1995;66:956–961.
9. Silva MV, Gomes DA, Leite FR, Sampaio JE, de Toledo BE, Mendes AJ. Sharpening of periodontal instruments with different sharpening stones and its influence upon root debridement—scanning electronic microscopy assessment. *J Int Acad Periodontol.* 2006;8:17–22.
10. Wilkins EM. *Clinical Practice of the Dental Hygienist.* 9th ed. Philadelphia, PA: Lippincott Williams & Wilkins; 2009.
11. Paquette OE, Levin MP. The sharpening of scaling instruments: II. A preferred technique. *J Periodontol.* 1977;48:169–172.
12. Paquette OE, Levin MP. The sharpening of scaling instruments: I. An examination of principles. *J Periodontol.* 1977;48:163–168.
13. Marquam BJ. Strategies to improve instrument sharpening. *Dent Hyg (Chic).* 1988;62:334–338.
14. Leiseca CB. Manual instrument sharpening. The best method may come as a surprise. *RDH.* 2010;30:2–5.

Section 6
Skill Application

STUDENT SELF-EVALUATION MODULE 23 INSTRUMENT SHARPENING

Student: ______________________ Instrument 1 = ______________________

Date: ______________________ Instrument 2 = ______________________

Instrument 3 = ______________________

Instrument 4 = ______________________

DIRECTIONS: Evaluate your skill level as: **S** (satisfactory) or **U** (unsatisfactory).

Criteria	1	2	3	4
Before sharpening, assesses the design characteristics of the working-end to be sharpened and describes these characteristics				
Selects an appropriate location for sharpening process (stable surface, good light source), prepares area for sharpening, and assembles armamentarium; maintains sterile technique				
Lubricates the sharpening stone				
Holds the instrument handle in a stable grasp				
Identifies the cutting edge to be sharpened				
Establishes a face-to-stone angulation between 70° and 80°				
Sharpens the cutting edge in sections: heel-, middle-, and toe-thirds				
Evaluates sharpness of entire length of cutting edge and, if necessary, sharpens any remaining dull sections of the cutting edge				
Uses magnification to evaluate the sharpened working-end and indicates if the design has been preserved successfully				

Module 24

Pain Control during Periodontal Instrumentation

Module Overview

This module discusses aspects of pain control during periodontal instrumentation including (1) pain control within the scope of dental hygiene care, (2) the need for pain control strategies during periodontal instrumentation, (3) strategies that can be employed by hygienists to allay patient fear, and (4) pain control modalities that can be useful for routine periodontal instrumentation.

Module Outline

Key Terms

Local anesthesia
Topical anesthesia
Infiltration injection
Regional nerve block injection
Nitrous oxide and oxygen inhalation sedation
Distraction techniques
Relaxation technique
Vasodilation
Vasoconstrictors
Potency of anesthetic
Duration of action of anesthetic
Protein binding
Computer-controlled local anesthetic delivery (C-CLAD)
Intrapocket local anesthesia
Transmucosal patches
Transcutaneous electrical nerve stimulation (TENS)

Learning Objectives

1. Explain the terms topical local anesthesia, infiltration injections, and regional nerve block injections.
2. Describe the need for pain control during periodontal instrumentation.
3. Explain the relationship between anxiety and perception of pain.
4. List strategies that can be useful to the dental hygienist to allay fear of pain.
5. List local anesthetic agents that are commonly used to control pain during periodontal instrumentation.
6. Explain factors to consider when selecting local anesthetic agents for use during periodontal instrumentation.
7. Explain the term intrapocket local anesthesia.
8. List some reasons for failure of local anesthetic agents.

Section I

Pain Control during Periodontal Instrumentation

INTRODUCTION TO PAIN CONTROL

1. Most patients are fearful about experiencing pain while undergoing dental procedures, including procedures such as periodontal instrumentation performed by a dental hygienist.
   a. *A fear of pain has often been cited as one of the primary reasons for patients failing to comply with recommendations for dental care of all types.*
   b. It is critical that members of the dental team recognize this patient fear, develop strategies for helping patients deal with fear of pain, and understand methods of controlling pain during recommended therapeutic procedures.
2. The most reliable means of providing painless periodontal instrumentation is the careful injection of a local anesthetic agent.
   a. Local anesthesia provides pain control in a small area of the body by injection of the site with an anesthetic drug.
   b. Local anesthetic—in dental terms—refers to an injection given in the mouth to cause a temporary loss of feeling in an area before performing a dental procedure. The patient remains awake but has no feeling in the area near the injection.
3. Most patients with periodontitis require thorough periodontal instrumentation as part of the nonsurgical therapy recommended to bring the disease under control.
   a. Without proper patient management, periodontal instrumentation may indeed cause pain, but wise patient management dictates that this procedure should always be performed painlessly.
   b. Additionally, for many patients, the thought of injections of local anesthetic can also cause fear of pain from the "shot," thus complicating the management of fearful patients.
   c. It should be noted that local anesthetic agents are the most common drugs used in dentistry, and for the large majority of patients, these agents have been demonstrated to be safe and effective when used correctly.
   d. Pain control with injections of local anesthetic agents can be an important aspect of nonsurgical periodontal therapy whether a dental hygienist or dentist performs the injections.

PAIN CONTROL WITHIN THE SCOPE OF DENTAL HYGIENE CARE

1. The scope of dental hygiene practice related to the administration of local anesthetics can be confusing because it varies from region to region. Regulations in different states in the United States or provinces in Canada determine whether dental hygienists are licensed to administer local anesthesia.
   a. Regulations pertaining to the administration of local anesthesia by dental hygienists are often described based on the intended mode of administration for the local anesthetic agent—that is, administration of topical applications, administration of infiltration injections, or administration of nerve block injections.

b. These three modes of administration will be discussed later in this chapter in the context of pain control during periodontal instrumentation, but a short orientation to these methods is outlined below.
   1. Topical anesthesia refers to the technique of applying an anesthetic agent to the surface of either the gingiva or mucosa, allowing the anesthetic agent to diffuse through the surface epithelium and block pain impulses from superficial nerve endings.
   2. Infiltration injection refers to the technique of injecting a local anesthetic agent into the tissues near the site where anesthesia is needed, allowing the anesthetic agent to diffuse through the deeper tissues near the site of injection and block pain impulses from the tissues near the site of injection.
   3. Regional nerve block injection refers to the technique of injecting local anesthetic agents near the site of a particular nerve branch, allowing the anesthetic agent to reach the nerve branch itself and block pain impulses from the entire nerve branch (anesthetizing an entire region of the mouth, such as one side of the mandible).

c. Related to the administration of local anesthesia by injection, regulations governing the practice of dental hygiene usually fall into one of three broad categories.
   1. Some do not allow dental hygienists to administer local anesthetic agent by injection.
   2. Some allow dental hygienists to administer local anesthetic agent by injection, but only using infiltration-type injections.
   3. Some allow dental hygienists to administer local anesthetic agent by injection using both infiltration and regional nerve block injections.

2. Although few adverse events have been reported for trained dental hygienists administering local anesthesia by injection, one justification cited for restrictions against injection of local anesthetic by dental hygienists is to ensure patient safety. Jurisdictions that limit dental hygienists to infiltration-type injections may make the least sense from a patient safety standpoint.
   a. Whereas it is true that gingiva and some teeth can be anesthetized using only infiltration into the tissues near the site, in some areas of the mouth it would require more actual local anesthetic agent to anesthetize a quadrant of teeth using infiltration anesthesia alone as compared to nerve block anesthesia.
   b. In general terms, the more local anesthetic agent administered, the greater the risk is to the patient.
   c. Another potential problem with attempting to use infiltration anesthesia to produce anesthesia in mandibular teeth is that for many mandibular posterior teeth, it is not possible to produce profound anesthesia of these teeth when a clinician is limited to infiltration alone.

3. Because of the variation in statutes and regulations governing the administration of local anesthesia by hygienists, each dental hygienist must become familiar with the rules of the jurisdiction governing the practice of dental hygiene in the individual state or province in which he or she is licensed.

NEED FOR PAIN CONTROL DURING PERIODONTAL INSTRUMENTATION

1. Despite the frequency of performing periodontal instrumentation in dental practices, the subject of pain during this procedure has not been investigated thoroughly.
2. Without the use of local anesthetic agents, many patients would indeed experience unnecessary pain during periodontal instrumentation. This is true for the use of both hand instruments and ultrasonic and sonic-powered instruments.
3. It should be noted that pain intensity experienced during periodontal instrumentation is dramatically different among patients and that pain intensity can even vary between different areas of the mouth in the same patient.
4. There are several clinical factors that make it more likely that an individual patient will experience pain during periodontal instrumentation. The wise clinician will evaluate individual patients for factors most likely to be associated with pain during periodontal instrumentation when planning this procedure.
   a. ***In general terms, the degree of pain experienced by a patient can be influenced by factors such as the level of inflammation in the periodontal tissues, the depth of the periodontal pockets in the sites being treated, and the location of the disease sites in the dentition.***
   b. Sites that bleed on gentle probing (one important sign of tissue inflammation) tend to produce more discomfort when instrumented than sites that exhibit minimal inflammation.
   c. Sites where probing depths measure 5 mm or greater tend to produce more discomfort than sites where there are shallower probing depths.
   d. Instrumentation of sites on the lingual surfaces of teeth tends to produce more discomfort than instrumentation of sites on the facial surfaces of teeth.
   e. In addition, patients who experience discomfort during initial periodontal examination are more likely to experience pain during periodontal instrumentation.

Section 2: Useful Strategies to Allay the Fear of Pain

Some patients with extreme fear require special management with antianxiety or sedative-hypnotic drugs; although these agents will not be discussed in this book, the administration of these drugs can include inhalation, oral, intramuscular, and intravenous routes. It is critical that the members of a dental team be aware of patient fears and address those fears.

DEALING WITH ANXIETY IN PATIENTS

1. Many patients come to a dental appointment with some level of anxiety, whether they show overt signs of anxiety or not. A patient may feel anxious before or during treatment.
2. Anxiety has a huge impact on the perception of pain (the higher the level of anxiety, the greater the pain sensitivity experienced by the patient), so minimizing patient anxiety is an important strategy.

3. Chairside manner is one key element in keeping the patient calm during any dental procedure requiring the management of pain. All patients should be approached with a calm and confident manner.
4. Patients should be informed about what to expect during a dental appointment to avoid unpleasant surprises during the treatment.
5. Patients should be reassured that a certain level of anxiety in a dental setting is normal. Helping a patient to realize that anxiety is normal may make the patient better able to deal with it.
6. It is frequently helpful to give a patient some sense of control over the procedure. Instructing the patient how to signal the clinician if he or she experiences discomfort is helpful in reducing anxiety. An example of a signal is the patient raising the left hand if uncomfortable.
7. There are numerous strategies that can allay some patient anxiety and reduce the risk of unnecessary discomfort during periodontal instrumentation; examples of these strategies are listed below and in Box 24-1.
   a. Evaluate the patient's emotional status prior to the procedure to identify patients who might need special management during periodontal instrumentation.
   b. Partner with the patient to improve self-care and reduce the level of inflammation in the tissues prior to scheduling an appointment for periodontal instrumentation.
   c. Use precise and gentle tissue manipulation during the procedure to increase patient confidence in the clinician.
   d. Monitor the patient for signs of pain or fear (such as facial expressions, pallor, or perspiration) throughout any procedure.
   e. Select properly sharpened instruments for use during the procedure because dull instruments inflict unnecessary tissue trauma and lead to the use of excessive force.
   f. Implement strategies to prevent pain prior to the procedure rather than attempting to minimize discomfort after it has begun.

Box 24-1. Strategies to Allay Patient Anxiety or Reduce the Risk of Unnecessary Discomfort during Periodontal Instrumentation

- Evaluate the patient's emotional status.
- Minimize the level of inflammation in the tissues.
- Use precise and gentle tissue manipulation.
- Monitor the patient for signs of pain or fear.
- Use properly sharpened periodontal instruments.
- Implement strategies to prevent pain prior to periodontal instrumentation.

NITROUS OXIDE AND OXYGEN INHALATION SEDATION

1. Nitrous oxide and oxygen inhalation sedation is a technique that uses a blend of two gases—nitrous oxide and oxygen (N_2O-O_2)—to relieve patient anxiety.
   - a. A fitted mask is placed over the nose and, as the patient breathes normally, uptake occurs through the lungs.
   - b. At the end of treatment, the gas is eliminated from the lungs after a short period of breathing oxygen and has no lingering effects.
2. Nitrous oxide and oxygen inhalation sedation is one technique that has been used successfully during periodontal instrumentation to allay fear.
   - a. Nitrous oxide and oxygen inhalation sedation can produce a state in which a patient is conscious and perfectly able to obey commands but feels a sense of well-being and remains relaxed.
   - b. Nitrous oxide and oxygen inhalation sedation is safe and effective when used appropriately in dealing with patients with mild-to-moderate anxiety.
3. The use of nitrous oxide and oxygen to allay fear provides several advantages to both the clinician and the patient. These advantages include quick onset of action, easy regulation of the concentration of the gases delivered, and rapid recovery following administration; this is the only form of sedation where a patient can drive an automobile after the procedure.
   - a. These advantages make this modality ideal for sedating patients during relatively short procedures such as periodontal instrumentation.
   - b. It should be noted that the use of nitrous oxide and oxygen sedation does not control pain from procedures such as periodontal instrumentation, although it is very effective in allaying mild-to-moderate patient anxiety.

DISTRACTION TECHNIQUES

1. Another technique that has been reported to reduce anxiety and discomfort during periodontal instrumentation is using distraction techniques (i.e., actively engaging a patient's mind on something other than the dental treatment).
2. Fear or anxiety can lower a patient's threshold for a pain reaction to a stimulus, thus altering how a patient's brain interprets a particular stimulus.
3. Examples of distraction techniques that can be used in a dental setting include allowing the patient to watch a patient-selected television program or listen to patient-selected music using a headset. Both of these types of activities have been demonstrated to be able to take the patient's mind off an actual dental procedure.
4. Although distraction techniques can be useful in managing some patients, for many patients, they do not appear to be reliable methods of controlling either anxiety or pain during periodontal instrumentation.

RELAXATION TECHNIQUES

1. A relaxation technique is a method used to reduce tension and anxiety. An example is deep breathing.
2. There are several relaxation strategies that have been recommended in attempts to elicit a relaxation response in dental patients. Relaxation techniques that have been used include guided imagery, deep breathing, progressive relaxation, and biofeedback.
3. Used in carefully selected patients, relaxation techniques can decrease heart rate, respiratory rate, and muscle tension.
4. Although relaxation techniques can produce a sense of calmness, in most patients, they do not appear to be adequate for the control of the discomfort produced during periodontal instrumentation.

Section 3: Pain Control Modalities for Periodontal Instrumentation

LOCAL ANESTHESIA ADMINISTERED THROUGH INJECTION

The most effective method for controlling pain during periodontal instrumentation is the administration of a local anesthetic agent by injection. Local anesthesia refers to the loss of sensation in a circumscribed area of the body resulting in the prevention of both the generation and the conduction of nerve impulses. In the simplest of terms, local anesthetic agents control pain by blocking pain impulses from reaching the brain.

1. Local anesthetic agents are the most important drugs used in dentistry. They are the safest and most effective drugs used in the prevention of pain that arises during periodontal procedures.
2. Historically, local anesthetic agents have been classified into types of agents described as either esters or amides.
   a. Currently, local anesthetic agents available in dental anesthetic cartridges are all of the amide type.
   b. The amide-type local anesthetic agents produce a lower incidence of allergic reactions in patients.
3. There are a number of local anesthetic agents available for use during periodontal instrumentation.
   a. Examples of commonly used amide local anesthetics agents that can be used for periodontal instrumentation include lidocaine, mepivacaine, prilocaine, articaine, and bupivacaine.
   b. It should be noted that other amide local anesthetics are available but less frequently used during periodontal instrumentation; examples of these include tetracaine, propoxycaine, and etidocaine.

4. Injectable local anesthetic agents used in dentistry produce varying degrees of vasodilation (i.e., dilation of blood vessels) at the site of injection.
   a. Vasodilators increase the flood flow at the injection site.
   b. Vasodilation at the site of injection facilitates the local anesthetic agent being carried away relatively quickly by the increased blood flow.
   c. This vasodilation effect of local anesthetic agents can decrease their duration of action, decrease their effectiveness, increase the blood level of the agent (increasing the risk to the patient), and increase the amount of bleeding at the site of the injection.
5. To counteract vasodilation effects of local anesthetic agents, other drugs called vasoconstrictors can be added to injectable local anesthetic agents used in dentistry.
   a. As the name implies, vasoconstrictors are chemical agents that constrict blood vessels.
      1. No matter how quickly an anesthetic agent can enter a nerve, the local blood vessels begin to absorb the anesthetic agent as soon as it is injected.
      2. In order to slow this process down, manufacturers of these solutions add a substance—a vasoconstrictor—that in low concentrations acts to cause the local blood vessels to constrict or narrow.
      3. This restricts the amount of blood and plasma entering and leaving the site of the injection and has the net effect of slowing the vascular absorption of the anesthetic solution. This keeps the unused anesthetic solution in place longer and prolongs the action of the drug.
   b. In addition to increasing the duration of action of the anesthetic agent, vasoconstrictors can increase the effectiveness of the agent, decrease bleeding at the site, and lower the blood level of the agent. Table 24-1 outlines some common vasoconstrictors used in local anesthetic agents intended for use during dental procedures such as periodontal instrumentation.
   c. Thorough periodontal instrumentation requires manipulation of periodontal tissues and can result in hemorrhage (or bleeding) during the procedure. Local anesthetic agents with vasoconstrictors can improve visibility of the site for the clinician by helping to control hemorrhage during the procedure.
6. When nerve block injections are used, it is also possible to supplement the administration of block anesthesia at a remote nerve branch site by injecting a few drops of local anesthetic agent containing a vasoconstrictor directly into the dental papillae in the site being treated to help control hemorrhage during the procedure.
7. To increase the safety for the patient, lower doses of vasoconstrictors are normally preferred. Lower doses produce fewer side effects, and using a higher dose of vasoconstrictor does not prolong the duration of action over lower doses.
8. Vasoconstrictors are contraindicated in some patients either because of the patient's health status or because of possible interactions with other medications that the patient is taking. Discussion of these contraindications is beyond the scope of this chapter, but these discussions can be found in any of the excellent textbooks related entirely to pain control.

TABLE 24-1. Vasoconstrictors Commonly Used in Dental Local Anesthetic Agents

Agent	Other Name	Concentrations Available in Dentistry		
Epinephrine	Adrenalin	1:50,000	1:100,000	1:200,000
Levonordefrin	Nordefrin	1:20,000		

SELECTION OF LOCAL ANESTHETIC AGENTS FOR PERIODONTAL INSTRUMENTATION

1. The selection of a specific injectable local anesthetic agent should be based on the type of procedure to be performed combined with several other critical factors. Examples of other critical factors for the dental hygienist or dentist to consider when selecting an injectable local anesthetic agent are discussed below and listed in Box 24-2.
   - **a.** Potency of the anesthetic agent is always an important factor in selection.
     1. Potency of the local anesthetic refers to the lowest concentration of drug that can actually block conduction of the pain impulse.
     2. Potency can be affected by lipid solubility of the drug, its inherent vasodilator effect, and its tissue diffusion properties.
   - **b.** Duration of action of the agent and the length of time that pain control is needed are other critical factors in selection.
     1. Duration of action is primarily determined by the protein-binding capacity of the anesthetic (the greater the binding, the longer the duration).

Box 24-2. Examples of Factors to Consider When Selecting a Local Anesthetic Agent

- Type of procedure to be performed
- Potency of the anesthetic agent
- Duration of action of the anesthetic agent
- The need for pain control following the office procedure
- Health status of the patient, including allergies and current medications

   - **a.** Protein binding refers to the binding of a drug to proteins in blood plasma. The interaction can also be between the drug and tissue membranes, red blood cells, and other components of the blood.
   - **b.** The amount of drug bound to protein determines how effective the drug is in the body.
     1. The bound drug is kept in the bloodstream, whereas the unbound components of the drug may be metabolized or extracted, making them the active part of the drug.

2. So, if an anesthetic agent is 90% bound to a binding protein and 10% free, then this means that 10% of the drug is active in the system and causing pharmacologic effects (pain control).

2. Duration of action can also be affected by an agent's inherent vasodilator effect and its tissue diffusion properties.
3. As already discussed, the duration of action of local anesthetic agents can be increased by combining the anesthetic agent with a vasoconstrictor.

c. The need for pain control following the office procedure is another factor to consider in selection.
   1. When continuing oral pain is expected as a result of a treatment procedure—as it might be following periodontal surgery—it is wise to consider this fact when selecting an anesthetic agent.
   2. Although lingering oral pain from periodontal instrumentation would not normally be expected, in some patients with a history of low tolerance for pain, this can be an important factor to consider.

d. Another factor to consider in selection is the health status of the patient, including a history of allergies and current medications being taken by the patient.

2. Table 24-2 provides an overview of common injectable dental local anesthetic agents along with the expected duration of action of each agent.
   a. Lidocaine and mepivacaine with vasoconstrictors are excellent choices of anesthetic agents for periodontal instrumentation because their protein binding is intermediate and their lipid solubility is also intermediate, resulting in an expected duration of action of a few hours.
   b. Bupivacaine would be a less ideal choice for routine periodontal instrumentation because the lipid solubility and protein binding are high, resulting in an expected duration of action of anesthesia of 4 to 9 hours. Such a long duration of action might be ideal for some periodontal surgical procedures but a bit excessive for most periodontal instrumentation procedures.
   c. An injectable amide local anesthetic agent, articaine, which has been available in Europe for over 30 years and was approved for US distribution in 2000, has been used for some periodontal procedures; one advantage to articaine that has been reported is that it can be metabolized quickly, thus reducing toxicity associated with repeated injections.

TABLE 24-2. Common Injectable Local Anesthetic Agents and Their Durations of Action

Duration	Agent	Duration of Soft Tissue Anesthesia
Short	Lidocaine 2%	1–2 hours
	Mepivacaine 3%	2–3 hours
Intermediate	Lidocaine 2% / 1:100,000 epinephrine	3–5 hours
	Mepivacaine 2% / 1:20,000 levonordefrin	3–5 hours
	Articaine 4% / 1:100,000 epinephrine	3–4 hours
	Prilocaine 4% / 1:200,000 epinephrine	3–8 hours
Long	Bupivacaine 0.5% / 1:200,000 epinephrine	4–9 hours

TYPES OF INJECTIONS OF LOCAL ANESTHETIC AGENTS

The administration of local anesthetic agents through injection in dentistry is usually described as being either regional block local anesthesia or infiltration local anesthesia.

1. **Regional Nerve Block Anesthesia**
   - **a.** As discussed in Section 1 of this chapter, regional nerve block local anesthesia refers to injections of local anesthetic agent into sites near nerve branches, allowing the local anesthetic agent to stop the transmission of pain impulses from the entire area of the oral cavity innervated by the nerve branch.
   - **b.** Using regional block local anesthesia for dental procedures can frequently result in fewer penetrations of the oral mucosa with the needle and use of smaller volumes of anesthesia compared with using strictly infiltration anesthesia.
   - **c.** Properly administered regional block local anesthesia can result in profound anesthesia for completely pain-free periodontal instrumentation.
   - **d.** Regional block anesthesia fits in with the standard dental hygiene protocol of performing quadrant or half-mouth procedures during periodontal instrumentation.
   - **e.** Only regional block anesthesia can produce profound anesthesia in mandibular posterior teeth in most patients because the thickness of the cortical plate in the mandible frequently precludes diffusion of infiltration anesthesia through the thick cortical bone.
   - **f.** Figures 24-1 and 24-2 and Table 24-3 provide an overview of nerve branches and the types of injections that might be used to produce anesthesia. Note that for most nerve branches supplying the jaws, nerve block anesthesia is the method of choice.
   - **g.** Specific techniques for administering nerve block anesthesia will not be discussed in this textbook, but there are many excellent textbooks available on this extensive topic.
2. **Infiltration Anesthesia**
   - **a.** Also as discussed in Section 1 of this chapter, infiltration local anesthesia refers to injections of local anesthetic agent in or near the site to be treated, allowing the local anesthetic agent to diffuse through the tissues and stop the transmission of pain impulses from the site. An example is the injection of anesthetic solution into an interproximal papilla before periodontal instrumentation.

b. Using infiltration local anesthesia would affect nerve impulses from the site while not affecting other areas innervated by a particular nerve branch.
c. Although there are distinct advantages to regional block anesthesia for most sites in the oral cavity, note that in Table 24-3, there are some sites where infiltration anesthesia is the method of choice.
d. Specific techniques for administering infiltration anesthesia will not be discussed in this textbook, but there are many excellent textbooks available on this extensive topic.

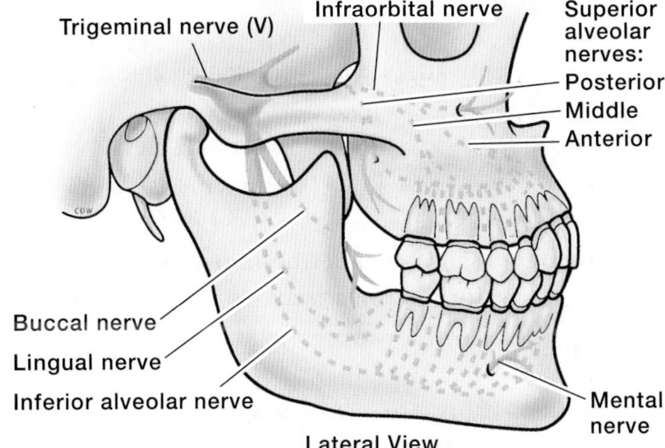

Figure 24-1. Nerve Supply to the Periodontium (Lateral View). The nerve supply to the periodontium is derived from the branches of the trigeminal nerve.

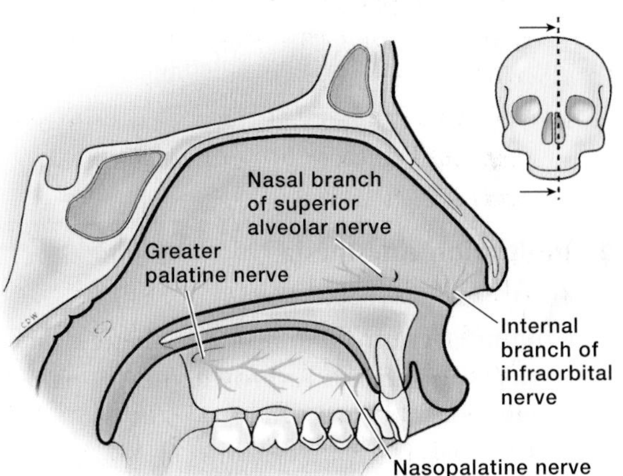

Figure 24-2. Nerve Innervation to the Palate.

TABLE 24-3. Producing Anesthesia for Periodontal Instrumentation Using Injection Local Anesthetics

Nerve Branch	Ideal Type of Local Anesthesia	Structures Affected
Greater palatine	Block anesthesia	Posterior palatal mucosa
Posterior superior alveolar	Block anesthesia	Maxillary posterior teeth Maxillary buccal mucosa
Infraorbital	Block anesthesia	Maxillary anterior mucosa
Anterior superior alveolar	Infiltration anesthesia	Maxillary anterior teeth
Nasopalatine	Block anesthesia	Anterior palatal mucosa
Inferior alveolar	Block anesthesia	Mandibular molars Mandibular premolars
Mental	Block anesthesia	Mandibular buccal mucosa
Incisive	Block anesthesia	Mandibular canine Mandibular incisors
Lingual	Block anesthesia	Mandibular lingual mucosa
Buccal	Infiltration anesthesia	Mandibular buccal mucosa

COMPUTER-CONTROLLED LOCAL ANESTHETIC DELIVERY

1. Computer-controlled local anesthetic delivery (C-CLAD) allows the dental hygienist or dentist to provide nearly painless delivery of local anesthetic agents to patients.
2. Using C-CLAD devices correctly can result in single-tooth anesthesia through injection into the periodontal ligament.
3. When a C-CLAD device is used to deliver anesthetic agent slowly, it can produce local anesthesia in a single mandibular molar tooth, which is not normally possible using standard injection techniques.

TOPICAL APPLICATION OF LOCAL ANESTHETICS

1. Topical anesthesia is a condition of temporary numbness caused by applying an anesthetic agent directly to the mucosal and gingival tissues with a cotton-tipped applicator. This technique has been used in dentistry for many years.

2. Application of topical anesthetic agents prior to injection can promote patient comfort during the initial penetration of a needle through the mucosa.
3. There are several topical local anesthetics available for use; one example is lidocaine in liquid or gel form, which can be applied prior to injection of local anesthetic agents. Use of these topical agents prior to injection can minimize patient discomfort during the injection.
4. It should be noted that using topical anesthetic agent applied to surface mucosa or gingiva does not normally result in the profound anesthesia of a site needed when performing periodontal instrumentation.

OTHER METHODS THAT MAY PRODUCE ANESTHESIA

1. **Intrapocket Local Anesthesia**
   a. Patient anxiety associated with injections of local anesthetic agent is an important concern, and there is a need for an effective substitute for injections to produce local anesthesia during periodontal instrumentation.
   b. There have been many attempts to develop effective alternatives for injectable anesthesia for use during procedures such as periodontal instrumentation.
   c. One alternative to injections of local anesthetic agents during periodontal instrumentation is the use of intrapocket local anesthesia. Intrapocket local anesthesia refers to placing a local anesthetic agent into a periodontal pocket, where it is allowed to diffuse through adjacent tissues.
      1. An example of intrapocket anesthetic application that has been used is a mixture of lidocaine and prilocaine (Oraqix); Oraqix is a 5% solution of 2.5% lidocaine and 2.5% prilocaine in a thermosetting gel.
      2. This technique involves placement of the gel into a periodontal pocket and can be useful in pain control during periodontal instrumentation in some adults; the most profound anesthesia following the application of this product occurs between 5 and 20 minutes.
      3. Though intrapocket anesthetic application of lidocaine/prilocaine gel produces less profound anesthesia than injections of local anesthetic agents, these gel applications have reduced the need for anesthetic injections during periodontal instrumentation in selected patients.
      4. For many patients in whom periodontal instrumentation can be expected to produce moderate-to-severe pain, these gel applications may not be adequate to control discomfort during these procedures.
   d. There have also been some attempts to use the anesthetic agent benzocaine as an intrapocket anesthetic agent.
      1. Benzocaine, however, is less effective in controlling pain during periodontal instrumentation than injections of lidocaine.
      2. More investigation is needed in the use of benzocaine as an intrapocket anesthetic agent during periodontal instrumentation.
2. **Transmucosal Patches**
   a. Another approach to avoiding injections is by using topical anesthesia delivered via patches placed directly on mucosal tissues; these patches are referred to as transmucosal patches.

   b. In attempts to use transmucosal patches, lidocaine-containing patches have been applied directly to the tissues at the site intended for treatment.
   c. Although more research is needed related to the use of these transmucosal patches during periodontal instrumentation, it does appear that this mode of administration of lidocaine can be substituted for injections in selected sites in some patients undergoing periodontal instrumentation.

3. **Transcutaneous Electrical Nerve Stimulation (TENS)**
   a. Other methods of producing anesthesia have been studied, but these need to be investigated thoroughly in the context of dental hygiene procedures. Using these methods may one day make it possible to produce needed anesthesia during a dental hygiene procedure without the use of an injection.
   b. One example of these other methods is a form of electronically delivered anesthesia called transcutaneous electrical nerve stimulation.
      1. The TENS technique offers one alternative to injections that uses a battery-powered device to send electrical impulses to the site to be treated, producing numbness.
      2. In this technique, a patient can control the level of electrical stimulation through a hand-held unit.

REVERSAL OF LOCAL ANESTHETIC EFFECTS

1. It is well known that the soft tissue effects of injected local anesthetic agents can last longer than needed for routine periodontal instrumentation.
2. The lingering "numbness" that can result for several hours is an annoying result of dental treatment for many patients.
3. *Studies have indicated that injection of the drug phentolamine mesylate at the end of a dental procedure into the same site as the original local anesthetic injection can induce a rapid return of sensation blocked by the local anesthetic by increasing vasodilation in the site and clearing the anesthetic agent from the site of the injection.*
4. Of course, the use of phentolamine mesylate to reverse local anesthetic numbness would require additional injections at the end of a clinical dental procedure.
5. Although more study of the use of this drug is needed in the context of dental hygiene procedures and other dental procedures, this medication may one day prove useful in the practice of dentistry, at least in selected patients.

FAILURE OF LOCAL ANESTHETIC AGENTS

1. Although administration of local anesthetic agents can be a safe and very effective mechanism for controlling pain during dental procedures, including periodontal instrumentation, all clinicians should recognize the fact that a few patients present special challenges by failing to develop profound anesthesia in the site intended.
2. The most common site for failure to develop profound anesthesia following injection of an agent using recommended techniques is in the region supplied by the inferior alveolar nerve.

3. There are a variety of reasons for this apparent failure of the anesthetic agent. Examples include inaccuracy of deposition of the agent at the intended site, variations in anatomy from patient to patient, variation among individuals in response to drugs, and status of the tissues at the site of deposition of the agent.
4. Additional injection techniques have been recommended for use in patients in whom the normally recommended injection techniques fail to produce profound anesthesia.
5. Although a detailed discussion of these additional techniques is beyond the scope of this book, examples of these methods include techniques such as intraosseous injections, periodontal ligament injections, and intraseptal anesthesia.

RECOMMENDED READING

Anderson JM. Use of local anesthesia by dental hygienists who completed a Minnesota CE course. *J Dent Hyg*. 2002;76:35–46.

Blanton PL, Jeske AH. Avoiding complications in local anesthesia induction: anatomical considerations. *J Am Dent Assoc*. 2003;134:888–893.

Canakci CF, Canakci V. Pain experienced by patients undergoing different periodontal therapies. *J Am Dent Assoc*. 2007;138:1563–1573.

Carroll D, Seers K. Relaxation for the relief of chronic pain: a systematic review. *J Adv Nurs*. 1998;27:476–487.

DiMatteo A. Efficacy of an intrapocket anesthetic for scaling and root planing procedures: a review of three multicenter studies. *Compend Contin Educ Dent*. 2005;26(suppl 1):6–10.

Donaldson D, Gelskey SC, Landry RG, Matthews DC, Sandhu HS. A placebo-controlled multi-centered evaluation of an anaesthetic gel (Oraqix) for periodontal therapy. *J Clin Periodontol*. 2003;30:171–175.

Friskopp J, Nilsson M, Isacsson G. The anesthetic onset and duration of a new lidocaine/prilocaine gel intrapocket anesthetic (Oraqix) for periodontal scaling/root planing. *J Clin Periodontol*. 2001;28453–28458.

Gunsolley JC. The need for pain control during scaling and root planing. *Compend Contin Educ Dent*. 2005;26(suppl 1):3–5.

Haas DA. An update on local anesthetics in dentistry. *J Can Dent Assoc*. 2002;68:546–551.

Hersh EV, Moore PA, Papas AS, Goodson JM, Navalta LA, Rogy S, et al. Reversal of soft-tissue local anesthesia with phentolamine mesylate in adolescents and adults. *J Am Dent Assoc*. 2008;139:1080–1093.

Hunt LC, George MS, Wilder R, Maixner W, Gaylord S. The effects of relaxation training on dental anxiety and pain perception during dental hygiene treatment. *J Dent Hyg*. 2005;4:17.

Jeffcoat MK, Geurs NC, Magnusson I, MacNeill SR, Mickels N, Roberts F, et al. Intrapocket anesthesia for scaling and root planing: results of a double-blind multicenter trial using lidocaine prilocaine dental gel. *J Periodontol*. 2001;72:895–900.

Kumar PS, Leblebicioglu B. Pain control during nonsurgical periodontal therapy. *Compend Contin Educ Dent*. 2007;28:666–669.

Laviola M, McGavin SK, Freer GA, Plancich G, Woodbury SC, Marinkovich S, et al. Randomized study of phentolamine mesylate for reversal of local anesthesia. *J Dent Res*. 2008;87:635–639.

Magnusson I, Geurs NC, Harris PA, Hefti AF, Mariotti AJ, Mauriello SM, et al. Intrapocket anesthesia for scaling and root planing in pain-sensitive patients. *J Peridontol*. 2003;75:597–602.

Malamed SF. Local anesthetics: dentistry's most important drugs, clinical update 2006. *J Calif Dent Assoc*. 2006;34:971–976.

Malamed SF, Gagnon S, Leblanc D. Efficacy of articaine: a new amide local anesthetic. *J Am Dent Assoc*. 2000;131:635–642.

Matthews DC, Rocchi A, Gafni A. Factors affecting patients' and potential patients' choices among anesthetics for periodontal recall visits. *J Dent.* 2001;29:173–179.

Milgrom P, Coldwell SE, Getza T, Weinstein P, Ramsay DS. Four dimensions of fear of dental injections. *J Am Dent Assoc.* 1997;128:756–766.

Moore PA, Boynes SG, Hersh EV, DeRossi SS, Sollecito TP, Goodson JM, et al. The anesthetic efficacy of 4 percent articaine 1:200,000 epinephrine: two controlled clinical trials. *J Am Dent Assoc.* 2006;137:1572–1581.

Perry DA, Gansky SA, Loomer PM. Effectiveness of a transmucosal lidocaine delivery system for local anaesthesia during scaling and root planing. *J Clin Periodontol.* 2005;32:590–594.

Roghani S, Duperon DF, Barcohana N. Evaluating the efficacy of commonly used topical anesthetics. *Pediatr Dent.* 1999;21:197–200.

Sisty-LePeau N, Boyer EM, Lutjen D. Dental hygiene licensure specifications on pain control procedures. *J Dent Hyg.* 1990;64:179–185.

Stoltenberg JL, Osborn JB, Carson JF, Hodges JS, Michalowicz BS. A preliminary study of intrapocket topical versus injected anaesthetic for scaling and root planing. *J Clin Periodontol.* 2007;34:892–896.

Svensson P, Petersen JK, Svensson H. Efficacy of a topical anesthetic on pain and unpleasantness during scaling of gingival pockets. *Anesth Prog.* 1994;41:35–39.

Tripp DA, Neish NR, Sullivan MJ. What hurts during dental hygiene treatment. *J Dent Hyg.* 1998;72:25–30.

Yagiela JA. Recent developments in local anesthesia and oral sedation. *Compend Contin Educ Dent.* 2004;25:697–706.

Module 25

Powered Instrument Design and Function

Module Overview

Powered instruments use the rapid energy vibrations of an electronically powered instrument tip to fracture calculus from the tooth surface and clean the environment of the periodontal pocket. This module presents principles of the design and function of powered instruments including sonic and ultrasonic devices.

Module Outline

Key Terms

Powered instruments
Fluid lavage
Acoustic microstreaming
Cavitation
Deplaquing
Dental aerosols
Sonic-powered instruments
Ultrasonic-powered instruments
Piezoelectric ultrasonic instruments
Magnetostrictive ultrasonic instruments
Standard-diameter tips
Slim-diameter tips
Frequency
Amplitude
Cleaning efficiency
Automatically tuned ultrasonic devices
Manually tuned ultrasonic devices
Fluid reservoirs
Active tip area

Learning Objectives

1. Discuss the history and technologic advances of powered instrumentation.
2. Compare and contrast the advantages and limitations of powered instrumentation.
3. Compare and contrast sonic and ultrasonic devices.
4. Compare and contrast automatically and manually tuned ultrasonic devices.
5. Compare and contrast standard-diameter and slim-diameter powered tip design.
6. Identify pretreatment considerations before the initiation of powered instrumentation.
7. Discuss medical and dental contraindications for powered instrumentation.
8. Discuss criteria for the selection of powered instrument tips.

Section I
Introduction to Powered Instrumentation

Powered instruments use a rapidly vibrating instrument tip to dislodge calculus from the tooth surface, disrupt plaque biofilm, and flush out bacteria from the periodontal pocket.[1,2] Powered devices consist of a handpiece that attaches to the dental unit or an electronic generator (Fig. 25-1) and interchangeable instrument tips (Fig. 25-2). Initially introduced in the late 1950s, powered instruments were bulky and limited to removing heavy, supragingival calculus deposits. Over the years, powered instrument design has evolved to a point that powered instrumentation now plays an indispensable role in periodontal debridement. Table 25-1 summarizes the evolution of powered instrument design.

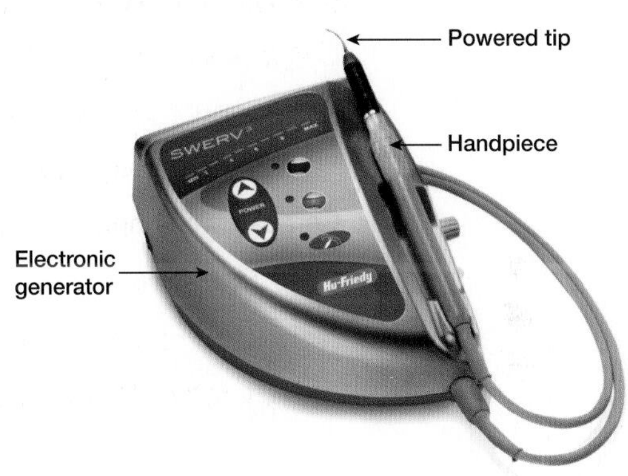

Figure 25-1. Electronic Generator, Handpiece, and Instrument Tip. This powered device consists of an electronic generator, a handpiece, and an instrument tip. (Courtesy of Hu-Friedy Manufacturing Co., LLC.)

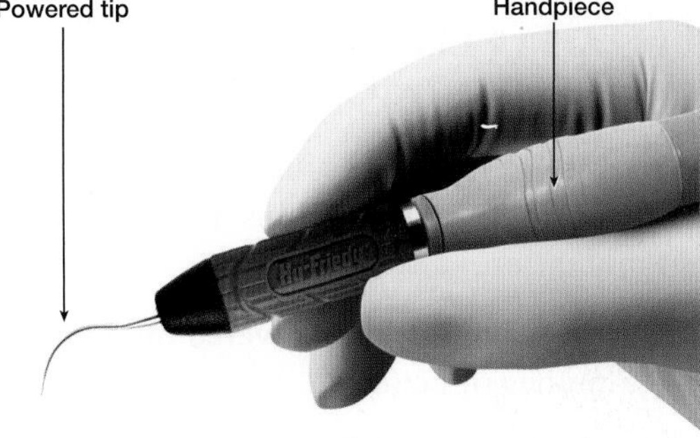

Figure 25-2. Interchangeable Instrument Tip. An interchangeable instrument tip inserted into the handpiece of a powered instrumentation device. (Courtesy of Hu-Friedy Manufacturing Co., LLC.)

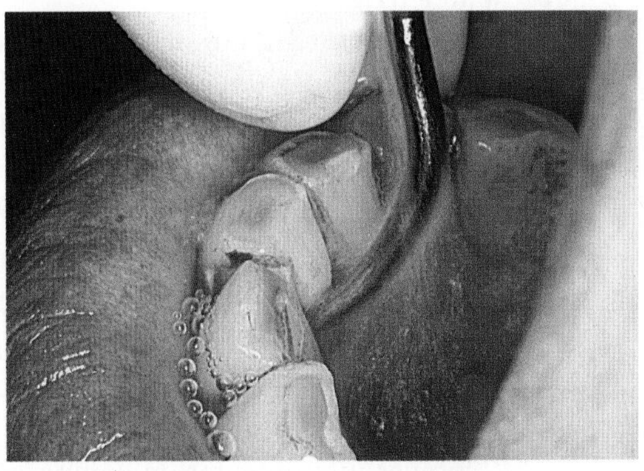

Figure 25-3. Powered Instrument Tip in Action. This photograph shows an activated powered tip. A constant stream of water is used to cool the rapidly vibrating powered instrument tip.

TABLE 25-1. A Time Line for the Evolution of Powered Instruments

Date	Event
Late 1950s	Development of the first electronically powered instruments.
1960s and 1970s	Powered instruments are used to remove heavy calculus deposits. The bulky design of the power instrument tip limits use to supragingival instrumentation or sites where the tissue allows easy subgingival insertion. The Gracey curet is the primary instrument for use within periodontal pockets.
Late 1980s	Slim-diameter instrument tips are developed for electronically powered devices. Slim-diameter tips are significantly smaller than the working-end of a standard Gracey curet.
1990s	Research studies establish that bacterial products are easily removed from the root surfaces, leading to a new approach to instrumentation and the conservation of cementum.
Today	Modern powered instrument tips have been shown to be as effective as hand instruments for removing subgingival calculus deposits, plaque biofilms, and bacterial products from periodontally involved teeth.

EFFECTIVENESS AND MODES OF ACTION OF POWERED INSTRUMENTS

Research investigations indicate that powered instrumentation is as effective as hand instrumentation in removal of calculus deposits, control of subgingival plaque biofilms, and reduction of inflammation.[3-5]

1. **Modes of Action: Powered Instrumentation.** Powered instruments have several modes of action.
   a. **Mechanical Removal.** Very rapid vibrations of the powered instrument tip create microfractures in a calculus deposit that result in deposit removal.
   b. **Water Irrigation**
      1. A constant stream of water exits near the point of an electronically powered instrument tip (Figs. 25-3 and 25-4). This water stream within the periodontal pocket is termed the fluid lavage.
      2. The water flowing over the instrument tip is needed to dissipate the heat produced by the rapid vibrations of the tip.
      3. Water irrigation also plays an important role in periodontal debridement. The water washes toxic products and free-floating bacteria from the pocket, provides better vision during instrumentation by removing blood from the treatment site, and creates acoustic microstreaming and cavitation.
      4. Research indicates that a greater area is cleaned when water is used for power instrumentation compared to power instrumentation without water.[6]

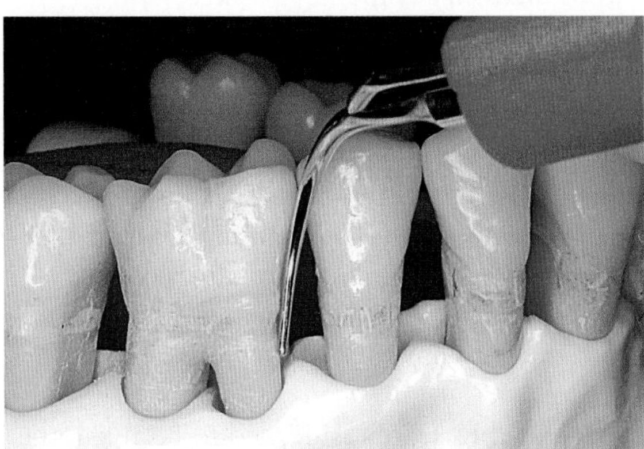

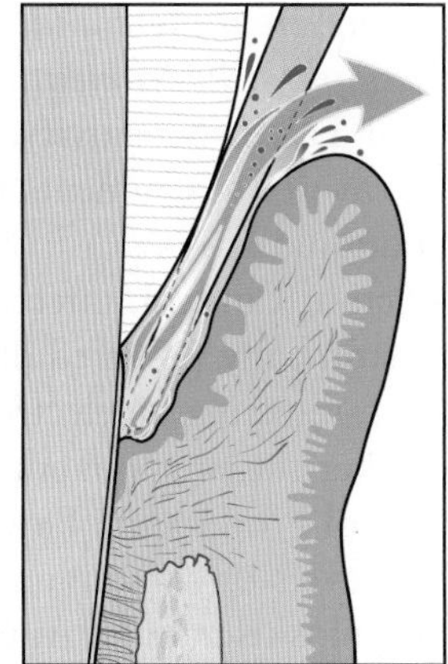

Figure 25-4. Pocket Penetration of Tip and Fluid Lavage. Slim-diameter instrument tips penetrate deeper into periodontal pockets and reach the base of the pocket better than hand instruments. The water lavage reaches a depth that is equal to the depth reached by the powered instrument tip.

c. **Acoustic Microstreaming of the Water Stream**
   1. Acoustic microstreaming is a swirling effect produced within the confined space of a periodontal pocket by the continuous stream of fluid flowing over the vibrating instrument tip. This intense swirling may play a role in the disruption of the subgingival plaque biofilms associated with periodontal disease.[6]
   2. The effect of acoustic microstreaming is limited to an area immediately surrounding the instrument tip. In order to most effectively remove plaque biofilm, the instrument tip must touch every part of the root surface.

d. **Cavitation of the Water Stream.** Cavitation is the formation of tiny bubbles in the water stream. When these tiny bubbles collapse, they produce shock waves that may alter or destroy bacteria by tearing the bacterial cell walls.[7]

2. Strengths of Powered Instrumentation

a. **Effective Removal of Calculus Deposits and Plaque Biofilms.** Powered instrumentation has been shown to be as effective as hand instrumentation. Powered instruments are especially effective in deplaquing—the disruption or removal of the subgingival plaque biofilm from root surfaces and the pocket space.
b. **Pocket Penetration.** Slim-diameter instrument tips penetrate deeper into periodontal pockets than hand instruments.[8–12]
c. **Access to Furcations.** Slim-powered instrument tips are more effective in treating class II and III furcations when used by experienced clinicians.[12–15]
d. **Irrigation (Lavage).** Water irrigation of the pocket washes toxic products and free-floating bacteria from the pocket and provides better vision during instrumentation by removing blood from the treatment site.[7,16,17]
e. **Shorter Instrumentation Time.** Several studies have shown that instrumentation time may be reduced when using powered instruments as compared to hand instruments.[1,3,5,8,18]

3. Limitations of Powered Instrumentation

a. **Clinician Skill Level.** The skill level of the clinician is the best predictor of the outcome of periodontal instrumentation regardless of whether a hand or powered instrument is used.
   1. Powered instrument is ineffective and may even be harmful if the clinician is not skilled in the technique. Powered instrumentation is just as technique sensitive as hand instrumentation.

2. ***A complete understanding of root anatomy is the key to successful periodontal instrumentation.***

b. **Reduced Tactile Sensitivity.** Clinicians experience less tactile sensitivity when using powered instruments than when using hand instruments.

c. **Occupational Risks**

1. **Infection Control.** Infection control can be compromised because some electronically powered devices have components that cannot be sterilized. When selecting an electronically powered device for purchase, consider whether the unit's handpiece and fluid reservoir bottles can be autoclaved.
2. **Aerosol Production.** Powered instruments have been shown to generate high levels of contaminated aerosols.
3. **Musculoskeletal and Auditory Damage.** Research is needed to establish the effect of powered instrumentation on musculoskeletal function and hearing.

d. **Contraindications for Powered Instrumentation.** Powered instrumentation is contraindicated for certain dental and medical conditions. Contraindications for powered instrumentation are summarized in Table 25-2.

TABLE 25-2. Contraindications for Powered Instrumentation
• **Communicable disease.** Individuals with communicable diseases that can be disseminated by aerosols (e.g., hepatitis, tuberculosis, respiratory infections).
• **High susceptibility to infection.** Individuals with a high susceptibility to opportunistic infection that can be transmitted by contaminated dental unit water or inhaled aerosols, such as patient with immunosuppression from disease or chemotherapy, uncontrolled diabetics, patients with organ transplants, and debilitated individuals with chronic medical conditions.[19,20]
• **Respiratory risk.** Individuals with respiratory disease or difficulty in breathing (e.g., history of emphysema, cystic fibrosis, asthma; history of cardiac disease with secondary pulmonary disease or breathing problem). The patient would have a high infection risk if he or she were to aspirate septic material or microorganisms from dental plaque into the lungs.[21]
• **Unshielded cardiac pacemaker.** The American Academy of Periodontology recommends that dental healthcare workers avoid exposing patients with cardiac pacemakers to magnetostrictive devices.[22] Piezoelectric ultrasonic devices do not interfere with pacemaker functioning.
• **Difficulty in swallowing or prone to gagging.** Individuals with multiple sclerosis, amyotrophic lateral sclerosis, muscular dystrophy, or paralysis may experience difficulty in swallowing or be prone to gagging.
• **Age.** Primary and newly erupted teeth of young children have large pulp chambers that are more susceptible to damage from the vibrations and heat produced by ultrasonic instrumentation.
• **Oral conditions.** Avoid contact of instrument tip with hypersensitive teeth, porcelain crowns, composite resin restorations, demineralized enamel surfaces, or exposed dentinal surfaces. Not for use with titanium implants, unless the working-end of the powered instrument is covered with a specially designed plastic sleeve.

OCCUPATIONAL RISKS OF POWERED INSTRUMENTATION

A significant occupational risk of powered instrumentation is the production of contaminated aerosols.[22] In addition to aerosol contamination, musculoskeletal and auditory damage are potential occupational risks of powered instrumentation.

1. **Contaminated Dental Aerosols and Powered Instrumentation**
   a. Overview of Dental Aerosols
      1. Dental aerosols are airborne particles that are composed of debris, microorganisms, and blood propelled into the air from the oral cavities of individuals treated throughout the day in a dental office.[23] Dental aerosols are defined as being particles smaller than 50 μm, with any particles larger than 50 μm being described as splatter.[24,25]
      2. The saliva, gingival tissues, nose, throat, and lungs of healthy patients contain large numbers of streptococci, staphylococci, gram-negative bacteria, and viruses.[26] Viruses include the common cold, influenza, and herpetic viruses.
      3. *Aerosols stay airborne and float on office air currents moving some distance from the point of origin.*[27] *Very small particles can remain suspended at the end of the procedure for many hours. Therefore, the risk of contamination continues long after the procedure is over.*
      4. Small aerosolized particles remain airborne and enter the nasal passage and are capable of penetrating deep into the respiratory tree.[28–30]

   b. Dental Aerosols and Powered Instrumentation
      1. The use of prophy angles, air-water syringes, and even hand instruments produces some splatter in the form of relatively large droplets.
      2. *Powered instruments and air polishers are the greatest producers of small-particle aerosol contamination in dentistry.*[31–38]
      3. Several studies show that blood is found routinely in the aerosols produced by powered instrumentation.[32,39,40]
      4. One study found a significantly greater prevalence of nasal irritation, running eyes, and itchy skin in a dental hygienist group who often use aerosol-generating instruments compared to a control group of clerical staff working in a hospital environment.[41]

   c. Preventive Measures for Powered Instrumentation
      1. Whenever powered instrumentation is used, the following steps should be followed: (a) barrier protection, (b) high-volume evacuation, and (c) preprocedural rinsing. Each of these adds a layer of protection for the clinician and others in the dental office. However, aerosols stay airborne after the procedure; therefore, the risk of contamination continues long after the procedure is over.
      2. Using a preprocedural rinse such as chlorhexidine or an essential oil mouthwash for approximately 1 minute prior to the beginning of treatment lowers the bacterial content of aerosols during powered instrumentation.[38,42,43] A preprocedural rinse, however, will not affect blood coming from the operative site or viruses coming from the respiratory tract. Using a preprocedural rinse should not be relied on to prevent airborne contamination.
      3. The use of a high-volume evacuator (HVE) has been shown to universally reduce airborne contamination by 90% to 98%.[40,42,43] Using an HVE is a mandatory infection control precaution during the use of an ultrasonic scaler.

   a. A saliva ejector does not function as an HVE. The small diameter of a saliva ejector keeps it from removing enough air to be effective in reducing aerosols.
   b. A large-diameter HVE may be held separately by an assistant or the hygienist, attached to the powered instrument tip, or attached to a dry-field device (an extraoral evacuator tip positioning device). Figure 25-5 shows an example of an HVE dry-field device.

2. **Other Potential Occupational Risks of Powered Instrumentation**
   a. **Musculoskeletal Damage.** Some studies suggest that dental hygienists may be in danger of nerve damage from dental instruments that cause vibration, such as powered instruments.
      1. One study found that about one-quarter of dental hygienists who use high-frequency powered instruments will develop a type of nerve damage that blunts the sense of touch and causes weakness.[44,45]
      2. A reduction in strength and tactile sensitivity was observed in women dentists and dental hygienists when compared with women dental assistants and medical nurses who were not exposed to vibration.[46]
   b. **Hearing Loss**
      1. Further research is necessary to confirm the effect of powered instrumentation on hearing.
         a. One study reports tinnitus, an early sign of hearing loss, in both clinicians and patients after powered instrumentation use.[47]
         b. A study by Wilson et al.,[48] however, found that the hearing ability of dental personnel does not differ from that of nondental controls, indicating that occupational exposure to powered instruments is not harmful to hearing.
      2. The use of hearing protection devices has been suggested for dental healthcare providers.
         a. Hearing protection devices, if used, must protect the dental professional from potential noise damage. At the same time, the clinician must be able to hear sufficiently to communicate with the patient.
         b. One option is to purchase custom earplugs, the same type of hearing protection used by many musicians for protection from occupationally induced hearing loss. Garner et al.[49] found that the "musician's style ear plug is perfectly suited to the dental environment and is an affordable and comfortable solution."

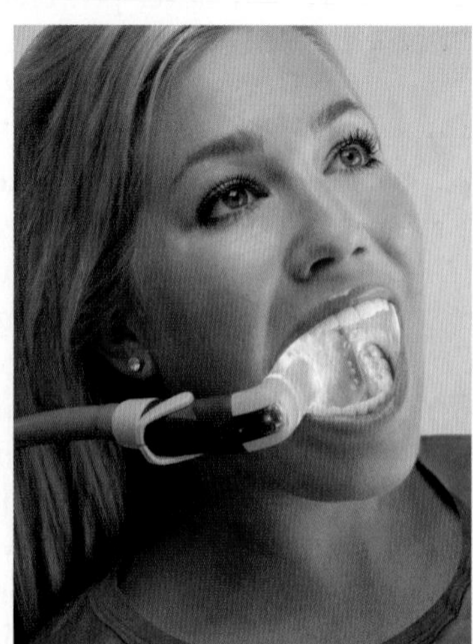

Figure 25-5. Evacuator Tip Positioning Device. The Isolite Dryfield Illuminator, a device that attaches to the high-volume evacuator (HVE), shows a significant reduction in the number of aerosolized particles that reach the breathing space of the clinician. In addition, the Isolite illuminates the oral cavity. (Courtesy of Isolite.)

Section 2
Types of Powered Devices

Powered instruments can be classified into two groups based on their operating frequencies: sonic and ultrasonic (Fig. 25-6).

1. Sonic-powered instruments operate at a relatively low frequency to 3,000 to 8,000 cycles per second and are driven by compressed air from the dental unit (Figs. 25-7 and 25-8).
2. Ultrasonic-powered instruments operate inaudibly at 18,000 to 45,000 cycles per second (kHz). Ultrasonic devices can be further categorized into magnetostrictive and piezoelectric based on the mechanism used to convert the electrical current used for energy to activate the tips.
    a. Piezoelectric ultrasonic instruments use electrical energy to activate crystals within the handpiece to vibrate the tip (Figs. 25-9 to 25-11).
    b. Magnetostrictive ultrasonic instruments transfer electrical energy to metal stacks made of nickel-iron alloy or to a ferrous rod (Figs. 25-12 and 25-13).

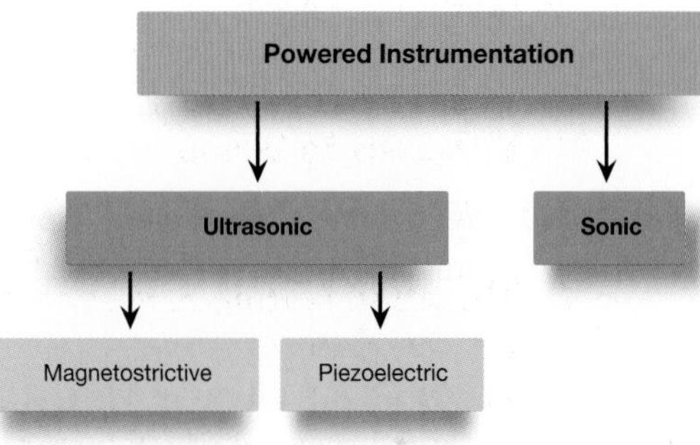

Figure 25-6. Types of Powered Devices. There are two types of powered instruments: ultrasonic and sonic. Ultrasonic-powered instruments may be magnetostrictive or piezoelectric.

SONIC DEVICES

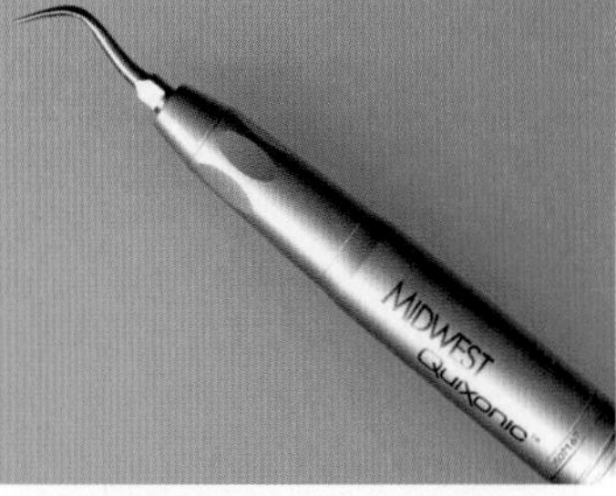

Figure 25-7. Sonic Device. Sonic devices consist of a handpiece (that attaches to the dental unit's high-speed handpiece tubing) and interchangeable instrument tips.

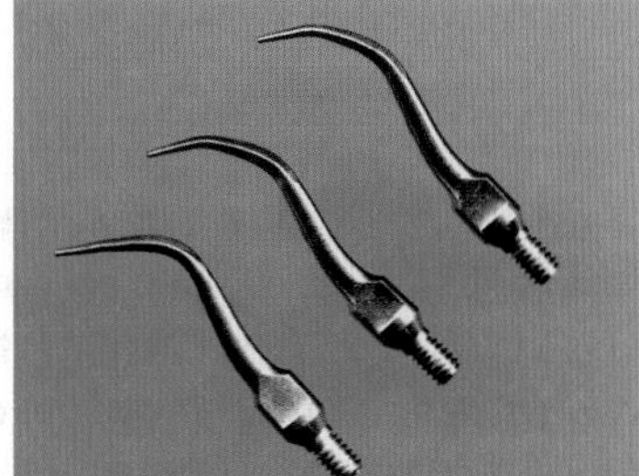

Figure 25-8. Instrument Tips. Examples of sonic instrument tips.

ULTRASONIC DEVICES

Piezoelectric Ultrasonic Devices

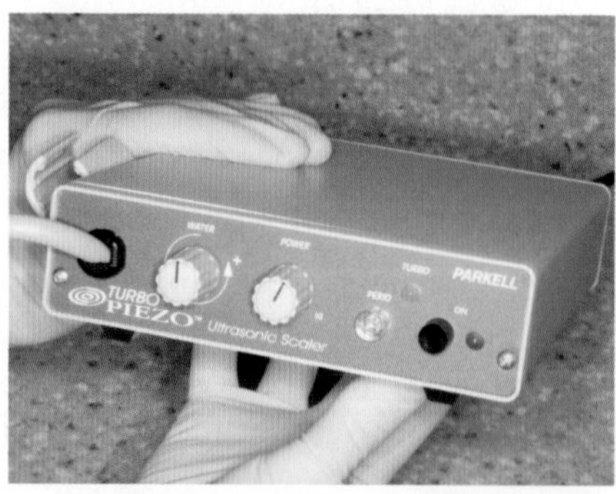

Figure 25-9. Piezoelectric Ultrasonic Device. Piezoelectric ultrasonic devices consist of a portable electronic generator, a handpiece, and instrument tips.

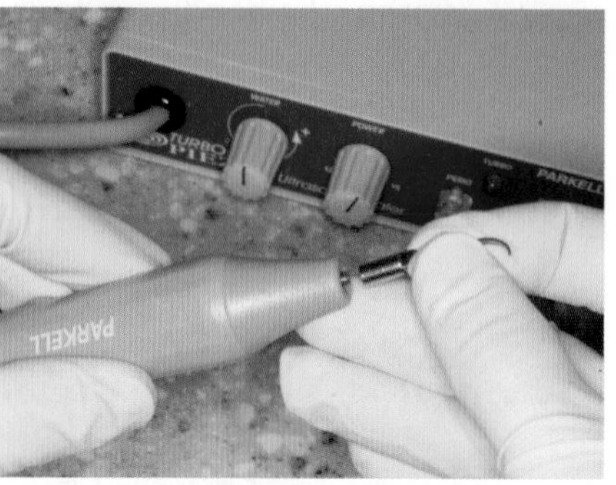

Figure 25-10. Piezoelectric Instrument Tips. Some piezoelectric devices have instrument tips that attach directly to the handpiece.

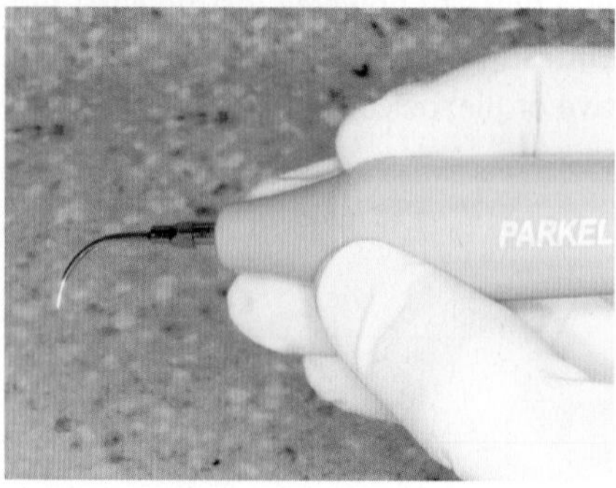

Figure 25-11. Piezoelectric Handpiece and Instrument Tip. An example of a piezoelectric ultrasonic handpiece and powered tip.

Magnetostrictive Ultrasonic Devices

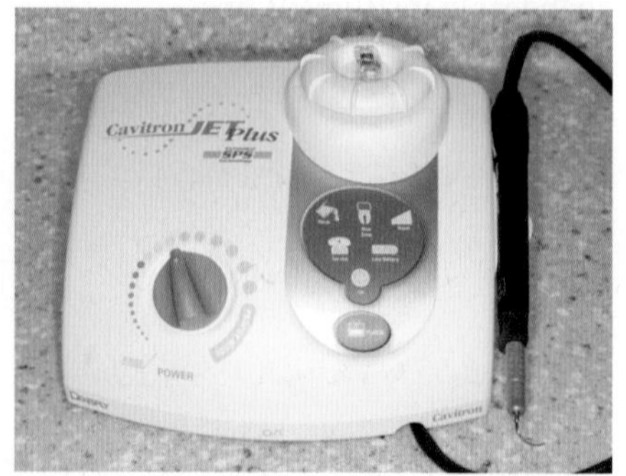

Figure 25-12. Magnetostrictive Ultrasonic Device. Magnetostrictive ultrasonic devices are comprised of a portable unit that contains an electronic generator, a handpiece, and interchangeable instrument inserts. Magnetostrictive devices are available in two different kilohertz (kHz) options: 25-kHz and 30-kHz devices. (Table 25.3)

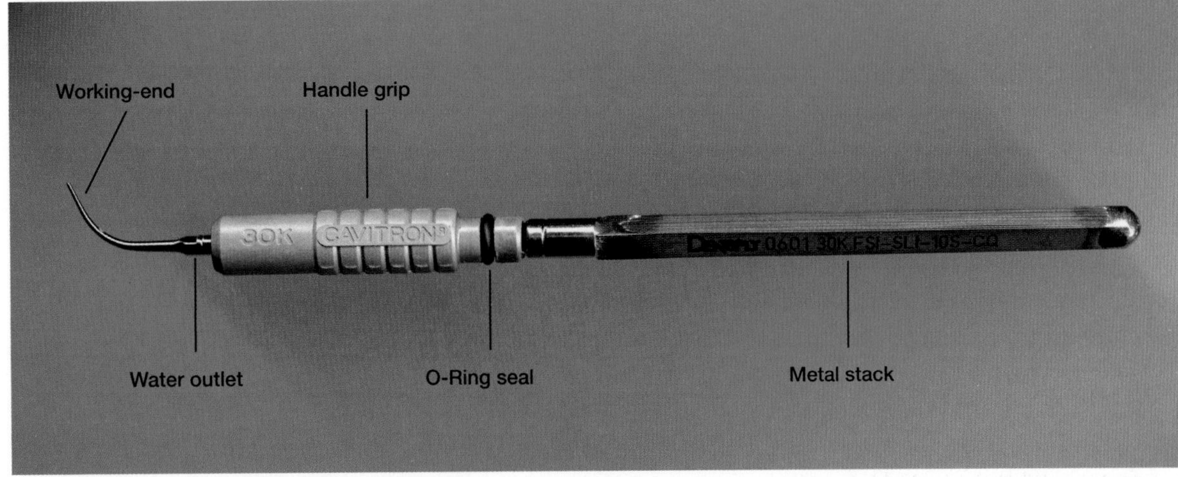

Figure 25-13. Magnetostrictive Inserts. Most magnetostrictive devices have removable instrument inserts that fit into a tubular handpiece. The components of a magnetostrictive insert are:

- Metal stack—converts electrical power into mechanical vibrations.
- O-ring—a seal that keeps water flowing through the insert rather than flowing out of the handpiece.
- Handle grip—portion of the insert grasped by the clinician during instrumentation.
- Water outlet—provides water to the instrument tip.
- Working-end—portion of the instrument insert used for calculus removal and deplaquing.

TABLE 25-3. Magnetostrictive Insert Frequency Options

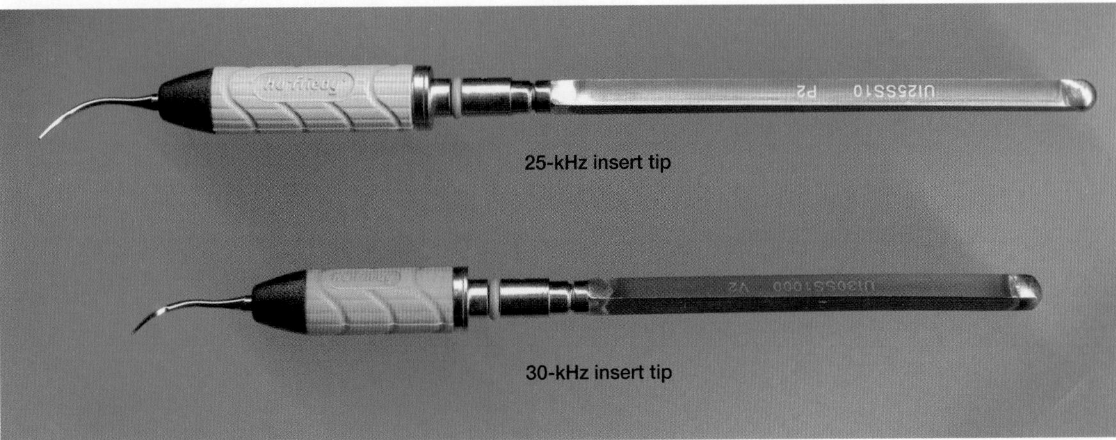

30-kHz Insert Tip	25-kHz Insert Tip
Works with 30-kHz devices only	Works with 25-kHz devices only
30,000 cycles per second	25,000 cycles per second
Shorter stroke length	Longer stroke length
About the same length as a hand instrument	Longer in length than a hand instrument

Section 3
Sonic and Ultrasonic Instrument Tips

As with the working-ends of hand instruments, there are a wide variety of instrument tip designs available for the various sonic and ultrasonic devices.

- Instrument tips from one device may not work with another manufacturer's handpiece.
- When purchasing an electronically powered device, one of the decisive factors should be the selection of instrument tips available for that device. The number of instrument tip designs offered for a particular device can vary from three to many different tip designs.
- Some electronically powered devices do not offer slim-diameter instrument tips. It is important to select a device that offers both standard-diameter and slim-diameter instrument tips.

POWERED INSTRUMENT TIP DESIGNS

The two basic types of powered instrument tips are standard-diameter tips and slim-diameter tips.

- Standard-diameter tips are larger in size and have shorter shank lengths than slim-diameter tips. These tips are comparable to sickle scalers and universal curets in function. Figure 25-14 shows several examples of standard-diameter tips.
- Slim-diameter tips are 40% smaller in diameter and have longer, more complex shanks than standard-diameter tips. These tips are comparable to area-specific curets in function. Figure 25-15 shows several examples of slim-diameter tips.

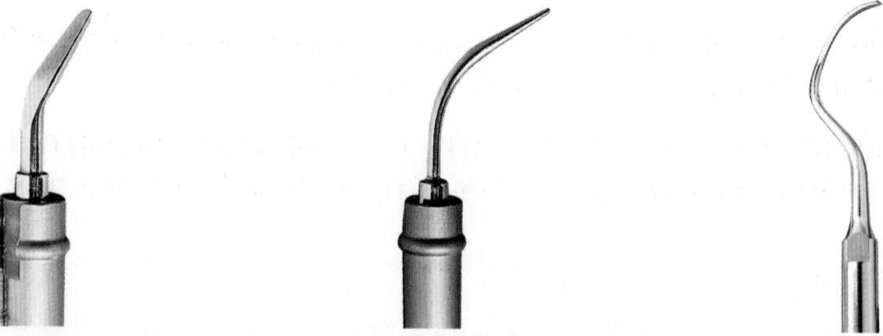

Figure 25-14. Standard-Diameter Powered Tip Designs. Several examples of standard-diameter powered instrument tips. (Left two photographs courtesy of Parkell, Inc.; right photograph courtesy of Hu-Friedy Manufacturing Co., LLC.)

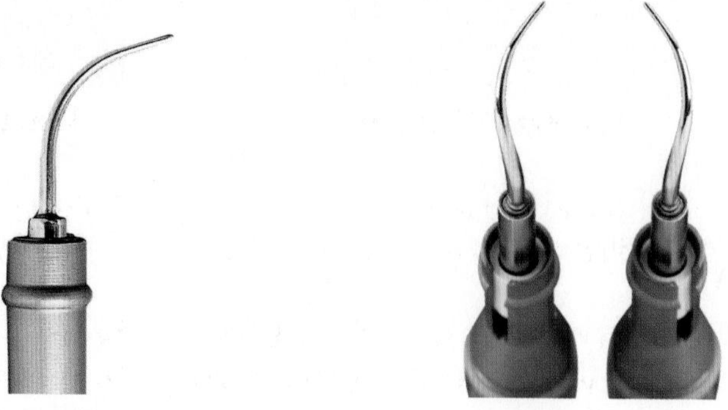

Figure 25-15. Slim-Diameter Powered Tip Designs. Slim-diameter tips come in straight, right, and left tip designs. (Photographs courtesy of Parkell, Inc.)

INSTRUMENT TIP WEAR AND REPLACEMENT

The working-end of the powered instrument should be inspected regularly for signs of wear. With use, the instrument tip is worn down. As the instrument tip wears, effectiveness decreases. Some companies provide instrument tip wear guides that facilitate evaluation of instruments.

1. A rule of thumb is that 1 mm of wear results in approximately 25% loss of efficiency.
2. Approximately 50% loss of efficiency occurs at 2 mm of wear, and the tip should be discarded at this point (Fig. 25-16).

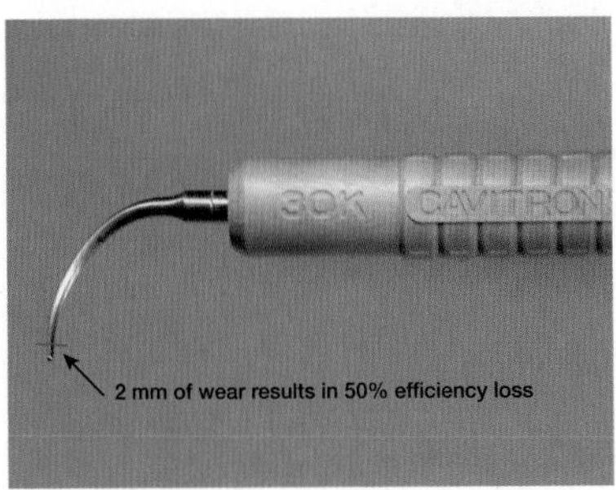
30K
2 mm of wear results in 50% efficiency loss

Figure 25-16. Tip Wear. Instrument tips should be evaluated for tip wear. Tips should be discarded after 2 mm of wear.

INSTRUMENT TIP SELECTION AND SEQUENCE FOR INSTRUMENTATION

Instrument tips vary in tip shape, diameter, length, and curvature (Fig. 25-4). Factors to be considered when selecting an instrument tip for a particular task include:

1. The extent and mode of attachment of calculus deposits (e.g., small-, medium-, or large-sized deposits; lightly adherent or tenacious)
2. The location of calculus deposits (e.g., deposits located above the gingival margin, 4 mm or less below the gingival margin, or more than 4 mm below the gingival margin)

TABLE 25-4. Instrument Tip Selection

Diameter	**Standard Diameter**	**Slim Diameter**
Characteristics	Standard diameter Shorter shank lengths	40% smaller in diameter Longer shank lengths
Use	Heavy deposit removal: supragingival use and for subgingival deposits easily accessed without undue tissue stretching	Light deposits and deplaquing Debridement of root concavities and furcation areas

Sequence for Use of Tips

1. A Combination of Inserts

a. Powered instrumentation requires a combination of standard-diameter and slim-diameter instrument tips (Table 25-5).
b. In addition to tip diameter, clinicians should consider the cross section of the tip.
   1. Tips that have a rectangular, trapezoidal, or beveled cross section are more effective for calculus removal.
   2. Tips that are round in cross section are most effective for removal of plaque biofilm (deplaquing).

2. Sequence of Tips

a. Powered instrumentation begins with standard-diameter tips and progresses to slim-diameter tips. Figure 25-17 summarizes tip selection and sequencing.
   1. Standard-diameter tips are used for moderate to heavy supragingival or subgingival calculus deposits.
      a) Standard tips have enough surface area to easily remove calculus deposits.
      b) Slim-diameter tips are not intended for the removal of moderate to heavy deposits.
      c) Examples of typical standard-diameter tips include beaver tail, triple bend, and universal tip designs.
   2. After instrumentation with standard-diameter tips, slim-diameter tips are used. Slim-diameter tips work well in removing light subgingival calculus deposits, plaque biofilm, and soft debris.

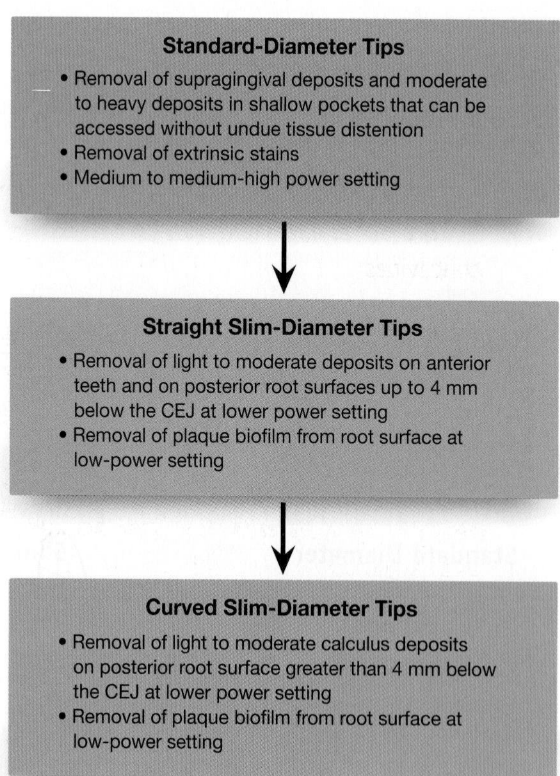

Figure 25-17. Sequence for Instrumentation. Powered instrumentation requires a combination of standard-diameter and slim-diameter instrument tips. (Key: CEJ = cementoenamel junction.)

TABLE 25-5. Common Instrument Tip Designs

Instrument	Description/Use
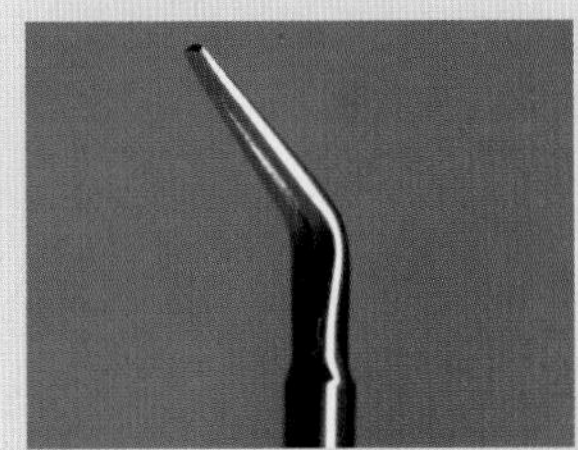	**Beaver Tail Tip:** • Broad bulky tip, resembling a beaver's tail • Supragingival: large-sized calculus ledges and stain; orthodontic cement
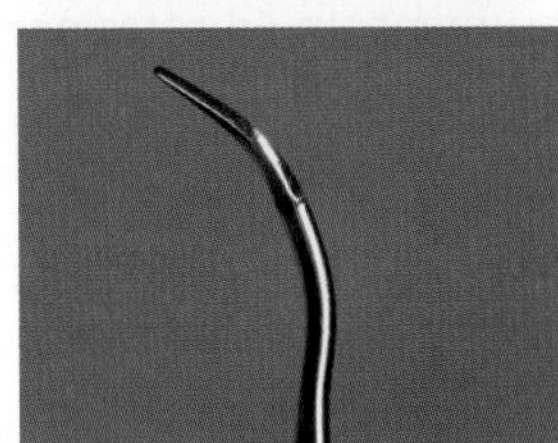	**Standard-Diameter Triple Bend Tip:** • Standard-diameter tip with shank bends that facilitate access to proximal surfaces and around line angles • Supragingival: small- to large-sized calculus deposits and stain
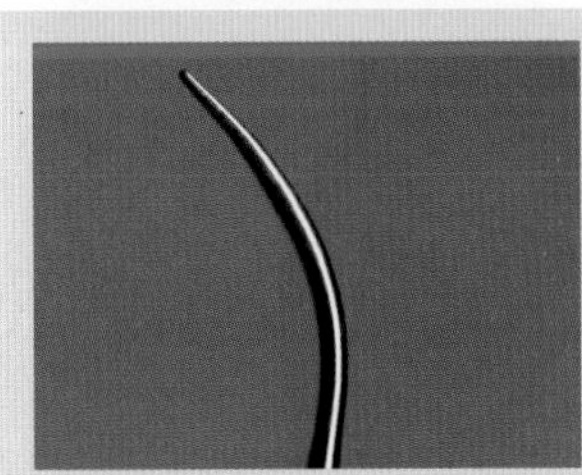	**Standard-Diameter Universal Tip:** • Standard-diameter tip with curved shank and tapered tip • Supragingival: small- to large-sized calculus deposits and stain • Subgingival: deposits accessed without undue tissue stretching
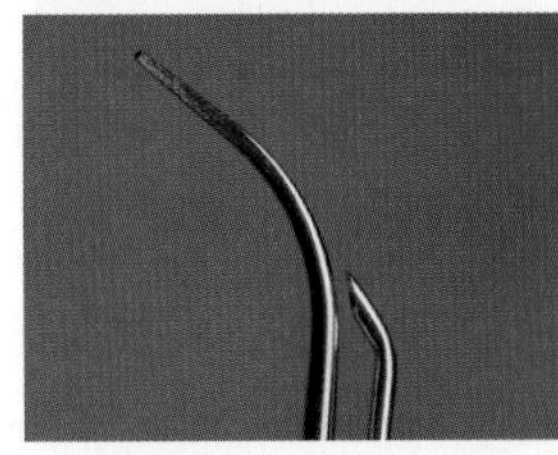	**Slim-Diameter Straight Tip:** • Slim-diameter tip with extended shank and tapered tip; similar in design to a calibrated periodontal probe • Subgingival: root surfaces located in periodontal pockets 4 mm or less in depth for calculus removal and deplaquing of root surfaces and concavities
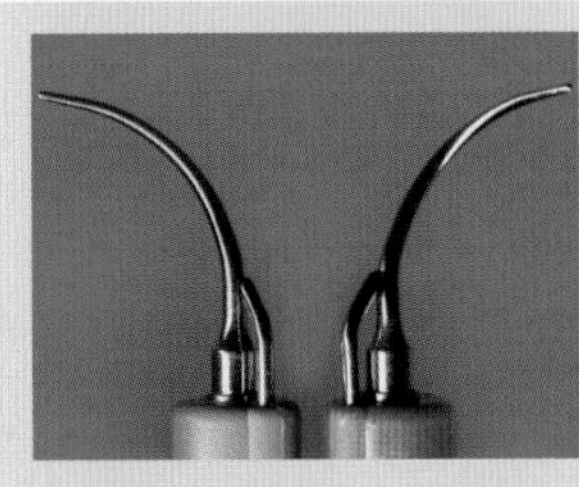	**Slim-Diameter Curved Tips (Right and Left):** • Slim-diameter tips with extended shank and tapered tip; similar in design to a furcation probe; enhanced access to interproximal areas and root surfaces • Subgingival: root surfaces located in pockets greater than 4 mm in depth for calculus removal and deplaquing of root surfaces, furcations, and concavities
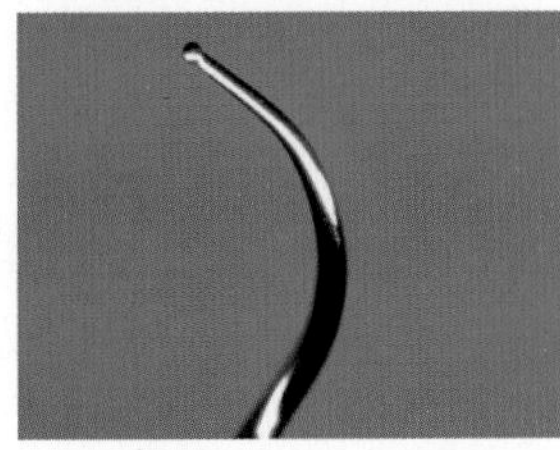	**Slim-Diameter Furcation Tips:** • Slim-diameter tips with a ball end • Subgingival: root surfaces located in periodontal pockets for deplaquing of furcation areas and root concavities

Section 4
Mechanisms of Action

How efficiently an electronically powered instrument removes a calculus deposit is determined by the instrument tip's vibration frequency, stroke length, and stroke motion, and the surface of the instrument tip in contact with the tooth.

FREQUENCY

Powered instruments use an electric current to produce rapid vibrations of the instrument tip. Frequency is the measure of how many times the electronically powered instrument tip vibrates per second (Fig. 25-18).

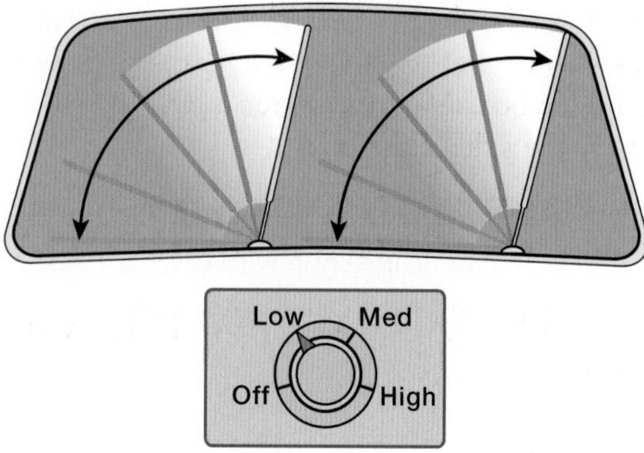

Figure 25-18. Frequency. The frequency of an electronically powered instrument can be compared to the settings for the windshield wipers on a car.

1. **Low Frequency.** When the wiper setting is on low, the wipers only go back and forth a few times in a minute. Similarly, when the frequency of a powered instrument is low, the instrument tip vibrates fewer times per second.
2. **High Frequency.** When the wiper setting is on high, the windshield wipers go back and forth many times in a minute. Correspondingly, when the frequency of a powered instrument is high, the instrument tip vibrates more times per second.

AMPLITUDE (STROKE)

Amplitude (stroke) is a measure of how far the instrument tip moves back and forth during one cycle. Ultrasonic powered devices have a ***power knob*** that is used to change the length of the stroke. Higher amplitude delivers a longer, more powerful stroke; lower amplitude delivers a shorter, less powerful stroke.

1. **Low Amplitude.** Using the example of a child on a swing, low amplitude would be a gentle push against the child's back, causing the swing to move forward a short distance before returning to its starting position (Fig. 25-19). Lower amplitude causes the instrument tip to move a shorter distance.
2. **Higher Amplitude.** Higher amplitude causes the instrument tip to move a longer distance. This is similar to a more forceful push against the child's back, causing the swing to travel a long distance before returning to its original position.

CLEANING EFFICIENCY

The cleaning efficiency of a powered instrument is determined by a combination of frequency and amplitude. Frequency determines the number of vibrations, whereas amplitude determines the length of each stroke. As an aid in understanding cleaning efficiency, imagine a boxer who is trapped in a wooden box. In order to escape, the boxer decides to try to punch through the side of the box.

1. **Low Frequency/Low Amplitude.** In the first instance shown in Figure 25-20A, the boxer is trapped in a narrow box, so that when he tries to punch the side of the box, his swing is hindered by the size of the box. He hits his elbow on the back of the box as he makes his punches. He is only able to make a few, short thrusts against the side of the box.
   - This example is similar to low frequency—few vibrations, or punches—combined with low amplitude—short strokes, or limited movement of the boxer's arm.
   - A combination of low frequency and low amplitude is ideal for disruption of plaque biofilm from the root surface (deplaquing).
2. **High Frequency/High Amplitude.** In the second example shown in Figure 25-20B, the boxer is trapped in a wide box. Now the boxer is able to pull his arm back to make many, long thrusts at the side of the box.
   - This example is similar to high frequency—many vibrations, or punches—combined with high amplitude—long strokes, or longer thrusts of the boxer's arm.
   - A combination of higher frequency combined with higher amplitude is ideal for the removal of tenacious calculus deposits.

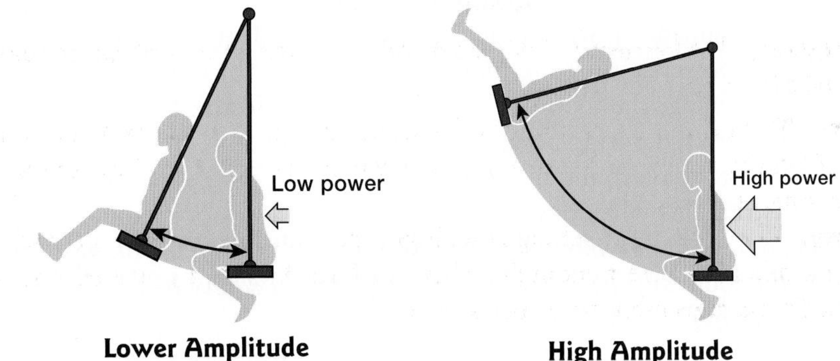

Figure 25-19. Amplitude. Low amplitude can be compared to a gentle push against the back of a child on a swing. High amplitude is comparable to a more forceful push against the child's back.

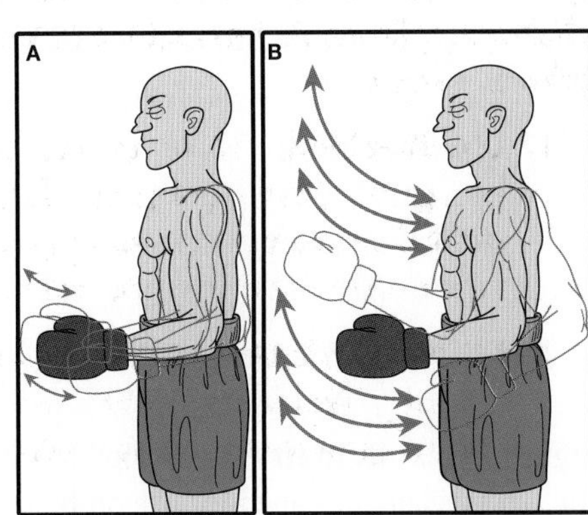

Figure 25-20. Cleaning Efficiency. Cleaning efficiency is determined by a combination of frequency and amplitude. A boxer trapped in a narrow box **(A)** can exert much less force per punch than the same boxer trapped in a wider box **(B)**.

CONTROLLING AMPLITUDE, FREQUENCY, AND WATER FLOW

Ultrasonic devices have controls that allow the clinician to adjust power and water flow. Some ultrasonic devices have a third control that allows the clinician to adjust the frequency. (Fig. 25-21)

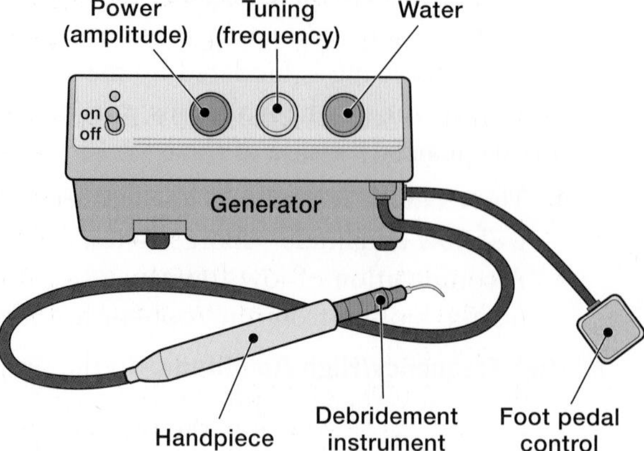

Figure 25-21. Manually Tuned Ultrasonic Device. Manual ultrasonic devices have three control knobs or buttons—power, tuning, and water—that allow the clinician to adjust the length of the stroke, tip frequency vibration, and water flow.

1. **Power Adjustment.** The power setting on magnetostrictive and piezoelectric ultrasonic devices determines the length of the stroke—the distance the instrument travels back and forth in one cycle.
   a. Higher power settings deliver a longer, more forceful stroke. Lower power settings deliver a shorter, less powerful stroke.
   b. Because the instrument tip strikes the tooth with more force at higher power settings, higher power settings are more uncomfortable for the patient and more likely to damage the tooth surface. The lowest effective power setting should always be used during powered instrumentation.
   c. A research investigation found no difference in the cleaning efficiency of ultrasonic instruments when operated at high-power levels or medium-power levels.[18] ***Therefore, to maximize patient comfort and minimize potential damage to the tooth surface, the power setting should rarely be placed above the medium setting.***
   d. ***Most slim-diameter tips cannot be used at higher power levels because of the risk of breakage.***
      1. Dentsply Cavitron makes two slim-diameter tips, called ThinSert tips, that are specially designed to withstand use on high power without danger of breaking.
      2. Parkell, Inc., makes the Burnett Power-Tip, which can be used on high power for removal of tenacious calculus (Fig. 25-22).

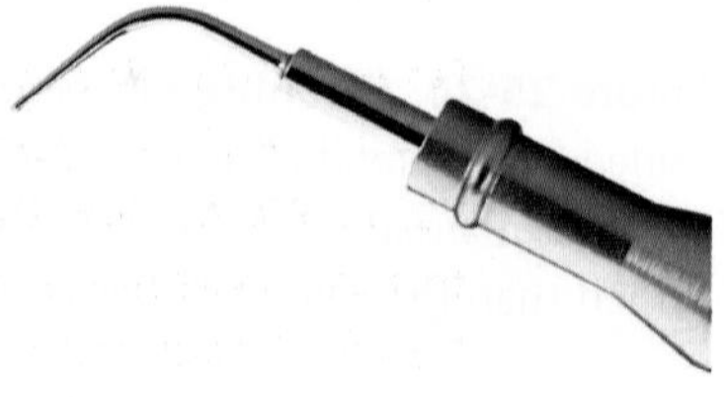

Figure 25-22. Burnett Power-Tip. The Burnett Power-Tip from Parkell, Inc., is specially designed for use on high-power settings for the removal of tenacious calculus deposits.

2. **Frequency Adjustment: Tuning.** Tuning on ultrasonic devices may be either manual or automatic.
   a. Automatically tuned ultrasonic devices have two control knobs or buttons—power and water—that allow the clinician to adjust the length of the stroke and the water flow.
      1. The power setting determines the length of the stroke and is generally kept to low or medium setting for patient comfort.
      2. The water flow is essential to dissipate the heat produced by the vibration of the tip.
      3. Automatic units allow the tip to vibrate at a frequency that produces the most effective calculus removal for the selected power setting.
   b. Manually tuned ultrasonic devices have three control knobs or buttons—power, tuning, and water—that allow the clinician to adjust the length of the stroke, tip frequency vibration, and water flow.
      1. Manual units allow the clinician to adjust the vibration frequency, power, and water.
      2. The tuning knob can be used to set the vibration frequency of the tip at a level above or below the resonant frequency.
      3. One problem with manual units is that an incorrectly tuned instrument will be ineffective in calculus removal. With manual units, the effectiveness of the powered instrument for calculus removal is dependent on the experience of the clinician in tuning the tip frequency.
3. **Water Flow**
   a. Magnetostrictive and piezoelectric ultrasonic instrument tips must be cooled by fluid to prevent overheating of the vibrating instrument tip. Fluid, usually water, is used as a coolant.
   b. Fluid constantly flows through the ultrasonic handpiece and disperses in a fine spray at or near the instrument tip.
   c. The clinician can adjust the volume of the water supplied to the instrument tip.
      1. Lower rates of water flow increase the heating of the handpiece and result in warmer water at the instrument tip.
         a. Too little water flow to the instrument tip can result in heat damage to the dental pulp.
         b. More water flow is recommended for calculus removal (Fig. 25-23A), and less water flow is needed for deplaquing (Fig. 25-23B).

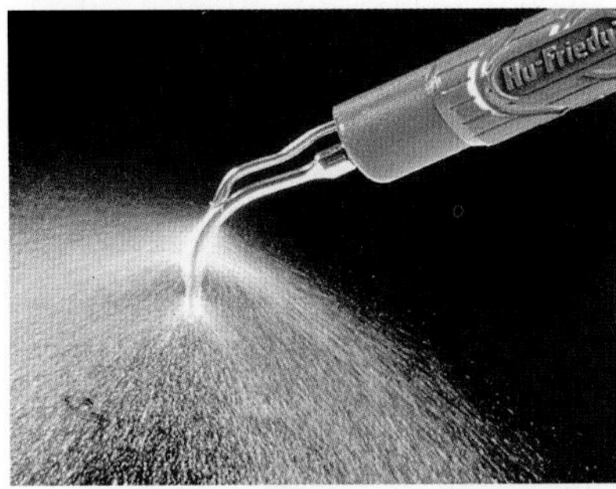

A

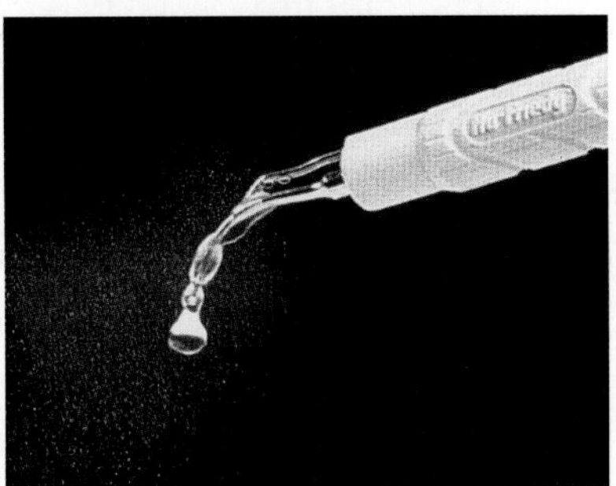
B

Figure 25-23. Water Flow. A. Water Flow for Calculus Removal: The instrument tip on the left is adjusted so that the water breaks into a fine mist at the instrument tip. **B. Water Flow for Deplaquing:** The instrument tip on the right is adjusted so that the water halo is smaller and water drips from the instrument tip. (Courtesy of Hu-Friedy Manufacturing Co., Inc.)

2. ***One of the most common mistakes made by beginning clinicians is using too little water. A warm handpiece is a sign of inadequate water flowing through the handpiece and instrument tip.***

d. Water is provided to the instrument tip through either external or internal fluid flow tubes. Figures 25-24 and 25-25 depict correct water flow adjustment for external and internal fluid flow tubes.

e. Changing from one powered tip to another during treatment may require adjustment of the water flow.[50]

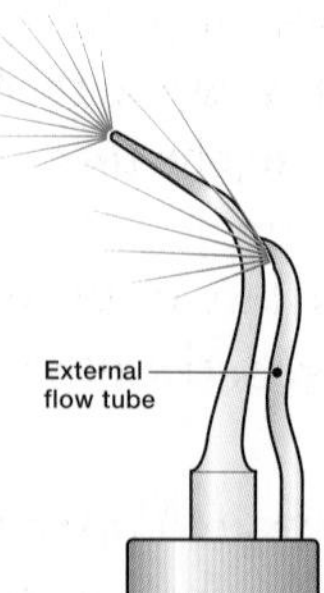

Figure 25-24. Water Adjustment for Tips with External Flow Tubes. For instrument tips with external flow tubes, the water flow should be adjusted so that the water breaks into a fine mist near the end of the external flow tube and at the very end of the tip.

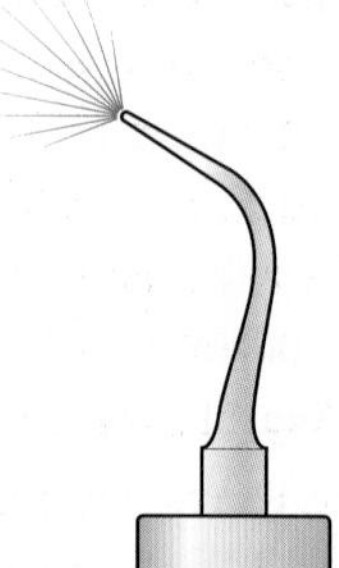

Figure 25-25. Water Adjustment for Tips with Internal Flow Tubes. For instrument tips with internal flow systems, the water flow should be adjusted so that the water breaks into a fine mist at the very end of the tip.

4. **Fluid Reservoirs and Powered Instrumentation.** Some ultrasonic devices have independent fluid reservoirs (bottles) that can be used to deliver distilled water or other fluid solutions to the instrument tip. Figure 25-26 shows one example of a fluid reservoir device.

   a. Solutions commonly used for irrigation include distilled water, sterile saline, stannous fluoride, and chemotherapeutic agents (antimicrobials), such as chlorhexidine.

   b. The use of chemotherapeutic agents with ultrasonic instruments has ***not*** been shown to enhance pocket depth reduction beyond that achieved by hand instrumentation or ultrasonic instrumentation with water.[16,22,51]

   c. Pathogenic plaque biofilms, which are found mainly in deep pockets (4 mm or greater), are highly resistant to antimicrobial agents and systemic antibiotics.[52,53] The only way to totally disrupt the biofilm is through mechanical removal. Control of bacteria in dental plaque biofilms is best achieved by the physical disruption of plaque.[54]

Figure 25-26. Fluid Reservoir Bottles. Fluid reservoirs are used to deliver distilled water, stannous fluoride, or chemotherapeutic agents to a magnetostrictive or piezoelectric-powered instrument tip. (Courtesy of Parkell, Inc.)

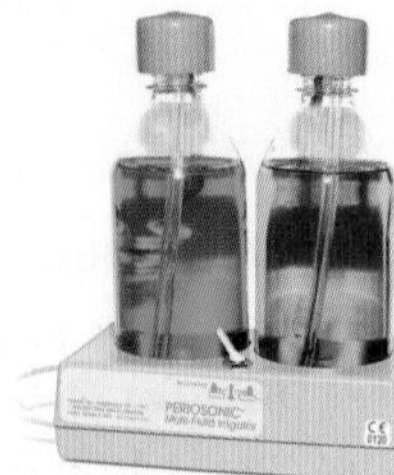

ENERGY DISPERSION BY THE WORKING-END SURFACES

Electronically powered instrument tips disperse energy vibrations from each surface of the working-end.[55] By adapting the appropriate tip surface, the clinician can control energy dispersion and patient sensitivity.

1. **Energy Output.** The face, back, lateral surfaces, and point of a powered instrument tip produce different amounts of energy.
   a. Point of the tip—produces the greatest amount of energy vibrations. ***The point of a powered instrument tip is never adapted directly on a tooth surface due to potential discomfort for the patient and damage to the root surface.***[56,57]
   b. Face of the tip (concave surface)—produces the second greatest amount of energy vibrations. The concave face of the tip is not adapted to the tooth surface because it would be difficult to adapt it correctly.
   c. Back of the tip (convex surface)—produces less energy than the face or the point.
   d. Lateral surfaces of the tip—produce less energy than the face or the point.
2. **Pattern of Tip Movement**
   a. In the past, researchers often photographed freely moving powered inserts—not adapted to a tooth surface—to determine the motion of the instrument tip. Tip motion of a freely moving powered tip varies from a lateral motion to an elliptical motion.
   b. The principle findings of a study by Lea et al.[58,59] show that the motion of a working (loaded) powered instrument tip is more dependent on the generator power setting and the shape of the instrument tip.
      1. Longer, slimmer probes are more prone to elliptical motion.
      2. Lea et al.[58,59] found that all powered instrument tips oscillate with an elliptical motion that may affect calculus removal and resulting tooth surface morphology.
3. **Adaptation of Powered Tips.** Clinicians should follow manufacturer's recommendations for instrument tip-to-tooth surface adaptation. In general, the following guidelines should be followed for powered instrumentation.
   a. ***The point of the tip and the face of the tip should never be directly adapted to a tooth surface*** (Fig. 25-27).
   b. The backs of most ultrasonic and sonic instrument tips can be adapted to the tooth surface, following the recommendations of the tip manufacturer (Fig. 25-28).
   c. Lateral surfaces of the tip. Adaptation of the lateral surfaces of the working-end is recommended with all sonic, piezoelectric, and magnetostrictive ultrasonic instruments.

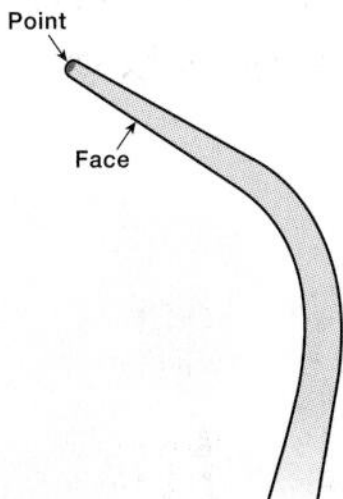

Figure 25-27. The Point and Face of a Powered Tip. The point or face of a powered tip should not be adapted to the tooth surface due to the high-energy output of these surfaces.

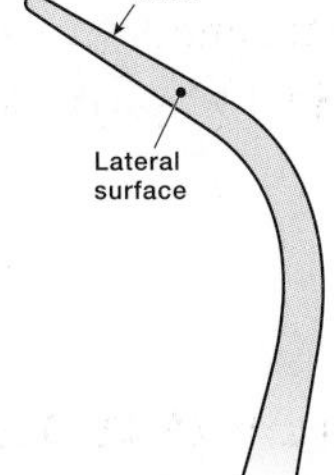

Figure 25-28. The Back and Lateral Surfaces. The back and lateral surfaces of a powered instrument tip are used for calculus removal and deplaquing of tooth surfaces.

ACTIVE TIP AREA

The portion of the instrument tip that is capable of doing work is called the active tip area. ***The power to remove calculus is concentrated in the last 2 to 4 mm of the length of a powered instrument tip.*** Figure 25-29 illustrates the active tip area of a powered tip.

1. The active tip area ranges from approximately 2 to 4 mm of the length of the instrument tip.
2. The higher the frequency of the powered device, the shorter the active tip area.
   a. For a 50-kHz device, the active tip area is 2.3 mm long.
   b. For a 30-kHz device, the active tip area is 4.2 mm long.
   c. For a 25-kHz device, the active tip area is 4.3 mm long.

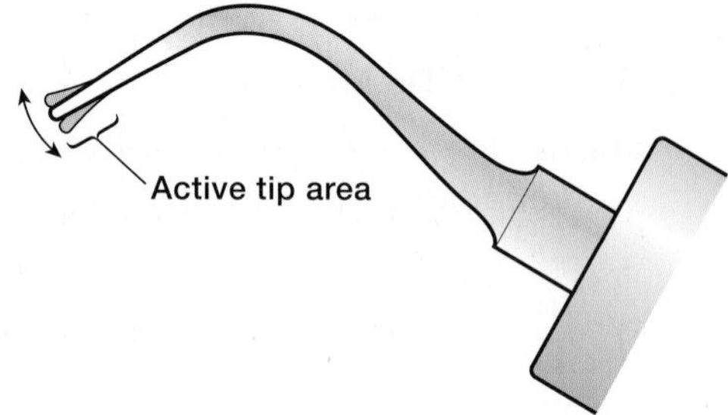

Figure 25-29. Active Tip Area. The power for calculus removal is concentrated in the active tip area (the last 2 to 4 mm of the tip).

POWERED TIPS FOR USE ON DENTAL IMPLANTS

Instruments used for the assessment and debridement of implant teeth should be made of a material that is softer than titanium because titanium is a soft metal that is easily damaged by metal instruments.

- Metal instruments, whether hand-activated or powered, may scratch the titanium implant surface, resulting in increased plaque biofilm retention, which in turn compromises periodontal health.
- Powered instrument tips fitted with a nonmetallic plastic or carbon tip are appropriate for instrumentation of dental implants (Fig. 25-30). Studies show no damaging effects from the use of plastic- or carbon-tipped powered instruments.[60–65]
- A study by Sato et al.[65] suggested that ultrasonic instruments fitted with nonmetallic tips are more effective than hand-activated plastic scalers in the removal of calculus deposits and plaque biofilms around a dental implant.

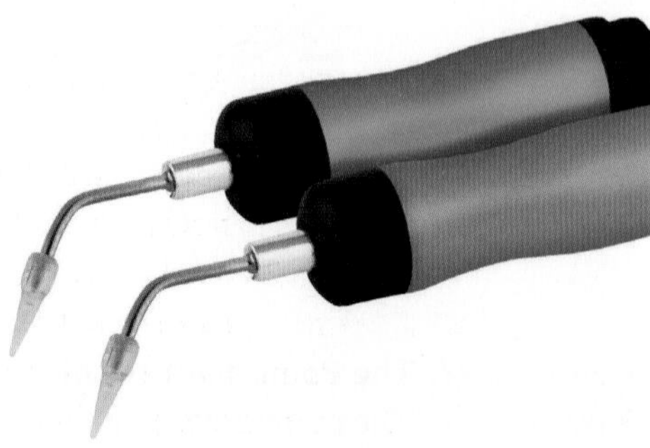

Figure 25-30. Powered Inserts for Instrumentation of Dental Implants. The GentleClean tips by Parkell, Inc., are examples of powered tips specially designed for use on dental implants. (Courtesy of Parkell, Inc.)

Table 25-6 presents a comparison of electronically powered and hand instrumentation.

TABLE 25-6. Presents a Comparison of Powered and Hand Instrumentation

Electronically Powered Instrumentation	Hand Instrumentation
• Several mechanisms of action: mechanical, water irrigation, acoustic microstreaming, and cavitation	• One mechanism of action: mechanical calculus removal
• Small size of instrument tip (0.3–0.55 mm)	• Larger size working-ends (0.76–1.0 mm)
• Easily inserted in pocket with minimal distention (stretching) of pocket wall away from the tooth	• Must be positioned apical to deposit, resulting in considerable distention of pocket wall
• Powered instrument tip can remove calculus deposit from above; working in an apical direction beginning at the gingival margin and moving toward the junctional epithelium	• Curet must be positioned beneath the deposit for removal; working in a coronal direction beginning at the junctional epithelium and moving toward the gingival margin
• Tissue trauma less likely, resulting in a faster healing rate	• Larger working-end with sharp cutting edge(s) more likely to cause tissue trauma
• No cutting edges to sharpen	• Frequent sharpening required
• Treatment outcomes dependent on the clinician's skill level with powered instrumentation and knowledge of root anatomy	• Treatment outcomes dependent on the clinician's skill level with hand instrumentation and knowledge of root anatomy
• High levels of aerosol production	• Low levels of splatter production

REFERENCES

1. Flemming T. Ultrasonics and periodontal pathogens. *Dimen Dent Hyg.* 2007;5:14, 16, 18.
2. Schenk G, Flemmig TF, Lob S, Ruckdeschel G, Hickel R. Lack of antimicrobial effect on periodontopathic bacteria by ultrasonic and sonic scalers in vitro. *J Clin Periodontol.* 2000;27:116–119.
3. Cobb CM. Clinical significance of non-surgical periodontal therapy: an evidence-based perspective of scaling and root planing. *J Clin Periodontol.* 2002;29(suppl 2):6–16.
4. Hallmon WW, Rees TD. Local anti-infective therapy: mechanical and physical approaches. A systematic review. *Ann Periodontol.* 2003;8:99–114.
5. Tunkel J, Heinecke A, Flemmig TF. A systematic review of efficacy of machine-driven and manual subgingival debridement in the treatment of chronic periodontitis. *J Clin Periodontol.* 2002;29(suppl 3):72–81.
6. Khambay BS, Walmsley AD. Acoustic microstreaming: detection and measurement around ultrasonic scalers. *J Periodontol.* 1999;70:626–631.
7. Walmsley AD, Walsh TF, Laird WR, Williams AR. Effects of cavitational activity on the root surface of teeth during ultrasonic scaling. *J Clin Periodontol.* 1990;17:306–312.
8. Dragoo MR. A clinical evaluation of hand and ultrasonic instruments on subgingival debridement. 1. With unmodified and modified ultrasonic inserts. *Int J Periodontics Restorative Dent.* 1992;12:310–323.
9. Rateitschak-Pluss EM, Schwarz JP, Guggenheim R, Duggelin M, Rateitschak KH. Non-surgical periodontal treatment: where are the limits? An SEM study. *J Clin Periodontol.* 1992;19:240–244.
10. Shiloah J, Hovious LA. The role of subgingival irrigations in the treatment of periodontitis. *J Periodontol.* 1993;64:835–843.
11. Walmsley AD, Laird WR, Lumley PJ. Ultrasound in dentistry. Part 2–Periodontology and endodontics. *J Dent.* 1992;20:11–17.
12. Young NA. Periodontal debridement: re-examining non-surgical instrumentation. Part I: a new perspective on the objectives of instrumentation. *Semin Dent Hyg.* 1994;4:1–7.
13. Bower RC. Furcation morphology relative to periodontal treatment. Furcation root surface anatomy. *J Periodontol.* 1979;50:366–374.
14. Bower RC. Furcation morphology relative to periodontal treatment. Furcation entrance architecture. *J Periodontol.* 1979;50:23–27.
15. Leon LE, Vogel RI. A comparison of the effectiveness of hand scaling and ultrasonic debridement in furcations as evaluated by differential dark-field microscopy. *J Periodontol.* 1987;58:86–94.
16. Nosal G, Scheidt MJ, O'Neal R, Van Dyke TE. The penetration of lavage solution into the periodontal pocket during ultrasonic instrumentation. *J Periodontol.* 1991;62:554–557.
17. Walmsley AD, Laird WR, Williams AR. Dental plaque removal by cavitational activity during ultrasonic scaling. *J Clin Periodontol.* 1988;15:539–543.
18. Chapple IL, Walmsley AD, Saxby MS, Moscrop H. Effect of instrument power setting during ultrasonic scaling upon treatment outcome. *J Periodontol.* 1995;66:756–760.
19. Wilkins EM. *Clinical Practice of the Dental Hygienist.* 9th ed. Philadelphia, PA: Lippincott Williams & Wilkins; 2005.
20. Daniel SJ, Harfst SA, Wilder RS. *Mosby's Dental Hygiene: Concepts, Cases and Competencies.* 2nd ed. St. Louis, MO: Mosby/Elsevier; 2008.
21. Suzuki JB, Delisle AL. Pulmonary actinomycosis of periodontal origin. *J Periodontol.* 1984;55:581–584.
22. Drisko CL, Cochran DL, Blieden T, Bouwsma OJ, Cohen RE, Damoulis P, et al. Position paper: sonic and ultrasonic scalers in periodontics. Research, Science and Therapy Committee of the American Academy of Periodontology. *J Periodontol.* 2000;71:1792–1801.
23. Bennett AM, Fulford MR, Walker JT, Bradshaw DJ, Martin MV, Marsh PD. Microbial aerosols in general dental practice. *Br Dent J.* 2000;189:664–667.

24. Holbrook WP, Muir KF, Macphee IT, Ross PW. Bacteriological investigation of the aerosol from ultrasonic scalers. *Br Dent J*. 1978;144:245–247.
25. Micik RE, Miller RL, Mazzarella MA, Ryge G. Studies on dental aerobiology. I. Bacterial aerosols generated during dental procedures. *J Dent Res*. 1969;48:49–56.
26. Harrel S. Contaminated dental aerosols. The risks and implications for dental hygienists. *Dimen Dent Hyg*. 2003;1:16, 18, 20.
27. Harrel SK, Barnes JB, Rivera-Hidalgo F. Aerosol and splatter contamination from the operative site during ultrasonic scaling. *J Am Dent Assoc*. 1998;129:1241–1249.
28. Harrel SK, Molinari J. Aerosols and splatter in dentistry: a brief review of the literature and infection control implications. *J Am Dent Assoc*. 2004;135:429–437.
29. Miller RL, Micik RE. Air pollution and its control in the dental office. *Dent Clin North Am*. 1978;22:453–476.
30. Molinari JA, Harte JA, Cottone JA. *Cottone's Practical Infection Control in Dentistry*. 3rd ed. Philadelphia, PA: Wolters Kluwer Health/Lippincott William & Wilkins; 2010.
31. Bentley CD, Burkhart NW, Crawford JJ. Evaluating spatter and aerosol contamination during dental procedures. *J Am Dent Assoc*. 1994;125:579–584.
32. Gross KB, Overman PR, Cobb C, Brockmann S. Aerosol generation by two ultrasonic scalers and one sonic scaler. A comparative study. *J Dent Hyg*. 1992;66:314–318.
33. King TB, Muzzin KB, Berry CW, Anders LM. The effectiveness of an aerosol reduction device for ultrasonic scalers. *J Periodontol*. 1997;68:45–49.
34. Legnani P, Checchi L, Pelliccioni GA, D'Achille C. Atmospheric contamination during dental procedures. *Quintessence Int*. 1994;25:435–439.
35. Logothetis DD, Gross KB, Eberhart A, Drisko C. Bacterial airborne contamination with an air-polishing device. *Gen Dent*. 1988;36:496–499.
36. Muzzin KB, King TB, Berry CW. Assessing the clinical effectiveness of an aerosol reduction device for the air polisher. *J Am Dent Assoc*. 1999;130:1354–1359.
37. Rivera-Hidalgo F, Barnes JB, Harrel SK. Aerosol and splatter production by focused spray and standard ultrasonic inserts. *J Periodontol*. 1999;70:473–477.
38. Trenter SC, Walmsley AD. Ultrasonic dental scaler: associated hazards. *J Clin Periodontol*. 2003;30:95–101.
39. Barnes JB, Harrel SK, Rivera-Hidalgo F. Blood contamination of the aerosols produced by in vivo use of ultrasonic scalers. *J Periodontol*. 1998;69:434–438.
40. Harrel SK. Clinical use of an aerosol-reduction device with an ultrasonic scaler. *Compend Contin Educ Dent*. 1996;17:1185–1193.
41. Basu MK, Browne RM, Potts AJ, Harrington JM. A survey of aerosol-related symptoms in dental hygienists. *J Soc Occup Med*. 1988;38:23–25.
42. Jacks ME. A laboratory comparison of evacuation devices on aerosol reduction. *J Dent Hyg*. 2002;76:202–206.
43. Klyn SL, Cummings DE, Richardson BW, Davis RD. Reduction of bacteria-containing spray produced during ultrasonic scaling. *Gen Dent*. 2001;49:648–652.
44. Cherniack M, Brammer AJ, Nilsson T, Lundstrom R, Meyer JD, Morse T, et al. Nerve conduction and sensorineural function in dental hygienists using high frequency ultrasound handpieces. *Am J Ind Med*. 2006;49:313–326.
45. Hjortsberg U, Rosen I, Orbaek P, Lundborg G, Balogh I. Finger receptor dysfunction in dental technicians exposed to high-frequency vibration. *Scand J Work Environ Health*. 1989;15:339–344.
46. Akesson I, Lundborg G, Horstmann V, Skerfving S. Neuropathy in female dental personnel exposed to high frequency vibrations. *Occup Environ Med*. 1995;52:116–123.
47. Coles RR, Hoare NW. Noise-induced hearing loss and the dentist. *Br Dent J*. 1985;159:209–218.
48. Wilson CE, Vaidyanathan TK, Cinotti WR, Cohen SM, Wang SJ. Hearing-damage risk and communication interference in dental practice. *J Dent Res*. 1990;69:489–493.

49. Garner G, Federman J, Johnson A. A noice induced hearing loss in the dental environment: an audiologist perspective. *J Georgia Dent Assoc.* 2002:17–19.
50. Koster TJ, Timmerman MF, Feilzer AJ, Van der Velden U, Van der Weijden FA. Water coolant supply in relation to different ultrasonic scaler systems, tips and coolant settings. *J Clin Periodontol.* 2009;36:127–131.
51. Slots J. Selection of antimicrobial agents in periodontal therapy. *J Periodontal Res.* 2002;37:389–398.
52. Costerton JW, Stewart PS, Greenberg EP. Bacterial biofilms: a common cause of persistent infections. *Science.* 1999;284:1318–1322.
53. Gilbert P, Das J, Foley I. Biofilm susceptibility to antimicrobials. *Adv Dent Res.* 1997;11:160–167.
54. Nield-Gehrig JS, Willmann DE. *Foundations of Periodontics for the Dental Hygienist.* 3rd ed. Philadelphia, PA: Wolters Kluwer Health/Lippincott Williams & Wilkins; 2011.
55. Hodges K, Calley K. Optimizing ultrasonic instrumentation. Magnetostrictive ultrasonic insert selection and correct technique in periodontal therapy. *Dimen Dent Hyg.* 2010;8:30, 32, 34–35.
56. Jepsen S, Ayna M, Hedderich J, Eberhard J. Significant influence of scaler tip design on root substance loss resulting from ultrasonic scaling: a laserprofilometric in vitro study. *J Clin Periodontol.* 2004;31:1003–1006.
57. Stach D. Powering the calculus away. *Dimen Dent Hyg.* 2005;3:18–20.
58. Lea SC, Felver B, Landini G, Walmsley AD. Ultrasonic scaler oscillations and tooth-surface defects. *J Dent Res.* 2009;88:229–234.
59. Lea SC, Felver B, Landini G, Walmsley AD. Three-dimensional analyses of ultrasonic scaler oscillations. *J Clin Periodontol.* 2009;36:44–50.
60. Bailey GM, Gardner JS, Day MH, Kovanda BJ. Implant surface alterations from a nonmetallic ultrasonic tip. *J West Soc Periodontol Periodontal Abstr.* 1998;46:69–73.
61. Kawashima H, Sato S, Kishida M, Ito K. A comparison of root surface instrumentation using two piezoelectric ultrasonic scalers and a hand scaler in vivo. *J Periodontal Res.* 2007;42:90–95.
62. Kawashima H, Sato S, Kishida M, Yagi H, Matsumoto K, Ito K. Treatment of titanium dental implants with three piezoelectric ultrasonic scalers: an in vivo study. *J Periodontol.* 2007;78:1689–1694.
63. Matarasso S, Quaremba G, Coraggio F, Vaia E, Cafiero C, Lang NP. Maintenance of implants: an in vitro study of titanium implant surface modifications subsequent to the application of different prophylaxis procedures. *Clin Oral Implants Res.* 1996;7:64–72.
64. Ruhling A, Kocher T, Kreusch J, Plagmann HC. Treatment of subgingival implant surfaces with Teflon-coated sonic and ultrasonic scaler tips and various implant curettes. An in vitro study. *Clin Oral Implants Res.* 1994;5:19–29.
65. Sato S, Kishida M, Ito K. The comparative effect of ultrasonic scalers on titanium surfaces: an in vitro study. *J Periodontol.* 2004;75:1269–1273.

Module 26

Powered Instrumentation Technique

Module Overview

Electronically powered instrumentation uses rapid energy vibrations of a powered instrument tip to fracture calculus from the tooth surface and clean the environment of the periodontal pocket. This module presents techniques for the use of powered instruments. Module 25, Powered Instrument Design and Function, should be completed before beginning this module.

Module Outline

Key Terms

Transverse tip orientation
Vertical tip orientation
Sweeping motions
Overhang removal

Learning Objectives

1. Identify pretreatment considerations before the initiation of powered instrumentation.
2. Discuss criteria for the selection of powered instrument tips.
3. Prepare a powered device for use.
4. Select appropriate instrument tips for a patient case.
5. Demonstrate correct adaptation of the active portion of a powered instrument tip.
6. Demonstrate correct technique for use of an ultrasonic device, including treatment room and patient preparation, patient/clinician positioning, armamentarium selection/setup, cord management, grasp, fulcrum, tip activation, tip insertion, stroke, and fluid evacuation.
7. Demonstrate the correct amount of stroke pressure and the different strokes used with an electronically powered instrument.

Section I
Fundamental Skills for Powered Instrumentation

As with hand-activated instrumentation, powered instrumentation relies on basic fundamental skills that are essential for success. This section discusses fundamental skills and techniques as they apply to powered instrumentation.

POSITION

- The clinician position used for powered instrumentation is the same as for hand instrumentation.
- Neutral seated or standing position is used throughout powered instrumentation.
- Position the patient in the normal supine position with his or her head turned to one side. The patient's head is positioned to the side so the water flow will pool in the corner of the mouth where it can be evacuated.
  - The patient turns toward the clinician for anterior sextants and posterior aspects facing away from the clinician.
  - The patient turns slightly away from the clinician for posterior aspects facing toward the clinician.

GRASP

- The handpiece is held in a modified pen grasp.
- A light relaxed grasp should be maintained for all powered instrumentation. Because the powered tip does all the work of calculus removal, lateral pressure is not needed to concentrate the force of instrumentation strokes.

FINGER RESTS

- An intraoral or advanced finger rest is critical for control during instrumentation.
- Intraoral fulcrums usually work best for supragingival calculus removal and instrumentation of normal sulci and shallow periodontal pockets.
- Advanced fulcrums are helpful when instrumenting deep periodontal pockets with slim-diameter tips with longer working-ends.

LATERAL PRESSURE

- Light lateral pressure is all that is needed with the powered tip against a calculus deposit or the tooth surface for deplaquing.
- In fact, moderate or firm pressure decreases the effectiveness of the instrument tip and can even stop the tip vibrations all together!
- Effective powered instrumentation requires a light touch. With proper technique, most patients do not feel the tip.

MOTION ACTIVATION

- Digital (finger) activation is recommended because the powered tip does all the work of calculus removal.
- Digital activation is excellent for applying the light stroke pressure needed for powered instrumentation.

ASSESSMENT/END POINT OF INSTRUMENTATION

- With any instrumentation technique, an explorer is still the instrument of choice to evaluate the final clinical end point of calculus removal.
- If the clinic or dental office has an endoscope, the clinician should consider using endoscopic evaluation of the root surface. The endoscope allows the clinician to observe the subgingival root anatomy and residual calculus following instrumentation.

ADAPTATION OF THE POWERED INSTRUMENT TIP

1. **Adaptation of Powered Tip Surfaces to the Tooth Surface.** Clinicians should follow manufacturer's recommendations for instrument tip-to-tooth surface adaptation. In general, the following guidelines should be followed for powered instrumentation.

   a. **The Point and Face of a Powered Tip**
      1. *The point or the face of a powered instrument tip should never be directly adapted to a tooth surface.* These surfaces of the powered tip are identified in Figure 26-1.
      2. Great caution must be taken with the point of the powered tip because not only is the ultrasonic motion high at the point, but also the surface area is very small, concentrating the ultrasonic energy.

   b. **The Back and Lateral Surfaces of a Powered Tip**
      1. The back surface of most ultrasonic and sonic instrument tips can be adapted to the tooth surface, following the recommendations of the tip manufacturer. With a magnetostrictive ultrasonic-powered insert, the back surface is most effective in breaking up calculus deposits.
      2. Adaptation of the lateral surfaces of the working-end is recommended with all sonic, piezoelectric, and magnetostrictive ultrasonic instruments. The lateral surfaces of an ultrasonic powered tip are the most effective for removal of tenacious calculus deposits.
      3. The last 2 to 3 mm of the back or lateral surface—the active portion—must be in contact with the tooth at all times and be adapted so that the point is not directed toward the root or against the soft tissue.

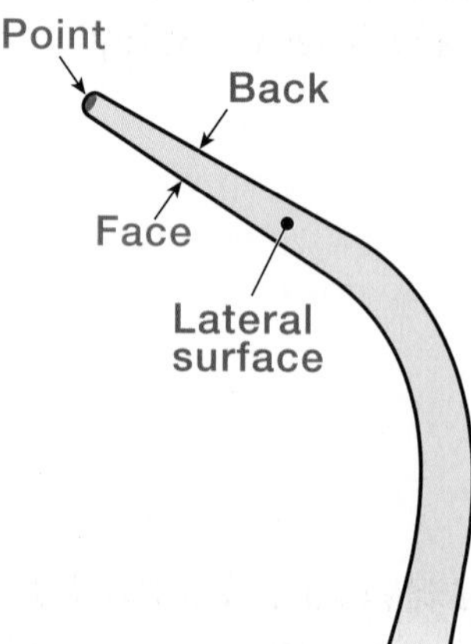

Figure 26-1. Instrument Tip-to-Tooth Surface Adaptation.

- The point or face of a powered instrument tip should not be adapted to the tooth surface.
- The back and lateral surfaces of most ultrasonic and sonic instrument tips are recommended for calculus removal and deplaquing.

2. **Orientation of the Powered Tip to the Tooth Surface.** There are two basic techniques for adapting a straight slim-diameter instrument tip to a tooth.
   - a. Transverse Tip Orientation ("Curet Position")
     1. With the transverse tip orientation, the length of the powered tip is positioned with the back or lateral surface in a transverse orientation—at a right angle—to the long axis of the tooth. This technique is shown in Figures 26-2 and 26-5.
     2. The tip is positioned in a similar manner to the working-end of a curet.
     3. A 0° angulation is maintained between the back surface—or lateral surface—of a powered tip and the tooth surface
     4. *The transverse tip orientation can be used when removing calculus deposits above or slightly below the gingival margin.*
   - b. Vertical Tip Orientation ("Probe Position")
     1. For the vertical tip orientation, the length of the powered tip is positioned with the back or lateral surface in a manner similar to that used with a calibrated periodontal probe. This technique is shown in Figures 26-3, 26-6, and 26-7.
     2. The back or lateral surface of the powered tip is adapted at a 0° angulation to the root surface.
     3. *The vertical tip orientation is used for calculus removal and deplaquing when instrumenting shallow or deep periodontal pockets.*

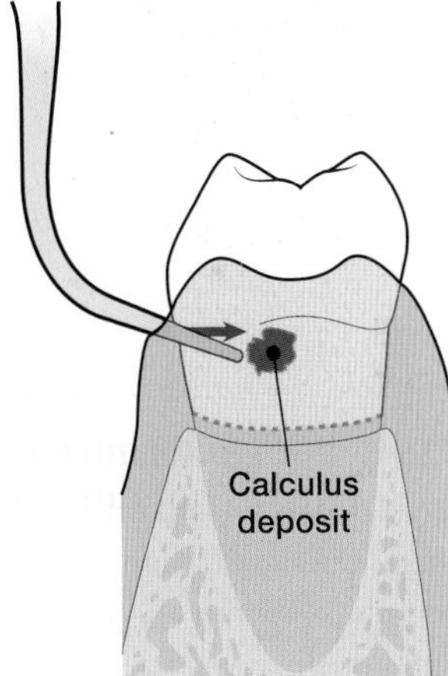

Figure 26-2. Transverse Tip Orientation, the "Curet Position." For a transverse orientation, the powered tip is positioned in a similar manner to a curet with the length of the back surface—or lateral surface—at a right angle to the long axis of the tooth.

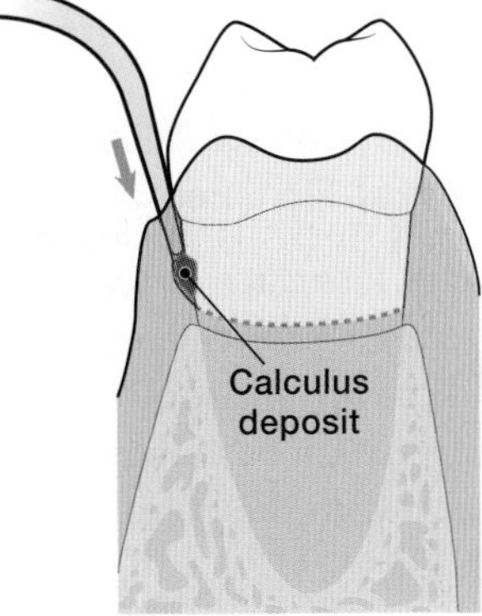

Figure 26-3. Vertical Tip Orientation, the "Probe Position." For a vertical orientation, the powered tip is positioned so the length of the back surface—or lateral surface—is positioned in a manner similar to that of a periodontal probe.

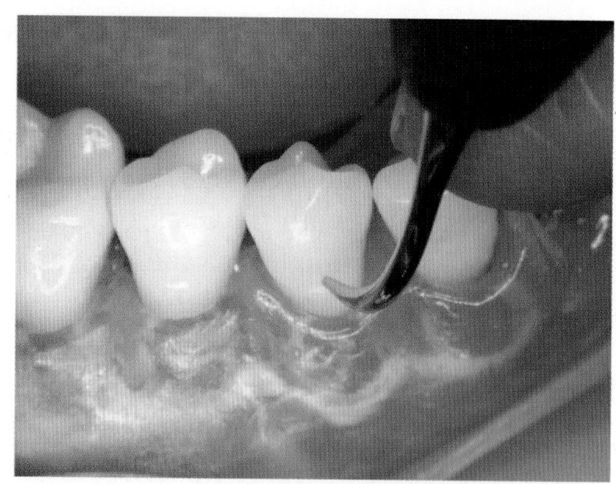

Figure 26-4. Incorrect Adaptation. The point of a powered instrument tip should *NOT* be adapted against a tooth surface. Using a powered tip in this manner can gouge cementum and dentin surfaces.

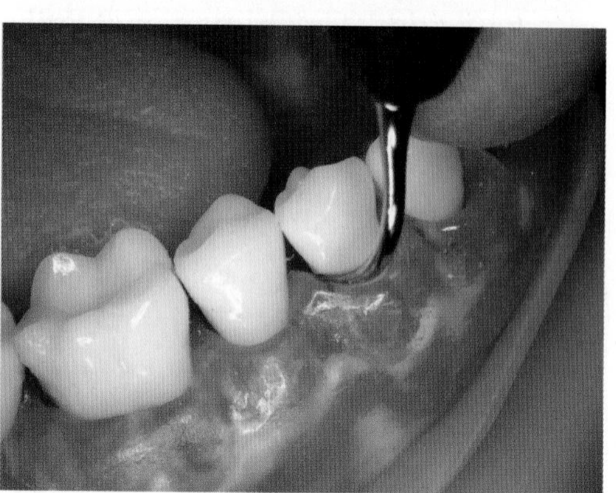

Figure 26-5. Correct Adaptation of Lateral Surface in a Transverse Tip Orientation. The photo shows correct adaptation of a lateral surface to the distal surface of the first premolar in a transverse tip orientation (similar to a curet).

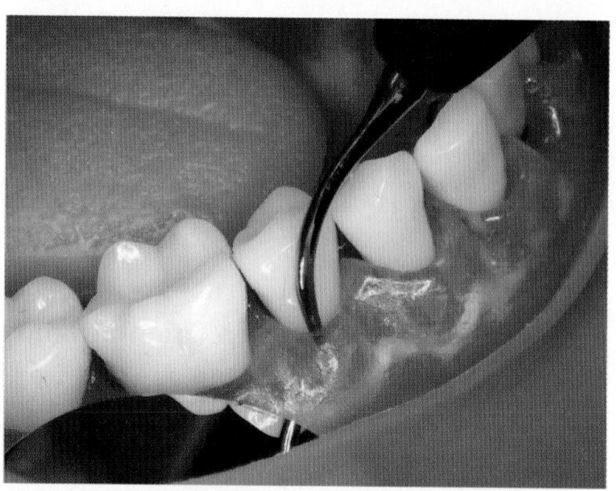

Figure 26-6. Correct Adaptation of a Lateral Surface in a Vertical Tip Orientation. A powered tip can be positioned in a similar manner to that of a calibrated periodontal probe with the length of a lateral surface against the tooth surface to be treated.

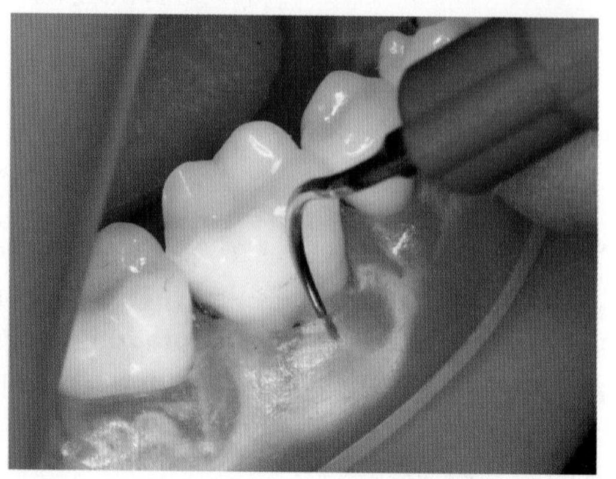

Figure 26-7. Correct Adaptation of the Back Surface in a Vertical Tip Orientation.

- The back surface of the powered tip is oriented correctly when its curvature (convex side) is in contact with the tooth surface to be instrumented.
- In this position, damage caused by hitting the root surface with the point of the powered tip can be avoided.

ANGULATION OF A POWERED TIP

- The tip-to-tooth surface angulation should be as close to 0° as possible and should never exceed 15°. So for example, when using the back of the powered tip, the back-to-tooth surface angulation should be as close to 0° as possible.[1,2]
- If the powered insert is used at an angulation greater than 15° to the root surface, the root surface will be gouged.

APPROACH TO CALCULUS REMOVAL

The technique used for calculus removal with a powered instrument tip is very different from that used with hand instruments.[3]

1. Calculus Removal Technique with a Curet

a. A curet—such as a Gracey extended shank curet—must be ***positioned apical to (below) the calculus deposit***—starting at the base of the pocket and working toward the cementoenamel junction (CEJ).

b. To be effective, the curet must be adapted at the proper angulation.

2. Calculus Removal with a Powered Instrument

a. A powered instrument tip works from the ***top of the deposit downward***—starting near the CEJ and working toward the base of the pocket.

b. There is no need to position the tip beneath the deposit. This is a great advantage when working in deep periodontal pockets. Figure 26-8 shows the technique used with a powered instrument tip and a hand-activated curet.

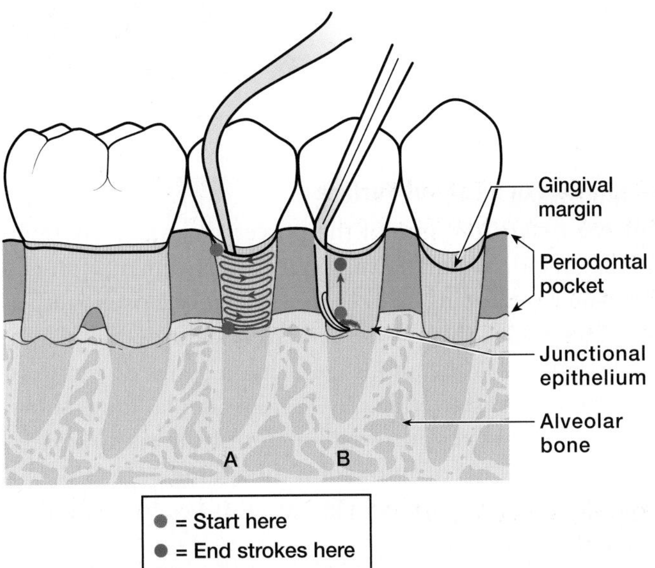

Figure 26-8. Different Techniques with a Powered Instrument Tip and a Hand-Activated Instrument.

A. Subgingival Calculus Removal with a Powered Instrument Tip. Calculus removal with a powered instrument tip takes place from the top of the deposit downward.

B. Subgingival Calculus Removal with a Curet. Calculus removal with a curet takes place from the base of the pocket upward toward the CEJ. Often, it is difficult to position the curet under calculus deposits near the base of the pocket.

MOVING THE INSTRUMENT TIP

1. Strokes for Calculus Removal

a. Powered instrument tips break up heavy calculus deposits by putting little microfractures in the deposit. ***The powered tip needs to be moved over the surface of a deposit for some time in order to allow the microfractures to develop. Slower, repetitive strokes are more effective in removing large or tenacious calculus deposits.***
b. The powered instrument tip should be kept moving at all times for effective debridement and patient comfort.
c. Overlapping vertical or oblique strokes are most effective for calculus removal. This overlapping stroke is always made with light pressure.
d. ***Horizontal sweeping strokes should be kept to a minimum during calculus removal because they tend to burnish the calculus until it is a smooth veneer on the root rather than remove it.***

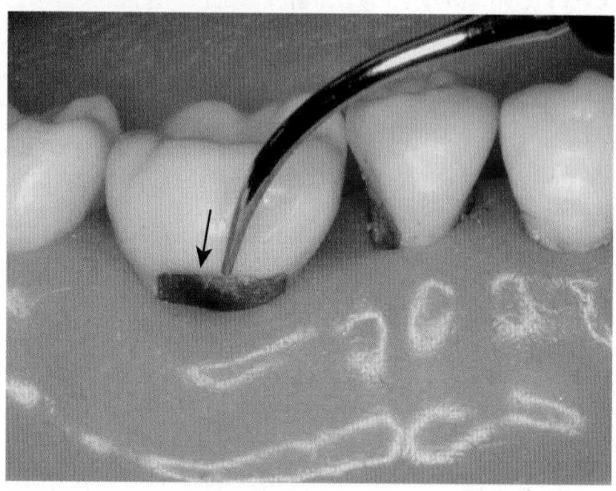

Figure 26-9. Motions for Calculus Removal.

- The first 2 to 4 mm of a powered tip are adapted to the coronal-most portion of the calculus deposit.
- ***The active portion of the lateral surface or back is moved against the coronal-most portion of the deposit in a series of light vertical or oblique push strokes.***
- Only gentle pressure is needed. Firm pressure greatly reduces the effectiveness of the instrument.

2. Strokes for Plaque Biofilm Removal

a. Technique for Deplaquing

1. Because only the first 2 to 4 mm of the powered tip actively remove the biofilm, thorough and systematic subgingival instrumentation is of great importance.[3] The overlapping strokes must be very close together in periodontal maintenance therapy to effectively debride the plaque biofilm.
2. Subgingival deplaquing is accomplished using a series of gentle sweeping motions over the root surface (Fig. 26-10). For deplaquing, short, overlapping strokes should cover every millimeter of the root surface using strokes in vertical, oblique, or horizontal directions.
3. The powered tip should be kept moving at all times for effective debridement and patient comfort.
4. The overlapping strokes can be a little faster than with hand-activated instrumentation because the purpose of debridement in periodontal maintenance therapy is to remove biofilm and lighter, newly formed calculus deposits.[4]
5. For biofilm removal, unnecessary loss of cementum from the root's surface should be avoided as much as possible by applying light force and selecting a lower power setting.[1–3]

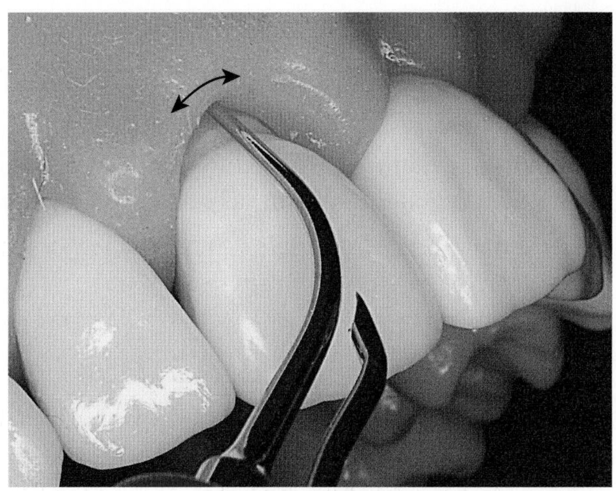

Figure 26-10. Sweeping Motions for Deplaquing.

- For subgingival deplaquing, a lateral surface or the back of the tip is adapted to the tooth surface and moved in a series of sweeping motions.
- It may be helpful for the clinician to imagine using the side of a crayon (rather than the point) to color the entire root surface (Box 26-1).

Box 26-1. Moving the Instrument Tip in Sweeping Motions

When using a powered instrument tip, imagine that the tip is a crayon. Your goal is to gently color the entire root surface using the ***side of a crayon tip***—rather than the point.

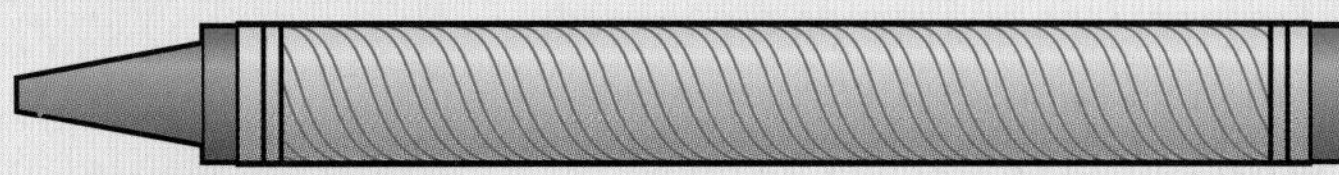

b. Deplaquing of Shallow Sulci: Is It Necessary?

1. Shallow sulci that are 3 mm or smaller and that are clinically normal with no inflammation and no detectable calculus may not require any instrumentation at all.
2. A systematic review of scaling and root planing outcomes clearly demonstrates that instrumentation of initially shallow sites (sulci) may cause attachment loss.[5]
3. *Normal sulci in the absence of inflammation are likely colonized by beneficial flora and need not be deplaqued.*

c. Deplaquing of Periodontal Pockets: Why Is It important?

1. Periodontal health cannot be achieved without the periodic removal or disruption of established plaque biofilm.[6]
2. Pathogenic plaque biofilms, which are found mainly in deep pockets (4 mm or greater), are highly resistant to antimicrobial agents and systemic antibiotics.[7,8] The only way to totally disrupt the biofilm is through mechanical removal.
3. Control of bacteria in dental plaque biofilms is best achieved by the physical disruption of plaque.[9] It is critical to cover every square millimeter of the root surface within a periodontal pocket with continuous, closely spaced, methodical overlapping strokes to mechanically disrupt and remove the plaque biofilm colonies. Ultrasonic instrumentation under low power is sufficient to accomplish this task.

Section 2
Use of Standard Tips for Calculus Removal

Standard-diameter tips are used for removal of medium-to-heavy calculus deposits. Standard tips are used on coronal tooth surfaces and for subgingival deposits easily accessed without undue tissue stretching.

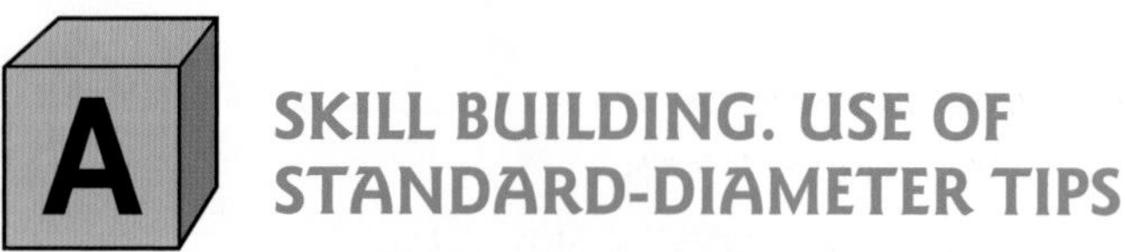

SKILL BUILDING. USE OF STANDARD-DIAMETER TIPS

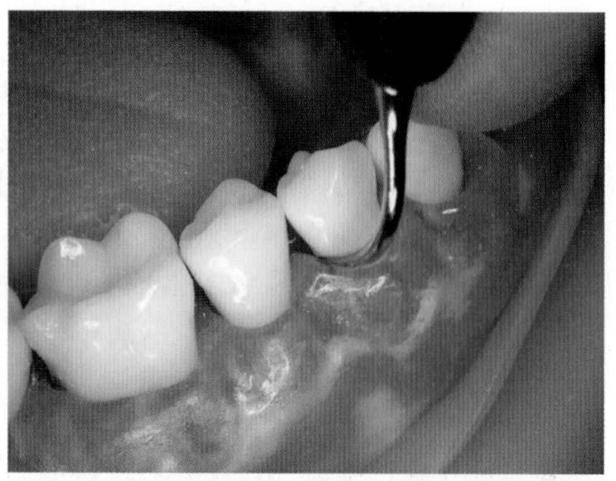

Figure 26-11. The Lateral Surface of a Standard Tip Adapted to a Proximal Surface. Use of a standard powered tip in a transverse (curetlike) orientation. A lateral surface of the tip is adapted to the distal surface of the first premolar for removal of a supragingival deposit.

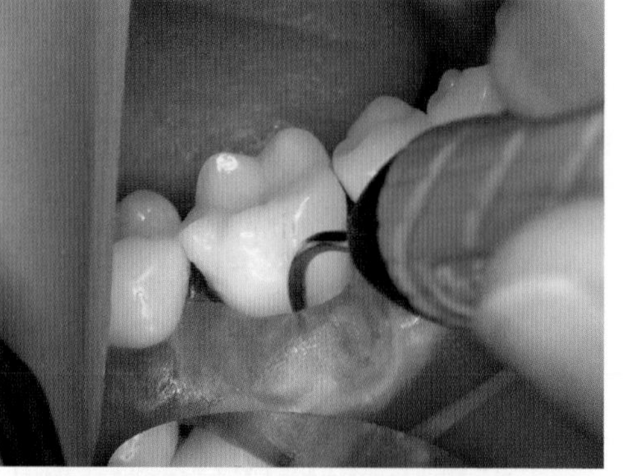

Figure 26-12. Lateral Surface Adapted to Facial Surface. Use of a vertical (probelike) orientation of a standard powered tip to the facial surface of a mandibular first molar tooth.

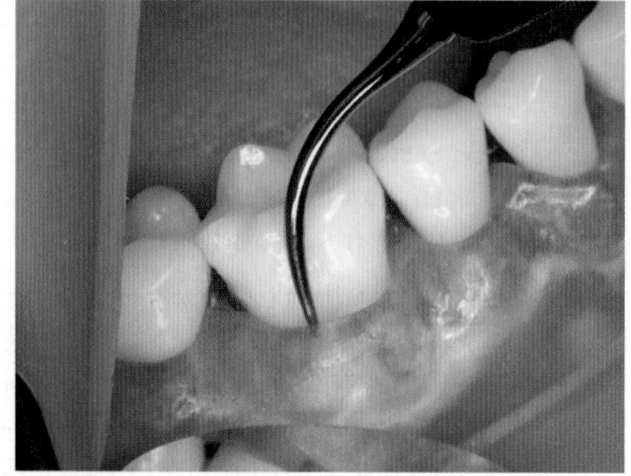

Figure 26-13. Lateral Surface Adapted to a Facial Surface. Adaptation of the lateral surface in a vertical (probelike) orientation is effective for calculus removal on facial or lingual surfaces.

REMOVING STUBBORN CALCULUS DEPOSITS

A common misconception among clinicians who are new to powered instrumentation is the belief that a single quick tap against a deposit will remove it. Powered instruments are very effective at removing calculus deposits, but they are not magic wands. Adequate time must be spent on a deposit to remove it. A calculus deposit will not vanish in a single stroke, but rather, the deposit will develop microfractures as it is exposed to the powered tip during a series of gentle strokes.

Effective strategies for removing stubborn calculus deposits include:

1. **Select the Proper Tip for the Task.** As with hand instruments, the instrument tip is selected based on the size and location of the calculus deposit.
   a. **Standard-Diameter Tips.** Use standard-diameter tips to remove moderate-to-heavy deposits above the gingival margin and in shallow pockets.
   b. **Straight Slim-Diameter Tips.** Use straight slim-diameter tips to remove light-to-moderate calculus deposits on anterior teeth and on posterior root surfaces up to 4 mm below the CEJ.
   c. **Curved Slim-Diameter Tips.** Use curved right and left slim-diameter tips to remove light-to-moderate calculus deposits on posterior root surfaces greater than 4 mm below the CEJ.
2. **Use a Tip That Can Withstand Medium Power.** Low power will not be effective in removing tenacious calculus deposits. The tip selected should be large enough to withstand a medium-power setting. Some powered tips are specially designed to withstand a high-power setting.
3. **Maintain Proper Control and Adaptation.** It is important to control the movement of the powered tip so that the 2- to 4-mm active tip area is adapted to the calculus deposit and many overlapping strokes cover each section of the deposit. Systematically remove the calculus in a horizontal zone a few millimeters down from the coronal-most edge. Repeat the process to remove the deposit in a series of horizontal zones.
4. **Attack the Deposit from All Directions.** Approach a deposit from a variety of directions. For example, interproximal deposits can be approached from both the facial and lingual aspects. Vertical and oblique strokes are most effective for medium calculus deposits. Horizontal strokes work well for deplaquing.
5. **Use the Correct Surface of the Powered Tip.** With a magnetostrictive powered tip, the back surface works best for removing heavy or moderate calculus deposits because this surface produces more energy vibrations. The lateral surfaces of a piezoelectric powered tip produce more energy and, therefore, are most effective in removing large or tenacious deposits.
6. **Change to a Different Tip.** Smooth powered tips that are round in cross section are less effective in removing stubborn calculus deposits. Larger tips with beveled edges or a straight edge with a corner perform better for removing heavy deposits.
7. **Begin with a Periodontal File.** Sometimes, it is most effective to use a hand-activated periodontal file to fracture a tenacious deposit and follow with a powered instrument tip.
8. **Increase the Power.** If all the above strategies fail to remove the deposit, it will be necessary to increase the power setting. In this instance, it would be best to use one of the powered tips that are specially designed to withstand a high-power setting, such as the Burnett Power-Tip by Parkell, Inc. (Fig. 26-14) or Dentsply's Cavitron ThinSert tip.

SMOOTHING AMALGAM OVERHANGS

Overhang removal is a recontouring procedure used to correct defective margins of restorations to provide a smooth surface that will deter bacterial accumulation. If a minor amalgam overhang is acting as a plaque biofilm trap, the excess amalgam can be removed using a specialized powered instrument tip for this purpose. The Burnett Power-Tip—from Parkell USA and designed by Dr. Larry Burnett of Portland, Oregon—is a unique slim-diameter tip that can withstand higher power settings and more lateral pressure than a conventional slim-diameter tip (Fig. 26-14). This tip is recommended for removal of tenacious calculus deposits, smoothing of amalgam overhangs, and removing orthodontic cement. The Burnett Power-Tip is ideal for smoothing overhanging amalgam restorations (Figs. 26-15 and 26-16). A conventional slim-diameter tip is not recommended for smoothing amalgam overhangs.

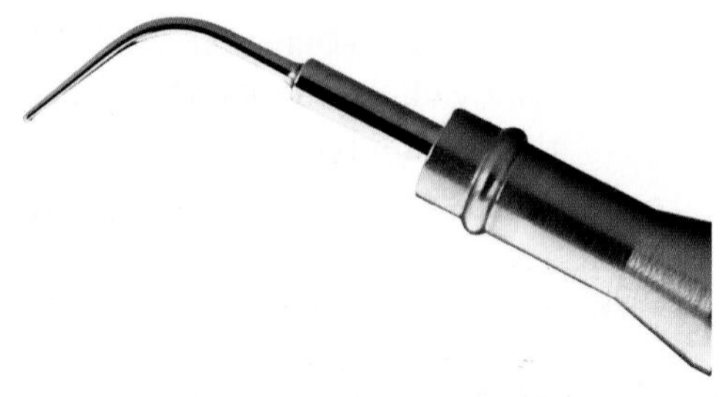

Figure 26-14. The Burnett Power-Tip. The Burnett Power-Tip is a unique slim-diameter tip that can withstand higher power settings and more lateral pressure than the typical slim-diameter tip. (Photograph courtesy of Parkell, Inc.)

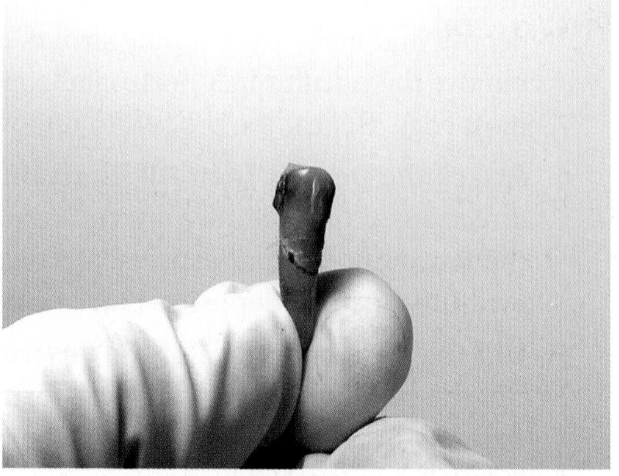

Figure 26-15. Amalgam Overhang. This tooth has an excess of amalgam protruding out from the surface of the tooth. If this tooth were still in the mouth, the amalgam overhang would retain plaque biofilm.

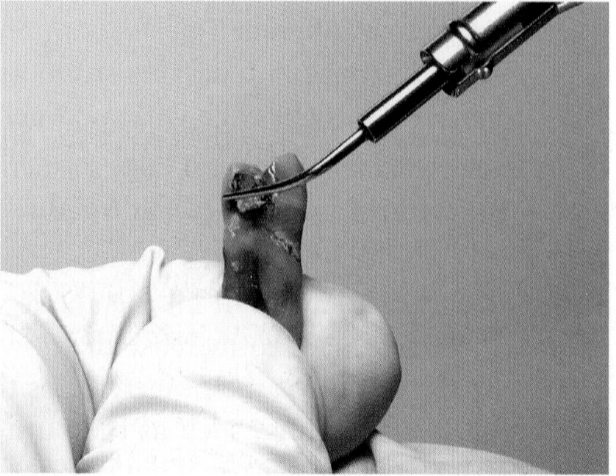

Figure 26-16. Smoothing the Overhang. The Burnett Power-Tip is placed apical to (below) the amalgam protuberance. Position the instrument tip in an oblique orientation to the tooth surface. Move the tip up and down over the amalgam protuberance to shave the amalgam surface. More lateral pressure than is normally used for powered instrumentation will be required for smoothing the amalgam. The goal is to have the amalgam restoration level with the root surface.

Section 3
Use of the Straight Slim-Diameter Tip

DESIGN CHARACTERISTICS OF THE SLIM-DIAMETER TIPS

Slim-diameter tips come in a set of three tips or inserts (Fig. 26-17). Use of all three slim-diameter tips is recommended to ensure that all areas of the root are thoroughly instrumented.

- The straight slim-diameter tip (Fig. 26-18) is used for anterior root surfaces and posterior root surfaces that are 4 mm or less apical to (below) the CEJ.
- The right- and left-curved slim-diameter tips are used for posterior root surfaces located more than 4 mm apical to the CEJ and root concavities and furcation areas on posterior tooth (Fig. 26-19).
- Slim-diameter tips are especially effective in reducing spirochetes and motile rods in class II and III furcations.[10]

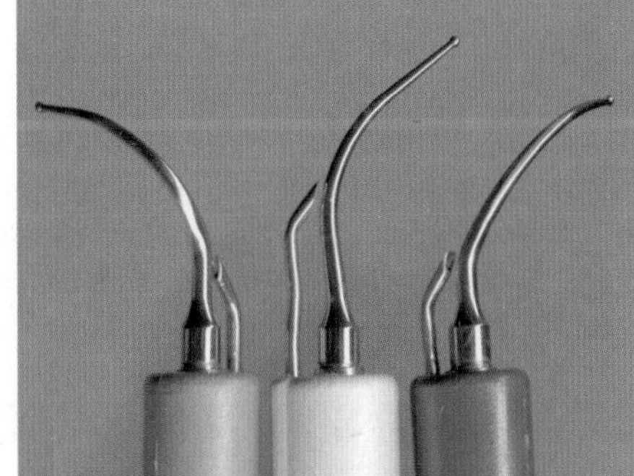

Figure 26-17. Set of Slim-Diameter Tips. Slim-diameter tips come in a set of three tips: a straight tip, a right-curved tip, and a left-curved tip.

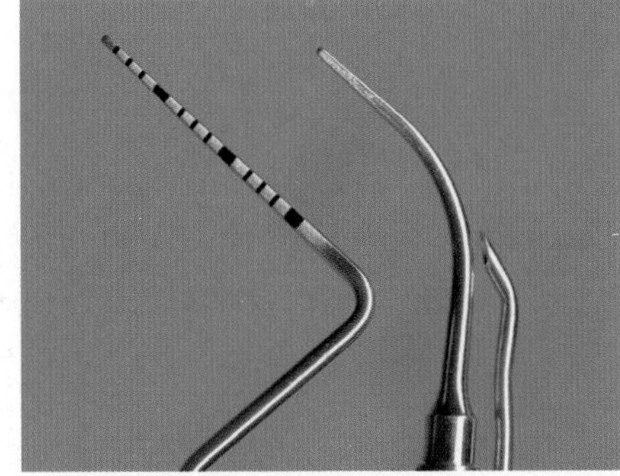

Figure 26-18. Straight Slim-Diameter Tip.

- The photograph shows a periodontal probe and a straight slim-diameter powered tip. Note that the working-ends of these two instruments are very similar in design.
- Straight slim-diameter powered tips are designed for use on anterior root surfaces and posterior root surfaces that are 4 mm or less apical to (below) the CEJ.

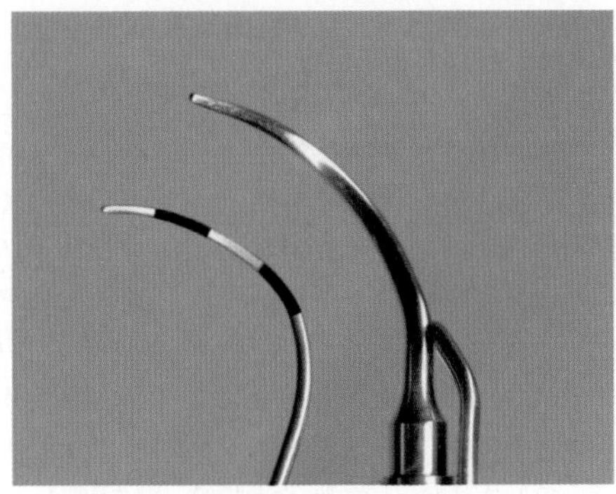

Figure 26-19. Curved Slim-Diameter Tips.

- The photograph shows a curved furcation probe and a curved slim-diameter powered tip.
- Curved slim-diameter tips are designed for use on posterior root surfaces located more than 4 mm apical to the CEJ.
- Curved tips adapt well to root curvatures, concavities, and furcation areas and reach calculus deposits under the contact areas of posterior teeth.

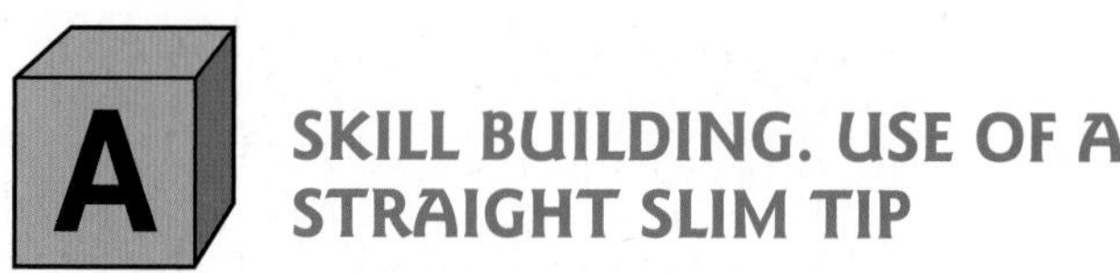

SKILL BUILDING. USE OF A STRAIGHT SLIM TIP

1. Use of Straight Slim-Diameter Tip on Anterior Teeth

- The straight slim-diameter instrument tip can be used on all surfaces of an anterior tooth.
- Because the roots of anterior teeth are not highly curved, the straight slim-diameter tip is effective for calculus removal even in deep periodontal pockets on anterior teeth.
- The straight tip can be used with either a vertical—probelike—orientation or a transverse—curetlike—orientation on the anterior tooth surfaces.

2. Use of Straight Slim-Diameter Tip on Posterior Teeth

- On posterior teeth, the straight slim-diameter instrument tip is recommended for use on root surfaces located 4 mm or less below the CEJ.
- Because the straight tip does not adapt well to root curvatures and concavities, the slim tip is reserved for use in normal sulci and shallow periodontal pockets on posterior teeth.
- The straight tip can be used with either a vertical or transverse orientation on the posterior tooth surfaces.

STRAIGHT SLIM TIP—VERTICAL ORIENTATION

Because the roots of these teeth are not highly curved, the straight slim-diameter tip is effective for calculus removal even in deep periodontal pockets.

STRAIGHT SLIM TIP—TRANSVERSE ORIENTATION ON ANTERIORS

The transverse—curetlike—orientation is effective for removing calculus deposits located above or slightly below the gingival margin on the mesial and distal tooth surfaces of anterior teeth.

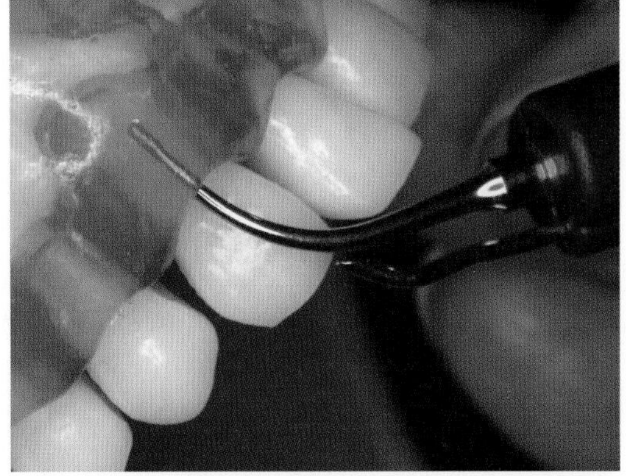

Figure 26-20. Vertical Orientation—with Lateral Surface of Tip. This photograph shows a straight slim tip positioned in a similar manner to a periodontal probe with the lateral surface against the root surface being debrided.

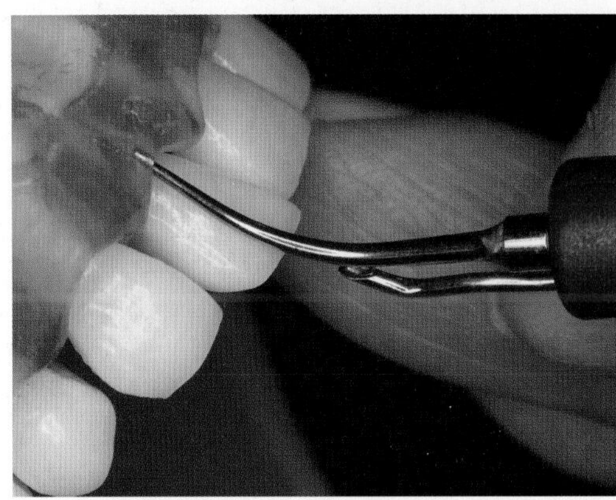

Figure 26-21. Vertical Orientation—with Back Surface of Tip. The back surface of a slim-diameter powered tip adapted to the facial surface of an anterior tooth.

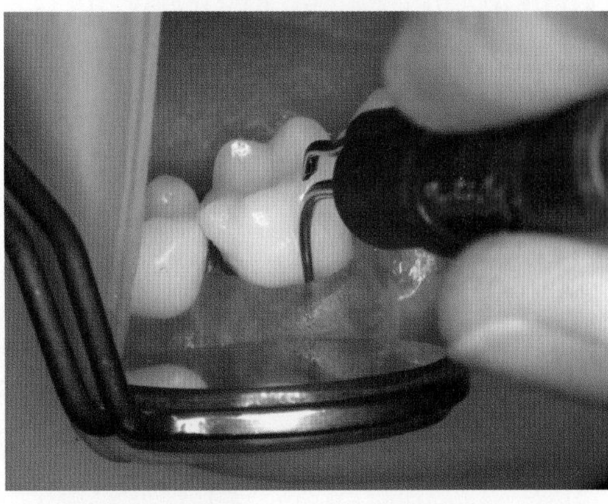

Figure 26-22. Vertical Orientation on a Posterior Tooth. On posterior teeth, the straight slim-diameter instrument tip is recommended for use on facial and lingual root surfaces located 4 mm or less below the CEJ.

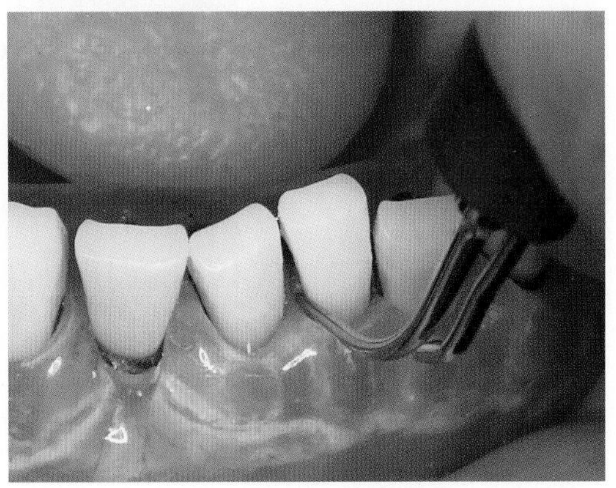

Figure 26-23. Transverse Orientation on an Anterior Tooth. The transverse, curetlike, orientation is very effective on proximal tooth surfaces to remove calculus deposits located beneath the contact areas.

Section 4
Use of the Curved Slim-Diameter Tips

The right- and left-curved powered tips are used for root surfaces located more than 4 mm below the CEJ. The back surface of these curved tips adapt well to the curved root surfaces of the posterior teeth.

- Curved tips come in right and left styles, and both tips are needed to instrument the entire dentition.
- Instrumentation is accomplished most efficiently by completing all surfaces with the right instrument tip before switching to the left instrument tip. For example, the clinician can use the right tip in a transverse orientation on the proximal tooth surfaces to remove deposits above and slightly below the gingival margin. Next, the right tip can be used in a vertical orientation for subgingival debridement of deep periodontal pockets.

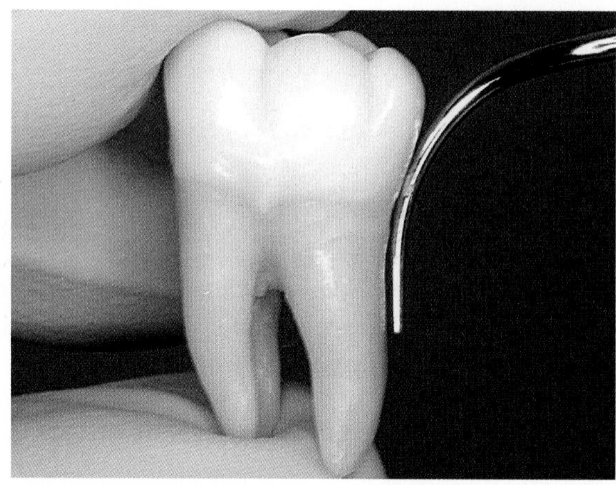

Figure 26-24. Curved Slim-Diameter Tips. Curved instrument tips were designed to facilitate adaptation to the curved root surfaces of posterior teeth. The back of the working-end adapts best to the curved root surfaces.

TIP IDENTIFICATION OF CURVED SLIM TIPS

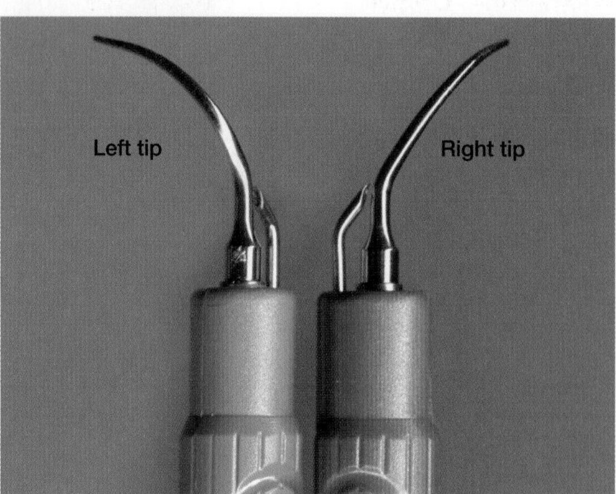

Figure 26-25. Identifying the Right- and Left-Curved Slim-Diameter Tips. A curved tip is identified as right or left by turning the insert so the point faces away from the clinician (with the back toward the clinician). With the insert in this position, the direction that a tip bends identifies it as a right or left tip. ***The terms "right" and "left" refer only to the bend in the design, not to a location for use in the mouth.***

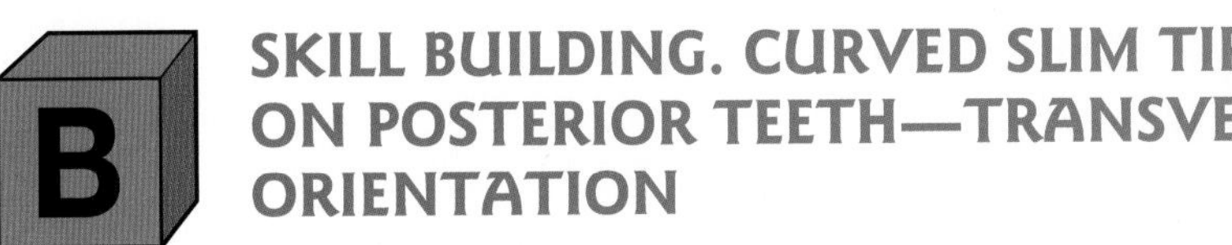

SKILL BUILDING. CURVED SLIM TIPS ON POSTERIOR TEETH—TRANSVERSE ORIENTATION

The curved slim tips can be used with the transverse (curetlike) orientation to remove calculus deposits above and slightly beneath the gingival margin from the mesial and distal surfaces of posterior teeth.

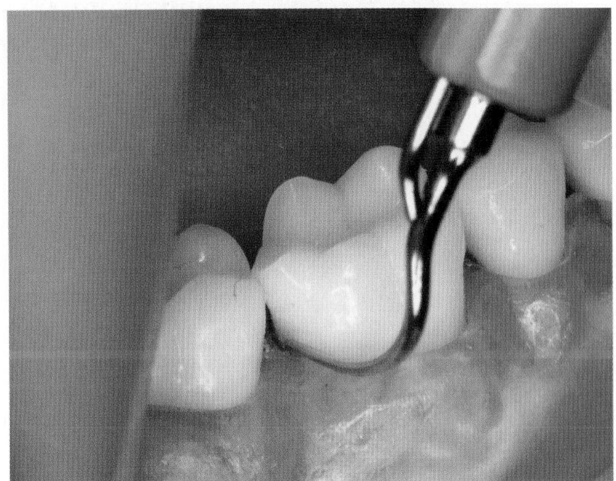

Figure 26-26. Transverse Orientation.

- Curved slim tips can be adapted to the mesial and distal surfaces using a transverse, curetlike, orientation.
- The transverse orientation of the instrument tip is excellent for removing deposits apical to the contact area and deposits in the area of the CEJ.

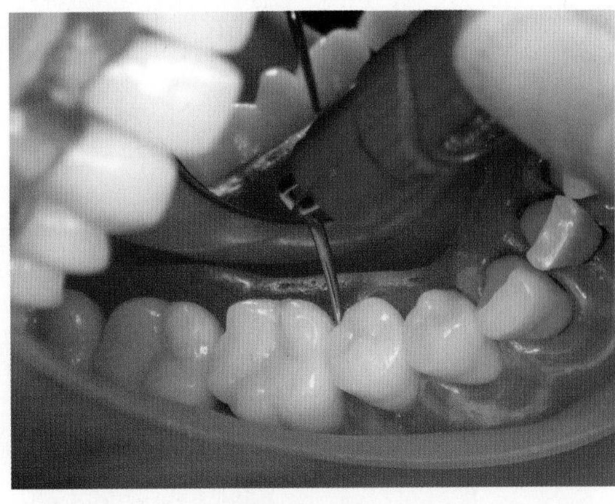

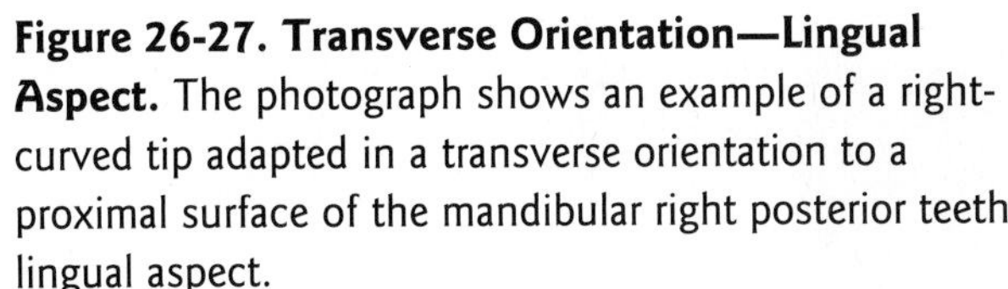

Figure 26-27. Transverse Orientation—Lingual Aspect. The photograph shows an example of a right-curved tip adapted in a transverse orientation to a proximal surface of the mandibular right posterior teeth, lingual aspect.

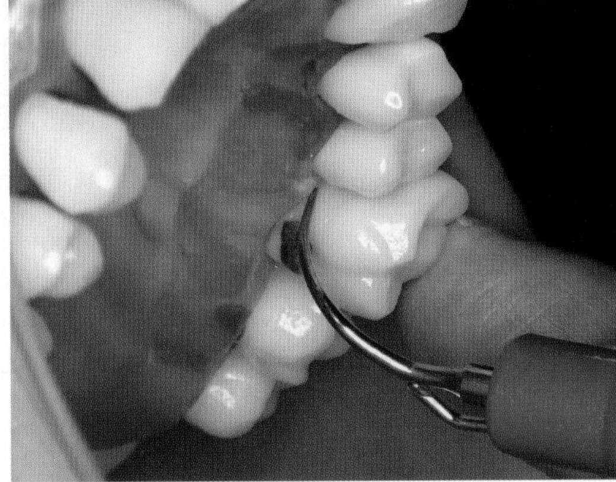

Figure 26-28. Transverse Orientation—Lingual Aspect. The photograph shows a right-curved tip adapted in a transverse orientation to the mesial surface of a maxillary first molar.

EFFICIENT SEQUENCE FOR USE OF TIPS IN A TRANSVERSE ORIENTATION

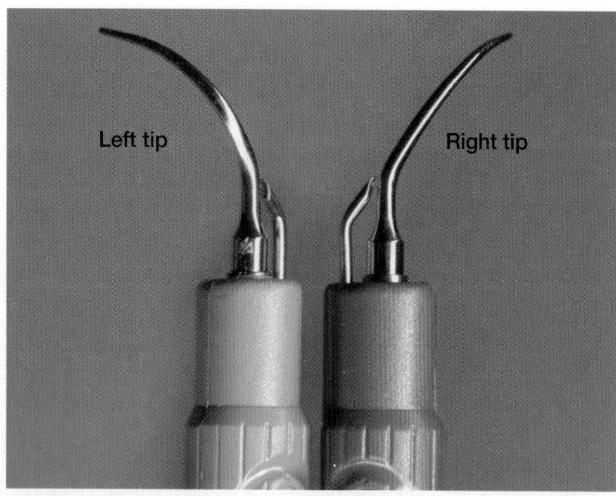

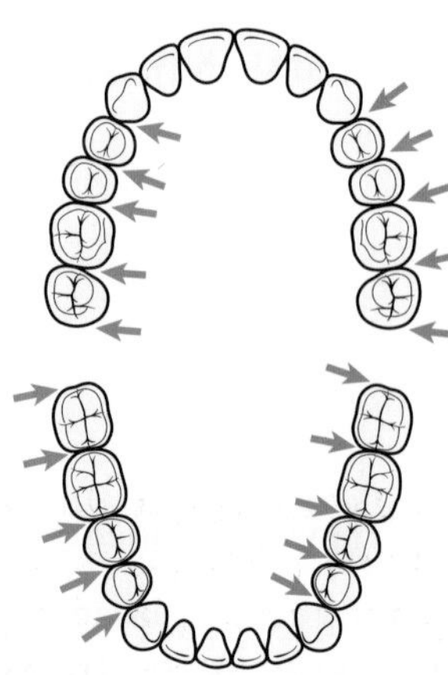

Figure 26-29. Use of the Left Tip in a Transverse Orientation.

- The photograph shows a set of right- and left-curved slim-diameter tips.
- On the illustration, the proximal surfaces indicated by the teal arrows can be debrided with the left slim-diameter tip using a transverse—curetlike—orientation. In this position, the tip can remove calculus deposits located above and slightly below the gingival margin.

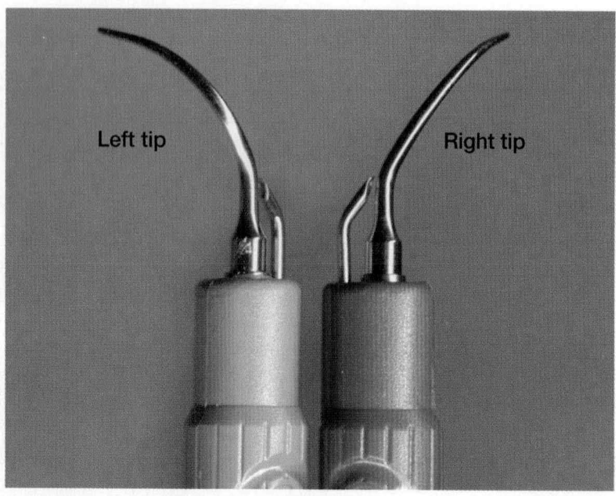

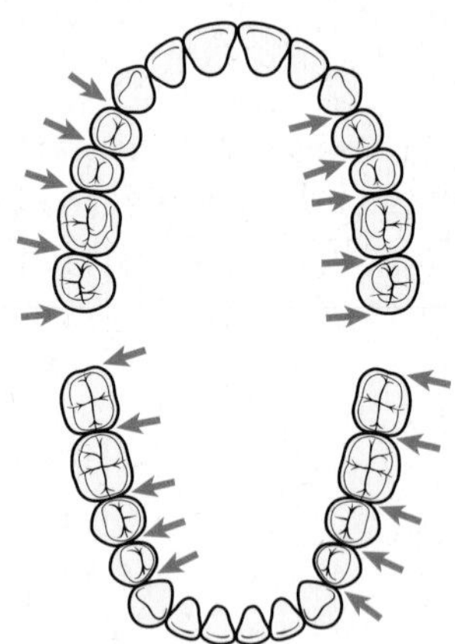

Figure 26-30. Use of the Right Tip in a Transverse Orientation.

- The photograph shows a set of right- and left-curved slim-diameter tips.
- On the illustration, the proximal surfaces indicated by the red arrows can be debrided with the right slim-diameter tip using a transverse—curetlike—orientation. In this position, the tip can remove calculus deposits located above and slightly below the gingival margin.

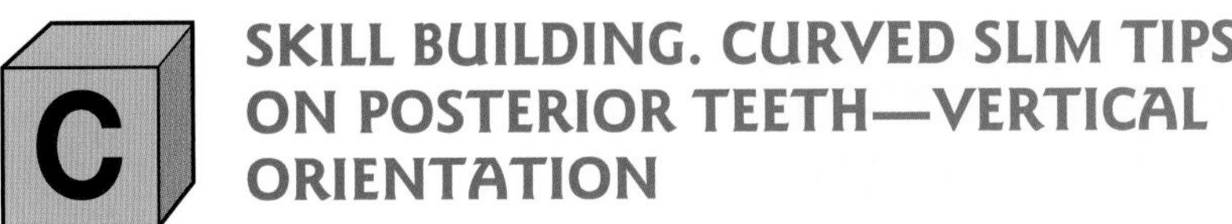

C SKILL BUILDING. CURVED SLIM TIPS ON POSTERIOR TEETH—VERTICAL ORIENTATION

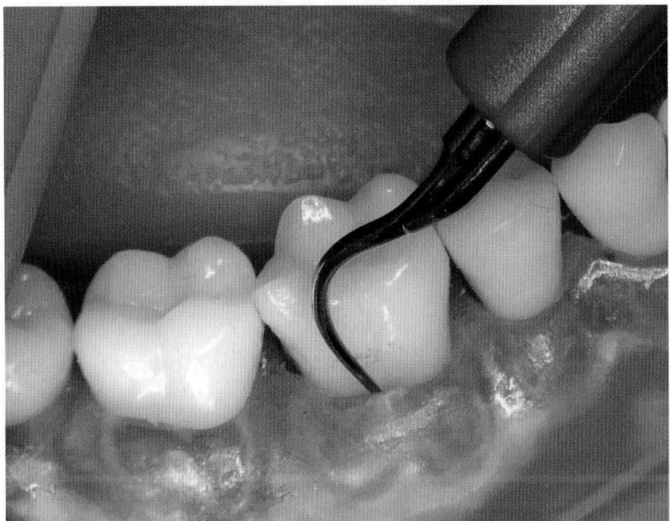

Figure 26-31. Vertical Orientation—with Lateral Surface. This photograph shows a curved slim tip positioned in a similar manner to a periodontal probe with the lateral surface against the tooth surface being debrided.

The back of a curved slim tip is very effective for debridement of the mesial surface of the root. The photographs in Figure 26-32 depict an efficient sequence for instrumentation inserting the tip at the mesiofacial line angle and moving back to the facial surface.

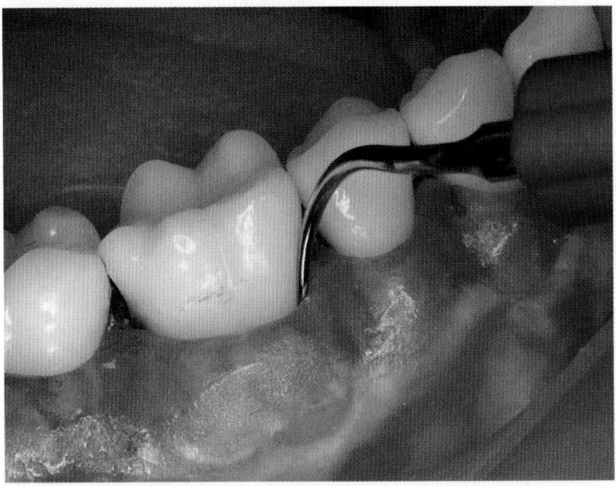

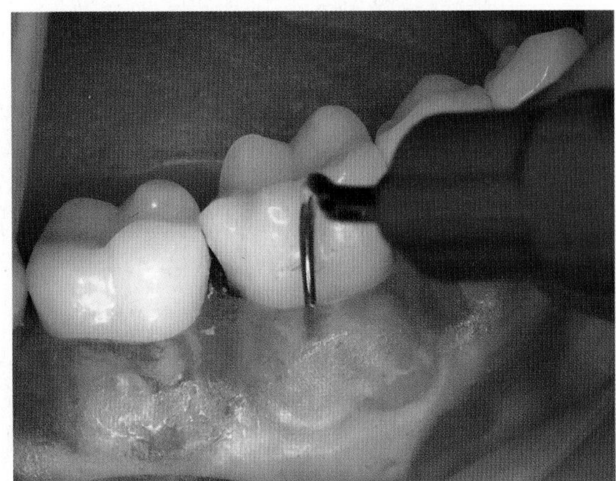

Figure 26-32. Adaptation of the Back of a Curved Tip.

- Insert the tip with the back surface against the mesial surface of the molar tooth.
- After instrumenting the mesial proximal surface, move the back onto the facial surface of the molar to debride this surface.

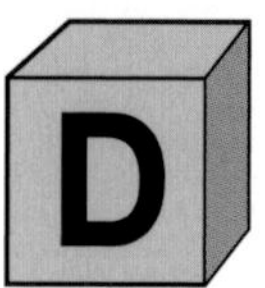

SKILL BUILDING. CURVED SLIM TIPS—VERTICAL ORIENTATION: CROSS ARCH FULCRUM FOR LINGUAL ASPECTS

The best adaptation to the lingual aspect of the mandibular and maxillary posterior teeth is achieved by adapting the back of the working-end to the tooth surface being treated. It can be difficult to adapt the back of the working-end to the lingual surfaces using a standard fulcrum. A cross arch fulcrum on the opposite side of the arch from the treatment area allows adaptation of the back of the instrument tip to the lingual aspects of the mandibular and maxillary arches.

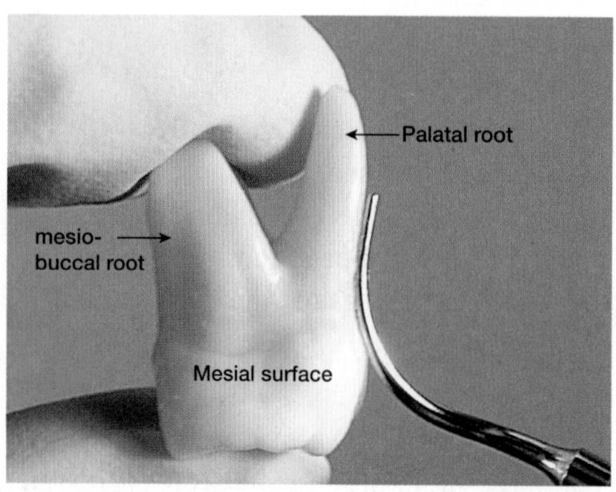

Figure 26-33. Palatal Roots of Maxillary Molars.

- On maxillary molars, the palatal root curves in a lingual direction.
- For this reason, the back surface of a curved slim tip adapts well to the palatal root.
- Use of a cross arch fulcrum facilitates adaptation of the back surface of a powered tip to the lingual aspect of the molar teeth.

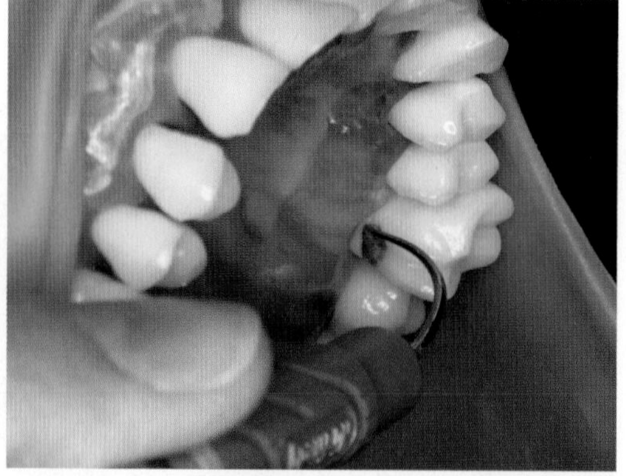

Figure 26-34. Cross Arch Fulcrum for the Lingual Aspects of the Maxillary Arch.

- The photo shows a cross arch fulcrum with the finger rest on the maxillary right posterior sextant.
- This cross arch fulcrum facilitates adaptation of the back surface of the tip to the lingual aspect of the maxillary left first molar tooth.

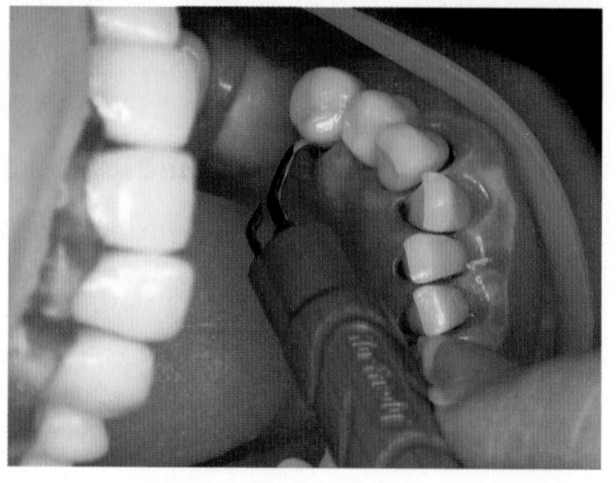

Figure 26-35. Cross Arch Fulcrum for the Lingual Aspects of the Mandibular Arch.

- In this example, a cross arch fulcrum is established on the mandibular anteriors.
- The powered tip is adapted in a vertical orientation to the lingual surface of the second premolar tooth.

EFFICIENT SEQUENCE FOR USE OF TIPS IN A VERTICAL ORIENTATION

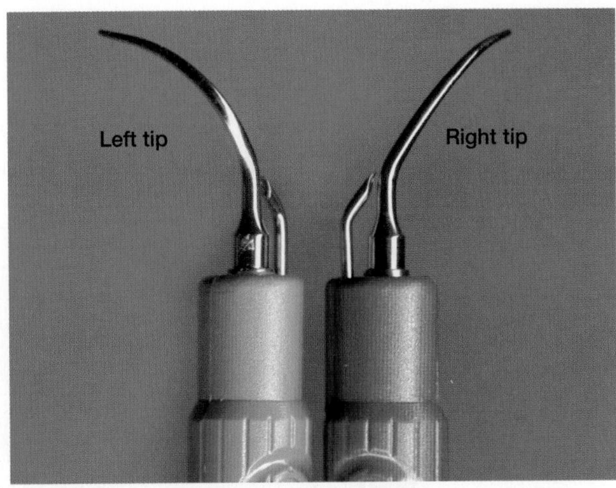

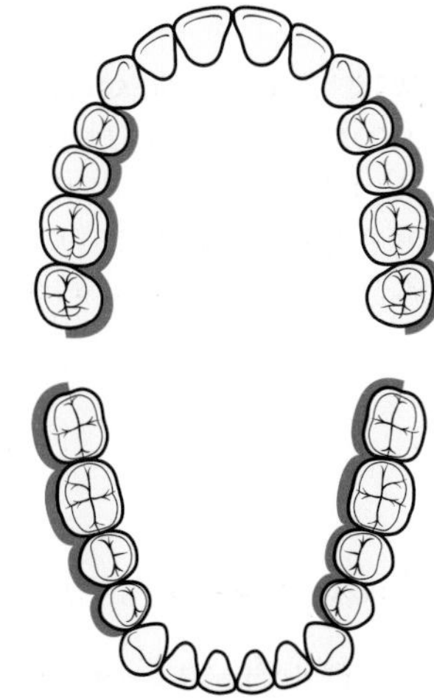

Figure 26-36. Utilization of a Right-Curved Tip.

- The photograph shows a set of right- and left-curved slim-diameter tips.
- On the illustration, the red line indicates the tooth surfaces that can be instrumented using the right-curved slim-diameter tip using a vertical—probelike—orientation.

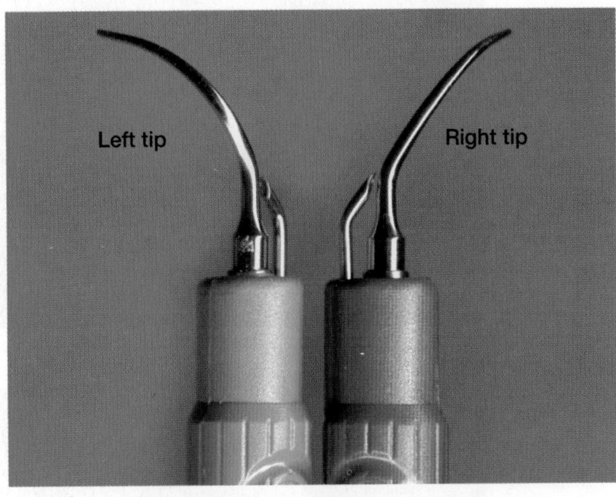

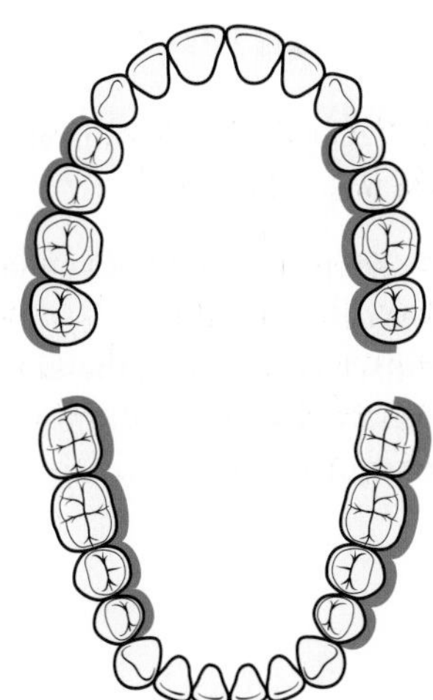

Figure 26-37. Utilization of a Left-Curved Tip.

- The photograph shows a set of right- and left-curved slim-diameter tips.
- On the illustration, the teal line indicates the tooth surfaces that can be instrumented using the left-curved slim-diameter tip using a vertical—probelike—orientation.

E SKILL BUILDING. CURVED SLIM TIPS—ACCESSING A FURCATION

Some manufacturers produce specialized powered tips with ball-tipped working-ends for use in the furcation areas of multirooted teeth.

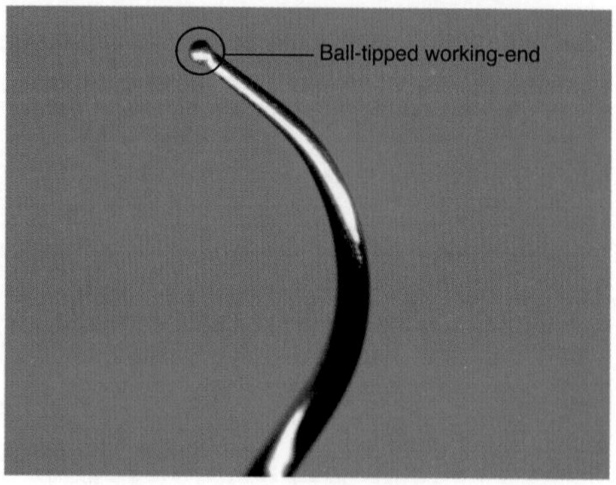

Figure 26-38. Ball-End Slim-Diameter Furcation Tip.

- Some slim furcation tips have a ball-end design.
- Furcation tips come in straight, right, and left designs.

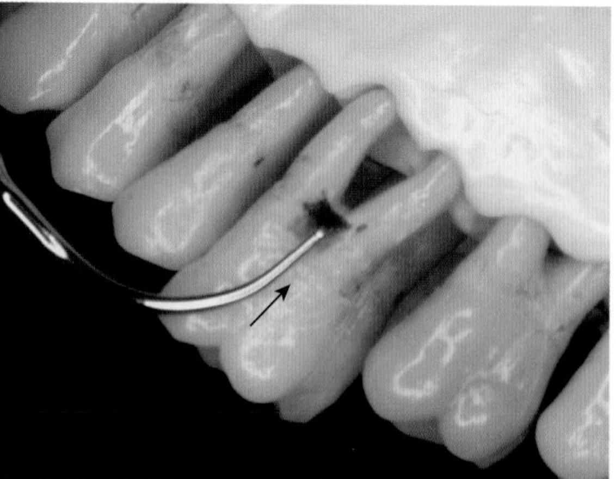

Figure 26-39. Locating a Furcation.

- The easiest way to locate the furcation area is to ***deactivate*** the powered tip (remove foot from foot pedal). Use of a deactivated instrument tip provides the clinician with improved tactile sensitivity.
- The tip is inserted beneath the gingival margin and moved in an oblique direction until the entrance to the furcation is detected.

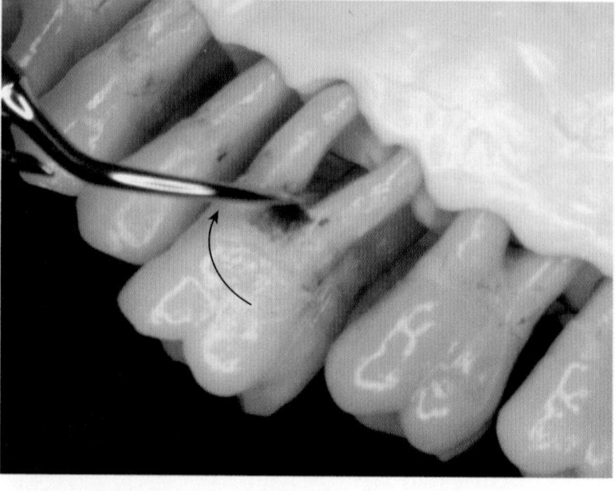

Figure 26-40. Enter the Roof of the Furcation Area.

- Once the entrance to the furcation area is located, the tip is turned while rotating the wrist. This twisting motion allows the tip to access the roof of the furcation.
- Once the tip is activated, the ball-end is rolled back and forth across the entire roof of the furcation area.

FURCATION ENTRANCES

Slim-diameter instrument tips are more effective than hand instruments in treating class II and III furcations.[11–13]

- Standard Gracey curets are too wide to enter the furcation areas of over 50% of all maxillary and mandibular molars.
- The average facial furcation entrance of maxillary and mandibular first molars is from 0.63 to 1.04 mm in width.
- The width of a standard Gracey curet ranges from 0.76 to 1 mm.
- The diameter of a modified slim-diameter instrument tip is 0.55 mm or less.

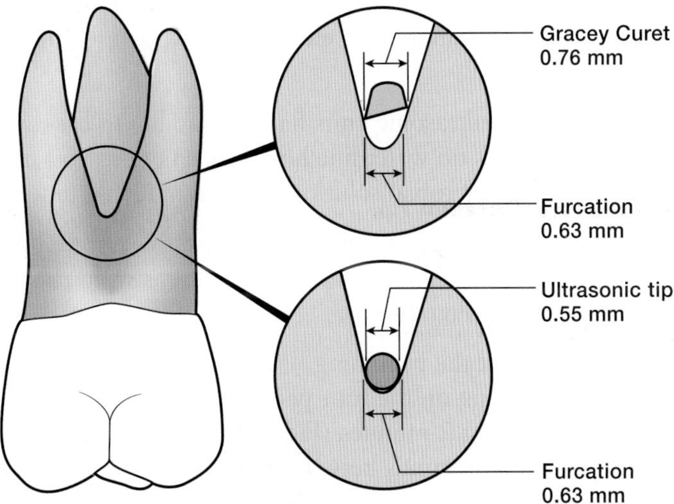

Figure 26-41. Furcation Entrances on a Maxillary First Molar.

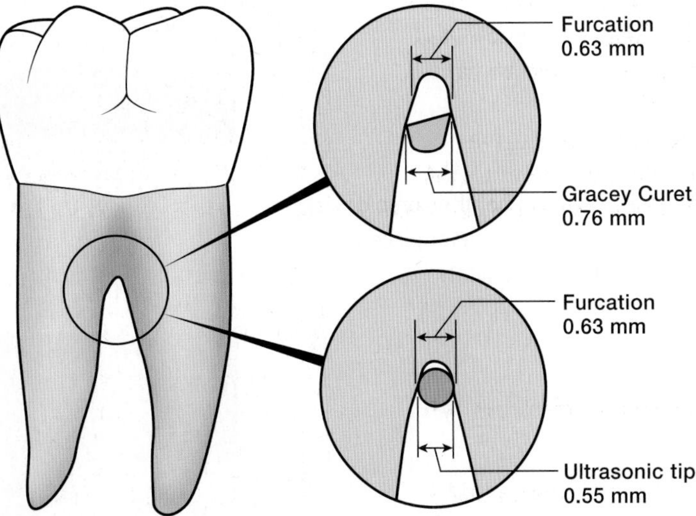

Figure 26-42. Furcation Entrances on a Mandibular First Molar.

Section 5
Treatment Preparation

FLUSHING OF WATER TUBING

Scientific investigations have shown that dental unit water lines may become significantly contaminated with microorganisms.[14,15] This contaminated water is delivered to electronically powered instruments, dental handpieces, and air/water syringes. Although water from a municipal water source is safe for drinking, the presence of even small numbers of organisms can present problems for dental unit water quality. Potable drinking water is defined as less than 500 bacterial colony-forming units per milliliter (CFU/mL). Water recovered from dental units connected to municipal water supplies may contain millions of bacterial colony-forming units per milliliter.

Options to control water tubing contamination of electronically powered devices include a combination of:

1. **Self-contained reservoirs.** Some ultrasonic units have the ability to use an independent reservoir bottle that requires no water line hook-up. The reservoir can be used to deliver distilled water or antimicrobial solution to ultrasonic instrument tip.
2. **Point-of-use filters.** Point-of-use filters are easily installed in existing dental unit water lines to physically reduce the numbers of microorganisms in the water flowing over the instrument tip (Fig. 26-43).
3. **Flushing of the water tubing.** At the beginning of each day, the handpiece water line should be flushed by stepping on the foot pedal and allowing water to flow through the handpiece for at least 2 minutes (Fig. 26-44). The water line should be flushed for a minimum of 30 seconds between patients. Flushing clears stagnant water from the tubing.

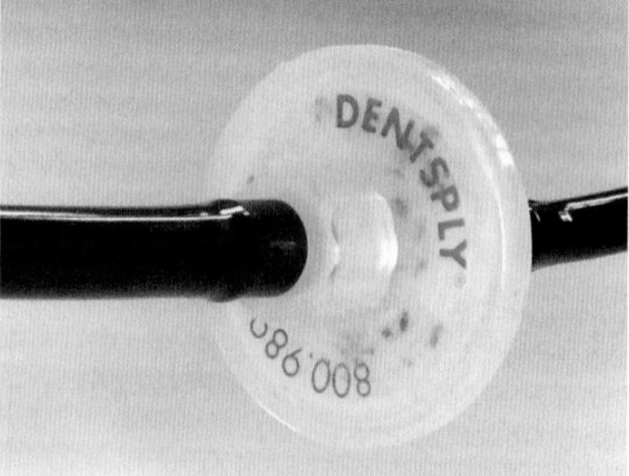

Figure 26-43. Point-of-Use Filter. Some ultrasonic devices have point-of-use filters preinstalled in the handpiece tubing that delivers water to the powered instrument.

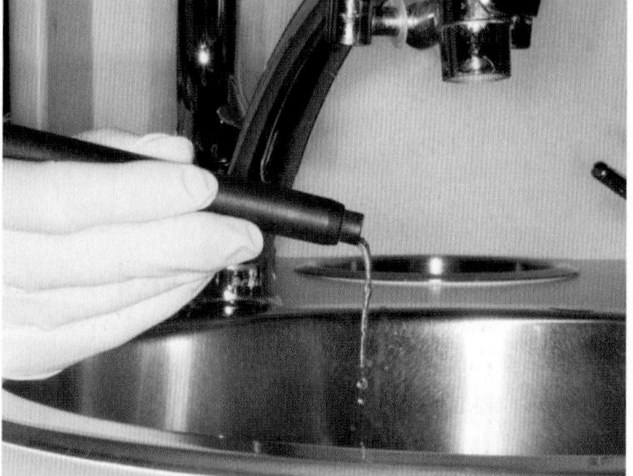

Figure 26-44. Flush Water Tubing. Flush water through the handpiece of an ultrasonic device or the water line of a sonic device for a minimum of 2 minutes at the start of the day and for 30 seconds between patients.

PREPARING THE CLINICIAN AND PATIENT

As with any treatment procedure, it is important to describe and explain powered instrumentation to the patient and obtain his or her informed consent for the procedure. The clinician should explain the purpose and functioning of powered instrumentation as well as the noise, water spray, and need for evacuation. The patient should be encouraged to ask questions.

Universal precautions must be used during ultrasonic instrumentation.

- The clinician should wear a gown with a high neck and long sleeves, mask, protective eyewear or a face shield, and gloves.
- A mask with a high bacterial filtration efficiency (BFE)[15] should be worn for powered instrumentation procedures. By definition, a mask with a high BFE will effectively filter out 98% of particles that are 3 μm or larger in size.
- Because of the high level of aerosols generated by powered instrumentation, masks should be changed every 20 minutes because a damp mask will not provide adequate protection.
- Personal protective gear for the patient should include a plastic drape, towel or bib, and protective eyewear. The patient may prefer to cover his or her nose with a flat-style mask to limit inhalation of aerosols.
- A preprocedural rinse is recommended to reduce the number of bacteria introduced into the patient's bloodstream and for control of aerosols into the surrounding environment. A 2-minute mouth rinse with either 0.12% chlorhexidine or an antiseptic mouth rinse, such as Listerine Antiseptic, is recommended for all patients prior to initiation of powered instrumentation.

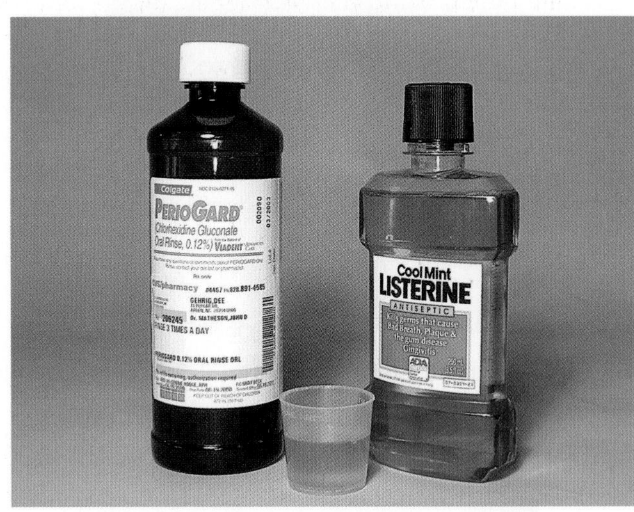

Figure 26-45. Preprocedural Rinses. Administering a preprocedural rinse is recommended to reduce the numbers of bacteria and other oral pathogens.

FLUID EVACUATION AND CONTAINMENT

Good fluid control is necessary to increase patient comfort and efficiency during powered instrumentation.

1. **Patient Positioning**
   a. The patient is positioned in a supine position with the head turned to the side and tipped slightly downward.
   b. Positioning the patient's head to the side causes the fluid generated by the instrument tip to pool in the corner of the mouth where it can be suctioned or evacuated.

2. **Evacuation for Reduction of Airborne Contamination**
   a. A large-diameter high-volume evacuator (HVE) or an extraoral "dry field" evacuator tip positioning device should be used for fluid control.
   b. The clinician may hold the HVE in the nondominant hand instead of a mirror. It may be helpful to shorten the length of the evacuation tip by cutting it in half for easier handling when working without an assistant.
   c. The powered tip should be deactivated occasionally to keep excessive amounts of fluid from pooling in the corner of the mouth.
3. **Cupping Techniques for Water Containment.** It can be very frustrating for the patient to have his or her face and hair sprayed with the water from the powered tip.
   a. Good water containment can be achieved through a combination of evacuation and use of the patient's lips and cheeks as fluid-deflecting barriers.
   b. When working on the mandibular anterior teeth, pulling the patient's lip up and out away from the teeth allows the lip to act as a barrier to deflect the water back into the mouth and as a "cup" to collect the water for evacuation. Figure 26-46 demonstrates this technique.
   c. A similar technique is used for the posterior teeth; holding the cheek away from the teeth creates a "cheek cup" to catch the water spray. This technique is shown in Figure 26-47.

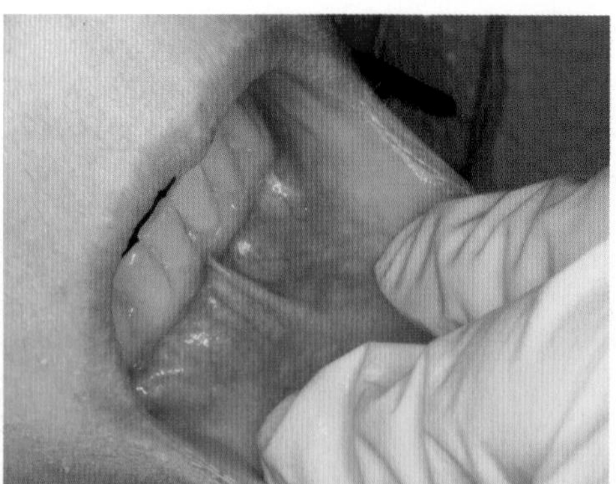
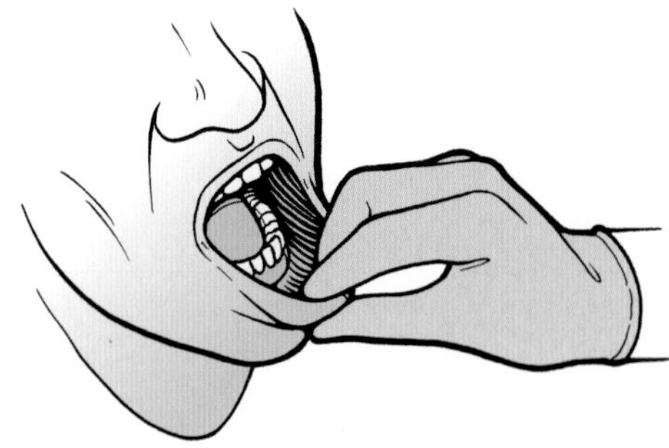

Figure 26-46. Fluid Control in Anterior Sextants. For anterior sextants, the lower and upper lips can be cupped to contain the water spray.

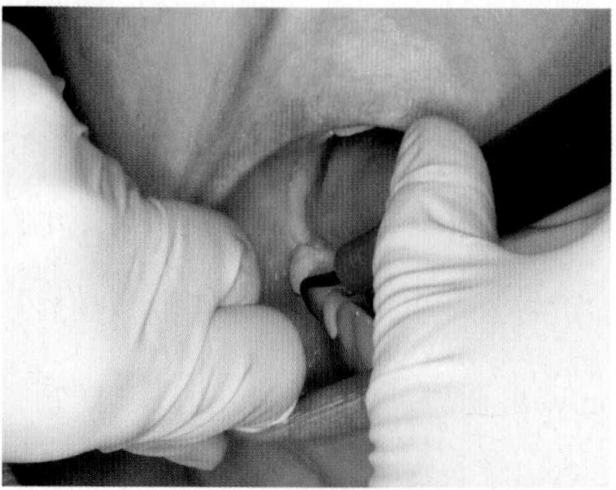
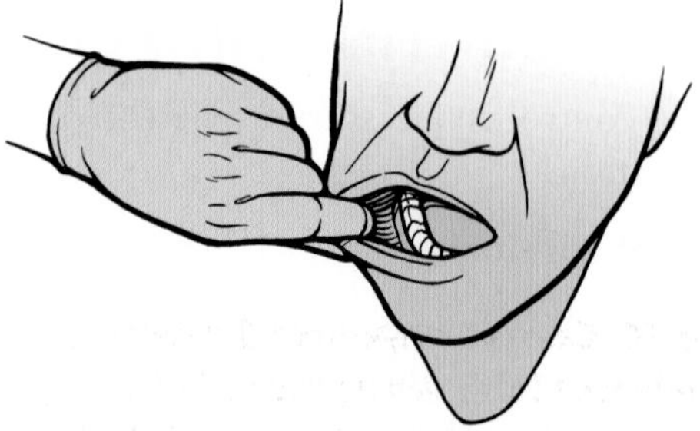

Figure 26-47. Fluid Control in Posterior Treatment Areas. For posterior treatment areas, hold the cheek between the thumb and index finger and pull out and up, or down, to form a cup.

HANDPIECE CORD MANAGEMENT

Some clinicians find that the cord tends to weigh down the end of the handpiece or causes the handpiece to twist during instrumentation. There are several techniques that are helpful in reducing the pull of the cord on the handpiece such as wrapping the cord around the forearm, running it between the little and ring fingers, or resting it in the palm of the hand around the thumb. These techniques are shown in Figures 26-48 to 26-50.

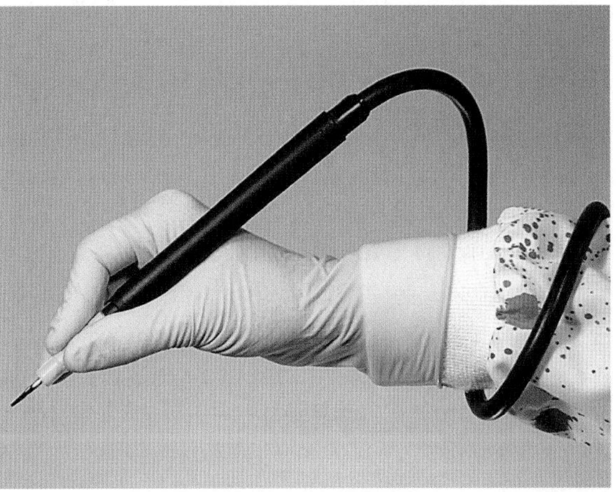

Figure 26-48. Cord Management Strategy 1. One technique for lessening the weight and pull of the handpiece cord is to wrap it around the forearm.

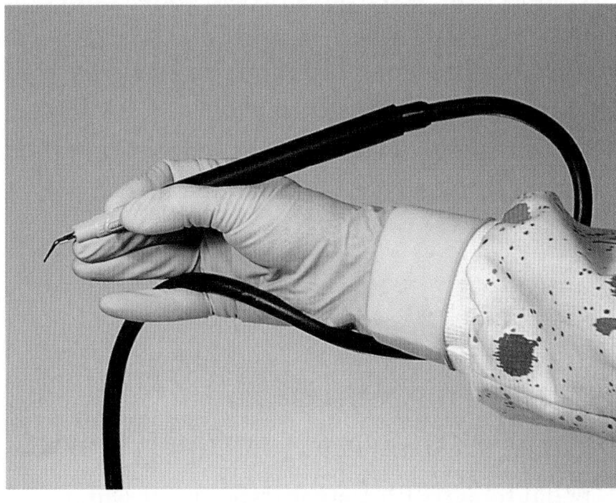

Figure 26-49. Cord Management Strategy 2. A second technique for handpiece cord management is to run the cord between the little and ring fingers.

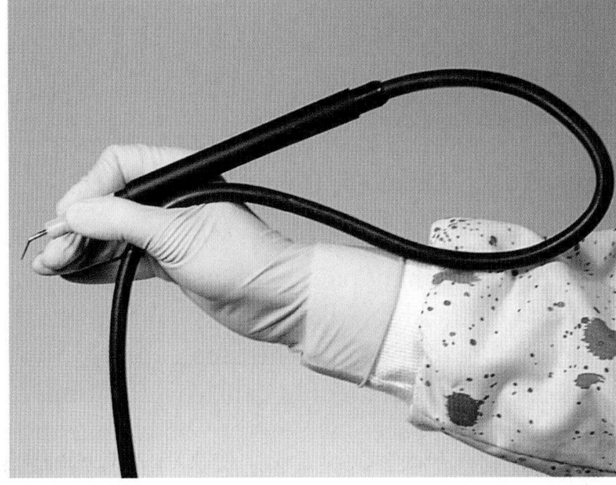

Figure 26-50. Cord Management Strategy 3. A third technique for lessening the pull of the handpiece cord is to rest it in the palm of the hand and loop it around the thumb.

SETUP FOR A PIEZOELECTRIC OR MAGNETOSTRICTIVE ULTRASONIC UNIT

Certain steps should be followed when setting-up an ultrasonic device. Follow the steps shown in Figures 26-51 to 26-58 to practice the recommended procedure for preparing an ultrasonic device for use.

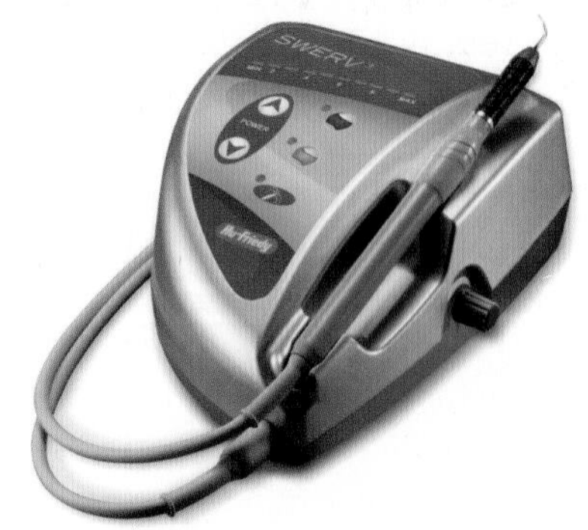

Figure 26-51. Locate Device on a Stable Surface.

- The ultrasonic device should be located on a stable countertop or cart so you will have easy access to the device at the dental chair.
- Place barriers over the control knobs on the power generator. (Courtesy of Hu-Friedy Manufacturing Co., LLC.)

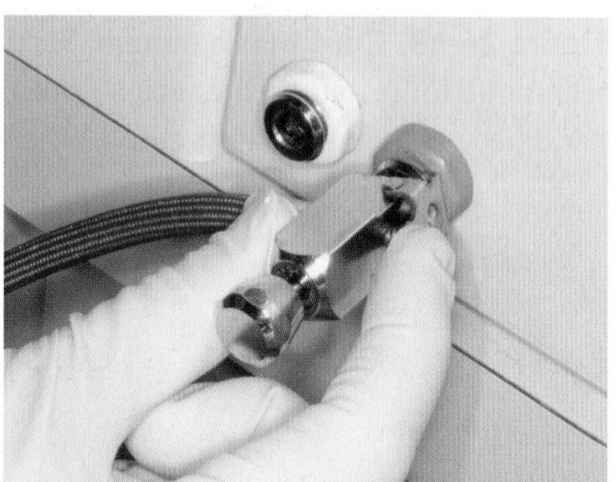

Figure 26-52. Connect the Water Hose.

- Connect the water hose to the water outlet on the dental unit.
- Turn on the dental unit and, if necessary, open the dental unit's water control knob.
- Or, if using a device with an independent fluid reservoir, attach the reservoir to the ultrasonic device.

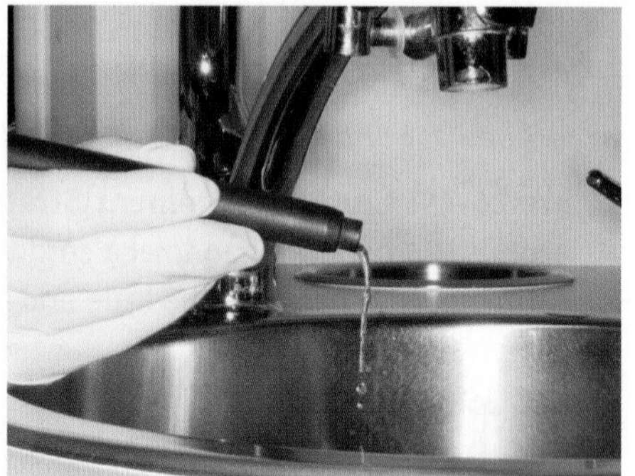

Figure 26-53. Flush the Water Tubing.

- Flush the water tubing of stagnant water by holding the handpiece or tubing over a sink and stepping on the foot pedal to activate a steady stream of water.
- At the start of each day, flush the tubing for a minimum of 2 minutes. Between patients, flush the tubing for at least 30 seconds.

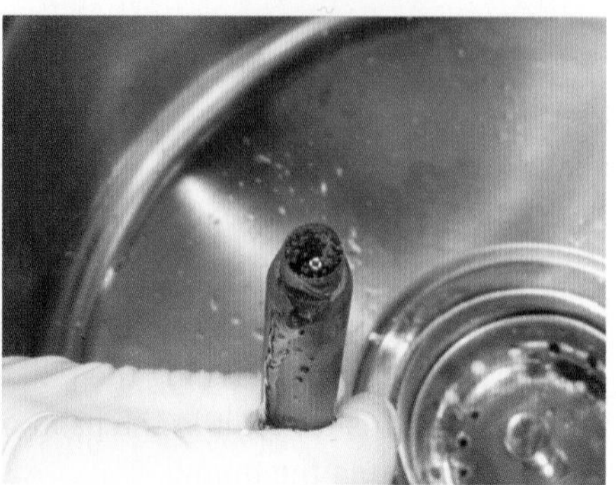

Figure 26-54. Expel Air from the Handpiece.

- Hold the handpiece upright and step on the foot pedal to fill the entire handpiece with water.
- While maintaining the handpiece in a vertical position, release the foot pedal. This step expels air bubbles from the handpiece that could cause overheating.
- Repeat this process whenever you change instrument inserts.

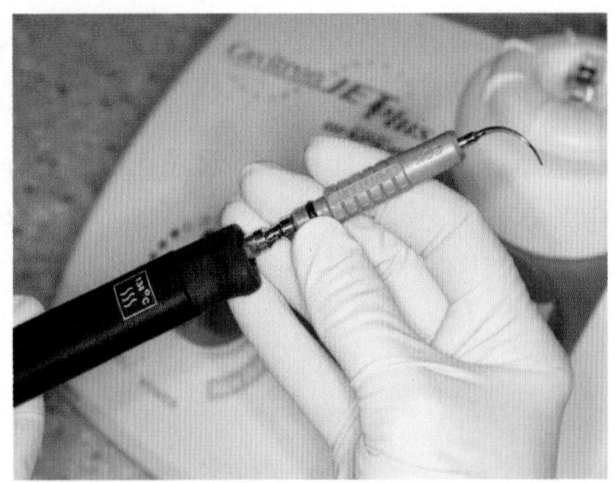

Figure 26-55. Lubricate the O-Ring and Seat the Insert.

- Use your fingertips to lubricate the o-ring with water from the handpiece.
- Grasp the insert grip, keeping your hand and fingers away from the working-end of the insert. Grasping or pushing against the working-end can bend the instrument tip.
- Gently twist the insert into the handpiece until it snaps into place.

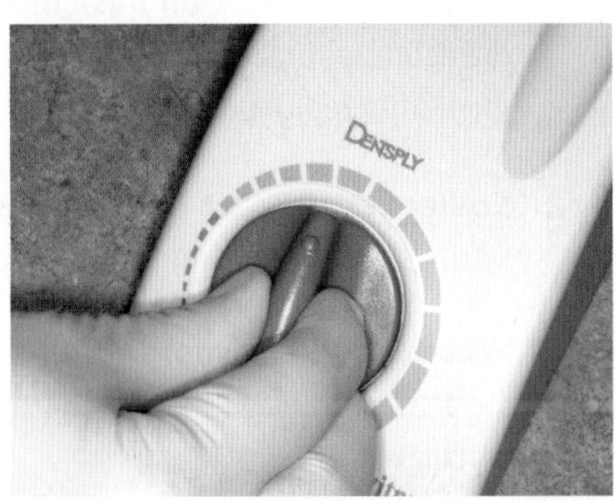

Figure 26-56. Adjust the Power Setting. Select an appropriate power setting for the particular tip you will be using (standard diameter, slim diameter) and the type of calculus deposit.

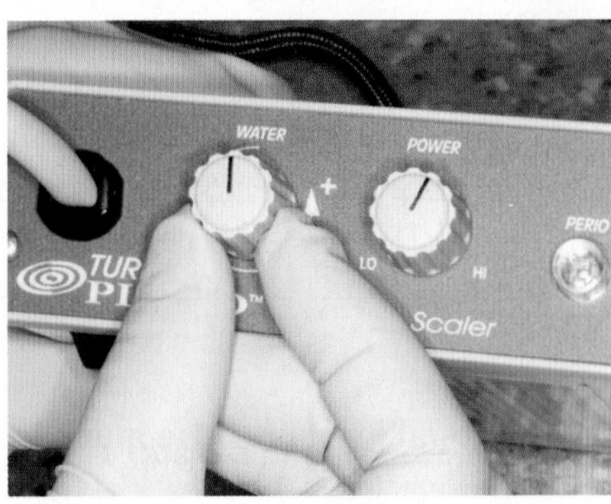

Figure 26-57. Adjust the Water Spray.

- A knob on the unit or on the ultrasonic handpiece controls the water spray.
- Adjust the water flow to create a light mist at the working-end.
- The water spray should be adjusted each time you change insert tips or the power level during instrumentation.

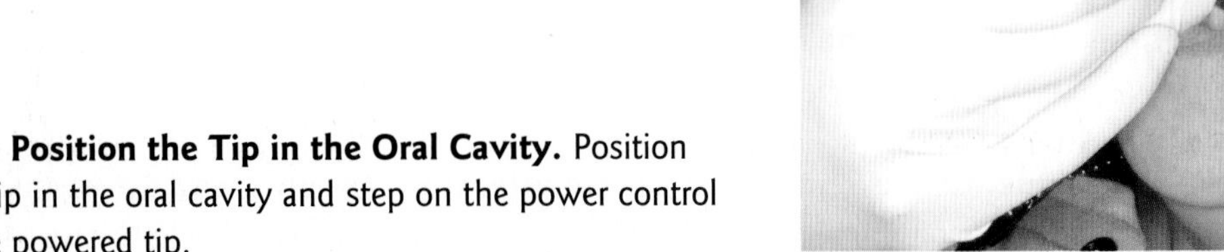

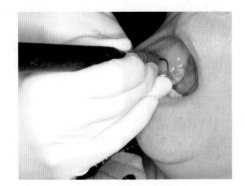

Figure 26-58. Position the Tip in the Oral Cavity. Position the powered tip in the oral cavity and step on the power control to activate the powered tip.

FUNDAMENTALS OF SONIC AND ULTRASONIC INSTRUMENTATION

Dr. Larry Burnett of Portland, Oregon—a master at electronically powered instrumentation—has developed what he refers to as his "secrets of powered instrumentation." Dr. Burnett's "secrets" are summarized in Table 26-1.

TABLE 26-1. Ten Secrets for Successful Powered Instrumentation
1. **Insert Selection. Don't ask more of an instrument tip than it can deliver.** Use a standard-diameter tip for large- or medium-sized calculus deposits. Use a slim-diameter tip for small- to medium-sized deposits.
2. **Power Setting. Set the power setting lower than you think is necessary.** Use medium-power settings for calculus removal and low-power settings for deplaquing.
3. **Water Flow. Use more water than you think is necessary.** Ensure that the water flow is hitting the active portion of the tip. Adjust the water until a halo of water surrounds the tip or until a rapid drip is achieved.
4. **Grasp. Use a lighter grasp than you think is necessary.** Powered instrumentation requires a light, related grasp similar to that used when probing.
5. **Finger Rest. Use a more stable finger rest than you think is necessary.** Use a stable standard intraoral finger rest or one of the extraoral fulcrums described in Module 20.
6. **Angulation. Use less angulation than with a hand instrument.** The angulation should be as close to 0° as possible and should never exceed 15°.
7. **Lateral Pressure. Use much less lateral pressure than with hand instrumentation.** Touch the lateral surface or back of the powered tip lightly (gently) against the deposit or tooth surface. Moderate or firm pressure decreases the effectiveness of the instrument tip and can even stop the tip vibrations all together! Powered instrumentation requires a light touch.
8. **Activation. Use more finger motion than you would with a hand instrument.** Digital (finger) activation is excellent for applying the light stroke pressure needed for powered instrumentation.
9. **Tip Motion. Never allow the instrument tip to be idle.** Keep the instrument tip moving at all times. Never continue to hold the tip on any one spot.
10. **Stroke Technique. Give each tooth adequate attention.** The powered tip needs to be moved over the surface of a deposit for some time in order to remove it. Slower, repetitive strokes are more effective in removing large or tenacious calculus deposits. Cover every millimeter of a root surface with overlapping, horizontal, vertical, and oblique brushlike strokes.

REFERENCES

1. Flemmig TF, Petersilka GJ, Mehl A, Hickel R, Klaiber B. Working parameters of a magnetostrictive ultrasonic scaler influencing root substance removal in vitro. *J Periodontol.* 1998;69:547–553.
2. Flemmig TF, Petersilka GJ, Mehl A, Hickel R, Klaiber B. The effect of working parameters on root substance removal using a piezoelectric ultrasonic scaler in vitro. *J Clin Periodontol.* 1998;25:158–163.
3. Petersilka GJ, Flemmig TF. Periodontal debridement with sonic and ultrasonic scalers. *Perio Periodont Pract Today.* 2004;1:353–362.
4. Stach D. Powering the calculus away. *Dimen Dent Hyg.* 2005;3:18–20.
5. Cobb CM. Non-surgical pocket therapy: mechanical. *Ann Periodontol.* 1996;1:443–490.
6. Sbordone L, Ramaglia L, Gulletta E, Iacono V. Recolonization of the subgingival microflora after scaling and root planing in human periodontitis. *J Periodontol.* 1990;61:579–584.
7. Costerton JW, Stewart PS, Greenberg EP. Bacterial biofilms: a common cause of persistent infections. *Science.* 1999;284:1318–1322.
8. Gilbert P, Das J, Foley I. Biofilm susceptibility to antimicrobials. *Adv Dent Res.* 1997;11:160–167.
9. Nield-Gehrig JS, Willmann DE. *Foundations of Periodontics for the Dental Hygienist.* 3rd ed. Philadelphia: Wolters Kluwer Health/Lippincott Williams & Wilkins; 2011.
10. Leon LE, Vogel RI. A comparison of the effectiveness of hand scaling and ultrasonic debridement in furcations as evaluated by differential dark-field microscopy. *J Periodontol.* 1987;58:86–94.
11. Bower RC. Furcation morphology relative to periodontal treatment. Furcation root surface anatomy. *J Periodontol.* 1979;50:366–374.
12. Holbrook WP, Muir KF, Macphee IT, Ross PW. Bacteriological investigation of the aerosol from ultrasonic scalers. *Br Dent J.* 1978;144:245–247.
13. Hou GL, Chen SF, Wu YM, Tsai CC. The topography of the furcation entrance in Chinese molars. Furcation entrance dimensions. *J Clin Periodontol.* 1994;21:451–456.
14. Atlas RM, Williams JF, Huntington MK. Legionella contamination of dental-unit waters. *Appl Environ Microbiol.* 1995;61:1208–1213.
15. Williams JF, Johnston AM, Johnson B, Huntington MK, Mackenzie CD. Microbial contamination of dental unit waterlines: prevalence, intensity and microbiological characteristics. *J Am Dent Assoc.* 1993;124:59–65.

Section 6
Skill Application

PRACTICAL FOCUS: ADAPTATION OF POWERED TIP

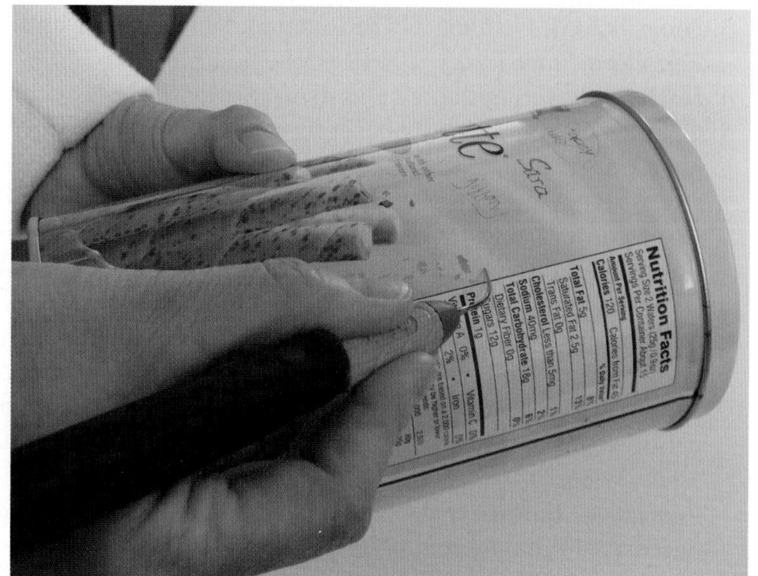

Figure 26-59. Painted Can Practice. Use a painted can to practice correct adaptation of a powered tip. Practice using the lateral surface and back of the tip to remove the paint from the can using light lateral pressure.

- The working-end of the tip should glide over the surface of the can in a smooth, even manner.
- If the tip skips off of the surface of the can (chatters), your technique is incorrect. If the tip gouges the surface of the can, your technique is incorrect.

PATIENT CASE: MR. BURLINGTON

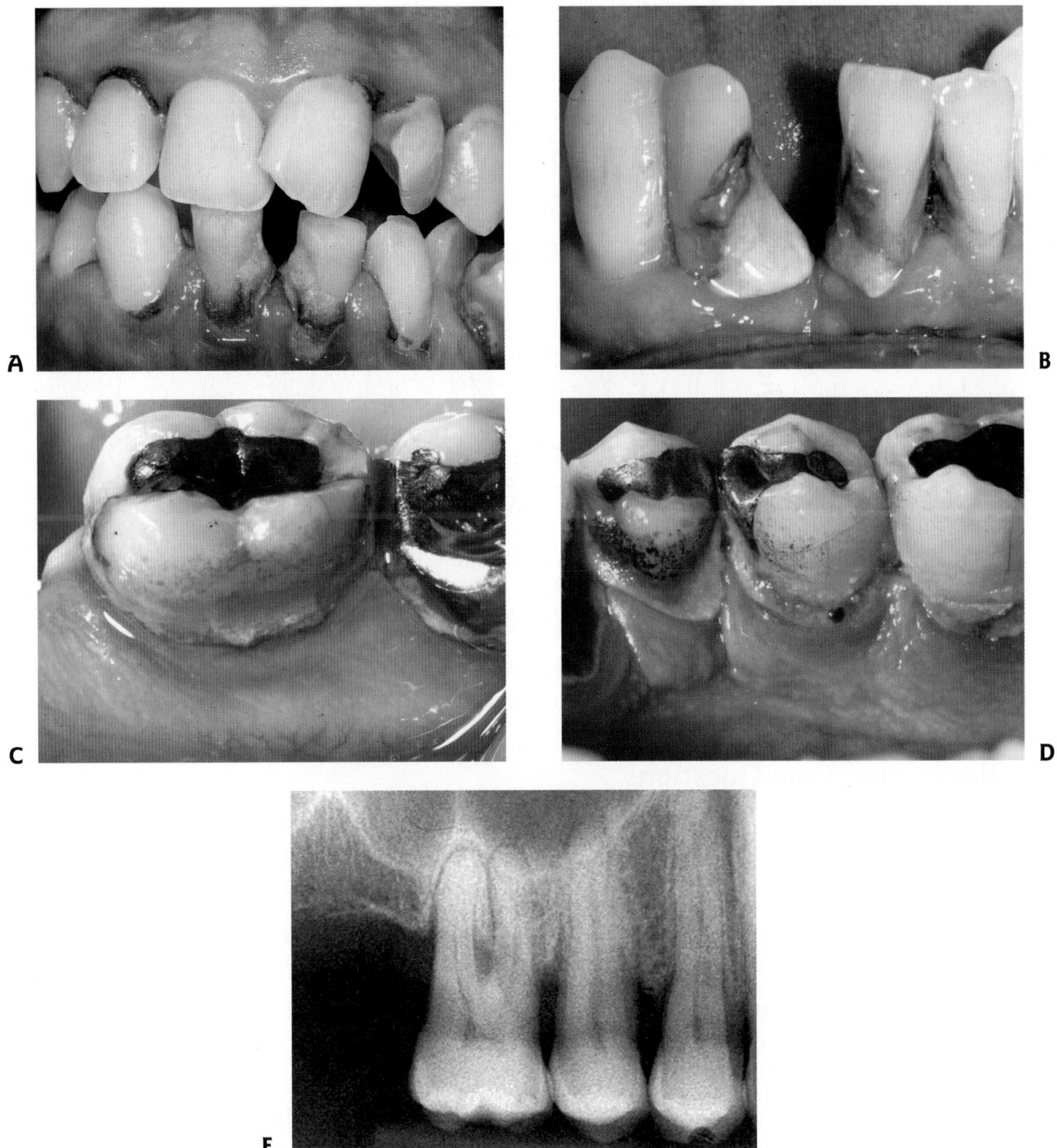

Figure 26-60, A–E. Intraoral Photos and Periapical Radiograph for Mr. Burlington.

Mr. Burlington: Assessment Data

1. Generalized heavy bleeding upon probing.
2. Deposits
   a. Medium- to large-sized supragingival calculus on all surfaces.
   b. Subgingival calculus deposits—medium-sized deposits on all surfaces.

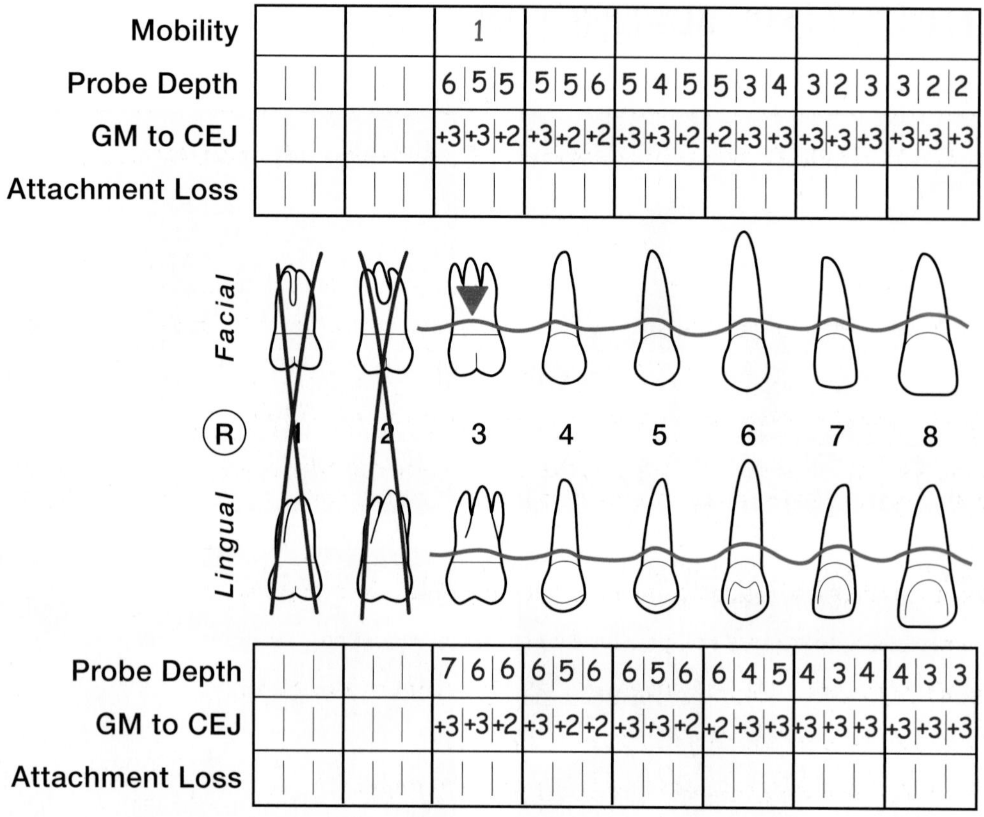

	1	2	3	4	5	6	7	8
Mobility			1					
Probe Depth			6 5 5	5 5 6	5 4 5	5 3 4	3 2 3	3 2 2
GM to CEJ			+3 +3 +2	+3 +2 +2	+3 +3 +2	+2 +3 +3	+3 +3 +3	+3 +3 +3
Attachment Loss								

	1	2	3	4	5	6	7	8
Probe Depth			7 6 6	6 5 6	6 5 6	6 4 5	4 3 4	4 3 3
GM to CEJ			+3 +3 +2	+3 +2 +2	+3 +3 +2	+2 +3 +3	+3 +3 +3	+3 +3 +3
Attachment Loss								

Figure 26-61. Mr. Burlington: Periodontal Chart for Maxillary Right Quadrant. (Key: GM = gingival margin; CEJ = cementoenamel junction.)

Mr. Burlington: Case Questions

1. *Use the information recorded on Mr. Burlington's chart to calculate the attachment loss on the facial and lingual aspects for teeth numbers 3 to 8.*
2. Do the assessment data indicate normal bone levels or bone loss in this quadrant? Do the assessment data indicate healthy sulci or periodontal pockets in this quadrant? Explain which data you used to make these determinations?
3. Do you expect to instrument any root concavities or furcation areas in this quadrant? If so, indicate which teeth will probably have root concavities and/or furcation areas to be instrumented.
4. Based on the assessment information, develop a calculus removal plan. Photocopy the "Calculus Removal Plan" form in Module 21 or create a similar form yourself on tablet paper.
   - **a.** Determine how many appointments you will need for calculus removal.
   - **b.** List the treatment area(s) to be completed at each appointment.
   - **c.** List appropriate hand and powered instruments for use at each appointment. Indicate the sequence the instruments will be used in and the size and location of the deposits each instrument will remove.

STUDENT SELF-EVALUATION MODULE 26 POWERED INSTRUMENTATION

Student: ______________________ Date: ______________________

DIRECTIONS FOR STUDENT: Evaluate your skill level as: **S** (satisfactory) or **U** (unsatisfactory).

Criteria	
Equipment Preparation	
Connects device to electrical and water sources; disinfects; applies barriers; flushes water line for 2 minutes	
Clinician and Patient Preparation	
Uses protective attire for self and patient; provides patient with preprocedural rinse	
Explains procedure to the patient, including purpose, noise, and water spray/evacuation; encourages patient to ask questions and provides appropriate answers; obtains informed consent	
Instrumentation Technique with All Tips	
Uses evacuation effectively, positioning patient's head and HVE to collect pooled water	
Adjusts power and water settings as appropriate for powered instrument tip	
Uses a gentle grasp and establishes an appropriate extraoral or intraoral fulcrum	
Correctly adapts working-end to the tooth surface being treated	
Keeps the tip in motion using light overlapping, multidirectional strokes	
Cups patient's lips and cheeks to collect water; deactivates tip occasionally to allow complete evacuation	
Universal or Straight Slim-Diameter Tip	
Demonstrates transverse orientation on maxillary anteriors, facial aspect	
Demonstrates vertical orientation on mandibular anteriors, lingual aspect	
Right- and Left-Curved Slim-Diameter Tips	
Identifies right and left tips	
Demonstrates correct tip adaptation with a lateral surface in a transverse orientation	
Demonstrates correct tip adaptation with a lateral surface in a vertical orientation	
Demonstrates correct tip adaptation with the back surface in a vertical orientation	
Demonstrates correct tip adaptation with the back surface using cross arch fulcrum for a posterior tooth	
Prepares device for next use; packages appropriate items for autoclaving	

Appendix I

Getting Ready for Instrumentation: Mathematical Principles and Anatomical Descriptors

Module Overview

This module contains a review of the mathematical principles and anatomical descriptors used in periodontal instrumentation. None of these concepts or terms is difficult; a brief review of these concepts will ensure a clear understanding of each principle or descriptor.

Module Outline

Key Terms

Angle	Perpendicular	Millimeter (mm)	Line angle
90° angle	Vertical	Midline	Aspects
Right angle	Oblique	Apical	Facial aspect
45° angle	Horizontal	Coronal	Lingual aspect
Parallel	Cross section	Zone	Sextant

Learning Objectives

1. Identify a 90° angle found in an everyday object. Create a 45° angle using two textbooks.
2. Draw two parallel lines. Draw two perpendicular lines.
3. Define the terms *vertical*, *oblique*, and *horizontal*.
4. Define the term *cross section*. Select an object and describe its shape in cross section.
5. Select a word from a page in a textbook. Measure the length of the word in millimeters.
6. Define the term *midline* as it relates to an anterior tooth.
7. Using a typodont tooth, demonstrate the terms *apical to* and *coronal to*.
8. Define the terms *midline*, *aspect*, and *sextant*.
9. Using a tooth model, name and identify (locate) the three zones on the tooth crown and the three zones on the tooth root.
10. Using a tooth model, name and identify (locate) the four line angles.
11. Using a tooth model, name and identify the three tooth surfaces included in the facial aspect of the tooth.

Section 1
Mathematical Principles

GEOMETRIC ANGLES

An angle is formed by two straight lines that meet at an end point. The size of an angle is measured in degrees using a protractor. The 90° angle and the 45° angle are common reference points in periodontal instrumentation. For example, the cutting edge of a periodontal instrument meets the tooth surface at an angle that is greater than 45° but less than 90°. Review the everyday examples of 90° and 45° angles shown below.

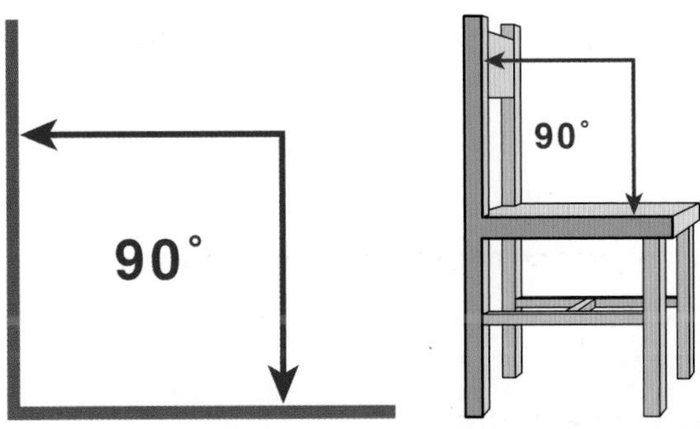

Figure A-1. A 90° Angle. The seat of this chair is at a **90° angle** to the chair back. A **right angle** is another term for a 90° angle.

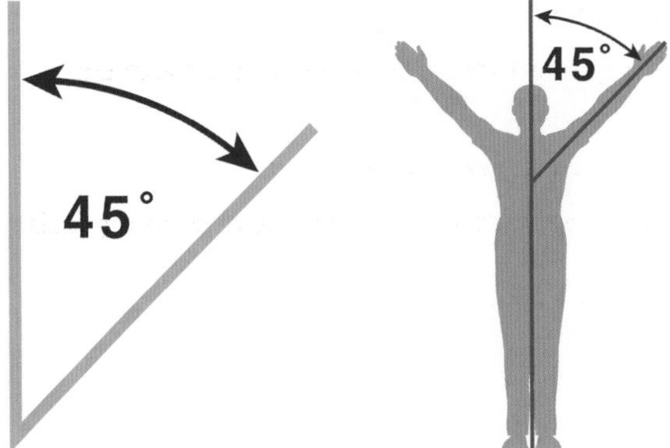

Figure A-2. A 45° Angle. This man is holding his arms at a **45° angle** to the midline of his body.

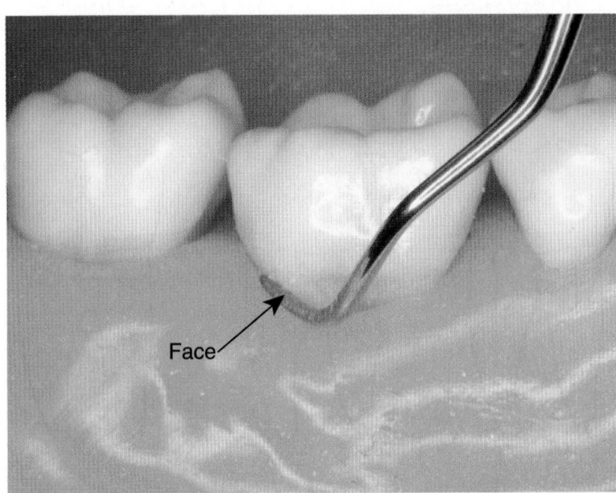

Figure A-3. Angulation for Calculus Removal. For effective calculus removal, it is important to establish the correct angulation between the cutting edge and the tooth surface. The correct angulation for calculus removal is an angle that is greater than 45° and less than 90°.

PARALLEL AND PERPENDICULAR

To correctly position a periodontal instrument, you will need to understand the terms *parallel* and *perpendicular*.

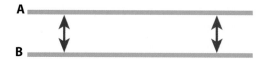

Figure A-4. Parallel Lines. Parallel lines are lines that run in the same direction and will never meet or intersect one another. Line A is parallel to line B.

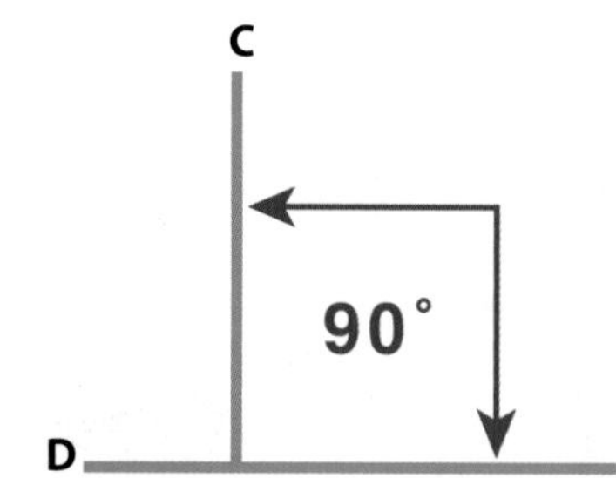

Figure A-5. Perpendicular Lines. Perpendicular lines are two lines that intersect (meet) to form a 90° angle. Line C is perpendicular to line D.

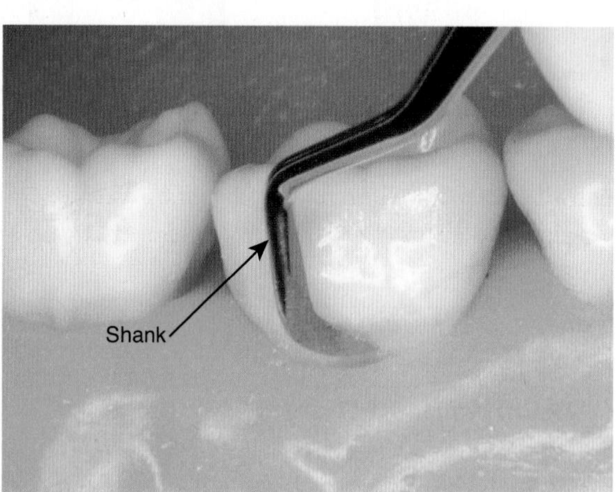

Figure A-6. Shank Position. The shank of this periodontal instrument is positioned parallel to the facial surface of this molar tooth.

LINES

The three orientations that lines may have are vertical, oblique, and horizontal. To correctly move the instrument over the tooth, you will need to understand these terms.

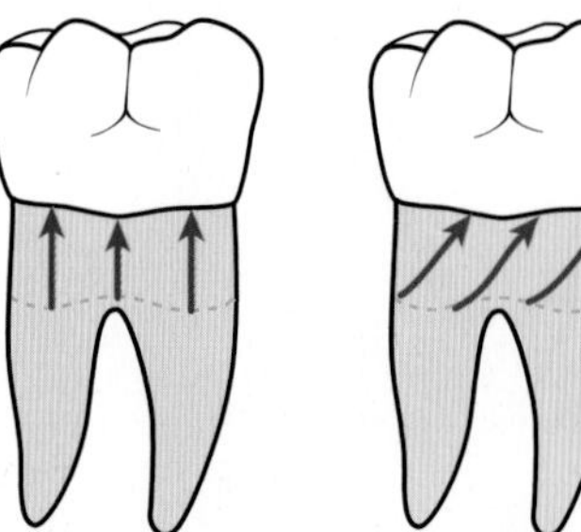

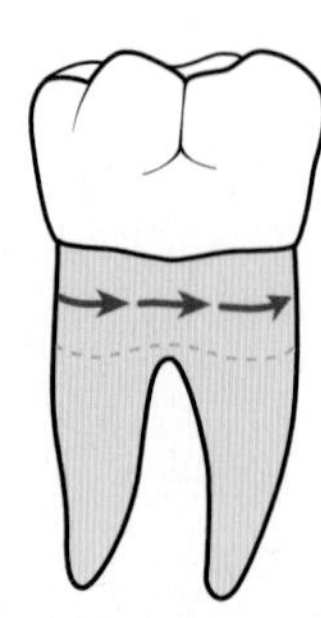

Figure A-7. Stroke Direction. During instrumentation, instrument strokes may be made across the tooth surface in a vertical, oblique, or horizontal direction. Horizontal instrumentation strokes also are referred to as circumferential strokes because these strokes are made around the circumference of the tooth.

CROSS SECTION

A cross section is exposed by cutting through an object, usually at right angles to its longest dimension. If you can imagine a knife cutting through a pencil at a 90° angle to its length, you will have a good idea of what a cross section looks like.

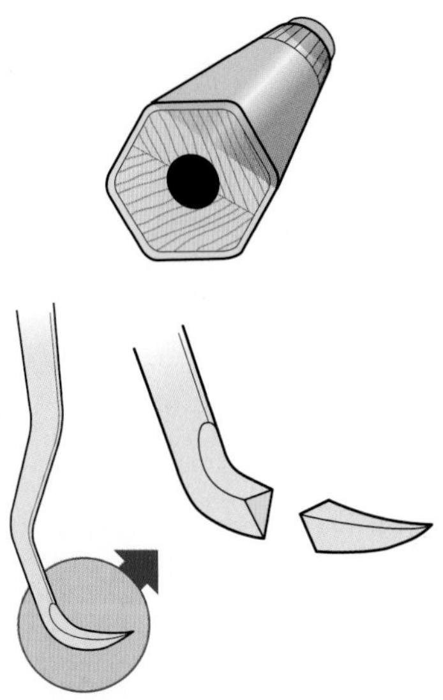

Figure A-8. Hexagonal Cross Section. A typical lead pencil is hexagonal in cross section.

Figure A-9. Triangular Cross Section. The working-end of certain periodontal instruments is triangular in cross section. Other periodontal instruments have working ends that are semi-circular in cross section.

MILLIMETER MEASUREMENTS

A millimeter is a unit of length equal to one thousandth of a meter or 0.0394 inch. The abbreviation for millimeters is "mm." The anatomical features of the teeth are often measured in millimeters.

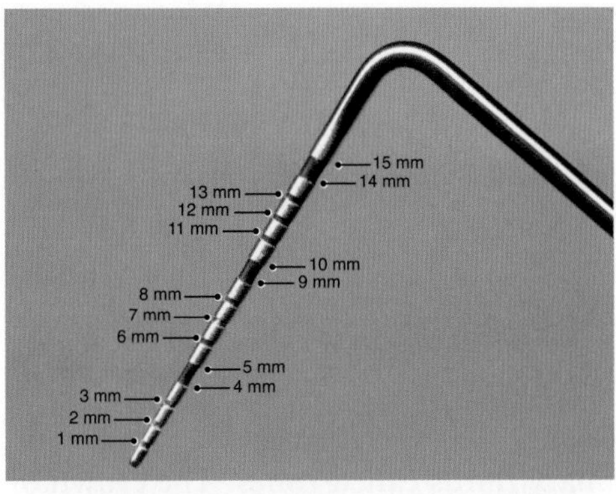

Figure A-10. A Periodontal Probe. A probe is a periodontal instrument that is similar to a miniature ruler. The probe is marked in millimeter units and is used for making intraoral measurements.

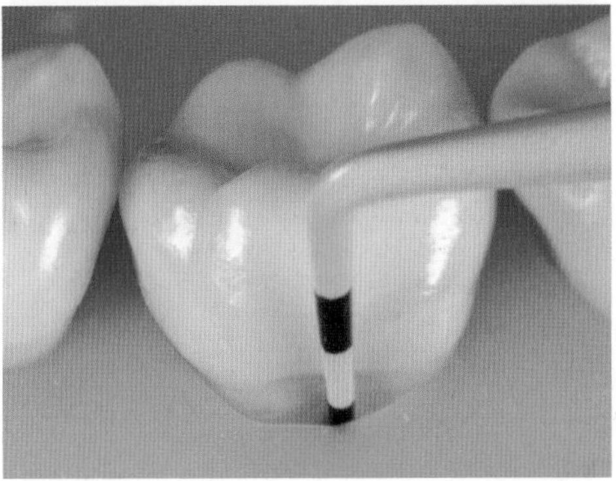

Figure A-11. Pocket Depth. Using a periodontal probe, the depth of a periodontal pocket is measured in millimeters. Periodontal pockets are 4 mm or greater in depth.

Section 2
Anatomical Descriptors

MIDLINE

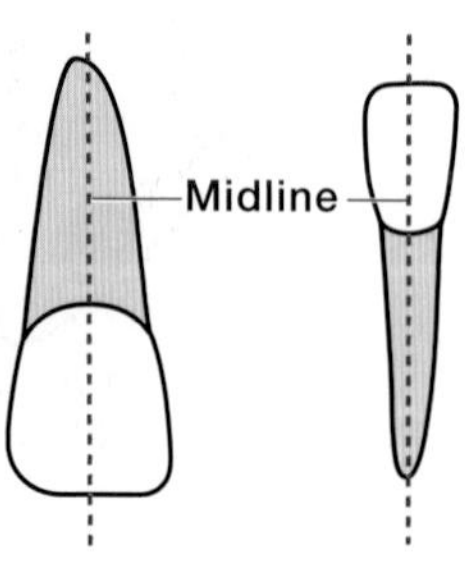

Figure A-12. Midline. A **midline** is an imaginary line that divides a tooth into right and left halves. Anterior teeth are divided into right and left halves for instrumentation.

APICAL AND CORONAL

If the working-end of an instrument moves in an apical direction, it is moved toward the tooth apex. If the working-end moves in a coronal direction, it is moved toward the tooth crown.

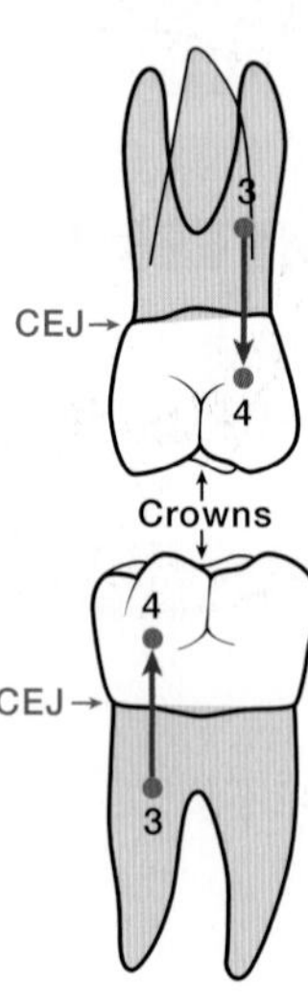

Figure A-13. Apical and Coronal.

- Apical. Point 3 is located apical to the cementoenamel junction (CEJ) on both illustrations.
- Coronal. Point 4 is coronal to the CEJ on both illustrations.

For both teeth shown here, moving from Point 3 to Point 4 is moving in a coronal direction. When removing calculus with a hand instrument, the cutting edge is placed apical to the calculus deposit, and the instrumentation stroke is made in a coronal direction.

ZONES AND LINE ANGLES

The crown and root of a tooth can be divided into three imaginary thirds called zones. The crown of a posterior tooth can be divided into surfaces at imaginary lines called line angles.

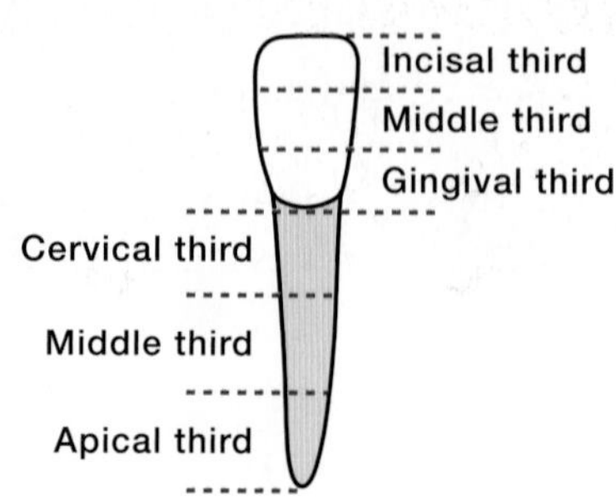

Figure A-14. Zones. The crown of a tooth may be divided into three imaginary zones: (1) the gingival third, (2) middle third, and (3) incisal or occlusal third. The root of a tooth may be divided into three imaginary zones: (1) the cervical third, (2) middle third, and (3) apical third.

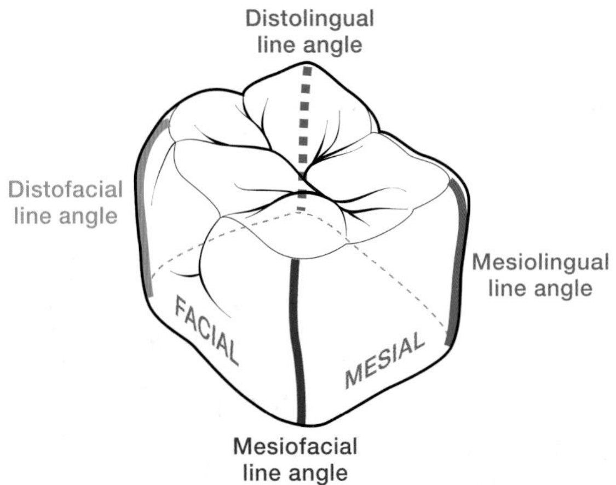

Figure A-15. Line Angle. A **line angle** is an imaginary line formed where two tooth surfaces meet. Instrumentation of a posterior tooth often is initiated at the distofacial or distolingual line angle of the tooth.

Each tooth has four line angles:

1. Mesiofacial line angle
2. Distofacial line angle
3. Mesiolingual line angle
4. Distolingual line angle

ASPECT

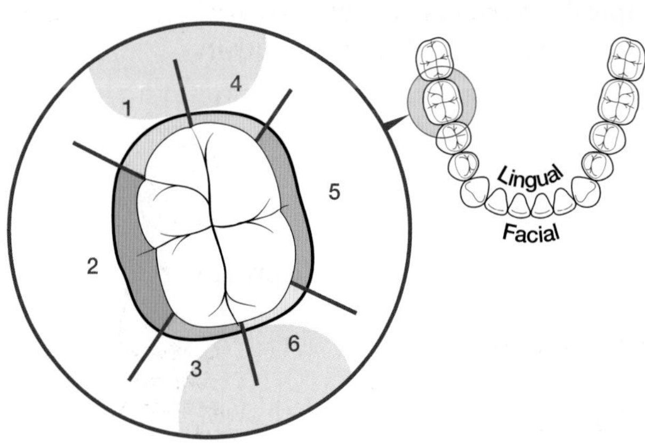

Figure A-16. Facial and Lingual Aspects. A tooth, sextant, quadrant, or dental arch may be divided into two **aspects**: (1) a facial aspect and (2) a lingual aspect.

The facial aspect of a tooth is subdivided into three areas: (1) distofacial area, (2) facial surface, and (3) mesiofacial area.
The lingual aspect of a tooth is subdivided into three areas: (4) distolingual area, (5) lingual area, and (6) mesiolingual area.

SEXTANT

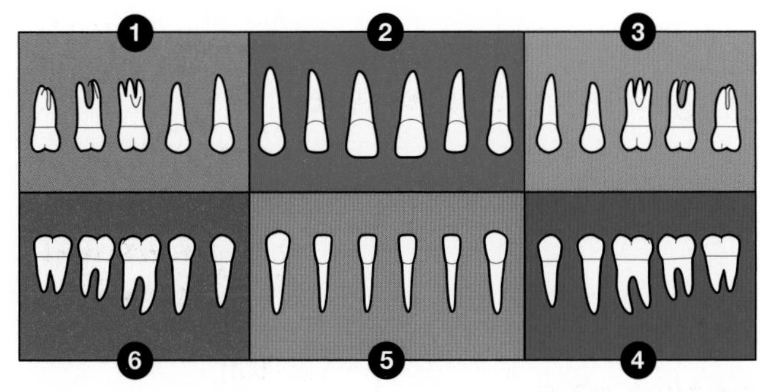

Figure A-17. Sextants. For purposes of identification, the dentition may be divided into six areas. Each area is referred to as a **sextant**. There are two anterior sextants and four posterior sextants in the dental arch:

1. Maxillary right posterior sextant
2. Maxillary anterior sextant
3. Maxillary left posterior sextant
4. Mandibular left posterior sextant
5. Mandibular anterior sextant
6. Mandibular right posterior sextant

Section 3
Skill Application

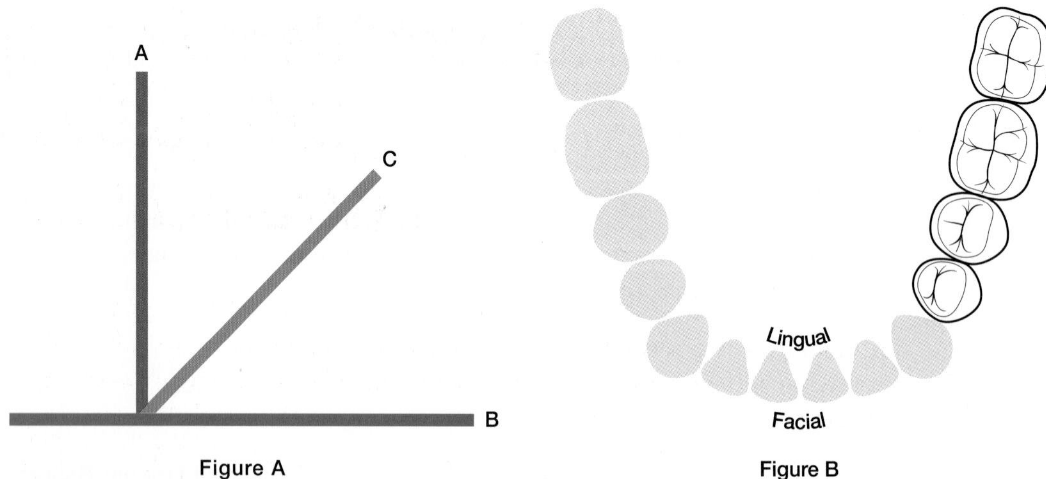

Figure A

Figure B

Questions 1 to 5 refer to **Figure A.** Directions: Circle the correct response.

1. Line A is:	vertical	horizontal	oblique
2. Line C is:	vertical	horizontal	oblique
3. Line(s) at 90° angle(s) to Line A:	B	C	both B & C
4. Line(s) at 45° angle(s) to Line C:	A	B	both A & B
5. Line(s) perpendicular to Line B:	A	C	both A & C
6. Shape of a baseball in cross section:	circular	triangular	rectangular
7. Shape of a pyramid in cross section:	circular	triangular	rectangular

8. On **Figure B,** color the *facial aspect* of the mandibular left sextant in red. Color the *lingual aspect* in blue.

Appendix 2

Problem Identification: Difficulties in Instrumentation

Module Overview

This module provides solutions for the most common instrumentation problems encountered by beginning clinicians. These problems are divided into seven categories:

Box A-1. DIRECTIONS FOR USE OF THE PROBLEM CHARTS

1. First, select the category ***that most closely describes the problem*** that you are having. Turn to the problem chart for that category.
2. The "Cause" column lists possible causes of the problem. In each category, the causes are listed in order from the most likely cause to least likely cause.
3. Read the "Solution" column for suggestions on how to correct the problem.

Problem Chart I: Can't See the Treatment Area!

Cause	Solution
Clinician seated in wrong "clock position" for treatment area	Refer to Positioning Summary Sheets
Patient positioned too high	Lower patient chair until the patient's mouth is below your elbow when you hold your arms against your side.
Patient head position	Mandibular arch = chin-down Maxillary arch = chin-up Aspect toward = turned slightly away Aspect away = turned toward
Not using indirect vision	A combination of direct vision and indirect vision is required in most treatment areas.
Using mirror, but still can't see	Be sure that you are using the mirror to fully retract the tongue or cheek away from the treatment area. If you can't see the treatment area in the mirror's reflecting surface, try rotating the mirror head slightly. Move mirror further away from treatment area. For mandibular lingual aspects, move mirror toward midline of the mouth. For maxillary anteriors, move mirror closer to the mandibular arch.
Finger rest too close to surface to be instrumented	Move rest slightly forward in the mouth so that your finger isn't covering up the surface to be instrumented.
Hand is blocking view	Swivel or pivot your hand and arm until you can see the treatment area.

Problem Chart 2: Can't Locate the Calculus!	
Cause	**Solution**
Middle finger not resting on shank	You will receive more tactile information if your finger is resting on the shank.
Using middle finger to hold the instrument (index finger is just "going along for the ride" rather than holding the handle)	Using the middle finger to hold the handle prevents it from detecting vibrations. The thumb and index finger should be across from one another. You should be able to lift your middle finger off of the shank and not drop the instrument.
Using "death grasp" on handle	Relax your fingers and grasp the handle as lightly as possible. Try working on a typodont without wearing gloves; if your fingers are blanched, you are holding the handle too tightly.
Not beginning strokes at the junctional epithelium	Be sure to insert the working-end to the base of the sulcus or pocket before initiating an assessment stroke. If you can't tell where the base is, get an instructor to help you.
Too few strokes, not overlapping strokes	When working subgingivally, use instrumentation zones and overlapping strokes to cover the entire root surface.
Not detecting calculus at line angles on posterior teeth	Position the working-end distal to the line angle with the explorer tip aimed toward the junctional epithelium (but NOT touching the junctional epithelium) and make short horizontal strokes "around" the line angle toward the front of the mouth.
Not detecting calculus at midlines of anterior teeth	Make small, controlled horizontal strokes at the midline on facial or lingual surfaces.

Problem Chart 3: Poor Illumination of Treatment Area!	
Cause	**Solution**
Unit light too close to mouth	Positioning the light close to the patient's mouth creates excessive shadowing and actually makes it harder to see. Light should be an arm's length above or in front of the clinician.
Patient's head positioned incorrectly for treatment area	Mandibular arch = chin-down Maxillary arch = chin-up Aspect toward = turned slightly away Aspect away = turned toward
Not using mirror for indirect illumination	Use mirror to direct light onto the treatment area.

Problem Chart 4: Can't Adapt Cutting Edge to Tooth Surface!	
Cause	**Solution**
Trying to adapt the middle-third of cutting edge	Usually only the tip-third or toe-third of the cutting edge can be adapted.
Using the wrong cutting edge for the tooth surface	Review the visual guidelines for the cutting edge selection for the instrument in question.
Using the wrong instrument for the task or area of the mouth	Review uses and applications of instrument classifications.
Finger rest too far away	Establish a finger rest near to the tooth to be instrumented.
Lower shank not parallel to facial or lingual surface of posterior tooth	On posterior teeth, the lower shank should be parallel to the tooth surface, but not touching it at any point.

Problem Chart 5: Can't Maintain Adaptation!

Cause	Solution
Incorrect grasp; not rolling instrument handle	Sloppy technique with grasp makes it difficult to control the instrument. As you work around the circumference of the tooth, roll the handle between your index finger and thumb to maintain adaptation.
Split grasp	Keep fingers together in the correct grasp position.
Fulcrum too close or too far away from tooth to be instrumented	Finger rest should be near (but not on) the tooth to be instrumented.
Fulcrum finger lifts off of the tooth as stroke is made	Fulcrum finger should be maintained in a straight, upright position throughout the stroke (acting as a "support beam"). Press down against the tooth with your fulcrum finger so finger can act as a "brake" to stop the stroke.
Tilting the instrument face away from the tooth surface during stroke (so lateral surface or back of working-end contacts tooth)	Maintain correct face-to-tooth surface angulation as you use a pull stroke to move the working-end in a coronal direction. Handle position should stay parallel to the tooth surface as you make strokes (it should not tilt away from the tooth surface).
Not pivoting on finger rest	On posterior teeth, pivot at line angles to maintain adaptation. In anterior sextants, as you work toward yourself, your hand and arm should gradually pivot closer to your body.

Problem Chart 6: Uncontrolled or Weak Calculus Removal Stroke!	
Cause	**Solution**
Instrument handle is supported solely by index finger and thumb	Handle should rest against the index finger or hand for support.
Split grasp—fingers not in contact	Keep fingers together in correct grasp position for control of strokes.
"Death grip" on handle	Use a firm grasp, but not a choking grasp.
Fulcrum finger lifts off of the tooth as stroke is made	Press down against the tooth with your fulcrum finger so finger can act as a "brake" to stop the stroke.
Fulcrum finger is relaxed and bent	Fulcrum finger should be straight and apply pressure against rest point on tooth (acting as a "support beam").
Stroke not stabilized; no lateral pressure with cutting edge against tooth surface	During a work stroke, the index finger and thumb should apply equal pressure against the instrument handle, and the fulcrum finger applies pressure against the tooth surface.
Wrist and arm not in neutral position	Assess patient position, clinician position, and arm position.
Using a push-pull stroke	Apply lateral pressure only when making a stroke away from the junctional epithelium.
Working too rapidly, strokes too fast	Pause briefly after each stroke. Make slow, controlled strokes.
On posterior teeth, lower shank not parallel—shank rocks on height of contour	On posterior teeth, the lower shank should be parallel to the facial or lingual surface, but not touching it at any point.

Problem Chart 7A: Missed Calculus Deposits! Deposits Missed at Midlines of Anterior Teeth

Cause	Solution
Not using horizontal strokes at midline of facial or lingual surface	Position the curet to the side of the midline with the toe aiming toward the junctional epithelium (but not touching the junctional epithelium). Make a series of short controlled horizontal strokes.
Not overlapping vertical strokes at midline	Position the working-end so that strokes will overlap for surfaces toward and away.
Not using a specialized instrument when indicated	Use an area-specific curet with a miniature working-end at midlines.

Problem Chart 7B: Missed Calculus Deposits! Deposits Missed at Line Angles of Posterior Teeth

Cause	Solution
Not using horizontal strokes at the line angles	Position the curet distal to the line angle with the toe aiming toward the junctional epithelium (but not touching the junctional epithelium). Make a series of short strokes around the line angle.
Not rolling handle to maintain adaptation to line angle	As you work around a line angle, it is necessary to roll the instrument handle between the index finger and thumb to maintain adaptation.

Problem Chart 7C: Missed Calculus Deposits! Deposits Missed on Proximal Surfaces	
Cause	**Solution**
Not using indirect vision	Beginning clinicians often have trouble learning to use indirect vision and so try to view all surfaces directly. Use of indirect vision is vital for proximal surfaces.
Not rotating reflecting surface to view proximal surfaces	This problem is common on lingual surfaces of anterior teeth. First, angle the mirror to view the surfaces toward you, and then turn the mirror to view the surfaces away from you.
Strokes not extended under contact area	Instrument at least one-half of a proximal surface from the facial and lingual aspects. Place curet between the papilla and the tooth surface. Adapt the working-end to the tooth surface and insert it to the junctional epithelium. (Do not "trace" papilla with working-end.)
Not rolling handle to maintain adaptation	As you work around a line angle and onto the proximal surface, make small, continuous adjustments in adaptation by rolling the handle.
Working-end not "aimed" toward surface to be instrumented	For distal surfaces of posterior teeth, the toe should aim toward the back of the mouth. Don't try to "back the working-end" onto the distal surface.

Glossary

Abscess of the periodontium—a localized collection of pus in the periodontal tissues.

Abutment post—a titanium post that protrudes through the tissue into the mouth and supports a crown or denture for replacement of a missing tooth or teeth.

Acoustic turbulence—the swirling effect produced within the confined space of a periodontal pocket by the continuous stream of fluid flowing over an electronically powered instrument tip. This intense swirling effect disrupts the plaque biofilm.

Active tip area—the portion of an electronically powered instrument tip that is capable of doing work. The active tip area ranges from approximately 2 to 4 mm of the length of the instrument tip.

Adaptation—the positioning of the first 1 or 2 mm of the lateral surface in contact with the tooth. Correct adaptation of the working-end to the tooth surface requires positioning the working-end so that only the leading-third of the working-end is in contact with the tooth surface.

Advanced fulcrum—a variation of an intraoral or extraoral finger rest used to gain access to root surfaces within deep periodontal pockets. Examples include the modified intraoral, cross arch, opposite arch, finger-on-finger, and finger assist fulcrums.

Aerosols—invisible airborne particles dispersed into the surrounding environment by dental equipment such as dental handpieces and electronically powered instruments. Microorganisms in the dental aerosols have been shown to survive for up to 24 hours. Also see *splatter*.

Air-powder polishing—a technique for extrinsic stain removal that uses a mixture of warm water, sodium bicarbonate powder, and air. The sodium bicarbonate powder is the abrasive agent used to remove stains from the tooth surfaces.

Alveolar bone—the bone that surrounds the roots of the teeth. It forms the bony sockets that support and protect the roots of the teeth.

Alveolar mucosa—the apical boundary, or lower edge, of the gingiva; it can be distinguished easily from the gingiva by its dark red color and smooth, shiny surface.

Amplitude—see *frequency*.

Angle—formed by two straight lines that meet at an end point. The size of an angle is measured in degrees using a protractor. The 90° angle and the 45° angle are common reference points in instrumentation.

Angulation—the relationship between the face of a calculus removal instrument and the tooth surface to which it is applied. For insertion beneath the gingival margin, the face-to-tooth surface angulation should be an angle between 0° and 40°. For calculus removal, the face-to-tooth surface angulation should be an angle between 45° and 90°.

Anterior surfaces away from the clinician—the surfaces of the anterior teeth that are farthest from the clinician.

Anterior surfaces toward the clinician—the surfaces of the anterior teeth that are closest to the clinician.

Apical—toward the tooth apex.

Area-specific curet—a periodontal instrument used to remove light calculus deposits from the crowns and roots of the teeth. Area-specific curets have long, complex functional shanks for root surface debridement within periodontal pockets. Each area-specific curet is designed for use only on certain teeth and tooth surfaces. These curets have only one working cutting edge that is used for calculus removal.

Aspect—a tooth, sextant, quadrant, or dental arch may be divided into two aspects: (1) a facial aspect and (2) a lingual aspect.

Aspects away from the clinician—the aspects of the posterior sextants that are farthest from the clinician.

Aspects toward the clinician—the aspects of the posterior sextants that are closest to the clinician.

Assessment stroke—an instrumentation stroke used to evaluate the tooth or the health of the periodontal tissues.

Attached gingiva—the part of the gingiva that is tightly connected to the cementum on the cervical-third of the root and to the periosteum (connective tissue cover) of the alveolar bone.

Automatically tuned—an ultrasonic device that does not allow the clinician to adjust the vibration frequency of the instrument tip. Also see *tuning* and *manually tuned*.

Back—the portion of the instrument working-end that is opposite the face. Sickle scalers have a pointed back, and curets have a rounded back.

Bacteremia—the presence of bacteria in the bloodstream. Bacteria from the oral cavity are introduced into the bloodstream during hand or powered instrumentation and polishing.

Balanced instrument—a periodontal instrument that has working-ends that are aligned with the long axis of the handle.

Basic extraoral fulcrum—an extraoral fulcrum in which the clinician's dominant hand rests against the patient's chin or cheek.

Bifurcation—see *furcation*.

Biofilm—a well-organized community of bacteria that adheres to surfaces and is embedded in an extracellular slime layer. Biofilms form rapidly on any wet surface and usually consist of many species of bacteria, as well as other organisms and debris.

Burnished calculus deposit—a calculus deposit that has had the outermost layer removed. Burnished calculus is difficult to remove because the cutting edge will tend to slip over the smooth surface of the deposit.

Calculus—mineralized bacterial plaque, covered on its external surface with a living layer of plaque biofilm. Because the surface of a calculus deposit is irregular and is always covered with disease-causing bacteria, dental calculus plays a significant role in causing periodontal disease.

Calculus removal stroke—an instrumentation stroke used to remove calculus deposits.

Calibrated periodontal probe—a type of periodontal probe that is marked in millimeter increments and is used to evaluate the health of the periodontal tissues.

Carious lesion—a decayed area on the tooth crown or root.

Cavitation—the formation of tiny bubbles in the water exiting from an electronically powered instrument tip; when these tiny bubbles collapse, they produce shock waves that destroy bacteria by tearing the bacterial cell walls. Also see *acoustic turbulence*.

Chlorhexidine stain—a yellowish brown stain on the cervical and proximal tooth surfaces, restorations, and the surface of the tongue caused by the use of antimicrobial mouth rinses that contain chlorhexidine.

Circuit scaling—see *gross scaling.*

Clinical attachment level (CAL)—the estimated position of the structures that support the tooth as measured with a periodontal probe. The clinical attachment level provides an estimate of a tooth's stability and the loss of bone support.

Clinical attachment loss (CAL)—the extent of periodontal support that has been destroyed around a tooth.

Closed angle—angulation of the working-end at an angle between 0° and 40° for insertion beneath the gingival margin into the sulcus or pocket.

Col—a valley-like depression in the portion of the interdental gingiva that lies directly apical to (beneath) the contact area of two adjacent teeth.

Color-coded reference marking—a colored band on the WHO probe located 3.5 to 5.5 mm from the probe tip. This reference marking is used when performing the PSR screening examination. Also see *Periodontal Screening and Recording System* and *WHO probe.*

Complex shank—a shank that is bent in two planes (front to back and side to side) to facilitate instrumentation of posterior teeth. Also termed a straight shank. See also *simple shank.*

Concavity—see *root concavity.*

Contra-angle—a prophylaxis angle that has a bend in the shank.

Coronal—toward the tooth crown.

Cross arch fulcrum—an advanced intraoral fulcrum in which the finger rest is established on opposite side of arch from the treatment area.

Cross section—formed by cutting through an object, usually at right angles to its longest dimension. A sickle scaler is triangular in cross section; a curet is semi-circular in cross section.

Curet—a periodontal instrument used to remove calculus deposits from the crown and roots of the teeth. Its working-end has a rounded back and rounded toe and is semi-circular in cross section. Also see *universal curet* and *area-specific curet.*

Cutting edge—a sharp edge formed where the face and lateral surfaces of a working-end meet. Cutting edges may be straight or curved. Also see *sharp cutting edge* and *dull cutting edge.*

Decay—See *dental caries.*

Dental calculus—mineralized bacterial plaque, covered on its external surface with a living layer of plaque biofilm. Because the surface of a calculus deposit is irregular and is always covered with disease-causing bacteria, dental calculus plays a significant role in causing periodontal disease.

Dental caries—a decayed area on the tooth crown or root.

Dental endoscope—an illuminated optic instrument that is inserted into the periodontal pocket to provide the clinician with direct vision of subgingival root conditions.

Dental implant—a nonbiologic (artificial) device surgically inserted into or onto the jawbone to (1) replace a missing tooth or (2) provide support for a prosthetic denture.

Dental mirror—the working-end of a dental mirror has a reflecting mirrored surface used to view tooth surfaces that cannot be seen directly.

Dentinal hypersensitivity—a short, sharp painful reaction that occurs when some areas of exposed dentin are subjected to a mechanical stimulus (touch of toothbrush bristles), thermal stimulus (ice cream), or chemical stimulus (acidic grapefruit).

Dentinal tubule—a long tunnel running through the dentin extending from the pulp chamber to dentinoenamel junction (in the crown) or the dentinocemental junction (in the root). This tube is filled with a cellular extension of the odontoblast called the odontoblastic process.

Deplaquing—the disruption or removal of the subgingival plaque biofilm and its products from root surfaces and the pocket space.

Design name—identifies the school or individual originally responsible for the design or development of a periodontal instrument or group of instruments.

Design number—a number designation that, when combined with the design name, provides an exact identification of the working-end of a periodontal instrument.

Digital motion activation—moving the instrument by flexing the thumb, index, and middle fingers. See also *motion activation* and *wrist motion activation.*

Drive finger—the finger used to turn the instrument handle while holding the instrument in a modified pen grasp. Either the index finger *or* the thumb acts as the drive finger to turn the instrument. The finger used to roll the handle determines the direction in which the working-end will turn.

Dull cutting edge—the rounded surface that results when metal is worn away from the cutting edge of an instrument.

Edema—abnormal swelling resulting from fluid accumulating in the tissues.

Electronically powered instrumentation—instrumentation using the rapid energy vibrations of a powered instrument tip to fracture calculus from the tooth surface and clean the environment of the periodontal pocket. Also see *sonic device, piezoelectric ultrasonic device,* and *magnetostrictive ultrasonic device.*

Endoscope—an illuminated optic instrument used to view the interior of a body cavity or organ. Also see *dental endoscope.*

Ergonomics—the science of adjusting the design of tools, equipment, tasks, and environments for safe, comfortable, and effective human use.

Evidence-based care—clinical care that is based on the best available scientific evidence.

Explorer—a fine wire-like periodontal instrument used to locate calculus deposits, tooth surface irregularities, defective margins, and carious lesions.

Explorer tip—the 1 to 2 mm of the side of the explorer working-end that is used for calculus detection.

Exposed dentin—dentin that has been exposed to the oral cavity due to an absence of the enamel or cementum that normally covers it. Dentin may be exposed on a tiny or extensive area of the tooth.

Extended lower shank—a shank that is 3 mm longer than a standard lower shank.

Extraoral fulcrum—a stabilizing point outside the patient's mouth (e.g., against the patient's chin or cheek). Also see *basic extraoral fulcrum.*

Extrinsic stains—stains that occur on the external (outer) surfaces of the teeth.

Face—the portion of the instrument working-end that is opposite the back; on sickle scales and curets, the face is bounded by the cutting edges.

Face at 90° angle to lower shank—a design characteristic of the cross sections of sickle scalers and universal curets. This design feature means that the working-end has two level cutting edges, both of which can be used for calculus removal.

Fibers of the gingiva—a network of fibers that brace the free gingiva against the tooth and unite the free gingiva with the tooth root and alveolar bone.

File—an instrument used to crush large calculus deposits. Its working-end has several cutting edges.

Finger assist fulcrum—an advanced fulcrum in which a finger of the nondominant hand is used to concentrate lateral pressure against the tooth surface and help control the instrument stroke.

Finger-like formation—a long, narrow deposit of calculus running parallel or oblique to the long axis of the tooth.

Finger-on-finger fulcrum—an advanced intraoral fulcrum in which the finger of the nondominant hand serves as the resting point for the dominant hand.

Finger rest—the place where the fulcrum finger rests and pushes against during instrumentation.

Flexible shank—an instrument shank that is thinner in diameter. Flexible shanks enhance the amount of tactile information transmitted to the clinician's fingers.

Fluid lavage—the action produced within the confined space of a periodontal pocket by the constant stream of fluid that exits near the point of an electronically powered instrument tip. This fluid lavage produces a flushing action that washes debris, bacteria, and unattached plaque from the periodontal pocket.

Free gingiva—the unattached portion of the gingiva that surrounds the tooth in the region of the cementoenamel junction (CEJ). The free gingiva is also known as the unattached gingiva or the marginal gingiva.

Frequency—how many times an electronically powered instrument tip vibrates per second.

Fulcrum—a stabilizing point for the clinician's hand during instrumentation. In periodontal instrumentation, the ring finger serves as the fulcrum finger acting as a "support beam" for the weight of the hand during instrumentation. Also see *intraoral fulcrum, extraoral fulcrum,* and *advanced fulcrum.*

Full mouth debridement—calculus removal that is completed in a single appointment or in two appointments within a 24-hour period.

Full mouth disinfection—full mouth debridement combined with the use of professionally applied topical antimicrobial therapy.

Functional shank—the portion of the instrument shank that allows the working-end to be adapted to the tooth surface. The functional shank begins below the working-end and extends to the last bend in the shank nearest the handle.

Furcation—the place on a multirooted tooth where the root trunk divides into separate roots. The furcation is termed a "bifurcation" on a two-rooted tooth and a "trifurcation" on a three-rooted tooth.

Furcation area—the space—apical to the root trunk—between two or more roots. In health, the furcation area cannot be probed because it is filled with alveolar bone and periodontal ligament fibers.

Furcation involvement—a loss of alveolar bone and periodontal ligament fibers in the space between the roots of a multirooted tooth.

Furcation probe—a type of periodontal probe used to evaluate the bone support in the furcation areas of bifurcated and trifurcated teeth.

Gingiva—the tissue that covers the cervical portions of the teeth and the alveolar processes of the jaws. Also see *free gingiva* and *attached gingiva.*

Gingival fibers—a network of fibers that brace the free gingiva against the tooth and unite the free gingiva with the tooth root and alveolar bone.

Gingival margin—the thin rounded edge of the free gingiva that meets the tooth.

Gingival pocket—a deepened sulcus that results from swelling of the gingival tissues.

Gingival recession—movement of the gingival margin from its normal position—usually with underlying loss of bone—resulting in the exposure of a portion of the root surface. In recession, the gingival margin is apical to the CEJ and the papillae may be rounded or blunted.

Gingival sulcus—the space between the free gingiva and the tooth surface.

Gingivitis—a bacterial infection that is confined to the gingiva. It results in damage to the gingival tissues that is reversible. Also see *periodontitis.*

Gross scaling—a method of planning multiple calculus removal appointments that advocated removing only the large-sized calculus deposits from the entire mouth at the first appointment. Gross scaling is no longer recommended because of the undesirable consequences that can result from incomplete calculus removal.

Handle—the part of a periodontal instrument used for holding the instrument.

Handle roll—the act of turning the instrument handle slightly between the thumb and index finger to readapt the working-end to the next segment of the tooth.

Horizontal—parallel to ground level; level with the ground.

Horizontal strokes—instrumentation strokes that are perpendicular to the long axis of the tooth; used (1) at the line angles of posterior teeth, (2) in furcation areas, and (3) within pockets that are too narrow to permit vertical or oblique strokes.

Implant—see *dental implant.*

Implant fixture—the portion of the implant that is surgically placed into the bone. The fixture will act as the "root" of the implant and needs a period of 3 to 6 months to be fully surrounded and supported by bone.

Indirect illumination—the use of the mirror surface to reflect light onto a tooth surface in a dark area of the mouth.

Indirect vision—the use of a dental mirror to view a tooth surface or intraoral structure that cannot be seen directly.

Insertion—the action of moving the working-end beneath the gingival margin into the sulcus or pocket. Curets are the primary calculus removal instruments for subgingival instrumentation. The working-end is inserted at an angle between 0° and 40°.

Instrumentation zones—a series of imaginary narrow tracts on the root surface used to assist the clinician in systematically removing calculus deposits from subgingival root surfaces. Each instrumentation zone is only as wide as the toe-third of the instrument's cutting edge.

Interdental gingiva—the portion of the gingiva that fills the area between two adjacent teeth apical to (beneath) the contact area.

Intraoral fulcrum—a stabilizing point inside the patient's mouth against a tooth surface.

Intrinsic stains—stains that occur within the enamel of the tooth and cannot be removed by polishing. Intrinsic stains may be endogenous (occurring during tooth development) or exogenous (acquired after tooth eruption).

Junctional epithelium—a specialized type of epithelium that attaches the gingiva to the tooth surface. The junctional epithelium forms the base of a gingival sulcus or periodontal pocket.

Knurling—texturing, as on the handle of a periodontal instrument.

Lateral pressure—the act of applying equal pressure with the index finger and thumb inward against the instrument handle to press the working-end against a calculus deposit or tooth surface prior to and throughout an instrumentation stroke.

Lateral surfaces—the surfaces on either side of the instrument face.

Leading-third—the portion of the working-end that is kept in contact with the tooth surface during instrumentation.

Ledge—a long ridge of calculus running parallel to the gingival margin.

Level of attachment—see *clinical attachment level.*

Limited use-life—an item that must eventually be discarded after a certain amount of use, such as a sickle scaler or curet. The working-end of a sickle scaler or a curet becomes worn and must eventually be replaced.

Line angle—an imaginary line formed where two tooth surfaces meet.

Long axis—an imaginary straight line that passes through the center of a tooth and divides the tooth symmetrically.

Long junctional epithelium—the primary pattern of healing that occurs after periodontal debridement; there is no new formation of periodontal ligament or bone.

Loss of attachment (LOA)—damage to the structures that support the tooth. Loss of attachment occurs in periodontitis and is characterized by (1) relocation of the junctional epithelium to the tooth root, (2) destruction of the fibers of the gingiva, (3) destruction of the periodontal ligament fibers, and (4) loss of alveolar bone support from around the tooth.

Lower cutting edge—the cutting edge of an area-specific curet that is used for periodontal debridement. Also see *working cutting edge.*

Lower shank—another term for the terminal shank; the portion of the functional shank nearest to the working-end. It provides an important visual clue when selecting the correct working-end of an instrument.

Lubricant—a substance, such as water or oil, applied to the surface of a sharpening stone to reduce friction between the stone and the instrument during sharpening.

Magnetostrictive ultrasonic instrument—an electronically powered device that uses the rapid energy vibrations of a powered instrument tip to fracture calculus from the tooth surface and clean the environment of the periodontal pocket. A magnetostrictive ultrasonic device is comprised of a portable unit that contains an electronic generator, a handpiece, and interchangeable instrument inserts. The instrument tip of a magnetostrictive instrument vibrates 18,000 to 42,000 cycles per second.

Magnification loupes—magnification of the treatment area through surgical telescopes that can be a technological aid during periodontal instrumentation.

Manually tuned—an ultrasonic device that has a tuning control knob or button that can be used to set the vibration frequency of the tip at a level above or below the resonant frequency. Also see *tuning* and *automatically tuned.*

Metal burs—minute pieces of metal that project from the cutting edge of an incorrectly sharpened instrument working-end.

Midline—an imaginary line that divides an anterior tooth into two equal halves.

Millimeter—a unit of length equal to one thousandth of a meter or 0.0394 inch. The abbreviation for millimeter is "mm."

Miniature working-end—a curet that has a *shorter, thinner working-end* and a *longer lower shank* in comparison to the design of a standard Gracey curet.

Mirror—the working-end of a dental mirror has a reflecting mirrored surface used to view tooth surfaces that cannot be seen directly.

Mobility—the loosening of a tooth in its socket. Mobility may result from loss of bone support to the tooth. Most periodontal charts include boxes for documenting tooth mobility. **Horizontal tooth mobility** is the ability to move the tooth in a facial–lingual direction in its socket. **Vertical tooth mobility** is the ability to depress the tooth in its socket.

Modified intraoral fulcrum—an advanced intraoral fulcrum that uses an altered point of contact between the middle and ring fingers in the grasp.

Modified pen grasp—the recommended grasp for holding a periodontal instrument. This grasp allows precise control of the working-end, permits a wide range of movement, and facilitates good tactile conduction.

Motion activation—the act of moving the instrument in order to produce an instrumentation stroke on the tooth surface. See also *wrist motion activation* and *digital motion activation.*

Moving instrument technique—a method of instrument sharpening accomplished by moving the working-end over a stabilized sharpening stone.

Moving stone technique—a method of instrument sharpening accomplished by moving a sharpening stone over the working-end of a stabilized instrument.

Mucogingival junction—the clinically visible boundary where the pink attached gingiva meets the red, shiny alveolar mucosa.

Multidirectional strokes—instrumentation strokes that are made using a combination of vertical, oblique, and horizontal strokes; used for assessment or debridement of a subgingival tooth surface.

Musculoskeletal disorder (MSD)—an injury affecting the musculoskeletal, peripheral nervous, and neurovascular systems that is caused or aggravated by prolonged repetitive forceful or awkward movements, poor posture, ill-fitting chairs and equipment, or a fast-paced workload.

Nabers probe—see *furcation probe.*

Neutral position—the ideal positioning of the body while performing work activities that is associated with decreased risk of musculoskeletal injury. It is generally believed that the more a joint deviates from the neutral position, the greater is the risk of injury.

Neutral wrist position—the ideal positioning of the wrist while performing work activities that is associated with decreased risk of musculoskeletal injury.

Nonworking cutting edge—a cutting edge on the working-end of an area-specific curet that is not used for calculus removal.

Oblique—line that has a slanting or sloping direction or position; inclined.

Oblique strokes—instrumentation strokes that are diagonal to the long axis of the tooth; used most commonly on facial and lingual surfaces.

Oblique technique—using the working-end of an electronically powered instrument with the lateral surface in an oblique—almost horizontal—orientation to the long axis of the tooth. The tip is positioned in a similar manner to the working-end of a curet.

Odontoblastic process—a thin tail of cytoplasm from a cell in the tooth pulp that enters a dentinal tubule and extends from the pulp to the dentoenamel or dentocementum junction.

Opposite arch fulcrum—an advanced intraoral fulcrum in which the finger rest is established on the opposite arch from the treatment area.

Overhang removal—recontouring procedures that correct defective margins of restorations to provide a smooth surface that will deter bacterial accumulation. If a minor amalgam overhang is acting as a plaque trap and preventing effective plaque control, the excess amalgam can be removed using a specialized powered instrument tip for this purpose.

Overhanging restoration—an area of a restoration where an excess of restorative material projects beyond the tooth surface.

Paired working-ends—a double-ended instrument with working-ends that are exact mirror images of each other. Also see *unpaired working-ends.*

Parallel lines—lines that run in the same direction and will never meet or intersect one another.

Pellicle—a thin coating of salivary proteins that attach to the tooth surface within minutes after a professional cleaning. The pellicle provides a sticky surface for attachment of plaque and dental calculus to the tooth surface.

Periodontal assessment—a fact-gathering process designed to provide a complete picture of a patient's periodontal health status.

Periodontal attachment system—a group of structures that work together to attach the teeth to the skull. The periodontal attachment system is comprised of the junctional epithelium, fibers of the gingiva, periodontal ligament fibers, and alveolar bone.

Periodontal debridement—the removal or disruption of bacterial plaque, its products, and plaque retentive calculus deposits from coronal surfaces, root surfaces, and within the pocket. Periodontal debridement includes instrumentation of every square millimeter of root surface for removal of plaque and calculus but does not include the deliberate, aggressive removal of cementum.

Periodontal disease—a bacterial infection of the periodontium. Periodontal disease that is limited to an inflammation of the gingival tissues is called *gingivitis*. Periodontal disease that involves the gingiva, periodontal ligament, bone, and cementum is called *periodontitis*.

Periodontal file—an instrument used to crush large calculus deposits. Its working-end has several cutting edges.

Periodontal ligament fibers—the fibers that surround the root of the tooth. These fibers attach to the bone of the socket on one side and to the cementum of the root on the other side.

Periodontal pocket—a deepened gingival sulcus where the junctional epithelium is attached to the root surface somewhere apical to (below) the cementoenamel junction. In periodontal pockets, there is destruction of alveolar bone and the periodontal ligament fiber bundles.

Periodontal probe—See *probe*.

Periodontal Screening and Recording (PSR) System—an efficient easy-to-use screening system for the detection of periodontal disease.

Periodontitis—a bacterial infection of all parts of the periodontium including the gingiva, periodontal ligament, bone, and cementum. It results in irreversible destruction (permanent damage) to the tissues of the periodontium. Also see *gingivitis*.

Periodontium—the functional system of tissues that surrounds the teeth and attaches them to the jawbone. These tissues include the gingiva, periodontal ligament, cementum, and alveolar bone.

Perpendicular lines—two lines that intersect (meet) to form a 90° angle.

Piezoelectric ultrasonic instrument—an electronically powered device that uses the rapid energy vibrations of a powered instrument tip to fracture calculus from the tooth surface and clean the environment of the periodontal pocket. A piezoelectric ultrasonic device is comprised of a portable electronic generator, a handpiece, and instrument inserts. The instrument tip of a piezoelectric instrument vibrates 24,000 to 34,000 cycles per second.

Pivoting—a swinging motion of the hand and arm carried out by balancing on the fulcrum finger. The hand pivot is used to assist in maintaining adaptation of the working-end.

Placement stroke—an instrumentation stroke used to position the working-end of an instrument apical to a calculus deposit or at the base of a sulcus or pocket.

Plaque biofilm—a well-organized community of bacteria that adheres tenaciously to tooth surfaces, restorations, and prosthetic appliances. Research investigations have shown that the primary cause of most periodontal diseases is the bacterial plaque biofilm.

Plaque retentive factors—conditions that foster the establishment and growth of plaque biofilms, such as calculus deposits and overhanging restorations.

Plastic instruments—instruments made of plastic that are used for the assessment and debridement of implant teeth.

Pointed junction—see *sharp cutting edge*.

Polishing—a cosmetic procedure to remove extrinsic stains from the enamel surfaces of the teeth. Stain removal is a nonessential procedure undertaken for aesthetic reasons—to improve the appearance of the anterior teeth. Also see *selective polishing*.

Position of the instrument face—refers to the position that the face of an instrument is placed in for the purpose of instrument sharpening.

Posterior aspects away from the clinician—the aspects of the posterior sextants that are farthest from the clinician.

Posterior aspects toward the clinician—the aspects of the posterior sextants that are closest to the clinician.

Precision-thin instrument tip—see *slim-diameter instrument tip*.

Preprocedural rinse—an antimicrobial or antiseptic mouthrinse before a treatment procedure to reduce the number of bacteria introduced into the patient's bloodstream and for control of aerosols into the surrounding environment.

Probe—a slender assessment instrument used to evaluate the health of the periodontal tissues. Also see *calibrated periodontal probe* and *furcation probe*.

Probing—the act of walking the tip of a probe along the junctional epithelium within the sulcus or pocket for the purpose of assessing the health status of the periodontal tissues.

Probing depth—a measurement of the depth of a sulcus or periodontal pocket. It is determined by measuring the distance from the gingival margin to the base of the sulcus or pocket with a calibrated periodontal probe.

Quadrant—one-fourth of the combined dental arches. There are two maxillary quadrants and two mandibular quadrants.

Recontouring—the process of removing metal from the back and toe to restore the curved surfaces of a curet's working-end.

Repetitive task—a task that involves the same fundamental movement for more than 50% of the work cycle.

Resonant frequency—the level at which a magnetostrictive instrument insert vibrates naturally. Also see *frequency*.

Retraction—use of a mirror head or finger to hold the patient's cheek, lip, or tongue so that the clinician can view tooth surfaces or other structures that are otherwise hidden from view by these soft tissue structures.

Right angle—another term for a 90° angle. The sides of a right angle are bounded by two lines that are perpendicular to each other and measure exactly 90°.

Right angle—a prophylaxis angle with a straight shank.

Rigid shank—an instrument shank that is larger in diameter and will withstand the pressure needed to remove heavy calculus deposits.

Ring—a ridge of calculus running parallel to the gingival margin that encircles the tooth.

Root concavity—a linear developmental depression in the root surface. Root concavities commonly occur on the proximal surfaces of anterior and posterior teeth and the facial and lingual surfaces of molar teeth. In health, root concavities are covered with alveolar bone and help to secure the tooth in the bone.

Root debridement stroke—an instrumentation stroke used to remove residual calculus deposits, bacterial plaque, and by-products from root surfaces.

Root planing—a treatment procedure designed to remove cementum or surface dentin that is rough, impregnated with calculus, or contaminated with toxins or microorganisms.

Rounded surface—see *dull cutting edge*.

Rubber cup polishing—a polishing technique that uses an abrasive polishing agent and a slowly revolving polishing cup to abrade stain from the tooth surfaces.

Scaling—instrumentation of the crown and root surfaces of the teeth to remove plaque, calculus, and stains.

Selective polishing—the practice of polishing only those stained tooth surfaces that have an objectionable appearance. Selective polishing stresses daily patient self-care for the removal of plaque biofilms. Also see *polishing*.

Self-angulated curet—a curet in which the face is tilted in relation to the lower shank, such as an area-specific curet. The tilted face causes one cutting edge to be lower than the other cutting edge on a working-end. This feature positions the working cutting edge in correct angulation to the root surface.

Sextant—one-sixth of the combined dental arches. There are two anterior sextants and four posterior sextants.

Shank—a rod-shaped length of metal located between the handle and the working-end of a dental instrument. Also see *complex, simple, rigid,* and *flexible shank*.

Sharp cutting edge—a fine line formed by the pointed junction of the instrument face and lateral surface. Also see *dull cutting edge, visual evaluation, tactile evaluation,* and *sharpening test stick*.

Sharpening—the procedure to restore a sharp cutting edge on a calculus removal instrument. Also see *sharp cutting edge, moving instrument technique,* and *moving stone technique*.

Sharpening stone—natural or synthetic stone made of abrasive particles that is used to restore a sharp cutting edge on a calculus removal instrument. Also see *stone angulation*.

Sharpening test stick—a plastic or acrylic rod used to evaluate the sharpness of a cutting edge.

Sickle scaler—a periodontal instrument used to remove calculus deposits from the crowns of the teeth. Its working-end has a pointed back and pointed tip and is triangular in cross section. Sickle scalers are available in anterior and posterior designs.

Simple shank—a shank that is bent in one plane (front to back). Also see *complex shank*.

Slim-diameter instrument tip—sonic or ultrasonic instrument tip that is smaller in size than the working-end of a Gracey curet.

Sonic-powered instrument—an electronically powered device that uses the rapid energy vibrations of a powered instrument tip to fracture calculus from the tooth surface. Sonic devices consist of a handpiece that attaches to the dental unit's high-speed handpiece tubing and interchangeable instrument tips. The instrument tip of a sonic device vibrates between 3,000 and 8,000 cycles per second (3 to 8 kHz).

Spicule—an isolated, minute particle or speck of calculus.

Splatter—airborne particles that land on people and objects. Unlike aerosols, splatter is often visible once it lands on objects such as eyewear, uniforms, skin, hair, or other surfaces.

Stabilization—the act of preparing for an instrumentation stroke by locking the joints of the ring finger and pressing the fingertip against a tooth surface to provide control for the instrumentation stroke.

Stone angulation—an angulation of the stone between 70° and 80° to the instrument face during instrument sharpening.

Stroke—how far an electronically powered instrument tip moves during one cycle. Another term for stroke is amplitude. Ultrasonic electronically powered devices have a *power knob* that is used to change the length of the stroke. Higher power delivers a longer, more forceful stroke; lower power delivers a shorter, less forceful stroke.

Subgingival instrumentation—the use of an instrument apical to (below) the gingival margin. Also see *supragingival instrumentation.*

Supine position—the position of the patient during dental treatment, with the patient lying on his or her back in a horizontal position and the chair back nearly parallel to the floor.

Support beam—descriptive term for the ring finger in the modified pen grasp. The ring finger supports the weight of the hand during instrumentation.

Supragingival instrumentation—use of an instrument coronal to (above) the gingival margin.

Surfaces away from the clinician—the surfaces of the teeth that are farthest from the clinician.

Surfaces toward the clinician—the surfaces of the teeth that are closest to the clinician.

Tactile evaluation—a method of evaluating cutting edge sharpness by testing the cutting edge against a plastic or acrylic rod known as a sharpening test stick. A dull cutting edge will slide over the surface of the stick. A sharp cutting edge will scratch the surface of the test stick. Also see *sharpening test stick* and *visual evaluation.*

Tactile sensitivity—the clinician's ability to feel vibrations transmitted from the instrument working-end with his or her fingers as they rest on the shank and handle.

Terminal shank—another term for the lower shank; the portion of the functional shank nearest to the working-end. It provides an important visual clue when selecting the correct working-end of an instrument.

Therapeutic procedure—a dental procedure used to maintain health or treat a disease to restore health.

Thin-diameter instrument tip—see *slim-diameter instrument tip.*

Thin veneer—a thin, smooth coating of calculus on a portion of the root surface.

Tip of working-end—a pointed working-end, such as found on a sickle scaler.

Tip-third of working-end—the portion of the working-end of a sickle that is kept in contact with the tooth surface during instrumentation. Also see *toe-third of working-end* and *leading-third of working-end.*

Tobacco stain—a tenacious dark brown or black stain on the teeth that results from cigarette or cigar smoking or the use of chewing tobacco.

Toe of working-end—a rounded working-end, such as found on a curet.

Toe-third of working-end—the portion of the working-end of a curet that is kept in contact with the tooth surface during instrumentation. Also see *tip-third of working-end* and *leading-third of working-end.*

Transillumination—the use of the mirror surface to reflect light through the anterior teeth.

Trifurcation—see *furcation.*

Tuning—adjusting the length of the stroke made by an electronically powered instrument. Also see *automatically tuned* and *manually tuned.*

Two-point contact—the method of correct adaptation of a periodontal file to the tooth with the working-end on the calculus deposit and the lower shank resting against the tooth. Two-point contact provides the additional stability and leverage needed when using a file.

Universal curet—a periodontal instrument used to remove calculus deposits from the crown and roots of the teeth. The working-end of a universal curet has a rounded back, rounded toe, and two working cutting edges, and is semi-circular in cross section. Universal curets are one of the most frequently used and versatile of all the debridement instruments.

Unpaired working-ends—a double-ended instrument with working-ends that are dissimilar, such as an explorer-probe combination. Also see *paired working-ends.*

Vertical—a line that is perpendicular to level ground; upright.

Vertical strokes—instrumentation strokes that are parallel to the long axis of the tooth; used on the mesial and distal surfaces of posterior teeth.

Vertical technique—using the working-end of an electronically powered instrument in a manner similar to that of a calibrated periodontal probe, with the point directed toward the junctional epithelium. The instrument tip is in a vertical orientation to the long axis of the tooth. The vertical technique is used for calculus removal and deplaquing when instrumenting shallow or deep periodontal pockets.

Visual—able to be seen by the eyes, especially as opposed to being registered by one of the other senses.

Visual evaluation—examination of a cutting edge to evaluate sharpness accomplished by holding the working-end under a light source, such as the dental light or a high-intensity lamp. A dull cutting edge will reflect light because it is rounded and thick. The reflected light appears as a bright line running along the edge of the face. A sharp cutting edge is a line—with no thickness—and does not reflect the light. Also see *tactile evaluation.*

Walking stroke—the movement of a calibrated probe around the perimeter of the base of a sulcus or pocket.

Water-cooled instrument tip—sonic or ultrasonic instrument tip that is cooled by a constant stream of water that exists near the point of the instrument tip.

WHO probe—the probe used with the Periodontal Screening and Recording (PSR) System for periodontal assessment. The WHO probe has a colored band (called the reference marking) located 3.5 to 5.5 mm from the probe tip. This color-coded reference marking is used when performing the PSR screening examination.

Working cutting edge—a cutting edge that is used for periodontal debridement. Universal curets have two working cutting edges per working-end; area-specific curets have one working cutting edge per working-end.

Working-end—the part of a dental instrument that does the work of the instrument. The working-end begins where the instrument shank ends.

Wrist motion activation—the act of rotating the hand and wrist as a unit to provide the power for an instrumentation stroke. See also *motion activation* and *digital motion activation.*

Index

Page numbers in *italic* designate figures; page numbers followed by "t" designate tables; page numbers followed by "b" designate boxes; (*see also*) designates related topics or more detailed lists of subtopics.

N

O

P

Q

R